D1300528

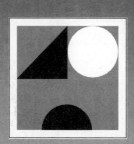

Primary Care Pediatrics

CAROL GREEN-HERNANDEZ, PhD, FNS, FNP-C
Editor-in-Chief, *Clinical Letter for Nurse Practitioners*
Associate Professor and Project Director
Primary Care Nurse Practitioner Program
The University of Vermont
Burlington, Vermont
and
Family Nurse Practitioner
In private practice for Healthcaring, Inc.
of Northern New England

JOANNE K. SINGLETON, PhD, RN, CS, FNP
Associate Professor
Pace University
School of Nursing
Department of Graduate Studies
Pleasantville, New York
and
Clinical Instructor (Voluntary)
Department of Family Practice
SUNY—Health Sciences Center at Brooklyn
Brooklyn, New York

DANIEL Z. ARONZON, MD, FAAP
Medical Director
The Children's Medical Group
Poughkeepsie, New York
and
President-Medical and Dental Staff
Senior Vice President of Medical Affairs
Vassar Brothers Hospital
Poughkeepsie, New York

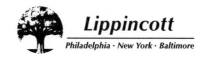
Lippincott
Philadelphia · New York · Baltimore

Acquisitions Editor: Jennifer Brogan
Managing Editor: Claudia Vaughn
Developmental Editors: Renee Gagliardi/Barclay Cunningham
Editorial Assistant: Susan Rainey
Project Editor: Nicole Walz
Senior Production Manager: Helen Ewan
Production Coordinator: Nannette Winski
Design Coordinator: Brett MacNaughton
Manufacturing Manager: William Alberti
Indexer: Ann Cassar
Interior Designer: Joan Wendt
Cover Designer: Deborah Lynam
Printer: Courier-Westford

9 8 7 6 5 4 3 2 1

Library of Congress Cataloging-in-Publication Data

Primary care pediatrics / Carol Green-Hernandez, Joanne K. Singleton, Daniel Z. Aronzon.
    p. ; cm.
    Includes bibliographical references and index.
    ISBN 0-7817-2008-7 (alk. paper)
    1. Pediatrics. 2. Primary care (Medicine) I. Green-Hernandez, Carol II. Singleton,
Joanne K. III. Aronzon, Daniel Z.
    [DNLM: 1. Pediatrics. 2. Primary Health Care. WS 100 P9517 2001]
RJ45 .P6656 2001
618.92—dc21
                                                                        00-056915

Care has been taken to confirm the accuracy of the information presented and to describe generally accepted practices. However, the authors, editors, and publisher are not responsible for errors or omissions or for any consequences from application of the information in this book and make no warranty, express or implied, with respect to the content of the publication.

The authors, editors, and publisher have exerted every effort to ensure that drug selection and dosage set forth in this text are in accordance with the current recommendations and practice at the time of publication. However, in view of ongoing research, changes in government regulations, and the constant flow of information relating to drug therapy and drug reactions, the reader is urged to check the package insert for each drug for any change in indications and dosage and for added warnings and precautions. This is particularly important when the recommended agent is a new or infrequently employed drug.

Some drugs and medical devices presented in this publication have Food and Drug Administration (FDA) clearance for limited use in restricted research settings. It is the responsibility of the health care provider to ascertain the FDA status of each drug or device planned for use in his or her clinical practice.

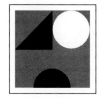

CONTRIBUTORS

Harvey W. Aiges, MD
Associate Chairman
Department of Pediatrics
North Shore University Hospital
Manhasset, New York

Aleksandra Alderman, MD
Medical Director, Consultant
REHAB Programs, Inc.
Poughkeepsie, New York

Phyllis W. Aldrich, AB, MA, SDA
Coordinator, Gifted Education
    Resource Center
Washington-Saratoga-Warren-
    Hamilton-Essex Board of
    Cooperative Education Services
Saratoga Springs, New York

Morton A. Alterman, MD
Associate Clinical Professor
Department of Ophthalmology
Albert Einstein College of Medicine
Bronx, New York

Daniel Z. Aronzon, MD, FAAP
Medical Director
The Children's Medical Group
Poughkeepsie, New York
and
President Medical and Dental Staff
Acting Vice President of Medical
    Affairs
Vassar Brothers Hospital
Poughkeepsie, New York

Richard Bachur, MD
Associate Clinical Director
Division of Emergency Medicine
Children's Hospital, Harvard Medical
    School
Boston, Massachusetts

Vincent P. Beltrani, MD
Associate Clinical Professor of
    Dermatology
Columbia Presbyterian Medical Center
New York, New York

Andrea Berne, RN, CPNP, MPH
Pediatric Nurse Practitioner
Private Practice
Brooklyn, New York

Fredrick Z. Bierman, MD
Chief, Division of Pediatric Cardiology
Schneider Children's Hospital
Long Island Jewish Medical Center
New Hyde Park, New York
and
Professor of Pediatrics
Albert Einstein College of Medicine
New York, New York

**Ann P. Bollmann, RN-C, MSN, FNP,
    RPA-C,**
Health Care Provider
Riverside Women's Health
Poughkeepsie, New York

**Particia A. Boltin, RN, MSN, MPH,
    CPNP**
Pediatric Nurse Practitioner
Pediatrics/Adolescents
Peekskill Community Health Center
Peekskill, New York

Janet Brandt, MS, RN, FNP
Family Nurse Practitioner
DOCS Physicians Affiliated with Beth
    Israel Medical Center
Valhalla, New York

Stephanie K. Brenner, RD, BS, MS
President of Autism Directory Service,
    Inc.
Poughquag, New York

Susan J. Brillhart, MSN, RN, CS, PNP
Clinical Coordinator, Medical Foster
    Care Program
Children's Aid Society
New York, New York

Dennis A. Cardone, DO
Assistant Professor, Director Sports
    Medicine Fellowship
UMDNJ – Robert Wood Johnson
    Medical School
New Brunswick, New Jersey

Rose Cassidy, RN, MS, FNP
Adult Nurse Practitioner
Hillside Medical Associates, Inc.
New Hyde Park, New York
and
Adult Nurse Practitioner/Pediatric
    Nurse Practitioner

Jamaica Hospital Center
Emergency Department
Jamaica, New York

**Margaret F. Clayton, MS, RN, CS,
    FNP**
Family Nurse Practitioner
Private Practice
Goldsboro, North Carolina

Penny Colbert-Kogan, RN, BSN
Legal Nurse Consultant
Pediatric Urology Nurse Clinician
Croton, New York

**Mardhie Coleman, RN, PICURN,
    PaedRN, BN, PhD (c) Nursing**
Research/Lecturer
School of Nursing
Edith Cowan University
Churchlands, Western Australia,
    Australia

Joseph P. Damore, Jr., MD
Departments of Pediatrics and
    Psychiatry
Memorial Sloan-Kettering Cancer
    Center
New York, New York

Mary Beth Damore, MD
Assistant Professor
Department of Pediatric Endocrinology
New York Medical College
Valhalla, New York

David M. De Iulio, MD, FAAP
Neonatologist (Hudson Valley
    Neonatology, PC)
Vassar Brothers Hospital
Poughkeepsie, New York

William J. DiScipio, PhD
Chief Psychologist
Westchester Jewish Community
    Services
and
Assistant Clinical Professor of
    Urology
Albert Einstein College of
    Medicine
Bronx, New York

Ellen Flynn, JD, MSN, CPNP
Pediatric Nurse Practitioner
Private Practice
Putnam Valley, New York

Pavel Fort, MD
Associate Professor of Clinical
   Pediatrics
NYU School of Medicine
and
Pediatric Endocrinologist
North Shore University Hospital
Manhasset, New York

Enitza D. George, MD
Assistant Professor
Department of Family Practice
State University of New York
Brooklyn, New York

**Goldie Gianoulis-Alissandratos, MS,
   FNP**
Dermatology Nurse Practitioner
Private Practice
New York, New York

Suzette T. Gjonaj, MD
Assistant Professor of Pediatrics
New York Medical College
Valhalla, New York

Evan R. Goldfischer, MD
Private Practice-Hudson Valley Urology
And
Director, Hudson Valley
   Comprehensive Stone Center
and
Surgeon, Vassar Brothers Hospital
Poughkeepsie, New York

Kenneth Steven Gottesman, MD
Assistant Clinical Professor of
   Pediatrics
Albert Einstein College of Medicine
Bronx, New York

**Carol Green-Hernandez, PhD,
   ANP/FNP-C**
Editor-in-Chief, *Clinical Letter for Nurse
   Practitioners*
Associate Professor and Project
   Director, Primary Care Nurse
   Practitioner Program
The University of Vermont
Burlington, Vermont
and
Family Nurse Practitioner
Private Practice
Healthcaring, Inc. of Northern New
   England

Jennifer Griswold, RN, MSN, PNP
Pediatric Nurse Practitioner
Department of Pediatrics
San Joaquin General Hospital
San Joaquin, California

Ann P. Guillot, MD
Professor
Department of Pediatrics
University of Vermont
Burlington, Vermont

Leah Harrison, RN, MS, CPNP
Associate Director
Child Protection Center
Montefiore Medical Center
The University Hospital for the Albert
   Einstein College of Medicine
Bronx, New York

Richard B. Heyman, MD
Adjunct Professor, Department of
   Pediatrics
University of Cincinnati College of
   Medicine
Cincinnati, Ohio

Jamie L. Hoffman-Rosenfeld, MD
Associate Professor of Clinical
   Pediatrics
Child Protection Center
Division of Community Pediatrics
Montefiore Medical Center
Department of Pediatrics
Albert Einstein College of Medicine
Bronx, New York

Stephen Paul Holzemer, PhD, RN
Dean, School of Nursing
Long Island College Hospital
Brooklyn, New York

Philip W. Hyden, MD, JD
Chief, Division of Child Protection
Assistant Professor of Pediatrics
NewYork-Presbyterian Hospital
Weill Medical College of Cornell
   University
New York, New York

Rosemary M. Jackson, MD
Assistant Professor of Pediatrics
State University of New York Health
   Sciences Center at Brooklyn
Brooklyn, New York

Ronald I. Jacobson, MD
Associate Clinical Professor of
   Neurology and Pediatrics
New York Medical College
Valhalla, New York
and
Pediatric Neurologist
Private Practice
White Plains, New York

Somasundaram Jayabose, MD
Chief, Pediatric Hematology-Oncology
Associate Professor of Pediatrics
New York Medical College
Valhalla, New York

Daniel M. Katz, MD
Attending Physician, Department of
   Urology
Vassar Brothers Hospital/St. Francis
   Hospital
Poughkeepsie, New York

**Nancy Kavanaugh, MS, RN, FNP,
   IBCLC**
Nurse Clinician/Lactation
   Consultant
The Mount Sinai-NYU Health System
New York, New York
and
Family Nurse Practitioner
Concordia College
Bronxville, New York

Eleanor M. Kehoe, RN, MS, PNP
Pediatric Nurse Practitioner
Maimonides Primary Care Center
Maimonides Medical Center
Brooklyn, New York

Jane Kiernan, PhD, RN
Part-time Faculty
Department of Nursing
Cayuga Community College
Auburn, New York

Renee Dellarose Kimball, MD
Gainesville Family Medicine Center
Gainesville, Georgia

Stanley J. Kogan, MD
Clinical Professor of Urology
New York Medical
   College/Westchester Medical Center
Valhalla, New York
and
Weil/Cornell University School of
   Medicine/New York Hospital
New York, New York

Stephen J. Kovacs, MD, FAAP
Director of Neonatology
Vassar Brothers Hospital
Poughkeepsie, New York

Catherine Koverola, PhD
Director of Mental Health and
   Research
Violence Intervention Program
USC School of Medicine
Department of Pediatrics
Los Angeles, California

**Linda J. Kristjanson, RN, BN, MN,
   PhD**
Professor
School of Nursing & Public Health
Edith Cowan University
Churchlands, Western Australia,
   Australia

Martin L. Kutscher, MD
Assistant Clinical Professor of
    Neurology and Pediatrics
New York Medical College
Valhalla, New York
and
Pediatric Neurologist
Private Practice
White Plains, New York

Dee L'Archeveque, MD
Assistant Director of the Emergency
    Department
Northshore University Hospital at
    Forest Hills
Forest Hills, New York

Jean Lavelle, RN, MSN, FNP
Family Nurse Practitioner
Stony Brook, New York

Herschel R. Lessin, MD, FAAP
Vice-President
The Children's Medical Group PLLC
Poughkeepsie, New York

Diana B. Lowenthal, MD, FAACP
Assistant Professor of Pediatrics
Department of Pediatrics
New York Medical College
Valhalla, New York

**Hendrika J. Maltby, RN, PhD,
    FRCNA**
Associate Professor
University of Vermont
School of Nursing
Burlington, Vermont

Keith P. Mankin, MD
Instructor
Harvard Medical School
and
Chief, Pediatric Orthopaedic Service
Massachusetts General Hospital
Boston, Massachusetts

Michele L. McLeod, MD
Pediatric Ophthalmologist
Attending Physician, Department of
    Ophthalmology
Manhattan Eye, Ear and Throat Hospital
New York, New York.

Wendy M. McKenney, MS, ARNP
Neonatal Nurse Practitioner
Department of Pediatrics
Dartmouth Hitchcock Medical Center
Lebanon, New Hampshire

Wendy M. McKinnon, MS
Clinical Assistant Professor of
    Pediatrics
College of Medicine
The University of Vermont
Burlington, Vermont

Mary Morahan, MSW, LCSW
Coordinator of Clinical Training
Violence Intervention Program
USC School of Medicine—Pediatrics
Los Angeles, California

Goldie Mulak, CSW, ACSW
Social Worker
Mount Sinai Medical Center
and
Teaching Assistant
Mount Sinai School of Medicine
Department of Community and
    Preventive Medicine
New York, New York

**Noreen Mulvanerty, RN, MS, CS,
    FNP**
Family Nurse Practitioner
Maimonides Medical Center
Department of Family Practice/ER
Brooklyn, New York

Roger Leo Nuñez, MD
Fellow, Family Practice Department
State University of New York
Health Science Center at Brooklyn
Brooklyn, New York

**Michelle E. Patrick, RN, BSN, MSN,
    CPNP**
Pediatric Nurse Practitioner
Children's Medical Group
Poughkeepsie, New York

Cynthia R. Pfeffer, MD
Professor of Psychiatry
Weill Medical College of Cornell
    University
New York, New York

Barbara Pisick, Med, RN, CS
Psychoanalytic
    Psychotherapist/Clinical Nurse
    Specialist
Private Practice
New York, New York

Thomas J. Powers, MD
Director, Division of Pediatric Primary
    Care
Department of Pediatrics
Maimonides Medical Center
Brooklyn, New York

William V. Raszka, Jr., MD, FAAP
Assistant Professor
Department of Pediatrics
The University of Vermont
Burlington, Vermont

Daniel A. Rauch, MD
Pediatric Residency Program Director
Assistant Professor of Pediatrics
Albert Einstein College of
    Medicine/Jacobi Medical Center
Bronx, New York

Keith Reinsdorf, MD
Sports Medicine Fellow
University of Medicine & Dentistry of
    New Jersey (UMDNJ)
Robert Wood Johnson Medical School
Department of Family Medicine
New Brunswick, New Jersey

Sue Robinson, RN, PhD(c)
School of Nursing & Public Health
Faculty of Communications, Health &
    Science
Edith Cowan University
Churchlands, Western Australia,
    Australia

Samuel A. Sandowski, MD
Director, Family Practice Residency
    Program
South Nassau Communities Hospital
Oceanside, New York

Maria Scaramuzzino, RN, MSN, PNP
Assistant Professor
Long Island College Hospital School of
    Nursing
and
Assistant Director of Nursing
Long Island Jewish Medical Center
New Hyde Park, New York

William T. Seed, MD
Private Practice
and
Associate Clinical Professor
Weill School of Medicine
New York-Presbyterian Medical Center
New York, New York

Jay E. Selman, MD
Assistant Clinical Professor of Neurology
Columbia University College of
    Physicians and Surgeons
New York, New York

Darsit K. Shah, MD
Assistant Clinical Professor
Department of Otalaryngology
Mount Sinai Medical Center
New York, New York

Marcey Shapiro, MD
Family Practice Physician
Private Practice
Albany, California

Pradeep Sharma, MD
Attending Physician
Vassar Brothers Hospital and St.
    Francis Hospital
Department of Pediatrics
Poughkeepsie, New York
and
Clinical Instructor
Department of Pediatrics
New York Medical College
Valhalla, New York

Joanne K. Singleton, PhD, RN, CS, FNP
Assistant Professor
Pace University
School of Nursing
Department of Graduate Studies
Pleasantville, New York
and
Clinical Instructor (Voluntary)
Department of Family Practice
SUNY—Health Sciences Center at Brooklyn
Brooklyn, New York

Elizabeth Dorsey Smith, EdD, CPNA, FAAN
Private Practice
and
Adjunct Professor
Hunter College, City University of New York
School of Nursing
New York, New York

Sunil K. Sood, MD
Associate Professor of Pediatrics
Schneider Children's Hospital
Albert Einstein College of Medicine
New Hyde Park, New York

Phyllis W. Speiser, MD
Professor
NYU School of Medicine
and
Director, Division of Pediatric Endocrinology
Professor of Clinical Pediatrics
North Shore-Long Island Jewish Health System
Manhasset, New York

Patricia J. Sterner, RN, MS, IBCLC
Lactation Consultant, Childbirth Educator
Maternal Child Health Care Center
Mount Sinai Hospital
New York, New York

Caroline Tassey, MS, CPNP
Children's Cardiac Center
Medical University of South Carolina
Charleston, South Carolina

Johanna Triegel, MD
Attending Pediatrician and Neonatologist
Vassar Brothers Hospital
Poughkeepsie, New York

Stella C. Laufer Turk, MS, CCC-A, FAAA
Director of Speech and Hearing Center
Clinical Lecturer
State University of New York, New Paltz
New Paltz, New York

Miriam T. Vincent, MS, MD (PhD Candidate)
Interim Chair, Family Practice
State University of New York
Health Science Center at Brooklyn
Brooklyn, New York

Robert A. Weiss, MD
Director, Pediatric Nephrology
Westchester Medical Center
and
Professor of Clinical Pediatrics
New York Medical College
Valhalla, New York

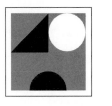

PREFACE

Pediatric primary care practitioners are specialists—they specialize in providing primary care to children. This includes health maintenance, disease prevention, education of new parents, helping parents to develop their parenting skills, helping children and adolescents to learn to care for themselves, identifying intra-familial stress, and teaching conflict resolution.

Pediatric providers specialize in the care of primary complaints in children, such as colds, fevers, earaches, sore throats, coughs, rashes, and minor injuries. Children are not little adults. Well-informed pediatric primary care *specialists* know more about the causes, microbiology, presentation, diagnosis, intricacies of management, and prognosis of middle ear disease in children than the ear, nose and throat "specialist."

In the area of chronic disease, pediatric primary care specialists are at the forefront, coordinating referrals and multi-specialty and multi-disciplinary treatment regimens, while preserving the family unit as the ultimate support group.

The goal of this text is to assist the primary care specialists in all of these areas. Our focus is clinical, practical, and factual. For example, classical pediatric texts devote reams to important yet obscure and rare metabolic neurodegenerative diseases, but only four or five pages to otitis media. Our aim is just the opposite. The old clinical adage reminds us that when we hear hoof beats to think of horses—not zebras. This text is focused on a detailed description of "horses"—those situations encountered everyday in a pediatric ambulatory care setting. These everyday pediatric concerns are covered in exquisite nuance and detail. Each chapter can stand alone as an enduring monograph. Our authors not only describe the factual aspects of a disease or problem, but how they think about it and the reasoning processes they go through to arrive at a sound diagnosis and plan of management.

Each of our authors spends the vast majority of their working day actually providing direct care. This text is dedicated to *all* of our current and future colleagues: nurse practitioners, physician assistants, family physicians, and pediatricians; as well as our students: nurse practitioner and physician assistant students, medical students, and pediatric and family practice residents—indeed, anyone who cares for children and adolescents. Welcome to pediatric primary care.

Because this book is for people in the trenches by people in the trenches, it is dedicated to all of us who devote long days and nights, caring for our most precious yet most vulnerable of assets—our children. Thus this dedication is underscored by our commitment to helping families help their children to achieve healthy growth and development. This commitment is the book's premise, for regardless of whether or not a pediatric patient has physical or emotional life challenges, that individual is still a child, and will be for only one special time in life. As we all know, once you grow up, you are grown up—and will be, life-long. It is imperative that all who minister to children remember that and, toward that end, strive to support healthy growth and development.

A final word about the route we took in creating this text. Like its predecessor, *Primary Care*, ours is an interdisciplinary text. To the best of our knowledge, *Primary Care* and *Primary Care Pediatrics* are the only interdisciplinary texts available. Our reason for taking an interdisciplinary rather than merely collaborative approach to this project was twofold.

First, like most providers today, the three of us practice pediatrics in an interdisciplinary environment, working on a regular basis with pediatricians, family and pediatric nurse practitioners, family physicians, and physicians assistants. Successful, salient pediatric primary care practice involves social workers, therapists, patients' schools, and—of course—families themselves in caring for children. We believe that involving providers from non-primary care disciplines in the writing of this book would strengthen content, giving the reader access to other players in the provision of pediatric health care. We included parents' voices as well, as it is important that all of us listen to their concerns while welcoming their ideas for co-managing illness in their children.

Second, it is our firmly held conviction that no one discipline has all the answers. There is just too much to learn, know, and apply to pediatric primary care nowadays. The "font" of knowledge is no longer the property of any one discipline—if indeed it ever was. Regardless of discipline, every provider practices from the same core of knowledge of pediatric primary care. Interdisciplinary teams really can deliver better primary care to children and their families. Just as every individual puts a different spin on information, so too does each health care discipline approach knowledge generation and application from a unique perspective. It is the interdisciplinary mix that makes such primary care practice stronger, often more supportive, and even fun. Whether authored by a medical or a nurse practitioner, a psychologist or a social worker, each chapter reflects a sound knowledge base, underscored by applicability to "on the fly" problems commonly encountered in pediatric primary care.

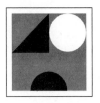

ACKNOWLEDGMENTS AND DEDICATIONS

Two books in 3 years, Joanne—I can honestly say that NOW I am pooped! What can I say—best friend, trusted colleague, and true "soul" sister. In for a penny, in for a pound, but together.

And to Danny—friend, colleague, and cheerleader extraordinaire. Without you this project not only would not have been as much fun, but might not have happened at all. *Merci, merci.*

Many thanks to our wonderful editorial team at Lippincott Williams & Wilkins—yes, Claudia Vaughn, this means you! You took the two-book ride with Joanne and me. Thank goodness you never ran out of petrol! Thanks, too, to Susan Rainey, Renee, Barclay ("just think of me as Renee-Two"), and the rest of the Lippincott gang. But most of all, thank you, Jennifer Brogan. Those planning sessions and late night drive-around talks gave me the confidence to undertake and complete my part of this project. I could not have done this without your belief in the project itself, your shared sense of the absurd, and your support. Lippincott is privileged to count all of you among its top employees.

Work in the real world must go on, even when some of us are not always around to help out. To all of my clinic colleagues—thanks for covering for me for low these many months while this project took shape. Many thanks to Pat Winstead-Fry at the University of Vermont. Your support in helping me to rearrange my teaching and scholarly commitments made it possible for me to complete what turned out to be a mammoth project. You are so much more than a terrific Interim Dean—you are a valued friend. And to my colleagues at that self-same University, especially my dear friend, colleague, and twin Dr. Brenda Hamel-Bissell, and my NP faculty colleagues Dr. Nancy Morris and Professor Carol Buck-Rolland—fellow friends of children. Thanks for being there when I needed a sounding board, support, or information.

And last but never least, I dedicate this book to my family. You are the center of my life, yet sometimes you all received short shrift while I was in the Implicate Whole. To Ed, my husband of 27 years—thanks for keeping the soccer balls, basketballs, baseballs, and horse hooves flying while I was typing, typing, typing. At least the kids had one viable parent while I was "otherwise engaged!" And to Ian and Gillian, my most precious children. Don't be in a hurry to grow up! Family first, all else after; always and in all ways.

CG-H

One never knows what will happen when you introduce two friends to each other. Thanks for letting me be in the middle of making this book happen. Carol, congratulations. We did it again; here's to some well-deserved rest and relaxation. Danny, now do you understand why we couldn't give you a better explanation of what to expect? You did a great job and can no longer claim rookie status.

Thanks to my colleagues at the Lienhard School of Nursing, Pace University for listening and offering suggestions, and to our Dean, Dr. Harriet R. Feldman for her oncoing encouragement and support of my scholarship.

Rolf, thanks from all of us for you negotiating savvy design suggestions; administrative assistance; and constant, unwavering support. Ed and Nancy, thanks for lending your spouses to this project. Jennifer and Claudia, it would not be a book without the both of you.

As I have said before, behind a successful woman is often a supportive man. I am fortunate to be such a woman and I thank Rolf. His untiring love and counsel has encouraged me once again to stay focused on the work at hand. To my son Andy, in so many ways working on this book has been a walk through the memories of watching you grow and develop. I am so proud of you. Thanks for always helping out. And to Lily, my pleasant distraction and calming influence.

JS

Thanks to Carol and Joanne for allowing a "rookie" to play with the "veterans." Thanks to the five-man room—MAB, FZB, MDS, and LBP—loyal friends for life. Thanks to my partners, colleagues, and brothers at CMG especially AB, LS, DF, and JH. Thanks to the Jacobi crew, AS, KK, SB, and HB; you've been both friends and role models. Thanks in advance to my "special friends" H&SE, and Z&MG for forgiving my absence both physically and mentally during these long months, and hopefully welcoming me back. Nina, Karl and Adam, and Mrs. E, thanks for putting up with my craziness. Mom and Grandpa—thanks for being with me all those nights—I think of you always, and hope that you are proud of me. Denise, Nicole, and Stephanie, whenever I felt discouraged or depressed, I thought of you and how lucky and proud I am to be your daddy. Most importantly, Nancy, as I sat glued to my desk, you held house and home together. You are my partner in love and in life—thank you.

DZA

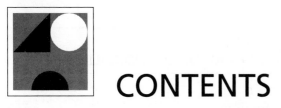

CONTENTS

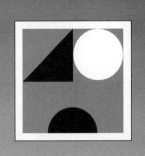

MULTIDISCIPLINARY PRIMARY CARE

Philosophy of Pediatric Primary Care

- CAROL GREEN-HERNANDEZ, PhD, FNP-C; DANIEL Z. ARONZON, MD, FAAP; and
JOANNE K. SINGLETON, PhD, RN, CS, FNP

INTRODUCTION

Pediatric primary care practitioners are specialists; they specialize in primary care. They specialize in health maintenance and disease prevention. They specialize in the education of new parents, the development of parenting skills, and the identification of intrafamilial stress and conflict resolution. They specialize in the care of primary complaints in children such as colds, fevers, earaches, sore throats, coughs, rashes, and minor injuries. They are specialists in managing the child with chronic disease, coordinating multispecialty and multidisciplinary treatment regimens, and preserving the family unit as the ultimate support group. Children are not little adults. Well informed pediatric primary care *specialists* know more about the causes, microbiology, presentation, diagnosis, intricacies of management, and prognosis of middle ear disease in children than the ear, nose, and throat "specialist."

Today's pediatric primary care practitioners come from various educational disciplines, backgrounds, ethnic groups, and cultures. The field still includes traditional medical practitioners in pediatrics, family practice, general practice, emergency medicine, and (for adolescents) obstetrics and gynecology. Over the last 35 years, individuals from the nursing profession also have joined pediatric primary care, so the field now includes certified pediatric, family, and neonatal nurse practitioners. Allied health professionals include physician assistants in various disciplines, psychologists, licensed social workers, audiologists, nutritionists, and physical, occupational, speech, and language therapists. Even more recently, practitioners of alternative and complementary medicine have become active in primary care. The settings for pediatric primary care are varied as well. Solo practices, single and multispecialty groups, public and private clinics, academic teaching centers, regional centers and small community hospitals, and rural and inner city facilities create a panorama of locales in which children receive primary care.

All pediatric primary care specialists realize that successes and failures in outcomes ultimately depend on the child's environment. On a "macro" level, society must do more to value its most important yet most vulnerable citizens. On a "micro" level, children must receive treatment within the context of their families. By creating a caring environment in which they clearly and effectively communicate health messages and where they support children and families in developing care-of-self skills, pediatric specialists may find that such practice yields positive outcomes. This chapter outlines methods for creating an environment that focuses on caring, communication, and care-of-self as tools for successful pediatric primary care.

CARING

The principle of caring in primary care is family focused, wherein the family and the primary care provider work in partnership to the greatest extent possible. This vision allows family members to be coparticipants in selecting and testing their health care plans, helping to ensure their continued involvement. The deliberate use of caring as an intentional therapeutic model can increase positive health outcomes. The clinician needs to use a holistic perspective, focusing on what the child and parents need not just physically, but also psychologically, spiritually, and emotionally.

Culturally Sensitive Caring

Because the intentionality is holistic, primary care based on professional caring necessitates a culturally sensitive approach, starting from the first moment of each family encounter. Most westernized countries are becoming increasingly diverse; so, too, are the populations that pediatric primary care is serving. This fact requires all practitioners to be culturally aware about what assessment and intervention strategies will work best to meet health care needs across cultural boundaries. Deliberate, culturally sensitive caring is especially important because western society is time-obsessed. For primary care providers, the time-driven demands of managed care further compound personal and professional demands. Issues of time are less troublesome when the clinician and family share a common language and customs, such as the handshake as a greeting, use of direct eye contact, and open discussion of "sensitive" topics, such as sexuality. When cultural norms and expectations differ, providers can quickly express caring through a simple touch on the arm, eye contact, and sitting kitty-corner rather than across from the family or separated by a barrier (eg, a desk or an examining table). Similarly, providers maintain professional caring when they do not break communication (both verbal and nonverbal) with the child and parents even when they are using a translator. All these measures can convey that the clinician is aware of and present for the family.

For the family whose culture would consider "getting right to the point" as rude or for whom language is a barrier, providers can express caring in other ways. For example, when working with Latino patients, Fontes (2000) suggests that professionals try to be helpful as soon as possible. The author asserts that providers should demonstrate caring and allow more time to build relationships with Latino clients. Providers can enhance these measures by increasing their knowledge of Latino cultures. Such involvement, however, requires time. Providers can simply and efficiently reconfigure the ongoing need for time—to acknowledge the humanity of the child and family, to build relationships, to be caring—through a calm and caring presence.

Coparticipative Relationships

The giving and receiving of caring require both provider and family to communicate their needs openly and honestly. The goal is a coparticipative relationship, in which both practitioner and family are equal members, with equal voices and equal responsibilities. This situation is the ideal, but sometimes the reality of developing and nurturing an open, coparticipative relationship with a child and family is impossible if they are unable to share this vision with the provider. The clinician must strive to support the family's participation in making and following the prescribed therapeutic regimen to the extent that circumstances allow. When efforts to support family functioning are successful, both provider and family are coactualized. That is, the very fact of giving and receiving caring inevitably changes both parties. Caring as a mutual experience helps both family and clinician to evolve as human beings.

The growth that derives from a caring, coparticipative practice means that the clinician collaborates with rather than controls the child and parents. Achieving this vision is a special challenge within the managed-care model and its accompanying constraints (eg, 10-minute office visits). The organized, formalized practice of primary care framed by the professional caring model requires that the clinician *learn* both how and how best to practice caring as a generic professional skill (Green-Hernandez, 1991a; 1991b; 1992; 1996; 1997; 1999).

Really listening to what families say and do not say is an important means of expressing caring. Doing so validates the importance of what the child and parent think is wrong or is needed. Taking a brief moment to inquire about how things are going at home, school, and with friends is not only important to history taking, but also helps to build a relationship. The provider can further these efforts by remembering to follow up at the next visit about what families previously shared. This work helps to forge links and build relationships between practitioner and family members.

Validation

Caring requires time and energy. Intentional, professional, therapeutic caring mandates that the provider be *involved* with the other person. The giving of caring, however, cannot be a one-sided effort. It must be reciprocal. The ability to continue to give professional caring depends on *receiving* caring in return, which validates the clinician as a human and as a professional who is deliberately trying to improve primary care through caring practice.

The continued ability to *give* caring depends on the provider's caring energy level. Validation is key to perpetuating this level. Receiving caring from people other than children and their parents can help providers to replenish the necessary energy reserves. Personal and collegial relationships that are marked by mutual caring and respect reinforce this cycle. Professional caring partnerships with colleagues provide a source for constant renewal. The support derived from collegial caring can fuel the sheer energy needed to practice primary care, with professional caring as the foundation for its delivery.

COMMUNICATION

Patients cannot perceive caring if it is not communicated to them in a way that they can understand. Communication is key to effective primary care, whether in taking a history or providing anticipatory guidance. However, communication is not a simple process. The provider must be aware of several important concepts to communicate *effectively* with children of differing ages and their parents. The health care practitioner with good communication skills and techniques

will enjoy improved outcomes, enhanced satisfaction, and a greater likelihood of financial viability and success. This section provides a framework for understanding and practicing effective communication in primary care pediatrics.

Communication, Quality, and Success

Mrs. H., a harried mother of four, has spent 30 minutes in a crowded waiting room, supervising her children, before a pleasant but uninterested LPN ushers her family into the examining room. Alex, her youngest child, has had a fever for 2 days. Dr. X enters the examining room, asks about the history, examines the child completely (albeit quickly), pronounces, "It's just a virus," and exits.

Was this care appropriate? From a strictly scientific viewpoint, the answer is yes. A history and physical were performed, and the correct diagnosis was established. Does this care represent quality? What are the possible results of such an encounter?

Upon returning home, Mrs. H. realizes that she did not understand what was wrong with Alex. She phones the practitioner. The explanation still is lacking. When Alex begins to run another temperature, Mrs. H. rushes him to the emergency room. Once there, after another long wait, the health care team evaluates Alex, draws blood, and obtains a chest x-ray. Results come back normal. The emergency room physician makes the diagnosis of upper respiratory infection and prescribes amoxicillin "to be safe."

What is the cost of this encounter to Mrs. H., to society, and to Alex, who has had an x-ray and blood work and is now taking an unnecessary antibiotic for 10 days? What is the likelihood of Mrs. H. returning to Dr. X's office? What is the likelihood of Dr. X surviving in practice? These questions are all obviously rhetorical. Clearly, however, the lack of effective communication during the initial primary care encounter adversely affected the family in this fictional scenario. More effective communication between clinician and family can and will result in better care, as defined by improved outcomes and higher satisfaction rates for both patients and providers.

Traditional View of Quality

Communication that improves outcomes enhances the traditional view of quality, defined by such things as accurate and prompt diagnoses and safe and effective treatments. Effective communicators will be more likely to ensure the patient's participation in designing a therapeutic plan, cooperating with treatment regimens, and returning for necessary follow-up. Providers practicing in the public sector, whose patients may represent a "captive audience," will reap the rewards of improved outcomes but equally important, will derive greater professional satisfaction. Similarly, clinicians whose practice is in the private sector will likely see improved outcomes linked to a stable base of patients. When people feel that their providers listen and treat them with care, they are more apt to choose to continue with such clinicians despite the vagaries of managed care.

A New Paradigm of Quality

In the various private sectors, clinicians have believed that by providing traditional "quality" primary care, they will be successful. That paradigm has changed. Today, patients and families, otherwise known as consumers, view technical quality (an accurate and prompt diagnosis, safe and effective treatments) care as a given. Improving all aspects of quality care is beyond the scope of this text and would be better addressed in a practice development or medical marketing book. Enhanced communication, however, certainly contributes to the consumer's new view of quality, thereby reinforcing the practitioner's or organization's continued economic viability. In the era of managed care (more aptly termed "managed competition"), the adage "no margin, no mission" has become increasingly relevant. Economic success not only ensures reasonable remuneration for the provider or organization, but also and more importantly ensures that the clinician or organization will continue to exist.

● **Clinical Pearl:** Health care consumers today measure quality in terms of accessibility, availability, waiting times, courtesy of staff, and attractiveness of surroundings. Perhaps highest on this list is the provider's ability to communicate effectively. What used to be the "niceties" of health care are increasingly becoming the "necessities."

Neophyte providers must learn how to become technically competent, feel professionally confident, and be reasonably cost efficient. Fortunately, for the most part, quality and the provision of cost-effective care go hand in hand. Over time and with experience, the pediatric provider will learn how to individualize professional caring for children and their families.

Techniques to Improve Communication

Enhanced communication is an essential ingredient of quality in primary care delivery, both in the traditional technical sense and in the newer paradigm of consumerism and economic viability. This section focuses on techniques of communication that the pediatric primary care specialist can use to foster quality care.

Preparing for "Show Time"

The health care setting, be it a private office or public clinic, is intimidating, threatening, and often less than comfortable for child and parent alike. All people have good and bad days; however, the appearance of a surly, argumentative, and gruff clinician will do little to allay fear or enhance communication. Whether a clinician was up for most of the previous night caring for a sick child or left home in the middle of a heated argument with a spouse or child is irrelevant. Providers are professionals, and when they set foot on the examining room stage, they must act professionally and leave personal problems outside. When a provider opens that examining room door or parts that cubicle's curtain, it is indeed "show time."

Maintaining a Professional Appearance

The pediatric primary care specialist must dress the part. The era of starched white coats is over. The office or clinic setting is strange enough for children, who are much more comfortable relating to a person who looks like everyone else. If a child is comfortable, he or she will be much more likely to submit cooperatively to the indignities of an examination.

No defined dress code exists for pediatric providers, but casual business attire comes closest. For males, a shirt and tie with slacks is usually appropriate, though some would argue that this might be too formal. For females, a blouse with a skirt or slacks is appropriate. The important thing is to appear neat, clean, and professional. Jeans, shorts, tee shirts, sneakers, and athletic apparel may be comfortable but fail to convey the image of a health care professional. Neatness counts: Hair, nails, makeup, and jewelry are best if understated. Cleanliness cannot be overemphasized. The first thing the clinician should do when entering the examination area is wash their hands.

Using Effective Greetings

If the provider is at all uncertain about whether a patient is new, an introduction is in order. The first step is to walk up to the parent, making eye contact and extending one's hand while saying, "Hi, I'm Steve Jones, the nurse practitioner" or "I'm Jennifer Diaz, the pediatrician." Wearing a name tag that delineates the clinician's name and discipline is very useful, because many parents will forget the practitioner's name. If the family is not new to the facility, the provider should greet parents by name, using the title that they prefer (eg, Mrs. Flynn or Sra. Ortez, rather than Ellen or Sarita). Greetings such as "Gee, its good to see you again" or "Long time no see, how have you been?"—and then listening for the response—convey welcome and warmth. By making the effort to express respect and genuine pleasure in seeing the family, the clinician conveys caring in a way that can powerfully transform communication dynamics.

The second step is to greet all children, even infants, by name in an age-appropriate fashion. The provider should make eye contact, at the child's level, and greet the patient in a fashion that validates his or her presence as an individual.

After the initial greeting, the clinician should segue into eliciting the history, asking questions, such as "How may I help you today?" instead of "Why are you here?" The former phrasing intimates a genuine desire to help; the latter is almost accusatory and may convey the message that the visit is a bother to the provider.

If a family has had to wait for services, which is often the case in many primary care settings, the clinician should apologize for the delay. Doing so acknowledges that the family's time is also valuable.

Making It Personal

At each encounter, the provider should attempt to have a brief exchange with the caregiver, patient, or preferably both that is unrelated to the reason for the visit. Taking a brief moment to inquire about how things are going at home, school, and with friends is not only important to history taking, but also helps to build a relationship. The provider can further this work by remembering to ask at the next visit, "How did the basketball game turn out?" or "Was the fair a lot of fun?" or "How did the piano recital go?" Similarly, the clinician should ask appropriate questions of the parent, such as "How's the new job going?" or "Are you over that cold you had the last time you were in with Timmy?"

Using Nonverbal Communication

Looking directly into the parent's or patient's eyes when talking and listening is perhaps the most effective way to convey understanding and caring. It also allows the provider to observe carefully how the other party is receiving and understanding the message. Spoken words represent only a fraction of the communication process. Posture, tone of voice, and facial expressions, to name a few, may reveal more about how a person feels than do actual words. Clinicians should remember that their posture, tone of voice, and facial expressions also convey more to the child or parent than what they actually say.

Listening and Acknowledging

Effective communication is a two-way street. All experienced providers occasionally feel the urge to interrupt a parent's long soliloquy about a child's bowel movement pattern. As much as possible, clinicians should avoid the temptation to interrupt abruptly. If providers acknowledge what parents are saying and use subtle affirmations, such as nodding, they may be able to use breaks in a conversation to direct the discussion to more productive areas.

Being Specific

Providers need to be specific. For example, if the results of an encounter suggest that a child has a virus, the clinician, if possible, should name the suspected virus, explain that antibiotics will not help, outline supportive care and fever control, estimate the duration of symptoms, and counsel the caregiver on when to return.

Sitting

If the provider has one hand on the doorknob while detailing instructions, he or she conveys impatience and lack of caring. Sitting down to explain treatment, even for a few seconds, conveys concern and caring.

Writing it Down

It has been said that an attentive, undistracted human being of average intelligence can only remember seven things at a time, under the best of circumstances. A health care facility probably represents the worst of circumstances. A worried parent, hearing that little Suresh has streptococcal pharyngitis, may hear very little else. Writing down simple instructions or handing out prepared instruction sheets will go a long way to ensure that Suresh gets all his medications, maintains his hydration, and returns if symptoms recur.

Keeping It Simple

"Dazzling them with verbiage" is a technique that many practitioners mistakenly use. The statement, "Your child has secretory otitis media with effusion secondary to acute otitis media" may be perfectly accurate, but unfortunately it is rather incomprehensible and frightening to most parents. A more meaningful explanation might be "Your child has some fluid in the middle ear space, which often follows an ear infection."

Asking About "Any Other Questions?"

While still seated, successful clinicians make it a point to close every encounter with this question. In doing so, they convey the message that they are caring, not rushed, and sincerely concerned about the child and family.

Following Up

It is 9 PM and Mrs. H. is worried about Alex. Although Steve Jones, the nurse practitioner, had explained that "it was a virus, and the fever might last a few days," she is still concerned, as most mothers would be. The phone rings in her home. It is Steve Jones, who inquires about Alex, reviews fever control, and reassures Mrs. H. that, although frightening, the fever will not hurt her son.

Given this scenario, is Mrs. H. likely to take Alex to the emergency room? Will Alex have to undergo unnecessary tests, x-rays, and treatments? Will Mrs. H. bring all her children to see Steve Jones? Will Mrs. H. tell her friends about that practice? Will that practice be successful?

Obviously, busy practitioners cannot make unsolicited calls to all patients that they see during the day. By selecting two or three encounters each day during which the child was a bit more ill or the parent a bit more concerned, however, the clinician can ensure important follow-up, while also effectively communicating caring and concern.

CARE-OF-SELF

Care-of-self, a new concept to the literature, is in its early stage of development (Singleton, 2000). Care-of-self is different from the less specific term "self-care" in two important ways. First, care-of-self recognizes and respects the delicate interplay of dimensions in the bio-psycho-social-spiritual being. This distinction is vitally important, because too often health care professionals focus on physical needs, overlooking or ignoring the individual's other interacting and inseparable needs. The second important distinction is that one cannot motivate another in care-of-self. Rather, one can only help to create an environment in which the other person can motivate himself or herself. While this difference may sound subtle, it is perhaps the key to positive patient outcomes and patient–provider satisfaction. The unfortunate misperception that health care providers can motivate their patients may foster passivity. Passivity is antagonistic to the idea of health promotion, in which health is an active process requiring the individual's intentional engagement.

Supporting Care-of-Self

How can providers support care-of-self for children? They can do so by directing their efforts toward the bio-psycho-social-spiritual person, which must be within the context of the child's family. In turn, community support is necessary. Children, because of their developmental needs, truly reflect the delicate interplay of the dimensions involved in care-of-self. Supporting care-of-self for children is synonymous with supporting healthy growth and development, which is at the core of working with children and their families. Care-of-self applies in all instances and is fundamental to health when health is recognized as an active process. Children are limited in care-of-self because of developmental stage. Providers, therefore, must support and entrust care-of-self to parents and other caregivers. As children mature, involving them in their own health may set the stage for continuation of care-of-self throughout their lives. When parents and other trusted adults fail to role model active participation in their own health, they place children at risk for repeating their example.

Using Anticipatory Guidance

Educating children and their families is an important strategy that the provider can use to encourage care-of-self to achieve positive health outcomes. To use the strategy of anticipatory guidance effectively, providers must approach each child and family based on their learning styles. Much has been written concerning how and how best primary care providers can offer anticipatory guidance in a busy office or clinic setting. The realities of managing this process can be especially challenging when little teaching time is available for the overall visit, let alone to evaluate learning needs for anticipatory guidance. The following material provides a guide for determining a patient's learning style, while also providing several teaching intervention techniques to help families understand healthy growth and development, health promotion, disease prevention, and episodic illness or disease management.

Effective Understanding

The parent's and child's ability to understand is critical to the family's success in participating in, developing, and carrying out a plan of care. The evaluation component of the plan's outcome is tied to this comprehension. Several key areas for evaluation include understanding the following:

- What is meant by healthy growth and development
- What is and is not healthy in diet, sleep, and social habits
- The difference between punishment and discipline
- Different parenting strategies

The provider also must evaluate the parents' understanding about the following:

- Episodic illness or, if applicable, disease process and course
- Symptoms and symptom management
- Child care strategies for symptom control
- Whom to call if a problem arises
- When it is appropriate to use over-the-counter medications, as well as safe and successful methods for administration of medication
- Use of medical equipment when indicated
- Awareness of possible/potential food–drug interactions
- Knowledge of when and how to seek further care
- Prior experience with the pediatric health care team

Learning Styles

Learning style is not a one-dimensional concept. Many learner-focused elements are involved, including the following:

- Reading comprehension and verbal understanding levels
- Developmental level
- Learning style
- Emotional status

Basic personality and learning style also influence the learner's ability to take in and use new information. Unin-vited information (information the parent or child may not wish or is unwilling to hear) may hinder its acceptance and integration.

Reading Levels and Content Understanding

Reading competency is categorized based on ascending complexity from level one to level five. Levels two to three in reading function, the average level for most North Americans, approximates eighth to ninth grade reading competency. When giving anticipatory guidance and other health information, providers should remember that approximately 20% of adults read at the lowest literacy level, which corresponds to below the fifth grade. Such individuals are considered functionally illiterate and are unable to read most magazines and newspapers, let alone interpret basic written instructions. Another 30% with marginal reading skills are able to follow very basic written directions that are worded clearly and simply.

Most available health care literature for patients generally is written at a sixth grade level. Literacy issues pose serious implications for health care delivery, because poor understanding of health and illness results in poor participation in with health care regimens. Individuals of low literacy exhibit more risk-taking behavior and experience increased health care costs over their lifetimes (Doak, Doak, & Root, 1996). Table 1-1 presents some basic differences between poor and skilled readers, with suggestions on how primary care providers can assist poor readers to understand written health-teaching materials.

While pediatric primary care providers must acknowledge the importance of child and parental levels of understanding, testing their reading skills and comprehension levels is unreasonable. A logical strategy is for clinicians to present written material to parents or child. Until they are certain that the recipient is capable of reading and understanding the material, wise practitioners should read some of the materials together with the family, using the directives provided in Display 1-1 to ensure that the content is usable. Clinicians also may wish to supplement commercially available written literature with their own written materials.

Meeting Learning Needs

Maximizing the "teachable moment" means that providers use every possible opportunity to convey their messages. In pediatric primary care, this message focuses on working with parents in all aspects of anticipatory guidance. These aspects include but are not limited to growth and development, discipline, personality development, self-esteem, health promotion, and disease prevention. Teaching and learning can be contagious. A health message may reach a parent or teenager, for example, through their children, family, or friends.

Table 1–1.   DIFFERENCES BETWEEN GOOD AND POOR READERS AND HOW TO MANAGE THE PROBLEMS

Skilled Readers	Poor Readers	Managing the Problems
Interpret meaning.	Take words literally.	Explain the meaning.
Read with fluency.	Read slowly, miss meaning.	Use common words, examples.
Get help for uncommon words.	Skip over the words.	Use examples; review.
Grasp the context.	Miss the context.	Tell context first; use visuals.
Persist with reading.	Tire quickly.	Use short segments, easy layout.

Doak et al., (1996).

DISPLAY 1–1 • Guidelines for Health Education Methods and Materials

- Set realistic objective(s):
    Limit the objective to what the majority of the target population needs now.
    Use a planning sheet to write down the objective and key points.
- To change health behaviors, focus on behaviors and skills:
    Emphasize behaviors and skills rather than facts.
    Consider placing key points first and last.
- Present context first (before giving new information):
    State the purpose or use for new content information before presenting it.
    Relate new information to the context of patients' lives.
- Partition complex instructions:
    Break instruction into easy-to-understand parts.
    Provide opportunities for small successes.
- Make it interactive:
    Consider including an interaction after each key topic. The patient must write, tell, show, demonstrate, select, or solve a problem.

Doak et al., (1996).

Keeping a selection of pamphlets in waiting rooms can help to ensure that patients pass on the "correct" version of messages to others. Providers also should have non-English versions of such material as appropriate to the patient population. An effective strategy for reaching parents of low literacy and young children is to use pictures illustrating health themes. Providers can mount such pictures in examining rooms. Adolescents should see materials related to safe sex and pregnancy prevention, smoking, alcohol and drug use, and disease prevention. Pediatric providers should consider periodically replenishing and updating literature and changing posters, so that patients and parents who visit the office frequently are exposed to more than one or two ongoing messages. Such messages may include, for example, information related to healthy babies, healthy diets and snacks, effective discipline, reading for fun, and exercise for fun. These simple acts can add interest to the family's wait, while reinforcing the messages that pediatric providers want to convey.

● **Clinical Pearl:** People will peruse material that is new to them. After that initial exposure, providers must continue to pique their interest if they are to reinforce health messages.

The "teachable moment" presents itself in many ways. For pediatric providers, learning to make the most of a teachable moment may help to create a climate that encourages children and their families to adopt healthy lifestyles. Through a caring and interactional environment, providers can encourage children and their families in the ongoing care-of-self.

BIBLIOGRAPHY

Singleton, J. K., Green-Hernandez, C., & Holzemer, S. P. (1999). The structure of primary care. In J. K. Singleton, S. A. Sandowski, C. Green-Hernandez, T. Horvath, R. V. DiGregorio, & S. P. Holzemer (Eds.), *Primary care* (pp. 3–7). Philadelphia: Lippincott Williams & Wilkins.

REFERENCES

Doak, C. C., Doak, L. G., & Root, J. H. (1996). *Teaching patients with low literacy skills.* Philadelphia: Lippincott-Raven.
Fontes, L. A. (2000). Working with Latino families on issues of child abuse and neglect. *The National Child Advocate, 3*, 1–7.
Green-Hernandez, C. (1997). Application of caring theory in primary care: A challenge for advanced practice. *Nursing Administration Quarterly, 21*(4), 77–82.
Green-Hernandez, C. (1992). Being there and caring: A philosophical analysis and theoretical model. In P. Winstead-Fry, (Ed.), *Rural health nursing.* New York: NLN Press.
Green-Hernandez, C. (1996). Engendering professional caring. *Staff Development Insider, 5*(1), 5, 7–8.
Green-Hernandez, C. (1991a). A phenomenologic investigation of caring as a lived experience. In P. Chinn (Ed.), *Anthology on caring.* New York: NLN Press.
Green-Hernandez, C. (1991b). Professional nurse caring: A conceptual model. In N. Watts et al. (Eds.), *Caring and nursing: Explorations in the feminist perspective.* New York: NLN Press.
Green-Hernandez, C. (1999). Family and cultural assessment measures in primary care. In J. K. Singleton, S. A. Sandowski, C. Green-Hernandez, T. Horvath, R. V. DiGregorio, & S. P. Holzemer (Eds.), *Primary care* (pp. 3–7). Philadelphia: Lippincott Williams & Wilkins.
Singleton, J. K. (2000). Nurses' perspective of encouraging clients' care-of-self in a short-term rehabilitation unit within a long-term care facility. *Rehabilitation Nursing, 25*(1), 23–29, 35.

CHAPTER 2

Assessment in Primary Care Pediatrics

• CAROL GREEN-HERNANDEZ, PhD, FNP-C

INTRODUCTION

The practice of pediatric primary care is family centered. Because of the complexities of care delivery in today's era of significant cost containment, providers must capitalize on this family-centered focus by making the family, to the fullest extent possible, partners in care delivery. Interactions that occur between the child and clinician and between parents and clinician have therapeutic potential. They provide an opportunity for relationships to develop; such relationships subsequently can improve patient outcomes as well as family and practitioner satisfaction (Tresolini & the Pew-Fetzer Task Force, 1994). Family-centered care thus recognizes and values the therapeutic potential of relationships (Singleton, Green-Hernandez, & Holzemer, 1999).

Assessment data, whether of pediatric providers, families, or cultural values and beliefs, are fundamental to the delivery of quality family-centered care. This chapter discusses the processes of self-assessment, family assessment, and cultural assessment.

SELF-ASSESSMENT THROUGH VALUES CLARIFICATION

For assessment of others to be successful, providers first must consider their own values and beliefs to ensure the delivery of appropriate and culturally sensitive primary care. Clinicians may find that clarifying personal values and beliefs assists them to discern possible sources for flawed assessment of children and their families. After discovering what they consider important, providers can focus on the personal values and beliefs that they share with the family. Values clarification may prove especially helpful when caring for families whose values, beliefs, and health behaviors differ from those of the provider. Although clinicians may find areas of value digression with the family, the process of self-reflection in values clarification can help prevent out-and-out conflict when strong differences emerge. Clearly, such conflict can jeopardize the therapeutic relationship. A sample values clarification tool and directions for its use are found in Appendix 2-1.

Values clarification can empower provider and family alike. The goal, of course, is to create and maintain primary care that is relationship centered. Such care must be both legal and ethical, while promoting self-actualization of the child and family (Green-Hernandez, 1997). Providers must be sensitive to both verbal and nonverbal cues and behaviors, including body stance, positioning, and use of eye contact. Similarly, maintenance of body space and use of touch can signal respect or lack of respect. The child's and family's feelings, values, and beliefs, including those per-

taining to health, are integral to all care management strategies in primary care. Children and their parents are not passive recipients of primary care; they are active partners. By using caring as a deliberate therapeutic model for communicating and working with children and their families (see Chap. 1), practitioners can avoid some of the value-laden conflicts that often emerge when primary care is provider controlled.

FAMILY ASSESSMENT

Like all open living systems, the family is an evolving entity. In the 21st century, the concept of a "typical" family eludes characterization. Today, the head of a family may be an emancipated minor, a single parent, two or more unrelated individuals, same-sex heads-of-household, or parents in a "traditional" or nuclear family. The family is what its members envision it to be. The key to family composition is that the group itself defines membership. This vision for family demography impacts family functioning. Evolving family structures and functions have implications for health promotion and illness management that present important challenges to primary care providers.

The following scenario provides an example of the need to use family-centered primary care within the context of family assessment:

A recent flu epidemic affected a 5-year-old boy and his three younger siblings. Their mother clearly is exhausted from caring for four sick little ones. Now recovered from flu, the 5-year-old comes to the practitioner's office in ketoacidosis. Following workup and emergency management, the clinician is faced with having to prepare the family for the child's diagnosis of type 1 diabetes.

The clinician needs to determine what the mother is feeling and what (if any) resources are available to support the family emotionally, physically, and financially through this crisis and beyond. The clinician also must assess the parents' and child's reading and comprehension levels to provide teaching that is understandable and, hence, usable. The provider needs to use a perspective that is sensitive to cultural and ethnic influences and to create an individualized plan that actually works for the child and family.

Caring theory as a foundation for family-centered pediatric primary care focuses on each individual family member and the family as a whole at the same time (Green-Hernandez, 1997; 1999). What happens to the child also happens to the family as a unit. Primary care delivered to the individual impacts the family as well. Whether integrating health promotion or confronting illness management, family members experience together the provider's professional caring for, communication with, and treatment of one of its members.

Historic View of Family-Centered Practice

Traditionally, primary care pediatric practitioners viewed the child as an individual who required treatment. They treated the family as an extension of the child, insofar as the child might communicate an illness to other members. Some enlightened providers also were concerned about the impact of illness or treatment requirements on family members, but by and large care delivery was individual rather than family focused. The primacy of individual rights and freedoms in western cultures further underscored these traditional health care practices.

A New Paradigm: Relationship-Centered Primary Care

Today the practice of primary care for children has moved toward a paradigm of family-centered health care. This clear and important vision is different from specialty practice, which emphasizes the individual. The family systems approach to primary care of children is at once both caring and respectful. The provider must remember that confidentiality must be at the forefront of care. Family-centered practice does not imply abandonment of the legal and ethical responsibilities the provider owes to the child and the parent(s) or caretaker(s).

Family-centered care is an optimum model for the practice of primary care to children. Providers recognize parents' feelings and responses to their child's health status. They view care management as important to the family's interactional function. Providers evaluate care given to the child within the context of other family members' responses to and connectedness with the child, while keeping in mind that the community is part of that connectedness. This kind of care delivery model is inherently more holistic than the traditional family practice model, wherein care is individual focused.

Assessment Data

Family assessment data help providers to deliver individualized, family-centered pediatric primary care. Such data can enhance the provider's understanding of the family and its needs both from individual and interpersonal perspectives. Display 2-1 summarizes important areas for collecting data in family assessment.

Providers should place family assessment data in the child's permanent record along with family demographic information. They should review such data annually, updating information as needed, because these data give valuable insights when the clinician interacts with the child and family. Data derived from a family assessment are quick and easy to obtain, especially when the provider combines a self-assessment questionnaire with interview content from the child's comprehensive history. In the case of multiple family members who are treated in the same practice, providers can copy the family assessment so that each person's chart contains this important information.

Family Assessment Tools

Family assessment tools provide contextual details about the objective information obtained in a standard genogram,

---

DISPLAY 2-1 • Areas for Family Assessment

- List information about the child and family, including immediate and extended members. Include individuals who, though perhaps not legally related, the patient may consider as part of the family matrix, including valued pets.
- Identify affectional and social networks of informal significance to the child. A matrix delineating the family's sources for immediate social support can be valuable in times of crisis. Its ready availability can enhance care delivery. Also identify distant or extended sources for social support because, in emergencies, the more sources of assistance known, the better the provider will be able to facilitate their implementation.
- Attempt to clarify life events of significance to the child and family. Examples include the child's own milestones (eg, grade progression) and family milestones (eg, births, deaths, marriages, remarriages, past and present informal domestic arrangements).
- Delineate important neighborhood factors to the child and family, including safety, stability, and social and economic variables that may affect health and well-being.
- How do family members make decisions affecting the group? Does each member have input? What resources (eg, financial, emotional, spiritual, professional) do they believe are available?
- What satisfaction(s) do members derive from family life? What stress(es) do they have?
- What does each member feel he or she contributes to the family?
- What is of importance to the family? Does a "higher power" support or guide them? What beliefs and value structures guide or do not guide them?
- What roles do gender and birth order play in family functioning, including member status? Are these variables sources for conflict? (Be clear about personal beliefs and values in collecting and analyzing this data. The provider must clarify differences—and even obvious conflicts—between personal and professional beliefs and values to maximize the provider's capability to analyze and use this data objectively and effectively).
- What (if any) change in cultural or ethnic identity has the family lost to or assimilated within a country's larger cultural expression? If loss has occurred, does it impact individual and family function and, in the wider arena, community identity? How has it affected health beliefs, health values, and in turn health function?

Green-Hernandez, C. (1999). Family and cultural assessment measures in primary care. In J. Singleton, S. Sandowski, C. Green-Hernandez, T. Horvath, R. DiGregorio, & S. Holzemer (Eds.), *Primary care.* Philadelphia: Lippincott Williams & Wilkins.

---

which providers collect during the child's history. They also can clarify immediate and extended familial relationships and social and community networks that might impact family-focused care. Such data help foster a coparticipative relationship between the provider and family to meet primary care needs (Artinian, 1994). Several published family assessment tools are available; Appendix 2-2 gives one example. Providers can use these instruments as they are or modify them to fit the needs of their practice.

The Family Circle

The Family Circle is a visual representation of a parent's, older child's, or adolescent's perception of the direction and importance of family relationships at a certain point and should be appended to the family assessment. The process for gathering a Family Circle diagram is quick and straightforward (Thrower, Bruce, & Walton, 1982). At a minimum, the clinician asks the parent to complete a Family Circle; alternatively, the provider gives each family member who is old enough a pen and paper. Each family member dates the paper and draws a large circle representing the family. The person then draws smaller circles inside or outside the large circle, representing the self, individual family members, and if desired, any other significant relationships, including pets. As each person constructs them, the circles suggest the emotional relationships inherent in the family matrix at that particular point. Each circle's size may indicate an individual's significance, while distance between circles may indicate the extent of affection one member feels toward that family member. The circles are not static. Anytime that the clinician perceives that family dynamics have changed is a good time to solicit a new diagram.

The parent may want to write a brief statement that describes personal feelings about the circles and their meaning. The provider and parent then discuss the Family Circle diagram together, with the parent confirming or explaining interpretation of the Circle. These subjective data can be extremely valuable to the provider's overall family assessment. Figure 2-1 illustrates a Family Circle for the family described earlier in this chapter. It helps to show what efforts may be needed to meet the child's and mother's needs, as well as those of other family members within the context of the wider community.

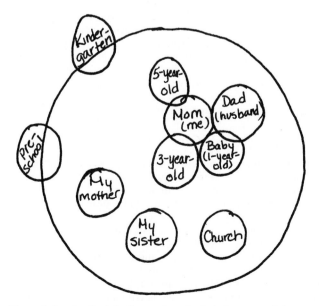

Figure 2–1 ■ Family circle diagram for a family facing type 1 diabetes mellitus.

CULTURAL ASSESSMENT

At its most basic level, cultural assessment is a clinical method for collecting and using data and supports the provider's understanding of the history, perspective, and world view of the child and family. Familial patterns of expression are part of a person's culture and ethnic identity; these patterns also can be placed within the context of the community at large. Cultural assessment is an outgrowth of family assessment. In all but homogeneous groups, both family and cultural assessments are logical precursors to a community appraisal.

Meaning of Culture

The first step in undertaking a cultural assessment is to clarify the meaning of culture. Culture embodies the beliefs, values, attitudes, customs, and ethnicity of a group. Cultural practices may be unique, because they derive from a group's particular world view. They also evolve over time. Were cultural practices and beliefs to remain completely static, their relevance would decrease, for people naturally grow and change due to life experiences and outside influences.

Culture can exert a powerful influence on family functioning. Gender roles and relevance of birth order, which are culturally influenced, can affect an individual's health behaviors and responses to life cycle events, including childbirth, aging, and illness. In turn, life cycle events influence both individual and family evolution. For example, the "sandwich generation" describes adult children who must balance caring for ailing parents against nurturing their own young children. Many such adults must negotiate this delicate balance while also working full-time outside the home.

A person's developmental stage also must be accounted for when examining culture and planning appropriate interventions. For example, the preschooler has very different eating requirements than the teenager. By the same token, variables such as athletic pursuits and peer influences will probably have more of an influence on the adolescent's ability to participate in a health regimen than will diabetic standards. In developing a therapeutic regimen, the caring provider works with children and families at their particular developmental stages.

Ethnic Influences on Culture

The notion of family varies among cultures, even when considered within the context of a country's "dominant culture." For example, cultural themes perpetuated by the television media of the 1950s and 1960s supported the view that family structure was nuclear and headed by a heterosexual, legally married couple. Extended family and friends enacted their roles indirectly rather than directly. Of course, reality always has been more complex than this view. In actuality, the dominant culture of many western countries is a montage of different cultures, each of which has different beliefs and values about family functioning. Multiculturalism is just that—many-cultured.

For example, families of African heritage often consider family to consist of both related and unrelated individuals in a kin and community structure. The family of English heritage may indeed most value the traditional nuclear structure. Families of Native American, Hispanic, Mediterranean, and Semitic backgrounds may function from a span of three or even four generations and also may include very close friends. Church, temple, or mosque may be central to such families and therefore serve a community function as well (Szapocznik & Kurtines, 1993; Markowitz, 1994; Green-Hernandez, 1999). In addition to including kin and close friends, many families of Asian ancestry include forebears as well as descendants in their vision of a kinship network (Berg & Jaya, 1993). Further enriching this picture of ethnic diversity, some cultures assign decision making to authority figures, such as a family or clan elder. The dominant culture sometimes supersedes the individual rights and privileges of a particular culture or ethnic group. This broader cultural view may conflict with an ethnic group's traditional view.

Provider–Family Differences and Impact on Health Care

Cultural differences can influence both the provider's and the family's values and beliefs about health, wellness, and personal responsibility for health management. In addition, the provider's own cultural beliefs and practices—not to mention family structure—may agree, disagree, or even strongly conflict with those of the family. Sometimes the provider's ethnic and cultural values are so different from those of the family that care delivery is threatened. For example, a clinical plan for type 1 diabetes management may be doomed if the provider does not prescribe it within a context that recognizes and values a family's dietary heritage. In relationship-centered primary care, the provider might best ensure success by working with the child and family to develop a management plan that reflects their dietary customs. Asking why this family does not just accept the standard diabetes management prescription and follow it, when in fact that plan may be culturally incongruent, can mean the difference between working with rather than against the family.

Verbal and Nonverbal Communication

Communication clearly improves when providers approach every interaction with awareness of the family's cultural and ethnic beliefs and values. Providers can enhance clinical practice when they know cultural expectations about use of touch or eye contact, personal space, and conversational pacing. Understanding the family's awareness of time and whether parents of older children expect to be included in examination or teaching also is helpful. When working with families whose language skills and abilities are different, providers may need to use nonverbal communication, including pantomime, to communicate information.

If nonverbal means prove inadequate, a language interpreter may be necessary. The ideal interpreter is a non-family member whose language skill is acceptable to both provider and family and who can interact effectively with the provider regarding health care information. A non-family member may be better able to communicate information objectively, because he or she is less likely to delete information perceived as embarrassing or private.

When a family member or close friend acts as interpreter for the parents or older child or adolescent, the clinician needs to be aware that the translator may "edit" the communication. Similarly, parents may edit what they otherwise would have told because of embarrassment when filtering their information through this person. Family translators also may be sources of possible violations of confidentiality. If family or close friends must act as translators, clinicians need to guard against possible "editing." They can do so by closely observing the parent, child, and translator as each speaks. Providers should avoid using staff members who have expertise in translation unless such service is part of their work assignment. Translating takes time and as such might place an employee under an undue burden relative to the employer's work expectations. In the case of older children, adolescents, or parents who are hearing-challenged, practitioners should obtain the services of a credentialed sign language interpreter.

Geographic Influences

Just as identifying the influence of ethnic heritage is important in cultural assessment, so too is recognizing the role of geography, whether urban, suburban, or rural. For example, rural dwellers share a cultural base that differs from what is found in urban and suburban areas. Most rural communities are composed of individuals who share a similar birthplace, ethnic heritage, and means of livelihood. The assessment for this community would differ from that done in an urban area, whose residents come from various ethnic traditions and are of varying socioeconomic levels. Non-native residents of each of these regions may appreciate and even try to assimilate into the native culture but will not be able to abandon fully their geographic culture of origin.

Traditionally, a dearth of services in rural, agrarian areas (few people, fewer services) meant that rural dwellers needed to develop self-reliance as much from necessity as from stubborn independence. A person's measure might derive more from physical endurance and native intuition than from social, educational, or economic advantages. Because cultural outcomes are at least partly a product of a lived world view, rural culture can be seen to reflect the traits of uncomplaining acceptance of that which one cannot change. Energy and purpose may emanate as much from the individual as from the wider community. Health care expectations typically are low among native residents of rural areas, where people are not accustomed to their providers making frequent specialty referrals or prescribing nonroutine, diagnostic testing. These attitudes are partly because of the decreased availability of referral services, including more of the "state-of-the-art" diagnostics (University of Vermont, College of Medicine, 1998).

The cultural context of urban life is distinctly different. A wide array of services emerges in a nonagrarian society. Oversupply may replace competition for services, necessitating further service differentiation. The result is increased demand for services and hence other-reliance rather than self-reliance (Kaslow, Celano, & Dreelin, 1995). Similar to urban life, modern suburban culture is fast-paced and replete with ready availability of goods and services. Residents of both urban and suburban areas generally have high expectations for health care delivery. Creative yet cost-effective models for urban and suburban primary care acknowledge this consumer expectation.

Influence of One's Own Origins

The place where one grew up can powerfully influence world view. For example, an urban or suburban youngster might spend leisure time in adult-supervised activities, including shopping or museum exploration. A rural child might spend many hours alone, exploring woods and fields. Urban residents typically do not hunt wild game for leisure, let alone for winter food. Native-born rural youngsters typically learn to or have family members who hunt. These childhood experiences bear directly on adult patterns of behavior. Demographics, including perceptions of socioeconomic status and class as well as educational levels, impact health care and health promotion delivery.

If providers move away from their childhood homes, they may find that local customs and values differ in their new locations from those of their childhood region. In such cases, rather than ignoring that differences exist, providers may find it helpful to examine the values and beliefs that emanated from their childhood homes. Even before they become enmeshed in the community, providers may want to identify, for example, the following:

- How does the community celebrate holidays?
- Is the community ethnically homogeneous or diverse?
- How does the community celebrate religious, patriotic, and other events?
- Do people reside nearby who share the provider's ethnic or religious background?
- How are local schools and services similar or different from those available to the provider while growing up?

Besides culturally ascribed beliefs and values, childhood experiences directly influence adult expectations. Where one grew up and at what educational or socioeconomic level can powerfully influence one's expectations for the community and its goods and services. The act of growing up and moving to a different geographic locale may not change the powerful effects of childhood experiences.

Of course, providers can successfully practice in areas other than their native homes. They may want to begin by reviewing their total life experiences, educational and economic heritage, and family customs. This process may assist with discerning similarities and differences in the values and traditions where they now practice. Such examination can assist the provider in clarifying personal expectations and helping to shed light on those of families and professional colleagues.

● **Clinical Pearl:** Application of primary care that is based on caring will be more successful if practice also is based on respect and honor. These attributes flow from the clinician's efforts to learn about a community's values. The clinician must recognize the importance of becoming knowledgeable about local ethnic groups, values and beliefs, festivals, and regional or religious traditions.

DISPLAY 2–2 • The Five Universal Value Orientations of Human Families

- A temporal focus for life, at least in relationship to important milestones. For some ethnic or cultural groups, this focus may be seasons of the year, while others value the progression of the calendar.
- Preferred or habitual blueprints for action in relationships.
- Standards for behavior in relationship to others.
- Connections to the world around us, within us, and beyond us.
- Beliefs about the innate nature of human beings.

Adapted from Ho, M. K. (1987). *Family therapy with ethnic minorities.* Rockville, MD: Aspen; Green-Hernandez, C. (1999). Family and cultural assessment measures in primary care. In J. Singleton, S. Sandowski, C. Green-Hernandez, T. Horvath, R. DiGregorio, & S. Holzemer (Eds.), *Primary care.* Philadelphia: Lippincott Williams & Wilkins.

DISPLAY 2–3 • Topical Areas Underscoring Cultural Assessment

- Country of origin (or, if native-born, region). How long the child/family have lived in this country/region
- Ethnic group and strength of ethnic feelings
- Sources of social support, including relevant family and friends (if applicable, ethnic community ties)
- Verbal and reading capability, and in what language(s)
- Method for nonverbal communication
- Religion—its relevance and practice demands
- Food choices; any taboos
- Personal economics—ability to meet the family's needs
- Health-illness notions and customs
- Beliefs, values, and customs surrounding birth, death, and sickness

Adapted from Lipson, J. G., & Meleis, A. I. (1985), In J. G. Lipson, S. L. Dibble, & P.A. Minarik, (1996). *Culture and nursing care: A pocket guide.* San Francisco: UCSF Nursing Press; Green-Hernandez, C. (1999). Family and cultural assessment measures in primary care. In J. Singleton, S. Sandowski, C. Green-Hernandez, T. Horvath, R. DiGregorio, & S. Holzemer (Eds.), *Primary care.* Philadelphia: Lippincott Williams & Wilkins.

Cultural Incongruence

Clearly, cultural incongruence can emerge when the provider's geographic, social, educational, and economic background differs from that of the community in which one is in clinical practice. This incongruence also may occur when family members live in a community that does not share their world view of the types and kinds of services needed and how they should be delivered. Does the family expect services that include house calls? Should care delivery be contractual, where both provider and parents agree on points of management? Does the family expect that the provider will direct needs assessment and care delivery? The answers to these questions depend on a variety of factors, including cultural and ethnic heritage, past and current socioeconomic background, geographic origin, and educational level of the provider and family. Health beliefs and values are shaped by the foregoing and, further, are influenced by past and present experiences of both traditional and complementary health care and its delivery.

Value Orientations in Family Life

Despite differences in the expression of family life in different cultures or in different geographic regions, five value orientations have been identified that all families universally share. An awareness of these value orientations can help the provider to deliver primary care that is sensitive to the family's core beliefs and values. Display 2-2 describes these value orientations.

Acknowledgment of the five value orientations can enhance the practice of primary care in today's complex, multicultural, and multiethnic society. Value orientations underscore the cultural assessment. Lipson, Dibble, and Minarik (1996) cite 10 topical areas that should underscore the cultural assessment (Display 2-3).

REFERENCES

Artinian, N. T. (1994). Selecting a model to guide family assessment. *Dimensions of Critical Care Nursing, 14*(1), 4–13.

Berg, I. K., & Jaya, A. (1993). Different and the same: Family therapy with Asian-American families. *The Journal of Marital and Family Therapy, 19*, 31–38.

Green-Hernandez, C. (1997). Application of caring theory in primary care: A challenge for advanced practice. *Nursing Administration Quarterly, 21*(4), 77–82.

Green-Hernandez, C. (1999). Family and cultural assessment measures in primary care. In J. Singleton, S. Sandowski, C. Green-Hernandez, T. Horvath, R. DiGregorio, & S. Holzemer (Eds.), *Primary care.* Philadelphia: Lippincott Williams & Wilkins.

Kaslow, N. J., Celano, M., & Dreelin, E. D. (1995). A cultural perspective on family theory and therapy. *The Psychiatric Clinics of North America, 18*(3), 621–633.

Lipson, J. G., Dibble, S. L., & Minarik, P. A. (Eds.) (1996). Culture and nursing care: A pocket guide. San Francisco: UCSF Nursing Press.

Markowitz, L. (1994). The cross-currents of multi-culturalism. *Family Therapy Networker, 4*, 18–27.

Singleton, J.K., Green-Hernandez, C., & Holzemer, S.P. (1999). *The structure of primary care.* In J.K. Singleton, S.A. Sandowski, C. Green-Hernandez, T. Horvath, R.V. DiGregorio, & S.P. Holzemer (Eds.), *Primary care* (pp. 3–7). Philadelphia: Lippincott Williams & Wilkins.

Szapocznik, J., & Kurtines, W. M. (1993). Family psychology and cultural diversity. *American Psychologist, 48*, 400–407.

Thrower, S. M., Bruce, W. E., & Walton, R. F. (1982). The family circle method for integrating family systems concepts in family medicine. *Journal of Family Practice, 15*, 451.

Tresolini, C. P., & the Pew-Fetzer Task Force. (1994). *Health professions education and relationship-centered care.* San Francisco: Pew Health Professions.

University of Vermont, College of Medicine. (1996). *Vermont AHEC proposal.* (Unpublished proposal). Burlington, VT: The University of Vermont.

A P P E N D I X   2 - 1

Values Clarification Tool

The individual is asked to respond in writing to each question in turn:

1. Write down three things you enjoy doing.
2. Record a place—either real or imaginary—where you go when you're feeling sad.
3. What is your most important *personal* achievement?
4. Record the three most pressing problems you face now, in order from worst to least.
5. Assume that you have only 1 year to live. You won't be handicapped or in pain because of your terminal status. What will you do? How will you use your time and abilities?
6. Assume that your last year is at an end. Write down three words you'd like others to remember you by; write down one word you do not want used to describe you after your death.

Interpretation of this tool:

- When you're having a hard time of it, plan to do some of the activities you enjoy, or go (either physically or mentally) to your "get-away" place.
- For item 4: You may not be able to solve your most difficult problem, but it's possible that you will be able to solve the second one in a reasonable time frame, such as 3 to 6 months. You may be able to resolve your least difficult issue now. Keep in mind that these are guidelines rather than an exact timetable for problem resolution.
- For item 6: Seek out friends and family who personify these attributes. Steer clear of anyone whose temperament puts you in mind of the characteristic you identified as unacceptable to you.

Adapted from Personal coat of arms, in King, E. C. (1984). *Affective Education in Nursing*, p. 31. Rockville, MD: Aspen; Green-Hernandez, C. (1999). Family and cultural assessment measures in primary care. In J. Singleton, S. Sandowski, C. Green-Hernandez, T. Horvath, R. DiGregorio, & S. Holzemer (Eds.), *Primary care*. Philadelphia: Lippincott Williams and Wilkins.

A P P E N D I X   2 - 2

Family Assessment Tool

Cultural heritage

For each family member:
   Age
   Relationship
   Degree of contact (if applicable):

Religion (if applicable)

Religious practices (if applicable)

Values
- What is important to each member?
- Is there any conflict in values, as between role in home, among family, compared to workplace?
   If yes, has the family resolved this conflict?
   If not, how is the family managing?

Ethnic/cultural traditions (if applicable)

Coping patterns

Stress management
- Day-to-day
- In times of increased stress

Caring for self
- How does each family member feel about himself or herself?
- What does each member do to take care of self?
- Does everyone do self-caring activities (eg, set aside some time for themselves each day)?
   If yes, what kinds of activities and their frequency?
   If not, why not?

Caring for others of importance to the family's members
- How does the family feel about them?
- Does family member help them with any of their care?
   If yes, how do they feel about this?
   How are they managing?
- Does the family want to continue in these activities?
   If yes, does anyone need any help?
   Is the family aware of resources and support services if needed or desired?

Family management
- Who is responsible for:
   Housework
   House maintenance (inside and out)
   Yard work
   Finances
   Pets (if applicable)
   Children (if applicable)
   Parent care (if applicable)

Family communication
- How does everyone communicate with one another?
- How do members feel about family communication?

Family support
- How do members feel about each other?
- Is there a particular member(s) they turn to in times of need?
   If yes, who?
- Does the family perceive that other resources are available to them if needed?
   If yes, who or what agency or church?

Income needs
- Which family member's income provides financial support?
- Are there gaps between family members' income needs and income available?
   If yes, explain.
   What are the usual work schedules for employed members?
   Is there any flexibility in these schedules?

School supports
- Which (if any) members attend school?
   If any, are they full- or part-time?
   What are their schedules?
   Is there any flexibility in these schedules?
- Are there any problems associated with schooling?
- What school supports would be available if needed?

Social and community supports
- In what social activities do members engage?
- Are there any problems or stressors associated with these activities?
- What social and community resources would be available if needed?

Logistical needs
- Does the family have reliable transportation available to them?
   If yes, and if not private transport, what is the schedule?
   Is there off-hour (ie, nights, week-ends, holidays) availability?
- What is the average distance the family travels for health care resources, including the primary care office? Are medical emergency services available?

Green-Hernandez, C. (1999). Family and cultural assessment measures in primary care. In J. Singleton, S. Sandowski, C. Green- Hernandez, T. Horvath, R. DiGregorio, & S. Holzemer (Eds.), *Primary care.* Philadelphia: Lippincott Williams and Wilkins.

CHAPTER **3**

Community-Based Primary Care Resources for Children

- STEPHEN PAUL HOLZEMER, PhD, RN; MARIA SCARAMUZZINO, MSN, RN, PNP; and JANE KIERNAN, PhD, RN

INTRODUCTION

This chapter provides a context for understanding the interconnectedness of children and families with the communities in which they live. Caring for children effectively, using appropriate resources is a global concern (Zotti, 1999; Morabia, 2000). This context underpins suggested community resources that pediatric primary care providers may want to use when working with children and their families. Additional community-based resources specific to the topic of discussion are found at the end of each remaining chapter in this text.

RESOURCE ALLOCATION: FEAST OR FAMINE?

Communities at the national, regional, and local levels make health-related resources available for treating illness and keeping people healthy. Many variables influence how resources are allocated. Primary care providers can influence some variables but cannot control others. For example, they cannot control the outbreak of a new pathogen, but they can modify and influence the public's response to a resulting epidemic. Providing community-based primary care resources to meet the needs of children and adolescents is particularly challenging because these age groups represent a vulnerable population. Factors contributing to this vulnerability and ways for providers to deal with them are discussed below.

Children's Health Issues May Be Ignored Until a Crisis

One major influence on resource allocation for health care involves the fact that many resources become allocated only in response to crisis, when groups initially affected by the situation in question demand action. For example, early in the acquired immunodeficiency syndrome (AIDS) pandemic, clinicians and people living with AIDS greatly increased the number and types of resources available to fight this disease. As more women, people of color, and children contract AIDS, funding for treatment and research may decrease if these aggregates cannot advocate successfully for what they need. Furthermore, when another major public health crisis occurs, it inevitably will trigger the restructuring of resource allocation, leaving people with AIDS in danger of losing needed resources.

Preventive Care for Children Is Undervalued

Another concern in resource allocation relates to how people value services. Many communities tend to develop more resources for illness care than for disease prevention or rehabilitation. Large medical centers devoted to cardiovascular, neoplastic, and other physical and psychological problems exist to cure illness, not to prevent it. The cost of illness care cripples efforts to move the concept of prevention beyond the philosophical to the real. This concern is especially important for the pediatric population, because much of pediatric primary care is directed toward health promotion and disease-prevention strategies.

Children Rely on Adults for Needed Resources

The needs of children and adolescents range from predictable and less common illnesses to complex physical, emotional, and social crises (Belcher, & Shinitzky, 1998; Britto et al., 1999; Xiaoming, Stanton, & Feigelman, 1999). Regardless of their individual concerns, all children and adolescents must rely on adults for needed resources; rarely are they able to negotiate for health resources themselves. Conflicts arise because many adults who identify and secure the needs of pediatric populations have no expertise in the care of children and adolescents. The scandal of lead poisoning provides an example in which children and adolescents were exposed to danger and not cared for properly by individual adults or society (Markowitz & Rosner, 2000). Because of the political power of the paint industry, children were and in some places continue to be exposed to lead paint.

Providers must exert serious efforts to guarantee sufficient resources for preventing illness while also treating and rehabilitating sick children and adolescents. Both traditional and complementary perspectives can play a part in this process (Ferris et al., 1998; Sikand & Laken, 1998). A master plan for meeting the needs of children and adolescents should be a primary goal for every well-functioning community. Politicians and others who make decisions about resource allocation may need guidance in meeting the needs of this special aggregate. Models of community assessment are useful in setting up a structure in which communities can allocate and distribute their resources and evaluate their benefits.

Children Are Unable to Negotiate for Resources

An increasing concern is the influence of special interest groups in shaping what services are available to the public. The reality is that resources are not available to provide all people with all health care needs. The traditionally silent voices of vulnerable groups (eg, children, mentally ill, homeless) are little match against the powerful voices of special interest lobbies, who strive to meet their own needs and achieve their own ends, sometimes at the expense of others.

These "others" obviously include vulnerable aggregates. For example, the politics of reproductive health and a woman's control over her body significantly influence the care that young women will receive. Some influential conservative political and religious groups want to limit access to some areas of women's health care (eg, genetic testing, in-vitro fertilization) for adolescents. If they succeed, emancipated minors may have difficulty negotiating for health care services if they do not have a system of adults who support their choices.

Contemporary decentralization of funding resources may be problematic. Some block grants, for example, while supporting the autonomy of communities to endorse programs they desire, do not provide for the checks and balances that protect groups who cannot negotiate for resources. If children and adolescents do not receive needed services, their health can be affected negatively as they move into adulthood. Failure to learn about or receive primary prevention measures related to health promotion and specific protection may result in serious acute and chronic illness in the future.

COMMUNITY-BASED PLANNING FOR COMPREHENSIVE SERVICES

The U.S. Department of Health and Human Services (1998) has developed an initiative to eliminate racial and ethnic disparities in health by the year 2010. Foci of this project include infant mortality, cancer screening and management, cardiovascular disease, diabetes, human immunodeficiency virus (HIV) infection, and child and adult immunizations. *Healthy People 2010*, created through public comment, attempts to move the public away from a preference for illness care toward designing appropriate preventive measures for comprehensive health care. The intention of this national prevention plan is to empower diverse populations to work together to improve health. One analogy compares this plan to a road map used by different lay and professional individuals, families, groups, and aggregates who are all working together to maintain health. Recipients and providers of care have developed the Pew Commission Competencies

TABLE 3–1. WORKSHEET COMBINING PEW COMMISSION COMPETENCIES AND CRITICAL HEALTH INDICATORS OF *HEALTHY PEOPLE 2010*

Competency	Infant Mortality	Cancer Screening	Cardiovascular Disease	Diabetes	HIV Infection	Immunizations
Embrace a personal ethic of social responsibility and service.						
Exhibit ethical behavior in all professional activities.						
Provide evidence-based, clinically competent care.						
Incorporate the multiple determinants of health in clinical care.						
Apply knowledge of the new sciences.						
Demonstrate critical thinking, reflection, and problem-solving skills.						
Understand the role of primary care.						
Rigorously practice preventive health care.						
Integrate population-based care and services into practice.						
Improve access to health care for those with unmet health needs.						
Practice relationship-centered care with individuals and families.						
Provide culturally sensitive care to a diverse society.						
Partner with communities in health care decisions.						
Use communication and information technology effectively and appropriately.						
Work in interdisciplinary teams.						
Ensure care that balances individual, professional, system, and societal needs.						
Practice leadership.						
Take responsibility for quality of care and health outcomes at all levels.						
Contribute to continuous improvement of the health care system.						
Advocate for public policy that promotes and protects the health of the public.						
Continue to learn and help others learn.						

(Bellack & O'Neil, 2000), which are requirements for successful primary care providers in the 21st century. Together, *Healthy People 2010* and the Pew Commission Competencies provide a template for identifying where community-based services for children exist and where they still need to be developed.

In planning comprehensive health care for children and adolescents, providers can combine the preventive strategies of *Healthy People 2010* with the expected health care provider competencies of the Pew Commission. For example, a provider who is considering the competency "improve access to health care for those with unmet health needs" might be inspired to partner with a local business to address diabetes management. The business might seek out the support of a recognized performer or athlete to conduct or sponsor a series of programs to children at different age levels about eating habits. For the competency of "continue to learn and help others learn" combined with the health concern "immunizations," the clinician could bring together students from schools of health professions to establish a phone bank to help parents keep appointments for vaccinations. Table 3-1 is a worksheet to help primary care providers, families, and community representatives identify areas where services need development or continued support.

Alliance for Health Model

The Alliance for Health model is one blueprint that provides a broad outline to evaluate needs in various aggregates (Holzemer & Arnold, 1998; Holzemer, Singleton, & Green-Hernandez, 1999). The five major components of the Alliance for Health model are as follows:

- Community-based needs
- Care management techniques
- Influences on resource allocation decisions
- Validation of services by the client
- Expertise of the interdisciplinary team

Display 3-1 identifies subcategories for assessment of the first three components. Patterns of morbidity and mortality are, for example, critical components of community-based needs. Knowing the patterns of disease, illness, and death are central to understanding the needs of the community. Similarly, the mix of patient problems is essential to understanding systems of case management. Finally, a population's values and beliefs will directly influence decisions about resource allocation. These first three components of the model rely on the last components for practical application. Validation of services by the client and, when necessary, a parent or guardian increases the probability that a treatment plan will succeed. Validation of services means that the patient and family find services acceptable, affordable, and culturally appropriate. The expertise of the interdisciplinary team directly influences how accurately and efficiently the patient–provider team works. This expertise is defined as the skill and success various disciplines have in working together with clients to solve health-related problems.

For visual effect, Figures 3-1 and 3-2 show interlocking circles that represent community-based needs, care management techniques, and influences on resource allocation. Careful assessment of these components is necessary to provide comprehensive health care. Figure 3-1 shows a well-integrated community as determined by the Alliance for Health model. Figure 3-2 shows a less integrated model,

which could represent a situation where an influx of children into a community has occurred, and their specific health needs are not well known. In such a situation (eg, high emigration or a natural disaster that caused displacement of people), specific community-based needs will need to be assessed. The existence of systems of care management and

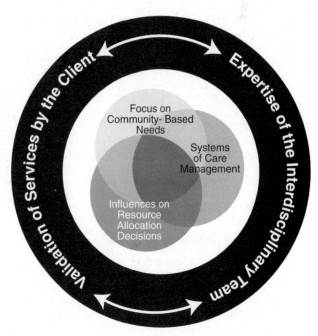

Figure 3–1 ■ The Alliance for Health model for community health assessment and care delivery in community-based pediatric care.

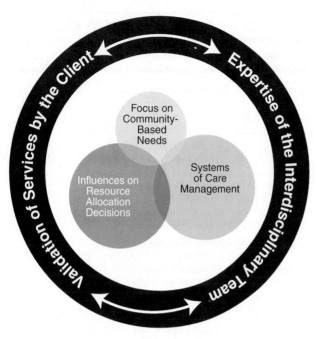

Figure 3–2 ■ A less integrated model for community health assessment and care delivery in community-based pediatric care.

methods for appropriate resource allocation are limited until needs are assessed adequately.

Combined Adult and Pediatric Services

Physically separating care of children and adolescents from care of adults will likely decrease the access to needed services. Limited money and time make double visits to care providers impractical for families. Such limitations are special concerns because integration and accessibility are two cornerstones of primary health care (Donaldson, Yordy, Lohr, & Vanselow, 1996). Some institutions have addressed the need for facility fiscal management by restricting the hours and location of primary care delivery, which may make securing services for adolescents and children problematic.

Combining the care of children and adolescents with that of adults who care for them is philosophically sound but not without difficulties. Challenges in combining services include finding times when the schedules of providers and patients mesh closely. In many situations, services need to be accessible when both caregiver and child are available. When services are combined, facilities may need to provide child care and supervision when adult caregivers need privacy (eg, during physical examinations or counseling). In some facilities, decentralization of support services like blood work and roentgen (x-ray) evaluations demands time away from work or school for the child and caregiver.

School-Based Services

An effective venue for primary or episodic pediatric primary care delivery is to provide it where children and adolescents go to school. The National Assembly of School-Based Health Care has developed principles to guide program planning. These principles, still under development, reinforce the need for comprehensive services, including physical, social, mental health, and health education needs. The most important

aspects about these competencies are that they vary closely with the growth and development needs of children and adolescents. Display 3-2 lists facts and principles that any group thinking about establishing school-based services should consider.

School-based health care can enhance privacy for children and adolescents when counseling is necessary. The setting may provide safety for confiding in providers about sensitive topics. Furthermore, providers can stress peer support of healthy behaviors in a way that encourages youth participation. Older peers can modify their own behaviors as necessary as they learn more about health and the effectiveness of peer support. Such students who are respected by younger students can serve as role models for healthy behaviors and risk reduction. Teachers also may obtain more accurate feedback from health-related programs that students support and make necessary changes so students eagerly participate in them.

Appropriate and Current Educational Materials

As discussed in Chapter 1, printed health-related information must be current and developed at the child's or adolescent's literacy level. Information used for adults often is not helpful and may even be inappropriate for children and adolescents. Developmentally appropriate material designed with the input of children and adolescents makes health-related information more contemporary and user friendly. When creating their own materials, clinicians need to take special care not to connect particular individuals with disease conditions due to confidentiality and privacy requirements. Providers may need to consider the religious and cultural beliefs of parents when developing health-related materials for children.

For non-English speakers and the deaf, professionally trained interpreters need to translate spoken and written language. Reliance on multilingual staff to translate accurately the concerns of children or their parents, except in emergencies, may be dangerous. Staff may place other patients in jeopardy if translation takes a long time. Using family members as interpreters also may be inappropriate, because the possibility of miscommunication or violation of privacy and confidentiality (eg, with reproductive health or disease evaluations) creates potentially serious legal issues. Chapter 2 explores this issue in greater detail.

Clinical Research Trials

Clinical trials are essential to developing better future treatments. Some patients and families, however, may feel that they must participate in clinical research trials for their own survival. They mistakenly may believe that experimental treatments being tested for efficacy and safety are the only treatments available or are superior forms of treatment. In fact, parents and minors need to know that they should not view research as treatment. Specific concerns of clinical research trials with children include assent versus informed consent, potential loss of privacy or control over the child's own body, and inability to negotiate out of a trial. Parents and guardians who act for the child may fear loss of services or a change in the level of care for their child if they do not participate in the clinical trial.

▲ **Clinical Warning:** Parents and minors need to know not to view research as treatment.

DISPLAY 3–2 • National Principles for School-Based Health Care

Principle #1: The school-based center and the school must be committed to operating with mutual respect and a spirit of collaboration. The school/school district should facilitate and promote the use of the center's services. Each school-based health center should form and maintain an advisory committee to provide input into the development and operation of the program. Advisory committee membership should include school staff, community members, health providers, and especially parents and students.

Principle #2: School-based health services should be developed based on local assessment of needs and resources. Schools having students with the highest prevalence of unmet medical and psychosocial needs should receive the top priority for the establishment of the centers. Once the center is open, the services should be available to all currently enrolled students, including children with special health care needs, and, if possible to out-of-school youth.

Principle #3: School-based health centers should be organized through school, community, health, mental health, social service, and legal service provider relationships. School-based health centers should provide services in keeping with state and local laws, regulations, and community practice.

Principle #4: The school-based health center should provide comprehensive primary medical, social, mental health, and health education services designed to meet the psychosocial and physical health needs of children and youth, including children with special health care needs in the context of their family, culture, and environment.

Principle #5: School-based health center services should be provided by a multidisciplinary team, which may include providers from the fields of medicine, nursing, social work, psychology, health education, nutrition, and law.

Principle #6: The school-based health center must arrange for 24-hour 12-month coverage to ensure access to services when school or the center is closed. This may be done through an on-call system staffed by its own staff or through a backup health facility.

Principle #7: The school-based health center must be integrated into the school health program, which includes environment and curriculum. The school-based health center should plan and coordinate its programs and services with school personnel, including nurses and counselors, and with other community providers that are also located at the school.

Principle #8: The school-based health center, in partnership with the school and other co-located service providers, should develop policies and systems to ensure confidentiality of services.

Principle #9: The school-based health center should be designed to complement services provided by existing health care providers or to serve as a medical home. For managed care plans, the school-based health center can function as the principal provider of primary care.

Principle #10: The school-based health center must coordinate care with the students' medical homes, including managed care providers, and with other medical providers, social service agencies, mental health providers, and other agencies, programs, and organizations.

Principle #11: The school-based health center must inform the community and the school, concerning the health needs of youth and children. The school-based health center should participate in the use of data collection instruments and distribute information on the who, what, and why of services provided.

National Assembly on School-Based Health Care
666 11th St., NW, Suite 735
Washington, DC 20005
Phone: (888) 286-8727 (202) 638-5872
Fax: (202) 638-5879

Providers must encourage parents or guardians to ask questions so that they are able to act in the child's best interest. The literacy level of parents and guardians must be assessed because some complex language still exists in informed consent and protocol documents. Parents, guardians, and emancipated minors are likely to have some immediate questions, while other questions may emerge over time. A list of questions, developed to help and not to overwhelm the client, is found in Display 3-3 (AIDS Treatment Data Network, 1999).

COMMUNITY RESOURCES

A number of variables can assist pediatric clinicians to secure and use community-based resources wisely. An orientation to this end is the belief that resource allocation decisions include the following:

- A philosophy of listening to communities
- Reflective analysis of practice to establish continuity of care
- Honest discussion of the limitations of continuity of care
- Partnership status of interdisciplinary team members
- Dedication to coalition building in the community

These variables provide focus for pediatric primary care providers. This focus can in turn give direction to clinicians, who can establish plans of care with children and families that use community-based resources to maximize their effect on health and wellness. Integrating these variables into pediatric practice can guide providers in developing creative and innovative relationships with the people and communities for whom they care.

To support the effort of developing a comprehensive plan, a beginning list of general internet resources and some examples of video and hard copy teaching resources is found below. Providers must verify resources and update them as necessary. Maintaining current resources spares patients and families distress when attempting to locate expired or out-of-date material.

General Internet Resources

Yonge, K. K. (1998). *The 110 best parenting sites*. Charleston, WV: Cambridge Educational. (See teaching resources below.)

DISPLAY 3–3 • Research Questions for Clinical Trials

- What is the name of this trial?
- What kind of trial is it (phase I, placebo-controlled)?
- Do I need to be in the hospital to be in this trial? If so, for how long?
- How often must I visit the site?
- What will happen on these visits?
- How long will each visit take?
- Is this trial being conducted at any other locations?
- Is there a location that is more convenient for me?
- Is there a site that has Spanish-speaking counselors?
- Is child care available at the site?
- Are there free laboratory tests or examinations at the site?
- Do I have to do anything while at home?
- Are there things I cannot do during the trial?
- Is this drug available outside of this trial? If so, where and how can I get it?
- When do I start the trial?
- How long will this trial last?
- What are the immediate side effects of this drug?
- What are the long-term effects of my using this drug?
- What if I have to miss a visit or forget to take the drug?
- How will I be helped to deal with side effects?
- What type of drug is being tested?
- How often must the drug be taken?
- How will the drug be given in this trial (pills, by shot)?
- Do I know what each drug looks like?
- Must the drug be taken in the hospital?
- Do I have to take the drug at the drug site?
- Can I take the drug at home?
- How will taking the drug affect my day-to-day life?
- Has this drug been used before? If so, for what conditions? What were the results?
- What other drugs are being used for this condition?
- How does the trial drug compare in safety and success?
- What is the evidence that this one works?
- What tests will be given before I start?
- Will these tests cost anything?
- Will I get the results of these tests?
- What tests will be given during the trial?
- Will I get the results of these tests? If so, when?
- How often will other tests be done?
- How often will the researchers tell me how I am doing?
- Is this trial confidential?
- Will anyone know about my health condition?
- How will information be coded to protect my privacy?
- Do the consent papers describe all of the risks and benefits?
- What written information will I be given?
- How often will the IRB review the trial?
- How will I be informed of any changes?
- What if the trial changes significantly?
- Will I be out into another trial?

- Will I receive an updated informed consent form to sign?
- Do I need health insurance?
- Do I need to have my own doctor to get into this trial?
- To what emergency room can I go?
- Who pays for medical care if I get sick from the drug?
- Do I have to pay for laboratory tests or other things?
- Will I be given any money for participating in the trial?
- Will I be given carfare for traveling to and from the site?
- Is child care money available?
- Will the sponsors of the drug supply it to me free?
- What happens when the drug is available by prescription?
- Will the treatment be available to me even if I leave?
- Can I take the drug on an empty stomach or must I take it with food?
- Are there any special foods that I need to eat?
- If I am already on a special diet, may I continue?
- Is there anything I shouldn't eat?
- Can I take nonprescription drugs?
- Are aspirin, cold tablets, or cough syrup okay?
- Can I use prescription drugs while I'm on this trial?
- Can I take other experimental drugs?
- Can I take drugs to prevent or treat opportunistic infections?
- Can I take drugs to prevent or treat other illnesses I may get (pain medications, methadone)?
- Can I drink alcohol?
- Are there any known interactions with drugs I take on a recreational basis (cocaine, heroin, X, K, others)?
- Will taking these during the trial disqualify me?
- What type of contraceptives can I use?
- Do I have to use contraceptives?
- Are contraceptives permitted or monitored?
- Are pregnant woman allowed in the trial?
- If I'm on placebo, can I get the drug if my condition worsens?
- Can I take the drug once the trial is over, even if the trial was declared a failure?
- How is the success of the trial defined by the protocol?
- How will decisions about stopping the trial be made?
- How is failure defined in the protocol?
- Will this be done even if I decide to leave the trial?
- Will my health be checked after I stop taking the drug?
- Will there be long-term follow-up on how I am doing?
- Will this be done even if I leave the trial before it is over?
- What if the entire trial is stopped early?
- How can I find out the results of the trial?
- Will I be able to participate in future trials of this drug?
- Will I receive the results of future trials using this drug?

A comprehensive listing of resources is provided in the categories of adoption, advice, anger, attachment parenting, baby care, books on parenting, breastfeeding, child abuse, daycare, discipline, disorders (eg, behavioral problems), education, family, fatherhood, games, grandparenting, health, missing children, motherhood, multiple births, parenting, pregnancy and childbirth, safety, shopping online, single parenting, and working parents.

Pediatric Points of Interest:
   http://www.med.jhu.edu/peds/neonatology/ search.html
   Categories are related to organizations, general and treatment information, articles, and reports.
All Kids Count: *www.allkidscount.org*
   This site provides immunization registry resources and best practices.

Department of Health and Human Resources initiative to eliminate racial and ethnic disparities in health: *www.raceandhealth.hhs.gov*
  Providers can access the specific measurable goals that have been set in the areas of infant mortality, cancer screening and management, cardiovascular disease, diabetes, HIV infection, and childhood immunizations.

Health Finder: *www.healthfinder.gov*
  Pairing "children" with a medical term like "cardiac" provides results in the categories of web resources and organizations.

American Academy of Pediatrics: *www.aap.org*
  This comprehensive internet resource guide includes state and federal advocacy sites; sites by issue that relate to, for example, diseases, social conditions, and parenting; and detailed information on all aspects of child and adolescent care.

Al-Anon Family Group Headquarters: *www.al-anon.alateen.org*
  Al-Anon/Alateen provides materials in many languages and services for many countries. The goal of services is to assist families to cope with the effects of alcoholism.

Kids Health at the AMA: *www.ama-assn.org*
  This site provides comprehensive information on parenting, childhood illnesses, and treatments. It lists special on-line resources for concerns of adolescents, parenting, and violence prevention and safety.

National Library of Medicine: *www.nlm.nih.gov*
  This site gives extensive resources in the categories of general/overviews, specific conditions/aspects, diagnosis, treatment, clinical trials, children, teenagers, organizations, Spanish language, and list of print publications.

Sudden Infant Death Syndrome and Other Infant Death (SIDS/OID): *http://sids-network.org*
  This site lists support services for families affected by SIDS/OID with special attention to sibling grief and SIDS-related topics like product safety, apnea monitoring, and use of vaccinations.

Pediatric Development and Behavior: *www.dbpeds.org*
  This independent web site was developed to promote better care and outcomes for children and families affected by developmental, learning, and behavioral problems.

National Safety Council: *www.nsc.org*
  Material focuses on traffic and road safety issues in both urban and rural settings. A primary message is to encourage youth to be responsible in their actions.

Healthy People 2010: *www.health.gov/healthypeople*
  Healthy People is the prevention agenda for the United States. Healthy People 2010 is the United States' contribution to the World Health Organization's "Health for All" strategy.

Teaching Resources

Primary care providers frequently find themselves in a position to facilitate the learning of their pediatric clients and their caregivers. The following resources may be of interest to the primary care provider:

Wisconsin Clearinghouse for Prevention Resources
University of Wisconsin-Madison
1552 University Avenue
P.O. Box 1468
Madison, WI 53701-1468
phone: (800) 322-1468
fax: (608) 262-6346

Many materials, available in both Spanish and English, are presented in simple, easy to understand format. *Young*

Children & Drugs: What Parents Can Do is a resource for parents to encourage discussion about avoiding drug use. *The Ritalin Riddle* explains the use of methylphenidate hydrochloride to treat attention deficit/hyperactivity disorder and explores the problems of overuse and illegal recreational use. *Great Expectations: Information About Drugs and the Unborn Child* explores the effects of inhaled, smoked, or injected drugs during pregnancy.

U.S. General Services Administration
Consumer Information Center
P.O. Box 100
Pueblo, CO 81002
phone: (888) 878-3256
fax: (719) 948-9724
web site: *www.pueblo.gsa.gov*

This center provides a *Consumer Information Catalog* of free and low-cost publications of consumer interest, published by organizations like the Food and Drug Administration and National Institutes of Health. Topics are health related, of general interest, and consumer friendly. *How to Give Medicine to Children* is a reprint article with clear safety tips. *Helping Your Overweight Child* is a sensitive pamphlet by the Weight-Control Information Network that takes a family approach to solving this problem.

Aquarius Health Care Videos
5 Powderhouse Lane
P.O. Box 1159
Sherborn, MA 01770
phone: (508) 651-2963
fax: (508) 650-4216
e-mail/web site: *aqvideos@tiac.net*
www.aquariusproductions.com

Health and healing videos under the topics of mental health, learning and developmental disabilities, relaxation, and stress reduction are available. *Rising to the Challenge: Friendships, Feelings, and Shared Experiences From Kids With Cancer* explores methods to support the needs of sick, dying, and recovering children and adolescents. *Ali* is a documentary following a young girl's battle with cancer. The emphasis on the entire family's response to this illness demonstrates the various needs of different members who live with cancer in the family.

Parlay International
Box 8817
Emeryville, CA 94662-0817
phone: 510-601-1000
(800) 457-2752
fax: (510) 601-1008
web site: *www.parlay.com*

Health education resources come in the form of sets of reproducible pages for teaching. *Children's Health*, 48 pages, includes topics such as lactose intolerance, lead poisoning, and safety. *Building a Family*, 96 pages, includes the comprehensive topics of family planning, pregnancy and childbirth, caring for baby, caring for mom, and family life. *Student Assistance: Resources for Troubled Youth*, 96 pages, covers essential topics like chemical dependency, eating disorders, tobacco, facts about drugs, mind and body (concerns), coping with change, and information for parents. Color brochures and posters also are available on many topics. Educators who use the material are encouraged to make as many copies for teaching as needed.

Films for the Humanities and Sciences
P.O. Box 2053
Princeton, NJ 08543-2053
phone: 609-275-1400
(800) 257-5126
fax: (609) 275-3767
web site: *www.films.com*

Basic and advanced educational material for professionals and lay people are available. Physiologic and psychosocial problems are explored in video and CD-ROM format. The video *Your Newborn Baby* reviews questions new parents may have about preparing for and experiencing birth and caring for the newborn. Expecting parents can use the material in childbirth classes or take it home and review it privately. Lay persons can view and easily understand the 45-minute video, a Cambridge Educational Production, in the short focus segments (by topic).

Fanlight Productions
4196 Washington Street
Suite 2
Boston, MA 02131
phone: (617) 469-4999
fax: (617) 469-3379
e-mail/web site: *www.fanlight.com*
fanlight@fanlight.com

Nursing and health care videos address a wide range of topics. *A Kid Called Troy* tells the story about a father and son living with AIDS and the supportive family and community who help them live life to the fullest. The video provides a clear picture of the many difficulties children with HIV experience. *There Was a Child,* a documentary about pregnancy loss, provides an excellent view of short-term and long-term coping with this loss. The video points out the insensitivity of some health care workers related to pregnancy loss. *No Fears, No Tears: B 13 years later* provides a follow-up of six children with leukemia and one child with bone cancer. It explores aggressive treatment and memories of its accompanying trauma and pain.

Center for the Prevention of Sexual and Domestic Violence
936 N 34th St., Suite 200
Seattle, WA 98103
phone: (206) 634-1903
fax: (206) 634-0115
e-mail/web site: *www.cpsdv.org*
cpsdv@cpsdv.org

Hear Their Cries: Religious Responses to Child Abuse is an educational video designed to help clergy and lay leaders recognize and respond to all forms of child abuse. Some themes include vulnerability of children, the need for religious leaders to intervene on their behalf in cases of abuse, and the importance of support from faith communities in the victim's healing process.

Cambridge Health and Physical Education
P.O. Box 2153, Dept. PE 17
Charleston, WV 25328-2153
phone: (800) 468-4227
fax: (304) 744-9351
web site: *www.cambridgeol.com/cambridge/*

When to Call the Doctor if Your Child is Ill deals with self-help methods for caring for children. The video demonstrates the use of system checklists to encourage accurate and complete reporting of systems. *For Dads Only* provides appropriate, solid information on baby care and day-to-day issues like eating, diapering, and bathing.

Resources for Gay, Lesbian, Bisexual, and Transgendered Youth

Gay, lesbian, bisexual, and transgendered children and adolescents experience a unique form of shame, guilt, isolation, and confusion when facing a predominantly heterosexual, intolerant society. Children and adolescents with other than heterosexual feelings or physical and emotional experiences should be referred to "gay-friendly" or "gay-sensitive" providers. The following references are suggested starting places for information gathering.

Homosexuality: Common Questions and Statements Addressed: *http://hcqsa.virtualave.net/ref.html*
Fountain of Youth: *http://www.thebody.com/poz/survival/9'98/resources.html*

Adolescent AIDS Program
Montefiore Medical Center
111 East 210th Street
Bronx, NY 10467
(718) 882-0322
e-mail: *adolaids@aecom.yu.edu*

Offers everything from case management to peer counseling and a newsletter, *Peer Power.*

Asian and Pacific Islander Coalition on HIV/AIDS (APICHA)
275 Seventh Avenue, Suite 1204
New York, NY 10001
(212) 620-7287
apicha@aidsinfonyc.com

Provides multilingual AIDS services and counseling with translations in more than 20 different languages.

Body Positive
19 Fulton Street, Suite 308B
New York, NY 10038
(212) 566-7333

Peer-led hotline, support groups, workshops, socials, a monthly magazine published in English, and a quarterly magazine published in Spanish.

Gay and Lesbian Latino AIDS Education Initiative (GALAEI)
1233 Locust Street
3rd Floor
Philadelphia, PA 19107-1906
(215) 985-3382
www.critpath.org/galaie

Bilingual support for gay, lesbian, bisexual, and transgendered Latino youth.

Hetrick-Martin Institute (HMI)
2 Astor Place
New York, NY 10003
(212) 674-2400
e-mail: *hmi@hmi.org*

Extensive AIDS peer education for gay, lesbian, bisexual, and transgendered youth.

HIV and AIDS Technical Assistance Program
131 Livington Street, Room 621
Brooklyn, NY 11201
(718) 935-5606
www.taproject.org

Offers grant to New York City public high school students to start HIV peer-to-peer prevention projects. Also helps teens in other cities develop new projects.

Lifebeat (Tour Outreach)
72 Spring Street, Suite 1103
New York, NY 10012
(800) AIDS-411
e-mail: *lbeat@aol.com*

Music-savvy peer counselors provide HIV information at rock concerts.

Midwest AIDS Prevention Project
429 Livernois
Ferndale, MI 48220
(888) ACONDOM
www.wwnet.net/~mapp

Peer-led prevention workshops and training.

National Network for Youth Safe Choices Hotline
1319 F Street N.W., Suite 401
Washington, DC 20004
(800) 878-AIDS
www.nn4youth.org

Technical assistance education and services for youth AIDS education workers.

National Youth Advocacy Coalition Bridge Project
1711 Connecticut Avenue N.W.
Suite 206
Washington, DC 20009
(202) 319-7596
www.nyacyouth.org

Specializes in the needs of gay, lesbian, bisexual, and transgendered youth.

Positively Kids
PO Box 4512
Queensbury, NY 12804
(518) 798-0915

Education and support in Spanish and English for families and people who serve children and adolescents with HIV.

Youth Aids Prevention Project (YAPP)
United Communities AIDS Network
1408 East State Street, Suite 100
Olympia, WA 98506
(360) 352-2375
www.ucan-wa.org

Sexuality workshops, educational theater, and street outreach programs designed especially for youth.

National AIDS Hotline
24 Hours: 800-342-AIDS
Spanish
8 AM to 2 AM, 7 days, (800) 344-7432
Deaf Access (TTY)
10 AM to 10 PM, Monday to Friday: (800) 243-7889

Teenage AIDS Hotline
6 PM to 12 AM, Friday and Saturday: (800) 440-8336

Teens Teaching AIDS Prevention
5 PM to 9 PM, Monday to Friday: (800) 234-Teen

REFERENCES

AIDS Treatment Data Network. (1999). *Should I join a clinical trial?* New York: Author.

Belcher, H. M., & Shinitzky, H. E. (1998). Substance abuse in children: Prediction, protection, and prevention. *Archives of Pediatric and Adolescent Medicine, 152,* 952–960.

Bellack, J. P., & O'Neil, E. H. (2000). Recreating nursing practice for a new century. *Nursing and Health Care Perspectives, 21,* 14–21.

Britto, M. T., Garrett, J. M., Dugliss, M. A., Johnson, C. A., Majure, J. M., & Leigh, M. W. (1999). Preventive services received by adolescents with cystic fibrosis and sickle cell disease. *Archives of Pediatric and Adolescent Medicine, 153,* 27–32.

Donaldson, M. S., Yordy, K. D., Lohr, K. N., & Vanselow N. A. (Eds.). (1996). *Primary care: America's health in a new era.* Washington, DC: National Academy Press.

Ferris, T. G., Saglam, D., Stafford, R. S., Causino, N., Starfield, B., Culpepper, L., & Blumenthal, D. (1998). Changes in the daily practice of primary care for children. *Archives of Pediatric and Adolescent Medicine, 152,* 227–233.

Holzemer, S. P., & Arnold, J. (1998). In M. Klainberg, S. Holzemer, M. Leonard, & J. Arnold (Eds.), *Community health nursing: An alliance for health.* New York: McGraw-Hill.

Holzemer, S. P., Singleton, J. K., & Green-Hernandez, C. (1999). In J. K. Singleton, S. A. Sandowski, C. Green-Hernandez, T. V. Horvath, R. V. DiGregorio, & S. P. Holzemer (Eds.), *Primary care.* Philadelphia: Lippincott Williams & Wilkins.

Markowitz, G., & Rosner, D. (2000). "Cater to the children": The role of the lead industry in a public health tragedy, 1900-1955. *American Journal of Public Health, 90,* 36–46.

Morabia, A. (2000). Worldwide surveillance of risk factors to promote global health. *American Journal of Public Health, 90,* 22–24.

Sikand, A., & Laken, M. (1998). Pediatricians' experience with and attitudes toward complementary/alternative medicine. *Archives of Pediatric and Adolescent Medicine, 152,* 1059–1064.

U.S. Department of Health and Human Services. (1998). *Healthy people 2010 objectives: Draft for public comment.* Washington, DC: Author.

Xiaoming, L., Stanton, B., & Feigelman, S. (1999). Exposure to drug trafficking among urban, low-income African American children and adolescents. *Archives of Pediatric and Adolescent Medicine, 153,* 161–168.

Zotti, M. E. (1999). Public health education for Liberian refugees. *Nursing and Health Care Perspectives, 20,* 302–306.

C H A P T E R 4

Complementary Therapies in Pediatrics

• MARCEY SHAPIRO, MD

INTRODUCTION

This chapter provides general information on a number of commonly used complementary modalities. The authors and publishers do not offer this discussion as a recommendation or endorsement of any of these approaches. Instead, the intention is to familiarize the reader with methods patients might already be using. Providers need to assess the use of complementary medicines as part of the patient's history, because such therapies may impact conventional treatments. Patients may not volunteer such information unless specifically asked. The efficacy of many complementary approaches is less well documented than that of conventional therapies. Providers should read the literature before suggesting any complementary approaches. The bibliography at the end of this chapter supports the material here and in the appendices and provides further readings for interested clinicans. Display 4-1 is a list of common pediatric problems and various modalities discussed in this chapter that sometimes are used to treat them.

ACUPUNCTURE, TRADITIONAL CHINESE MEDICINE, AND KANPO

Traditional Chinese medicine (TCM) refers to the Chinese herbal tradition, certain therapeutic massage techniques (eg, tui na), and the kind of acupuncture practiced in China. Many would argue that these practices are "traditional" in name only, because Communist ideology intentionally excludes many concepts from other schools of thought that conflict with current political doctrine. TCM in North America, which derives from the contemporary Chinese system, also excludes these other schools of thought. One of the best known pre-Communist systems is five elements acupuncture, also known as traditional acupuncture. J. R. Worsley, who has established schools in Miami, Maryland, and Great Britain, has popularized this method, which focuses more on the emotional and spiritual dimensions of health.

Chinese herbal medicine generally does not use individual herbs alone but combines herbs in various formulas. Diagnosis in TCM is empirical; symptoms for physical ailments include emotional components. TCM practitioners rely on physical diagnostic signs to ascertain patterns of disharmony, including pulses, tongue, body odor, and sweat patterns. The wide variety of schools of training in TCM makes regulation difficult.

Acupuncture is one commonly used modality of TCM. Although children may find the needles frightening, they usually tolerate their actual use quite well. For young or scared children, acupressure (tui na) or laser acupuncture may be more appropriate. Practitioners trained in different methodologies have different beliefs about point locations, depth of needling, and applications. Still, some movement has been made toward comprehensive, standardized licensure. In many states, the title LAc connotes licensure by a state regulatory board. NCCA certification is the national board examination, which several states recognize as a prerequisite for licensure. NCCA-certified individuals are entitled to practice acupuncture without another medical degree.

Medical acupuncture is the term used when conventionally trained practitioners, such as medical doctors (MDs), osteopaths (DOs), and nurse practitioners, complete basic training in acupuncture. Several states have mandated that physicians complete a minimum number of hours of additional training to practice acupuncture among the therapies they offer. As of this writing, however, most states do not require any specific training for physicians practicing acupuncture.

A doctorate in Chinese medicine is signified by the letters OMD, which indicates training in both acupuncture and Chinese herbal medicine. Currently, the only training programs that offer this degree are in Asia and the Pacific.

Kanpo, traditional Japanese medicine, is similar to TCM in using the practices of acupuncture, herbs, and physical manipulation. Typically the depth of needling in Kanpo acupuncture is less than in TCM, which may make Kanpo easier for children to tolerate. Meridian therapy, also developed in Japan, emphasizes working with the channels of energy flow or meridians to restore or maintain health.

AROMATHERAPY

Aromatherapy is a branch of healing that uses essential oils and perfumes for physical therapeutics, spiritual development, and cosmetic purposes. This ancient practice was described in the oldest of Sanskrit Vedic documents about 5000 years ago. Ancient Egyptians, Chinese, Greeks, and Romans, as well as Medieval and Arabic physicians, religious authorities, and perfumers, were familiar with the properties of essential oils.

The term "aromatherapy" is relatively recent, coined by a French perfumer, Rene-Maurice Gattefosse, in the 1920s. Gattefosse became interested in the dermatologic and especially antiseptic properties of essential oils after burning his hand during a laboratory explosion. To treat the burn, he immediately immersed his hand in pure lavender essential oil. He found that the injury healed in hours rather than days without scarring or infection. Dr. Jean Valnet, a surgeon, later studied Gattefosse's work and used essential oils to treat injured soldiers during World War II. These therapies were so effective that Valnet continued to use aromatic oils in all areas of his medical practice after the war. In 1964 he published *The Practice of Aromatherapy*, which is still available in English translation.

DISPLAY 4–1 • Conditions for Which Alternative Therapies May Be Used

---

Acne: aromatherapy, ayurveda, botanical/herbal, homeopathy, naturopathy, nutritional therapy, TCM

Attention deficit hyperactivity disorder (ADHD): aromatherapy, ayurveda, botanical/herbal, homeopathy, massage/bodywork: craniosacral, Ortho-Bionomy; naturopathy; nutritional medicine; osteopathy; TCM

Allergies: aromatherapy, ayurveda, botanical/herbal, homeopathy, naturopathy, nutritional medicine, osteopathy

Anemia: aromatherapy, ayurveda, botanical/herbal, homeopathy, naturopathy, nutritional medicine

Asthma: acupuncture, aromatherapy, ayurveda, botanical/herbal, chiropractic, homeopathy, massage/bodywork: craniosacral, lymphatic drainage, Ortho-Bionomy, shiatsu; naturopathy; nutritional medicine; osteopathy; TCM

Bedwetting: acupuncture, aromatherapy, ayurveda, botanical/herbal, homeopathy, naturopathy, osteopathy, TCM

Bites: aromatherapy, botanical/herbal, homeopathy, naturopathy

Breast-feeding support: acupuncture, aromatherapy, ayurveda, botanical/herbal, homeopathy, massage/bodywork: craniosacral, lymphatic drainage, infant massage, Ortho-Bionomy, shiatsu; naturopathy; nutritional therapies; osteopathy; TCM

Bronchitis: acupuncture, aromatherapy, ayurveda, botanical/herbal, homeopathy, massage/bodywork: lymphatic drainage; naturopathy; nutritional therapies; osteopathy; TCM

Celiac disease: acupuncture, aromatherapy, ayurveda, botanical/herbal, homeopathy, naturopathy, nutritional therapies, osteopathy, TCM

Colds/flu: acupuncture, aromatherapy, ayurveda, botanical/herbal, homeopathy, massage/bodywork: lymphatic drainage; naturopathy; nutritional therapies; osteopathy; TCM

Colic: aromatherapy, ayurveda, botanical/herbal, homeopathy, naturopathy, nutritional therapies, TCM

Conjunctivitis: aromatherapy, ayurveda, botanical/herbal, homeopathy, naturopathy, nutritional therapies, TCM

Constipation: acupuncture, aromatherapy, ayurveda, botanical/herbal, homeopathy, massage/bodywork: craniosacral, lymphatic drainage, infant massage, Ortho-Bionomy, shiatsu; naturopathy; nutritional therapies, osteopathy, TCM

Coughs: acupuncture, aromatherapy, ayurveda, botanical/herbal, homeopathy, massage/bodywork: lymphatic drainage; naturopathy; nutritional therapies; TCM

Cradle cap: aromatherapy, ayurveda, botanical/herbal, homeopathy, massage/bodywork: infant massage; naturopathy; nutritional therapies; TCM

Diaper rash: aromatherapy, ayurveda, botanical/herbal, homeopathy, naturopathy, nutritional therapies, TCM

Diarrhea: acupuncture, aromatherapy, ayurveda, botanical/herbal, homeopathy, naturopathy, nutritional therapies, TCM

Earaches: acupuncture, aromatherapy, ayurveda, botanical/herbal, chiropractic, homeopathy, massage/bodywork: lymphatic drainage; naturopathy; nutritional therapies; osteopathy; TCM

Eczema: acupuncture, aromatherapy, ayurveda, botanical/herbal, homeopathy, naturopathy, nutritional therapies, TCM

Failure to thrive: aromatherapy, ayurveda, botanical/herbal, chiropractic, homeopathy, massage/bodywork: craniosacral, infant massage, Ortho-Bionomy; naturopathy; nutritional therapies; osteopathy; TCM

Headaches: acupuncture, aromatherapy, ayurveda, botanical/herbal, chiropractic, homeopathy, massage/bodywork: craniosacral, lymphatic drainage, Ortho-Bionomy, shiatsu; naturopathy, nutritional therapies; osteopathy; TCM

Insomnia: acupuncture, aromatherapy, ayurveda, botanical/herbal, chiropractic, homeopathy, massage/bodywork: craniosacral, Ortho-Bionomy, shiatsu; naturopathy; nutritional therapies; osteopathy; TCM

Jaundice: acupuncture, aromatherapy, ayurveda, botanical/herbal, homeopathy, naturopathy, nutritional therapies, TCM

Nightmares: acupuncture, aromatherapy, botanical/herbal, homeopathy, naturopathy, TCM

Parasites: ayurveda, botanical/herbal, naturopathy, nutritional therapies, TCM

Pharyngitis: acupuncture, aromatherapy, ayurveda, botanical/herbal, homeopathy, massage/bodywork: craniosacral, lymphatic drainage; naturopathy; nutritional therapies; osteopathy; TCM

Sinusitis: acupuncture, aromatherapy, ayurveda, botanical/herbal, homeopathy, massage/bodywork: lymphatic drainage; naturopathy; nutritional therapies; osteopathy; TCM

Skin diseases (various): acupuncture, aromatherapy, ayurveda, botanical/herbal, homeopathy, massage/bodywork: infant massage, lymphatic drainage, shiatsu; naturopathy, nutritional therapies, osteopathy, TCM

Teething: aromatherapy, ayurveda, botanical/herbal, homeopathy, naturopathy, TCM

Toothache: acupuncture, aromatherapy, ayurveda, botanical/herbal, homeopathy, naturopathy, TCM

Varicella (chickenpox): acupuncture, aromatherapy, ayurveda, botanical/herbal, homeopathy, naturopathy, TCM

Vomiting: acupuncture, aromatherapy, ayurveda, botanical/herbal, homeopathy, naturopathy, nutritional therapies, TCM

Warts: ayurveda, botanical/herbal, homeopathy, naturopathy, nutritional therapies, TCM

The biochemist Marguerite Maury, Valnet's student, later published her own text that expanded the range of aromatherapy to include spiritual and emotional balancing. She incorporated much traditional knowledge of aromatics in massage. Since that time, the body of knowledge has continued to grow. A wide variety of books on numerous aspects of aromatherapy is available, including well-known works by Robert Tisserand and Shirley Price.

Production of essential oils occurs through a steam distillation process (usually of flowers or leafy plant matter). The oils are very concentrated extractions from the oil fraction of plants and usually are not used without the guidance of an experienced practitioner. Very few essential oils are taken internally; most are diluted in a neutral oil (eg, olive or sesame) and are applied topically in small amounts or inhaled with a diffuser or steam.

Both practitioners and patients should be very careful with essential oils. Almost all are toxic in large doses. In the home, families should keep essential oils out of children's reach. Because essential oils smell good, children are naturally attracted to them, yet ingestion can cause serious morbidity and might even be fatal.

▲ **Clinical Warning:** Families should regard essential oils in the home as prescription drugs and keep them out of children's reach. Ingestion can be toxic.

Essential oils should never be applied in the noses of children younger than 5 years. Practitioners should not use undiluted essential oils (except a bit of lavender or tea tree oil) on a child's skin. They must use all oils cautiously on sensitive or broken skin. Oils for a child's bath should be much more diluted than for an adult's. Typically, not more than four to five drops are used. Similarly, oils for massage on a child should be one-quarter to one-half the strength of those massaged on an adult. Practitioners should give inhalations to children only briefly, initially around 30 seconds. If well tolerated, they can repeat these brief inhalation treatments several times. They should use essential oils orally only with extreme caution and preferably not at all. When used with children, oils should be extremely dilute and given under the guidance of an experienced practitioner.

Appendix 4-1 provides brief and general guidelines for some essential oils commonly used in the pediatric population. Training in aromatherapy is urged before prescribing any of these oils; reading these guidelines does not constitute training. These notes are not intended to provide instruction in aromatherapy or to advocate the use of these agents.

AYURVEDA

Ayurveda, the traditional medicine of India, is an ancient, complex, and complete medical system that involves diet and nutrition, herbal medicine, massage and bodywork, meditation, and contemplation. Students of Ayurveda usually train for practice over 4 years. Many brief courses and popular books, however, provide a sampling of the wisdom of this healing tradition. Currently, no board in the United States certifies or licenses Ayurvedic practitioners. Most Ayurvedic practitioners have either trained in India or studied with a teacher who trained in India.

Ayurveda has its roots in the Vedas, the revered ancient scriptures of Hinduism. The major written texts that are the foundation of Ayurvedic practice are the *Charaka Samita* and the *Sushruta Samita*. The underlying principles are the three dosas (pronounced "doshas") or constitutional types that are the foundation for each individual's unique physiology. They are *Pitta* (eg, oil, heat, fire), *Vata* (eg, air, nervous system), and *Kapha* (eg, water, muscles). Though each person is thought to possess elements of all three dosas, typically one or two predominate. Ayurvedic therapy focuses on harmonizing the elements while respecting each individual's unique constitution.

In children as in adults, any dosa may predominate, but children are believed to have a healthy predominance of Kapha that supports their growth and development. Many Ayurvedic approaches are effective for children; application

of the dietary principles of Ayurveda may be particularly helpful.

Pancha karma, thought to be among the oldest of Ayurvedic practices, is a system of cleansing and restorative therapies. It includes ways to support, cleanse, purge, and nurture the body to achieve balance and eliminate excess dosas. Pancha karma practice pays attention to the individual's homeostasis, the seasons, the phases of the moon, and the times of day. It can be quite extreme; a qualified practitioner should guide anyone undergoing this healing method, especially children and adolescents.

BOTANICAL OR HERBAL MEDICINE

Every traditional society has an herbal pharmacopoeia; herbal medicines have been around about as long as humans. For most of history, herbal medicines were virtually the only available treatments. Many botanicals commonly used today were used hundreds and even thousands of years ago. For example, the ancient Egyptian Ebers Papyrus (1552 BC) lists more than 700 prescriptions, including aloes, opium, caraway, coriander, dill, juniper berries, gentian, and peppermint. The Bible mentions many botanicals. In his writings, Hippocrates discusses about 400 single herbs used as medicinal substances. According to Galen, Hippocrates prepared his own medicines and practiced pharmacy as well as medicine. He also believed strongly in diet as essential to recovery. Galen himself wrote more than 500 medical works; several of his surviving texts discuss 141 herbal remedies and their actions.

Pharmacognosy, the earliest scientific approach to botanical medicine, arose in the 18th and 19th centuries both in Europe and North America. It grew out of western thought and paradigms, stressing an analytical approach, seeking a mechanism of action, and applying active principles for each medicinal substance. Its reductionistic model was similar to contemporary orthodox medicine. The basic work from this tradition led to the isolation of many current botanically derived drugs, such as digitalis, cocaine, and morphine. The major texts of pharmacognosy include Felter and Lloyd's *King's American Dispensatory* and Ellingwood's *American Materia Medica Therapeutics and Pharmacognosy*, both of which have been in continuous publication since the late 19th century.

Asia has a rich, unbroken written herbal tradition. Chinese herb books are known as Bun Cao, the first of which was the Shun Nun Bun Cao (approximately 150 AD). This text discusses the actions of 365 herbs. By 600 to 700 AD, various Chinese Materia Medica listed 800 medicinal herbs. In 1596, Li Sher Chen published a Materia Medica listing approximately 2000 herbs. As recently as 1972, approximately 5700 herbs were in the various Chinese Materia Medica; however, fewer than 1000 of these are commonly used. Most practitioners typically use 300 to 500 herbs.

Each Native American tribe has an herbal tradition. Many such traditions are oral, but some are written texts, such as the Badianus manuscript of the ancient Incas. Coca, chinchona (quinine), wintergreen, bloodroot, lobelia, goldenseal, mayapple (podophyllum), and echinacea are among significant North American medicinal plants.

Scientific evidence of the safety and efficacy of commonly used herbs is mounting. The chemical constituents of many commonly used herbs have long been established. A great deal of research is being done regarding specific herbs and specific phytochemical constituents. Popular herbs, such as gingko and echinacea, have quite a bit of literature supporting their use. Ayurvedic herbs are among the most well studied, because the Indian government has long supported solid research about their use. In Europe, phytomedicine (plant medicine) is widely accepted. For example German physicians wrote over 2 million prescriptions for echinacea alone in 1998.

No independent licensure exists for herbalists anywhere in North America. For lay herbalists, a peer review guild, the American Herbalist Guild, has fairly high standards for admission, and members can exhibit the title AHG with their names. Primary care providers should check carefully into the training and experience of herbalists. Although many lay herbalists are outstanding, others claim titles like "master herbalist" after only a few weekends of classes. Herbs are potentially wonderful allies in healing patients, but some are dangerous and toxic as well. Practitioners should be sure to understand the nuances of herbal therapeutics, just as they would understand medications before prescribing them.

Appendix 4-2 provides brief general guidelines for some herbs commonly used in the pediatric population. Training in herbal medicine is urged before any of these herbs are prescribed. Reading these guidelines does not constitute training. These notes are not intended to provide instruction in herbal medicine or to advocate the use of these agents.

CHIROPRACTIC

The term chiropractic, derived from the Greek, refers to treatment by manipulation. David Daniel Palmer developed this therapeutic and preventive system of healing around 1895. He discovered that manipulation of the spinal vertebrae could improve health not only in people with back pain, but also for those with conditions as diverse as heart disease, asthma, and headaches. He theorized these effects resulted from the existence of spinal subluxations, or subtle vertebrae displacements, that affected nerve conduction. Because spinal nerves innervate every body tissue and organ, even partial disruption of flow could have wide-ranging effects. Optimal health, then, would depend on unrestricted nerve impulse conduction. Later, other chiropractors devoted much study and research to the manipulation of peripheral joints to alleviate more distal structural problems.

Today, most chiropractors use a number of modalities. Some advise patients about diet and nutritional supplements and provide in-office massage, ultrasound treatment, acupuncture, and hydrotherapy. Many order laboratory tests, and most use x-rays in diagnosis.

Chiropractic is quite popular throughout the United States. Every state has independent professional licensure boards regulating who may practice chiropractic. They restrict the title to those who have completed a 4-year chiropractic college and passed proficiency examinations. Most states, however, do not regulate additional training required for the practice of other modalities under a chiropractic license, such as acupuncture and nutritional counseling.

Much research has validated the effectiveness of chiropractic for structural problems, such as back pain. Early studies by the Workman's Compensation Administration found that patients treated by chiropractors for job-related injuries healed twice as quickly as patients who received orthodox medical care. Recent studies regarding chiropractic for other conditions, such as asthma, have failed to demonstrate any benefits. Because chiropractic traditionally was unpopular with the medical establishment, some animosity exists between conventional physicians and chiropractors. This situation, however, has been shifting toward greater cooperation in recent years.

FLOWER REMEDIES

Flower essence therapy is a safe and gentle form of treatment thought to be particularly suitable for children. Dr. Edward Bach, a London physician, developed flower essence therapy. He had a successful private practice in bacteriology and homeopathy; throughout the 1920s, however, he became disillusioned with both allopathic and homeopathic medicine, because he felt that both dealt with the results and not the causes of disease. In 1930, Bach left his home, family, and medical practice to embark on a period of itinerant wandering. During this time, he lived very simply, mostly in nature, and gave his services away for free. He relied greatly on his intuition and observations of personality and illness. Bach felt the true cause of disease was conflict between the soul and the mind. Over several years, he developed a system of healing that relied on inner attunement to the energy of flowers. The 38 remedies he developed are called the Bach flower remedies; they address the emotional and spiritual causes that Bach believed were responsible for all physical and emotional illnesses. Many still enthusiastically use these original remedies today; other providers have expanded this body of knowledge.

In making flower essences, practitioners first connect with the vibration of the plant and ask permission to take a few flowers. Generally they choose flowers in full bloom, often at midsummer. Then providers are intuitively guided to the appropriate flowers that wish to become medicine. Practitioners infuse them in pure water in the sunlight, until they feel that the essence is ready (usually when the flowers wilt). They then decant the essence and add food-grade alcohol as a preservative. They then dilute the essence in a manner similar to homeopathic dilution. A few drops of a flower essence are enough for one dose.

Many courses train practitioners to work with flower essences. No board or body, however, certifies competency or sets minimum standards for practice. This is as Bach himself would have preferred, because he conceived his healing system as one that would be quite accessible to lay people. Because the preparations are essentially homeopathic high dilutions, virtually no danger exists in using these remedies, even if one chooses an incorrect remedy. Flower remedies are considered to be safe for children and infants.

HOMEOPATHY

Homeopathy is a broad system of medicine practiced by numerous individuals from various backgrounds. Samuel Hahnemann, a German physician, was the founder of modern homeopathy. He expounded the "law of similars," which is based on the principle that "like cures like." That is, homeopathic doses that cause symptoms in a well person can cure the same symptoms in an ill person. So, for example, homeopaths might treat vomiting with ipecac (nux vomica), bee stings with apis mellifica (bee venom), and insomnia with coffea cruda (coffee).

Homeopaths believe that symptoms are the body's attempt to restore homeostasis and thus should not be suppressed. In fact, the term "healing crisis" refers to the therapeutic activity of an appropriate remedy that temporarily exacerbates symptoms as the body corrects itself. In homeopathic thought, the suppression of symptoms by allopathic medicine actually may cause further imbalance.

Homeopathy is one of the most challenging types of complementary medicine for conventionally trained medical practitioners to accept, because it is based on a different paradigm of health and illness. Practitioners discover and elaborate on remedies by "provings." This method requires that practitioners give substances to be "proved," some of which may be toxic (eg, mercury) to healthy individuals, who then meticulously record symptoms caused by their administration. Currently, Hahnemann and his successors have proven about 2000 remedies.

According to homeopathic principles, potentization occurs with increasing dilution, so the most dilute remedies are the most powerful. Frequently no actual molecules of the original substance remain in the remedy after successive dilutions. Remedies are prepared through decussation, which includes dilution and vigorous shaking at each stage. A 6x or 6c (the terms are used interchangeably) has been successively diluted and shaken six times. A 6x is a low potency, 30x is an average potency, and 100x, 200x, and 1 million x are high-potency extractions. Lower potencies typically are used for acute physical problems and many children's remedies. Higher potencies are chosen more frequently for chronic or severe illness and psychological disturbance. Current homeopathic theory postulates that these remedies work by the principles of quantum physics rather than biochemistry, so efficacy is not ideally evaluated biochemically, especially initially.

Different forms of homeopathy are practiced worldwide. Classical homeopathy is an exacting and rigorous discipline that usually requires several years of training. Any individual, including a child, receives only one constitutional remedy at any given time. The homeopathic interview is painstaking and specific, eliciting broad information about symptoms, personality traits and preferences, food cravings, favorite colors, sleep patterns, and other diverse characterizations. Classical homeopaths also may advise patients to avoid all other therapies, including conventional medications, when using constitutional remedies. Homeopathy also is practiced as a form of first aid, where just a few matching symptoms are considered enough to select for an appropriate remedy. Other methodologies combine remedies simultaneously (combination remedies) or blend potencies of the same remedy (homaccords).

Because of the variety of approaches, some contention exists among practitioners about what constitutes homeopathy, who should be allowed to practice it, and what training is appropriate. Very few states license homeopathy, and in those, only medically trained practitioners (eg, MDs or DOs) may administer remedies. Nonetheless, in reality, most oral homeopathic remedies are available over the counter, and many lay people and practitioners prescribe them. In fact, relatively few physicians have embraced homeopathic prescribing, although recently the number has grown.

The literature contains some favorable studies of homeopathy. For example, a study of diarrhea in Nicaraguan children was done with randomization to two groups. One received appropriate hydration alone, while the other received identical hydration plus a homeopathic remedy. Although all the children recovered, those in the homeopathy group recovered twice as rapidly as those who received hydration alone.

Homeopathy is considered to be especially effective for children, because their constitutions are more pure and respond well to energetic medicine. In infants and young children, homeopathic remedies typically are given in liquid form. Pellets can be crushed and put into liquid for small children (usually hands should not touch them) if necessary. Older children, who can suck on small candies, can take the pellets, which typically are prepared in a pleasant lactose base. Homeopathy is considered to be extremely safe, precisely because, by Avogadro's number, no molecules of the original substance actually are given. Thus, an incorrect remedy usually will have no effect rather than cause ill effects. This is especially true of milder remedies.

Display 4-2 lists some remedies commonly used for children, although many remedies might be appropriate in a variety of circumstances. The authors and publisher do not endorse homeopathy or these remedies. Training in homeopathy is urged before prescribing any of these remedies; reading these guidelines does not constitute training.

MASSAGE/BODYWORK

Numerous types of bodywork and massage are considered appropriate for the pediatric population. Some of the more useful and popular forms are discussed below, but this list is by no means exhaustive. Generally, bodywork modalities have been little studied for efficacy. The gentler modalities especially are presumed safe for most patients, because they are noninvasive or minimally invasive. Most forms of bodywork are contraindicated in patients with lymphatic cancers or metastatic disease, because massage theoretically could spread the illnesses. Providers need to read the literature before suggesting these complementary approaches.

Acupressure

Acupressure refers to a number of related techniques that rely on the hands to manipulate acupuncture points and meridians for therapeutic benefits. Many of these techniques are used with children; unlike acupuncture, needles are not used. Some gentle techniques promote overall health; others are used more frequently for more serious illness. A few better known forms are outlined below.

Amma, a strong Japanese form of acupressure similar to the Chinese tui na, uses rubbing, percussing, and vibrating points. Amma is used for treatment of serious illness in internal medicine and pediatrics.

Bagua is a type of practice using 36 types of manipulation of acupressure points for therapeutic efficacy. Its indications are similar to Amma and Tui Na.

Do-in®, a self-massage acupressure technique, is especially popular with parents and children. It is gentle and applied typically for gradual change of chronic conditions, mild concerns, and self-care.

Jin shin Jyutsu is a technique developed in Japan by Jiro Mai. Typically, practitioners hold single points for several seconds and in certain sequences to treat various problems. Jin Shin Jyutsu can be applied for musculoskeletal or certain internal medicine and pediatric concerns. A number of styles of Jin Shin have developed, including Jin Shin Do®.

Shiatsu, a popular Japanese form of acupressure, means literally "finger pressure." The focus is on sequential application of pressure in the meridians. It is one of the more gentle forms of acupressure and can be used for specific musculoskeletal conditions or to promote overall well-being.

Tui Na, a Chinese form of acupressure, includes deep point palpation, rubbing, kneading, and strong stimulation. One of the more therapeutic forms of acupressure, it is used often for treatment of serious illness in internal medicine and pediatrics.

Craniosacral

Craniosacral, a gentle type of bodywork, developed out of osteopathic discoveries of the early 20th century. William

---

DISPLAY 4–2 • Homeopathic Remedies

Aconite: colds, especially febrile; croupy cough at onset; otitis externa; rubella; vomiting; acute nervous upset from fright

Apis mellifica: insect bites, including bee stings; breathing difficulty similar to early anaphylaxis; ovarian pain, especially if stinging quality (like ovulatory pain)

Arnica: topically applied for bruises, strains, sprains; homeopathic pellets also administered for the same indications and bleeding and shock; toxic when used in other than homeopathic preparation but safe in homeopathic preparations

Arsenicum album: asthma, fever, gastroenteritis from tainted food, vomiting

Belladonna: bedwetting; colds; otitis media (especially in right ear); fever, headache; overexposure to sun; pharyngitis with tonsillar swelling; rubella; teething

Bryonia: colic, especially with constipation; constipation, especially with dry stools; vomiting

Calcarea carbonica: colic, especially if child has dairy intolerance

Calcarea phosphorica: pharyngitis, especially if tonsils are chronically enlarged

Calendula: diaper rash, minor burns, including sunburn, minor scrapes and cuts

Cantharis: burns, urinary tract infection and burning pain

Carbo vegetalis: bloating, gas, gas pains, indigestion

Chamomilla: colic; crankiness; diarrhea; otitis media; menstrual cramps, especially if moodiness and crankiness; teething

Colocynthis: colic with abdominal distention, diarrhea, menstrual cramps

Causticum: bedwetting, especially if early in the night; burns; warts, especially at fingertips

Ferrum phosphoricum: early otitis media, pharyngitis, especially if the tonsils are chronically enlarged

Gelsemium: colds; flu; headaches, especially frontal or after heat and sun; stage fright

Hepar sulphuris: boils, colds (especially with yellow phlegm), croup, pharyngitis (especially if pain in ears with swallowing)

Hypericum (tincture): burns

Ipecac: vomiting

Iris versicolor: migraines

Kali bichromicum: headache, especially sinus type

Kali bromatum: acne

Kali muraticum: pharyngitis, especially with coated tonsils and mucus; mononucleosis

Ledum: acne, preventive for insect bites

Magnesia phosphorica: earache, menstrual cramps relieved by heat

Mercuris vivus: colds, diarrhea, pharyngitis

Nature muraticum: colds, especially if watery drainage or stuffy nose with clear or white mucus; constipation; moody, depressed, sullen adolescents

Nux vomica: burping; constipation; diarrhea; headache, especially in back of head or from rich food; rhinitis; stomachaches, especially due to emotional upsets and anger; vomiting

Phosphorus: diarrhea

Pulsatilla: colds, especially with white drainage; menstrual cramps; insomnia; constipation or diarrhea; otitis externa

Rhus Tox: chickenpox, poison ivy, sprains and strains, especially after acute phase

Sepia: bedwetting, nightmares

Silica: teething

Spongia tosta: croup, especially if not resolved from aconite; dry cough; sensation of phlegm stuck in throat

Sulfur: acne; constipation, especially if stools are dry and hard to eliminate; diarrhea, especially if stools change consistency a lot; irritable bowel

Symphytum: mending broken bones

Verbascum: otitis media, especially left side

Sutherland observed that the bones of the skull move in relationship to one another. Sutherland's work was controversial with many of his contemporaries, who believed that the bones of the skull fuse at the sutures by age 35 and therefore cannot move. Since that time, a mounting body of scientific evidence has supported Sutherland's findings and the efficacy of the therapies. Nonetheless, some circles still do not accept his work.

Craniosacral may be used to treat a diverse range of conditions, including otitis media, hyperactivity, headaches, cerebral palsy, and epilepsy. Craniosacral practitioners palpate the craniosacral system through gentle touch, often initially at the occiput, to sense the wavelike rhythm of the cerebrospinal fluid. From working with this rhythm and correcting restrictions detected at various cranial bones, the whole organism can shift and self-correct. This type of manipulation uses no force; instead, it applies a very subtle touch to the cranium and facial bones.

Several popular variations of craniosacral exist. The first is the structural approach used by osteopaths, medical doctors, and physical therapists who have been trained in this area. It is called cranial osteopathy, and practitioners may be located by contacting osteopathic medical societies or the Cranial Academy in Tucson, Arizona. All osteopathic colleges teach the rudiments of this system, but cranial osteopaths typically have undertaken significant extra study beyond their required courses.

In the 1970s, John Upledger, an osteopathic physician, developed an approach to craniosacral work that relied on gently manipulating the meninges. The Upledger Institute teaches this approach by levels. Completion of each level denotes competency to provide care at that level. Practitioners may be located through the Upledger Institute. In most large communities, finding practitioners who are trained in these techniques is easy. For purposes of insurance billing, a licensed practitioner is required to provide or directly supervise these services.

Lymphatic Drainage

Lymphatic drainage refers to a number of specific therapies that address problems of lymphatic congestion or stasis. These typically gentle techniques assist in the circulation of lymph, thus helping the body eliminate cellular wastes and toxins and supporting proper immune function. Frederic Millard (1922), a Canadian osteopath, and Emil Vodder, a Danish massage therapist (1932), pioneered the techniques. Today many varieties of lymph drainage are used, and because they are so effective at relieving various symptoms, the techniques are common practice in Europe and have gained much recognition in the United States. Movement toward standardization of training requirements for practitioners is underway in a number of states. Medicare and many other insurers reimburse appropriately trained practitioners who perform lymphatic drainage. Problems amenable to lymphatic drainage are numerous; they range from severe (eg, postsurgical lymphedema) to minor (eg, lymphatic congestion seen in children with frequent otitis or head colds who present with "shotty adenopathy").

Healing Touch

Healing touch refers to both ancient and modern practices that address and treat subtle levels of body energy disturbance. For example, therapeutic touch, a healing technique developed by Doris Kreiger and Dora Kunz, combines many traditional techniques performed worldwide. Therapeutic touch corrects imbalances and relieves blockages in the aura, or energy field, of the body. Typically practitioners do not touch the body directly unless a traumatic injury has occurred. Instead, they hold their hands near the patient's body and use intuition, intention, and hand motions to diagnose and correct disturbances in the energy field. Therapeutic touch is popular with many doctors and nurses. Because it is noninvasive, it can be used in many settings, including the home, clinic, and even acute care hospitals.

Infant Massage

Infant massage refers to a group of techniques drawn from various worldwide traditions to stimulate good health and balance in babies. Typically these techniques are mild and gentle and can be taught to parents and caregivers. They facilitate bonding and help parents and caregivers to participate in their children's well-being.

Ortho-Bionomy

Ortho-Bionomy is a gentle, effective approach to somatic reeducation that uses comfortable positioning and relaxing movements to unlock tension, relieve pain, promote structural balance, reduce stress, and increase personal awareness and well-being. It is gaining popularity in the United States.

A British osteopath, Arthur Lincoln Pauls, built on the work of an American osteopath, Lawrence Jones. In an article published in 1964 entitled "Spontaneous Release by Positioning," Jones describes that pain and tension can be relieved in a few minutes by slowly and carefully exaggerating an abnormal body posture to make the patient maximally comfortable. He found that the muscle spasm that had been holding the bones in an abnormal position would spontaneously relax without forceful manipulation. From these principles, his study of Judo, and his own observations, Pauls developed the phased reflex techniques of Ortho-Bionomy. They encompass positional release and energetic techniques that enable clients to understand, consciously experience, and even participate in their own capacity to self-correct. The key to effectiveness lies in reflex activity and in the proprioceptive nervous system. The slow movements, gentle positions, and slight compressions in this system stimulate the proprioceptors at a pace that allows the client to be present consciously and attuned to the stored experience within these movement patterns. Proprioceptively, the client is offered alternative and more functional patterns.

Ortho-Bionomy is compatible with any system of traditional medicine. The name Ortho-Bionomy is a trademark held by the Society of Ortho-Bionomy International, which strictly enforces who may use the title. Thus, competency and consistency in the therapy is ensured if a registered practitioner is selected. Training requirements for a registered basic practitioner are 500 hours of teaching and client contact organized and supervised by the Society. Senior practitioners complete an additional 500 hours of training. Some physicians, osteopaths, nurses, lymph drainage therapists, physical and occupational medicine therapists, and bodyworkers currently practice Ortho-Bionomy®. For an appropriately licensed individual, such as a licensed massage therapist, physical therapist, or physician, insurer billing is done through physical medicine coding, such as neuromuscluar reeducation. Common pediatric problems that Ortho-Bionomy addresses include scoliosis, sports injuries, sprained ankles and wrists, shin splints, rotator cuff injuries, tendonitis, joint pain and restricted motion, surgical sequelae, cerebral palsy, abdominal and digestive discomfort, hyperactivity, thoracic outlet syndrome, whiplash, and contractures of paraplegia or quadriplegia.

NATUROPATHY

Naturopathy is actually a multidisciplinary approach encompassing a wide variety of healing modalities. Emphasis in naturopathy is placed as much on the patient's interconnected social, physical, and emotional environment as on specific disease etiology. In fact, much naturopathic treatment aims to prevent rather than treat illness. Both prevention and treatment are directed toward restoration of the individual's harmony and balance. Therapeutic interventions to restore homeostasis emphasize natural modalities, such as acupuncture, homeopathy, spinal manipulation, hydrotherapy, dietary and nutritional modifications, and herbal medicine.

Naturopathy as practiced by graduates of the four department of education-accredited colleges is currently licensed in only 11 states. Graduates of naturopathic schools, however, practice throughout the United States, sometimes under other licenses (eg, acupuncture), if they have completed appropriate training. The scope of practice allowed by licensure varies among states from the ability to prescribe only vitamins, homeopathics, and herbs in some locales to broader leeway, including the ability to perform minor surgery and prescribe certain pharmaceuticals, such as oral contraceptives and antibiotics. Naturopathy shares some similarities with conventional medical education, especially in the basic sciences, but naturopathy views pathogenesis from more of a multisystem approach.

Unfortunately, the naturopathic community disagrees about what constitutes naturopathy and who may practice under that title. Graduates of accredited 4-year naturopathic colleges are usually represented by the American Association of Naturopathic Physicians. This group advocates that the title naturopath be reserved for graduates of these colleges and is pushing for licensure in other states. Many other licensed practitioners, however, call themselves naturopaths. For example, the American Naturopathic Medical Association is actually a group of holistic MDs, chiropractors, physician assistants, nurse practitioners, and nurses who possess training in both orthodox and natural medicines. This group opposes restricting the title of naturopath to those who have graduated from accredited naturopathic colleges. The situation is further complicated because some schools provide mail-order degrees with scant training and oversight. No national board oversees credentialing or competency. Consensus is probably long in the future.

NUTRITIONAL AND FUNCTIONAL MEDICINE

Nutrition, of course, means the application of dietary principles to maintain health. Nutrition has been taught in schools in the United States for generations, yet notions of what constitutes proper and even ideal nutrition have evolved considerably in recent decades. Seminal research has indicated that standards such as the recommended dietary allowances for nutrients may well be the minimum that most (but not all) individuals require to prevent frank disease but may be quite inadequate for optimum function. Much has been learned about specific nutrients, their interrelationships, and their contributions to human health. Thinking has shifted about the roles of both macronutrients (ie, proteins, fats, and carbohydrates) and micronutrients (ie, vitamins, minerals). The entire field illuminating the contributions of phytochemicals and phytonutrients is another recent development.

Advances have occurred in diagnosing functional rather than clinical deficiencies. Acknowledgment has been given that each person is biochemically individual, so no one dietary program is appropriate for all people. Wide variation, for example, is found in different people's bodies in terms of the functional capacity of detoxification mechanisms. An individual, based on observations and measurements of various parameters, can get an increasingly accurate picture of his or her constitutional strengths and weaknesses and can then devise a program most supportive to his or her unique physiology.

This area is important in pediatrics. Some children's illnesses are quite amenable to dietary or lifestyle changes. Also, the health habits children and teens build will serve them throughout their lives. Early intervention can mean prevention.

Functional medicine, an emerging branch of wellness medicine, is designed to optimize the patient's function through dietary and lifestyle modification as well as nutritional intervention and supplementation when appropriate. It is based on the principle that although disease may not be present, individuals can make lifestyle choices that produce optimal wellness rather than just freedom from illness. If an illness exists, similar choices might help the individual to mitigate the severity of the illness or eliminate it completely. The field is growing rapidly for several reasons. In the 1980s and 1990s, many research studies and data contributed to the growth of information and therapeutic interventions in this field. Much has been learned, for example, about specific genes that code for predisposition to certain illnesses. Research also has been directed at modifying gene expression through nutrition and lifestyle modification. Also, knowledge about nutrition and the relationships of specific nutrients in human health has exploded.

OSTEOPATHY

Osteopathy is a branch of medicine founded in the United States by physician Andrew Taylor Still. Dr. Still opened the first school of osteopathy in Kirksville, Missouri, in 1892 to provide a model of care that he felt improved treatments for his patients. His work combined the conventional medical practices of his day with training in manual manipulation, hydrotherapy, and increased focus on nutrition. The movement was successful: By the time of Still's death, more than 5000 osteopaths were practicing in the United States. Today 16 osteopathic medical colleges are in the United States, and more are abroad. The scope of practice for osteopaths is the same as for traditional physicians. They can write prescriptions, order tests, and perform surgery. Many, but not all, also work with physical manipulation. Referrals specifically for the physical medicine approach of osteopathy should be directed toward those who practice osteopathic manipulations. A subset of osteopaths specializes in cranial manipulation; they are referred to as cranial osteopaths.

A central tenet of osteopathy is correction of physical restrictions to optimize health. Thus, initial examination usually includes assessment of nutritional status and the musculoskelatal system, as well as evaluation of any pathology. Regarding structure, examinations include assessment of joint motion, posture, gait, overall flexibility (including joints and tendons), muscle energy, and muscle tone. During treatment, osteopaths may use a number of therapeutic techniques, including gentle cranial manipulations, isometrics or isotonics of a muscle of muscle group, range of motion exploration, positional releases, or velocity adjustments. They also may explore diet and nutrition during treatment and prescribe therapeutic diets.

Pediatric patients often are quite amenable to osteopthic treatments. Osteopathy can be used to as an approach for many illnesses that are often treated with drugs or surgery. A few examples of conditions for which a patient or provider might consider osteopathy include allergies, chronic or acute otitis media, scoliosis, immune dysfunction, and headaches. Osteopathic manipulation also can be applied with other therapies in conditions like asthma, respiratory infections, or urinary tract problems.

BIBLIOGRAPHY

Anderson, R. (1997). *Wellness medicine*. New Canaan, CT: Keats Publishing.

Bach, E. & Wheeler, J. (1979). *The Bach Flower Remedies*. New Canaan, CT: Keats Publishing.

Balick, M., & Cox, P. (1996). *Plants, people, and culture: The science of ethnobotany*. New York: Scientific American Library.

Barral, J. P., & Mercier, P. (1988). *Visceral manipulation*. Seattle, WA: Eastland Press.

Barral, J. P. (1989). *Visceral manipulation II*. Seattle, WA: Eastland Press.

Borrall, J. P. (1991). *The thorax*. Seattle, WA: Eastland Press.

Bartram, T. (1995). *Encyclopedia of herbal medicine*. Grace Publishers.

Bensky, D., & Barolet, R. compil. and translation (1990). *Chinese herbal medicine: Formulas and strategies*. Seattle, WA: Eastland Press.

Bensky, D., & Gamble, A. (1986). *Chinese herbal medicine: Materia Medica*. Seattle, WA: Eastland Press.

Bisset, N. G., & Wichtl, M. (Eds.) (1994). *Herbal drugs and phytopharmaceuticals*. Boca Raton, FL: CRC Press.

Blumenthal, M. (Ed.) (1998). *The German commission E monographs*. Austin, TX: American Botanical Council.

Bone, K. (1997). *Clinical application of ayurvedic and Chinese herbs*. Warwick, Australia: Phytotherapy Press.

Brennan, B. A. (1988). *Hands of light: A guide to healing through the human energy field*. New York: Bantam Books.

Brinker, F. (1998). *Herbal contraindications and drug interactions*. Sandy, OR: Eclectic Medical Publications.

Bronner, F. (Ed.) (1995). *Nutrition and health: Topics and controversies*. Boca Raton, FL: CRC Press.

Buckle, J. (1997). *Clinical aromatherapy in nursing*. Singular Publishing.

Burton Goldberg Group. (1994). *Alternative medicine*. London, OR: Future Medicine Publishing.

Chancellor, P. (1980). *Handbook of Bach flower remedies*. New Canaan, CT: Keats.

Clavey, S. (1995). *Fluid physiology and pathology in traditional Chinese medicine*. London: Churchill Livingstone.

Colbin, A. (1996). *Food and healing* (2nd ed.). New York: Ballantine Books.

Connely, D. (1979). *Traditional acupuncture: The law of the Five Elements*. Columbia, MD: Centre for Traditional Acupuncture.

Cooksley, V. (1996). *Aromatherapy*. Paramus, NJ: Prentice Hall.

Coulter, C. (1986). *Portraits of homeopathic medicines: Psychospiritual analysis of selected constitutional types*. Washington, DC: Wehawken Book.

Coulter, H. (1981). *Homeopathic science and modern medicine*. Berkeley, CA: North Atlantic Books.

Damian, P., & Damian, K. (1995). *Aromatherapy scent and psyche*. Rochester, VT: Healing Arts Press.

De Smet, P. A. G. M. et al. (Eds.) (1993). *Adverse effects of herbal drugs* (vols. 2 & 3). Berlin: Springer-Verlag.

Dintenfass, J. (1971). *Chiropractic: A modern way to health*. New York: Harcourt, Brace, Jovanovich.

Duke, J. (1992). *Handbook of biologically active phytochemicals and their activities*. Boca Raton, FL: CRC Press.

Duke, J. (1985). *Handbook of medicinal herbs*. Boca Raton, FL: CRC Press.

Duke, J. (1992). *Handbook of phytochemical constituents of GRAS herbs and other economic plants*. Boca Raton, FL: CRC Press.

Ellis, A., Wiseman, N., & Zmiewski, P. (1985). *Fundamentals of Chinese medicine*. Brookline: Paradigm Publications.

Ellis, A., Wiseman, N., & Boss, K. (1991). *Fundamentals of Chinese acupuncture*. Brookline: Paradigm Publications.

Erasmus, U. (1994). *Fats that heal, fats that kill*. Burnaby, B.C., Canada: Alive Books.

Fan, W. J. W. (1996). *A manual of Chinese herbal medicine: Principles and practice for easy reference*. Boston: Shambhala.

Felter, H. W. (1994). *The eclectic Materia Medica: Pharmacology and therapeutics*. Cincinnatti: Eclectic Medical Publications.

Fratkin, J. (1986). *Chinese herbal patent formulas*. Boulder, CO: Shya Publications.

Galland, L. (1997). *The four pillars of healing*. New York: Random House.

Garrison, R. H., & Somer, E. (1985). *The nutrition desk reference*. New Canaan: Keats Publishing.

Gehin, A. (1981). *Atlas of manipulative techniques for the cranium and face*. Seattle, WA: Eastland Press.

Golan, R. (1995). *Optimal wellness*. New York: Ballantine Books.

Gottschall, E. (1997). *Breaking the vicious cycle: Intestinal health through diet*. Baltimore and Ontario: Kirkton Press Ltd.

Grieve, M. (1971). *A modern herbal* (2 Vols.). New York: Dover.

Griggs, B. (1981). *Green pharmacy: The history and evolution of Western herbal medicine*. Rochester: Healing Arts Press.

Hadady, L. (1998). *Asian health secrets*. New York: Crown Publishers.

Harper, J. (1997). *Body wisdom: Chinese and natural medicine for self-healing*. London: Thorsons.

Hoffer, A., & Walker, M. (1994). *Smart nutrients: A guide to nutrients that can prevent and reverse senility*. Garden City Park: Avery Publishing Group.

Huang, K. C. (1993). *The pharmacology of Chinese herbs*. Boca Raton: CRC Press.

Hyne Jones, T. W. (1985). *Dictionary of the Bach flower remedies*. Saffron Walden, UK: C.W. Daniel.

Jouanny, J. (1990). *The essential of homeopathic Materia Medica*. Bordeaux: Laboratories Boiron.

Junemann, M. (1998). *Enchanting scents*. Wilmot, WI: Lotus Light Press.

Kapoor, L. D. (1990). *Handbook of ayurvedic medicinal plants*. Boca Raton: CRC Press.

Kaptchuk, T. (1984). *The web that has no weaver*. New York: Congdon and Weed.

Kirby, D., & Dudrick, S. (Eds.). (1994). *Practical handbook of nutrition in clinical practice*. Boca Raton: CRC Press.

Kuwaki, T. (1990). *Chinese herbal therapy: A guide to its principles and practice*. Long Beach: Oriental Healing Arts Institute.

LaWall, (1927). *4000 years of pharmacy*. Philadelphia: Lippincott.

Lawless, J. (1992). *The encyclopedia of essential oils*. London: Element Books.

Levy, J. B. (1974). *Common herbs for natural health*. New York: Schocken Books.

Lifshitz, F. (Ed.) (1994). *Childhood nutrition*. Boca Raton: CRC Press.

Lu, H. C. (1987). *Chinese herbs with common foods*. New York: Kodansha International Ltd.

Maciocia, G. (1990). *The foundations of Chinese Medicine*. London: Churchill Livingstone.

Magoun, H. (1976). *Osteopathy in the cranial field* (3rd ed.). Kirksville, Missouri: The Journal Printing Company.

Moore, M. (1989). *Medicinal plants of the Desert and Canyon West*. Santa Fe: Museum of New Mexico Press.

Moore, M. (1979). *Medicinal plants of the Mountain West*. Museum of Santa Fe: New Mexico Press.

Moore, M. (1993). *Medicinal plants of the Pacific West*. Red Crane Books.

Murphy, R. (1993). *Homeopathic medical repertory*. Pagoda Springs, CO: Hahnemann Academy of North America.

Murray, M. (1995). *The healing power of herbs*. Rockland, CA: Prima Publishing.

Nadkarni, K. M. (1976). *Indian Materia Medica* (2 vols.). Bombay: Popular Prakashan.

Newall, C., Anderson, L., & Phillipson, J. D. (1996). *Herbal medicines: A guide for health professionals*. London: The Pharmaceutical Press.

Newman Turner, R. (1984). *Naturopathic medicine*. Wellingborough, UK: Thorsons.

Ody, P. (1993). *The complete medicinal herbal*. New York: Dorling Kindersly.

Overmyer, Luann (1997). *"Ortho-Bionomy" paper* presented at Fifth National Conference on Integrative Medicine and Wellness in Allied Health. San Francisco.

Panos, M., & Heimlich, J. (1980). *Homeopathic medicine at home*. Boston: Houghton Mifflin.

Pitchford, P. (1993). *Healing with whole foods: Oriental traditions and modern nutrition*. Berkeley: North Atlantic Books.

Price, S. (1994). *Practical aromatherapy*. London: Harper Collins.

Reynolds, J. E. F. (Ed.). (1993). *Martindale: The extra pharmacopoeia* (13th ed). London: The Pharmaceutical Press.

Romm, A. (1996). *Natural healing for babies and children*. Freedom, CA: The Crossing Press.

Ryman, D. (1993). *Aromatherapy: The complete guide to plant and flower essences for health and beauty*. New York: Bantam Books.

Ryman, D. (1984). *The aromatherapy handbook*. London: Century Hutchinson.

Samuelson, G. (1992). *Drugs of natural origin*. Stockholm, Sweden: Swedish Pharmaceutical Press.

Schilcher, H. (1997). *Phytotherapy in paediatrics*. Stuttgart: Medpharm Scientific Publishers.

Schumlick, P. (1994). *Ginger: Common spice and wonder drug*. Brattleboro, VT: Herbal Free Press.

Scofield, A. G. (1981). *Chiropractic*. Thorsens.

Sharma, C. H. (1976). *A manual of homeopathy and natural medicine*. New York: E. P. Dutton & Co.

Spiller, G. (Ed.) (1992). *Dietary fiber in human nutrition* (2nd ed.). Boca Raton: CRC Press.

Stanway, A. (1987). *The natural family doctor*. New York: Simon and Schuster.

St. Clare, D. (1997). *The herbal medicine cabinet: Preparing natural remedies at home*. Berkeley: Celestial Arts.

Svoboda, R. (1989). *Prakruti: Your ayurvedic constitution*. Albuquerque, NM: Geocom Ltd.

Tang, W., & Eisenbrand, G. (1992). *Chinese drugs of plant origin*. Berlin: Springer-Verlag.

Tisserand, R. (1985). *The art of aromatherapy*. Saffron Walden, UK: C.W. Daniel.

Tisserand, R., & Balacs, T. (1998). *Essential oil safety: A guide for health professionals*. London: Churchill Livingstone.

Tiwari, M. (1995). *Ayurveda: Secrets of healing*. Twin Lakes, WI: Lotus Press.

Tyler, V. E. (1993). *The honest herbal*. Binghamton, NY: Haworth Press.

Walton, W. (1972). *Textbook of osteopathic diagnosis and technique procedures* (2nd ed.). Colorado Springs: The American Academy of Osteopathy.

Werbach, M. R. (1993). *Nutritional influences on illness* (2nd ed.). Tarzana: Third Line Press.

Wood, M. (1997). *The book of herbal wisdom: Using plants as medicines*. Berkeley: North Atlantic Books.

Wood, M. (1992). *The magical staff*. Berkeley: North Atlantic Books.

Wren, R. C. (1988). *Potter's new cyclopedia of botanical drugs and preparations*. Essex, GB: C. W. Daniel Company.

Wu, Y., & Fischer, W. (1997). *Practical therapeutics of Traditional Chinese Medicine*. Brookline: Paradigm Publications.

Yen, K. Y. (1992). *The illustrated Chinese Materia Medica*. Tipai: SMC Publishing.

A P P E N D I X   4 - 1

Aromatherapy:
Selected Oils Commonly Used in Pediatrics

Discussion	Uses	Major Constituents	Safety/Efficacy	Contraindications
Bergamot particularly helps many skin conditions and urinary tract infections. It is useful for acute and chronic depression and anxiety. It is not a stimulant but a mild sedative used over time and in combination with other therapies.	Acne, anorexia, antidepressant, antiseptic, antiviral, boils colitis, cystitis, diarrhea, herpes simplex virus type 1, insomnia, varicella	Limonene, linalool, linalyl acetate, bergapten	Use only very diluted. Terpeneless oil generally is advised because it is safer.	Avoid exposure to sunlight for 12 h after use. Do not use on sensitive, diseased, or damaged skin or children younger than 2 y.
Chamomile, a very gentle oil, is popular worldwide and for all ages. It is used frequently in pediatrics because it addresses many problems and is well liked and quite safe. It is excellent in a bath for skin conditions, anxiety, or insomnia.	Anti-inflammatory, antiseptic, colic, colitis, cystitis, diarrhea, dry skin, eczema, insomnia, menstrual cramps, stomachache, teething, urticaria	Chamazulene, isodol, famesine, matricin, pinocarvine, bisbaloxides A, B, and C, chamaviolin, spiroethers; esters, sesquiterpenes, flavenoids, coumarins	Do not use in the eye.	None known (unless child is allergic to chamomile)
Eucalyptus, a well-known oil and flavoring found in cough drops and chest rubs, makes an excellent steam inhalation for upper respiratory ailments. It is antiseptic and anti-inflammatory.	Analgesic, antibacterial, antiviral, bronchitis, colds, cough, cystitis, diuretic, expectorant, headache, herpes simplex virus type 1, insect repellents, sinusitis	Cineol	Use with caution on mucous membranes. Eucalyptus induces the p450 system and may decrease the efficacy of other drugs.	Do not use on sensitive, diseased, or damaged skin or with children younger than 2 y. Do not apply to the faces of children younger than 5 y.
Helichrysum is among the most frequently used "children's oils." It is good for sensitive skin and is used in baths and skin massages (dilute) even for infants. It blends well with other children's oils like chamomile, lavender, and mandarin. It is particularly useful for coughs, because it is a gentle expectorant, anti-inflammatory, and antispasmodic.	Anti-inflammatory, antispasmodic, allergies, asthma, bronchitis, croup, eczema, psoriasis, stomachache, whooping cough	Geraniol, linalol, nerol, neral acetate, pinene	Generally recognized as safe.	None known.
Lavender lifts spirits and increases courage, fortitude, and sense of purpose. Usually used as aroma-therapy or in baths or steams, lavender can be taken internally as tea. The tea is very tannic and usually combined with other herbs.	ADHD, anxiety, asthma, depression, headache, stress	Camphor, cineol, linalyl acetate, linalool, beta-ocimene	Oil official in Austria, Egypt, France, Hungary, Mexico, Switzerland, former Yugoslavia.	Use with caution if child has a history of seizure disorders.
Mandarin, particularly popular for the pediatric population, is used for all types of stomach upsets. In France, it is known as "the children's remedy."	Constipation, diarrhea, hiccups, indigestion, stomachache	Limonene, methyl anthralinate, geraniol, citral, citronellal	Generally recognized as safe.	None known.

(continues)

A P P E N D I X   4 - 1

Aromatherapy:
Selected Oils Commonly Used in Pediatrics *(Continued)*

Discussion	Uses	Major Constituents	Safety/Efficacy	Contraindications
Melissa, a lemony-scented essential oil extracted from lemon balm, is very expensive. Adulteration is common.	Asthma, cough, croup, eczema, shock	Citral, citronellal, linalol	Very small amounts (1–3 drops in a bath) are typically used.	Do not use on sensitive, diseased, or damaged skin or on children younger than 2 y. Do not use in glaucoma.
Neroli oil is distilled from flowers of the bitter orange. Cosmeticians highly value its excellence for all skin types. When dilute, its fragrance is used in many massage oils and skin preparations. It is great for children suffering from acute or chronic anxiety, especially helpful in stomachache or diarrhea from "nervous stomach."	Antispasmodic, anxiety, diarrhea, dry skin, indigestion, insomnia, stomachache	Linalol, d-limonene (largest constituent), nerol, nerolidol, geraniol, jasmone, bergapten esters	Avoid exposure to sunlight for 12 h after using.	None known.
Peppermint oil, most popular for children as a tea, can be used in older children as an inhalation for colds and flu. It is used topically as an analgesic and given in enteric-coated capsules for digestive upset.	Analgesic, colds, cough, flatulence, irritable bowel, stomachache	Carvone, cineol, limonene, menthol, menthone, isomenthol, neomenthol, menthyl acetate, menthofuran, pugelone.	Use with caution if child has a history of seizure disorder. Use less than 3% concentration, if at all, on mucous membranes.	Avoid oral administration if child has G6PD deficiency. Use only in children older than 4 y. because it can cause laryngeal or bronchial spasm in younger children.
Rose was probably the first essential oil ever distilled. It is found in many pediatric preparations, probably because this scent is associated with love. Rose soothes upsets and skin conditions and is a powerful tonic for the nervous system and internal organs.	Anxiety, depression, dry skin, eczema, failure to thrive, grief, insomnia, stomachache	Citronellol, farnesol, geraniol, nerol, phenlyl ethanol, stearopten.	Generally recognized as safe. Because of high cost, high possibility of adulteration exists.	None known.
Rosemary oil has been appreciated as a medicinal plant for at least 2000 y. The essential oil fraction of rosemary contributes most to its culinary and medicinal virtues, specifically the phenolic acids, such as rosmarinic acid. It has several uses in aromatherapy.	Analgesic, antiflatulent, anti-inflammatory, antiseptic, anti-spasmodic, acne, asthma, bronchitis, colic, dandruff, eczema (bath), headache, indigestion, pharyngitis, sinusitis, stimulant (mild)	Essential oil: esters (2%–5%): bornyl acetate, free alcohols (up to 18%): especially borneol, linalol, citranellol; phenolic acids: (including rosmarinic)	Use with caution if child has a history of seizure disorder.	Do not use on sensitive or damaged skin. Official in pharmacopoeia of Austria, Belgium, Czechoslovakia, Germany, Hungary, Mexico, and Switzerland.
Tea tree is native to Australia, and most historical information about its use comes from Aboriginal Australians, who used it broadly.	Antibacterial, anti-fungal, antiviral, antiseptic	Cineol, pinene, terpineol	Generally recognized as safe.	None known.

A P P E N D I X   4 - 2

Common Herbal Remedies

Discussion	Uses	Precautions/Contraindications
Alfalfa, most effective as a nutrient supplement, derives a rich array of vitamins and minerals from the earth. It is excellent as a nutritionally supportive herb in chronic illness. Most often used in combination with other herbs in daily tonic tea blends, it can help in convalescence from any serious illness. It is used postpartum and to nourish mother and breast-feeding baby.	Anemia, appetite stimulant, colitis, convalescence, hyperacidity, nutritional support	Like most legumes, alfalfa contains coumarins, so caution is needed when using it while taking blood thinners (eg, coumadin). It also can cause photosensitivity.
Aloe vera is a wonderful, soothing remedy for mild burns (including sunburn). It is most effective as a fresh leaf, although gel helps. Evidence supports its use as an anti-infective. Studies have shown fresh aloe works as well as silver sulfadiazine in inhibiting common bacteria that infect burns. Aloe contains anti-inflammatory constituents. It is a popular laxative, but caution is to be emphasized. Its active laxative components are from the anthraquinone glycoside family, which directly irritate the bowel wall. It is definitely habit-forming. Many (even children) take aloe juice daily as a bowel "tonic." Doing so tends to irritate the mucous membranes of the GI tract over time, leading to dependence and decreased colonic muscle tone. It usually is not advised for children younger than 12 y. Aloin-free preparations should be safer, because the irritating anthraquinones are in the aloin fraction.	Antiseptic, burns, constipation	Aloe should be avoided in pregnancy, breast-feeding, in the presence of hemorrhoids or inflammatory bowel disease, such as ulcerative colitis, Chron's disease, and irritable bowel syndrome. Internal use should be limited.
Anise, a stimulant digestive aid, is safe in infants and children for nausea, gas, and colic. Anise passes into breast milk, a good way to deliver it to colicky infants. It also increases flow of breast milk. It is used as a flavoring agent with other herbs to make their taste more pleasant. Anethol is important as a respiratory tract antiseptic and decongestant expectorant, making anise good for babies and children with colds.	Asthma, colds, colic, flatulence, upper respiratory tract infections	None known.
Ashwaganda is often called the ayurvedic ginseng. Unlike ginseng, ashwaganda is suitable for all ages and is used especially in the pediatric population for poor weight gain and failure to thrive. Milk fortified with this herb is advised for children of all ages. In a double-blind study of normal 8–12 y olds it was shown to increase body weight, total plasma proteins, and mean corpuscular hemoglobin. It is also given to lactating moms to enhance breast milk and nourish an infant who is not thriving.	Fatigue, convalescence, memory, nervine, failure to thrive, infants and children, lactation, muscles: ataxia	None known.
Astragalus has been widely studied for its ability to enhance the immune system. It is used specifically to strengthen resistance to infections, often for babies, children, and adults who get frequent colds and ear infections. Research has shown that the polysaccharides and saponins in astragalus are responsible for its immunostimulating properties. Astragalus has been shown to increase the cytotoxicity of natural killer cells in a similar manner to alpha-interferon. It also activates macrophages. It increases production of interleukin-2, thus enhancing splenic lymphocyte activity, and affects levels of cyclic GMP and AMP in the spleen, liver, and blood. In TCM, astragalus is frequently found in combinations	AIDS, allergies, asthma, bronchitis, convalescence, hepatitis, HIV, immune enhancement, otitis media: chronic, recurrent, and serous, sinusitis-chronic, upper respiratory tract infection, chronic	None known.

(continues)

A P P E N D I X   4 - 2

Common Herbal Remedies *(Continued)*

Discussion	Uses	Precautions/Contraindications
for people who are convalescing, weak, debilitated, or have chronically poor digestion. It also is excellent and safe in improving endurance in athletes.		
Burdock, a gentle and safe herb used in pregnancy and for infants and small children, is helpful for constipation and various skin conditions. It increases the flow of bile. As bile is a natural laxative, burdock is safe and non-habit forming. It is also useful as an antimicrobial in cystitis, likely because of its polyacetylenes, some of which contain sulfur.	Acne, boils, constipation, hives, psoriasis, urinary tract infection	None known.
Calendula is used topically in many creams, gels, and lotions. It is also taken internally, most often combined with other herbs, as an anti-inflammatory. It speeds wound healing and takes the sting out of insect bites. It is useful in healing burns, cuts, and lacerations. It acts as an antiseptic and anti-inflammatory. Studies in rats have indicated its effectiveness as a topical antibiotic against Staphylococcus aureus. For burns, the gel is preferred, applied liberally. As an antifungal, it can be used orally for thrush or topically for diaper rash, including candidal. As a bath, it soothes and moistens dry skin and eczema.	Anti-inflammatory, baths, burns (topical), diaper rash (including fungal), eczema, eyes: inflammation, compress of tea, thrush, wounds and wound healing (topical)	None known.
Cascara sagrada, one of the very few herbs still official in the U.S. pharmacopoeia, is an excellent occasional laxative, largely because of the significant presence of anthraquinone glycosides that directly stimulate activity of the colonic mucosa. The complete mechanism of action is not fully established. Anthrones are formed during the interaction of anthraquinones with intestinal flora. These anthrones are cytotoxic, and part of mechanism of action of anthraquinone-containing laxatives may be this cytotoxicity. Anthraquinone-containing plants also increase free water secretion from the colon into the feces.	Constipation, laxative, cathartic	Do not use in intestinal obstruction, inflammatory bowel disease, or for children younger than 12 y. It has synergistic effects with standard diuretics, increasing potassium loss. It decreases bowel transit time and therefore absorption of some drugs. Do not use with cardiac glycoside-containing drugs. It is contraindicated in lactation. Prolonged use can promote dependence and severe potassium depletion. Carcinogenicity is possible.
Catnip, most famous as a stimulant/sedative for cats, is **not** intoxicating or addictive in humans but can cause mild stimulation or sedation. A cup of iced catnip tea is a mild stimulant, providing a pleasant temporary lift without jumpiness. Hot, steeped catnip tea or infusion is a mild-to-moderate sedative/antispasmodic. Warm catnip is wonderful for colicky babies, as it relieves intestinal cramps and gas, relaxes the smooth muscle of the intestinal wall, and helps the baby fall asleep. Catnip is also good for stomach upset, nausea, and stomach flu in older children and adults. It combines well with ginger, chamomile, and licorice. Hot catnip preparations also relax the uterine smooth muscle, relieving painful menstrual cramps.	Colic, diarrhea, flatulence, headache, insomnia, menstrual cramps, nausea	For babies, use only very small amounts. The national poison control hotline reports that a few times each year, frantic parents call who have given their babies catnip tea and who then cannot awaken the babies. The babies have all eventually awakened unharmed, but this must certainly be a terrifying experience for the parents.
Chamomile is a particularly versatile and gentle herb. It soothes infant colic, digestive upsets, gas, poor digestion, and diarrhea. It is a useful antiviral and anti-infective. Its essential oil fraction, flavenoids, and sesquiterpene lactones all contribute substantially to its pharmacology. Components of the essential oil fraction are	Antibacterial, antiflatulent, antifungal, anti inflammatory, anti spasmodic, anxiolytic, carminative, sedative, mild	Occasional allergies in susceptible individuals, most commonly those allergic to asters and chrysanthemums.

(continues)

A P P E N D I X   4 - 2

Common Herbal Remedies (Continued)

Discussion	Uses	Precautions/Contraindications
particularly responsible for the anti-infective (including antifungal) properties. The flavenoids, particularly apigenin and luteolin have demonstrated significant anti-inflammatory activity. The ester bisbalol has been found to help heal inflammatory processes in the GI tract. The essential oil azulene (chamazulene) is antiseptic, anti-inflammatory, and pain relieving. In a study of noncomplicated children's diarrhea, a preparation of chamomile with pectin plus rehydration was examined versus placebo plus rehydration. The diarrhea ended significantly more quickly in the pectin/chamomile group than in the placebo group and parent enthusiasm was high in the treatment group.		
Dandelion is a mild diuretic because of its high potassium content. It increases the flow of bile. Because bile is a natural laxative, dandelion is safe for a constipated baby or child. Its other hepatobiliary uses mostly relate to the liver. It is safe for use during acute and chronic hepatitis, will help cool inflammation, supports bile production, and increases glutathione levels.	Constipation, diuretic (mild), hepatitis, urinary tract infections	Mild diuretic and laxative. High in potassium so replaces this nutrient. Generally regarded as safe.
Dill, best known as a culinary herb, has therapeutic properties, mostly enhancing digestion. Dill seed is an excellent remedy for gas pain and colic. It is safe as a tea even for infants. It is also a traditional tonic to increase breast milk. Dill is good for mild constipation in infants, either as a tea or via the breast-feeding mother but will not help severe constipation other than to relieve some gas and bloating. Dill weed is good for breaking up mucus.	Fruit/Seed: bloating, colic, constipation, flatulence, lactation Weed: mucous congestion	None known.
Echinacea, a native North American plant, is one of the most popular and widely used herbs in the United States. Its mechanism of action is nonspecific activation of the immune system, although understanding of this is incomplete. Research has shown that echinacea activates natural killer cells, increases circulating levels of alpha-interferon, stimulates fibroblasts, and activates macrophages, thus increasing phagocytosis. The caffeic esters, including echinoside, are antibacterial and antiviral. The polyacetylenes are thought to contribute to the herb's bacteriostatic and antifungal activity. Fairly well studied, it is used to prevent and treat colds and flu.	Antibiotic, antiseptic, immunostimulant, antiviral, lymphatic congestion	Generally use of echinacea is avoided in people with autoimmune disorders, like SLE.
Elder flower/berry dries mucus and cools inflammation. Research has shown its powerful immunostimulating properties, supporting its traditional use as a tonic for frequent bronchial and lung infections and asthma. The immunostimulant action is attributed, at least in part, to sambucin. The berries are mildly laxative. They are safe for children and breast-feeding moms and are usually quite popular because of their sweet flavor. Elder flower water is used in skin and eye preparations and for freckles and acne.	Allergies, apthous ulcers, bronchitis, colds, constipation, cystitis, eye inflammation, fevers, influenza, laryngitis, laxative, sinusitis	Teas should be strained to avoid ingesting large amounts of the seeds

(continues)

A P P E N D I X   4 - 2

Common Herbal Remedies *(Continued)*

Discussion	Uses	Precautions/Contraindications
Eyebright is used to treat a variety of external eye ailments and irritations. This gentle herb has a relatively high tannin content that can be irritating if used over a long period. It also is taken internally as a tea, infusion, or tincture for allergies and asthma.	Allergies, allergic rhinitis, asthma, blepharitis, conjunctivitis, styes	Avoid in babies under 6 mo due to tannins.
Fennel seed, a dried fruit, is excellent as a diluted tea for infant colic. It is both anti-inflammatory and antispasmodic. Older children with gas pains may chew the seeds whole or take them as a tea with peppermint. Its antiflatulent effects are due mostly to certain constituents in the plant's essential oil fraction.	Anti-inflammatory, anti-spasmodic, blepharitis, colic, conjunctivitis, diuretic, flatulence, lactation	Fennel is very weakly estrogenic due to the constituent estragole.
Garlic is a remarkably potent and versatile herb. Much of its activity is secondary to sulfur-containing compounds in both the inert and volatile oil fraction. These compounds give garlic its characteristic odor, so odorless preparations are generally less active. Garlic is a broad spectrum anti-infective with significant activity against many bacteria. It also is an important antiviral, antifungal, and antihelminthic. As a food, it is a digestive stimulant, helpful in emulsifying fats. It is useful in mucous GI tract problems, but caution should be taken when using it with chronic inflammation. It is often taken preventively for traveler's diarrhea or at the first signs of infectious diarrhea. It is also used for respiratory tract infections and is eaten by breast-feeding mothers when babies have thrush. Garlic does pass into breast milk, and is, of course, safe. It may protect against cancers.	Antibiotic, antifungal, antiseptic, antiviral, diaphoretic, expectorant warming, stimulant, mucolytic, colds, flu, gastroenteritis, thrush	
Ginger root is recognized worldwide for its warming, decongestant, and soothing properties. Ginger relieves cramps, colic, and GI spasms. It assuages some menstrual cramps.	Anti-inflammatory, colic, flatulence, menstrual cramps, motion sickness, nausea, upper respiratory tract infections	Increases menstrual flow; do not use for cramps if flow is already very heavy.
Goldenseal has a broad spectrum of antimicrobial action, largely due to berberine alkaloids. It is antifungal as well, apparently blocking the actions of some bacterial toxins including those of *Vibrio cholera* and *Escherichia coli*. As a bitter root, stimulates flow of bile and saliva. It is a useful eyewash for treating chlamydial conjunctivitis, blepharitis, and corneal abrasion.	Antifungal, antibacterial, antiseptic, stops bleeding, anti-inflammatory (topically), conjunctivitis	Large doses may interfere with B vitamin metabolism and can cause digestive upset.
Hyssop is typically selected for relief of viral pharyngitis and acute upper respiratory tract ailments.	Bronchitis, colds, expectorant, pharyngitis, sinusitis	Avoid in seizure disorder. It is not good for long-term use because there is some chronic toxicity, especially from pinocamphene and other camphors.
Licorice root has been used for thousands of years, and much recent scientific research substantiates its traditional uses. A main component, glycyrrhizin, is responsible for its effectiveness in suppressing coughs. Glycerrhizin also has been demonstrated as effective in healing gastric ulcers and preventing aspirin-induced ulcers in rats. It aids in healing ulcers through its mucilaginous components. Another constituent,	Anti-inflammatory, aphthous ulcer, asthma, bronchitis, cough, expectorant, heartburn, hepatitis, laxative, liver disease (hepatoprotective), gastritis, pharyngitis	Because of the ACTH-like effects, avoid high doses in hypertension, borderline hypertension, and renal disease.

(continues)

A P P E N D I X   4 - 2

Common Herbal Remedies *(Continued)*

Discussion	Uses	Precautions/Contraindications
glycyrrhetic acid, has affinity for binding to kidney aldosterone receptors. Thus, long-term moderate to frequent use may lead to sodium retention and elevated blood pressure. Licorice has been demonstrated to have immunomodulating effects, inducing interferon and inhibiting growth of HSV 1. Clinical studies have shown its protective effects against hepatotoxins, such as strychnine and carbon tetrachloride. It also is a mild laxative and promotes urination.		
Marshmallow root is a safe and gentle mucilaginous demulcent that helps loosen and moisten thick mucus in sinusitis, colds, and bronchitis. It settles queasiness during bouts of acute gastroenteritis and can be used by children with inflammatory bowel disease. It is safe for long-term use, but may have mild diuretic effects.	Bronchitis, gastroenteritis, inflammatory bowel disease, laryngitis, pharyngitis, sinusitis, urinary tract demulcent	Prescription medications should be taken at least 1 h before or 2 h after marshmallow root, because the herb may decrease absorption of drugs.
Milk thistle, once used for liver congestion and hematologic problems, became popular in the 1970s after studies indicated its significant hepato-protective and hepatoregenerative benefits. Its Silymarin complex increases glutathione stores in liver, stabilizes membrane, and acts as an antioxidant. Silymarin also increases de novo hepatocyte synthesis, stimulating ribosomal protein synthesis. Milk thistle is safe to use even in the acute phase of hepatitis.	Hepatitis, poisoning, hepatoprotective, laxative (mild), kidney protective, increases bile solubility	None known.
Mullein is a safe herb for asthma. It decreases phlegm, strengthens the lungs, and helps keep bronchi open yet is not a stimulant. It is safely used with other herbs and pharmaceuticals to treat numerous respiratory tract problems. Mullein also works topically as a local anti-inflammatory.	Asthma, bronchitis, cough, expectorant, hay fever, mucilage	None known.
Nettle has lots of vitamins and minerals. Nettles have been promoted for seasonal allergies/rhinitis. The freeze-dried form gives significant relief to 40%–50% of people with hay fever. Nettles also have effectively treated eczema, often in conjunction with other herbs, as a tea or in baths. They are a good lung tonic for children with asthma, especially if phlegm is chronic. Very high in vitamin K and bioavailable iron, nettles are useful for chronic bleeding problems and nosebleeds. They nourish the blood and connective tissue.	Allergies, anemia, asthma, astringent, bleeding, colitis, diuretic, eczema, nosebleeds	Generally regarded as safe.
Oat straw, useful for a wide variety of nervous disorders is calming and relaxing but not sedating. Safe and nonaddictive, it promotes sleep. It also helps a wide variety of skin eruptions, probably because of its high silica content. A bath of oat straw is less drying to eczematous skin than colloidal oatmeal, but still quite soothing.	Anxiety, convalescence, eczema, insomnia	None known.

(continues)

A P P E N D I X   4 - 2

Common Herbal Remedies *(Continued)*

Discussion	Uses	Precautions/Contraindications
Peppermint, well liked by children and adults, settles upset and nervous stomachs, helps dispel gas and bloating, and eases belching. It is used for nausea and vomiting and can be quite helpful in acute gastroenteritis. Peppermint tea is a great headache remedy and is safe for administration to children. Peppermint inhalation treatments are particularly good for sinusitis, cough associated with bronchitis, and acute pneumonia. Menthol from tea or infusion passes into breast milk, a safe and effective way to treat colic in breast-feeding infants.	Belching, bloating, bronchitis, colic, cough, flatulence, gastroenteritis, headache, influenza, nausea	Avoid daily use because of high tannins. Avoid in chronic dyspepsia.
Raspberry leaf (red) is a very old herb. In addition to its uses in pregnancy, it is an important remedy for gastroenteritis and diarrhea. This great remedy for babies and children is safe, nutritive, and mildly flavored. It can be mixed in tea blends with other herbs, such as chamomile. It is cooling and makes a refreshing rehydration drink in the summer, especially when mixed with other nutritive herbs like rose hips, lemon balm, and alfalfa.	Apthous ulcers, diarrhea, menstrual cramps, nausea, gastroenteritis	None known.
Saint John's Wort is commonly used for depression and seasonal affective disorder. Reasonably well studied in adults, its pharmacology and mechanisms of action are still under debate. Early studies focused on hypericin as the main active constituent, but it now appears that the pharmacology is complex. Biflavones are known to be sedative, as is the antibiotic constituent hyperforin, which also is active against gram-negative and gram-positive bacteria. Hyperforin probably is partly responsible for mild SSRI effects. Hypericin potentiates binding at GABA-a receptors, benzodiazapene receptors, and 5HT-1 serotonin receptor. Hypericin and psuedohypericin show *in vitro* activity against herpes simplex types I and II, influenza, EBV, and vesicular stomatitis virus. Saint John's Wort has not been studied in children but is approved and used in Europe in children older than 6 y. There have been no reports of serious adverse effects.	Arthritis, antiviral, antidepressant, antispasmodic, anti-inflammatory, depression	The herb can cause photosensitivity and occasional GI upset.
Usnea actually is a group of mosses. It is rich in anti-infective components and helps break up phlegm and congestion. Some evidence has shown that usnic acid is effective against tuberculosis. It also can be used topically to eliminate candidal diaper rash and as a soak or poultice for other fungal infections (eg, ringworm, athlete's foot).	Antibacterial, antifungal, athlete's foot, bronchitis, ringworm, sinusitis, diaper rash	None known.
Wild cherry bark, with a pleasant cherry flavor, probably suppresses cough in aqueous extracts secondary to hydrocyanic acid.	Cough	It should not be taken often because of trace amounts of cyanide.

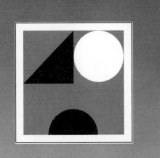

PROMOTING HEALTH AND NORMAL GROWTH AND DEVELOPMENT

Genetic Preconception and Prenatal Counseling

- WENDY C. MCKINNON, MS; ELIZABETH DORSEY SMITH, EdD, RN; and WILLIAM T. SEED, MD, FAAP

P A R T   1   ▲

Genetic Counseling

- WENDY C. MCKINNON, MS

INTRODUCTION

The financial and societal costs resulting from genetic conditions are significant. Last estimates of the incidence of genetic disease in newborns were between 5% and 6% (Baird, Anderson, Newcombe, & Lowry, 1988). Although current estimates are unavailable, past studies show that 52% of pediatric hospitalizations (Hall, Powers, McIlvaine, & Ean, 1978), 42% of pediatric deaths (Roberts, Chavez, & Court, 1970), and 11.5% of adult inpatient admissions (Emery & Rimoin, 1990) were attributable to genetic conditions. Preconception genetic risk assessment may direct screening and testing for unsuspected genetic disorders in individuals of childbearing age, helping to provide a more accurate assessment of risks for future offspring (Cohn, Miller, Gould, Macri, & Gimovsky, 1999).

Historically, the primary goal of genetic counseling was prevention of birth defects. In this era of increasing genetic information, however, expanded knowledge and enhanced reproductive choice should be the goals. The value of preconception genetic counseling must not be overlooked. With regard to congenital malformations, birth defects, and many inherited conditions, education and counseling before conception and subsequent organogenesis allow couples to make informed decisions regarding possible risks and to assess the possibilities that best fit their individual circumstances. They often will miss such opportunities if they wait until the first prenatal visit (Hogge & Hogge, 1996).

Individuals and couples will likely have different reactions to genetic information depending on the specific condition, its severity, prenatal testing options, disease treatment options, and personal experience with the condition. Reproductive options include the following:

- Not bearing children
- No intervention during pregnancy
- Prenatal diagnosis, with the option of terminating an affected fetus
- Alternative reproductive options, such as ovum or sperm donation or preimplantation diagnosis

FAMILY HISTORY

A thorough and appropriately detailed family history is an important part of genetic counseling. A three-generation pedigree significantly influences risk assessment for future offspring and reveals an individual's risk for significant heritable medical problems. The provider should inquire about a family history of birth defects, neural tube defects, recurrent miscarriages, stillbirths, mental retardation or developmental delay, consanguinity, early deaths, and specific genetic disorders (eg, cystic fibrosis [CF], fragile X syndrome, neurofibromatosis). If a family history of an apparent heritable disorder exists, the preconception period allows time to collect medical records, document the reported history, and refer the woman or couple to a clinical geneticist or other specialist. If a specific diagnosis is made, then the parties can discuss risks of recurrence, options for possible prenatal diagnosis, and available treatment options.

The provider should ask about late-onset disorders in the family, such as Huntington's disease, Alzheimer's disease, hereditary breast or ovarian cancer syndrome, and hereditary nonpolyposis colon cancer syndrome. Individuals may want to consider predisposition genetic testing before starting a family to determine whether they are at risk. Genetic counseling before and after the test is extremely important for individuals interested in predisposition genetic testing. The National Society of Genetic Counselors has outlined the important elements of such counseling in its position statement (McKinnon et al., 1997).

ETHNICITY AND GENETIC CONDITIONS

Couples from certain ethnic populations may be at increased risk for having offspring with specific autosomal recessively inherited conditions. Common conditions are discussed in the following sections.

Thalassemias

The thalassemias are a heterogeneous group of genetic disorders characterized by absent or decreased production of normally functioning hemoglobins. Normal red blood cells contain a combination of three hemoglobins: hemoglobin A (Hb A), hemoglobin A_2 (Hb A_2), and hemoglobin F (Hb F). Each of these hemoglobins is composed of two α- and two non-α (β-, δ-, or τ-) -globin chains. Two α-globin genes are on chromosome 16, providing four copies in normal individuals; the β-, δ-, and τ-globin genes are on chromosome 11.

Normally, production of α- and non–α-chains is balanced: Hb A is $\alpha_2\beta_2$, Hb A$_2$ is $\alpha_2\delta_2$, and Hb F is $\alpha_2\tau_2$.

In both α- and β-thalassemias, a decreased number of globin chains results in microcytosis and ineffective erythropoiesis and hemolysis. Varying degrees of microcytic hypochromic anemia ensue (Dumars et al., 1996). If Hb A$_2$, Hb F, or both are increased, then the diagnosis is β-thalassemia. If Hb A$_2$ and Hb F are normal and ferritin is normal or high, then α-thalassemia is the likely diagnosis. Providers must be aware that unusual structural variants also can occur (Dumars et al., 1996).

Couples of Mediterranean (eg, Southern Italy, Greece) descent are at increased risk for having a child with β-thalassemia (Olivieri, 1999). Couples of Southeast Asian (eg, Laos, Thai, Cambodia, Hmong) descent are at increased risk for having a child with α-thalassemia. Couples of East Indian and Middle Eastern ancestry are at increased risk for having a child with either α- or β-thalassemia or sickle cell disease (discussed below). A simple first-line screen for both types of thalassemia is a complete blood count with red blood cell indices.

● **Clinical Pearl:** Carriers of thalassemia have a mild anemia and a low mean corpuscular volume (MCV). An MCV less than 80 should prompt further evaluation. Providers should offer individuals with a low MCV hemoglobin electrophoresis for quantitative Hb A$_2$ and Hb F. Measurement of ferritin in such individuals also is important to rule out iron-deficiency anemia.

Sickle Cell Anemia

Sickle cell anemia (SCA) is a hemoglobinopathy in which an inherited structural abnormality occurs in one of the globin chains. A change of one amino acid from glutamic to valine in the hemoglobin molecule alters the molecule's configuration, causing the cells to sickle and obstruct blood flow in small vessels. Episodes of vaso-oclusive crisis and chronic anemia characterize SCA because the red blood cells tend to become deformed under conditions of decreased oxygen tension.

● **Clinical Pearl:** People of African American ancestry are at increased risk for having a child with SCA. The carrier state (sickle cell trait) is found in approximately 1 out of every 10 African Americans, and incidence of SCA in this population is 1 in 400. To identify carriers of sickle cell trait, providers should obtain a hemoglobin electrophoresis.

Cystic Fibrosis

Cystic fibrosis is an autosomal recessive, chronic illness characterized primarily by pulmonary insufficiency and pancreatic dysfunction. One of every 25 individuals of northern European ancestry is a carrier for CF, resulting in 1 in 2500 affected births in this population. CF results from an abnormality in the CF transmembrane receptor gene. Normally, this gene produces a protein that is crucial to the proper transport of salt and chloride across cell membranes. When this transport is disrupted, the body produces excessive amounts of thick mucus, which leads to breathing problems and lung infections. Diarrhea and poor digestion also occur. Individuals with CF have an increased risk for infertility. Male infertility primarily results from congenital bilateral absence of the vas deferens (CBAVD). Up to 82% of males with isolated CBAVD have been found to have an identifiable CF mutation in one or both chromosomes (de Braekeleer & Ferec, 1996).

Severity of CF varies greatly. Some affected individuals manifest symptoms at birth, others later in childhood, and still others in young adulthood. Carrier screening for CF involves DNA mutation analysis. The detection rate is approximately 90% among individuals of northern European ancestry and 97% among Ashkenazi Jews, but it is lower among individuals of other ethnic backgrounds. This detection rate varies depending on the number of mutations that a laboratory screens. Therefore, even with a negative carrier screen, a chance still exists that the individual is a carrier.

In April 1997, the National Institutes of Health (NIH) convened a consensus conference regarding carrier genetic testing for CF. The panel concluded that the following people should be offered testing:

- Adults with a positive family history of CF
- Partners of individuals with CF
- Couples planning a pregnancy
- Couples during early pregnancy as a screening test for CF in the fetus

The American College of Medical Genetics (ACMG), however, disagrees with the NIH's recommendations to offer CF genetic testing to all couples who are planning a pregnancy or are pregnant. They believe this recommendation to be premature until two requirements are readily available:

- Adequate educational, genetic counseling, and other support systems
- Adequate experience with the sensitivity and specificity of the testing for CF mutations in the ethnic and racial groups being served

The ACMG emphasizes that widespread genetic testing for CF is not simple and should be offered only by a provider who is familiar with the tests and their interpretation (www.faseb.org/genetics/acmg/pol-32.htm, 1997).

Lysosomal Storage Diseases

Couples of Ashkenazi Jewish ancestry are at increased risk for having offspring with autosomal recessive lysosomal storage diseases, such as Tay Sachs disease (TSD), Canavan's disease (CD), Gaucher's disease (GD), and Niemann-Pick disease (NPD). In addition, approximately 1 in 40 individuals of Ashkenazi Jewish ancestry carries an abnormality in either the *BRCA1* or *BRCA2* gene. These mutations are associated with autosomal dominantly inherited breast and ovarian cancers (Tonin et al., 1996). Several laboratories offer carrier testing, often as a panel, for these diseases.

Tay-Sachs Disease

Tay-Sachs disease is a progressive, neurologic disease that begins in infancy. Among Ashkenazi Jews, approximately 1 in every 30 individuals is a carrier for TSD, and the incidence of TSD in this population is 1 in 3600. TSD results from a deficiency of the enzyme hexosaminidase A (Hex A), which is crucial to the normal functioning of the central nervous system (CNS). Deficiencies of Hex A cause fatty substances to accumulate in the nerve cells and other organs. Typically, a baby with TSD develops normally for several months, but a progressive deterioration then begins, causing blindness, deafness, seizures, and paralysis. Children with TSD usually die by age 5 years, but some survive longer. Unfortunately, no treatment is available for TSD. Carrier screening is done through an enzyme assay that measures Hex A activity in the blood; however, this test is not reliable in pregnant women. Hex A in the leukocytes or platelets should be measured in pregnant women. TSD carrier testing also can be done with DNA mutation analysis; however, this technology has limitations. Therefore, the most reliable method for routine TSD carrier testing is Hex A level enzyme analysis, rather than DNA testing (Natowicz & Prence, 1996).

Couples of French Canadian ancestry, specifically from the Bas-St. Laurent and Gaspesie regions of Quebec, appear to be at increased risk for having a child with TSD, owing to a founder effect. Population studies have suggested that individuals of French Canadian ancestry living in southern New England (eg, Connecticut, Rhode Island, Massachusetts) are likely to have migrated from northern Quebec. The carrier frequencies for TSD among such individuals appear to be similar to those of the Ashkenazi Jewish population, suggesting that carrier testing is appropriate in this region (Prence, Jerome, Triggs-Raine, & Natowicz, 1997). Individuals of French Canadian ancestry living in northern New England (eg, Vermont, New Hampshire, Maine) are less likely to be from northern Quebec, and an increased carrier frequency for TSD has not been found in this population. Thus, routine carrier testing is not indicated for this region (Palomaki, Williams, Haddow, & Natowicz, 1995).

Canavan's Disease

Canavan's disease is a progressive, neurologic disease that usually results in death before age 10 years, although some children with CD survive until their teens or early 20s. Three variants of CD exist: congenital, infantile, and juvenile. The infantile form is the most common, with onset beginning at age 3 to 6 months. One in 40 individuals of Ashkenazi Jewish ancestry is a carrier for CD, and the incidence of CD in this population is 1 in 6400.

A deficiency of the enzyme aspartoacylase, which is crucial to normal functioning of the CNS, results in CD. Typically, babies with CD appear normal at birth, but a progressive deterioration begins after several months, resulting in mental retardation and hypotonia, which progresses to spasticity, blindness, seizures, and feeding problems. No effective treatment is available. Carrier testing for CD involves DNA mutation analysis. The detection rate is 98% in Ashkenazi Jews but is lower in individuals of partly Jewish or non-Jewish ancestry (Matalon, 1997).

Gaucher's Disease

Gaucher disease is a condition that occurs in three clinically distinct forms, classified by age of onset, severity, and presence of neurologic involvement. Type I, the most common and mildest form of GD, usually has onset in adulthood and does not have neurologic manifestations. One of 12 Ashkenazi Jews is a carrier for type 1 GD, which translates to a 1 in 576 incidence in this population. Types 2 and 3 are much rarer, have earlier onset, and include neurologic involvement. They occur in all ethnic groups, and incidences are not increased among Jews.

All three types of GD result from deficiency of the enzyme glucocerebrosidase, which is necessary for the breakdown of glucocerebroside. In type 1 GD, glucocerebroside accumulates in the bone marrow, spleen, and liver, causing these organs to enlarge, with subsequent bone and joint pain, anemia, and impaired blood clotting. Type 1 is treatable through enzyme replacement. DNA testing for type 1 detects 95% of carriers in the Jewish population. Providers must remember that type 1 GD can be mild with late onset, and carrier screening may identify affected individuals who are asymptomatic (Grabowski, 1997).

Niemann-Pick Disease

Niemann-Pick disease consists of a group of clinically distinct inherited disorders. Type A, progressive and neurogenerative with onset in infancy, is most common among Ashkenazi Jews, with a carrier frequency of 1 in 90 and an incidence of 1 in 32,400 in this population. Type B has delayed onset, usually is not neuronopathic, and is found in all populations. Types C, D, and E also exist.

All forms of NPD result from deficiency of sphingomyelinase, which is necessary for the metabolism of sphingomyelin. In type A, accumulation of sphingomyelin in the bone marrow, CNS, and other organs leads to organ enlargement, failure to thrive, rapid neurologic deterioration, and death by age 4 years. Patients with type B may survive into adolescence or adulthood, depending on the degree of neurologic involvement. No effective treatment is available for NPD. DNA-based carrier testing in the Ashkenazi Jewish population can identify approximately 95% of carriers of type A (Schuchman & Miranda, 1997).

Hereditary Breast and Ovarian Cancer

Approximately 5% to 10% of all cases of breast and ovarian cancer are inherited, with two genes, *BRCA1* and *BRCA2*, primarily responsible. Three specific mutations in these two genes account for most cases of hereditary breast and ovarian cancer in the Ashkenazi Jewish population. Approximately 1 in 40 individuals of Ashkenazi Jewish heritage carries one of these three mutations. When a personal or family history of breast or ovarian cancer is present, the probability that one of these three mutations also exists increases (Tonin et al., 1996).

While these three mutations account for most hereditary breast and ovarian cancer in the Jewish population, some families that clearly have inherited breast and ovarian cancer by pedigree analysis do not have one of these mutations. These families may have mutations in other parts of *BRCA1* or *BRCA2* or in another gene that has yet to be identified (Schubert et al., 1997). Genetic testing for inherited breast and ovarian cancer should occur only after pretest genetic counseling and informed consent, followed by post-test genetic counseling and psychosocial support (McKinnon et al., 1997).

GENETIC CONDITIONS AND PRIOR PREGNANCY HISTORY

In the following situations, the provider should refer the couple for genetic counseling to discuss recurrence of risks and options for prenatal diagnosis:

- For women who have had complications in previous pregnancies, the provider should consider screening for mutations in the thrombophilia genes. One study (Kupferminc et al., 1999) identified mutations in the factor V gene (factor V Leiden), which encodes methylenetetrahydrofolate reductase, and the prothrombin gene. This study also found deficiencies in proteins S and C, antithrombin III, and anticardiolipin antibodies. Another study showed that carriers of factor V Leiden have a higher risk for fetal loss, particularly miscarriage, than noncarriers (Meinardi et al., 1999).

- For couples who have had a child with a neural tube defect, the woman must increase folic acid supplementation (see later discussion).
- For couples who have had a child with a chromosomal trisomy, the recurrence risk in a subsequent pregnancy is 1% or the woman's age-related risk, whichever is higher.
- For couples who have had a child with one or more congenital anomalies, the recurrence risk depends on the etiology. The couple should consult a clinical geneticist to determine the correct diagnosis.
- For couples who have had multiple recurrent miscarriages, karyotyping of both partners can help rule out a translocation or other chromosome rearrangement, which is the etiology in approximately 5% of cases (Bick, Madden, Heller, & Toofanian, 1998).
- For couples who have had a fetal demise or stillbirth, the provider should review the autopsy (if available) and consult a clinical geneticist for the possible diagnosis.

● **Clinical Pearl:** Kupferminc et al. (1999) found that women with serious obstetric complications (eg, preeclampsia, abruptio placentae, fetal growth retardation, and stillbirth) have an increased incidence of mutations, predisposing them to thrombosis.

GENETIC CONCERNS RELATED TO AGE

Providers should educate women and their partners about age-related risk factors and available tests during the preconception period. Such tests include screening (eg, triple marker screening test and ultrasound) and diagnostic tests (eg, chorionic villus sampling and amniocentesis). Please see the Appendix on Prenatal Screening.

Maternal Age

Providers should offer genetic counseling to women age 35 and older because of the increased risk for chromosomal abnormalities associated with older maternal age. Down syndrome is the most common chromosomal trisomy, but couples should realize that other chromosomal trisomies are associated with increasing maternal age, some of which are more life-threatening than Down syndrome (trisomy 13 and 18) and some less (sex chromosome abnormalities).

● **Clinical Pearl:** Although all women are at risk for having a child with a chromosomal anomaly, women over 35 years routinely are offered prenatal diagnosis for such anomalies. After a woman is 35, her risk for losing a pregnancy from an amniocentesis is less than the risk of identifying a chromosomal abnormality (Hect & Hook, 1996).

Paternal Age

Increased paternal age has been linked with autosomal dominant genetic diseases (eg, neurofibromatosis, achondroplasia, Apert's syndrome, Marfan syndrome) appearing as new mutations in their offspring. Estimates are that the absolute frequency of such diseases resulting from new mutations among offspring of fathers age 40 years or older is between 0.3% and 0.5%. This risk is similar in magnitude to the risk of Down syndrome in offspring of mothers who are 35 years or older. No specific prenatal tests screen for new dominant mutations. Genetic counseling is recommended for couples in whom advanced paternal age is a concern (McIntosh,

Olshan, & Baird, 1995; American College of Obstetricians and Gynecologists, 1997).

MATERNAL HEALTH

Certain medical conditions in women, including diabetes, epilepsy, and phenylketonuria (PKU), may increase the risk for congenital malformations in their offspring. Women with specific genetic conditions, such as CF, Marfan syndrome, myotonic dystrophy, neurofibromatosis, and hereditary hemorrhagic telangiectasia, will likely benefit from preconception genetic counseling.

Infants of mothers with poor glucose control during organogenesis have a twofold to threefold higher risk of birth defects than offspring of nondiabetic mothers. Good glucose control preconceptionally can reduce the risk of birth defects to a level comparable to that of the general population (Janz et al., 1995; Casele & Laifer, 1998; Herman, Janz, Becker, & Charron-Prochownik, 1999).

Women with epilepsy of unknown etiology, even with the factored risk of many anticonvulsant medications, have a twofold increased risk for congenital malformations in their offspring. Specific defects related to maternal epilepsy include cleft lip or palate, congenital heart defects, and neural tube defects.

A less commonly recognized situation is the risks posed by maternal PKU. Over the past decades, successful screening and institution of a low phenylalanine diet in newborns with PKU have resulted in an increased number of women with PKU who are now of childbearing age. In the past, dietary restriction was discontinued when children with PKU reached adolescence. During pregnancy, however, phenylalanine easily crosses the placenta, causing intrauterine growth retardation and subsequently severe mental retardation and microcephaly. Data suggest that normalizing serum phenylalanine levels before conception results in children with normal intelligence and no increased rate of birth defects (Rouse et al., 1997; Kirby, 1999).

FOLIC ACID SUPPLEMENTATION

The benefits of folic acid are many but are primarily associated with a 70% reduction in neural tube birth defects, which occur between the 23rd and 28th days of development. Adequate folic acid levels are best obtained from supplements. Evidence suggests that folic acid supplementation during critical periods of organogenesis is associated with a reduction in both the occurrence and recurrence of neural tube defects, congenital heart defects, obstructive urinary tract anomalies, limb deficiencies, orofacial clefts, and pyloric stenosis (Hall & Solehdin, 1998). Current recommendations from the CDC are for all women of childbearing age (regardless of whether they are currently planning pregnancy) to take 0.4 mg of folic acid daily. If one partner has a neural tube defect or the couple has had an affected child, the female partner should take 4 mg of folic acid daily during the preconception period and throughout the first trimester (Morrow & Kelsey, 1998; Locksmith & Duff, 1998).

● **Clinical Pearl:** All women of childbearing age should take folic acid supplements of 0.4 mg and consume a diet rich in folate daily. Because many pregnancies are unplanned, women should not wait to begin supplementation until they initiate plans for conception.

REFERENCES

American College of Medical Genetics. (1997). Statement on genetic testing for cystic fibrosis. www.faseb.org/genetics/acmg/pol-32.htm.

American College of Obstetricians and Gynecologists (ACOG). (1997). Committee opinion, Advanced paternal age: Risks to the fetus. *International Journal of Gynecology and Obstetrics, 59,* 271–272.

Baird, P. A., Anderson, T. W., Newcombe, H. B., & Lowry, R. B. (1988). Genetic disorders in children and young adults: A population study. *American Journal of Human Genetics, 42*(5), 677–693.

Bick, R. L., Madden, J., Heller, K. B., & Toofanian, A. (1998). Recurrent miscarriage: Causes, evaluation, and treatment. *Medscape Women's Health, 3*(3), 2.

de Braekeleer, M., & Ferec, C. (1996). Mutations in the cystic fibrosis gene in men with congenital bilateral absence of the vas deferens. *Molecular Human Reproduction, 2,* 669–677.

Casele, H. L., & Laifer, S. A. (1998). Factors influencing preconception control of glycemia in diabetic women. *Archives of Internal Medicine, 158*(12), 1321–1324.

Cohn, G. M., Miller, R. C., Gould, M., Macri, C. J., & Gimovsky, M. L. (1999). Impact of genetic counseling on primary and preventive care in Obstetrics and Gynecology. *Journal of Reproductive Medicine, 44,* 7–10.

Dumars, K. W., Boehm, C., Eckman, J. R., Giardina, P. J., Lane, P. A., & Shafer, F. E. (1996). Practical guide to the diagnosis of thalassemia. *American Journal of Medical Genetics, 62,* 29–37.

Emery, A. E. H., & Rimoin, D. L. (eds.) (1990). *Principles and practice of medical genetics* (2nd ed.). New York: Churchill Livingstone.

Grabowski, G. A. (1997). Gaucher disease: Gene frequencies and genotype/phenotype correlations. *Genetic Testing, 1,* 5–12.

Hall, J. G., Powers, E. K., McIlvaine, R. T., & Ean, V. H. (1978). The frequency and financial burden of genetic disease in a pediatric hospital. *American Journal of Medical Genetics, 1*(4), 417–36.

Hall, J., & Soledtidin, F. (1998). Folic acid: It's a good preventative medicine. *Contemporary Pediatrics, 15*(7), 119–135.

Hect, C. A., & Hook, E. B. (1996). Rates of Down syndrome at live-birth by one year maternal age intervals in studies with apparent close to complete ascertainment in populations of European origin: A proposed revised rate schedule for use in genetic and prenatal screening. *American Journal of Medical Genetics, 63,* 376–385.

Herman, W. H., Janz, N. K., Becker, M. P., & Charron-Prochownik, D. (1999). Diabetes and pregnancy. Preconception care, pregnancy outcomes, resource utilization and costs. *Journal of Reproductive Medicine, 44*(1), 33–38.

Hogge, J. S., & Hogge, W. A. (1996). Preconception genetic counseling. *Clinics in Obstetrics and Gynecology, 39,* 751–762.

Janz, N. K., Herman, W. H., Becker, M. P., Charron-Prochownik, D., Shayna, V. L., Lesnick, T. G., Jacober, S. J. (1995). Diabetes and pregnancy: Factors associated with seeking preconception care. *Diabetes Care, 18*(2), 157–165.

Kirby, R. B. (1999). Maternal Phenylketonuria: A new cause for concern. *Journal of Obstetric, Gynecologic and Neonatal Nursing, 28*(3), 227–234.

Kupferminc, M. J., Eldor, A., Steinman, N., Many, A., Bar-Am, A., Jaffa, A., Fait, G. (1999). Increased frequency of genetic thrombophilia in women with complications of pregnancy. *New England Journal of Medicine, 340,* 9–13.

Lemke, A. A., Dayal, S., & Geibel, L. J. (1998). Preconception genetic counseling: Three years of experience at a community-based health center. *Journal of Genetic Counseling, 7,* 71–85.

Leuzzi, R. A., & Scoles, S. (1996). Preconception counseling for the primary care physician. *Medical Clinics of North America, 80,* 337–369.

Locksmith, G. J., & Duff, P. (1998). Preventing neural tube defects: The importance of periconceptional folic acid supplements. *Obstetrics and Gynecology, 91,* 1027–1034.

Matalon, R. (1997). Canavan disease: Diagnosis and molecular analysis. *Genetic Testing, 1,* 21–24.

McIntosh, G. C., Olshan, A. F., & Baird, P. A. (1995). Paternal age and the risk of birth defects in offspring. *Epidemiology, 6*(3), 282–288.

McKinnon, W., Baty, B., Bennett, R., Magee, M., Neufeld-Kaiser, W. A., Peters, K. F., Sawyer, J. C., & Schneider, K. A. (1997). Predisposition genetic testing for late-onset disorders in adults. A position paper of the National Society of Genetic Counselors. *Journal of the American Medical Association, 278,* 1217–1220.

Meinardi, J. R., Middeldorp, S., de Kam, P. J., Koopman, M. M., van Pampus, E. C., Hamulyak, K., Prins, M. H., et al. (1999). Increased risk for fetal loss in carriers of the factor V Leiden mutation. *Annals of Internal Medicine, 130*(9), 736–739.

Moos, M. K., Bangdiwala, S. I., Meibohm, A. R., & Cefalo, R. C. (1996). The impact of a preconceptional health promotion program on intendedness of pregnancy. *American Journal of Perinatology, 13*(2), 103–108.

Morrow, J. D., & Kelsey, K. (1998). Folic acid for prevention of neural tube defects: Pediatric anticipatory guidance. *Journal of Pediatric Health Care, 2,* 55–59.

Natowicz, M. R., & Prence, E. M. (1996). Heterozygote screening for Tay-Sachs disease: Past successes and future challenges. *Current Opinion in Pediatrics, 8,* 625–629.

Olivieri, N. F. (1999). The ?-Thalassemias. *New England Journal of Medicine, 341*(2), 99–109.

Palomaki, G. E., Williams, J., Haddow, J. E., & Natowicz, M. R. (1995). Tay-Sachs disease in persons of French-Canadian heritage in northern New England. *American Journal of Medical Genetics, 56,* 409–412.

Prence, E. M., Jermone, C. A., Triggs-Raine, B. L., & Natowicz, M. R. (1997). Heterozygosity for Tay-Sachs and Sandhoff diseases among Massachusetts residents with French Canadian background. *Journal of Medical Screening, 4,* 133–136.

Roberts, D. F., Chavez, J., & Court, D. M. (1970). The genetic component in child mortality. *Archives of Disease in Children, 45,* 33–38.

Rouse, B., Azen, C., Koch, R., Matalon, R., Hanley, W., de la Cruz, F., Trefz, F., Friedman, E., & Shifrin, H. (1997). Maternal Phenylketonuria Collaborative Study (MPKUCS) offspring: Facial anomalies, malformations, and early neurological sequelae. *American Journal of Medical Genetics, 69*(1), 89–95.

Schubert, E. L., Mefford, H. C., Dann, J. L., Argonza, R. H., Hull, J., & King, M. C. (1997). BRCA1 and BRCA2 mutations in Ashkenazi Jewish families with breast and ovarian cancer. *Genetic Testing, 1*(1), 41–46.

Schuchman, E. H., & Miranda, S. R. P. (1997). Niemann-Pick disease: Mutation update, genotype/phenotype correlations, and prospects for genetic testing. *Genetic Testing, 1,* 13–19.

Swan, L. L., & Apgar, B. S. (1995). Preconceptual obstetric risk assessment and health promotion. *American Family Physician, 51,* 1875–1885.

Tonin, P., Weber, B., Offit, K., Couch, F., Rebbeck, T. R., Neuhausen, S., Godwin, A. K. (1996). Frequency of recurrent BRCA1 and BRCA2 mutations in Ashkenazi Jewish breast cancer families. *Nature Medicine, 2*(11), 1179–1183.

Wallace, M., & Hurwitz, B. (1998). Preconception care: Who needs it, who wants it, and how should it be provided? *British Journal of General Practice, 48*(427), 963–966.

PART 2 ▲

Preconception and Prenatal Counseling

- ELIZABETH DORSEY SMITH, EdD, RN,
  and WILLIAM T. SEED, MD, FAAP

INTRODUCTION

Preconception and prenatal counseling and care can significantly affect the outcome of a pregnancy and the beginning of the newborn's life. Women usually are more amenable to changing their life patterns while they are pregnant (Scheibmeir & O'Connell, 1997), even though they may resume deleterious patterns and habits postpartum. Challenges for primary care providers are to obtain accurate histories, offer anticipatory guidance, and monitor pregnant women carefully, assisting them with momentous choices.

PRECONCEPTION COUNSELING

Preconception counseling is a significant yet all too often neglected component of health care. More than 50% of pregnancies in the United States are unplanned and often unintended; thus, many pregnancies begin without the essential preconception counseling that can optimize both maternal and fetal health. Primary care providers, dedicated to the promotion and maintenance of health, can make a substantial difference by addressing preventive care issues before conception occurs. This chapter is based on the premise that pregnancy is a planned event.

Providers should recognize that preconception services are unavailable in many communities due to social, economic, and medical barriers. Lemke, Dayal, and Geibel (1998) report their successful implementation of a preconception genetic counseling program in a community-based health center in Chicago that primarily serves women from minority and low-income backgrounds. More innovative ways to reach at-risk populations must be created as well (Moos, Bangdiwala, Meibohm, Cefalo, 1996; Wallace & Hurwitz, 1998).

Preconception counseling allows time for individuals and couples to prepare appropriately for a future pregnancy (eg, stop medication, improve health, obtain accurate family history). Counseling women of childbearing age before they become pregnant about genetic, medical, psychological, and environmental risk factors that could affect obstetric outcomes gives individuals more reproductive choices (Swan & Apgar, 1995; Leuzzi & Scoles, 1996).

Issues and Objectives

The issues to address before planning a pregnancy include the following:

- Is the woman (and her partner) in good general health?
- Does the woman (or her partner) wish to become pregnant and become a parent?
- Is the woman and/or her partner able to be responsible for the infant(s)?
- What resources are available in this event?
- What are the specific guidelines regarding the woman's physical and emotional well-being?

The objectives of preconception counseling include the following:

- Assess the woman (couple) for readiness for parenthood (eg, desire to be pregnant, desire to be a parent).
- Evaluate risk factors for genetic disorders.
- Assess the woman's general health status.
- Obtain the woman's history of chronic diseases (eg, diabetes, eating disorders, asthma, hypertension, epilepsy, lupus, substance use or abuse, kidney disease, hepatitis, human immunodeficiency virus [HIV] status, mental illness).
- Determine the woman's use of medications and chemicals (eg, insulin, dilantin, oral contraceptives, antivirals, folic acid, alcohol, cigarettes, cocaine, opiates).
- Discuss chemical or other teratogen exposure in the workplace, home, or environment.
- Obtain a history of abuse (physical, sexual, or verbal).
- Discuss nutrition, diet, and weight issues.
- Screen for disease and immunization status.
- Promote wellness by explaining healthy activities and medications (eg, folic acid supplementation [0.4 mg] 1 month before and for at least the first 12 weeks of pregnancy, Centers for Disease Control and Prevention [CDC], 1992]).

▲ **Clinical Warning:** Physiologic preparation for pregnancy is essential before conception because the first trimester is the vulnerable period when organogenesis occurs.

PRENATAL COUNSELING

Prenatal counseling, extremely important to a pregnancy's outcome, is defined as anticipatory guidance after a pregnancy ensues. A woman is more likely to contact her primary care providers after becoming pregnant than before she conceives. Ideally, the initial prenatal visit should occur during the first trimester (after the woman misses two periods), but it may happen anytime during pregnancy.

Issues and Objectives

One aspect of prenatal counseling involves the decision to maintain a pregnancy. Pregnancy and parenthood are choices that require decision making on the part of a woman and, if he or she is involved, her partner. Providers need to explain the available options, including the following:

- Maintain the pregnancy, become a parent, and raise the child.
- Maintain the pregnancy, and place the infant for adoption.
- Terminate the pregnancy.

The primary care provider needs to take a complete health history of both parents (if available), including present health status, past history (including reproductive history), family history (including genetic history), social history, environmental history, nutritional status, and medication and drug history. The provider first must assess and then convey to the woman or couple the relative risks for the mother, pregnancy, and fetus.

Pregnant women and their partners require anticipatory guidance throughout the pregnancy, which varies according to trimester (Table 5-1). This information is predicated on the notion that pregnant women make regular health care visits. Visits may be more frequent if the woman has a chronic disease or complications of pregnancy. If the magnitude of these problems is extensive, then consultation with or referral to an obstetrician or other specialists is essential. See Table 5-2 for a prenatal visit schedule.

Teratogens

According to Stevenson, "A teratogen can be defined as any agent capable of causing abnormal development in the fetus. Both environmental and chemical agents are included" (1998, p. 333). Teratogens may act directly on the developing fetal structure or indirectly, affecting a maternal structure, such as the placenta. The most commonly identified teratogens are drugs (prescription, over-the-counter, and street), chemicals and other solvents (eg, scavenger gases in operating rooms and radiation), and infectious agents (eg, rubella and cytomegalovirus). TORCH is an acronym that assists providers in identifying some agents for which screening is needed (Table 5-3). The significant issue in relation to any teratogen is the time during gestation at which the insult occurs. "Gestational age at the time of potential teratogen exposure is critical, with the second through the eighth week being the most critical because this is the time when organogenesis occurs" (Stevenson, 1998, p. 333). The fetus also is vulnerable to insults from teratogens throughout the remainder of the pregnancy. For example, after 34 weeks' gestation, sulfonamides may cause hyperbilirubinemia, and ibuprofen has been associated with the closing of the fetal ductus arteriosis (Briggs, Freeman, & Yaffe, 1994). Table 5-4 lists common teratogens and their deleterious fetal effects.

Medications

The Food and Drug Administration (FDA) has classified medications based on their risk to the fetus (Table 5-5). This FDA intends this classification to warn providers and consumers about the possible effects of drugs on fetal development. Most research in this area has been based on results from prospective animal studies and retrospective historical data (eg, the thalidomide tragedy, in which use of thalidomide caused an epidemic of phocomelia [short limbs] in the offspring of women who took the drug). For obvious ethical reasons, prospective human studies on pregnant women are prohibited.

Drugs, Alcohol, and Tobacco

Pregnant women who use or abuse alcohol or drugs pose major management difficulties during pregnancy. Many addicts do not participate in their own health care. Often their addiction, not the pregnancy, is their primary objective. Very few addiction treatment facilities are available for assisting pregnant women.

Cigarettes have deleterious effects on the size of the fetus (Bragg, 1997). Maternal consumption of alcohol, even in small amounts, can cause fetal alcohol syndrome (FAS). A baby with FAS presents with dysmorphic features, eipcanthal folds, broad nasal bridge, hypoplastic maxilla, microcephaly, abnormal palm creases, growth retardation (both intrauterine and after birth), and CNS problems (eg, cognitive difficulties and impulsivity). According to Kenner and D'Apolito (1997), behavioral problems, CNS dysfunction, and safety issues are concerns for children with FAS. Children with FAS are born most frequently to women who have

had a longstanding addiction to alcohol with associated liver and kidney damage; however, some infants are affected when a woman has only had one or two drinks during a pregnancy. Because accurate prediction is not possible, pregnant women need to avoid all alcohol. The federal government requires bars to post a sign warning pregnant women of alcohol's potential harmful effects.

Research has demonstrated that children who are exposed to heroin, other opiates, and cocaine have problems with language and social skills and neurologic development (Kenner & D'Apolito, 1997). Other street drugs affect the neurologic development of the fetus. Infants who are born addicted need to be detoxified at birth. Drug-addicted mothers are, by definition, not considered able to care appropriately for their infants and usually are reported to state child protective services. The status of methadone as a treatment for opiate addiction is coming under a great deal of scrutiny, because the program basically substitutes one drug for another. Methadone detoxification is more difficult than heroin detoxification for the fetus.

Chemicals and Solvents

Chemicals and solvents have been implicated in spontaneous abortions and congenital anomalies. In the past, the workplace was often the culprit in exposure. Women of childbearing age frequently were prohibited from working in specific settings unless their reproductive risk was eliminated (Hewitt & Tellier, 1998). Presently, most workplaces remove or contain the chemical or offending agent (eg, filtering of scavenger gases out of operating rooms).

Chemicals are found in many occupational settings, both urban and rural. Health care providers need to take careful occupational histories of women and assess fetal risks based on the data. They should consider obtaining safety data sheets for specific workplace exposures and consulting a teratogen information service for data on risks of exposure during pregnancy. If a significant risk exists, providers must discuss (preferably in the preconception period) ways to reduce exposure (eg, wear proper safety gear, avoid skin exposure or inhalation) as well as the possibility of a temporary job transfer.

Infectious Agents

Hepatitis B Virus

Hepatitis B virus (HBV) is the most prevalent chronic viral infection in the world (CDC, 1991). The incidence of those carrying hepatitis B surface antigen (HbsAg) is increasing substantially in the United States (Bader, 1997). One reason is because immigration from Asian, African, and Mediterranean countries to North America has increased, and these population groups have a carrier state prevalence rate of 10% to 15%.

Infection with HBV is spread through contaminated objects (eg, needles) or sexual activity that causes blood and other body fluids to cross mucous or percutaneous membranes. Contaminated objects, including condoms and diaphragms, can transmit HBV for 1 week or longer. Perinatal infection is the primary means of transmission of HBV.

According to Corrarino (1998), HBV infection in the mother poses no increased risk of anomalies, low birth weight, or spontaneous abortion in the infant; however, HBsAg carrier status in the pregnant woman is highly associated with perinatal transmission. Without vaccination, 90% of children of HbsAg-positive mothers will become chronic carriers (Kane, 1997). Women who acquire HBV during pregnancy have an increased risk of transmitting HBV to their

TABLE 5–1.   ANTICIPATORY GUIDANCE: FETAL DEVELOPMENT AND MATERNAL CHANGES THROUGHOUT PREGNANCY

Gestational Week	Physiologic Development	Physical Changes
First Trimester 1–2 wk (zygote) 3–5 wk (embryo) 6 wk 7 wk 8 wk 9 wk 10 wk 11 wk 12 wk	• Cells begin to multiply. • Digestive system forms. • Germ layers differentiate. • Trophoblasts appear. • HCG is sealed; HCG secretion increases. • Amnionic fluid develops. • Chorionic villi are developing. • Central nervous system and brain are forming. • Heart starts beating. • Genitourinary system develops • Genitourinary system develops. • Eyes, ears, limbs, respiratory system, muscles, and circulation begin to develop. • Placenta is developing. • Limb buds appear. • Umbilical cord is organizing. • Organogenesis begins. • Hands, feet, and fingers are developing. • Genital organs are forming but are not well differentiated. • Eyelids are developing. • Secretion of HCG decreases. • Placenta secretes estrogen and pregnanediol. • Kidneys develop. • Respiratory movements are visible. • Gender distinction is visible. • Teeth are forming. • Skeleton is ossifying.	*Changes observed by the woman herself:* • Amenorrhea • Enlarging breasts—tender and tingling • Fatigue with altered metabolic state • Urinary frequency • Nausea and vomiting (morning sickness) *Changes observed by the examiner:* • Enlarging breasts • Uterus increasing and beginning to rise out of pelvic cavity • Chadwick's and Goodell's signs positive • Positive pregnancy tests based on secretion of HCG by fourth to fifth week *Metabolic activities* • Shift in H_2O metabolism • Increased sodium and potassium retention • Blood sugar first decreases in fifth to sixth week then gradually rises to end of the trimester • Increased glomerular filtration • Increased nitrogen retention • Increased free fatty acids • Slightly decreased BMR
Second Trimester 13 wk 14 wk 15 wk 16 wk 17 wk 18 wk 19 wk 20 wk 21–24 wk	• Muscles begin to contract slightly (4 in long). • Placental and fetal weights are equal. • External genitalia are easily observable. • Lanugo appears. • Hair develops on head. • Muscles are contracting more actively. • Fetus is 6 in long, and weighs ¼ lb. • Skeleton is observed on x-ray and seen easily on sonography. • Meconium is collecting, and vernix is developing. • Iron is stored; enamel and dentine are deposited. • Fetus undergoes a rapid growth spurt. • Fetal heart can be heard with stethoscope. • Fetus is 10 in long and weighs ¾ lb. • Hair is visible on head and face. • Amniotic fluid continues to collect. • Fetus is 12 in long and weighs 1¼ lb.	• Pigment changes occur (eg, areolas, linea nigra, chloasma). • Uterus becomes an abdominal organ. • Striae gravidarium begins at end of this trimester. • Fetal movement is palpated by both the woman (quickening) and examiner. • Uterine soufflé—equal to maternal pulse rate (blood rushing through uterine artery). • BMR is increasing. • Blood volume and cardiac output increase. • Total plasma-protein decreases related to blood volume increase and physiologic anemia. • Blood pressure decreases. • Nitrogen storage increases. • Free HCL in gastric juices decreases. • This is the period of greatest weight gain.

Emotional Changes	Tests	Interventions
Discovery of pregnancy—response may be • Ambivalence • Joy • Guilt • Shame • Fear • Anger	*B1 Tests* • HCG • CBC differentiation • STDs *Urine* • HCG • U/A *Sonogram* • Picture of fetus and observation of the beating of fetal heart *Fetal EKG* • At 12th week can hear beating of the fetal heart	• Encourage early health care supervision. • Explain physiologic changes to woman and her fetus. • Begin to educate her regarding other changes. • Provide atmosphere to discuss feelings and home situation, especially with respect to planning of pregnancy and support of significant others. • Identify abuse risk for both woman and fetus (eg, chemical abuse, teratogens and domestic violence). • Discuss danger signs with respect to pregnancy. • Give nutritional counseling, including supplements. • Explain "old wives tales" that are inaccurate (eg, knife under bed cuts pain of labor).
• Hormonal shifts cause mood swings. • Woman accepts pregnancy; egocentricity increases. • Changes in sexual desire (some women increase, some women decrease).	• Blood pressure readings monthly • U/A monthly • Hgb—Hct monthly • Sonograms as needed • Amniocentesis as needed • Screening for sickle-cell anemia	*Gastrointestinal (eg, burping, heartburn, constipation)* • Suggest increasing water intake and avoid eating gaseous foods. *Cardiovascular (eg, varicosities; hemorrhoids; prevention of chenemia)* • Elevate legs when possible. • Avoid constipation as possible. • Use witch hazel soaks for comfort. • Take iron supplements as needed. *Genitourinary* • Prepare woman for normal changes, such as increased vaginal secretions, decreased urinary frequency; and Braxton-Hicks contractions. *Skeletal/muscular (eg, backache)* • Pelvic girdle changes due to softening of the cartilaginous tissues between bones; therefore, prepare woman for more give when walking and exercising. • Promote healthy level of exercise. • Discuss importance of posture and supportive positioning. *Respiratory* • Advise that increase in shortness of breath is normal, and she should rest as needed.

(continues)

TABLE 5–1.   ANTICIPATORY GUIDANCE: FETAL DEVELOPMENT AND MATERNAL CHANGES THROUGHOUT PREGNANCY *(Continued)*

Gestational Week	Physiologic Development	Physical Changes
Third Trimester 25–28 wk	• Skin is shiny. • Fetus has "old man" appearance. • Subcutaneous fat is stored. • Testes descend (male). • Fetus is 14 in long and weighs more than 2 lb (viable).	*Changes noted by woman and examiner* • Continued gastrointestinal discomforts • Continued pregnancy "waddle" • Frequency—uterus pressing on the bladder • Colostrum expression from the breasts *Changes noted by examiner on pelvic examination*
29–32 wk	• Large amounts of calcium are stored. • Nitrogen storage increases. • Amniotic fluid decreases.	• May notice cervical dilation *General physiologic* • Cardiac output remains high 28–32 weeks; largest hemodynamic burden
33–36 wk	• Fetus is 16 in long and weighs 3.5 lb. • Iron, nitrogen, and calcium storage accelerate.	• Decreasing plasma protein • BMR increasing
37–40 wk	• Fetus is 18 in long and weighs more than 5 lb. • Lightening occurs 2–4 wk before delivery. • Fetal HgB increases. • Placenta weighs 1–2 lb. • Fetus is 20 in long and weighs between 7–7.5 lb.	• Glomrulofiltration rate increases

fetuses. Risk for transmission is greatest in the third trimester. Without vaccination, all infants of HBV-infected mothers will be infected. The CDC recommends HBV screening for all pregnant women and administration of hepatitis B vaccine to all infants as per the current recommendations of the American Academy of Pediatrics (AAP) (see Chap. 13, Immunizations).

The younger the age at which a child contracts HBV, the greater the child's risk for developing chronic HBV and associated complications. Efforts to diminish or eradicate HBV are necessary to decrease associated morbidity (liver, cancer, and cirrhosis) and mortality (Committee on Infectious Disease, 1997). Women who present at delivery without antepartal care need to be screened for HbsAg. Infants should be vaccinated within 12 hours. If the mother's test comes back positive, the infant needs to receive hepatitis B immune globulin (HbIG) within 18 hours after birth to provide protection for 3 to 6 months. This combined treatment increases the effectiveness of the prevention strategy (CDC, 1991).

Varicella

Varicella, or chickenpox, can have devastating effects on the fetus, with possible multisystem damage (CDC, 1996). Risks to the fetus are greatest if exposure to varicella occurs before 20 weeks' gestation (Katz, Kaller, McMahon, Warren, & Wells, 1995). Cataracts, deafness, and microcephaly may result from the exposure. Providers must screen for history of varicella in every woman of childbearing age; if the history is negative or equivocal, providers should then draw titers. They should offer vaccination to vulnerable nonpregnant women. Immunosuppression is a contraindication for the vaccine. After vaccination, women must avoid pregnancy for 3 months. They also must avoid contact with all pregnant women, regardless of trimeseter (Cottrell & Carter, 1998). If a woman contracts varicella during pregnancy, particularly the first trimester, she requires administration of varicella zoster immune globulin, which lasts about 3 weeks. Acyclovir is the treatment of choice for these women, but its use carries risks.

Emotional Changes	Tests	Interventions
		Promote and explain:
		• Need for rest and emotional stability
		• Need for maternity clothes
		• Nutritional counseling
		• Prevention of infections
		• Avoidance of ill people
		• Immunizations
		• Adequate dental care
		• Safe sex practices
		Discuss signs of danger:
		• Bleeding, pain, fever
		• Excessive and rapid weight gain (seen at end of trimester)
		• Headache and visual problems (seen at end of trimester)
		• Increasing edema (seen at end of trimester)
		• Signs of pending labor (ie, contractions that continue; rupture of membranes)
Emotional	• Visits to doctor closer together—once a week in last month	• Continue with the anticipatory guidance and the education of the third trimester.
• Increase in mood swings	• Blood pressure readings each visit	• Prepare for childbirth—offer education classes and health care.
• Increasing egocentricism	• U/A	• Repeat education regarding danger signals (headache, visual disturbances, excessive edema, elevated blood pressure, hyperflexia).
• Thoughts about self and future baby	• Sonograms as needed	• Educate for preparation for newborn at home.
• Baby of the imagination—naming and relating to fetus; expecting a perfect baby	• Litmus paper test for amniotic fluid	
• Fears of death and pregnancy outcome		

Health care workers need to know their status with respect to varicella and varicella zoster if they are working either with pregnant women or immunosupressed patients. Health care workers who do not have antibodies against varicella zoster need to be vaccinated. After receiving the vaccine, health care workers should avoid vulnerable populations for at least 6 weeks, which may affect their work assignments. They need to caution patients who might have varicella to avoid using the waiting room and exposing others.

Sexually Transmitted Infections

Sexually transmitted infections that can have teratogenic effects include HIV, *Neisseria gonorrhoea*, *Chlamydia trachomatis*, syphilis, and human papillomavirus. These diseases often are identified in pregnant women addicted to drugs (see earlier section). All require treatment to prevent untoward fetal effects. For example, the application of silver nitrate or an antibiotic to a newborn's eyes (usually a state regulation) prevents blindness caused by *N. gonor-*

rhoea, regardless of whether it has been diagnosed in the mother.

Infection with HIV is an especially significant concern. According to the CDC (1994) and the World AIDS Conference (1998), HIV-positive women have a 25% risk of transmitting HIV to their babies through vertical transmission. Use of treatments such as zidovudine (AZT) and cesarean section can lower the risk to less than 2%. AZT or other drugs alone will lower the risk to approximately 8%. Unfortunately, breast-feeding remains a significant mode of mother-to-infant transmission (United Nations AIDS statement, 1998). According to Fowler, Bertolli, and Nieburg (1999), the method of feeding is a real dilemma for poor women, especially African Americans in the United States. In 1998, perinatal transmission accounted for 91% of cases of acquired immunodeficiency syndrome (AIDS) in children younger than 13 years (CDC HIV/AIDS Report, 1998).

African American and Hispanic children are disproportionately represented in the HIV-positive population, as are African American and Hispanic adults. For women, hetero-

Table 5–2 PRENATAL VISIT SCHEDULE

Visit Scheduled	Assessed Each Visit
• Every month through 32nd week	• Weight gain, urine for protein & glucose, vital signs, especially BP and palpate abdomen
	• Pelvic examinations on initial visit and during last month
• Every 2 weeks through 36th week	
• Every 1 week until delivery	
More visits if pregnancy warrants	

Adapted from author teaching materials

sexual sex is responsible for 75% of cases of AIDS. Cases of HIV are increasing for young women between 15 and 24 years.

Because of the advances in treatment and prevention of transmission, screening for and treating pregnant women with HIV early in a pregnancy are essential. Treating affected newborns is just as vital. Most states now have laws that will permit the immediate treatment of newborns.

Chronic Diseases and Conditions

Chronic diseases can affect pregnancy in many ways. Some of the most common diseases and conditions that affect pregnancy are diabetes mellitus, cardiac disease, hypertension, epilepsy, systemic lupus erythematosus (SLE), and kidney disease.

Diabetes Mellitus

Because it increases the body's metabolic rate, pregnancy significantly alters insulin needs, which require very close monitoring and stabilization. Some women develop gestational diabetes and need careful monitoring. Some patients with gestational diabetes do not develop full-blown diabetes after the pregnancy is over. Women with type I diabetes often have difficulties becoming pregnant. After pregnancy occurs, the fetus of a diabetic woman is often large but immature in the third trimester. Careful monitoring of both maternal and fetal status is necessary to determine appropriate delivery time. Women with diabetes need to be referred to both an endocrinologist and a perinatologist for a consultation and, if possible, endocrine comanagement throughout pregnancy.

Cardiac Disease

The major effects of cardiac disease are seen primarily during the second trimester (when the hemodynamic burden is highest) and at delivery. The pregnant woman with cardiac disease needs a referral to a cardiologist and a perinatologist. Depending on the severity of the disease, the primary care provider may continue to care for the woman in conjunction with other specialists. Labor is another potential crisis for this woman because of the increased exertion. Careful monitoring is necessary.

Hypertension

Chronic Hypertension

A woman with chronic hypertension is at risk for coexisting problems during pregnancy. Chronic hypertension and many of its sequelae are evident before the 24th week of pregnancy. Edema, blood pressure above 140/90 mmHg, and other symptoms (eg, blurry vision, headache) are all signs that require careful monitoring and control for both maternal and fetal well-being. Medications for hypertension, such as diuretics or β-adrenergic blocking agents, may be prescribed during pregnancy. It is important that blood pressure be controlled, even given the risks related to medication. In addition, recent investigation of hypertension-complicated pregnancies has revealed that maternal blood vessels in the placentas are not able to adjust to fetal needs (Scalafia, 1999). Often, these mothers are at risk for long-term cardiovascular disease. Unfortunately, chronic hypertension can precipitate a pregnancy-induced hypertension (PIH; preeclamptic) incident for the pregnant woman.

Pregnancy-Induced Hypertension

Pregnancy-induced hypertension occurs after the 24th week of pregnancy, with blood pressure elevated to 140/90 mmHg or higher. Edema, significant weight gain, hyperflexia, and proteinuria are all signs of preeclampsia. Headaches, blurry vision, and jitteriness are accompanying symptoms, which can indicate the need for bed rest. Medication (eg, diuretics) to lower the blood pressure is essential at this juncture. Also, if necessary, medication (eg, magnesium sulfate) may be given to combat the hyperflexia and prevent convulsions. The onset of seizures means that the woman has become eclamptic. Both preeclampsia and eclampsia can deleteriously affect the woman and the health status of the fetus. Delivery of the fetus usually reverses the course of PIH. Preeclampsia and eclampsia also can occur up to 6 weeks postpartum.

TABLE 5–3. AGENTS THAT MUST BE SCREENED IN PREGNANCY

	Agent	Effect	Source
T O	Toxoplasmosis	Blindness, growth retardation, central nervous system calcification, jaundice	Undercooked meat
R	Rubella	Cataracts, congenital heart disease, deafness, mental retardation	Respiratory transmission
C	Cytomegalovirus (CMV)	Microcephaly, erythroblastosis, thrombocytopenia, chorioretinitis, deafness, mental retardation	Sexually transmitted
H	Herpesvirus	Disseminated neonatal infection	Sexually transmitted
S	Syphilis	Underdeveloped; bullous rash on palms and soles, nasal sniffles, abnormality of faces (bridge of nose and eyes), mental retardation	Sexually transmitted

Adapted from author teaching materials

TABLE 5–4. KNOWN TERATOGENS THAT CAUSE HUMAN MALFORMATIONS

Teratogen	Classification	Effects on Embryo/Fetus
Drugs		
Testosterone	Male hormone	May cause virilization of female fetus, ambiguous genetalia with hypertrophy of clitoris and fusion of labia
Estrogens dielhyistibestrol (DES), stilbestrol	Female hormone	Cause a variety of genital malformations in females and changes in males. Genital cancer may occur in female offspring of mothers who took DES during pregnancy.
Cyclophosphamide (Cytoxan)	Antineoplast and immunosuppressant (folic acid antagonist)	Blocks synthesis of DNA, RNA, and protein. During pregnancy it is used only when potential benefits to fetus because it causes many major congenital deformities.
Busulfan (Myleran)	Antineoplast (tumor-inhibiting)	May cause skeletal deformities, corneal opacities, cleft palate, organs, and stunted growth
Methotrexate (Amethopterin, (Mexate)		Multiple skeletal deformities of face, skull, limbs, and vertebral column
Aminopterin	Antineoplast	May result in death of conceptus during embryonic period. Multiple skeletal and other congenital malformations occur if fetus survives
Phenytoin (Dilantin)	Anticonvulsant	Causes fetal hydantoin syndrome: IUGR, mental retardation, microcephaly, inner epicanthic folds, ptosis of the eyelids, depressed nasal bridge, phalangeal hypoplasia
Warfarin (Coumadin)	Anticoagulant	Nasal hypoplasia, mental retardation, microcephaly, optic atrophy, chrondroplasia punctata
Lithium carbonate (Cibalith, Eskalith, Lithane, Lithobid)	Psychotropic drugs (used to control manic episodes of manic depressive psychosis)	May cause a variety of malformations, particularly involving heart and great vessels
Thalidomide	Antiemetic in early pregnancy (no longer available)	Absence of one or more limbs, meromelia and other limb deformities; and malformations of the heart, gastrointestinal system, and external ear
Alcohol	Drug	Fetal alcohol syndrome: IUGR, mental retardation, microcephaly ocular anomalies, joint abnormalities, short palpebral fissures
Isotretinoin (Accutane)	Antiacne agent	Causes a wide range of abnormalities (CNS, CV, craniofacial defects, thymus gland abnormalities and microcephaly, hydrocephaly) and blindness
Ribavirin (Virazole)	Antiviral	Malformation of skull, palate, eye, jaw, and GI tract
Tetracycline	Antibiotic (anti-infective)	Hypoplastic tooth enamel, bone and tooth anomalies
Maternal Disease		
Herpesvirus	Infection	Microcephaly, microphthalmia, retinal dysplasia, mental retardation
Rubella virus (German measles)	Infection	Cataracts, cardiac malformations, deafness, glaucoma, chorioretinitis
Cytomegalovirus	Infections	Abortion during embryonic period, IUGR, microphthalmia, chorioretinitis, blindness, microcephaly, mental retardation, deafness, cerebral palsy, cerebral calcifications, hepatosplenomegaly (enlargement of liver and spleen)
Toxoplasma gondii (contracted by eating raw or poorly cooked meat; infects cats; causes toxoplasmosis)	Protozoan infections (intracellular parasite)	Oocyst of contaminated cat crosses human placent, causing microcephaly, microphthalmia, hydrocephaly
Treponema pallidum (causes syphilis)	Spirochete infection	Hydrocephaly, deafness, mental retardation, Hutchinson's teeth, saddle nose, poorly developed maxilla
Syphilis	Infection	Deformed nails; osteochondritis at joints of extremities; abnormal epiphyses
Varicella zoster (chickenpox)	Infection	Skin and muscle defects; limb abnormalities; eye anomalies
Diabetes mellitus	Carbohydrate intolerance	CNS and cardiac defects
Phenylketonuria	Inforn error in metabolism	Microcephaly; mental retardation
Chemical Agents		
Lead	Heavy metal	CNS anomalies; mental retardation
Methyl mercury	Metal compound	CNS anomalies; microcephaly blindness
Radiation		
High-level radiation therapy, radioiodine, atomic weapons	Radiation	Microcephaly, mental retardation, skeletal deformities

Source: May, K. A. & Mahlmeister, L. (1994). *Maternal and neonatal nursing: Family-centered care* (3rd ed.). Philadelphia: Lippincott. Reprinted with permission.

TABLE 5–5.   1979 FOOD AND DRUG ADMINISTRATION (FDA) CLASSIFICATION OF MEDICATIONS INTO ONE OF FIVE CATEGORIES WITH REGARD TO POSSIBLE FETAL RISK

Teratogen: Any agent capable of causing abnormal development in the fetus—both environmental and chemical agents can be teratogenic

Category A	Category B	Category C	Category D	Category X
Drugs for which controlled human studies have not demonstrated fetal risk when taken during any trimester. There are very few category A drugs.	Drugs for which animal studies have not demonstrated a fetal risk but for which there have not been controlled studies in pregnant women.	Drugs for which studies in animals have produced adverse fetal effects, but for which there are no controlled studies in humans. Drugs in this category should be used only if the benefit outweighs the potential risk. Many drugs taken during pregnancy are in this category.	Drugs for which there is evidence of fetal risk, but for which maternal benefits of use outweigh potential fetal risk.	Drugs for which the risk to the fetus clearly outweighs any potential maternal benefit. Drugs in this category are contraindicated in women who are or may become pregnant.
Example: multivitamin supplements	*Example:* penicillin	*Example:* acyclovir	*Example:* phenytoin	*Example:* isotretinoin

From: Food and Drug Administration

HELLP Syndrome

HELLP syndrome is a complication of PIH, featuring the combination of hemolysis (H), elevated concentration of liver enzymes (EL), and low platelet counts (LP). Patients with HELLP have a fulminating disease and may be eclamptic. Referral to a perinatologist (high-risk) obstetrician is warranted. Morbidity and maternal and fetal mortality are very much at risk if fulminating PIH is not treated appropriately.

Epilepsy

Epilepsy is another chronic disease that may affect a woman's ability to become pregnant. Because pregnancy alters the body's metabolism, it also alters levels of antiepileptic medications. Serum levels of the drugs will decline even as the maintenance dose remains stable. To increase serum levels to therapeutic levels, the provider must increase the dose and monitor the woman regularly as the pregnancy progresses. The goal is for the woman to remain seizure free. Seizures themselves have not been associated with birth defects, but decreased oxygen levels can cause problems during the last month of pregnancy and during labor.

Affected women should take antiepileptic drugs throughout pregnancy and should not discontinue them abruptly. Taking more than one drug poses a greater risk of deleterious effects to the fetus. A woman with epilepsy has a 4% to 6% risk of having an infant with anomalies; however, 90% of women with epilepsy have normal infants (Women's Epilepsy Institute, Epilepsy Foundation, 1998). The anomalies that do occur could possibly be related to the antiepileptic medications, the type of disease, or the gene related to epilepsy.

Rest is essential for the pregnant woman with epilepsy. Providers should refer these women to a neurologist and perinatologist and can work with these specialists in providing care. Careful monitoring and consultation with a collaborating neurologist and perinatologist are essential.

Systemic Lupus Erythematosus

Systemic lupus erythematosus (SLE) affects the connective tissue of the body and therefore affects the major organ systems. Often, women with SLE have difficulty becoming pregnant, and those who do may have difficulty maintaining the pregnancy. Because this disease is autoimmune, the body's reaction to pregnancy may be less than hospitable. Multisystem failure is a threat. Early diagnosis and referral to a medical specialist are essential. Potential fetal effects are cardiac arrythmias and thrombocytopenia.

Kidney Disease

Kidney failure or being a kidney transplant survivor does not preclude pregnancy or carrying it to successful completion. Careful monitoring and referral to appropriate medical specialists are required. Women taking medications for rejection need careful follow-up. It is more important for the pregnant woman to remain on the medication and, if on dialysis, continue with the regimen than to terminate therapy because of the pregnancy.

Selection of an Infant Care Provider

Choosing an infant care provider is a major decision for the family and will most certainly affect the development of the family and infant. In the United States, health care availability is high, but the need for preventive care for infants has not been significantly emphasized. The average number of well-child visits during the first year of life is eight, but for adults who do not participate regularly in their own health care, the risk for providing suboptimal infant care increases. Providers may need to develop outreach programs to increase health care to infants who they believe may fall into this risk category.

As a pregnancy progresses, the woman needs to become familiar with resources available for infant care. Visiting a pediatric provider encourages the pregnant woman and her partner to discuss their concerns and to become acquainted with the practice. When options are available, the woman or couple can make informed choices. Clinical issues to discuss include the following:

- The philosophy of the practice and the provider's vision of parenting

- The provider's views on feeding (breast versus bottle) and the support available to parents
- The provider's views on circumcision
- Care in hospital and throughout the first year, including discharge and first follow-up visit
- Philosophy and practices with respect to childhood vaccinations
- Practices with respect to quick child care, including availability, phone access, and sick visits
- Philosophy with respect to the use of antibiotics and other medications
- Testing for vision and hearing
- Discussion of parental expectations of provider and provider's expectations of parents
- Discussion of the pregnancy
  - Was the pregnancy planned?
  - What is the obstetric history?
  - Were there any complications?
- Supports available to the woman/couple
- Concerns of the woman/couple

Business issues to discuss include the following:

- Finances, insurance for both well-child and ill-child visits
- Practical information about the practice with respect to access, hours, telephone availability, and who will see the infant regularly (group versus individual practices and how to maintain continuity of care)
- After-hours coverage
- Admitting privileges and practices with respect to hospitalization
- How the child will be supported—personal finances of the parents or public assistance. Many states are requiring public assistance families to be in a health maintenance program.

COMMON CONCERNS AND ISSUES IN PRECONCEPTION AND PRENATAL CARE

Ethical Issues

When caring for and counseling pregnant women, health care providers need to confront their beliefs and value systems. Not all pregnant women want to become parents; some want to place their infant for adoption. Not all pregnant women want to maintain a pregnancy; some opt for an abortion. Abortion is a central political issue in North America. Technology has made pregnancy possible for many people who otherwise would not experience it. In vitro fertilization, egg and sperm donors, and surrogate motherhood are examples of the technological revolution. Each of these situations raises issues with which segments of the population have ethical concerns. Health care providers need to know where their values lie and what relationships they are willing to develop with pregnant women. Genetics also presents many issues about which providers need to be knowledgeable and comfortable.

Teenage Pregnancies

Teenage pregnancy is a significant public health problem. According to the United States Department of Health and Human Services, between 1991 and 1996, the rate of teenage pregnancy showed a decline for all ethnic groups. A 21% drop for African Americans decreased the rate to the lowest level ever reported for this group. In 1995, the teenage pregnancy rate fell in all 50 states and Washington, DC. The national campaign to Prevent Teenage Pregnancy reported 54.7 births per 1000 to adolescents during 1996.

The problems arising from teenage pregnancy are multiple. Teenagers are less likely than older women to receive timely prenatal care. They are more likely to smoke and more likely to give birth to low birth weight infants (Lifelines, 1998). Because of these issues, infants of teenage mothers often have difficulties. Poverty is a frequent concomitant issue in the mother–baby dyad, bringing with it a multitude of health and psychological problems for the infant's development and the teenager's continued development. According to Koniak-Griffin, Matherage, Anderson, & Verzemnieks (1999), early intervention programs can lower premature birth rates.

Physical Abuse

Violence against women and pregnant women in particular is a situation for which primary providers need to screen. It is critically important to examine the pregnant woman's torso and limbs at each visit. Provision for private interaction between the pregnant woman and the clinician is necessary. A woman in an abusive situation must be provided privacy from both her children and her partner (McFarland & Gondoff, 1998) so that a plan can be developed for her safety and that of her children. Some states may require reporting, much like child abuse, but many do not; it then becomes the woman's decision to report the abuser and seek orders of protection. If children are involved, then a report can be made, but this may leave the woman's safety at risk.

If the woman's provider is male, the need for chaperoned pelvic examinations is essential. In the interview setting, if the provider is male, a female's presence protects both the pregnant woman and the provider. Even if no abuse occurs, a woman may report an abusive interaction. The presence of two providers, male and female, may be cumbersome and not cost-effective but may need to be considered.

COMMUNITY RESOURCES

American Academy of Pediatrics
PO Box 927
141 North Point Boulevard
Elk Grove Village, IL 60009-0927

American Society of Human Genetics (ASHG)
9650 Rockville Pike
Bethesda, MD 20814-3998
Telephone: (301) 571-1825
Fax: (301) 530-7079
http://www.faseb.org/genetics

Centers for Disease Control and Prevention
1600 Clifton Road NE
Atlanta, GA 30333
(800) 311-3435

Epilepsy Foundation
4351 Garden Center Drive
Landover, MD 20785
(800) 332-1000

GeneTests

GeneTests is a directory of laboratories providing testing for genetic disorders. Laboratories are listed by disease name. Both research and diagnostic laboratories are included.

GeneTests is restricted to health care professionals, who must register with GeneTests to receive a password.

http://www.genetests.org

Juvenile Diabetes Foundation
381 Park Avenue South
New York, NY 10016
(800) 533-8590

March of Dimes
Birth Defects Foundation
1275 Mamaroneck Avenue
White Plains, NY
(914) 997-4460

National Coalition for Health Professional Education in Genetics (NCHPEG)
http://www.nchpeg.org
National Society of Genetic Counselors (NSGC)
233 Canterbury Drive
Wallingford, PA 19086-6617
Telephone: (610) 872-7608
Fax: (610) 872-1192
E-mail: NSGC@aol.com
http://members.aol.com/nsgcweb/nsgchome.htm

Online Mendelian Inheritance in Man (OMIM)
http://www3ncbi.nlm.nih.gov/omim/

This database is a catalog of human genes and genetic disorders authored and edited by Dr. Victor A. McKusick and his colleagues at Johns Hopkins and elsewhere. It was developed for the World Wide Web by the National Center for Biotechnology Information (NCBI). The database contains textual information, pictures, and reference information. It also contains copious links to NCBI's Entrez database of MEDLINE articles and sequence information.

Organization of Teratology Information Services (OTIS)
PO Box 144270
Salt Lake City, UT 84114-4270
Telephone: (801) 328-2229)
Fax: (801) 538-6510
http://orpheus.ucsd.edu/otis/index.html

Planned Parenthood Foundation
810 Seventh Avenue
New York, NY 100
(212) 261-4300

The Population Council
1 Dag Hammarshjold Plaza
New York, NY 100
(212) 339-0500

Reproductive Toxicology Center (Reprotox)
Columbia Hospital for Women Medical Center
2440 M Street, NW, Suite 217
Washington, DC 20037-1404
Telephone: (202) 293-5137
Fax: (202) 778-6199
http://reprotox.org/

REFERENCES/BIBLIOGRAPHY

Bader, T. (1997). *Viral hepatitis.* Seattle, WA: Hogrefe & Huber.
Bragg, E. (1997). Pregnant adolescents with addictions. *Journal of Obstetric, Gynecologic, and Neonatal Nursing, 26*(5), 577–584.

Briggs, G., Freeman, R., & Yaffe, S. (1994). *Drugs with pregnancy and addiction.* Philadelphia: Williams & Wilkins.
Centers for Disease Control. (1991). Hepatitis B virus: A comprehensive strategy for eliminating transmission in the United States through universal childhood vaccination. *Morbidity and Mortality Weekly Report, 40,* 171.
Centers for Disease Control. (1992). Recommendations for the use of folic acid to reduce the number of cases of spina-bifida and other neural tube defects. *Morbidity and Mortality Weekly Report, 41,* 1.
Centers for Disease Control. (1994). AIDS statistics and pregnant women. *Morbidity and Mortality Weekly Report, 43,* 20.
Centers for Disease Control. (1996) Prevention of varicellar: Recommendations of the advisory committee on immunizations (ACIP). *Morbidity and Mortality Weekly Report, 45,* 26–27.
Centers for Disease Control. (1998). Young people at risk-epidemic shifts further toward young women and minorities. *Fact sheet.* July.
Committee on Infectious Disease. (1997). *The 1997 red book report of the Committee on Infectious Disease* (24th ed.). Evanston, IL: American Academy of Pediatrics.
Corrarino, J. (1998) Perinatal hepititis B: Updates and recommendations. *Maternal Child Nursing, 23*(5), 246–251.
Cottrell, B., & Caiter, C. (1998) Chicken pox and child bearing. *AWHONN: Lifelines, 2*(4) 33–38.
Fowler, M. G., Bertolli, J., & Nieburg, P. (1999). When is breastfeeding not best? The dilemma facing HIV-infected women in resource-poor settings. *Journal of the American Medical Association, 282*(8), 781–783.
Hall, J., & Solehdin, F. (1998). Folic acid for the prevention of congenital anomalies. *European Journal of Pediatrics, 157,* 445–450.
Hewitt, J., & Tellier, L. (1998). Risk of adverse outcomes in pregnant women exposed to solvents. *Journal of Obstetric, Gynecologic and Neonatal Nursing, 27*(5), 521–531.
Kane, M. (1997) Hepatitis viruses and the neonate. *Clinics in Perinatology, 24,* 181–191.
Katz, V., Kaller, J., McMahon, N., Warren, M., & Wells, S. (1995). Varicella during pregnancy: Maternal and fetal effects. *Western Journal of Medicine, 163,* 446–450.
Kenner, C., & D'Apolito, K. (1997). Pregnant adolescent with addictions. *Journal of Obstetric, Gynecologic and Neonatal Nursing, 26*(5), 597–599.
Koniak-Griffin, D., Matherage, N., Anderson, E., & Verzemnieks, I. (1999). An early intervention program for adolescent mothers: A nursing demonstration project. *Journal of Obstetric, Gynecologic and Neonatal Nursing, 1,*
McFarland, J., & Gondoff, E. (1998). Preventing abuse during pregnancy: A clinical protocol. Recommendations. *Maternal Child Nursing, 23,* 22–26.
National Institute of Health. (1998). Presentation at World AIDS Conference.
Rowland, R., Kenner, C., Greene, D., & Pohorecki, S. (1998). The lived experience of women who undergo prenatal diagnostic testing due to elevated maternal serum alpha-fetoprotein screening. *Maternal Child Nursing, 23*(4), 180–186.
Scalafia, C. (1999). Perinatal pathology at The New York-Presbyterian Hospital evaluates compromised pregnancies. *Network newsline,* February 6.
Scheibmeir, M., & O'Connell, K. (1997). In harm's way: Childbearing women and nicotine. *Journal of Obstetric, Gynecologic, and Neonatal Nursing, 26*(4), 477–484.
Serafine, M., & Broom, B. (1998). Predicting low-risk pregnant women's attendance at a preterm birth prevention class. *Journal of Obstetric, Gynecologic and Neonatal Nursing, 27*(3), 279–287.
Standing Committee on the Scientific Evaluation of Dietary Reference Intakes. (1998). *Institute of Medicine Dietary reference intakes for Thiamin, Riboflavin, Niacin, Vitamin B6, Folate, Vitamin B12, Pantothentic need, Biotin, and Choline.* Washington, DC: National Academy Press.
Stevenson, A. (1998). Teratogens. *Maternal Child Nursing, 23*(6), 333.
United Nations AIDS statement (1998).
Women's Epilepsy Institute, Epilepsy Foundation. (1998). *Epilepsy and pregnancy,* 1-25. Landover, MD: Epilepsy Foundation.

C H A P T E R 6

Adoption

• JOHANNA TRIEGEL, MD

INTRODUCTION

Adoption has been a way to create families for thousands of years, despite the common belief that adopting children is less desirable than bearing and raising biologic offspring. Adoption in fact may be the only way to create a family for parents unable to have children. Adoption also provides families for children who, because of birth parent relinquishment, poverty, or abandonment, might otherwise grow up in foster care, orphanages, or even on the street. Adoption can, and usually does, work well for everyone involved. Both adoptive parents and birth parents can derive profound satisfaction from knowing that their child has grown up to become a happy, productive adult.

The emphasis in this chapter is on supporting the child and his or her adoptive parents. For convenience only, parents are referred to in the plural, though many adoptive parents are single. The aim of this chapter is to review common problems adoptive families face so that the primary care provider will be able to help such families succeed.

TODAY'S ADOPTIVE FAMILY

Adoption traditionally has been thought of as a way for an infertile couple to have and raise a child. This perception, however, excludes a large number of families with adopted children. The reality of adoption today is that:

- Many children are adopted by relatives, foster parents, and nontraditional families, such as single, gay, or lesbian parents.
- Biologic children may already be present in the family.
- The adopted child usually is not a newborn and may have come from abroad.

Who Is Adopted?

Between 110,000 and 120,000 children are adopted every year in the United States (National Committee for Adoption, 1989). Of these, about half are adopted by relatives (including stepparents) and half by nonrelatives. In the United States, about 1.5 million families (or 2.2% of all U.S. families) have at least one adopted child (Adoption in the U.S., 1996). These data are only approximations, however, because states are not required to report their statistics to any federal agency.

Adoptees Born in the United States

Approximately 50% of adopted infants born in the United States are adopted without agency assistance. Most of these are open adoptions to some degree, with varying degrees of contact maintained among the birth parent(s), adopted child, and adoptive parents. Fewer than 50% of domestic adoptions are infants; the rest are older children and children with so-called special needs (Stolley, 1993). Children with special needs make up about 25% of domestic adoptions. These children may have disabilities, serious medical conditions, or psychological problems. They also may be older (over age 5), part of a sibling group, or members of a minority group (National Committee for Adoption, 1989).

At any one time, approximately 500,000 children are in foster care in the United States. Many more children are available for adoption than actually are placed. Children in foster care generally are more difficult to place than infants. Reasons for this include older age, race, the presence of sibling groups, a history of maternal substance abuse and neglect, or a history of long placement in foster or multiple homes. The average length of stay in foster care before adoption is 4 to 5 years. Approximately 90% of children adopted from foster care are adopted by their foster parents, a few of whom are biologic relatives. Thus, these children may have had long relationships with their adoptive families (Adoption Medical News, 1996).

Adoptees Born in Other Countries

About 15,000 children are adopted from other countries each year. Most are infants, with very few of them younger than 4 to 6 months old. Despite constant challenges due to changing economic and political factors and abrupt closings and openings of adoption programs, the number of international adoptions has risen every year and probably will continue to increase. At the same time, the countries of origin for most of these children have changed almost completely. In 1989, the most common country of origin was Korea, followed distantly by Colombia, India, the Philippines, and Chile. In 1998, the two most common countries of origin were Russia and China, followed by Korea and more distantly by Guatemala and Romania (Personal Communication, Immigration and Naturalization Service and U.S. Department of Justice, 1999). In general, children now are most likely to come from Eastern Europe and the former Soviet Union, East Asia, and Central and South America, with smaller numbers from Southeast Asia, India, and Africa. This mix probably will continue to change. On the whole, children adopted from abroad are more likely to come from very poor developing countries than they were a decade ago. They often have experienced prolonged institutional care, with limited access to good nutrition and medical care.

Russia and Eastern Europe

The number of children adopted from Russia and Eastern Europe was small until 1992, but increased steadily over the next several years. This region has now become the most popular area for adoption. These children are more likely to be older infants or toddlers. Virtually all have been in institutions for some time (often for long periods) before placement. These youngsters may be part of sibling groups. One of the most challenging aspects of adopting children from Russia and Eastern Europe is the frequency of abandonment and maternal alcohol abuse. In one study of children adopted from Eastern European orphanages, maternal alcoholism was listed in 17% of referral documents, while fetal alcohol syndrome (FAS) was found in 2.4% of referrals (Johnson et al., 1996).

China

The number of children adopted from China was small until 1993 to 1994. Since then, adoptions have increased rapidly, largely because of abandonment resulting from China's one-child policy, rather than social or medical issues. Almost all Chinese children available for adoption are girls. Their health usually is quite good, largely because of early placement with adoptive families. Since reorganization of the Chinese adoption system in 1997, however, children have been slightly older on arrival and may have more problems related to longer periods in large orphanages. These problems may include developmental delay (generally transient, with resolution seen sometime after placement) and attachment disorders due to institutionalization. Parents must be older than 30. They may be single (although single men must be over 40). Older parents must be willing to accept older infants and toddlers.

Korea

Adopted children have come from Korea for many years and generally have been healthy. The number of children available from Korea, while higher prior to the early 1990s, has remained in the range of 1600 to 1800 per year (U.S. Immigrations and Naturalization Service). Korea has a high standard of living and excellent medical care, and the children often have quite complete accompanying medical records. Children are cared for in foster homes or orphanages and may be normal developmentally except for some gross motor delay from being carried on the backs of caretakers. This "piggybacking" is a cultural norm for Korean child raising.

Who Adopts?

Because restrictions on parental eligibility have relaxed over the last 20 to 30 years, the range of people seeking to adopt has broadened considerably. Today's adoptive parents include the following:

- Married couples with primary or secondary infertility
- Relatives of the adopted child
- Foster parents, who may have other foster or biologic children
- Single women or men
- Gay or lesbian couples
- Older parents
- Parents with disabilities
- People who choose adoption over biologic parenting

Although generalizing about such a diverse group is difficult, it usually is true that adoptive parents are older than biologic parents and are of higher socioeconomic status.

PREPARING POTENTIAL PARENTS FOR ADOPTION

The provider often is the first person that a family approaches with questions about adoption. The provider has a wonderful opportunity to offer support and insight during a long and complicated process that can be emotionally and finan-

cially draining. There are many things to discuss with parents, including readiness for adoption and lifestyle issues. Readiness for adoption includes issues related to motivation, infertility, acceptance of children with special needs or from different ethnic and racial backgrounds, and gender preferences. Lifestyle issues involve health, finances, emotional stability, work, family obligations, and health care.

Readiness for Adoption

Ideally, parents are exploring adoption because they want above all to love and parent a child. They do not view adoption as inferior to biologic parenting. They think of the adopted child as the child they have always wanted. They accept that the child most likely will not look like them and may have an entirely different temperament.

Acceptance of Infertility

If the parents are considering adoption because of infertility, acceptance of their infertility and the loss of a biologic relationship with their child is essential. Usually this means that they have stopped fertility treatments. Some adoption agencies require that parents have not just stopped treatment, but also are using birth control.

Considering Children With Special Needs

Some parents express an interest in adopting a child with a medical problem or fall into a group likely to be offered a child with special needs (eg, older parental age or single marital status). Such individuals must consider carefully the lifelong implications of such a placement and their ability to meet that child's needs. Parents should evaluate honestly their feelings and abilities, recognizing that adoption involves a great deal of uncertainty and that problems may be either better or worse than described in referral documents. The clinician should be as objective and supportive as possible and prepared to describe the range of problems that parents may encounter.

Parents who want a healthy child should never feel pressured to adopt a child who has a problem that they cannot handle. Having the parents review a special needs checklist (Display 6-1) may be an extremely useful starting point for discussion about children with special needs. This checklist also can assist the provider in gauging the parents' understanding of the risks of adoption.

● **Clinical Pearl:** The clinician can assist the family by avoiding extremes when describing problems and their ranges. Connecting descriptions to local sources for referral and support also can help the parents make informed decisions.

Ethnic, Racial, and Gender Issues

Most children from abroad are of a different racial or ethnic background than parents who are adopting. Parents need to consider carefully such differences. If parents are planning an interracial or international adoption, unresolved feelings about infertility may come painfully to the foreground after the adoption is complete. The parents may be the recipients of many embarrassing, intrusive, and even offensive questions if the child obviously is not biologically related (eg, of a different skin color). Complete strangers may feel entitled to discuss the parents' infertility without invitation and to question the parents' relationship to their child.

For many reasons, adoptive parents frequently express a distinct preference for adopting a boy or a girl. This may

---

DISPLAY 6–1 • Special Needs Checklist

	Yes	Maybe	No		Yes	Maybe	No
Family/birth parent history				Burns (needing surgery)	___	___	___
Mental illness, birthparent				Cleft lip/cleft palate	___	___	___
other family member	___	___	___	Dwarfism	___	___	___
Mental retardation, birth	___	___	___	Orthopedic defects,			
parent				correctable	___	___	___
other family member	___	___	___	not correctable	___	___	___
Drug or alcohol use	___	___	___	Spina bifida	___	___	___
History of prostitution or	___	___	___	Rickets	___	___	___
STDs				Heart defect, minor (murmur)	___	___	___
History of homelessness	___	___	___	major (surgery)	___	___	___
History of incest	___	___	___	Sickle cell disease	___	___	___
History of physical or sexual	___	___	___	Thalassemia	___	___	___
abuse				Hemophilia	___	___	___
Birth history				Diabetes	___	___	___
Prematurity	___	___	___	Kidney disease	___	___	___
Birth defects	___	___	___	Epilepsy	___	___	___
Infection at birth	___	___	___	Developmental problems			
Abandonment	___	___	___	Vision, partial	___	___	___
Infectious diseases				blind	___	___	___
Tuberculosis	___	___	___	Hearing impaired	___	___	___
Hepatitis B	___	___	___	Deaf	___	___	___
Syphilis	___	___	___	Cerebral palsy	___	___	___
HIV/AIDS	___	___	___	Hyperactivity	___	___	___
History of meningitis	___	___	___	Learning disability	___	___	___
Polio	___	___	___	Speech problems	___	___	___
Medical conditions				Emotional problems, mild	___	___	___
Severe birthmarks or	___	___	___	severe	___	___	___
disfigurements							

---

limit their options to some degree, and the provider may need to discuss gender and race preferences.

● **Clinical Pearl:** The provider should help the family to consider questions such as the following:

- How will your family accept a child of another race?
- Can you handle the public attention (both good and bad) that such children receive?
- Will you be able to recognize and deal with racism directed toward your child?
- How do you feel about incorporating your child's heritage, including customs and holidays, into your family?
- Will opportunities exist for your child to network with others of his or her ethnic or racial background?
- How do you feel about your child growing up and marrying someone of his or her race or a different race?

▲ **Clinical Warning:** Some prospective parents (such as older or single parents) may have difficulty finding healthy infants in North America. They may consider an international adoption in an effort to avoid a special needs placement. Both the family and the provider must appreciate that children from abroad may be older and at risk for problems arising from extreme poverty, nutritional deficiencies, lack of medical care, and prolonged institutional care, including severe behavioral and emotional problems. Most come with virtually no birth or family history and no likelihood of ever obtaining such information.

Lifestyle Issues

The beginning of the adoption process is a good time for a thorough evaluation of the parents' health, especially if they are older or single. Parents are required to have a medical evaluation as part of their dossier, but this often is done in a very cursory fashion because of the parents' desire to move quickly through a large volume of paperwork. The wise provider will address health issues at the beginning of the adoption process.

Some other issues the provider may want to address include financial stability, emotional and financial support, plans for work and child care, and the presence of other family obligations, such as care of an elderly relative. This consideration is especially important for single parents.

Parents should be sure that their health insurance covers dependent children, even those who have preexisting medical conditions. The Health Insurance Act of 1996 (P.L. 104-191, known as the Kennedy-Kassebaum Bill) bans group health insurance carriers from excluding adopted children because of preexisting conditions as long as such children have been included in the insurance plan within 30 days of adoption. It also allows parents to obtain coverage without having to wait until an open enrollment period and has "portability provisions" for when the parent changes insurance plans or jobs.

ASSISTING THE FAMILY AT THE TIME OF PLACEMENT

Adoption usually is a very slow process, but eventually parents will have a referral for a child. At this time, they may return to their provider for advice about a particular child's health or special needs. Parents may seek an opinion about a prospective placement but with very scant information about the child. They are entitled to as much information as they need to make a decision about placement, but at times they may suspect that the information they have received is incomplete. Information that parents should seek at the time of placement is outlined in Display 6-2.

Considerations Related to the Child's Age and Origin

Most parents are quite realistic and understand the limitations of the information they receive and the risks involved. They expect the provider only to give as honest an assessment as possible and to provide some insight into problems they may encounter. They also may seek information about specific medical problems or support groups of people with similar experiences. The provider must appreciate that potential medical and psychological issues differ markedly for each child. Some particulars depend on the child's history and country of origin.

Infants Adopted in the United States

Because these adoptions usually are open to some degree, substantial information may be available about biologic and family history, pregnancy, and delivery. The birth mother usually (but not always) has received adequate prenatal care. Medical problems typically have been identified. A western-trained clinician almost certainly will have examined the child, and the results of that examination are known. If the placement occurs at birth, however, congenital anomalies may not yet have been detected.

Older Children Adopted in the United States

These children are likely to have been in some kind of temporary placement and tend to be older, because toddlers rarely are available for adoption. Their basic nutritional needs probably have been met, and they most likely have had some past medical care. Medical records frequently are available, although they may be incomplete. Any handicaps

---

probably are being treated. Most North American-born adoptees either are healthy or have defined diagnoses with accompanying information.

These children may have had some level of comfort and affection if they only had one or two placements in foster homes. Some children, however, have been in many foster homes or are isolated from biologic family members, including siblings. They may have a history of abuse or neglect and may be quite emotionally troubled.

▲ **Clinical Warning:** Children in foster care have a high prevalence of chronic medical problems, emotional and behavioral disorders, mental health problems, and educational needs. They usually have received inadequate preventive services, including immunizations. Information about older children adopted from foster care should be as complete as possible, because this may affect the amount of the adoption subsidy from the state. The provider should be aware that records are likely to be incomplete if the child is older, has known diagnoses, or has been in multiple placements. It may be particularly difficult to assess such things as maternal alcohol and substance abuse or physical or sexual abuse of the child.

Infants Adopted From Another Country

These infants rarely are newborns. They may be younger than 6 months but usually are closer to 1 year old. They may have medical problems, such as poor nutrition, restricted growth, parasite infestation, lack of medical care, and incomplete or absent immunizations, as well as adjustment problems resulting from institutional care. They may have experienced extreme poverty, only slightly improved by orphanage care, or may come from a background of abandonment and significant alcohol or other substance abuse. These children usually have no available family history or medical records.

Older Children Adopted From Another Country

In addition to the problems infants from abroad may experience, these children may have endured more prolonged periods of abuse, neglect, and institutionalization. They may have had little or no schooling and some period of street life. On the other hand, they may have received relatively good care. Living conditions can range from small foster homes (or the child's own family) to crowded, poor orphanages.

Medical Considerations at the Time of Placement

The provider should provide a differential diagnosis for any significant finding that does not yet have a specific diagnosis. The provider also may need to outline a worst possible scenario based on the information given to allow the parents to make a realistic decision about the placement.

Children Born in the United States

The following are some medical and social issues that may be encountered in U.S.-born adopted children, with which the provider should be very familiar:

- Maternal alcohol or substance abuse
- FAS
- Behavioral and emotional problems related to abuse, neglect, and abandonment

---

> **DISPLAY 6–2 • Information to Seek at the Time of Referral**
>
> 1. Birth family medical history, including the following:
>   Medical illnesses
>   Mental health history
>   History of genetic disorders
>   Ethnic origin
>   History of substance abuse of birth parents
>   Assessment of risk for infection with HIV,
>   hepatitis B and C, STDs
> 2. Birth history, including the following:
>   Results of the physical examination, including
>   height, weight, and head circumference
>   Results of any screening tests of mother or child
> 3. Immunization records
> 4. Dental records
> 5. History of illnesses, injuries, and hospitalizations
> 6. Allergies and medications
> 7. Consultants' evaluations, including educational and
>   behavioral
> 8. Chronology of placement in foster care
> 9. History of past abuse or neglect
> 10. Reasons for relinquishment or termination of
>   parental rights

- Attachment disorders
- Attention deficit/hyperactivity disorder

Children Born in Other Countries

The problems parents can anticipate in children from other countries differ in many ways from those of children born in the United States. Although the number of internationally adopted children is fairly small, these children often have medical problems that are unfamiliar and challenging to western providers.

Parents who seek their clinician's opinion about a child just placed with them may have few records or brief videotapes to view. They rarely have enough information to make truly informed decisions. Medical information provided may be difficult to interpret or wrong, but the provider should advise parents never to ignore a diagnosis made in a foreign country. The provider should look carefully for clues in the referral papers or videos to substantiate any listed diagnoses. It is especially important to look for objective findings that cannot be attributed to prolonged institutional care.

Parents have the right to obtain as complete information as possible and should not immediately accept a referral without further inquiry. Minimally, they should get a date of birth (or estimate), current measurements (height, weight, and head circumference), the results of a recent physical examination, and an estimation of the child's developmental progress.

Chronologic Age and Growth

A child adopted from abroad may have an assigned birth date estimated by the adoption workers in that country. If the child is an infant, the assigned date usually is accurate enough for evaluation of growth and development. Occasionally, an older child will have a birth date that appears suspicious because the child is small for age. The opposite also may occur; a child may appear to be of appropriate size for age, but is in fact older and small. Such problems occur because of a deliberate underestimation or under-reporting of age to facilitate placement.

▲ **Clinical Warning:** Children with psychosocial growth retardation due to prolonged institutionalization usually fall behind 1 month of growth for every 3 to 4 months of institutionalization. Weight usually is affected less than height. These children are very likely to have a dramatic growth spurt after arrival in their new homes. If weight is markedly affected, the provider should consider malnutrition as well, although overt nutritional growth failure is much less common than deficiencies of specific nutrients, such as iron or vitamin D.

● **Clinical Pearl:** The most important measurement is that of head circumference. A small head may suggest inaccurate dating or severe impairment of growth due to maternal alcohol abuse or malnutrition, neurologic disorders, or prematurity. Serious language, cognitive, and social delays may accompany severe growth retardation, for which the provider and parents should look carefully.

The provider should review what information was used to estimate age, including pregnancy history, measurements at birth, or other physical findings. A short delay in growth in an infant may be due to incorrect gestational age rather than true growth failure. Subsequent measurements can be plotted on standardized growth charts for initial comparison. Korean and Chinese children follow growth curves in infancy similar to U.S. children, even in institutional care; children from the Indian subcontinent tend to be somewhat smaller. Growth charts specific for Korean, Chinese, and Indian children are available from the University of Minnesota International Adoption Clinic, identified in the Community Resources section at the end of this chapter.

Development

Not only do these children come from high-risk backgrounds (abandonment, poverty, alcohol abuse, neglect, physical and sexual abuse, inadequate medical and prenatal care, prematurity, or physical handicaps), but they also may have significant health problems due to prolonged orphanage life. Both parents and provider should look for specific clues from the documents and videos that suggest diagnoses (such as FAS) that will make catch-up unlikely after placement with the family.

● **Clinical Pearl:** Although parents naturally are very concerned about their child's intellectual, emotional, and social development, it is almost impossible to determine from referral information whether a child is normal. In fact, parents should assume that a child adopted from abroad will not be developmentally normal, because virtually all institutionalized children will be delayed in one or more areas by age 1 year.

Medical Diagnoses

Children from abroad may come with specific medical diagnoses that are difficult for the provider to understand because of obscure, unfamiliar terms or use of familiar terms that differ from western practice. This is especially true for children from Eastern Europe and the former Soviet Union. For example, children from Russia may have the diagnosis of perinatal encephalopathy, a term with ominous connotations to western providers. Russian physicians use this term much more loosely to describe a child at risk for neurologic impairment. Likewise, a Russian child may come with findings unfamiliar to western providers, such as oligophrenia or intracranial hypertension syndrome.

● **Clinical Pearl:** Sometimes false or exaggerated diagnoses are made to satisfy local requirements for placement abroad. The provider should search the record or video for confirmatory or contradictory evidence, gaps in the history, or problems not mentioned in the list of diagnoses. If the provider cannot reassure the family that a diagnosis is either questionable or false, the clinician may want to consult a specialist experienced in interpreting medical information from abroad for confirmation. No diagnosis should be disregarded in the absence of specific contradictory evidence.

One of the most difficult situations in which adoptive parents find themselves is the referral of a child with an obscure, frightening diagnosis accompanied by incomplete information. If the child has a serious or frightening diagnosis, the report should include the physical findings or laboratory results leading to the diagnosis. It also should include a description of what the child can do and how the child compares with other children of the same age. It may be helpful to send the referring agency a list of developmentally related questions that can be answered with "yes" or "no." The parents should take time to investigate, obtain consultations, and talk with other families with similar referrals. If they still have substantial worries after adequate time to reflect and research or if they feel pressured to accept a placement that they think they cannot handle, they should consider saying no.

Adoptive parents dread this event above all else. They probably have waited a long time for this referral and already feel a bond with the child in the tiny photograph or brief video. They feel guilty about "rejecting" this child and worry that it will jeopardize their chances for another referral. The provider can help the parents by reframing the discussion in terms of what is best for this child, including the possibility that another family may have more resources to handle this problem.

Preplacement Testing

Parents may be offered the opportunity to test the child for specific medical conditions, such as hepatitis B and human immunodeficiency virus (HIV), before placement. They may ask the provider for advice about the interpretation or desirability of such testing, as well as the long-term implications of these conditions.

Hepatitis B

Hepatitis B is a common infection in most countries placing children for adoption in the United States. It also is common in institutional settings. Although infected adults and older children usually clear the virus from their bodies, infants infected in the neonatal period have an approximately 90% risk of becoming chronic carriers. These children are at higher risk of developing cirrhosis and hepatocellular carcinoma as adults (Conjeevaram & DiBisceglie, 1995). Despite these grim facts, there are many reasons to be encouraging to parents:

- Most children are asymptomatic in childhood.
- Medical therapy is advancing quite quickly.

Children who are hepatitis BsAg positive do not pose a substantial risk to others (except for parents or other long-term caregivers, who can be vaccinated) and should not be excluded from daycare settings or school or denied medical or dental care.

Despite the high prevalence of infection (8%–10% on the Asian subcontinent, 2%–7% in eastern Europe and northern China), the incidence of infection in most adoptees has not been high. For example, the incidence of hepatitis B infection in Chinese children has been 2.5% to 5% (Johnson, 1996).

The children usually are healthy, have normal or only slightly elevated liver function tests, and are hepatitis D negative. With good nutrition and avoidance of liver toxins, such as alcohol and raw shellfish, they should continue to be quite healthy in later childhood and adulthood.

▲ **Clinical Warning:** Parents who are offered the opportunity to test their children abroad before formal adoption procedures should consider carefully whether they want the test. In some countries, the risk of infection with hepatitis at the time of testing due to contaminated equipment is quite real, and the reliability of the testing also may be of concern. Both false-positives and false-negatives have been reported. Positive tests may stigmatize children unfairly and make them unadoptable. Such tests do not by themselves diagnose chronic infection. A good general rule to follow is that if the results of the test will not change the parent's mind about adoption, it should not be done.

Human Immunodeficiency Virus

The World Health Organization estimates that 25.5 million adults and 2.4 million children were infected with HIV worldwide at the end of 1996, while 40 million people will be infected by the year 2000 (AIDS and Adoption, 1997). To date, the highest rates of infection have been reported in Sub-Saharan Africa and Asia, including Thailand, Vietnam, Cambodia, and India. It appears likely that rates in India, China, and Indonesia will increase markedly over the next several years. Of particular concern is the high risk of infection in women between 14 and 24 years of age (AIDS and Adoption).

To date, international adoptees have had a low rate of infection, but there are still issues of concern. U.S. law does not require testing of immigrants younger than age 16, although embassy officials in countries like Thailand may request testing if it was not done. Parents may be reasonably counseled to not request testing in most instances. If risk factors are present, however, such as residence in a high prevalence or urban area or a history of intravenous drug use, sexually transmitted infections, or homelessness, testing may be advisable. Both parents and the provider are advised to keep track of current trends in HIV infection worldwide, because things will undoubtedly change and most likely not for the better. Refer to the chapter on HIV and acquired immunodeficiency syndrome for more information.

▲ **Clinical Warning:** Before testing the child for HIV in his or her country of origin, parents should be reminded of the following:

- The test may be wrong.
- There may be infectious risks in testing.
- A positive test may be false because it reflects maternal antibody.
- U.S. law prohibits immigration of a person with known HIV infection, so the child may become unadoptable.

Syphilis

Despite problems of inadequate history, unreliable testing, and the continued high incidence of syphilis worldwide, the rate of infection in international infant adoptees has been very low. Diagnoses of late, unsuspected congenital syphilis are rare. Parents should be reassured that testing is reliable, and treatment is effective. Older children may be positive because of infection due to sexual abuse (both before relinquishment for adoption and after placement in an institution) or occasionally because of infection with other treponemes, such as yaws and pinta.

▲ **Clinical Warning:** If either a child or his or her birth mother was treated for syphilis abroad, it is important to obtain as much information as possible about the regimen used, including the specific dosage of the antibiotic, to assess adequacy of treatment.

Preparing Family and Friends

Many parents have not yet discussed their plans with family or friends out of fear that something will go wrong during the adoption process. At the same time, they have thought about adoption for a long time and have come to terms with issues such as the lack of a biologic relationship to their child, racial differences, and the change in lifestyle that accompanies becoming a parent. They now are excited and happy to finally have a child. They may be surprised by the reaction of friends and family, who may be unprepared, disapproving of single parenthood, ambivalent about a child of another race or with a disability, or concerned about the child's social history. Parents need help to prepare for a less than enthusiastic first response from loved ones. They can be reassured that most concerns disappear quickly, and that typically family and friends will welcome their new child.

▲ **Clinical Warning:** Parents should be advised to resist the temptation to tell friends and family everything that is known about their child. This is especially true for sensitive information that parents will want to tell their child themselves when the time is right. Parents almost certainly will regret it when the child learns something from someone else at the "wrong" time or manner. In addition, family members may bring up parts of the child's past to explain specific behaviors years later, even though such information may be quite irrelevant or none of their business.

Helping the Parents Become Educators

One of the parents' most important roles is that of educator to those around them, including their child, extended family, important people in the child's world (such as teachers and primary care providers), and often complete strangers. Unless the child is of similar ethnic background and looks like the parents, the fact of adoption will be obvious to the world before the child understands the difference between adoptive parents and birth parents. Adoptive families quickly learn that even complete strangers feel entitled to comment on a child's being adopted, as if the child is uncomprehending. Their remarks can be breathtakingly insensitive. ("How much did she cost?" "How could his mother give up such an adorable child?") Parents should start practicing their responses early so that they will be prepared for these inevitable awkward situations.

One of the most effective ways to encourage the acceptance of adoption is the use of "positive adoption language." Parents already should have learned most of these terms and should practice them regularly. Providers are especially encouraged to become fluent in positive adoption language. Parents who hear providers refer to birth parents as "real" or "natural" parents will quickly leave their practices. Table 6-1 provides a framework for differentiating positive from prejudicial language.

Table 6-1. POSITIVE VERSUS NEGATIVE ADOPTION LANGUAGE

Positive Language	Negative Language
Birth parent	Real parent
Biologic parent	Natural parent
Birth child	Own child
My child	Adopted (or own) child
Born to unmarried parents	Illegitimate
Make an adoption plan	Give away
To parent	To keep
Waiting child	Adoptable child
Parent	Adoptive parent
International adoption	Foreign adoption
Child placed for adoption	An unwanted child
Court termination	Child taken away
Child with special needs	Handicapped child
Was adopted	Is adopted

From OURS magazine, May/June 1992

Travel Preparation

Most parents who adopt internationally are required to travel to the child's country of origin for weeks or even months. Parents should assume that medical care abroad for themselves and the child will be hard to obtain, unfamiliar, or inadequate. They need to come prepared to meet their basic medical needs. They also may need one or more immunizations listed in Display 6-3, depending on the area to which they will travel, the expected duration of stay, and the time of year of their trip.

▲ **Clinical Warning:** The provider should make every effort to see the family promptly after referral and before travel to allow several weeks for immunizations to be effective.

The following are some specific medical problems that the family and provider may need to consider:

- Diphtheria occurs in all states of the former Soviet Union. Parents traveling to these areas should have a booster if needed.
- Hepatitis B vaccine is indicated for parents adopting a child known to be positive for the disease; if parents anticipate a prolonged stay in an area of high prevalence, such as Asia, Romania, Russia, or South America; or if exposure through medical treatment seems likely.
- Malaria prophylaxis is indicated for most countries to which adoptive parents travel. Malaria is prevalent in tropical and subtropical areas; it occurs as far north as northern India, Mexico, and China and as far south as Argentina. The most virulent form, *P. falciparum*, is especially prevalent in Africa. Chloroquine alone is effective in preventing malaria in areas such as temperate South America, most of Central America, North Africa, and the Caribbean, but chloroquine-resistant strains are common in most other areas. Mefloquine is the recommended malaria prophylaxis in such cases, but patients with known hypersensitivity to the medication or with a history of epilepsy, psychiatric disorders, or cardiac conduction abnormalities should not use it. Doxycycline is a good alternative, but patients should be warned about skin photosensitivity, causing intense sunburn. Mefloquine resistance has been detected in northern Thailand, where doxycycline is recommended. Patients who cannot take either mefloquine or doxycycline can use chloroquine and proguanil. The latter is not available in the United States but can be obtained in Canada, Europe, and many African countries.

DISPLAY 6–3 • Recommended Vaccinations for Travel Preparation

Tetanus and diphtheria booster (Td)*
Hepatitis A vaccine*
Hepatitis B vaccine*
Typhoid vaccine (endemic rural areas for more than 6 wk)
Yellow fever vaccine (rural areas of Panama and tropical South America)
Rabies vaccine (if animal exposure is very likely)
Measles vaccine (if born after 1957)
Polio vaccine
Malaria prophylaxis
Japanese encephalitis (rural areas of east and southeast Asia)

*Recommended for almost all travelling parents.

- Cholera is prevalent in most of Africa, Central and South America, east and southeast Asia, and the Indian subcontinent. This prevalence usually is limited to rural areas, to which parents rarely travel. Specific prophylaxis is not available.
- Yellow fever is present in tropical areas of South America and Africa. Vaccination may be required for entry to those areas.
- Typhoid fever occurs in rural areas of Asia and Central and South America. Travelers are at risk during long stays in these areas.
- Tick-borne encephalitis and Lyme disease occur in Central and western Europe.
- Japanese encephalitis vaccination is required only if a stay of longer than 4 weeks is planned during the rainy season in endemic areas of India, China, Japan, and southeast Asia.
- For more details about malaria prophylaxis, the provider may want to consult an infectious disease specialist, travel clinic, or the Centers for Disease Control and Prevention (see the Community Resources section at the end of this chapter).

Parents may also ask for advice about a medical travel kit, because medical care may be very difficult to find or involve unfamiliar terminology or treatment. A sample kit is outlined in Display 6-4.

● **Clinical Pearls:**

- Scabies and lice are very common among institutionalized children. The clinician should have some good quality pictures of scabies to show parents so that they have an idea of what the rash looks like. Parents should be informed that persistent itching does not signify failure of treatment and can be treated with hydrocortisone until they return.
- Antibiotics in powdered form can be extremely useful for both impetigo and otitis. Otitis media is a common occurrence in newly adopted children and can make a long flight back miserable and painful. There is probably no real reason to withhold a prescription for an antibiotic out of fear that the parents will overtreat or undertreat an infection.

Unless the provider has adopted abroad, it is hard to appreciate the isolation and helplessness parents feel with a hot, screaming child who has an earache or other illness in a hotel room in a provincial Chinese city. The provider may want to advise parents to seek medical attention if at all possible and to treat their child with the advice of a local provider. Oral rehydration solution may be extremely useful, especially in powdered form, because it is virtually impossible for a child with diarrhea to take as many bottles of solution as are needed. WHO solution contains 3.5 g of NaCl, 2.5 g of NaHCO$_3$, 1.5 g KCl, and 20 g of glucose in 1 liter of bottled water, and most pharmacists can obtain it.

EVALUATING THE NEWLY ADOPTED CHILD

Parents should be advised to plan for an initial evaluation by their provider 1 to 2 weeks after the child arrives in the family, although most families will be in the office in 1 to 2 days. Display 6-5 includes a list of recommended evaluations, which may be completed over several visits. Depending on

---

DISPLAY 6–4 • Sample Medical Travel Kit

- 1% to 2.5% hydrocortisone cream
- Insect repellent containing DEET if travelling to malaria-prone areas (30%–35% strength for adults, 6%–10% for children)
- Permethrin solution for bed nets (malaria) and clothing (ticks)
- Sun block, sunglasses, and hat
- OTC antidiarrheal medication, such as loperamide
- An antibiotic for traveler's diarrhea
- 5% permethrin cream (Elimite) for scabies
- 1% permethrin (Nix) for head lice
- An antibiotic, such as amoxicillin in powdered form, with instructions
- Topical antibiotic cream, such as mupiricin
- Child's decongestant/antihistamine preparation, with instructions
- Oral rehydration solution, preferably in powder form
- Adult's and child's acetaminophen or ibuprofen
- Extra prescription medication for parents
- Written prescriptions for medications and corrective lenses
- General first aid supplies: Bandaids, thermometers, emergency dental fillings, emollient creams, tongue depressor, and so forth
- Iodine tablets and water filter (only if bottled water is not available)
- Your favorite child care guide in paperback

DISPLAY 6–5 • Evaluation of the Adopted Child

1. A complete physical examination, including the following:
   - Presence of dysmorphic features
   - Assessment of growth and age
   - Documentation of bruises and scars already present
   - Genital examination if suspicion of history of sexual abuse
   - A developmental examination, including language assessment
2. Vision and hearing screening appropriate for age
3. Dental evaluation
4. Complete blood count
5. Urinalysis
6. Hepatitis profile, including HBsAg, anti-HBs, anti-HBc, anti-HC
7. HIV-1 and -2 screening, PCR or viral culture if infant
8. Mantoux skin test with Candida control
9. Stool for ova and parasites (three specimens)
10. VDRL
11. Lead level*
12. Thyroid screening† or state newborn screening test
13. Chemistry profile, including Ca, P, and alkaline phosphatase

---
*Especially eastern Europe, Russia, and China.
† Especially Russia, China, Mongolia, and Tibet.

the child's condition as well as country of origin. The provider should use clinical judgment in deciding the order and the extent of the evaluation based on the child's condition and country of origin. Many of the tests performed abroad may need to be repeated.

Immunizations

Many adopted children arrive with a record of at least some immunizations (usually DT or DPT, polio, and BCG). Many children have low or no antibodies to diphtheria and tetanus when tested, however, indicating improper storage or administration of the vaccines or incorrect records. This is less likely to occur if the child received vaccines in a clinic or hospital rather than at an orphanage.

▲ **Clinical Warning:** In almost all cases, it is prudent to start immunizations over again according to the American Academy of Pediatrics' (AAP's) recommendations for children not immunized in the first year of life (AAP, 1997).

Age

Review of the child's paperwork at referral and documentation of the results of the initial examination are the only steps indicated for the first examination of the child of unknown age. There is no reason to consider an age assignment until the child has been with the family for at least 1 year. Waiting allows for catch-up growth and for a period of observation of the child's development. Infants with uncertain birth dates usually do not need their assigned dates changed. Older children may need age assignment later based on bone or dental age and evaluation by professionals, such as teachers.

▲ **Clinical Warning:** Children who have had growth failure due to prolonged institutionalization and neglect may be at risk later for precocious puberty or obesity. Chapters 22 and 60 provide more information on these topics.

Developmental Delay

Virtually all adopted children will have some degree of delay on placement, especially those who were in institutional or foster care for a year or more. Fortunately, most children catch up very quickly. In the absence of specific risk factors, such as neurologic abnormalities or a history of severe maternal alcohol use or intrauterine infection, an observation period within the family is reasonable to allow for recovery. Serial developmental examinations should show rapid progress. Until that time, the provider should remember that many states' early intervention programs cover children at risk due to prolonged institutionalization.

Rickets

Rickets is a relatively common finding among institutionalized children and children from other countries. It most often is due to nutritional deficiencies. It also is a frequent finding in the child's medical records, especially if the child is from Russia, Romania, or China or was born prematurely. Children may have mild to severe symptoms, including bowed legs, enlarged joints, craniotabes, growth failure, fractures, delayed or defective dentition, excessive sweatiness, weakness, hypotonia, or seizures. Most children respond well to treatment with a balanced diet and oral vitamin D supplementation. Children who do not respond to treatment or whose physical or laboratory findings suggest

liver or kidney disease may need further evaluation by an appropriate subspecialist.

▲ **Clinical Warning:** The provider should not forget the possibility of abuse when evaluating fractures.

Gastrointestinal Disorders and Diarrhea

As in the general pediatric population, viral infections are the most common problem encountered in adopted children. Specific pathogens, such as *Salmonella, Shigella, Yersinia,* and *Campylobacter,* are less common but may be seen in children coming from orphanages or shelters, especially those from India. Protozoal infections with *Giardia* or *Entamoeba histolytica* are fairly common, although children usually are asymptomatic. These infections should be detected in stool specimens for ova and parasites. Worms are unusual except in children who have lived on the streets for some time.

Tuberculosis

Tuberculosis (TB) is still a common infection in institutions and in most countries from which international adoptees come. BCG vaccination is a common practice outside the United States and will be quite obvious by the scar on the child's upper arm. BCG is not completely effective in preventing disease, however, and TB occurs in international adoptees. If the child is well and BCG was given within the past year, the provider may choose to wait a year after BCG to retest. If the child has symptoms suggestive of TB, a positive protein derivative should be done immediately.

▲ **Clinical Warning:** All international adoptees (as well as selected American-born children) should be screened with a Mantoux test with a *Candida* control. Any vaccinated child with a Mantoux positive greater than 10 mm (or 5 mm in an HIV-infected child) should be evaluated for TB. Multiple drug-resistant strains have been reported worldwide, especially in Argentina, southeast Asia, India, Russia, and the Baltic States, so consultation with an infectious disease specialist may be desirable.

Cytomegalovirus

Internationally adopted children have been shown to excrete cytomegalovirus (CMV) at approximately the same rate as infants and toddlers in day care in the United States (30%–50%) (Adoption Medical News, 1996). Routine screening of adoptees is not recommended. The provider should recommend only good hand washing after contact with urine and oral secretions. A child who is toilet-trained presents no risk to the caregiver. A child with specific symptoms suggesting CMV infection during pregnancy or birth should be evaluated. These symptoms include hearing loss, growth retardation, retinitis, intracranial calcifications, and mental retardation.

● **Clinical Pearl:** Primary CMV infection in pregnancy is less common in developing countries because of a higher incidence of infection later in childhood.

Hepatitis B

Hepatitis B is a fairly common problem among adoptees from virtually all countries. It is especially prevalent in India, China, Korea, southeast Asia, Russia, and eastern Europe.

All children should be screened on arrival and 3 to 6 months later with a hepatitis B profile.

● **Clinical Pearl:** Children who are negative on initial screening may be vaccinated against hepatitis B.

Any child who is positive on initial screening should have a repeat screening 6 months later to determine if he or she is a chronic carrier. Infants who are positive on initial screening are very likely to be persistently positive on retesting. Chronically infected children should be evaluated with the following:

- A complete hepatitis B panel, including e antigen and anti-HBe
- Screening for hepatitis D, especially if from eastern Europe, the Amazon region, or the South Pacific
- Liver function tests, including aspartate transaminase (AST) and ALT
- Urinalysis

▲ **Clinical Warnings:**

- Chronic carriers of hepatitis B should be followed subsequently with a yearly physical examination, liver enzymes, and complete blood count and with hepatitis B testing every 3 years until age 10. About 1% of chronic carriers revert to negative every year. Referral to a pediatric gastroenterologist for evaluation and management should be considered, particularly if the child exhibits failure to thrive, an AST greater than 150, and elevated alpha-fetoprotein or abnormalities on ultrasound (Conjeevaram & DiBisceglie, 1995).
- Family members of a child who is positive for hepatitis B on first screening should be vaccinated because of an increased risk of transmission to household members. Studies have shown that this risk is almost entirely confined to the caretakers.

Other Concerns

Abnormal hemoglobins, such as hemoglobin E and Hemaglobin Constant Spring, commonly are found in immigrants from southeast Asia and will be detected on hemoglobin electrophoresis. Microcytosis may be found in children from south and southeast Asia with alpha or beta thalassemia trait; these children do not need iron therapy unless iron deficiency also is present. G6PD deficiency commonly is seen in Asian and Mediterranean populations. High fevers may be seen in children with specific exotic infections (eg, malaria or drug-resistant *Salmonella typhi* in children from Vietnam). Iodine deficiency and hypothyroidism have been reported in some inland rural areas of China, Mongolia, and Tibet. Lead toxicity can be seen in poor, rapidly industrializing countries without environmental regulations. Recurrent, severe abdominal pain may be seen in children with malabsorption, parasites, constipation, overeating, ulcers, adjustment reactions, or *Helicobacter pylori*. Hepatitis C has been seen in both China and eastern Europe.

ASSISTING THE FAMILY AFTER ARRIVAL

For some time after the child's arrival in the new family, both parents and provider are preoccupied with resolving any health issues. Attention also must be given to the adjustment of both parent and child to a new and stressful situation.

Careful, gentle exploration of stresses early on can yield tremendous benefits to the entire family. The following section discusses some common adjustment problems for which the clinician can provide anticipatory guidance.

The Parents' Adjustment

After the initial excitement and joy at their child's arrival, many adoptive parents begin to express fears about not being able to love or bond with their child in the way that they hoped. Lack of sleep, fatigue after a long journey, unfamiliarity with their child's temperament, and concern about health and adjustment problems may cause parents to worry that they are incompetent and will not be able to love their child. They may even think that they have made a mistake. It is very important to reassure parents of the following:

- Most parents' fantasies about their children, whether adopted or biologic, clash with reality.
- Almost all adoptive parents have these fears to some degree.
- Love for a child usually develops over time and with increasing intensity.
- The vast majority of parents report years later that adoption was successful, even in the presence of severe adjustment and behavioral problems at the beginning.

The provider should reassure parents that separation of the child from their adoptive family does occur, but very infrequently. As for any new parents, the provider also should encourage them to reserve as much time as possible for themselves, both individually and as a couple.

● **Clinical Pearls:**

- The provider should strongly advise parents to talk openly about their fears and to seek counseling if needed. The provider should encourage an open dialogue between the parents and an adoption social worker. This professional can be a lifesaver to the family at this time and, in addition, can be of tremendous support and encouragement years later, as the family progresses through their adoption journey.
- Parents should be very careful to avoid overstimulation during the first few months after placement, including too frequent or intense contact with extended family, friends, or neighbors. This can be extremely fatiguing for both parents and child.

A key issue for parents is maternity or paternity leave after adoption. Many adoptive parents do not yet feel like "real" parents and have guilt or anxiety about taking appropriate leave from work after their child's arrival. Stress may be compounded by the time already taken for travel, the financial pressures of a costly adoption, and the perception (often correct) that their employers or coworkers do not view them as "real" parents who are entitled to family leave. The provider should encourage parents to take as much time now as possible to ease the transition to family life. Adoptive parents are their child's "real" parents.

The Child's Adjustment

Children adopted as young infants fit into families and interact with their parents in the first year or two much like nonadopted infants. Adoptive and biologic parents can be equally loving and nurturing, allowing for the same development of trust and attachment. Adoptive parents may even think at this point that being adopted will not make any difference to their child because the initial adjustment was so successful.

The adjustment of the older adopted child may range from quite untroubled to prolonged bizarre and disruptive behavior, with most adjustments falling in the mild to moderate degree of severity. Common problems that occur in the older child who was institutionalized include sleeping disorders (especially fear of sleeping alone); feeding problems (preoccupation with availability of food or going to the grocery store, hoarding food, gorging); hypersensitivity or hyposensitivity to noise, visual events, tastes, and smells; insensitivity to pain; clumsiness; self-stimulating behavior, such as rocking; fear of abandonment or abuse; and excessive friendliness due to lack of early attachment. The sensitive parent can usually cope with these problems in the following ways:

- Providing a quiet, structured environment with limited stimulation, new experiences, and numbers of toys
- Adjusting activities to the child's developmental level
- Tolerating strange behaviors as long as they are not dangerous
- Seeking counseling early

Most early adjustment problems extinguish gradually over time. Many parents believe that the older the child is on entry to the new family, the longer the adjustment will take. Sometimes a child who appeared to have an initially smooth adjustment may start acting out and testing their parents later. Parents need reassurance that this may represent the child's delayed attempt to bond with them. Parents should discuss issues of concern with their adoption social worker. Support groups that deal with adoption issues also may prove helpful. Information about such support groups is available from local and state or provincial adoption agencies.

Transracial Issues

Many social challenges await the family that adopts a child from a different ethnic or racial heritage. Social challenge readily translates into prejudice, especially if parents are Caucasian and their child is not. Parents who choose this road must be prepared to travel it with their child. This means that parents need to help their child combat racism while at the same time helping him or her to develop strong self-esteem. Strategies for achieving these tasks include adoption support activities, involvement in ethnically centered groups, and teaching their child how to prepare for and deal with racism.

● **Clinical Pearl:** The provider should encourage families who adopt transracially to seek out support.

Strong sources of support can include an adoption social worker as well as, for example, church members of their child's ethnic/racial heritage. Several studies speak positively about the outcomes of transracial adoption. Schaffer and Lindstrom (1991) describe a study of 300 midwestern American multiracial families composed of Caucasian parents and children of African American heritage. Although race was a complicating factor for the children as they grew up, such issues more often arose in the outside world, not from within their families. Several excellent publications are available that can guide parents; these are suggested in the Resources section at the end of this chapter.

Preserving Ethnic Identities

As in any family, the family whose children are adopted will create its own special routines and customs. Especially for families whose members are ethnically and racially diverse, the provider should encourage exploration of their child's customs, rituals, and, if feasible, language of ethnic origin. The addition of a specific ethnic custom can proclaim to both child and family that the child's presence adds beauty and uniqueness to the family. The family also may find that incorporating some aspect of an important ethnic festival into the family calendar increases their child's happiness and self-esteem. Planning for such activities may require that the parents read ethnically oriented books and, if available, participate in activities organized by local members of their child's ethnic heritage. The provider should encourage these efforts. In addition, a referral to an adoption social worker can provide parents with access to any available local resources.

The public library may own adoption-related and culture-specific books and language tapes. The clinician also can point the family toward local/regional colleges and universities, which are rich resources for possible connections to cultural experts and sometimes exchange students from a child's country of origin. Like-minded families can join together to plan and run a culture-specific adoption group focused on one particular ethnic or racial cohort. The addition to the group of a college faculty member or student who shares the ethnicity of the group's children can provide a strong cultural anchor. Similarly, an adult adoptee can be an important role model and support person for children.

Birthdays and Coming Home Day Anniversaries

Most cultural groups commemorate an individual's birth in annual celebration. Children in particular eagerly anticipate their "special" day. Adopted children are no different in this regard, of course, but the provider should keep in mind that, in general, the child's day of birth was not attended by any family members. This fact of adopted life is most acute for the youngster whose birthday was assigned arbitrarily. The provider's empathy for this situation can be well expressed by describing for parents an addition to the traditional birthday celebration, that is, the "gotcha day." Whereas everyone has a "birth" day (arbitrary or not), the adopted child also has the anniversary of the day when he or she joined the family. The "gotcha day" (the anniversary of the day we "got" you) can be a special day of child-centered activities and family fun. Some families have planned activities; others opt for a family party. The provider who encourages the adopted family to commemorate the anniversary of their child's homecoming supports them in their celebration of family strengths and bonds.

Issues as the Adopted Child Grows

Adoption usually is a very successful way to build a family. Parents experience the joy and feeling of fulfillment that nurturing a child brings, helping the child to become a happy, productive adult. Children receive the benefit of a safe, permanent home with warm, loving parents. Most parents bristle at the idea that adoption is an inferior way to have and raise children, but they would not dispute that it is a different way.

Adoption is based on the experience of loss, and the sense of loss remains pervasive and quite profound throughout the child's life. The ability to deal successfully with loss and grief at different developmental stages is key to the child's health and happiness.

● **Clinical Pearl:** The most important issue is that the child comes to the adoptive family with the experience of the loss of both birth parents and genetic roots.

Many adoptive parents often will have had a similar experience of loss because of their inability to have a biologic child. Coping with issues of separation and loss associated with adoption becomes a permanent part of both the child's and parents' lives. These issues recur during each developmental stage as the child develops a deeper appreciation of the meaning of that loss.

The third member of the "adoption triangle" is the birth mother and, less commonly, the birth father, who also must learn to cope with the experience of loss. Because American adoptions are likely to be open, at least to some degree, the birth mother may know something about the child's new family and may have met the adoptive parents. She also may be somewhat involved in her child's upbringing. On the whole, birth parents usually find that an open or semi-open arrangement helps them accept their decision for adoption and to move on with their lives. The adoptive parents themselves may find that maintaining some degree of contact helps them resolve their frequently ambivalent feelings about the birth parents.

Infancy and Early Childhood

The concept of "being adopted" usually is thought to mean little to infants and young children. Older preschoolers usually know the word "adoption" and have a positive, warm feeling about it, because parents portray adoption in a loving way that emphasizes the happiness that it has brought to them. The child may be quite vague about the existence of a birth mother and the birth process itself and may even think that all children are adopted. Adoption plays a major role in infancy and early childhood, however, in the development of bonding, attachment, and a sense of belonging.

Bonding occurs primarily in the first few months of life and involves the consistent satisfaction of a child's needs for food, warmth, and dry clothing. It allows the child to develop a sense of trust in the caretaker and the ability to trust others. Bonding may fail to develop in infancy for many reasons, including illness, institutionalization, and the inability to sense or to express needs. Adopted children who live in large orphanages with few attendants may not have had their needs met and may not have learned to trust their caretakers. They then have no feeling of trust to transfer to the parents. Some children in foster or orphanage care may have had needs met before they were fully aware of them; for example, being fed before they were hungry or being changed before they realized they were wet. The feeling of having needs satisfied by someone with whom they could bond did not develop.

Attachment is an affectionate link between parent and child that develops throughout the first year of life. A variety of mutually pleasurable interactions (playing, smiling, singing, hugging) allows the child to develop a feeling of self-worth. Attachment may be inhibited by the child's sense of not belonging. This can happen in a variety of situations: parents fear that they are unable to love an adopted child and hold back; parents are afraid that the birth mother will change her mind; or the child does not meet the parents' need to have someone like them—a need of which the parents may be unaware. Parents may have difficulty attaching because of unrealistic expectations of family life; residual

feelings of anger after a long, difficult adoption process; or return of grief over the inability to have a biologic child. Children who are placed in adoptive families after they have begun to experience separation anxiety may have quite intense problems becoming attached to their new parents.

A sense of belonging within a family provides a safe base from which children can develop a sense of identity and, eventually, separate from their parents. Children need to identify with their parents and recognize their own unique characteristics and abilities. In biologic families, the sharing of physical attributes, talents, and mannerisms with members of both the immediate and extended family reinforces this sense of likeness. Adoptive parents usually are unable to take advantage of these similarities and may choose instead to emphasize shared interests, tastes, habits, or mannerisms that children acquire simply by living with them.

Preschoolers often do not realize that most families are not created by adoption and may have a difficult time when people use terms such as "real child" and "real parents." Confusion about whether they are "real" or "fake" may lead them to question their identity and place in their families. This can be very threatening to preschoolers, who like to find ways in which they belong. If a child is of a different race than the parents, the issue of difference may be thrust on them quite publicly—often in places such as the grocery store. Strangers will often ask direct and uncomfortable questions about where the child came from, how much the adoption or the child cost, or what is known about the "real" parents. Adoptive parents should learn not to answer these questions in any detail and to redirect the conversation until the stranger gets the point. (Whose child is she? Mine. Where did you get her? I picked her up at my babysitter's. How much did she cost? Oh, she's priceless.) The parents also might want to turn to the child and ask for permission to answer such questions. Parents may want to educate the stranger asking the questions or explain the benefits of adoption, but they should not forget that the most important audience is their child, who desires a feeling of belonging and has a right to privacy.

Children begin to appreciate racial differences by 3½ years of age. Children of color may experience the first episodes of racism at this time. Racism may occur in quite benign or condescending ways, such as comments made about how cute Asians are or a stranger touching a child's skin or hair. The child also may start to notice stares or disapproving glances. Parents may find that they need to discuss racism at an earlier age than they anticipated. Non-minority parents may not anticipate this because they tend to talk about racism later (after an experience with racism) than minority parents (who start before).

Most experts agree that preschoolers who are adopted early in life have adjustments and developments similar to other children of their age and that issues related to adoption tend to emerge during the school years. From that time on, the fact of being adopted is a central issue in the child's life. Parents and health care professionals may make the mistake of thinking that adoption is the key issue in an otherwise ordinary childhood adjustment, as well as thinking that it is not a concern at all, when it very well may be.

Middle Childhood (6–10 Years)

Middle childhood represents a major leap forward in the child's development. Children move beyond egocentrism and develop empathy and the beginnings of a moral conscience. Concrete thinking gives way to more logical thinking. Relationships with peers and the need to belong to a group become more important. Middle childhood also represents a difficult time for children in understanding and accepting adoption. They begin to recognize that adoption is different from birth. From 7 to 8 years of age, they begin to appreciate that "family" usually is defined by blood relationships rather than by with whom one lives. They may have to come to terms with the existence of birth parents and possibly even birth siblings. Logical thinking allows them to understand the double meaning of the term "chosen child." For their birth parents to have chosen them, someone else first had to reject them.

Adopted children in middle childhood see more ways in which they are different from others. Their friends also may notice differences and may distance themselves from adopted children because they "lost" their parents, a situation that children at this age find very frightening. For the first time, adopted children may hear negative remarks about themselves and about adoption. An increased racial awareness and sensitivity about not looking like other family members may interfere with the development of the child's self-esteem.

One of the major life events of middle childhood is the start of kindergarten and first grade. All children and parents have to deal with the separation issues that occur at this time, but the problem is especially acute for adopted children. They are learning about the loss of their first parents and are struggling with the "chosen child" dichotomy at the same time they are adjusting to being away from home and family all day. Parents need to reinforce the child's feelings of belonging, continue to talk about adoption issues, and encourage the child to talk about school experiences.

Parents may find that they need to educate their children's teachers about adoption. This may include instruction about positive adoption language, encouragement of a multicultural curriculum, and modification of common grade-school projects, such as drawing family trees or bringing in baby pictures, which the child may not have.

Children in middle childhood will use a variety of defense mechanisms to cope with their grief for the lost family. Children who were adopted as infants and who have no bad memories of past living situations may fantasize about what their birth parents were like and what their lives would be like if they were still with them. Children who have experienced frequent moves or abuse may use anger and disruptive behavior as coping mechanisms.

By age 8, children's understanding of adoption becomes much more sophisticated. Their appreciation of the implications of being adopted is deeper. At the same time, their attitudes toward adoption may become negative, with behavioral, emotional, and academic problems becoming more common.

From ages 9 to 12, children develop greater independence and involvement with the outside world, moving increasingly away from their parents. Parent—child conflicts increase. The fantasy of the "perfect parents" becomes an important mechanism to cope with their ambivalent feelings about their parents. ("These people are so awful and mean, they can't be my 'real' parents. They'd be much kinder and wiser and would understand me much better.") As children grow older, they realize that they can have both good and bad feelings about their parents and that perfect parents are just a fantasy. Adopted children may have trouble relinquishing this fantasy because, after all, they do have another set of parents. They may be unable to stop thinking about how much better life would be with them.

Adolescence

Adolescence usually is considered to begin at about age 11 and is characterized by the child's attempts to develop more independence and a distinct identity. Children become much more social and involved with peer groups, to whom they look for a sense of belonging and approval. Adolescents also are very preoccupied with abstract concepts of morality and philosophy.

Developing an independent identity requires children to come to terms with past events so that they can start planning for the future. During early adolescence, adoptees may experience a return of the grief they felt over the loss of their birth parents. Later in adolescence, they may have trouble with separation and development of unique identities because of their inability to differentiate themselves from the "other" set of parents whom they do not know. In an attempt to move as far away as possible from their adoptive parents, adopted children may move instead toward an identity based on their perceptions of their birth parents, whether good or bad. They may assume negative characteristics that they know or imagine their birth parents to have. For this reason, it is critical that the adoptive parents come to terms with whatever negative feelings they may have about the birth parents so that they can present a balanced picture of them to their child, pointing out the birth parents' good qualities as well as failings.

Adopted children who are members of a racial or ethnic minority may experience disturbing instances of racism during adolescence, especially when they are trying to find a comfortable peer group with whom to belong. Although they may have been subjected to teasing during middle childhood, now they may find themselves perceived as more different from than similar to their peers, and they may be quite unprepared for rejection. They also may encounter more overt racism when they begin dating, including what they perceive as racist reactions from parents.

If adopted children have had little or no contact with their birth parents, adolescence often is a time when they express a desire to search for them. Although establishing contact with the birth parents may be very helpful in resolving feelings of grief and developing a more positive sense of self, the search process usually is very frightening for all involved.

▲ **Clinical Warning:** Most adoption experts recommend that children not undertake a search until they have worked through the normal developmental issues of adolescence. For most people, this means that search activities begin after secondary school. Some children may express an interest in the search but are not in fact ready to meet their birth parents. They may find that an imaginary correspondence with their birth parents helps them express their unanswered questions and fears.

● **Clinical Pearl:** The provider should refer the adolescent who asks about the search process to a competent adoption social worker. This individual can assist the adolescent and family in many ways, from providing needed support to pointing them to resources and support groups. He or she can encourage parents to support their child during the process of searching and to make clear that the child will always be part of their family.

Adolescence can be a very disturbing time for parents because of their children's rebelliousness and idealization of the birth parents. As with any adolescent, parents should be alert for behaviors that suggest more serious problems. These include truancy, delinquency, running away from home, abuse of drugs or alcohol, self-mutilation, abuse of others (including family members or pets), suicidal ideation or attempts, association with gangs or cults, or involvement with street life. In such instances, adoption issues often are involved. The clinician needs to refer such youths for intensive professional therapy. The family as a whole may benefit from family therapy. Schafer and Lindstrom (1996) report that their own and others' research demonstrates that adoptive families are quicker to improve in family therapy and are better at maintaining their improvement, compared with other matched samples of families who seek help. Chapter 25 provides further insight into the issue of adolescent problem behavior.

● **Clinical Pearl:** The provider should become familiar with post-adoption resources in the area. He or she should offer the adolescent information about these resources. If specific supports, such as teen groups, are not available, the clinician can work with the local adoption social worker network to make such services available. Support groups composed of other adopted teens can be a valuable and safe place for resolving some adoption and identity issues.

Early Adulthood and Beyond

The experience of being an adopted child remains a part of the adult forever, even if it appears that most issues have been resolved successfully. Sometimes the experience expresses itself only as a feeling of something missing. Inability to resolve feelings of loss and grief may affect the adoptee's ability to establish intimate, loving relationships and to cope with the loss of friends and loved ones during life. Unresolved issues about adoption may remain dormant for years, only to resurface during major life changes, such as marriage, the birth of a child, or the death of a parent. Such life events can bring with them new understanding and new questions. At each major life change, the adoptee may again feel the need to search for birth parents or, at an older age, birth siblings, to resolve some of these questions. Such a search may assist the adult adoptee to feel in control, helping him or her to understand and come to terms with what it means to be adopted.

> "He allowed himself to be swayed by his conviction that human beings are not born once and for all on the day their mothers gave birth to them, but that life obliges them over and over again to give birth to themselves" (Garcia Marquez, 1988).

REFERRAL POINTS AND CLINICAL WARNINGS

The provider should remember that issues of self-esteem arise in most middle and high school children as part of their normal progression toward adulthood. Self-discovery for adopted children usually contains the added dimension of a genetic unknown, because they rarely know much about their biologic families. Reasons for eye color, health history, and personality traits are all typically "hidden" from adopted children and their families. This "great unknown" is just one more stressor for adolescent adoptees to address when they are already struggling with the same issues of maturity as their friends. The clinician can provide much-needed reassurance to teenagers and their parents during this challenging life phase. Referral to an adoption social worker can provide insight and support for the child and family. This individual also is skilled at supporting the search process if and when the child decides to look for biologic parents. Most adoption experts recommend that search not be undertaken until the child has worked through the normal developmental issues of adolescence. For most people, this means that search activities begin after secondary school.

COMMUNITY RESOURCES

Multiple adoption resources are available on the web for prospective and adoptive parents and their children. Using any standard search engine and typing in the words www.adoption.org will begin the search process. Available hyperlinks include those for adoption agencies (domestic and international), birth and adoptive parents, adoptees, search, chat groups, books and magazines related to adoption, and adoption organizations. Other selected resources include the following:

American Adoption Congress (information for search for adult adoptees and birth parents)
Box 44040
L'Enfant Plaza Station
Washington, DC 20026

Adoption Council of Canada (information and educational services)
Box 8442 Stn. T
Ottawa, Ontario K1G 3H8
(613) 235-1566

Adoption Council of Ontario
134 Clifton Rd.
Toronto, Ontario M4T 2G6

Adoptive Families of America (source of support and information)
2309 Como Avenue
St. Paul, MN 55108
(800) 372-3300
Fax (612) 645-0055

This organization also publishes a magazine, Adoptive Families (formerly OURS magazine), which is a good resource for culture camps, ethnic reunions, and motherland visits. Ask for a catalog of dolls and books for all ethnic and racial groups.

In Canada: Adoptive Parents Association of Alberta
Box 6496
Bonnyville, Alberta T9N 2H1
(403) 826-5625

Chosen Child: International Adoption Magazine
Subscription Dept.
246 S. Cleveland Ave.
Loveland, CO 80537

The on-line publication, www.chosenchild.com, uses parent-written articles and pieces from adoption educators to inform and support families and their children. An especially valuable feature is the column Reflections, in which young adult adoptees reflect on their own experiences, both positive and negative.

Korean American Adoptee Adoptive Family Network (KAAN)
www.KAANET@aol.com

Founded by a young Korean adult adoptee, this organization hosts symposiums and workshops for adoptees and their families. Its website provides information for subscribing to KAAN's weekly e-mail, with its myriad hyperlinks to related sites, including Korean cultural websites.

Report of Foreign Adoption (a comprehensive annual report with updates on foreign adoption)
International Concerns Committee for Children
911 Cypress Drive
Boulder, CO 80303
(303) 494-8333

National Resource Center for Special Needs Adoption
Spaulding for Children
16250 Northland Drive, Suite 120
Southfield, MI 48075
(810) 443-7080

Parent Network for Post-Institutionalized Children
P.O. Box 613
Meadow Lands, PA 15347
(412) 222-1766

The following health-related organizations can provide necessary health information for adoptive families:

Hepatitis B Coalition News
Immunization Action Coalition
1573 Selby Avenue, Suite 234
St. Paul, MN 55104
(612) 647-9009
http://www.immunize.org

B-Informed
Hepatitis B. Foundation
700 East Butler Avenue
Doylestown, PA 18901
(215) 489-4900
http://www2.hepb.org/hepb

Centers for Disease Control and Prevention
Travel and Health Updates
http://www.cdc.gov/travel
http://www.cdc.gov/travel/rx'malar.html (malaria information)
Traveler's hotline: (877) FYI-TRIP
Fax information line: (888) 232-3299
Malaria Hotline: (404) 332-4555

Centers for Disease Control and Prevention, Hepatitis Branch
Mailstop G-37
1600 Clifton Road, NE
Atlanta, GA 30333
(888) 443-7232
http://www.cdc.gov/ncidod/diseases/hepatitis/hepatitis.htm

Adoption/Medical News
2001 "F" Street, NW
Suite 302
Washington, DC 20009

International Adoption Clinic
University of Minnesota Hospital and Clinics
Box 211, 420 Delaware St. SE
Minneapolis, MN 55455
(612) 624-1164
Fax (612) 624-8176

The following publications can provide valuable insights as well:

Barnett, E. D., & Miller, L. C. (1996). *International adoption: The pediatrician's role.* Contemporary Pediatrics, 13, 29–46.
Brodzinsky, D. M., Schechter M. D., & Henig, R. M. (1992). *Being adopted: The lifelong search for self.* New York: Doubleday Books.
Cantor, R., & Cantor, J. (1995). *Special needs schooling: Early intervention years.* Praeger.
Dorris, M. (1989). *The broken cord.* New York: Harper and Row.
Edelstein, S. (1995). *Children with prenatal alcohol and/or other drug exposure: Weighing the risks of adoption.* Los Angeles: CWLA Press.
Hopson, D. P., & Hopson, D. S. (1993). *Raising the rainbow generation: Teaching your children to be successful in a multicultural society.* St. Paul, MN: Adoptive Families of America.
Jewett, C. (1994). *Helping children deal with separation and loss.* The Boston: Harvard Common Press.
Lancaster, K. (1996). *Keys to parenting an adopted child.* New York: Barron's.
Lifton, B. J. (1994). *Journey of the adopted self (A quest for wholeness).* New York: Basic Books.
Melina, L. (1998). *Raising adopted children.* Solstice Press.
Miller, M., & Ward, N. (1996). *With eyes wide open, a workbook for parents adopting international children over age one.* St. Paul: Children's Home Society of MN.
Opening and closing Pandora's box: A manual for child and adolescent health care professionals. New York: Children of Alcoholics Foundation.
Schaffer, J., & Lindstrom, C. (1991). *How to raise an adopted child.* New York: Plume-Penguin.
Streissguth, A. (1997). *Fetal alcohol syndrome: A guide for families and communities.* Paul Brooks Publishing (800-638-3775).
van Gulden, H., & Bartels-Rabb, L. M. (1995). *Real parents, real children: Parenting the adopted child.* Crossroad Publishing Company.

REFERENCES

Adoption in the U.S. *USA Weekend,* February 11, 1996.
Adoption Medical News, Vol II, No.5, Adoption Advocates Press, May 1996.
AIDS and Adoption. (1997). *Adoption Medical News,* 3(3).
American Academy of Pediatrics. (1997). Red Book, Committee on Infectious Diseases (24th ed.). Elk Grove, IL: Author.
Conjeevaram, H. S., & DiBisceglie, A. M. (1995). Management of chronic viral hepatitis in children. *Journal of Pediatric Gastroenterology and Nutrition, 20*(4), 365–375.
Garcia Marquez, G. (1988). *Love in the time of cholera* (p. 165). Penguin Books.
Johnson, D. et al. (1996). Health status of eastern European orphans referred for adoption. *Pediatric Research, 39*(4) part 2, #791.
Johnson, D. E., & Hostetter, M. K. (1996). Medical supervision of internationally adopted children. *Pediatric Basics, 77,* 10–17.
National Committee for Adoption. (1999). *Adoption factbook, III.* Washington, DC: Author.
Schaffer, J., & Lindstrom, M. C. (1991). *How to raise an adopted child.* New York: Plume-Penguin.
Stolley, K. S. (1993). Statistics on Adoption in the United States. *The Future of Children, II,* 24–42.
U.S. Immigrations and Naturalization Service. Immigration Visas Issued to Orphans Coming to the US. (*http://travel.state.gov/orphan'numbers.html*).

The Decision to Breast-feed

• NANCY KAVANAUGH, MS, RN, FNP, IBCLC, and PATRICIA STERNER, MS, RN, IBCLC

INTRODUCTION

Throughout history, most women have breast-fed their infants. As the birthing process moved into the hospital setting and became more sterile, however, mothers were separated from their infants, and medical advice on breast-feeding disappeared. Mothers in industrialized areas, adopting "modern" methods, opted to use well-advertised infant formulas instead of breast milk. Women in suburban and then rural areas followed this decision. By 1971, only 25% of mothers left the hospital breast-feeding their infants, and only 14% continued 2 months postpartum (Martinez & Nalezienski, 1981).

In the 1970s, a surge in breast-feeding promotion occurred, and by 1979, 52% of mothers left the hospital breast-feeding, with 19% continuing 6 months postpartum (Martinez & Nalezienski, 1981). The number of women initially breast-feeding declined from a high in 1982 of 61.9% to an apparent low in 1991 of 51%.

The report *Healthy People 2000*, issued in 1990 by the United States Department of Health and Human Services, stated a goal for 75% of infants to be breast-feeding at hospital discharge, and 50% of infants to continue breast-feeding for 6 months postpartum by the year 2000. This goal has not been met, but between 1988 and 1997, breast-feeding during the early postpartum period increased for all targeted groups. By 1997, the initiation rate had risen to an average of 62% across all categories of women, with 26% continuing through 6 months (NCHS, 1999). Breast-feeding of 5- to 6-month old infants increased somewhat between 1988 and 1996 for all targeted groups, except Native Americans and Alaska Natives (Department of Health and Human Services, 1999).

BREAST-FEEDING PROMOTION

Most women decide how they will feed their babies before conception occurs. Factors that positively influence the success and duration of breast-feeding include support systems (Kessler, Gielen, Diener-West, & Paige, 1995), intended duration (found to be a strong predictor of actual duration; Scott & Binns, 1999), and early initiation (Yamauchi & Yamanouchi, 1990). The number-one reason that mothers stop breast-feeding is the perception that they are producing insufficient breast milk. For some mothers-to-be, the decision not to breast-feed is permanent and unchangeable from before the baby is born.

Positive factors that influence a woman's decision to breast-feed include the following:

- Individual counseling and prenatal education classes (Reifsnider & Eckhart, 1997; Duffy, Percival, & Kershaw, 1997)
- Feeding preference of the significant other and family (Wiemann, DuBois, & Berenson, 1998; Scott & Binns, 1999)
- Higher level of education (Riva et al., 1999; Carbonell, Botet, Figueras, Alvarez, & Riu, 1998)
- Contact with a peer counselor (Schafer, Vogel, Viegas, & Hausafus, 1998; Humphreys, Thompson, & Miner, 1998; Marrow et al., 1999)

Breast-feeding promotion is the process of empowering a woman to believe that she can nourish her infant. Many organizations have come forward to take strong stands in support of breast-feeding. In addition, the provider can discuss with prospective parents the many benefits of breast-feeding for both mother and infant.

Current Recommendations

The current recommendation for breast-feeding from the American Academy of Pediatrics (AAP) is that " human milk is the preferred feeding for all infants, including premature and sick newborns. It is recommended that breast-feeding continue for at least the first 12 months, and thereafter for as long as mutually desired" (AAP, 1997). The AAP further suggests the following:

- Breast-feeding should begin as soon as possible after birth, preferably within the first hour of life.
- Rooming-in for the mother and newborn should be continuous during the postnatal period to facilitate breast-feeding.
- The woman should breast-feed the infant on demand in response to signs of hunger, such as increased alertness or activity, mouthing, or rooting. She should not use the infant's crying as an indicator to nurse.
- The woman should refrain from giving supplements, such as formula or water, to breast-feeding newborns unless medically indicated.
- The woman should express human milk when direct breast-feeding is not possible.
- Breast-feeding should be exclusive for about the first 6 months after birth, after which time the woman can add iron-enriched solid foods to complement the breast milk diet.
- A trained observer should formally evaluate and document breast-feeding performance during the first 24 to 48 hours following delivery and again at a follow-up visit 48 to 72 hours after discharge (AAP, 1997).

The position of the American Dietetic Association (ADA) is as follows:

Public health and clinical efforts to promote breast-feeding should be sustained and strengthened. ADA strongly encourages the promotion and advocacy of activities that support longer duration of successful breast-feeding, in order to optimize the indisputable nutritional, immunological, psychological, and economic benefits. The establishment of breast-feeding for at least six months, but optimally for at least one year, as a cultural norm supported by medical, social, and economic practices is a fundamental cornerstone of true promotion of wellness (position of the ADA: Promotion of breast-feeding, Adopted by the House of Delegates, March 16, 1997).

The Association of Women's Health, Obstetric and Neonatal Nurses (AWHONN) supports breast-feeding as the optimal method of infant feeding. In its position paper, AWHONN states its commitment to work

in support of the Healthy People 2000 initiative to raise the initiation of breast-feeding to 75% and the six-month rate of breast-feeding to 50%.... AWHONN recognizes that cultural beliefs and values may influence the choice to breast-feed; therefore, health care providers should integrate culturally sensitive information into all aspects of breast-feeding promotion" (AWHONN Position Statement, 1995).

To promote breast-feeding further, the World Health Assembly adopted the WHO/UNICEF International Code of Marketing of Breastmilk Substitutes in 1981 to ensure safe and adequate nutrition by protecting and promoting breast-feeding. The Code prohibits all promotion of bottle feeding and establishes requirements for labeling and information on infant feeding (Resolution WHA34.22).

Clinicians should be aware that baby food companies may not do any of the following:

- Promote their products in hospitals, shops, or to the general public
- Give free samples to mothers or free or subsidized supplies to hospitals or maternity wards
- Give gifts to health workers or mothers
- Promote their products to health workers (Any information that companies provide must contain only scientific facts.)
- Promote foods or drinks for babies
- Give misleading information

The Baby Friendly Hospital Initiative

In 1991, WHO and UNICEF launched The Baby Friendly Hospital Initiative, a global program designed to protect, promote, and support breast-feeding in the birth setting. "Ten Steps to Successful Breast-feeding," published in 1989, is the centerpiece of this initiative and is based on scientific and clinical research data. It was modeled after Wellstart International Model Hospital Breastfeeding Policies (Powers, Naylor, & Wester, 1994). The designation "Baby Friendly" identifies facilities that have established optimal lactation management for the nursing dyad. In 1997, Baby Friendly USA was started with the sole mission of promoting the Baby Friendly program in the United States. The following statement is from a joint WHO/UNICEF document published in 1989:

Every facility providing maternity services and care for newborn infants should support the following ten steps to successful breast-feeding:

1. Have a written breast-feeding policy that is routinely communicated to all health care staff.

2. Train all health care staff in skills necessary to implement this policy.
3. Inform all pregnant women about the benefits and management of breast-feeding.
4. Help mothers initiate breast-feeding within a half-hour of birth.
5. Show mothers how to breast-feed, and how to maintain lactation even if they should be separated from their infants.
6. Give newborn infants no food or drink other than breast milk, unless medically indicated.
7. Practice rooming-in: allow mothers and infants to remain together 24 hours a day.
8. Encourage breast-feeding on demand.
9. Give no artificial teats or pacifiers (also called dummies or soothers) to breast-feeding infants.
10. Foster the establishment of breast-feeding support groups and refer mothers to them on discharge from the hospital or clinic.

Participants at the WHO/UNICEF policymakers' meeting on "Breastfeeding in the 1990s: A Global Initiative" adopted the Innocenti Declaration in 1990. The declaration stated that all women should "be enabled to practice exclusive breast-feeding and all infants should be fed exclusively on breast milk from birth to 4–6 months of age."

Benefits to the Mother

The following are benefits of breast-feeding to the mother that providers should discuss with women who plan to become or are pregnant:

- Breast-feeding protects against breast and ovarian cancers (Romieu, Hernandez-Avila, Lazcano, Lopez, & Romero-Jaime, 1996; Stuver, Hsieh, Bectove, & Trichopoulos, 1997).
- Exclusive nursing (only) delays the return of the menstrual cycle (Labbok et al., 1997).
- Breast-feeding requires no shopping, preparing, cleaning up, or sterilizing.
- The mother is able to bond closely with the infant (Uvnas-Moberg & Erikson, 1996).
- Breast-feeding is economical (Heinig, 1998; Ball & Wright, 1999).
- Breast-feeding empowers the woman (Kavanaugh, Meier, & Zimmerman, 1997).
- Women who breast-feed have a lower risk of postpartum hemorrhage.
- Breast-feeding provides an antistress effect (Uvnas-Moberg, 1998).

Benefits to the Baby

The following are benefits of breast-feeding to the baby that providers should discuss with women who plan to become or are pregnant:

- Breast-feeding protects against gastrointestinal (GI) infection and diarrheal disease (Beaudry, Dufour, & Marcuox, 1995; Dewey, Heinig, & Nommsen-Rivers, 1995).
- Breast-fed infants have a lower risk of developing necrotizing enterocolitis (Convert et al., 1995; Bernt & Walker, 1999).
- Breast-feeding protects against otitis media (Aniansson et al., 1994).
- Breast-feeding enhances the immune response (Pabst et al., 1997; Ellis, Mastro, & Picciano, 1997; Hanson, 1998).

- Breast-feeding enhances vaccine responses (Lteif & Schwenk, 1998).
- Breast-feeding protects against *Haemophilus influenzae* (Silverdal et al., 1997).
- Breast-feeding protects against childhood cancers (Shu et al., 1995).
- Breast-fed infants have a lower risk of heart disease in later life (Routi et al., 1995).
- Breast-feeding protects against respiratory infections (Wright, Holberg, Taussig, & Martinez, 1995; Cushing et al., 1998).
- Breast-feeding enhances neurologic and cognitive development (Wang & Wu, 1996; Horwood & Ferguson, 1998).
- Infants who are breast-fed have a decreased incidence of allergies (Saarinen & Kajosaari, 1995).

ANATOMY AND PHYSIOLOGY OF LACTATION

The breasts or mammary glands are exocrine glands that store their secretions extracellularly. The mammary glands go through numerous changes during pregnancy to prepare for the infant's arrival. By 16 weeks' gestation, the breasts are capable of full lactation (Lawrence & Lawrence, 1999).

Hormonal Influences

Estrogen, progesterone, and prolactin contribute to lobular tissue and duct growth and proliferation. After birth, estrogen and progesterone levels fall dramatically, but prolactin levels remain high. The fall of plasma progesterone initiates lactation. Retained uterine placental tissue can delay or reduce milk production.

During pregnancy, prolactin, which also is essential for the synthesis and secretion of human milk, rises. It drops slightly before birth, and then rises again when the infant suckles at the breast. When stimulated, the sensory nerve endings of the nipple and areola send messages to the hypothalamus and anterior pituitary, which in turn stimulate the release of prolactin. Prolactin surges are very important in the early weeks of milk production. In later weeks, the infant's consumption of milk from the breasts regulates milk production. Prolactin levels are highest at night. They also are higher when a woman is feeding multiple infants or using a pump with two collection containers to release milk from both breasts at the same time. Maternal serum prolactin levels remain high if more than eight feedings occur in 24 hours (Cox, Owens, & Hartman, 1996).

Oxytocin is another essential hormone in breast-feeding. Stimulation of the nipple and areola by the baby's suckling releases oxytocin from the posterior pituitary gland. Myoepithelial cells that surround the alveoli, where the milk is synthesized, respond to oxytocin by contracting and ejecting milk into the ductules and ducts to the lactiferous sinuses so the infant can receive the milk. Oxytocin also may be released when the mother sees, smells, hears, or touches her baby (Newton, 1992). Placing the mother and baby skin to skin right after delivery also elevates oxytocin (Nissen, Lilja, Widstrom, Uvnas-Moberg, 1995). Prolactin, on the other hand, only is released by nipple or breast stimulation.

Human Milk

Human milk is a species-specific, live fluid that changes in composition with each feeding and from day to day.

Lawrence & Lawrence (1999) note that milk contains more than 200 constituents. The milk at the beginning of a feeding differs from the milk at the end. Milk composition also depends on the mother's diet and her own individual variations. Volume varies at different times of the day. Unless the mother is severely malnourished, however, the mother's nutritional status does not appear to affect milk volume.

Colostrum

Colostrum is present at birth. For 1 to 5 days postpartum, the breasts secrete this thick, yellow fluid. Colostrum is higher in protein and lower in fat and carbohydrates than are transitional milk and mature milk. It contains high levels of immunoglobulins, especially immunoglobulin A (IgA), which "is the most important immunoglobulin in milk, not only in concentration but in biologic activity" (Lawrence & Lawrence, 1999). A "mucosa-protecting non-inflammatogenic secretory immunoglobulin," IgA protects against *Vibrio cholerae*, enterotoxogenic *E. coli*, *Campylobacter*, *Shigella*, and *Giardia liamblia*, to name a few pathogens (Hanson, 1998). Maternal malnutrition affects immunoglobulin concentrations.

Colostrum also contains high levels of the iron-binding protein lactoferrin, which is known to have a bacteriostatic effect on many organisms. Colostrum helps with the passage of meconium and with the establishment of *Lactobacillus bifidus* flora, which inhibits certain pathogenic bacteria in the gut. Vitamin E, an antioxidant that helps protect lung tissue and the eyes, is two to three times higher in colostrum than in mature breast milk (Lawrence & Lawrence, 1999). Sodium is higher in colostrum than in mature milk. Sodium that remains high in mature milk may indicate lactation problems. Colostrum has a mean energy of 67 kcal/dL, whereas mature milk has 75 kcal/dL (Lawrence & Lawrence, 1999).

Transitional Milk

Transitional milk is produced between the colostrum and mature milk stages. It gradually changes to mature milk from 7 days to 2 weeks postpartum. Immunoglobulin levels, total protein, and fat-soluble vitamins decrease. Lactose, fats, and water-soluble vitamins increase. Milk prolactin is high in transitional milk and then declines steadily throughout the breast-feeding duration.

Mature Milk

Mature milk is made up of mostly water and about 10% solids. The water is important for the infant's temperature regulation. Breast-feeding infants in hot climates do not require supplemental water, because breast milk meets their water requirement needs.

Lipids provide a good source of energy. They make up about 50% of the calories in mature human breast milk and about 3% to 5% of total milk composition (Lawrence & Lawrence, 1999). The total fat content usually increases during a feeding and with the stage of lactation. The baby's gestational age at birth and the mother's diet and diurnal rhythm impact the lipid content. Ninety-eight to 99% of the fat in milk is made up of triglycerides that are broken down into fatty acids, which the intestines absorb easily. Unsaturated fatty acids and monoglycerides inactivate lipid-enveloped viruses, such as herpes simplex, Semliki Forest, and influenza. Breast milk is an important source of long chain polyunsaturated fatty acids, which are considered very important for brain development. DHA, one essential fatty acid found in breast milk, is essential to visual development and may be especially important to preterm infants and the development of visual acuity and retinal responses to light (Carlson, 1999).

Adrenocorticotropic hormone (ACTH), a peptide hormone that can cross the intestinal barrier, is found in breast milk. ACTH influences the production of cortisol, a hormone that induces change in the microvillus membrane in the intestine, which in turn favors the colonization of nonpathogenic microbes in the gut. Cortisol also helps the intestinal barrier mature, which is important because the primary cause of necrotizing enterocolitis is an immature intestinal barrier (Bernt & Walker, 1999).

Growth hormone (GH), found in milk, may help GI tract function. GH also may play a role in preventing or delaying GI allergies. Nucleotides and their derivatives, which appear in higher concentrations in human milk than in cow's milk–based formula, appear to have significant effects on the immune and GI systems (Carver, 1999).

Lactose, the most abundant carbohydrate found in human milk (about 7 gm/dL), is synthesized in the mammary gland. Lactose easily breaks down into simple sugars, essential for providing accessible energy for the infant. Other carbohydrates found in small amounts include peptides, monosaccharides, and more than 80 neutral and acid oligosaccharides. The functions of the oligosaccharides are not understood fully, but they do play an important role in enhancing defenses against viruses, bacteria, and their toxins (Coppa et al., 1999). They also have a role in promoting the growth of bifidogen flora and indirectly providing protection against GI infections in newborns.

Human milk proteins constitute 0.9% of breast milk. Breast milk has a ratio of 40:60 of casein/whey protein. Casein in human milk forms soft, easily digested curds. When whey (mainly alphalactabumin and lactoferrin) is taken into the stomach, it also forms soft, easily digested curds. In later lactation, the ratio of casein to whey is 50:50 (Lawrence & Lawrence, 1999). Many other components in human breast milk support the newborn nutritionally and provide immunologic, anti-inflammatory, and antiallergic properties that promote optimal health in the infant.

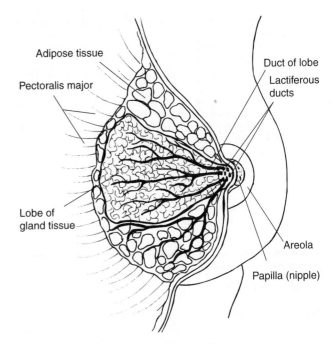

Figure 7–1 ■ Anatomy of breasts.

PRENATAL BREAST ASSESSMENT

Breast examination is a routine component of the initial antepartum examination during the first prenatal appointment (Fig. 7-1). At this time, the primary care provider has an opportunity to discuss breast-feeding and examine the breast for potential problems in breast function or anticipated latch-on difficulties (Table 7-1). It is recommended to repeat this examination at 28 weeks.

Size and symmetry of the breasts have little impact on milk production. The provider looks to ensure that the breasts have increased in size (even slightly) and that a venous pattern appears over the breasts. Wide spacing (greater than 2 inches between breasts), narrow tubular shape, and breasts that only cover two rib spaces are potential indicators of low future supply (Huggins, 1999). Qualities that facilitate latch-on are protractility and compressibility of the nipple and areolar tissue. The provider performs the pinch test on each breast, compressing the breast between the first two fingers, and placing the thumb behind the areola. When compressing the tissue, the provider observes the nipple. The normal nipple appears everted during compression. Underlying adhesions can retract or invert a nipple. A retracted nipple appears to be pulled back at the

base or edges. An inverted nipple appears folded in from the center. The clinician also assesses the breasts for previous surgeries and resultant interruption of ducts. The provider looks closely at the areolar border, which is a popular site for insertion/removal of implants, excision of cysts, and correction of nipple inversion. If augmentation has been performed, the provider asks the patient about the appearance of the breasts before the surgery. Recent nipple inversion, change in skin texture, and marked asymmetry may be signs of carcinoma and require follow-up (Petok, 1995).

THE DELIVERY ROOM EXPERIENCE

Research has shown that events in the delivery room have major effects on the success and duration of breast-feeding. Health care professionals should emphasize the importance of skin-to-skin contact during this critical time. The mother may request that her delivery attendant place the newborn on her bare skin, rather than on her gown or sterile drapes. Providers can dry, suction, and assess the newborn while the baby is on the mother's abdomen. They can perform the common delivery room routines of taking footprints, applying bracelets, and performing eye prophylaxis while the infant is in the mother's arms or delay these procedures until the mother has had time to enjoy skin-to-skin contact and nurse her baby. Prolonged holding of the newborn accustoms the mother to handling her baby. It also gives her the opportunity to keep the newborn near her breast and observe for feeding cues.

Initiation of Breast-feeding

In the first hour after delivery, newborns tend to be very alert and awake. They generally are eager to nurse, provided the mother did not receive narcotics during labor. Many believe

Table 7-1.   BREAST-FEEDING: BREAST ASSESSMENT

Finding	Potential Problem	Plan
Dense areola	Difficult latch on	Wear shells between feedings.
		Pump before latch on.
Retracted or inverted nipple	Difficult latch on	Wear shells between feedings.
		Perform Hoffman technique four to six times per day.
		Pump before latch on.
		Fully pump after feeding.
		Attempt to develop milk supply and to provide milk to baby if not latching well or at all.
Wide-set breasts	Potential for low supply	Conduct early follow-up after delivery.
		Pump after feeding to encourage her supply 5 minutes on each breast.
No breast enlargement during pregnancy	Potential for low supply	Conduct early follow-up after delivery.
		Pump after feeding to encourage her supply, 5 minutes each breast.
Reduction surgery	Potential for low supply	Conduct early follow-up after delivery.
		Apply ice packs to breasts as needed to relieve fullness from milk that cannot move out of the breasts. If the baby is supplemented, the mother pumps after feeding to encourage her supply.

that a long administered epidural with fentanyl as an additive sedates the newborn as well as the mother (Hale, 1999) due to fentanyl's long half-life. If the newborn does not show feeding cues, provider and mother should focus on socializing the newborn to the breast. Discussion of positioning and latch-on techniques can take place later, when the mother is better able to sit up and handle her newborn. If a newborn does not latch on in the delivery room, providers can teach hand expression to the mother so that the infant can taste the colostrum, and the woman can stimulate her breast. Viewing colostrum as it is expressed from the breast is a very powerful moment for the new mother and her partner or family. It validates that the breast will work, that something really is there, and that the baby will not starve if unsupplemented.

If delivery has been by cesarean section, providers should assist the mother to breast-feed her newborn in the recovery room. Most of these mothers need extra assistance unwrapping the newborn for skin-to-skin contact and positioning the baby at the breast. After the mother has had the opportunity to take in the birth experience, emphasis shifts from bonding and skin-to-skin contact to correct positioning and latch-on techniques and frequent offering of the breast.

Mechanism of Sucking

The infant is born with a sucking reflex. To assess this reflex, the practitioner places a finger in the infant's mouth with the pad of the finger against the palate. As the infant sucks, the provider can feel where the tongue places against the finger as it moves through the suck cycle. The tongue extends beyond the lower gum line and cups the finger. The end of the tongue presses against the joint of the finger and the pressure moves along the tongue like a wave as the infant retracts the tongue into the mouth. This mechanism of suck can change when an infant is fed with a bottle. On digital examination, the bottle-fed infant no longer extends the tongue. The tongue remains in the mouth and the back of the tongue presses up and down during the suck cycle. Imagine that the tongue is closing and opening the end of the rubber nipple to control the flow of the bottle. This change in suck reflects a preference for the easier mechanism, which is bot-

tle feeding. When an infant has this suck preference, yet the mother wants to breast-feed, the breast-feeding becomes most difficult.

COMMON CONCERNS RELATED TO BREAST-FEEDING

In North American society, many women grow up never having seen another woman breast-feed. It is much harder to do something that one has never viewed. The following are common and important topics that providers should discuss with breast-feeding women.

Positioning

Two positions are easiest to use in the first weeks of breast-feeding: transitional position (also called cross-cradle) (Fig. 7-2) and football position (Fig. 7-3). After the mother masters these positions and latch-on technique is good and consistent, then she can use any position she wants, for she will have established her newborn at the breast.

Transitional Position

The following are the steps in transitional positioning for breast-feeding:

1. Place one pillow behind the mother's back and one on her lap. Nursing pillows that wrap around the mother's body are very helpful because they do not slip out and fall off her lap. If the mother is nursing twins or multiples, larger foam wrap-around pillows are available.
2. Place the baby very close to the mother's body, tummy to tummy. Her elbow holds the baby close to her body.
3. The mother grips the baby's head firmly behind the ears with the first two fingers and thumb.
4. Instruct the mother to sandwich the breast at midbreast, holding the hand in a "u" shape under the breast. She holds the hand in place, but relaxes it during the feeding.

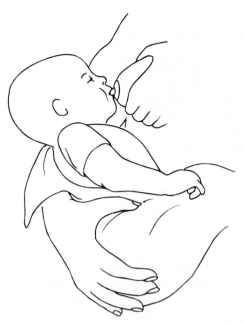

Figure 7–2 ■ Example of transitional position for breast-feeding.

After breast-feeding is established, she can remove the hand after the initial latch on.

5. The mother slowly taps the nipple on the baby's lower lip. *The mother should wait for a wide open mouth.*
6. Quickly and firmly, the woman presses the baby's shoulders to the breast using pressure from the heel of her hand. She centers the nipple during this process. (She presses the baby quickly to the breast because as the baby feels something crossing over the lower lip, the baby clamps down. If the mother has moved slowly, then the baby will have latched onto the tip of the nipple.)

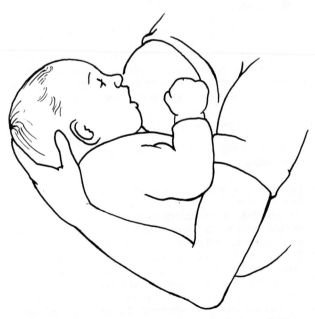

Figure 7–3 ■ Example of football hold position for breast-feeding.

7. The baby's head should be in a "sniff" position at the breast, with the chin and cheeks buried into and the nose just touching the breast. The mother should not have to retract breast tissue from the baby's nose area. If the nose is too close to the breast, the woman is placing too much pressure on the baby's head and should transfer more pressure to the shoulders, allowing the head to lean back. She should keep a two-finger space beneath the chin. It may be helpful to instruct the mother to aim the baby's chin into the breast, allowing it to touch first as the baby is pressed to the breast.

Football Hold

The following are the steps for positioning for the football hold for breast-feeding:

1. Place two pillows behind the mother's back and stack two pillows next to her. If she is in an armchair, then stuff one pillow next to her in the armchair. The space behind her back is very important; this is where the baby's body will be. If she is using a circular pillow, then pull it around to her side, and place a pillow behind her back as well.
2. Place the baby on the back very close to the mother's body. Slide the baby back until the baby's chin is just behind the mother's nipple. The mother places her breast on top of the baby's chest.
3. Describe to the mother that the baby is like a clutch bag on the rush hour train. She places her wrist under the baby's back, and grips the baby's head from behind the ears. She holds the baby close to her body with her forearm and elbow.
4. The mother places her hand under the breast, flattening her fingers against the breast with the thumb on top. She sandwiches the breast for the latch on and holds the hand in place, but relaxes it during the feeding. After breast-feeding is established, she can remove the hand after the initial latch on.
5. She slowly taps the nipple on the baby's lower lip. *The mother should wait for a wide open mouth.*
6. Quickly and firmly, the mother presses the baby to the breast, using pressure from the heel of her hand on the baby's shoulders.
7. The baby's nose just touches the breast; the chin and cheeks are buried into the breast tissue. The mother uses her wrist to adjust the baby's head.
8. Look for the space under the chin.

Latching on

Incorrect latch on to the breast is the number-one cause of nipple soreness. Nipple soreness in turn contributes to a mother's decision to supplement or wean. Many women imagine that the newborn will instinctively know how to breastfeed and latch on correctly and that their job will be merely to hold their newborns near the breast. Latch on to the breast, however, is a learned skill that the mother must teach the infant. The infant will develop a preference for how the mother teaches latch on. Shallow latch is incorrect and will influence the infant to prefer only a small amount of the breast in his or her mouth. The longer the infant is allowed to latch on incorrectly, the more difficult it will be to change this pattern. In the early weeks of feeding, a shallow latch on may be indicated by prolonged, frequent feedings.

When the infant latches on, nipple placement in the infant's mouth should be where the hard and soft palates

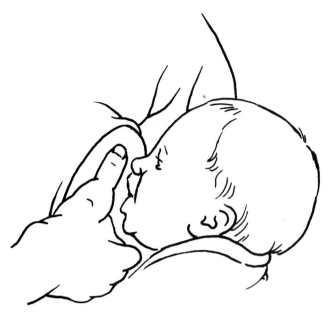

Figure 7–4 ■ Correct latch-on.

meet (Fig. 7-4). Pressure in this area of the mouth stimulates the palate and sucking reflex. Ideally, as infants grasp the nipple and areola, they draw the tissue into the mouth, forming a teat. Some infants are better able to do this than others. The emphasis is on depth. If the mother has a wide, rounded breast or a short nipple, deep latch on becomes more difficult. The mother may need to compensate by pressing the infant more firmly to the breast during latch on. If the mother has a very long nipple, she also must press more firmly, because the infant must reach the lactiferous sinuses, the ducts located beneath the areola. The infant must cover approximately a half-inch depth of the areola.

When a baby is latched onto the breast correctly, the mother may feel some discomfort as the baby begins suckling. This discomfort should disappear within 30 to 60 seconds. The baby begins with a rapid suckling pattern that helps to elicit the milk ejection reflex. As the milk fills the lactiferous sinuses, the baby's suckling pattern changes to suck-swallow. The swallow sounds like a short forced breath. During the feeding, milk volume decreases and the baby's suckling pattern changes. The baby takes more and more sucks before swallowing. It is best to allow the baby to end the session at the breast. The baby may fall asleep at the breast. Ideally, the baby lets go of the breast. Feedings are never timed. The mother should watch the baby, not the clock. When a baby is hungry, the baby demonstrates feeding cues, such as hand to mouth activity, hands held in fists, and rooting. As the baby becomes satiated, the hands open and fall away from the face. At the end of a feeding, the baby's hands should be open and held at sides, with the baby relaxed.

Breast Shells and the Hoffman Technique

Breast shells are plastic domes that pregnant women begin to wear inside the bra usually at the end of the second trimester. Women gradually build up to wearing them all day and evening. Inside the dome is an opening that fits over the nipple and places pressure on its base. Breast shells are used to improve problems of nipple inversion, nipple retraction, and dense areola. They also are helpful when a mother is engorged, because they soften the areola and facilitate latch on. Breast shells sometimes are confused with nipple shields, a rubber or silicone nipple shape that is placed over the mother's nipple and areola. The shield has small holes in it, through which the baby latches onto and suckles. The problem with nipple shields is that they decrease stimulation of the areola and therefore lower prolactin levels, subsequently decreasing the mother's milk supply. The baby often develops a preference for the shield and may then refuse the breast. In special cases, some professionals briefly use shields as a last resort. If a breast shield is used for infant feeding, the mother–infant couple requires close follow-up and weekly weight checks of the infant.

The Hoffman technique also may be prescribed. Hoffman (1953) suggested a nipple exercise for the treatment of nipple inversion. The mother places a finger from each hand on either side of the areola. She gently presses inward and pulls fingers away from the nipple. She repeats this several times vertically and then horizontally. The woman performs this exercise three to four times each day starting at 36 weeks.

Foremilk Versus Hind Milk

Woolridge and Fisher (1988) describe milk composition during the course of a feeding. The foremilk is low in calories and high in volume, quenching the baby's initial thirst. As the feeding progresses, the volume decreases, and the fat and calorie count increase. The hind milk, which comes from the breast last, is high in calories and fat and low in volume. Mothers frequently question how long it will take for the baby to get to the hind milk. No research is available on the timing of hind milk. Each baby will feed at his or her own rate, and the mother may eject milk at her own rate. Hence the reasoning for allowing the baby to lead, feeding on the first breast until finished. If the baby wants to nurse on the second breast, the mother switches the baby over. If the baby is satiated, the second breast is for later. This pattern of one breast per feeding may be a preferred management technique for certain problems.

The foremilk also is high in sugars. When a baby nurses for a short time on both breasts at each feeding, the baby may get a lot of foremilk, but little hind milk. This high-sugar, low-fat mix causes loose green stools and GI discomfort. A mother with a copious milk supply may inadvertently have this same dilemma. The solution is to nurse the baby on one breast per feeding. Doing so will increase the milk's fat content and somewhat slow the mother's supply. As the mother transitions to this pattern, she may need to pump a small amount of milk from the second breast to be comfortable until the next feeding. She should decrease the amount that she pumps gradually. The provider should reassure the mother that her body will regulate itself to this pattern.

Basic Nipple Care

After feeding, the woman should hand express some colostrum or milk and apply it to her nipple and areola. She should then air dry the breast for 10 to 15 minutes. These measures are considered preventive and also healing for nipple soreness. Application of wet tea bags, warm saline soaks, warm water compresses, and USP-modified lanolin after feeding also are reported to relieve nipple pain (Lavergne, 1997; Buchko et al., 1994). A recent trend is the use of hydrogel pads, which women wear between feedings.

Growth Spurts

A growth spurt is a sudden change in the nursing pattern, created by the infant's need for more milk. Growth spurts can happen at any time but are expected at 3 and 6 weeks and at 3, 6, and 9 months. (Some infants experience one at 2 weeks as well.) The nursing pattern of a growth spurt often is described as increased frequency but shorter duration of feeding. The mother may complain of being up all night, nursing constantly all day, being overwhelmed, or suddenly losing her milk supply. Growth spurts commonly last 1 to 2 days. Appropriate interventions are to reassure the mother that this pattern is normal and to encourage her to eat, drink, and rest well.

Pumping

Expressing milk from the breast to feed in a bottle to the infant is discouraged for the first 2 to 3 weeks so that the newborn has an opportunity to learn to breast-feed well first. The newborn uses a different sucking action on the breast than on the bottle nipple. Early introduction of bottles and pacifiers is linked with breast-feeding difficulties and early weaning. Windows exist between 2 to 3 weeks and at 6 weeks in which the mother may use one bottle of expressed milk per day so that the infant also will learn to take a bottle. If the mother waits beyond 6 weeks to introduce a bottle, her baby may then refuse to take it, preferring the breast. Some mothers are able to exclusively nurse their infants throughout the first year, choosing not to use bottles at all.

The provider instructs the mother to wait until feeding time draws near and then to express the milk from her breasts and place it in a bottle. It is best when several family members as well as the mother offer bottles so that the infant learns that food comes from others as well. A most important concept for the mother to understand is that everyday her body produces the same amount of milk, give or take an ounce. Many women fail to grasp this concept, which is the source of many breast-feeding difficulties. If the mother pumps and then stores several ounces of milk from her breast, and this is not her normal routine, the baby will be deprived of that food. If the mother gives the baby artificial milk and therefore skips a feeding, milk that does not belong in the breast will remain. This can lead to plugged ducts or, over time, a decreased milk supply (Humenick & Van Steenkiste, 1983). The number-one reason women stop breast-feeding is lack of confidence in their milk supply. Formula company gifts emphasize this message. When maternity wards distribute formula on discharge, women receive a subtle message that they will not produce enough to feed their children adequately. Studies show that if a new mother has formula in her home after discharge from the hospital birthing center, she will use it. She will also go on to purchase that same brand.

Stockpiling

Stockpiling extra milk in the freezer gives the new mother flexibility, enhances her feelings about her milk supply, and prepares her to return to school or work if she chooses. The provider should instruct the mother to pump after a morning feeding because the mother has higher prolactin levels overnight and her supply is enhanced at this time of day. Pumping extra milk at the same time every day is best, because the body has an internal clock and can be trained to pick up production at this time.

Instructions to give to the mother are as follows:

- Pump 1 oz/d for 2 to 3 days, then increase.
- Pump 2 oz/d for 2 to 3 days, then increase.
- Pump 3 oz/d for 2 to 3 days and so forth.

Women's individual responses will vary. Some are barely able to get to 3 oz; others are able to store 5 to 7 oz/d in this manner. They store milk in the freezer for future use. Placing small containers of milk in a large plastic freezer bag further protects the milk from freezer damage. If she takes milk from the freezer for use, the mother must pump and replace this milk. The clinician should remind the mother about growth spurts.

Returning to Work

The number of women in the workforce who have small children is growing. Mothers who work part time report greatest satisfaction. Health care providers have an opportunity to encourage new mothers to continue breast-feeding after they return to work. Employers are beginning to recognize the unique needs of the pumping employee, and some provide special rooms or breast pumps as a benefit. Arrangements work best when a mother returns to work part time for several weeks or, if this option is not available, returns to work for 1 or 2 days only before having a day off. In this way, the mother can rectify any difficulties she may be experiencing with pumping, child care, or coordination of her new routine. The emphasis is on stockpiling as much milk as possible before returning to work. The only necessary preparation is a mother who is comfortable using a breast pump and a baby who can take a bottle. There is no need to rehearse the work schedule for days or weeks.

Weaning

The decision to wean may be sudden or planned. When sudden, as a result of difficulty with lactation or dissatisfaction with the nursing experience, the patient will find it therapeutic to explore the difficulties she is facing. Unrealistic expectations of the birth experience and the immediate postpartum period often contribute to dissatisfaction with breastfeeding. Very often, the needed intervention is validation that it is normal to feel overwhelmed, need a nap every day, have crying episodes, feel disappointed about her experience, or not feel immediate love for the baby. This validation empowers the new mother and helps her to realize that she is normal. She might then continue breastfeeding a little longer. Mothers often report specific points over the first 8 weeks at which they feel better physically and emotionally: 3 weeks, 6 weeks, and 8 weeks.

Sudden weaning, often referred to as "cold turkey," is not recommended, because it is exquisitely painful. If the baby is younger than 6 months and is to be weaned onto formula, the mother should add 1 oz of formula per day, thereby decreasing her breast milk supply by 1 oz/d. If she begins to experience uncomfortable fullness, she can level off for a day or two and then continue to decrease. Dropping an entire feeding at a time is not recommended; doing so may leave 4 to 8 oz of breast milk in the breasts that do not belong there. This certainly is uncomfortable and may lead to plugged ducts. If the mother is unable physically or emotionally to continue to breast-feed during weaning, she can pump down her supply. In this process, the mother pumps every 3 to 4 hours and measures all milk for 24 hours to determine her supply level. She then continues to pump each day but decreases the amount pumped over 24 hours by an ounce or two each day. She also spaces the number of hours between pumpings. Very often the mother will underestimate her body's ability to produce milk. In the last days of weaning, pumping or feeding every other day for a week works best. Mothers often report a lump or plugged duct in the first weeks after their babies have weaned completely. Applying ice and taking ibuprofen are appropriate interventions.

If a baby is older than 6 months and has started solids, the weaning experience is different. This scenario may be considered the natural process of weaning, as the woman continually adds solids as complementary foods to the breast-feeding diet, but continues breast-feeding through 12 months. If the mother plans to discontinue breast-feeding, she adds formula to the diet with solids, and the formula complements the solids through 12 months. The provider discusses with the mother the infant's ability to take adequate amounts of formula from a cup or bottle before she begins weaning the baby. The mother offers solids before instead of after the breast (which is the preferred pattern if the mother is continuing to breast-feed). After establishing this pattern, the woman increases the amount of formula she adds to the diet by 1 oz/d.

Weaning a toddler is accomplished by distracting the toddler from the normal routine of predicted nursing times, delaying feedings, and offering alternatives. In this way, the milk supply decreases gradually, and the toddler loses interest. In many countries, the norm is to continue breastfeeding for 2 to 4 years. Mothers of nursing toddlers may feel intense social pressure to wean when they are not ready to do so. Discussion of the motivation to wean is important. If the mother is ambivalent, the provider should encourage her to continue to breastfeed until she feels certain that the timing is right. The goal of health care providers is to encourage mothers to breast-feed for as long as possible. More breast milk over a longer period provides increased health benefits to both the mother and baby.

Maintaining Supply

Providers can suggest many methods that mothers can use to maintain their milk supply:

- Discuss how precious breast milk is and how difficult it is to provide extra. The woman should defrost or warm only the amount the baby needs.
- Provide caregivers with a log to record the amount of breast milk the baby takes during the workday.
- At the end of each day, the mother should compare the amount she used for the baby and the amount pumped. These amounts should be equal. If the baby has used more milk than the mother has pumped, then the mother should try to pump after feeding the baby at home to make up the difference. This attention to detail is most important in maintaining her supply.
- Before leaving in the morning, the mother pumps just after she feeds the baby so that she will be comfortable longer, leave more milk for the baby, and need less pumping time at work. A time saver is to nurse the baby on one breast while simultaneously placing a quiet electric pump on the other breast.
- The longer the mother's workday is, the more times she should pump at work. Some mothers are able to pump

at work only once, with a pump before and after her workday at home.
- If the mother's supply tends to dip at the end of the week, extra nursing over days off will help to improve the supply.
- While pumping at work, looking at the baby's picture, massaging the breast, and performing deep breathing exercises (such as Lamaze) will improve the woman's response to the pump.

For mothers who are unable to pump at work, pumping after or during most feedings at home will maximize the milk supply, necessitating only minimal use of formula. The woman practices this routine at home for several weeks, gradually shifting the milk supply from the working hours by increasing what she pumps during "home time."

COMMON CONDITIONS RELATED TO BREAST-FEEDING

Mastitis

Mastitis, an inflammation of the breast, is a common condition, occurring in 20% to 33% of breast-feeding women (Amir, Harris, & Andriske, 1999). Although it can occur anytime, including in women who have never been pregnant, mastitis occurs most frequently during the second or third week postpartum (Inch & Fisher, 1997). Mastitis often follows an oversupply or inadequate drainage of milk (Amir et al., 1999). If the woman does not transfer milk to the baby or pump it, the duct may become obstructed, resulting in a small, hard, warm, tender lump. Within about 12 to 24 hours, the internal ducts and ductules become inflamed, and the breast becomes swollen, hard, tender, and hot. If the obstructed duct is not treated, "infectious mastitis" follows "inflammatory mastitis" within 24 to 48 hours (Amir et al., 1999).

Thomsen, Espersen, and Maigarrd (1984) identified three clinical states of human milk: milk stasis, noninfectious inflammation, and infectious mastitis. Milk stasis was identified by $<10^6$ leukocytes and $<10^3$ bacteria/mL of milk. In noninfectious inflammation, breast milk had $>10^6$ leukocytes and $<10^3$ bacteria/mL. Infectious mastitis had $>10^6$ leukocytes and $>10^3$ bacteria/mL of milk. The current definition of mastitis includes fever of 101.3°F or more, chills, flulike aching, systemic illness, and pink, tender, hot, swollen, wedge-shaped area of the breast (Lawrence & Lawrence, 1999). In light of the literature, Amir et al. (1999) recommend a reexamination of the minimum level of fever in favor of 100°F.

Causes

Breast milk stasis caused by infrequent or missed feedings, skipped night feedings, tight clothing, or abrupt weaning can result in inflamed tissue. The body produces approximately the same amount of milk every day. An overabundant milk supply or an infant with a short frenulum also may cause milk stasis. The built-up milk can leak from the distended alveoli into surrounding tissue and bloodstream. Bacteria, usually *Staphylococcus aureus*, infects the inflamed tissue. *Escherichia coli*, *Streptococcus*, and other pathogens also can be responsible. Many people have small amounts of *S. aureus* on their skin. When a woman's nipple is cracked or cut, bacteria have a direct route into the ductile system. An exhausted and stressed mother also is at risk for developing mastitis.

Prevention

The provider should encourage the mother to position the baby at the breast carefully to avoid traumatizing the nipples. The provider should advise her to rest when possible, drink plenty of fluids, and eat a well balanced diet. She should feed the baby frequently and regularly, which includes night feeding. She should avoid early bottle and pacifier use (Walker, 1999). If the mother is weaning her baby, she should do so over a period of time (Mohrbacher & Stock, 1997). If she wears a bra, it should fit well. The clinician should advise the mother not to sleep wearing her bra. Clothing should not bind. The provider should remind the mother not to carry heavy objects against the breasts or to carry heavy shoulder bags with straps that cross across the breasts. She should respond quickly to early warning signs of milk stasis.

If a tender area or a plugged duct develops, the mother should apply warmth, then massage behind the tender area. She should breast-feed, positioning the infant's nose or chin directed toward the tender area. The mother should continue to massage the affected area while breast-feeding. Frequent feedings with the baby effectively draining the breast discourages milk stasis and inflamed tissue. If the baby is not able to latch on or to drain the breast well, the mother may want to hand express or pump. If the plugged duct does not resolve within 48 hours, therapeutic ultrasound once a day for two days is recommended (Newman, 1998). For some women, one capsule of lecithin (1200 mg) three to four times a day may help prevent recurrence of blocked ducts (Newman, 1998).

Usually the mother is treated with a 7- to 14-day course of antibiotics. Many practitioners are unfamiliar with non-infectious mastitis and assume that all mastitis requires antibiotics (Amir et al., 1999). When treating infectious mastitis with antibiotics, relief usually occurs within 24 to 48 hours. Choosing an antibiotic that is appropriate for both the mother and the infant is very important. The recommended antibiotics are dicloxicillin, cephalosporins, amoxicillin-clavulanic acid, and nafcillin. For patients who are allergic to penicillin, erythromycin is prescribed. Sulfa drugs, such as trimethoprim-sulfamethoxazole DS, sometimes are ordered but should not be used if the infant is younger than 1 month. The clinician should emphasize to the mother the need to finish the course of treatment, because antibiotic-resistant strains of bacteria are more likely to develop when treatment stops too soon. Premature cessation of antibacterial treatment is the most common reason for recurrent mastitis (Riordan & Auerbach, 1999). Recurrent mastitis can lead to an abscess, which may need to be surgically incised.

Because of the importance of keeping the breast drained, the mother should continue to breast-feed (Thomsen et al., 1984). The baby should suckle on the unaffected side first while the affected side "lets down." The mother must empty the affected breast either by feeding or pumping. Bed rest is mandatory (Lawrence & Lawrence, 1999). A key to preventing further damage is to check for a good latch.

If the infant and mother are separated or the infant is unable to latch on well because of illness or some other problem, the mother should express or pump her milk. If mastitis develops in the first or second week, milk stasis secondary to poor milk transfer may be the problem. Careful evaluation of the infant's latch and suck is important. The provider should reassure the mother that the breast milk is not harmful to the baby. Mother and clinician should discuss strategies for getting more rest.

Treatment

Providers should recommend the following measures to provide comfort when a woman experiences mastitis:

- Apply warm moist packs or cool packs over the affected area, based on what is most comfortable (Lawrence, 1997). Heat is soothing, and warmth increases blood flow. Also, the woman can bend over in the shower to increase drainage through warmth and gravity (Biancuzzo, 1998).
- Take ibuprofen to reduce pain and inflammation.
- Drink water to replace body fluids lost through fever. Water helps the body get rid of toxins.
- Increase protein intake to build and repair cells damaged by bacteria.
- If discomfort persists, treatment may need to be changed.

Pump the affected breast three times per day immediately after a feeding to empty it completely.

Mammary Candidosis

Candida albicans normally is colonized in the mouth, intestines, and vagina, where it can overgrow and cause infection. Lactation professionals have noted infection of the breast tissue with *C. albicans* to be a significant, although largely unstudied, problem.

Causes

Maternal history may reveal a history of vaginal yeast infections, recent antibiotic use, or yeast infection (groin or foot) in her partner. The baby may have oral thrush or a fungal diaper rash, or the mother may report that the baby has increased intestinal gas and seems colicky. Early nipple trauma from incorrect latch on allows *C. albicans* to penetrate the tissue through microscopic skin breaks (Odds, 1994). The mother most often presents with significant nipple pain; the skin may or may not be intact. The nipple is often a bright pink, sometimes the only visual symptom in the mother–baby dyad. The nipple also may appear bright red, shiny, or eczematous with sloughing skin (Heinig, Francis, & Pappagianis, 1999). White plaques may appear on the nipple folds or in a fissure or crack (Auerbach & Riordan, 2000). Many affected mothers state that increased milk is leaking from the breasts between feedings. They describe the nipple pain as burning, especially after feedings. The level and intensity of pain are much greater than in a mother with a cracked or bruised nipple. Diagnosis and treatment usually are based on symptoms and history rather than laboratory findings. Culturing the skin by use of a moistened cotton-tipped or polyester sponge swab is possible. Heinig, et al. (1999) suggest initially washing the area with 60% ethanol (alcohol) solution to minimize bacterial contamination before collecting the sample, although the author reports this practice to be unpopular with patients. *C. albicans* can survive at least 24 hours on a moist swab (Odds, 1988). Skin sampling may be used for direct microscopic examination as a screening tool for superficial candidosis. A scraping is taken of the affected skin, and the sample is immersed in 10% to 15% potassium hydroxide (or Gram's staining) (Crisey, Lang, & Parish, 1995).

Treatment

Treatment focuses on ridding the dyad of infection and preventing reinfection by environmental sources. Mother and baby receive treatment simultaneously, usually for 2 weeks. The mother uses Nystatin or Mycolog cream, which she rubs into the breast after each feeding. The baby receives oral nystatin. Breast care, which includes gently rinsing the nipples with a cotton ball and water, should occur after every feeding and before application of the antifungal cream. The woman should change breast pads frequently. Because the breast pad itself may be an irritant, the woman may wear sterile pads instead. Exposing the breasts to sunlight for 10 minutes a day and frequently airing the breasts also are helpful.

Any symptomatic family members in the home also require treatment. In the early postpartum period, the woman may apply antifungal cream to the labia for vaginal itching. A diet low in sugar helps inhibit yeast growth. The woman should eliminate sweets and fruit juices from the diet and limit fermented foods, such as wine, beer, pickles, and vinegar. Family members should wash underwear, towels, shirts, and bed linens in hot water, adding a cup of white vinegar to the rinse cycle. They should boil all breast pump parts, bottles, bottle nipples, and pacifiers after each use. If the baby puts toys in the mouth, family members also must cleanse toys appropriately.

The clinician emphasizes hand washing to all family members (no antibacterial soap). Washing the baby's hands regularly also is important. Treatment with acidophilus and garlic can inhibit yeast growth. Ecchinacea can enhance the immune system. All treatment modalities should continue until 1 week after symptoms disappear.

Nipple Soreness

Many women experience some nipple soreness when they initiate breast-feeding. Numerous factors enter into pain perception, and some pain may be related to the newness of the experience. When soreness persists beyond the first 7 to 10 days or is excruciating; nipples crack, bleed, or bruise; or a woman expresses a desire to stop breast-feeding because of the pain, the provider must perform an assessment and initiate a plan of care. The most common cause of nipple soreness is improper positioning and latch on; correction usually brings relief in 2 to 3 days. A stripe of redness or cracking over one or both nipples is a classic sign of a shallow latch on. One-sided soreness is most common on the side where the woman uses the less dominant hand for latch on or if one nipple is different (eg, shorter, retracted, less protractile) from the other. Another diagnostic tool is to observe the nipple immediately after the baby has been nursing. A line of compression over the nipple is a good indicator of shallow latch on; this line often matches in contour the sore stripe or crack on the breast. A shallow latch on or the nipple rubbing against the palate may cause a blister or abrasion. Very often observing a latch on and making simple corrections solves most soreness problems.

White Spot

Women often describe a white spot on the surface of the nipple as exquisitely painful. The spot may balloon into a small blister or bleb during a nursing session and then shrink after the feeding. The mother also may describe breast pain in a quadrant of the breast, which may result from milk trapped in a duct. Lawrence (1999) hypothesizes that a small bleb represents a small pressure cyst formed at the end of the duct from milk seeping into this very elastic tissue. Abrasion of the nipple or poor positioning at the breast may cause a blister. Conservative treatment consists of warm saline soaks after feeding and application of lanolin. An alternative that brings immediate relief is to allow the baby to nurse for a short time to draw out the blister. The baby is then removed and the blister is broken with a sterile needle. The baby is then returned to the breast to continue nursing.

Bacterial Infection of the Nipple

Current research on treatment for bacterial infection of the nipple is unavailable. When a nipple is traumatized in the early days of breastfeeding, microscopic breaks in the skin expose the tissue to potential invasion by organisms. A new trend is to treat cases that do not respond to basic nipple care and correct positioning or that are not fungal with a course of antibiotics.

REFERENCES

American Academy of Pediatrics. (1997). Breastfeeding and the use of human milk. *Pediatrics, 100*, 1035–1039.

American Dietetic Association. (1997). Position of the American Dietetic Association: Promotion of breastfeeding. *Journal of the American Dietetic Association, 97*, 662–666.

Amir, L. H., Harris, H., & Andriske, L. (1999). An audit of mastitis in the emergency department. *Journal of Human Lactation, 15*, 221–224.

Aniansson, G., Alm, B., Andersson, B., Hakansson, A., Larsson, P., Nylen, O., Peterson, H., Rigner, P., Svanborg, M., Sabharwal, H., et al. (1994). A prospective cohort study on breast-feeding and otitis media in Swedish infants. *Pediatric Infectious Disease Journal, 13*(3), 183–188.

Association of Women's Health Obstetric and Neonatal Nurses. (1995). *Position statement: Breastfeeding*. Washington, DC: Author.

Auerbach, K. G., & Riordan, J. (2000). *Clinical lactation: A visual guide*. Sudbury, MA: Jones & Bartlett.

Ball, T. M., & Wright, A. L. (1999). Health care costs of formula feeding in the first year of life. *Pediatrics, 103*(4), 870–876.

Beaudry, M., Dufour, R., & Marcuox, S. (1995). Relation between infant feeding and infections during the first six months of life. *Journal of Pediatrics, 126*, 191–197.

Bernt, K. M., & Walker, W. A. (1999). Human milk as a carrier of biochemical messages. *Acta Paediatr, Suppl 430*, 27–41.

Biancuzzo, M. (1998). Mastitis: Painful and preventable. *Childbirth Instructor, Nov/Dec*, 10–12.

Buchko, B. L., Pugh, L. C., Bishop, B. A., Cochran, J. F., Smith, L. R., & Lerew, D. J. (1994). Comfort measures in breastfeeding, primiparous women. *Journal of Obstetric, Gynecologic, and Neonatal Nursing, 23*(1), 46–52.

Carbonell, X., Botet, S., Figueras, J., Alvarez, E., & Riu, A. (1998). The incidence of breastfeeding in our environment. *Journal of Perinatal Medicine, 26*(4), 320–324.

Carlson, S. E. (1999). Long-chain polyunsaturated fatty acids and development of human infants. *Acta Paediatr, Suppl. 430*, 72–77.

Carver, J. D. (1999). Dietary nucleotides: Effects on the immune and gastrointestinal systems. *Acta Paediatr, Suppl. 430*, 83–88.

Convert, R. F., Barman, N., Domanico, R.S., et al. (1995). Prior enteral nutrition with human milk protects against intestinal perforation in infants who develop necrotizing enterocolitis. *Pediatric Research, 37*, 305A. Abstract.

Coppa, G. V., Pierani, P., Zampini, L., Carloni, I., Carlucci, A., & Gabrielli, O. (1999). Oligosaccharides in human milk during different phases of lactation. *Acta Paediatr Suppl. 430*, 89–94.

Cox, D. B., Owens, R. A., & Hartman, P. E. (1996). Blood and milk prolactin and the rate of milk synthesis in women. *Experimental Physiology, 81*, 1007–1020.

Crisey, J. T., Land, H., & Parish, L. C. (1995). *Manual of medical mycology*. Oxford, England: Blackwell Science.

Cushing, A. H., Samet, J. M., Lambert, W. E., Skipper, B. J., Hunt, W. C., Young, S. A., & McLaren, L. C. (1998). Breastfeeding reduces risk of respiratory illness in infants. *American Journal of Epidemiology, 147*(9), 863–870.

Dewey, K. G., Heinig, M. J., & Nommsen-Rivers, L. A. (1995). Differences in morbidity between breast-fed and formula-fed infants. *Pediatrics, 126*, 696–702.

Duffy, E., Percival, P., & Kershaw, E. (1997). Positive effects of an antenatal group teaching session on postnatal nipple pain, nipple trauma and breastfeeding rates. *Midwifery, 13*(4), 189–196.

Ellis, L. A., Mastro, A. M., & Picciano, M. I. (1997). Do milk-borne cytokines and hormones influence neonatal immune cell function? *Journal of Nutrition, 127*, 9855–9885.

Hale, T. W. (1999). Anesthetic medications in breastfeeding mothers. *Journal of Human Lactation, 15*(3), 185–194.

Hanson, L. A. (1998). Breastfeeding provides passive and likely long-lasting active immunity. *Annals of Allergy Asthma Immunology, 81*, 523–537.

Heinig, M. J. (1998). Breastfeeding and the bottom line: Why are the cost savings of breast feeding such a hard sell? *Journal of Human Lactation 14*(1), 87–88.

Heinig, M. J., Francis, J., & Pappagianis, D. (1999). Mammary candidosis in lactating women. *Journal of Human Lactation, 15*(4), 281–288.

Hoffman, J. B. (1953). A suggested treatment for inverted nipples. *American Journal of Obstetrics and Gynecology, 66*, 346.

Horwood, L. J., & Fergusson, D. M. (1998). Breastfeeding and later cognitive and academic outcomes. *Pediatrics, 101*(1), E9.

Huggins, K. (1999). *Lecture: The slow gaining infant.* International Lactation Consultant Association Conference, Scottsdale, AZ.

Humenick, S. S., & Van Steenkiste, S. (1983). Early indicators of breast-feeding progress. *Issues in Comp Pediatric Nursing, 6*, 205–215.

Humphreys, A. S., Thompson, N. J., & Miner, K. R. (1998). Intention to breastfeed in low-income pregnant women: The role of social support and previous experience. *Birth, 25*, 169–174.

Inch, S., & Fisher, C. (1995). Mastitis: Infection or inflammation. *The Practitioner, 239*, 472–476.

Kavanaugh, K., Meier, P., & Zimmerman, B. (1997). The rewards outweigh the efforts: Breastfeeding outcomes for mother of preterm infants. *Journal of Human Lactation, 13*(1), 15–21.

Kessler, L. A., Gielen, A. C., Diener-West, M., & Paige, D. M. (1995). The effect of a woman's significant other on her breastfeeding decision. *Journal of Human Lactation, 11*(2), 103–109.

Lavergne, N. A. (1997). Does application of tea bags to sore nipples while breastfeeding provide effective relief? *Journal of Obstetric, Gynecologic, and Neonatal Nursing, Jan-Feb 26*(1), 53–58.

Lawrence, R. A. (1997). A review of the medical benefits and contradictions to breastfeeding in the United States. *Maternal and Child Health Technical Information Bulletin.*

Lawrence, R. A., & Lawrence, R. M. (1999). *Breastfeeding: A guide for the medical profession.* St Louis, MO: Mosby-Year Book.

Labbok, M. H., Hight-Laukaran, V., Peterson, A. E., Fletcher, V., von-Hertzen, H., & Van-Look, P. F. (1997). Multicenter study of the Lactational Amenorrhea Method (LAM): I. Efficacy, duration, and implications for clinical application. *Contraception, 55*, 327–336.

Lteif, A. N., & Schwenk, A. F. (1998). Breast milk: Revisited. *Mayo Clinic Proceedings, 78*, 760–763.

Marrow, A. L., Guerrero, M. L., Shults, J., et al. (1999). Efficacy of home-based peer counseling to promote exclusive breastfeeding: A randomized controlled trial. *Lancet, 353*, 1226–1231.

Martinez, G. A., & Nalezienski, J. P. (1981). 1980 update: The recent trend in breastfeeding. *Pediatrics, 67*, 260–263.

Mohrbacher, N., & Stock, J. (1997). *The breastfeeding answer book.* Schamburg, IL: La Leche League International.

Newman, J. (1998). Blocked ducts and mastitis. http://www.btlrc.com/newman/breastfeeding/mastitis.htm

Newton, N. (1992). The quantitative effect of oxytocin (Pitocin) on human milk yield. *Annals of the New York Academy of Science, 652*, 652.

Nissen, E., Lilja, G., Widstrom, A. M., & Uvnas-Moberg, K. (1995). Elevation of oxytocin levels early postpartum in women. *Acta Obstetricia Et Gynecologia Scandinavica, 74*, 530.

Odds, F. C. (1994). Candida species and virulence. *ASM News, 60*(6), 313–318.

Odds, F. C. (1988). *Candida and candidosis.* London: Bailliere Tindall.

Pabst, H. F., Spady, D. W., Pilarski, L. M., Carson, M. M., Beeler, J. A., & Krezolek, M. P. (1997). Differential modulation of the immune response by breast or formula feeding of infants. *Acta Pediatr, 86*, 1291–1297.

Petok, E. S. (1995). Breast cancer and breastfeeding: Five cases. *Journal of Human Lactation,* 205–209.

Powers, N. G., Naylor, A. J., & Wester, R A. (1994). Hospital policies crucial to breastfeeding success. *Seminars in Perinatology, 18*(6), 517–524.

Reifsnider, E., & Eckhart, D. (1997). Prenatal breastfeeding education: Its effect on breastfeeding among WIC participants. *Journal of Human Lactation, 13*, 121–125.

Riordan, J., & Auerbach, K. (1999). *Breastfeeding and human lactation.* St Louis, MO.: Jones and Bartlett.

Riva, E., Banderali, G., Agostoni, C., et al. (1999). Factors associated with initiational duration of breast feeding in Italy. *Acta Paediatr, 88*(4), 411–415.

Romieu, I., Hernandez-Avila, M., Lazcano, E., Lopez, L., & Romero-Jaime, R. (1996). Breast cancer and lactation history in Mexican women. *American Journal of Epidemiology, 143*(6), 543–552.

Routi, T., Ronnemaa, T., Lapinleimu, H., Salo, P., Viikari, J., Leino, A., Valimaki, I., Jokinen, E., & Simell, O. (1995). Effect of weaning on serum lipoprotein(a) concentration: The STRIP baby study. *Pediatric Research, 38*, 522–527.

Saarinen, U. M., & Kajosaari, M. (1995). Breastfeeding as prophylaxis against atopic disease: Prospective follow-up study until 17 years old. *Lancet, 346*, 1065–1069.

Schafer, E., Vogel, M. K., Viegas, S., & Hausafus, C. (1998). Volunteer peer counselors increase breastfeeding duration among rural low-income women. *Birth, 25*(2), 101–106.

Scott, J. A., & Binns, C. W. (1999). Factors associated with the initiation and duration of breastfeeding: A review of the literature. *Breastfeeding Review, 7*(1), 5–16.

Shu, X.-O., Clemens, J., Zheng, W., Ying, D. M., Ji, B. T., & Jin, F. (1995). Infant breastfeeding and the risk of childhood lymphoma and leukemia. *International Journal of Epidemiology, 24*, 27–32.

Silfverdal, S. A., Bodin, L., Hugosson, S., Garpenholt, O., Werner, B., Esbjorner, E., Lindquist, B., & Olcen, P. (1997). Protective effect of breast feeding on invasive *Haemophilus influenzae* infection: A case-control study in Swedish preschool children. *International Journal of Epidemiology, 26*, 443–449.

Stuver, S. O., Hsieh, C. C., Bectove, E., & Trichopoulos, D. (1997). The association between lactation and breast cancer in an international case-control study: A re-analysis by menopausal status. *International Journal of Cancer, 71*, 166–169.

Thomsen, A. C., Espersen, T., & Maigarrd, S. (1984). Course and treatment of milk stasis, noninfectious inflammation of the breast, and infectious mastitis in nursing women. *American Journal of Obstetrics and Gynecology, 149*, 492–495.

U.S. Department of Health and Human Services. (1991). *Healthy People 2000: National Health Promotion and Disease Prevention Objectives.* Washington, DC: Public Health Services, DHHS publication PHS 91-50212.

Uvnas-Moberg, K., & Eriksson, M. (1996). Breastfeeding: physiological, endocrine and behavioral adaptations caused by oxytocin and local neurogenic activity in the nipple and mammary gland. *Acta Paediatrica, 85*(5), 525–530.

Uvnas-Moberg, K. (1998). Oxytocin may mediate the benefits of positive social interaction and emotions. *Psychoneuroendocrinology, 23*(8), 819–835.

Walker, M. (1999). Mastitis in lactating women. La Leche League International, Inc., 298, 1–16.

Wang, Y. S., & Wu, S. Y. (1996). The effect of exclusive breastfeeding on development and incidence of infection infants. *Journal of Human Lactation, 12*, 27–30.

Wiemann, C. M., DuBois, J. C., & Berenson, A. B. (1998). Racial/ethnic differences to breastfeeding among adolescent mothers. *Pediatrics, 101*(6), E11.

Woolridge, M. W. (1986). The anatomy of infant sucking. *Midwifery, 2*, 164–171.

Woolridge, M. W., & Fisher, C. (1988). Colic, "overfeeding," and symptoms of lactose malabsorption in the breast-fed baby: A possible artifact of feed management? *Lancet, 2,* 382.

World Health Organization. (1981). *International Code of Marketing of breast-milk substitutes.* Geneva: Author.

World Health Organization/United Nations Children's Fund. (1989). *Protecting, promoting and supporting breastfeeding—The special role of maternity services. A joint WHO/UNICEF Statement.* Geneva, Switzerland: Author.

Wright, A. L., Holberg, C. J., Taussig, L. M., & Martinez, F. D. (1995). Relationship of infant feeding to recurrent wheezing at age 6 years. *Archives of Pediatric and Adolescent Medicine, 149,* 758–763.

Yamauchi, Y., & Yamanouchi, I. (1990). Breastfeeding frequency during the first 24 hours after birth in full-term neonates. *Pediatrics, 86,* 171–175.

Healthy Growth and Development of the Newborn/Infant

• RENEE DELLAROSE KIMBALL, MD

INTRODUCTION

The first year of a child's life is one of the most exciting periods of growth, development, and exploration both for infant and parents. It is an exciting time of "firsts." The primary care provider is seen not only as the physical expert but also as an expert in mental health, development, parenting, and other psychosocial issues. Most of the questions parents bring to the primary care provider during office visits concern psychosocial or "nonillness" issues. The expectation that primary care providers are sources of information, support, and understanding for psychosocial and developmental concerns mandates that the health professions produce primary care providers who are adept and comfortable responding to and counseling parents about such issues.

GROWTH AND DEVELOPMENT

A discussion of "normal" must consider an individual's variability throughout the day or week and according to culture. Individual variability means the individual's different responses as he or she adapts to environmental changes. An example of individual variability to environmental stimuli can be seen when comparing an introverted child's quiet withdrawal in social situations to an extroverted child's attention-grabbing antics. Cultural variability is vast and includes philosophy, expectations, and traditional practices. A classic example of cultural variability is an Asian family investigated for child abuse when marks are noted on a child's back that are a result not of abuse, but of the tradition of "cupping" to rid disease. Thus, what is normal must be interpreted in the context of each particular individual in each particular environment.

Although all children go through orderly, predictable sequences of neurodevelopment and physical growth, both intrinsic and extrinsic factors make each baby unique. Gross generalizations can be made to help illustrate the child's progress during this time. Physical growth changes depending on stage of life. Prenatally, the growth of the head predominates, reaching the peak in the third trimester. The mother's prepregnancy weight and pregnancy weight gain and placental function and gestational age at birth primarily determine the infant's birth weight. During infancy, the growth of the trunk predominates, and weight gain continues at a rapid but less steep rate. Fat content in infancy accelerates until approximately age 9 months. Development progresses from generalized reflexes to stimuli (Table 8-1), to voluntary discrete actions that are asymmetric and precise toward stimuli (eg, grasping with one hand and examining with the other). Developmental control progresses from

cephalad to caudal and proximal to distal. Development also progresses from dependence to independence.

Development frequently is divided into four categories for discussion: gross motor, fine motor, cognitive, and social. Table 8-2 outlines the common milestones for each category and their expected age of mastery. Social development varies most because it depends more on environmental than genetic factors and represents the steps necessary to form interpersonal relationships. Delays in achieving milestones should be assessed in the context of the domains affected. One mild delay affecting only one domain may be monitored carefully, while delays affecting several domains are more worrisome. Development delayed 30% from expected norms should prompt referral for formal evaluation (Johnson & Blasco, 1997). The scope of developmental pediatrics encompasses not only motor skills, but also the mental, sensory, and emotional function of a child. Parents are not reliable historians for retrospective development but are highly reliable for current accomplishments.

● **Clinical Pearl:** A delay in achieving milestones does not always indicate an abnormality, because there is no age at which failure to achieve a skill is abnormal. Most late talkers and walkers turn out to be normal. Likewise, achieving a milestone at a given time does not always indicate normalcy. A child with cerebral palsy or Down syndrome may meet early milestones on or ahead of schedule. Developmental testing is not a substitute for the physical examination. Testing is merely an adjunct to aid in forming a complete picture about the patient.

HISTORY AND PHYSICAL EXAMINATION

The purpose of the periodic scheduled well child visit is the promotion of wellness and the prevention of disease through anticipatory guidance, evaluation of growth and development, and immunizations. The American Academy of Pediatrics (AAP) recommends a preventive health care schedule for healthy, appropriately growing and developing children. If a child is not well physically or developmentally, more frequent and sophisticated visits are required. The recommended schedule for well child visits and immunizations is summarized in Table 8-3.

History

History taking and anticipatory guidance during the first year should concentrate on general health since the last visit, prevention of injury and illness, nutrition, infant care issues, parent–infant interactions, family relationships, community interactions, and any parental concerns. A wealth of evi-

Table 8–1. PRIMITIVE REFLEXES AND PROTECTIVE RESPONSES

Reflex	Description	Appearance	Disappearance
Moro startle*	Hold and support the infant in the supine position. Then lower the infant's entire body about 2 ft. Suddenly stop. Two part response: The arms, hands, and fingers abduct and extend, while the legs flex and abduct; then the arms return to clasping at midline as the baby cries.	Birth	5 mo
Palmar grasp*	All fingers flex to grasp object pressing on palm when placed from ulnar side.	Birth	3 mo
Plantar grasp*	All toes flex to grasp object pressing on sole at base of toes.	Birth	8–15 mo
Stepping*	While supporting the infant upright, touch the dorsal surface of one foot on a table edge. The hip and knee flex as if the child is stepping up onto the table; alternate stepping movements follow as examiner moves infant forward.	Birth	2 mo
Asymmetric tonic neck reflex*	With infant supine, turn head to one side. The arm and leg on the side, the head is facing extended while the opposite arm and leg flex.	2 wk	6 mo
Propping†	With infant seated, gently tilt infant to one side. The head rights back toward midline, the arm extends protectively, and the opposite arm and leg make equilibrium countermovements.	6 mo	Persists
Parachute†	Suspend the infant prone and slowly lower the head first toward a surface. The infant extends its arms and legs, and the fingers spread as if breaking a fall.	8–10 mo	Persists

*Normal is inconsistent or transient. Abnormal is strong, sustained reflexes.
†Normal is easy to elicit. Abnormal is markedly slow to appear.

TABLE 8–2. EARLY DEVELOPMENTAL MILESTONES*

Age (Mo)	Gross Motor	Fine Motor	Cognitive	Social
1	Holds up head when prone	Holds hands tightly fisted	Fixes and follows face	Makes throaty sounds
2	Holds chest up when prone	Holds hands unfisted half the time	Tracks horizontally past midline	Shows social smile, coos
3	Head partly lags when child pulls to sitting	Bats at objects Sustains grasp if an object is placed on ulnar side of palm	Regards small objects	Babbles Echoes speaker immediately
4	Rolls front to back Shows no head lag	Reaches for objects when supine	Mouths objects Shakes rattles Turns head to localize voice	Laughs out loud Listens to speaker then verbalizes back Makes gutteral sounds (ahh, goo)
5	Rolls back to front Sits with pelvic support	Transfers objects from hand to mouth to hand	Attains objects he or she reaches for Turns head to localize inanimate noise	Makes "raspberries" Smiles/vocalizes to mirror
6	Sits propped on hands (tripod)	Transfers objects hand to hand Makes immature rake	Looks for dropped toy Removes cloth covering face	Discriminates strangers (stranger anxiety begins)
7	Sits without support Does a commando crawl		Bangs/shakes toys Attempts to hold object in each hand	Imitates speech sounds
8	Gets into sitting position from supine	Shows scissor grasp Holds block in each hand	Pulls string to pull toy in closer Plays peek-a-boo	Says "dada" inappropriately Responds selectively to own name
9	Pulls to stand Crawls	Shows inferior pincer grasp Uncovers hidden objects	Rings bell	Says "mama" inappropriately Waves goodbye
10	Cruises Walks with two-hand support	Points with index finger Shows pincer grasp	Bangs two cubes together Looks at pictures in book	Says "dada" or "mama" appropriately Comprehends no
11	Stands alone Walks with one-hand support		Uncovers toy under cup	Says first word (other than "mama" or "dada")
12	Walks independently	Shows fine pincer grasp Attempts two-block tower		Follows one-step commands Indicates desire by pointing with index finger

*Other sources may have slightly different achievement ages.

TABLE 8–3.   RECOMMENDED WELL CHILD VISIT SCHEDULE AND POINTS OF IMPORTANCE

Age	History	Physical Examination	Health Promotion and Disease Prevention	Labs and Immunizations
Prenatal	Parental questions Preparation Review of risk factors Feelings toward baby	None unless provider also doing OB care	Breast-feeding Circumcision Safety (car seat, water temperature, smoke detectors) Support systems Community resources and referral if needed	None unless provider also doing OB care
Newborn	Congratulations Prenatal course Delivery review Family response and support	Complete physical examination Gestational age assessment Congenital anomalies Birth trauma	Car seat (rear facing, back seat) Back to sleep position Hot water heater <120° F *No* smoking near the baby Smoke detectors on each floor of house Breast-feeding instruction Expected weight loss Formula with iron Umbilicus and circumcision care Visit limitations Crowd avoidance until infant is 2.5 mo Sibling rivalry	Newborn screening for metabolic disorders
1–2 wk	Infant personality Consolability Infant's cues Nutrition review Postpartum blues	Complete physical examination Signs of abuse Developmental observations Parent–child interaction	Car seat (rear facing, back seat) Back to sleep position No smoking near the baby Breast-feeding instruction Expected weight gain Formula with iron Skin, nail care Temperament Consoling techniques— impossible to spoil Family/pet response to new baby Visitors welcome	
1 mo	As above	As above	As above Sunscreen Signs of illness Temperature taking No bottle to bed Colic, crying Pacifiers, thumbs Bowel movements Stimulation, play Couple and family time Sibling attention Partner's and family's help	
2 mo	Infant schedule Nutrition review Hearing or vision concerns Family adaptation	As above	As above Family planning Contact with friends, community Child care	DTaP, Hib, IPV
4 mo	As above Child care issues Family and couple time	As above	As above Fall precautions (rolling over) May begin infant cereal/solids No honey Daily/bedtime routine	DTaP, Hib, IPV
6 mo	As above Babyproof home	As above	As above Stranger anxiety Childproof home, accident precautions First aid/CPR/syrup of ipecac Water safety Comfort objects Brush teeth Allow exploration Self-comfort Play groups	DTaP, Hib Hepatitis B #1 Lead risk

(continues)

TABLE 8–3.   RECOMMENDED WELL CHILD VISIT SCHEDULE AND POINTS OF IMPORTANCE *(Continued)*

Age	History	Physical Examination	Health Promotion and Disease Prevention	Labs and Immunizations
9 mo	Household routines Nutrition review Discipline Family and couple time	As above	As above Separation anxiety Manipulative behavior Lower crib mattress Cup use Table foods Family meal time Self-feeding Distraction as discipline Gait and shoes	Hepatitis B #2
12 mo	As above	As above	As above Switch to whole cow's milk Picky eater Role model Expression of feelings	Hib #4, IPV #3, Hepatitis #3, Varicella Lead level, Hemoglobin

dence supports the immense role the family plays in shaping a child's physical, emotional, mental, and behavioral health. Family dysfunction is a strong risk factor for childhood disorders. Prenatal and postnatal visits may allow for observations that help identify families at risk. During all well child care visits, observation of the parent–child interaction is important. The parents' manner of handling and holding the infant, their response to the infant's discomfort, and their affect when speaking of the infant should be noted to identify maladaptive nurturing that contributes to health problems. Often stressors at home are seen in the office as somatic symptoms; in severe cases, this may present as failure to thrive. An emotionally deprived infant will not produce growth hormone, but once the infant is given attention that provides both physical and emotional warmth, growth begins again as growth hormone is produced.

Physical Examination

Before approaching the infant to do the physical examination, the primary care provider first should observe the infant at rest or play. The child should become acclimated to the primary care provider. A gentle, friendly approach with a quiet voice and interaction at the child's level for both age and development are important. A complete physical examination with the infant unclothed is essential at each visit. The infant is examined in parts, with areas exposed and covered to avoid chill. The primary care provider progresses from areas needing a child's cooperation (lungs) to painful or unpleasant areas (ears). The examining table is convenient, but a parent's arms or lap will provide security for the young infant. The primary care provider should face the parent with the knees touching the parent's to create a makeshift table on which the entire examination can be performed.

Neonate-Specific Considerations (Birth–30 Days)

The care of a new family ideally begins prenatally to help build rapport and to focus on the particular family's concerns, fears, and desires regarding the upcoming birth. For a family that is new to the primary care provider's practice, the prenatal visit also begins the relationship and provides an opportunity to foster trust in the primary care provider before birth. This is particularly important if a problem

arises prenatally or perinatally, because establishing rapport is difficult in times of urgency or stress. This also is an opportune time to review the effects of environmental tobacco smoke on the fetus and on children in the home (Display 8-1) (AAP, 1997a).

Gestational age is essential for evaluating whether an infant's developmental progress and growth are appropriate and for predicting increased risks of morbidity or mortality. Gestational age also allows for a description of a newborn's fetal growth pattern and size in three categories. Small for gestational age (SGA) is a weight percentile less than 10th, appropriate for gestational age is 10th to 90th percentile, and large for gestational age (LGA) is more than 90th percentile. SGA and LGA newborns are predisposed to increased risks, which are compounded further if such infants are born premature (< 37 weeks' gestation) or postterm (> 41 weeks' gestation). To this end, various scoring systems have been

---

DISPLAY 8–1 • Environmental Tobacco Smoke Hazards

Infants who live with smokers are doubly likely to have bronchitis or pneumonia in first 5 years of life.

They are four times more likely to be admitted for bronchitis and pneumonia.

They are 1.5 times more likely to have acute nasopharyngitis and sinusitis in first 5 years.

Risk for recurrent otitis media during first year of life is significant.

Infants who live with smokers are 50% to 60% more likely to develop middle ear effusion requiring myringotomy and tubes.

Symptoms are more frequent and severe in asthmatic children who live with smokers.

Risk of SIDS is increased.

Infants who live with smokers have greater ratio of total cholesterol to high-density lipoprotein (HDL) and lower HDL levels by adolescence.

Risks for lung cancer, leukemia, and lymphoma as an adult are increased.

Source: American Academy of Pediatrics. (1997). *AAP policy statement: Environment and tobacco smoke.*

developed to assess physical and neurologic signs of maturity. The Ballard exam (Fig. 8-1), a common tool used for this purpose, is accurate to within 2 weeks of assigned gestational age.

The APGAR score is unique to the newborn (Table 8-4); it indicates the newborn's in utero, intrapartum, and immediate postnatal experience. It estimates the severity of respiratory and neurologic depression at 1 minute and 5 minutes of age. The 1-minute APGAR score is less predictive than the 5-minute score for residual neurologic damage. A cord-blood pH less than 7.20 is the direct measurement of perinatal asphyxia.

Vernix covers the infant at birth, protecting the baby from amniotic fluid. Vernix consists of sebum and cornified epidermis and is removed by the bathing process in the nursery. Lanugo is the fine silky hair seen on the newborn, particularly on the shoulders and back. It usually is shed by 10 to 14 days of life. Transient puffiness lasting 2 to 3 days, which has no identifiable cause, is of no concern and can be seen in the newborn's eyelids, hands, feet, legs, pubis, genitalia, or sacrum.

Physiologic jaundice is due to numerous factors and is present in two thirds of infants by 48 hours after birth. Jaundice begins in the face and progresses caudally. It is most eas-

NEUROMUSCULAR MATURITY

NEUROMUSCULAR MATURITY SIGN	SCORE						RECORD SCORE HERE
	0	1	2	3	4	5	
Posture							
Square window	90	60	45	30	0		
Arm recoil	180	100-180	90-100	90			
Popliteal angle	180	160	130	110	90	<90	
Scarf sign							
Heel to ear							

TOTAL NEUROMUSCULAR MATURITY SCORE

SCORE

Neuromuscular _____

Physical _____

Total _____

TOTAL MATURITY SCORE	GESTATIONAL AGE (WEEKS)
5	26
10	28
15	30
20	32
25	34
30	36
35	38
40	40
45	42
50	44

GESTATIONAL AGE (weeks)

By dates _____

By ultrasound _____

By score _____

PHYSICAL MATURITY

PHYSICAL MATURITY SIGN	SCORE						RECORD SCORE HERE
	0	1	2	3	4	5	
Skin	gelatinous red transparent	smooth, pink, visible veins	superficial peeling &/or rash; few veins	cracking, pale area, rare veins	parchment, deep cracking, no vessels	leathery, cracked, wrinkled	
Lanugo	none	abundant	thinning	bald areas	mostly bald		
Plantarcreases	no crease	faint red marks	anterior transverse creases only	creases anterior 2/3	creases cover entire sole		
Breast	barely perceptible	flat areola, no bud	suppled areola 1-2mm bud	raised areola 3-4mm bud	full areola 5-10mm bud		
Ear	pinna flat, stays folded	sl. curved pinna; soft with slow recoil	well-curved pinna; soft but ready recoil	formed and firm with instant recoil	thick cartilage, ear stiff		
Genitals (male)	scrotum empty, no rugae		testes descending, few rugae	testes down, good rugae	testes pendulous, deep rugae		
Genitals (female)	prominent clitoris and labia minora		majora and minora equally prominent	majora large, minora small	clitoris and minora completely covered		

TOTAL PHYSICAL MATURITY SCORE

Figure 8–1 ■ Ballard scoring assessment tool. (From Ballard, J.L., Novak, K.K., Driver, M. [1979]. A simplified score for assessment of fetal maturation of newly born infants. *Journal of Pediatrics*; 95: 769–774).

Table 8–4. APGAR SCORE

Finding	0 Points	1 Point	2 Points
Heart rate	0	<100	>100
Respiratory rate	0	Grunting	Normal
Color	Blue	Acrocyanosis	Pink
Reflex to nasal suction	0	Grimace	Cough/sneeze
Tone	Limp	Some flexion	Full flexion

ily seen in the sclera, particularly in dark-skinned infants. Jaundice that presents within the first 24 hours is pathologic and must be investigated appropriately to rule out hemolytic disease, liver disease, or severe infection. Newborns have an increased red blood cell mass per kilogram, shorter red blood cell life span, and an immature liver with decreased hepatic uptake and conjugation. Newborns also have decreased intestinal catabolization of unconjugated bilirubin and increased hydrolyzation of conjugated bilirubin to the unconjugated form. The result is more unconjugated bilirubin in the intestine for reabsorption. These combined factors result in increased enterohepatic circulation of bilirubin. Physiologic jaundice is associated with a relatively rapid increase in indirect bilirubin, which usually peaks at a mean unconjugated bilirubin of 5 mg/dL by 3 to 4 days and then declines to adult levels by 11 to 14 days (Gartner & Lee, 1999). The peaks and rate of resolution, however, vary by race and mode of feeding, suggesting that "normal" physiologic jaundice also may have to be interpreted within the context of an individual and situation. Bilirubin levels are the same from birth to 4 days in breastfeeding and formula-fed infants but diverge at 5 to 6 days. Bilirubin levels decline rapidly to adult levels in formula-fed infants, while they decline slower in breastfed infants, with two thirds of these infants having an elevated bilirubin level at 8 weeks (Gartner & Lee, 1999). African American and Caucasian infants reach a peak bilirubin level at 2 to 3 days, while Asian infants reach a peak at 4 to 5 days.

Jaundice seen in breastfeeding infants may be described as either "early onset," due to inadequate milk and calorie intake and representing an exaggeration of physiologic jaundice, or "breast milk" ("late onset," "prolonged") caused by not yet identified factors in transitional and mature milk. Early-onset breastfeeding jaundice may precede breast milk jaundice. Both processes result in increased enterohepatic circulation from increased intestinal bilirubin absorption. The AAP discourages the interruption of breastfeeding in healthy term newborns with early-onset breastfeeding or late-onset breast milk jaundice. Early-onset jaundice can be prevented by establishing optimal breastfeeding through frequent nursing (> 10 nursings in 24 hours) and careful observation to identify and correct any suckling difficulties. Taking the infant off the breast will result in decreased breast stimulation, a decreased milk supply, and continuation of the problem. Formula supplementation is not recommended unless the serum bilirubin is greater than 20 mg/dL or the infant is experiencing significant starvation or dehydration. These infants can continue to nurse at the breast while using a supplemental nursing system to obtain sufficient calories while continuing to suckle and stimulate breast milk production. A supplemental nurser is a device in which a bottle filled with formula is hung around the mother's neck with one or two small, soft, pliable tubes attached to the end of the bottle with the other ends at the mother's nipples. As the baby suckles at the breast, he or she also sucks on the tubes, thus receiving both breast milk and formula during a feed-

ing. Glucose water supplementation is not indicated, because it does not decrease bilirubin levels (bilirubin is excreted through the stool, not the urine). It also negatively affects the volume of breast milk by interfering with nursing. These infants should be evaluated 48 to 72 hours after discharge from the hospital to ensure that successful breastfeeding has been established.

Infants who have breast milk jaundice may have elevated unconjugated bilirubin levels that persist for 3 to 4 weeks and sometimes up to 12 weeks of life. In the infant with prolonged hyperbilirubinemia, breast milk jaundice is a diagnosis of exclusion. Infants with breast milk jaundice are thriving, vigorous, and gaining weight appropriately without clinical or laboratory signs of disease. The peak bilirubin occurs between days 5 and 15 in these infants. Cessation of nursing will lead to a precipitous drop in serum bilirubin; however, this is not recommended, because the bilirubin concentration will decline on its own.

Prolonged hyperbilirubinemia has other causes besides breast milk jaundice that should be ruled out. These include hemolytic disease of the newborn; polycythemia; glucuronyl transferase defects; metabolic disorders, such as hypothyroidism and galactosemia; hematomas; and intestinal obstruction. Workup of a jaundiced infant often includes total, indirect, and direct bilirubin levels; complete blood cell count with peripheral smear; blood type, Rh, and antibody profile (mother and newborn); direct and indirect Coombs'; and reticulocyte count (>5% suggests hemolysis). Treatment levels are based on studies from Caucasian, formula-fed infants. The concern about neonatal jaundice stems from its action as a cell toxin that can be deposited in various tissues, ultimately causing necrosis of the cells. The evidence for kernicterus is based on studies of preterm, low–birth-weight infants or those with hemolytic disease. In determining the effect on normal term infants without hemolysis, several collaborative long-range studies were done. These studies found that hyperbilirubinemia had little or no effect on IQ, mental development, neurologic abnormality, speech, language, or hearing tests at least to a total serum bilirubin level of 20 in term babies without hemolysis. This does not mean that infants will not have toxicity due to bilirubin if they have other risk factors (eg, acidosis, hypoxia, anoxia, or sepsis). Treatment consists primarily of phototherapy when the total serum bilirubin reaches 15 to 20 mg/dL and can be discontinued when the total serum bilirubin drops below 14 to 15 mg/dL (Bland, 1996). Breastfeeding can continue throughout phototherapy. Phototherapy can be accomplished safely in the low-risk infant with a Wallaby blanket, even as an outpatient, to reduce adverse effects on breastfeeding, mother–infant relationship, and cost.

Considerations for All Infants (Birth–12 Months)

Growth charts of height, weight, and head circumference should be done at all well child visits to monitor ongoing growth. Normal growth is one of the most reassuring findings during a well child examination, because it implies health, adequate nutrition and genetic makeup, and absence of major chronic disease. A pattern of growth abnormalities can help narrow the differential diagnosis of growth failure. Congenital, constitutional, familial, or endocrine causes of growth abnormalities appear as a decrease in the height curve before or at the same time as the decrease in the weight curve so that the weight-to-height curve is either normal or increased. Starvation initially appears as a decrease in weight and weight-for-height curves. In chronic starvation, there is a decrease in the height curve and possibly a return toward normal weight-for-height curve.

Measurements and Temperature

Length should be measured with the child in the supine position until he or she is 24 to 36 months. Birth lengths average 18 to 22 in (45–55 cm), and length increases 30% by age 5 months and 50% by the first birthday. Weight should be measured on an infant scale using ounces or grams. Birth weights average 5 lb 8 oz to 8 lb 13 oz (2500–4000 g), and weight generally doubles by 4 to 5 months and triples by 12 months. Based on Department of Health, Education, and Welfare growth charts with reference percentiles, a healthy term infant can be expected to gain approximately 1 oz/d for the first 3 months of life and 0.5 oz/d for the remainder of the first year. Weight often is considered the fifth vital sign in children. A weight that falls off the growth curve often is the first sign of a psychosocial or physical disorder. Head circumference should be measured at each visit until the child is 24 months old. Correct placement is essential for accurate data interpretation. The measuring tape should be placed snugly around the head at the occipital protuberance and the supraorbital prominence to find the largest circumference. Birth head circumferences average 13 to 14 in (33–35 cm) and are usually two thirds of adult size by age 2 years. Delayed growth suggests premature suture closure or microcephaly, while too rapid growth suggests hydrocephalus or intracranial mass. Chest circumference is not universally done.

Accurate measurement and monitoring of body size are especially important in infants, because deviations may be the first or only sign of disease, such as in chronic renal disease, hyperthyroidism, or parental deprivation syndrome. All infant measurements should be plotted on the appropriate growth curve for comparison with population means. The most important aspect of the growth curve is following the individual's progress. Any curve within the 5th to 95th percentiles is "normal." Values that begin to deviate from the infant's growth curve history are of concern (ie, is the child falling off or rising above the curve). Growth parallel to but below the 5th or above the 95th percentile is more than likely normal; however, an increased prevalence of developmental disabilities associated with many genetic syndromes is found in these two groups. Knowing the stature of the parents is helpful when assessing deviation from the norm. Rectal temperature is the most accurate means of assessing core body temperature in infants.

● **Clinical Pearl:** The body temperature of infants and young children is more variable and higher than that of adults. In normal infants, the average rectal temperature usually does not fall below 99°F and may be as high as 101°F in the afternoon after a busy or anxious day. Conversely, young infants may have normal or subnormal temperatures even with severe infections.

Skin, Hair, and Nails

Newborns have very little subcutaneous fat at birth, a large body surface area, and an inability to shiver. Thus, they are predisposed to hypothermia. Infants lose four times more body heat per unit weight than adults do (Seidel et al., 1997). Body fat is only 12% at birth but increases fairly rapidly to 25% at 6 months and then less rapidly to 30% by 12 months. Infants also are at increased risk of dehydration due to high surface area, turnover rate, and relative amount of body water. Infants have 80% body water at birth; this amount does not drop to the adult level of 60% until after the first birthday.

Infant skin lacks coarse terminal hair and appears much smoother and softer than adult skin. Newborn skin also lacks appocrine function, and eccrine function does not begin until after the first month of life. Thus, infant skin is less oily than adult skin.

The color of an infant's skin is inversely related to the amount of subcutaneous fat: the less fat, the more red and transparent the skin. Dark-skinned infants often appear less pigmented at birth than they will look when they are 2 to 3 months old. Skin color can be estimated by looking at the scrotum and nail beds.

Acrocyanosis (cyanosis of the hands and feet) is normal in newborns and in older infants who are chilled. Central cyanosis should be investigated for an underlying cardiac defect. Other color and common neonatal and infant skin conditions are listed in Table 8-5.

Skin creases can give clues to maturity and are associated with certain abnormalities. The older the baby is, the more creases will appear on the palms and soles. One of the best known abnormal palmar creases is the Simian crease frequently seen in trisomy 21; however, it also may be seen in normal children.

Skin turgor should be inspected to assess nutritional and hydration states. Severe dehydration or malnutrition will result in prolonged skin tenting. Tenting in an infant is best observed by pinching a fold of skin on the abdomen or thigh.

No matter how much hair is on the infant's head at birth, most hair is lost (transient plagiocephaly) by age 2 to 3 months and replaced by permanent hair. Permanent hair may be of a different texture or color than the birth hair.

Lymphatics

The infant's immune system is immature at birth, leaving the baby vulnerable to serious infections during the first few months of life. This is true even though the amount of lymphoid tissue is greater than during adulthood. Lymph nodes usually are not palpable in infants but do respond briskly to mild stimuli, such as viral infections or infections in the associated drainage area (eg, otitis media), particularly in the cervical and postauricular chains. It is not unusual to find these nodes enlarged in children younger than 2 years. Generally, discrete, movable, and nontender nodes less than 1 cm in the cervical, axillary, or inguinal chains or less than 0.5 cm elsewhere are of little concern.

Head and Neck

An infant's skull consists of seven soft bones separated by sagittal, coronal, and lamboidal sutures. The sutures allow the skull to expand, permitting brain growth, and can be palpated as ridgelike lines until age 6 months. At this time, they usually become nonpalpable. The fontanelles are located at the intersection of the sutures and begin to ossify in the first year of life (Fig. 8-2). The fontanelles should feel

Table 8–5.   COMMON NEONATAL AND INFANT SKIN FINDINGS

Finding	Description
Cutis marmorata	Mottled appearance of body and extremities in response to changes in ambient temperature; more common in prematurity, Down syndrome, and hypothyroidism; resolves spontaneously
Harlequin (dyschromia)	Sharp demarcation down the midline, with dependent side of the body more red than the other; seen in normal infants or associated with intracranial pathology; resolves within hours
Mongolian spots	Flat, bluish black to slate gray spots on the posterior trunk and legs; most often seen in normal newborns of African American and Asian heritage; usually resolve by preschool age; inexperienced examiner may confuse them with ecchymosis
Café au lait patches	Coffee-colored patches; may be associated with neurofibromatosis if multiple and >1 cm in diameter
Miliaria/prickly heat	Irregular, red, macular, or papulovesicular pruritic rash from occlusion of sweat ducts during heat and high humidity; overdressed infants prone to it during summer months; treatment is decreased heat and clothing and cool soaks
Milia	Small (1–2 mm), white, discrete papules on face in first 2–3 mo from plugged sebaceous glands; resolves spontaneously
Sebaceous gland hyperplasia	Numerous tiny yellow macules and papules on the face from androgen stimulation prenatally, disappearing quickly by 1–2 mo
Neonatal acne	Open and closed comedones in typical acne distribution from androgen stimulation; occurs in 20% of infants and resolves spontaneously by 1–2 mo
Seborrheic dermatitis/cradle cap	Chronic, relapsing, erythematous scaling lesions near sebaceous glands (scalp, back, intertriginous, diaper area); scalp lesions can be adherent, thick, yellow, and crusted "cradle cap"; treatment is mild to midpotency topical corticosteroids as needed; scalp scales can be softened with mineral oil and brushed out, then hair can be shampooed with 1% selenium sulfide (be sure to avoid eyes)
Erythema toxicum	Erythematous base with central wheals or vesicles from unknown cause appearing at 2–3 d in 50% of newborns and resolving spontaneously within 1 wk; not found on palms or soles
Acropustulosis	Recurrent pruritic vesiculopustules on hands and feet; general course lasts 7–10 d and recurs every few weeks or months; usually resolves by 2–3 y; unknown etiology and no specific therapy; can use antihistamines for pruritus
Pustular melanosis	Recurrent crops of brown vesicles and pustules on neck, face, palms, and soles appearing at birth or shortly thereafter; vesicles/pustules shed within a few days, leaving a scaling brown macule; usually resolves without scarring in 3–4 mo; unknown etiology and no specific therapy
Reddened patches due to rich capillary bed	Examples include strawberry hemangiomas, cavernous hemangiomas, nevus flammeus, nevus vasculosus, and telangiectatic nevus; usually disappear by 1 y but may recur
Irritant diaper dermatitis	Results from chafing or prolonged contact with feces or urine; skin is erythematous with glazed appearance and wrinkled surface sparing the creases; treatment is mild topical corticosteroid, covered by moisture barrier emollient (Zinc oxide) in addition to frequent diaper changes or allowing the area to be open to air
Candidal diaper dermatitis	Results from *Candida* infection (usually from feces); skin is diffusely erythematous with a peripheral scale and satellite pustules involving the creases; treatment is topical anticandidal creams with or without concomitant mild topical corticosteroid
Atopic dermatitis (eczema)	Chronic, inherited, >80% present by 12 mo (usually around 3 mo); often associated with other atopic diseases (asthma, hay fever); skin is erythematous with scaling or vesicles, usually symmetrical on cheeks, scalp, and lateral extensor areas of legs with generalized xerosis; treatment is mild to midpotency topical corticosteroids until improvement, then emollients and limited bathing times; antihistamines can be used for pruritus; skin lesions tend to improve with age

somewhat depressed and have minimal pulsation. The posterior fontanelle usually closes by 2 months; the anterior fontanelle may remain open until 18 to 24 months, though in 90% of infants it closes by 7 to 19 months. An anterior fontanelle that is greater than 4 to 5 cm in diameter or bulging with marked pulsation may indicate increased intracranial pressure, either from infection or hydrocephalus. This clinical sign, however, often is not present in infants younger than 3 months and thus should not be used to predict the presence of meningitis. Ultrasound of the skull is recommended in infants suspected of having an intracranial lesion or a rapidly enlarging head circumference on serial examinations.

Birth-related findings can be identified during the newborn examination and are described in Table 8-6 and Figure 8-3. The head, face, and neck are inspected for shape, symmetry, and abnormalities that may give clues to congenital or chromosomal disorders. Asymmetry of the head, or a "flat spot," is common in infants due to positioning, particularly because the "Back to Sleep" campaign has increased the number of infants who sleep in the supine position. If a thorough examination does not reveal any other abnormalities when a flat spot is found, parents should try changing the infant's positions over a 4- to 6-week period (Liptak & Serletti, 1998). Position changes can be accomplished easily by alternating the infant's line of vision to outside activities during supine sleeping (ie, turn the infant so that the head is at the other end of the crib). Prone positioning is encouraged during awake times to stimulate upper body strength and development and limit the time spent supine. If the asymmetry resolves, positional deformity is extremely likely, and no further workup is required. If the asymmetry persists, a

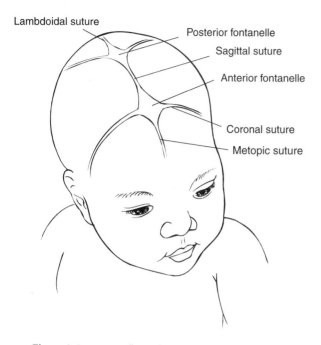

Lambdoidal suture

Posterior fontanelle

Sagittal suture

Anterior fontanelle

Coronal suture

Metopic suture

Figure 8–2 ■ Fontanelles and sutures on the infant's skull.

plain radiograph or computed tomography scan of the head should be obtained to examine the sutures, which should be patent.

The neck should be inspected and palpated to check for muscle tone and masses. Torticollis may be present and is easily treated with physical therapy. A cystic mass in the upper neck may be a thyroglossal duct or branchial cleft cyst. A mass in the lower portion of the sternocleidomastoid muscle may represent a hematoma. A mass over the clavicle that changes size with respiration may be a cystic hygroma.

Eye

Infants are hyperopic when born, with visual acuity of 20/200 and a field of vision only about the distance from a cradled arm to a parent's face. Visual acuity, dependent on nervous system maturation, continues to develop and matures enough for an infant to be able to discern colors by 8 months. Most children do not achieve 20/20 acuity until 6 years. Infants begin to have voluntary control of the eye muscles at 5 to 6 weeks but are unable to see a single image until around 9 months due to incomplete coordination. Visual acuity can be assessed through observation of the infant's reaction to the environment (eg, focusing on a face,

tracking objects, or responding to a bright light). Nystagmus in any direction is common at birth, but persistence after several days may indicate blindness. Infant lacrimal ducts begin carrying tears at 2 to 3 months. A blocked nasolacrimal duct is common and identified by constant tearing or accumulation of mucous material at the inner canthus. Most blocked ducts result from incomplete development. The majority of blocked ducts spontaneously open by age 6 months, while the remainder open by 12 months when development is complete. Massage of the sac (with or without a warm compress) at the root of the nose with the proximal end blocked may result in spontaneous opening of the duct. If the condition persists for more than 1 year, referral to an ophthalmologist for probing can be pursued.

The external eye structures; the size, eyelid, sclera, conjunctiva, pupil, and iris of each eye; and the distance between the eyes are inspected (AAP, 1996a). Abnormalities in any of these may be associated with various syndromes. For all infants, the red reflex should be elicited with an ophthalmoscope to observe for symmetry, any opacities, and white or dark spots in the red circle, which may indicate congenital cataracts or retinoblastoma. Congenital glaucoma should be ruled out by checking the cornea's diameter (<1 cm is normal). Eye color does not stabilize until age 6 years, and in about 10% of individuals it continues to change into adulthood (Bito et al., 1997). For more information, see Chapter 52.

Strabismus is the inability to focus both eyes on an object simultaneously. This normally may be seen intermittently up to 6 months of age as the infant develops extraocular muscle control. It can be detected by an asymmetric light reflex test or with the cover test, in which the examiner detects the child's dominant eye by watching the movement of the infant's eyes while they focus on a near object. The nondominant eye will move to focus if the dominant eye is covered. Amblyopia (reduced visual acuity) occurs in the nondominant eye as a result of suppressing its image to avoid diplopia.

▲ **Clinical Warning:** Any hint of constant or persistent intermittent squint in a child older than 6 months warrants referral to an ophthalmologist. Failure to detect and treat strabismus and its resultant amblyopia within the first few years of life can lead to permanent visual loss.

Ear, Nose, and Throat

The ear, nose, and throat area is a frequent site of congenital malformations and should be examined thoroughly. Fetal insults during the first trimester (when the inner ear is developing) may result in impaired hearing. Prematurity also increases the risk for hearing impairment. Children who experienced these conditions require close follow-up and

Table 8–6.   BIRTH TRAUMA TO HEAD

Term	Findings	Resolution
Molding	Overlapping cranial bones as a result of mechanical forces exerted by the birth canal	2–3 d
Caput succedaneum	Subcutaneous edema over presenting part of head	2–3 d
	Scalp soft and margins ill defined	
	Crosses suture lines	
Cephalhematoma	Subperiosteal blood	Weeks to months
	Scalp firm and margins well defined	
	Does not cross suture lines	

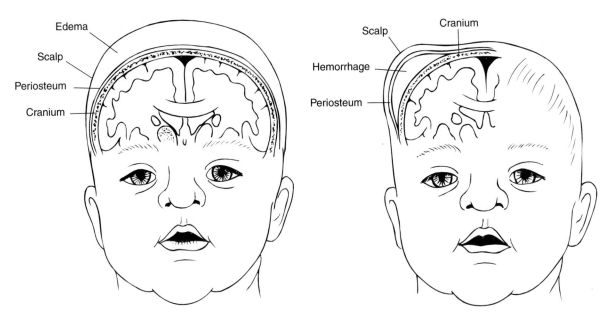

Figure 8–3 ■ (A) Caput succedaneum. (B) Cephalhematoma. Note that the swelling does not cross suture lines.

testing. The Joint Committee on Infant Hearing has recommended universal screening for hearing loss in the newborn period. Hearing can be assessed, though not completely accurately, by observing the infant's response to the environment. Signs of normal hearing may include display of the startle reflex to a loud noise, changes in the respiratory pattern to sound, and turning toward and localizing sound.

● **Clinical Pearl:** Parental perception of their child's hearing usually is correct. Concerns from a parent should prompt investigation.

The external ear should be examined for shape, presence of landmarks, and position. Abnormalities of the external ear often are associated with renal disorders. The external canal is short with a downward curve, so examination may require traction of the pinna down to straighten the canal to view the tympanic membrane.

● **Clinical Pearl:** Assessing the tympanic membrane of an infant younger than 3 months is fraught with difficulty and at best a challenge for even the most experienced provider.

The eustachian tube has three functions: equilibration of pressures in the middle ear, protection from nasopharyngeal secretions, and provision of a route for drainage of middle ear secretions into the nasopharynx. Dysfunction of the eustachian tube's ability to equalize pressure results in a greater negative middle ear pressure than normal. When the eustachian tube then opens, nasopharyngeal secretions may be aspirated into the middle ear. Obstruction of the eustachian tube also can result in impaired drainage of middle ear secretions, creating an environment conducive to infection. In children, the eustachian tube is wide and short with a more horizontal lie and poorer equilibration function than found in adults, placing the child at increased risk for otitis media. As the child grows, the eustachian tube lengthens, reducing the predilection to otitis media.

Infants are obligate nose breathers. Patent nares, therefore, are essential. They can be assessed after delivery by alternating compression of the nares and observing the respiratory

pattern or by passing a small catheter into each nare to the posterior nasal opening to detect choanal atresia. Maxillary and ethmoid sinuses are very small at birth. The frontal sinus does not develop until early childhood, and the sphenoid sinus does not fully develop until puberty. The lips should be complete without a cleft. Sucking calluses on the upper lips or circumoral cyanosis may be present at birth but should not persist. The buccal mucosa should be pink, and white patches should be scraped with a tongue blade to see if they are adherent, indicating thrush (candidiasis), or nonadherent, indicating milk deposits. The infant may be exposed to *Candida* in the birth canal, but infection often does not show up as thrush until the second week of life. Thrush often is associated with candidal diaper rash, because the gastrointestinal (GI) system may serve as a reservoir. Treatment consists of nystatin suspension for 7 to 10 days or crystallized lactobacillus solution by mouth. All pacifiers, bottle nipples, and teething rings should be boiled daily to prevent reinfection. Breastfeeding moms may develop candidal infection on their nipples from the infant. Mothers with *Candida* should apply mycostatin suspension to the nipple after nursing. Thrush is not an indication to discontinue breastfeeding.

Salivation increases at a greater rate than swallowing control, so an infant commonly drools between 2 and 6 months. Infants have 20 deciduous teeth that begin to calcify by 3 months of age but do not erupt until they are calcified enough to withstand chewing (generally between 6 and 24 months). Newborns may have natal teeth, which pose a choking threat if loose and should generally be removed. Epstein pearls may be seen on the gum line; these pearl-like retention cysts will disappear in 1 to 2 months. The tongue should be examined for size, such as in macroglossia, which may be associated with congenital hypothyroidism or other anomalies. Ankyloglossia (tongue-tied) also may be seen, but feeding or speech problems are not expected if the tongue is able to protrude beyond the alveolar ridge. Frenulectomy rarely is indicated. Both the hard and soft palates should be examined for clefts and shape. Cleft of the palate may occur with or without cleft of the lip. High arching and narrow palates are associated with congenital anomalies and affect tongue placement, leading to feeding and speech problems.

● **Clinical Pearl:** The palates should be palpated with the examiner's fingerpad, and the strength of the infant's suck can be assessed at this time. A strong coordinated suck should be expected. A weak suck may be associated with congenital anomaly, illness, or sedation. A gag reflex should be elicited as well.

Chest and Lungs

The change in the newborn's lungs from collapsed alveoli prenatally to functional air exchange sacs postnatally is rapid. Blood flow through the lungs increases as the blood is rerouted from the placenta with clamping of the umbilical cord. The increased blood flow causes the pulmonary arteries to expand and relax, creating a decrease in resistance of the pulmonary circulation compared with the systemic circulation, which causes closure of the foramen ovale within minutes. The increased oxygen in the pulmonary arterial blood stimulates contraction and closure of the ductus arteriosus within 24 to 48 hours. These changes complete the transformation from fetal to extrauterine circulation.

The respiratory rate should be counted for a full minute to get an accurate count, because the rate may vary appreciably each moment. Infants use their diaphragms predominantly, so the abdomen is synchronous with chest movements during respiration. Age-appropriate rates are found in Table 8-7. The rate depends on numerous factors, including room temperature, fever, feeding, and sleep. The newborn rate may be depressed because of the transfer of drugs given to the mother during labor or more rapid than usual if the baby was delivered by cesarean section. Periodic breathing, vigorous respiratory effort followed by apnea lasting 10 to 15 seconds, diminishes as the fetus matures and resolves within a few hours after birth in the term infant. Apnea periods lasting longer than 20 seconds are seen in premature infants and some term infants, which may put them at risk for sudden infant death syndrome (SIDS). Respiratory distress is detected by stridor (inspiratory high pitch as a result of proximal respiratory obstruction), grunting (positive and expiratory pressure [PEEP] to keep alveoli open), accessory muscle use (intercostals or sternoclavicular), or nasal flaring.

The chest wall should be inspected for size and shape, including nipple placement and number. Supernumerary nipples are seen 11 times more commonly in African Americans than in Caucasians; they are more often associated with congenital abnormalities in Caucasians if present. Infants of both sexes may have enlarged breast buds, usually 1 to 3 cm, as a result of transferred maternal estrogen during pregnancy. The breasts also may express a small amount of clear or milky white fluid. Both conditions usually resolve by 2 to 4 weeks, rarely extending beyond age 3 months. No treatment is required. Palpation of the chest should focus on identifying birth trauma, such as crepitus, tenderness, or

swelling around a fractured clavicle, which occurs in 1% to 3% of vaginal deliveries. Greenstick type fractures are the most common in infants. The thick periostium around the clavicle prevents severe displacement and angulation, so complications such as pneumothorax are highly unusual.

● **Clinical Pearl:** Most fractured clavicles will be asymptomatic with minimal physical examination findings. They heal very well within 2 to 3 weeks and generally require no specific treatment. Percussion of the chest is unreliable as the infant's thorax is too small to isolate changes in pitch.

Expansion of the chest should be symmetrical unless a diaphragmatic hernia or pneumothorax compromises one lung. Auscultation is sometimes difficult, because the small size of an infant's chest results in hyper-resonance and transmission of sounds from one area to another. Any asymmetry of sound should prompt investigation.

● **Clinical Pearl:** Sneezing is frequent and not always indicative of a problem or infection.

▲ **Clinical Warning:** Transient coughing can occur when drinking a new consistency or feeding too rapidly. This problem should resolve as the infant becomes accustomed to a new feeding pattern. Persistent coughing is always significant and should signal an investigation of respiratory disease or gastroesophageal reflux.

Tracheomalacia, lack of rigidity of the trachea, may present as "noisy breathing" or wheezing in infancy. This condition generally is benign and resolves as the child gets older. Fixed lesions, such as vascular rings, tracheal stenosis, or foreign body, should be ruled out in cases of recurrent or persistent stridor.

Heart

The circulatory system in children is very dependent on respiratory function. Most alterations are responses to respiratory changes as can be seen at birth (described previously). The right and left ventricles are equal in size at birth. The left ventricle grows as its work increases postnatally, finally reaching the adult ratio, compared with the right ventricle, of 2:1. Cardiac abnormalities may cause subtle findings in young infants, such as tiring easily or increased breathing effort during feeding, perioral or prolonged cyanosis during feeding or crying, hepatomegaly from congestion, or lack of expected weight gain. Thus, examination of heart function involves the skin, lungs, and liver in addition to cardiac auscultation as described elsewhere in this chapter. Cyanosis distinguishes the two types of congenital heart disease, and the timing of its appearance helps to distinguish between the types of cyanotic heart disease, as seen in Table 8-8.

The heart rate should be counted for a full minute to get an accurate count. Age-appropriate rates are found in Table

Table 8–7.   NORMAL VITALS IN INFANCY

Age	Respiratory Rate (Breaths per Minute)	Heart Rate (Beats per Minute)	Blood Pressure (Average)
Newborn	30–60	120–170	75/40
1–6 mo	30–40	85–160	96/60
6–12 mo	24–30	75–160	100/60

Each increase of 1°F above normal temperature increases respiratory rate by 4 breaths per minute and heart rate by 10 beats per minute.

TABLE 8–8.   CONGENITAL HEART DISEASE

Early Neonatal Cyanosis (Around Birth)	Late Cyanosis (Usually Within First Year)
Severe pulmonary stenosis	Pure pulmonary stenosis
Tetralogy of Fallot	Tetralogy of Fallot
Tricuspid atresia	Eisenmenger complex
Severe septal defect	Large septal defects
Transposition of great vessels	

8-7. The rate may be highly variable, particularly in the young infant, and it changes with feeding, fever, sleeping, or waking. Persistent tachycardia of more than 185 beats per minute should prompt proper investigation. The apical pulse is felt at the fourth or fifth intercostal space at the midclavicular line due to the horizontal placement of the infant's heart. The position becomes more vertical as the child grows and reaches adult positioning by 7 years. Serious medical conditions, such as cardiomegaly or a tension pneumothorax, can displace the apical pulse.

Heart sounds are commonly split. In infants, S2 is higher pitched and more discreet than S1, though infant heart sounds are difficult to evaluate due to the rapid rate and transmission of respiratory sounds across the small chest.

● **Clinical Pearl:** Listening during feeding or pinching the nares briefly may allow discrimination between a murmur and a respiration.

At some point, nearly 90% of children will have a heart murmur (McCrindle et al., 1996), though only 4% to 5% of murmurs are related to cardiac pathology. Murmurs (Table 8-9) are common in the first 2 days of life during the transition from fetal circulation, as are innocent murmurs of childhood. Pathologic murmurs can be either congenital or acquired. One quarter of patients will have extracardiac anomalies as well (McCrindle et al., 1996). In one third of infants with severe cardiac anomalies, a murmur may not be present until the infant is several weeks old (McCrindle et al., 1996). These patients present with poor weight gain, developmental delay, increased respiratory or heart rate, or cyanosis. This is evidence of the importance of checking for a murmur at birth, 1 week, and 6 weeks of age. Please refer to Chapter 56 for further information of specific conditions.

● **Clinical Pearl:** Persistent resting tachypnea should prompt quick investigation because it is present in 90% of infants with serious cardiac pathology. Pathology is suggested when a murmur is loud, pansystolic, late systolic, diastolic or continuous, a single accentuated S2, S4 gallop, or ejection or midsystolic click is heard.

Pressing on the liver to increase right atrial pressure may cause a left-to-right shunt through a patent ductus arteriosus (PDA) or septal defect to disappear or a right-to-left shunt to intensify. A common congenital heart abnormality is the ventricular septal defect (VSD) with an incidence of 1.5 to 2 in 1000 (higher if positive family history, congenital rubella, and chromosomal disorder). A VSD may close spontaneously in 20% to 50% of the cases, by the end of the first year congestive heart failure or other complications may occur in the remaining patients with moderate or large defects. Please refer to Chapter 56 for further information on specific conditions.

▲ **Clinical Warning:** If a murmur does not sound clearly innocent, consulting a cardiologist to determine if the murmur is benign and requires no further intervention is often more cost effective (McCrindle et al., 1996; Swenson et al., 1997) than ordering multiple expensive tests. Tests that may help in accurately making the diagnosis, in concert with a complete history and physical examination, include chest x-ray, electrocardiogram, and 2D M-mode echocardiogram.

Palpation of the pulses is an important aspect of the cardiovascular examination as well. The brachial, radial, and femoral pulses are easily palpated and should be compared. Weaker pulses than expected are indicated by decreased cardiac output or peripheral vasoconstriction, while a bounding pulse may indicate a large left-to-right shunt from a PDA. A weaker or absent femoral pulse compared to the radial pulse suggests coarctation of the aorta.

Capillary refill also gives information related to circulation. Infants have a very rapid capillary refill time (less than 1 second). Capillary refill is noted by compressing the ball of the thumb and counting the seconds until return of blood flow or a "blush." Slower refill times indicate significant dehydration or hypovolemia as a result of peripheral vasoconstriction; however, peripheral vasoconstriction can occur in cool ambient environments in otherwise healthy infants. Acrocyanosis, cyanosis of the hands and feet that is common in newborns and can occur during early infancy, also can obscure observation of the blush.

Table 8–9.   DISTINGUISHING INNOCENT FROM PATHOLOGIC HEART MURMURS IN CHILDREN

Type	Shape	Timing	Grade	Other Findings
Transitional	Ejection	Systolic	I–II	No other signs or symptoms Disappears by 24–36 h of age
Innocent	Ejection Flow	Systolic	<III	No other signs or symptoms Physiologic splitting of S2 Vibratory or musical in character
Pathologic	Ejection Plateau Diamond	Late systolic Holosystolic Diastolic continuous	≥III	Loud, single S2 S4 or S4 gallop Ejection or midsystolic click Cyanosis Resting tachypnea Often noncardiac anomalies present

Abdomen

As the fetus matures, the GI tract develops in a cephalocaudal direction. The GI tract is able to adapt to extrauterine life by 36 to 38 weeks' gestation; however, it does not achieve mature functioning until the child is 2 to 3 years old. Examination should be done when the infant is relaxed and quiet to prevent contracted abdominal muscles. It can be done between cries when the infant takes a breath, because the abdomen should be soft on inspiration. The examiner also can relax the abdomen by holding the infant's legs flexed at the hip and knee with one hand while examining with the other.

The shape and contour should be noted. The infant's abdomen should be rounded and dome-shaped, because the musculature is not fully developed. The chest and abdomen should move synchronously during respiration. An abdomen that protrudes above the chest suggests a mass, organ enlargement, or lower tract distension, while an abdomen that is schaphoid may be due to upper intestinal obstruction. Pulsation in the epigastric area and visible superficial veins are common in the infant, but distended veins may indicate vascular or abdominal obstruction.

The newborn umbilical cord should be inspected for the presence of two arteries and one vein. A single umbilical artery may be associated with congenital anomalies. Any intestinal structure in the umbilical cord or visible through a transparent membrane is an omphalocele. The remaining umbilical cord should fall off by 3 weeks if it is kept dry; this can be done by using an alcohol swab during cleaning and folding the diaper down at the stump to prevent moisture from trapping. The stump should be examined at subsequent visits for signs of infection or umbilical hernia. An umbilical hernia causes more "discomfort" for parents than children, primarily because of the hernia's appearance and parental concerns about resolution. They are 6 to 10 times more common in African American infants and also are associated with Down syndrome and hypothyroidism (presumably secondary to hypotonia) (Zitelli & Davis, 1997). The size of the hernia should be measured at the umbilical opening rather than the width of the protruding contents. The maximum umbilical opening usually occurs by 1 month and spontaneously closes within the first 3 years (Zitelli & Davis, 1997). Surgery thus is deferred until the child is at least 3 to 4 years old or if the opening is greater than 5 cm. The use of pressure dressings (taping a quarter over the belly button) is not useful and may cause contact dermatitis.

Bowel sounds should be present by 1 to 2 hours after birth. No bruits or venous hums should be heard on auscultation unless a renal artery stenosis or renal arteriovenous fistula is present. The abdomen may be more tympanic than expected due to the tendency of infants to swallow air when feeding or crying.

The infant's abdomen should be palpated for organomegaly or masses. The liver edge usually is just below the right costal margin but may extend to 1 to 2 cm below in infants and toddlers. Hepatomegaly is considered when the liver extends more than 3 cm below the right costal margin and suggests infection, liver disease, or cardiac failure. Often hepatomegaly is the first sign of congestive heart failure, and the span of the liver can be used to gauge the effectiveness of therapy. Masses in the abdomen may represent feces, intussusception, pyloric stenosis, or bladder distention; in more than 75% of neonates, they are renal in origin (Zitelli & Davis, 1997). Tenderness to palpation can be difficult to gauge in the infant; however, changes in behavior (such as change in cry pitch, grimacing, or drawing up of the legs) may be indicators.

Genitalia

The genitalia can aid in gestational age assessment, and they reflect the influence of maternal hormones in the early weeks of life. The newborn genitalia should be examined for any abnormality in development or ambiguity. Any genital ambiguity should be investigated expeditiously before a gender is assigned.

At birth, the female genitalia may be swollen and prominent with a protruding vascular hymen. These effects will resolve in a few weeks. The clitoris may appear large initially; this appearance usually does not have significance. The hymen should have a small (0.5 cm) crescent-shaped opening in the midline. An imperforate hymen is rare but may cause problems later in childhood and adolescence. A white vaginal discharge, which may be mixed with blood, is a common finding during the first month of life due to the effects of maternal hormone withdrawal. Labial adhesions may be seen and are often asymptomatic. The adhesions may need to be broken down, however, by highly effective estrogen creams or gentle mechanical separation (if it does not cause significant trauma) to allow urine to pass. Doing so will prevent recurrent vulvovaginitis and urinary tract infections.

In males, the penis should be inspected for placement of urethral opening, anomalies, and projection when erect. The urethra should be slit-like, near the tip of the glans. Hypospadias is misplacement of the urethral meatus to the ventral surface of the glans or shaft of the penis. There is a 5% to 7% familial tendency for hypospadias, and the infant should be examined carefully for other genital anomalies (Seidel, 1997). A circumcision should not be done until after correction of hypospadias. The urinary stream in an infant should be uninhibited, strong, and with good caliber. Abnormalities in the urinary stream may indicate urethral meatal stenosis. A hooked or downward projection of the penis indicates a chordee or tethering and may be associated with hypospadias. Separation of the prepuce from the glans begins in the third trimester and is complete in 90% of uncirumcised boys by age 5 to 6 years. Forceful retraction of the foreskin in an uncircumcised infant should not be done, because it results in tears of the prepuce, which can cause binding adhesions. The circumcised neonate should be inspected for bleeding, ulceration, and inflammation.

Circumcision is the removal of the foreskin. Circumcision remains an elective procedure to be decided by the parents based on the pros and cons and personal and religious beliefs (Table 8-10). Though evidence has been questioned in terms of methodology, reports have shown that uncircumcised males are at increased risk for balanitis, penile cancer, human immunodeficiency virus infection, and urinary tract infections and that their female partners are at increased risk for cervical cancer (AAP, 1999a). Appropriate hygiene, which can be taught, and behaviors later in life significantly decrease the incidence of these problems in uncircumcised men but do not eliminate them entirely. Conversely, circumcision is a surgical procedure with a quoted complication rate of 0.2% to 0.6%; most complications are minor (AAP, 1999a). The AAP recently amended their position on circumcision, stating "Existing scientific evidence demonstrates potential medical benefits of newborn male circumcision; however, these data are not sufficient to recommend routine neonatal circumcision" (AAP, 1999a). If the parents desire circumcision after informed consent, then procedural analgesia should be provided in the form of EMLA cream application 60 to 90 minutes prior to the procedure, dorsal penile nerve block, or the most effective midshaft circumferential subcutaneous ring of lidocaine without epinephrine.

Table 8–10. PROS AND CONS OF CIRCUMCISION

Pros	Cons
Decreased risk of UTIs up to age 5 y	Risks, though rare and usually minor: bleeding, infection, unacceptable cosmetic result, improper healing
Decreased risk of penile cancer	Foreskin has possible protective action against meatitis during infancy
Slightly decreased risk of STIs, including HIV	Possible decreased penile sensation during sexual activity
Decreased incidence of foreskin infection (balanitis)	
Prevention of phimosis	
Ease in genital hygiene	

Source: American Academy of Pediatrics. (1999). *AAP policy statement: Circumcision position statement.*

The scrotum of a full-term male infant should be pendulous with rugae and a midline raphe. It usually appears large compared with the rest of the genitalia. The infant's testes are palpated and in the newborn are about 1 cm in diameter. The testes begin to descend from the retroperitoneal space through the inguinal canal into the scrotum during the third trimester. They may be arrested at any point or follow an abnormal path. Occlusion of the inguinal canal with a finger from the nonexamining hand can help prevent retraction of the testicle into the canal or abdomen during the cremasteric reflex. If either testicle is not palpable, it should be pushed toward the scrotum starting at the upper inguinal ring. If the testicle can be pushed into the scrotum, regardless of whether it retracts back into the canal, it is considered descended. An exaggerated cremasteric reflex is the cause of retractile testes. These testes eventually stay in the scrotum permanently and are not at risk for the complications associated with true undescended testes. A testicle that either cannot be pushed into the scrotum or that is not palpable at all is considered undescended, ectopic, or cryptorchid. Deterioration of cryptorchid testes begins around age 1 year if the testes are not relocated into the scrotum. These testes are associated with infertility, testicular cancer, torsion, and associated hernias. Spontaneous descent after age 6 months is unlikely, so surgical relocation into the scrotum is recommended at around age 1 year. When orchidopexy is performed between 0 and 2 years of age, 90% of men will be fertile (AAP Policy Statement, 1996).

Any scrotal mass that is not the testicle or spermatic cord should be evaluated to determine if it is solid or filled with fluid. Most scrotal masses in infants are hernias or hydroceles. Transillumination is helpful in distinguishing between solid and fluid masses. Hernias are often reducible by pushing the mass back through the external inguinal canal. Hydroceles transilluminate. Hydroceles may be communicating (open tunical vaginalis) or noncommunicating. In communicating hydroceles, mothers may state the scrotum changes size with every diaper change. Noncommunicating hydroceles are the most common and generally resolve spontaneously by 6 months. Communicating hydroceles usually require surgical closure because they may be associated with inguinal hernia.

Rectum

The infant usually passes the first meconium stool sometime within the first 24 to 48 hours of life, indicating anal patency. Lack of stool after this time frame should arouse suspicion of anal atresia, cystic fibrosis, or Hirschsprung's disease. Newborns often stool after each feeding due to the gastrocolic reflex; the stooling patterns of older infants vary widely. The internal and external sphincters are under involuntary reflexive control because spinal cord myelination is incomplete. Voluntary control of the external sphincter is not achieved until 18 to 24 months. External inspection should be performed for masses, redness, fissures, or fistulae. A small anal fissure due to straining or passing of a large stool is the most common cause of bloody stools in an otherwise well infant. The baby should be treated with a mild stool softener to allow healing. Topical steroids are of uncertain use for anal fissures in infants. Asymmetric creases can be seen in congenital dislocation of the hips, and lack of the "anal wink" (contraction of anal sphincter after light touch) may indicate a spinal cord lesion. Rectal examinations are not performed on infants unless a particular problem exists. If an examination is necessary, use of the fifth finger is indicated.

Musculoskeletal System

During infancy and childhood, bones form from cartilage as it calcifies along a specific timed sequence. Thus, ligaments and joints are stronger than bones until adolescence. When injury occurs, fractures result rather than sprains. Skeletal anomalies can result from either genetic abnormalities, fetal insults, or mechanical forces in utero.

Observation of posture and spontaneous generalized movements can provide much information regarding the musculoskeletal system. Symmetry of extremity movements, creases, and proportions are noted. Muscles should be palpated for tone. Any spasticity or flaccidity should be noted. All bones should be palpated for their presence, fractures, dislocations, crepitus, masses, or tenderness.

Developmental dysplasia of the hip (DDH) is both difficult to diagnose and disabling if left untreated. DDH is not always detectable in the newborn examination; as a result, a high index of suspicion and a good clinical examination are indicated at each visit during the first year of life. Most softly positive or equivocal findings will resolve by 2 to 4 weeks; the remainder will require intervention. Increased risk factors in light of equivocal results should prompt earlier referral or ultrasonography (if the child is younger than 6 months) or radiography (if the child is older than 6 months) of the infant's hips. These risk factors include female sex (female newborn risk is 19/1000), breech presentation (female newborn risk is 120/1000 versus male newborn risk of 26/1000), or family history (female newborn risk is 44/1000 versus male newborn risk of 9.4/1000) (AAP, 2000a). If either Barlow's or Ortolani's sign is grossly positive, referral to an orthopedist is indicated. The earlier the child receives treatment, the better the outcome. The Barlow-Ortolani maneuver has become the standard test for detecting hip dislocation or subluxation. The Barlow (dislocation) portion is positive if the femoral head can be dislocated out of the acetabulum. The Ortolani (reduction) portion is positive if a palpable, sometimes audible, "clunk" occurs with reduction of the femoral head into the acetabulum. As the hip musculature increases in strength, decreased abduction of the hip becomes the positive finding as the click becomes less obtainable (see Fig. 8-4 for description of the maneuver).

Congenital clubfoot is apparent at birth and consists of three deformities: the foot in plantar flexion, the hindfoot in fixed inversion, and the forefoot in adducted supination. Etiology is believed to be multifactorial; treatment consists of manipulation and serial casting for progressive correction. Screening for other musculoskeletal deformities is part of each examination and includes genu varum (bow-legged), genu valgum (knock-kneed), intoeing, and other torsional deformities of the lower extremity. Infants stand and walk with a wide stance and are bowlegged up to 20 degrees until 18 months. All infants (and children up to 3 years old) appear flat-footed due to adipose tissue in the arch and have some degree of metatarsus adductus from intrauterine positioning. Watchful waiting is appropriate, because most torsional deformities are physiologic secondary to in utero positioning and are expected to resolve after 6 to 12 months of independent walking. Persistent torsion is rare but may require further investigation and treatment. (For more information, see Chap. 59.) During the newborn period, the hands should open periodically, though infants usually hold them in a fisted position with the thumb inside the fingers. Progressive fine motor development follows.

Spine

The overlying skin is inspected for small defects, pilonodal tufts of hair, or masses near the spine, which may signal a sinus tract, occult spina bifida, or meningocele respectively. With the infant's trunk flexed, the spinal processes are inspected for deformities.

Neurologic System

Growth and myelinization of the CNS are most rapid during the last trimester of pregnancy and through the first year of life but continue until ages 12 to 15 years. Insult at any time during this period of explosive growth can have profound effects on CNS function. Primitive reflexes, such as grasp, moro, and suck (see Table 8-1), are present at birth, and motor development is observed through integrated successive milestones as described previously. Neurologic disorders often are suspected as a result of failure to reach a milestone rather than from an abnormal finding on examination. Primitive reflexes also give clues to neurologic disorders in their timely appearance, disappearance, and symmetry of movement. Consequently, the neurologic examination is intimately tied to developmental assessment. Issues not covered in the development section are described below.

The infant's level of responsiveness to the environment and stimuli should be observed. Of concern would be an infant who is lethargic, drowsy, irritable, or noninteractive with parents or examiner. The quality of the infant's cry should be evaluated as well. A loud, angry cry is expected, while a high-pitched, whiny, or catlike screech suggests a CNS deficit. Fine, high-frequency tremors of the arms and legs can be seen in the newborn; if present after 4 days of life, they may signal a CNS disease. Asymmetry in movements of the extremities at any time should prompt appropriate examination for CNS or peripheral nervous system deficits, birth injuries, or congenital anomalies.

The patellar tendon reflex is present at birth, while the Achilles' and brachioradial tendon reflexes appear at 6 months. The corticospinal pathways are not developed fully, so the absolute presence, absence, or exaggerated response to deep tendon reflex (DTR) testing has very little diagnostic significance unless a different response is obtained from previous testing in a particular infant (Seidel et al., 1997). DTRs often are brisk (3+) in the infant and gradually become the expected 2+ by 6 months of age (Seidel et al., 1997). General observation of the infant's movements and responses is more informative than testing tendon reflexes; however, hypoactive DTRs are seen in muscular dystrophies and lower motor neuron lesions, while hyperactive DTRs are seen with hypocalcemia and upper motor neuron lesions. Several beats of ankle clonus are common and nonpathologic. The Babinski reflex (fanning toes, dorsiflexed great toe) is present and nonpathologic until 24 months. Tests of sensory function are difficult to perform and interpret in young children, but observations can be made through symmetric withdrawal of extremities to stimuli. Cranial nerves are examined and interpreted as in the adult, with observation of spontaneous movement and response to stimuli. Table 8-11 gives examples of things to assess in the infant when observing cranial nerve function.

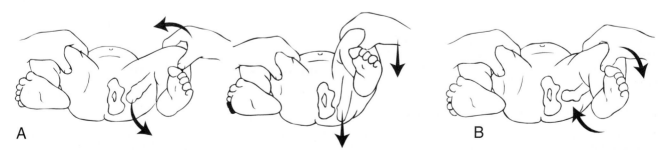

Figure 8–4 ■ Barlow-Ortolani test for DDH. (A) Barlow test should be done first. With the index finger over the greater trochanter and the thumb near the lesser trochanter, abduct the flexed hip to 90°, then adduct to midline with gentle posterior pressure. (B). The Ortolani maneuver is basically reduction of the hip dislocated by Barlow or one that is dislocated at rest. With the hand in the same position as for Barlow, starting with flexed hip in adduction, abduct (externally rotate) the hip and apply pressure to the greater trochanter with the index finger.

Table 8–11.   CRANIAL NERVE ASSESSMENT CLUES IN INFANCY

Cranial Nerve	Observation
CN I, III, IV, VI	Closes eyes in response to bright light
	Extraocular movement tracking of object
	Gazes at parent's or examiner's face
	Doll's eye maneuver (eye muscle function)
CN V	Rooting reflex
	Sucking reflex
CN VII	Symmetry of facial movements during crying or smiling
CN VIII	Response to loud noise by startle, blink, or looking for noise with eyes or turning head
	Doll's eye maneuver (vestibular)
CN IX, X, XII	Gag reflex
	Coordinated suck and swallowing while feeding (also a cerebellar function)

PLAN

A well child is one who has not developed important health problems physically, emotionally, or socially and who is growing and developing as expected. For these children, the AAP recommends routine screening and immunization schedules. New immunization recommendations come out yearly. Primary care providers should consult them, because new vaccines are continually developed and recommended either to replace or be given in addition to current vaccines. See Chapter 13 for in-depth information on immunizations.

Children at risk for health problems, either due to prematurity, congenital anomalies, or dysfunctional family situations, require more intensive intervention. The approach to these children often requires a multidisciplinary team effort.

SCREENING

Screening procedures are part of preventive heath care. In addition to the thorough physical examination performed in the newborn period and at each periodic well child visit, several other procedures are recommended. To allow the child to do his or her best when assessing development, screening tests should be performed when the child is well and familiar with the setting and the clinician. The most commonly used screening test is the Denver Developmental Screening Test II (DDSTII). Screening tests are not appropriate for children at obvious risk for developmental delay (eg, those with cerebral palsy, premature birth, or spina bifida).

Metabolic and Hematologic Screening

In the newborn period, state-specific screening for metabolic and hematologic disorders is completed to ensure prompt diagnosis and treatment and to improve prognosis and prevent many avoidable consequences of such diseases as phenylketonuria and hypothyroidism. Babies whose mothers have blood type O or are Rh negative have their blood typed and a Coombs' test performed to identify hemolysis secondary to incompatibility. Other selected groups should

be screened appropriately during this time as well. After the newborn period, further laboratory studies can be performed as indicated.

Hearing

Risk factors only identify approximately 50% of infants with significant congenital hearing loss (AAP, 1999b). The AAP recently endorsed the Joint Committee on Infant Hearing's recommendations for universal screening of hearing loss in the newborn period by either evoked otoacoustic emissions or auditory brainstem response. For more information, see Chapter 53.

Vision

Vision cannot be adequately tested in children younger than 3 years; however, attention to an infant's eyes should begin in the newborn nursery as described previously. Concerns that arise during examination, from parental history, or because an infant is at risk from previous complications necessitate a referral to an ophthalmologist.

Lead Poisoning and Anemia

Screening for lead poisoning usually is done at the 9- to 12-month visit, when children become mobile and are at risk of ingesting lead-contaminated objects. At particular risk are homes built prior to 1960, when lead-based paint and lead-soldered plumbing pipes were used. Lead intoxication causes microcytic anemia, abdominal pain, malaise, and behavioral changes. If untreated, problems can progress to coma and death when blood lead levels climb high enough (near 60–70 μg/dL). Chronic low-grade lead intoxication can be seen at levels less than 15 μg/dL and often is asymptomatic. It has been found, however, to disturb cognition and is linked to lower IQ scores in affected children (AAP, 1998a).

Screening for iron deficiency anemia also is done in this age group, because the infant's iron stores become depleted by 5 months, and nutritional sources are started. Chronic iron deficiency also has been associated with lower IQ scores and some behavioral changes (primarily irritability). Complicating the picture is that lead poisoning and iron deficiency often coexist in the same patient with additive behavioral and cognitive effects.

ANTICIPATORY GUIDANCE

Anticipatory guidance should take up most of the well child visit. At this time, most questions will be answered, and parents will be educated about what to expect in the interval between their next appointment.

Common Questions and Concerns

When given the chance, most parents will ask questions regarding their concerns. Open-ended questions focusing on the most common areas of concern promote parental involvement. Once a parent has raised a concern, the primary care provider must address it to reassure the parents and educate them. It is unacceptable to ignore the concern. Passive acknowledgment of the problem (eg, asking further questions but not offering any suggestions or reassurance) also is unacceptable. Concerns may be brought up at any time during the interaction, so the primary care provider should be sure to pick up on signals and take advantage of the opportunity to build a relationship with the parents and to educate them about their incredible bundle of joy. The concerns usually are not problems that would be found in the Diagnostic and Statistical Manual of Mental Disorders, which includes mental retardation, developmental coordination disorders, communication disorders, and pervasive developmental disorders (eg, autism), but rather are issues disruptive to the child, parents, or family as a whole. These types of issues have the potential to interfere with the child's optimum functioning, development, and relationships.

Successful well child care is achieved through a partnership between the parents and primary care provider that assists each child to develop to his or her full potential physically, mentally, and emotionally. Once parents raise a concern, the primary care provider needs to obtain additional information. Depending on the nature of the concern, the appropriate response may be giving information: reassurance for normal variations or specific suggestions for the management of abnormal behavior. Written information should be provided and reviewed to reinforce health or behavioral intervention, counseling, or referral. Many parental "overconcerns" are really clues to deeper anxieties or problems with the parent–child relationship. They should be explored after the parent has been reassured about the current concern.

Nutrition

Ensuring adequate nutrition is especially important during childhood when explosive growth occurs. Infants require 110 to 120 kcal/kg/d for the first 6 months and 95 to 100 kcal/kg/d for the remainder of the first year. By comparison, an adult needs 35 to 40 kcal/kg/d (Park et al., 1998). Fortunately, in industrial countries, nutritional deficiencies are uncommon today due to the increase in breast-feeding and nutritionally adequate commercial formulas.

Neonate

Breast milk not only has the ideal quantity and quality of nutrients needed to optimize growth and development, but also protects against infection and chronic diseases across the life span (Display 8-2). The latest AAP recommendation for infant nutrition (AAP, 1997b) states that breast milk is the optimum choice and should be the infant's exclusive diet for the first 6 months. During the next 6 months, breast milk should be continued with solids until the child is 12 months old and thereafter as long as the nursing dyad desires. Before recommending cessation of breast-feeding due to mother or infant illness or medication taken by the mother, the primary care provider should check with any number of resources. There are very few contraindications or circumstances in which breast-feeding cannot occur or continue. Breast-feeding ideally is initiated within the first hour of birth and then every 2 to 3 hours ad lib. Encouraging "rooming in" to avoid delays in nursing can facilitate this. Nursing infants do not require supplemental formula or glucose water. Colostrum is sufficient and will be replaced with milk within the first few days. Every effort should be made to ensure a supportive and friendly environment to promote continued success for mothers who choose to breast-feed. For more information, please see Chapter 7.

Commercial formulas, though containing the minimum RDA of vitamins, are not equivalent to breast milk in either content or benefits. Parents should be aware of the appropriate method of preparing the formula to avoid overdiluting or underdiluting it, which can result in undernutrition or electrolyte imbalances. There is no role for the use of low-

DISPLAY 8–2 • Benefits of Breast Milk for Infant, Mother, and Environment

Breast milk always is conveniently packaged, ready, and the right temperature. Packing for a trip is a snap. Night feedings are easier (no extra hand or going to the kitchen to warm a bottle while the baby is crying, a late sign of hunger).

The average IQs of breast-fed babies are about 10 points higher.

Breast-fed babies are admitted to the hospital 10 times less frequently during the first 18 months.

Breast-fed babies have fewer ear infections, diarrheal infections, blood infections, and meningitis.

Breast-fed babies have fewer cases of pneumonia and bronchitis.

Breast-fed babies have decreased allergic diseases.

Breast-fed babies are six to eight times less likely to experience childhood lymphoma.

Breast-fed babies are at a 25% decreased risk for premenopausal breast cancer as adults.

Breast-fed babies have fewer cases of urinary tract infections, necrotizing enterocolitis, and botulism.

Breast-fed babies have reduced risks for SIDS, type 1 diabetes mellitus, inflammatory bowel disease, and other chronic digestive diseases.

Incidence of breast cancer in breast-feeding women is decreased by 25%. Breast-feeding mothers also are at decreased risk for uterine and ovarian cancer and have fewer hip fractures from osteoporosis.

iron formulas in infants (AAP, 1999c). They carry unacceptable risks of iron deficiency anemia, its associated symptoms, and possibly nonreversible reduction in cognitive ability. Most infants who are not breastfed are given cow's milk-based formula, but in the last decade, the use of soy milk-based formula has risen to approximately 25% of formula use (AAP, 1998b). Soy protein-based formulas use a soy protein isolate to reduce indigestible carbohydrates and antiginicity. All are iron and zinc fortified, thus meeting the AAP guidelines for vitamin, mineral, and electrolyte specifications. In appropriate for gestational age, full-term infants with normal renal function, soy protein-based formula provides appropriate energy and minerals for equivalent growth, development, and bone mineralization as compared with those achieved with cow's milk-based formula. The aluminum content of soy protein-based formulas is 600 to 1300 ng/mL (compared with 4–65 ng/mL in breast milk). Aluminum is deposited in the CNS and competes with calcium for absorption. It contributes to reduced skeletal mineralization (osteopenia). For this reason, soy protein-based formulas are not appropriate for preterm infants, infants with intrauterine growth retardation, and infants with reduced renal function (AAP, 1996b). Soy formulas have been marketed for recovery from acute gastroenteritis and transient lactase deficiency because they are lactose-free. Studies, however, have shown that after immediate rehydration, most infants can be managed with continued breast-feeding or cow's milk-based formulas with no difference in rate of recovery (AAP, 1998c).

The iron in breast milk is highly bioavailable, and supplementation is unnecessary until 6 months. At this time, iron requirements can be met with solid foods. Iron-fortified formula should be used in nonbreast-fed infants or as a supplement in infants who are not exclusively breast-fed.

● **Clinical Pearl:** Studies have found no difference between frequency or consistency of stool or other gastrointestinal symptoms (eg, colic, gas, or spitting up) between infants fed formula with iron compared with those fed formula without iron (AAP, 1999c). The same was true when soy formulas were compared with cow's milk formulas. All formula-fed infants should receive formula with iron, whether soy or cow's milk based. There is also little evidence supporting the use of soy-based formula to help reduce colic or cow's milk protein-induced enteropathy or enterocolitis, because up to 60% of cow's milk allergic infants are also allergic to soy. In these instances, a predigested amino acid-based formula should be used.

Vitamins usually are unnecessary if an infant is obtaining appropriate nutrition, except for the following indications. The amount of vitamin D in breast milk depends on the mother's diet and exposure to the sun. These factors are highly variable, but vitamin D deficiency rickets has occurred in infants of darker skinned mothers, especially during winter months. Consequently, a conservative recommendation has been made for all breast-fed infants to receive vitamin D supplementation through the first 6 months.

One to Three Months

Breast-feeding or iron-fortified formula feeding should be the exclusive diet of infants in this age group as described previously. Vitamin D supplementation of breast-fed infants should continue.

Cow's milk should not be introduced until after the infant's first birthday because of its effects on nutritional iron and the accompanying increased risk of developing chronic medical conditions. Intestinal blood loss has been found to increase 30% in infants fed whole cow's milk, leading to a nutritionally significant loss of iron in the stool. The high levels of calcium and phosphorus and low concentration of ascorbic acid in whole cow's milk interfere with the bioavailability and intestinal absorption of iron from other sources. These two factors may put infants at risk for iron deficiency anemia throughout the first year of life. In young infants, iron deficiency anemia is associated with lower IQ and subtle behavior differences and may lead to long-term behavioral changes that are not reversed even with correction of anemia. Cow's milk also has high concentrations of sodium, potassium, chloride, and protein, producing a high solute load (two to three times that of cow's milk-based formula) to the kidney, which narrows the margin of safety when dehydration is a concern. Strong evidence also is accumulating that links early exposure to bovine antigens and whole soy proteins with development of atopic conditions and type 1 diabetes mellitus in susceptible individuals (Vaarala et al., 1999).

Four to Six Months

Breast-feeding or iron-fortified formula feeding should continue with introduction of solids in this age group. Vitamin D supplementation of breast-fed infants should continue as well.

The introduction of solids depends on the infant's needs and development rather than strict timetables. Infants do not nutritionally require solid foods until after 6 months of age. Introduction of solids before then can increase an infant's risk of developing food allergies. This is due to the immature gut's ability to absorb large protein molecules, which serve as antigenic stimuli to the baby's immune system.

● **Clinical Pearl:** Numerous studies have failed to show any evidence to support the practice of feeding young infants cereal to get them to sleep through the night (Bainbridge et al., 1996). Sleeping through the night results as a combination of CNS maturation, individual biorhythms, and temperament. Only about 50% of infants sleep through the night by 4 to 5 months of age, regardless of feeding method or supplementation.

Once an infant's neurologic development has progressed sufficiently to allow for coordinated movement of the tongue and mouth, solid foods may be introduced. The usual tradition is to begin with rice cereal (rice is least allergenic), progressing to thickened cereal as the infant learns to swallow it. There is nothing magical, however, about infant cereal. It is best to follow the infant's cues and offer foods in which he or she is interested. Meat is actually the best source of iron for infants. Cereal should not be added to bottles due to the risk of choking. Other foods can then be introduced, not necessarily in any particular order, but individually every few days to observe for allergic reaction or intolerance.

● **Clinical Pearl:** Mashed home foods are adequate or commercial baby foods can be chosen if care is taken to avoid those high in sodium (the RDA for sodium for infants is 17.6 mg/kg/d) (Food and Nutrition Board, 1989). Parents can prepare food in a food processor, then fill the wells of an ice cube tray and freeze them. This is a convenient way to make and store home-made baby food in perfect serving sizes. At mealtime, the cubes can be popped out, defrosted, and warmed up before serving.

Six to Nine Months

Breast-feeding or iron-fortified formula feeding should continue with introduction of solids in this age group. Vitamin D supplementation can be discontinued.

As infants get older, they begin to exert independence and want to feed themselves. They should be encouraged to do so. Table foods may be started between 7 and 9 months in the form of finger foods, which include chunks of bananas, well-cooked pasta, scrambled eggs, crunchy toast, and pea-sized pieces of meat. Infants often swallow food without chewing well and are unable to grind food between their teeth until 4 years of age. Infants should never be left unattended while eating and should never be given round or hard, smooth foods than can cause choking. Such choke foods include popcorn, chunks of peanut butter, hard candies, raw carrots, grapes, and raisins. Parents should encourage self-feeding, understanding that the amount that goes into the baby will be less than that which goes everywhere else. As long as the baby continues to grow and develop appropriately, there is no reason to worry about how much the infant actually eats. Self-feeding is a developmental task that infants relish and at some point will accomplish. At this point, the baby's intestines will be impermeable to large protein molecules and the need to wait 4 to 5 days between new foods becomes unnecessary. Fruit juice should be limited to less than 12 oz/d to avoid large consumption of empty calories. Infants who consume too much fruit juice eat fewer required nutritious foods, resulting in obesity, short stature, and chronic diarrhea. No restriction of fat or cholesterol is recommended for infants younger than 2 years due to the need for high-energy intakes to accommodate rapid growth and continued CNS development (Bainbridge et al., 1996).

In children 6 months to 3 years old, fluoride is provided using fluoride drops in areas in which the fluoride level in the water supply is low, an infant is breast-fed and does not receive fluoridated water, or a prediluted liquid formula is used that does not contain fluoride (AAP, 1995). Fluoride should *not* be administered to infants younger than 6 months, whether they are breast-fed or formula fed. Please see Table 8-12 for age-dependent fluoride doses.

Nine to Twelve Months

Breast-feeding or iron-fortified formula feeding should continue with table foods in this age group as described previously. Fluoride supplementation should continue as indicated.

Stooling

Parents often are concerned about the frequency and consistency of stooling in their infants and the normal grunting sounds associated with defecation. Bowel movements vary so much that it is hard to define too many or too few. Frequent, loose bowel movements after every feeding are common in very young infants. Breast-fed infants tend to have loose, seedy, yellow bowel movements, which unaware parents may interpret as yellow diarrhea. Conversely, a bowel movement every few days also is a normal pattern seen in many infants; it becomes more of the normal pattern for breast-fed infants by 1 to 3 months of age. An individual infant may vary each day as well. Parents need reassurance about the wide range of "normal" stooling patterns. Concern is needed when constipation truly is present, defined by infrequent, hard, pellet-like stools with associated pain on defecation or other findings on examination that raise concern. Straining and grunting are part of learning to coordinate bearing down and allowing the rectum to relax to have a bowel movement. They are not signs of pain or difficulty. As long as the stool remains soft, parents should be reassured. No evidence supports the belief that iron-fortified formulas cause constipation. Studies have shown no difference in the number of stools per day and frequency of hard or firm stools between those drinking no-iron and those drinking iron-fortified formulas (AAP, 1999c). Given the potential long-lasting harm iron deficiency can cause, only iron-fortified formulas should be used if the infant is not breast-feeding.

Pacifier

The use of a pacifier is quite common. Infants have a basic need to suck and will do so on any number of objects they can get into their mouths, including their hands or blankets.

Table 8–12. DIETARY FLUORIDE SUPPLEMENTATION SCHEDULE (REVISED 1994)

Age of Child	Fluoride in Home Water (Parts/Million)		
	<0.3	0.3–0.6	>0.6
0–6 mo	0*	0	0
6 mo–3 y	0.25	0	0
3–6 y	0.5	0.25	0
6–16 y	1	0.5	0

*mg of fluoride/day. Jointly endorsed by the American Academy of Pediatrics, the American Academy of Pediatric Dentistry, and the American Dental Association.

There are several concerns regarding use of pacifiers. First is the imprinting of oral gratification for frustration. The infant is frustrated, cries, and gets the pacifier to calm down. Some argue this leads to unhealthy eating habits later in life for comfort as a result of nonsubstitive sucking or oral stimulation. Some evidence also suggests that infants who use a pacifier in the latter part of the first year of life have increased ear infections, though this relationship is unclear (AAP, 2000b). The use of a pacifier is associated with difficulty breast-feeding due to nipple confusion in some infants; thus, it should be avoided at least during the critical time of breastfeeding initiation and establishment of a successful nursing dyad. Also is the issue of midnight search parties for the pacifier if it should fall out of the infant's reach. Parents frequently are encouraged now, for a number of reasons, to avoid the use of pacifiers and to encourage the infant to learn self-comforting techniques, such as crying, sucking the fist or a comfort object, or holding a blanket or stuffed toy.

Injury Prevention

Among children younger than 1 year, airway obstruction (eg, suffocation, choking, and strangulation) is the leading cause of unintentional injury-related death, followed by motor vehicle occupant injury, fires and burns, drownings, falls, and poisonings (Centers for Disease Control and Prevention, 1998). Parents should be counseled on risks so they can baby-proof their home to decrease the risk of unintentional injury.

Airway obstruction may occur internally as a result of choking on food or small objects. Small children are especially prone to choking because of the small size of their airways and their natural curiosity that causes them to put objects in their mouths. Airway obstruction may result from materials that block or cover the external airways (suffocation), such as plastic bags. Infants are at increased risk for suffocation because of their inability to lift their heads or remove themselves from tight places (eg, from between a mattress and a wall). External airway obstruction also may occur when an item such as a window blind cord, drawstring, necklace, or pacifier string becomes wrapped around an infant's neck and interferes with breathing (strangulation).

Auto safety is another concern. Child safety seats are extremely effective when correctly installed and used in passenger cars, reducing the risk of infant death by 71% (National SAFE KIDS Campaign, 1999). All 50 states require the use of child safety seats for all children. Infants should ride in rear-facing safety seats until they are 1 year old and weigh 20 lb. The safest place for children is in the rear seat. A rear-facing safety seat should never be placed in the front seat of a car with a passenger air bag (AAP, 1996c).

Water safety is an issue for all ages. Infants can drown in just a few inches of water. More than 50% of infant drownings occur in bathtubs (National SAFE KIDS Campaign, 1999). Drowning in infants also can occur in toilets and buckets. Infants should never be left alone around water in the home (eg, bathtubs, toilets, buckets) or around open bodies of water (eg, lakes or swimming pools).

Scalding burns in younger children usually result from spills of hot foods or liquids. The provider should counsel parents not to hold small children while the adults are consuming hot liquids. Hot tap water accounts for nearly 25% of all scald burns and for more deaths and hospitalizations than other hot liquid burns (National SAFE KIDS Campaign, 1999). These tap water burns usually occur in the bath and thus tend to cover a larger portion of the body. The younger the child, the thinner is his or her skin, so water will burn infants at lower temperatures and more severely than older children or adults. A child exposed to tap water at 140°F for 3 seconds will sustain a third-degree burn (National SAFE KIDS Campaign, 1999). The provider should instruct parents to set the hot water heater no higher than 120°F and to check the bath water before putting an infant in it.

As infants become increasingly mobile, falls are common. Their curiosity that leads them to climb on furniture, tables, and other objects places them at risk for falling off or backwards. Parents should secure unsteady tables and heavy objects because infants, when pulling themselves to standing, also may pull down objects on themselves, resulting in serious injury. Parents should block off stairs to prevent serious falls. A major health hazard to discuss with parents is the use of infant walkers. In 1993 alone, the National Electronic Injury Surveillance System of the U.S. Consumer Products Safety Commission recorded 25,000 children between 5 and 15 months treated in emergency rooms for injuries associated with the use of infant walkers. Eleven related deaths occurred between 1989 and 1993. Stairs are implicated in 75% to 80% of injuries and account for nearly all severe injuries, including closed head injuries and fractures. Gates are not protective enough to prevent falls. In one study, more than one third of falls occurred while stair gates were in place. Walkers have been found to impede crawling and may delay walking by a few weeks. No evidence exists of persistent abnormal gait or motor development as a result of walker use. Due to the considerable risk of harm and even risk of death with no benefit, parents should be advised to avoid all mobile infant walker use (Smith et al., 1997).

Another risk from an infant's natural curiosity and exploring is the possibility of poisoning. All household products and medications should be locked out of sight and reach. The poison control center number should be kept at the telephone, and syrup of ipecac should be available in the home. Syrup of ipecac should not be used until the poison control center instructs the parent to do so. This is important to avoid further damage from some ingestions when emesis occurs. Another source of poisoning to which younger children are more prone is carbon monoxide poisoning. This most often occurs in the winter months as a result of unvented supplemental heaters, poorly ventilated fireplaces, or gas leaks. A carbon monoxide detector can be used to assess risk and avoid this potential poisoning.

Common Conditions

The visit to the primary care provider also is the time to review common conditions or issues for each age group and how to handle them.

Spitting Up

Feeding and gastrointestinal problems commonly are major concerns of parents. Spitting up during or after feeding occurs frequently, usually with burping, and generally causes the infant no discomfort. This is a developmental issue, because the lower esophageal sphincter does not become fully functional until nearly the end of the first year. The analogy of a full, untied balloon that leaks with increased abdominal pressure or overdistention (ie, the stomach with decreased lower esophageal sphincter function) can be used to explain this process to parents. Recommending a firmer nipple or smaller holes to prevent feeding too fast or swallowing air may help. Overfeeding may be the culprit; in this case the parents should try to interpret their infant's cues and provide appropriate comfort (diaper change, cuddling, pacifier/fist) rather than feeding whenever the infant cries.

Gastroesophageal Reflux

Complicated, or pathologic, reflux occurs less frequently than spitting up and is associated with failure to thrive, aspiration, and even apnea. Investigation may include barium swallow (which identifies abnormality in 50% of cases) (Zitelli & Davis, 1997). Modified milk scan, esophageal pH probe, or esophageal manometry may identify more persistent or difficult presentations. In mild cases, treatment is conservative with small, frequent feedings and maintenance of an upright position for 30 to 60 minutes after feeding. Adding rice cereal to milk in a bottle (breast or formula) to thicken the consistency often is recommended at a ratio of 1 tablespoon/oz. Pharmacologic intervention is required if complications are severe or resistant to conservative measures. Medications then used include prokinetic agents (metoclopramide [Reglan]) and the H_2 blockers (ranitidine [Zantac], cimetidine [Tagamet]).

Vomiting

Vomiting is uncomfortable for the infant and requires investigation. Pyloric stenosis often presents at 3 to 6 weeks. It is characterized by persistent, projectile, nonbilious vomiting and may progress to failure to thrive. A pyloric "olive" mass in the epigastrium and visible intestinal peristaltic waves after feeding often are found clinically. Ultrasound or barium swallow can confirm the diagnosis; treatment is pyloromyotomy. Another pathologic cause of vomiting seen in infants 3 to 12 months is intussusception or invagination of a portion of bowel into itself. The onset can be dramatic as an apparently well child suddenly begins crying inconsolably, with acute intermittent abdominal pain, distention, and vomiting. Pain seems to subside but then returns; subsequent stools may be mixed with blood and mucus (red currant jelly). Etiology is unknown in this age group. A sausage-shaped mass usually can be palpated, and abdominal films often reveal obstruction. A barium or air contrast enema confirms the diagnosis and often reduces the intussusception with a less than 5% recurrence rate. If an enema fails to reduce the obstruction or it recurs, immediate surgery is required.

Colic

Colic and crying spells are trying for any parent and thus often are brought to the primary care provider's attention during visits. Almost all babies have a fussy period in the early evening lasting 1 to 2 hours, but colic is characterized by paroxysms of crying, pulling up of legs as if abdominal pain is present, and irritability. It also lasts for much longer periods. Colic affects 10% to 20% of infants and generally starts at a few weeks of age. It spontaneously resolves sometime before 3 to 4 months. Excessive crying causes the infant to swallow air, resulting in abdominal distention and flatulence. This is probably why antigas drops have been given in an attempt to provide relief and presumably stop the crying. Unfortunately, no evidence has proven the etiology of colic or the effectiveness of antigas medications and so they should be avoided (Lucassen et al., 1998). If milk intolerance is suspected, a short trial of predigested formulas, such as Alimentum or Nutramigen, should be considered. Soy formula should not be substituted.

Colicky infants eat, gain weight well, and have normal physical examinations. Counseling parents to arm them with knowledge as to cause, what is and is not known, and duration of colic is of more value than switching to soy formula. Parents also should be counseled on what nonpharmacologic methods they can try. Motion, as in car rides, carriages, or any device that makes motion, appears anecdotally to be of benefit. Also, holding the infant across the lap belly down to put gentle pressure on the abdomen may provide relief. Infant massage has had some success as well and can be found in various books. One method is a 5-minute, three-part massage at each diaper change. Long strokes are done with the parent's palm from chin to diaper area in a hand after hand pattern so that one hand is always stroking the infant's trunk, and this is followed by a gentle "riding a bicycle" motion with the infant's legs. The last step is a clockwise circle massage around the belly button. Parents should be reassured that colicky infants are basically healthy, that excessive crying is not harmful to the infant, and that the episodes will end eventually.

▲ **Clinical Warning:** Many providers still prescribe drugs, such as paregoric, for colic. Controlled studies have consistently failed to show benefit from these medications, and they may actually cause respiratory distress.

Illness

On average, children have six to eight colds per year the first 2 years of life; this number is higher if the child is enrolled in daycare (Appropriate use of antibiotics for URIs in children, 1998). As a result, parents may feel like their child is always sick and worry that something is wrong immunologically. Infants have limited immune function and must develop immunity to each infectious particle they encounter. Nursing infants have fewer colds than non-nursing infants due to the passive transfer of antibodies (primarily secretory IgA), other proteins, and immune cells in mother's milk. The vast majority of infants with colds are well children. Fewer than 5% of children with recurrent infections have an immunodeficiency; the unusual site of infection, unusual infectious agent, or unusually severe infection to a common agent often readily identifies such children. Parents often want to be able to do something to help ease their children's symptoms and, as a group, spend an enormous amount of money on over-the-counter cold medications. For more information, see Chapter 30.

● **Clinical Pearl:** Of those studies that can be found that specifically examine the young child (ages 6 months to 5 years), no evidence suggests that an antihistamine-decongestant combination, or each separately, reduces cold symptoms. The risks to using over-the-counter medications are the cost, side effects (such as sedation or hyperactivity), and accidental ingestion or overdose. Consequently, parents should be encouraged to increase fluids, use vaporizers, and avoid cold medications in this age group (Clemens et al., 1997; Katcher, 1996).

Failure to Thrive

Failure to thrive is a common problem, with an incidence ranging from 5% to 10% in children in the first year of life. The vast majority of cases are nonorganic in etiology and result from a dysfunctional psychosocial environment or interaction (Identification and Management of FTT, 2000). For more information, see Chapter 23.

Child Abuse

Child abuse is unfortunately too common. Approximately 10% of children younger than 5 years who are seen for trauma have inflicted injuries (Herman-Giddens et al., 1999). Legal definitions vary among states, but inflicted rather than accidental injury generally is considered as abuse. Neglect falls under this category as well. All primary care providers should specifically look for, note, and report any signs of child abuse or neglect at each patient encounter to protect children. Unfortunately, the number of children who die from abuse is vastly underreported by as much as 60% (Herman-Giddens et al., 1999). Early recognition and reporting of child abuse may help to prevent subsequent homicides. Findings that should prompt further investigation are bruises in sites not usually hurt during falls, burns, rope marks or other unusual markings on the skin, and fractures.

Sudden Infant Death Syndrome

The definition of SIDS is a sudden death in an infant in which no cause of death can be identified after a thorough investigation. Each year more than 5000 infants die of SIDS in the United States. It is the most common cause of death in infants 1 week to 1 year of age. Deaths from SIDS peak at age 3 months. Most SIDS deaths occur between ages 1 and 5 months, with a slightly higher incidence in males. African Americans and Native Americans have two to three times higher rates (AAP, 2000b).

The loss of an infant to SIDS is devastating for parents, families, and their health professionals. The etiology is still unknown, though theories that have been proposed include abnormal (or immature) respiratory control, suffocation, prolonged QT syndrome, or a combination of intrinsic and extrinsic factors that tragically includes intentional injury. Identifying a group of infants at increased risk is difficult, though many theories have been proposed. Prone sleeping seems to be associated with impairment of airway protection reflexes (such as swallowing and behavioral arousal) and may explain the increased risk of SIDS in the prone position (Jeffery et al., 1999). Other identified risks include male sex, young maternal age, twins, low socioeconomic status, maternal smoking, maternal alcohol use, and bottle feeding (l'Hoir et al., 1998).

Unfortunately, testing with a pneumogram or home monitoring of infants at perceived risk has not decreased the incidence of SIDS (AAP, 2000b). Modifiable risk factors that have been identified and addressed include maternal smoking, prematurity, and sleeping position; these have impacted the incidence of SIDS. Maternal smoking is associated with almost a three times increased risk of SIDS. The risk of household smoke exposure compounds maternal smoking risk. In households where more than 40 cigarettes per day are smoked, there is a 7.5 times increased risk (Fleming et al., 1996). The "Back to Sleep" campaign, with its increased public education, has been reported to have decreased the incidence of SIDS by 40% in the United States (Willinger et al., 1998). No evidence has shown that supine sleeping results in delayed motor milestones outside the normal range of development (Davis et al., 1998). The risk of SIDS is reduced by placing an infant on the side to sleep (as compared to prone sleeping) but is much less effective than placing the infant on the back to sleep, so side sleeping is not recommended either. The risk of SIDS in infants placed on the side to sleep who were found prone at the time of death was 21 times the risk of those infants placed on the side who remained on the side or rolled to supine (Fleming et al.,

1996). These recommendations are for sleeping, and the parents should be advised to have some "tummy time" during play for development of the upper trunk and neck.

The family bed is a concept that many societies practice. After western societies became industrialized, solitary infant sleeping emerged. Benefits of the family bed that have been described include coordination of infant and parent sleep cycles; improved sleeping, breathing, and waking of infants; and rapid availability of the mother for breastfeeding. Some studies have found an increased risk of SIDS in infants who share a family bed; others have not. These studies have been debated in terms of their control of confounding factors. The only clear, evidence-based recommendations on bedsharing that can be made are that soft bedding, comforters, and pillows should not be around the infant. The infant should be placed in the supine position, regardless of where he or she sleeps.

Management of SIDS unfortunately is limited to supporting the surviving parents and, no less so, the surviving siblings. Parents will need counseling on risks for subsequent children and avoidance of overprotection, leading to the "vulnerable child" syndrome. This syndrome is characterized by a disruption in the parent–child relationship, with the parents being so overprotective and restrictive that the child has difficulty with separation, displays infantile behavior, is overconcerned with minor injuries, and underachieves at school.

COMMUNITY RESOURCES

Numerous resources are available today to help parents with parenting because, unfortunately, babies do not come with instruction books, and the close-knit large extended family is becoming less common. It is helpful for parents to have somewhere to turn when questions arise. This empowers and supports parents to promote healthy growth and development of their children.

Books

Briggs, G.G., Freeman, Freeman, R.K., Yaffe, S.J. (1998). *Drugs in pregnancy and lactation* (5th ed.) A reference guide to fetal and neonatal risk. Baltimore, MD: Williams & Wilkins.

Eisenberg, A., Murkoff, H.E., Hathaway, S.E. (1996). *What to expect the first year.* New York: Workman Publishing.

Eisenberg, A., Murkoff, H.E., Hathaway, S.E. (1996). *What to expect the toddler years.* New York: Workman Publishing.

Eisenberg, A., Murkoff, H.E., Hathaway, S.E. (1996). *What to expect when you're expecting.* New York: Workman Publishing.

Green, M. (1996). Bright futures. *Guideline for health supervision of infants, children and adolescents pocket guide.* Arlington, VA: National Center for Education in Maternal and Child Health.

Hale, T. (2000). *Medications and mother's milk* (9th ed.).Pharmasoft Medical Publishing.

Mohrbacher, N., and Stock, J. *The breast feeding answer book.* Schaumburg: La Leche League.

Schneider McClure, V. (j1989). *Infant massage: A handbook for loving parents.* Schaumburg: La Leche League International.

Organizations

American Academy of Family Physicians
8880 Ward Parkway
Kansas City, MO 64114
Phone: (816) 333-9700
http://www.aafp.org

American Academy of Pediatrics National Headquarters
141 Northwest Point Boulevard
Elk Grove Village, IL 60007-1098
Phone: (847) 228-5005
http://www.aap.org

American SIDS Institute
6065 Roswell Road, Suite 876
Atlanta, GA 30328

American Society for Deaf Children
1820 Tribute Road, Suite A
Sacramento, CA 95815

National Federation of the Blind
1800 Johnson Street
Baltimore, MD 21230

Pediatric/Adolescent Gastroesophageal Reflux Association
P.O. Box 1153
Germantown, MD 20875-1153

Web Sites

- Old Wives Tales and Other Pediatric Myths (*http://members.aol.com/tireswing/index.html*)
- The Virtual Children's Hospital (*http://vch.vh.org/*)
- Why Breast Feed web site (*http://www.erols.com/cindyrn/index.htm*)

REFERENCES

American Academy of Pediatrics. (1995). Committee on Nutrition: Fluoride supplementation for children: Interim policy recommendations. *Pediatrics, 95*(5), 777.

American Academy of Pediatrics. (1996a). AAP policy statement: Aluminum toxicity in infants and children (RE9607). *Pediatrics, 97*(3), 413–416.

American Academy of Pediatrics. (1996b). AAP policy statement: Timing of elective surgery on the genitalia of male children with particular reference to the risks, benefits and psychological effects of surgery and anesthesia (RE9610). *Pediatrics, 97*(4), 590–594.

American Academy of Pediatrics. (1996c). AAP policy statement: Selecting and using the most appropriate car safety seats for growing children: Guidelines for counseling parents (RE9618). *Pediatrics, 97*(5), 761–762.

American Academy of Pediatrics. (1996d). AAP policy statement: Eye examination and vision screening in infants, children and young adults (RE9625). *Pediatrics, 98*(1), 153–157.

American Academy of Pediatrics. (1997a). AAP policy statement: Environmental tobacco smoke: A hazard to children (RE9716). *Pediatrics, 99*(4), 639–642.

American Academy of Pediatrics. (1997b). AAP policy statement: Breastfeeding and the use of human milk (RE9729). *Pediatrics, 100*(6), 1035–1039.

American Academy of Pediatrics. (1998a). AAP policy statement: Screening for elevated blood lead levels (RE9815). *Pediatrics, 101*(6), 1072–1078.

American Academy of Pediatrics. (1998b). AAP policy statement: Soy protein-based formulas: Recommendations for use in infant feeding. *Pediatrics, 101*(1), 148–153.

American Academy of Pediatrics. (1998c). AAP policy statement: Cholesterol in childhood. *Pediatrics, 101*(1), 141–147.

American Academy of Pediatrics. (1999a). AAP policy statement: Circumcision policy statement. *Pediatrics, 103*(3), 686–693.

American Academy of Pediatrics. (1999b). AAP policy statement: Newborn and infant hearing loss: Detection and intervention. *Pediatrics, 103*(2), 527–530.

American Academy of Pediatrics. (1999c). AAP policy statement: Iron-fortification of infant formulas. *Pediatrics, 104*(1), 119–123.

American Academy of Pediatrics. (2000a). AAP clinical practice guideline: Early detection of developmental dysplasia of the hip (AC0001). *Pediatrics, 105*(4), 896–905.

American Academy of Pediatrics. (2000b). AAP policy statement: Changing concepts of SIDS: Implications for infant sleeping environment and sleep position (RE9946). *Pediatrics, 105*(3), 650–656.

American Academy of Pediatrics. (1996). AAP policy statement: Timing of elective surgery on the genitalia of male children with particular reference to the risks, benefits, and psychological effects of surgery and anesthesia (RE9610). *Pediatrics, 97*(4), 590–594.

Bainbridge, R. R., Mimouni, F. B., Landi, T., et al. (1996). Effect of rice cereal feedings on bone mineralization and calcium homeostasis in cow milk formula fed infants. *Journal of the American College of Nutrition, 15*(4), 383–388.

Bito, L. Z., Matheny, A., Cruickshanks, K. J., et al. (1997). Eye color changes past early childhood. *Archives of Ophthalmology and Otology, 115*, 659–663.

Bland, H. E. (1996). Jaundice in the healthy term neonate: When is treatment indicated? *Current Problems in Pediatrics,* 355–363.

Centers for Disease Control and Prevention. (1998). CDC surveillance summaries. *Morbidity and Mortality Weekly Report, 47*(SS-2), 15–30.

Clemens, C. J., Taylor, J. A., Almquist, J. R., et al. (1997). Is an antihistamine-decongestant combination effective in temporarily relieving symptoms of the common cold in preschool children? *Journal of Pediatrics, 130*(3), 463-6.

Davis, B. E., Moon, R. Y., Sachs, H. C., et al. (1998). Effects of sleep position on infant motor development. *Pediatrics, 102*, 1135–1140.

Dowell, S. F., Phillips, W. R., The Pediatric URI Consensus Team. (1998). Appropriate use of antibiotics for URIs in children: Part II. Cough, pharyngitis, and the common cold. *American Family Physician, 59*, 1335–1344.

Fleming, P. J., Blair, P. S., Bacon, C., et al. (1996). Environment of infants during sleep and risk of the sudden infant death syndrome: Results of 1993-5 case-control study for confidential inquiry into stillbirths and deaths in infancy. *British Medical Journal, 313*, 191–195.

Food and Nutrition Board. (1989). *Recommended daily allowances* (10th ed.). National Academy Press.

Gartner, L. M., & Lee, K. S. (1999). Jaundice in the breastfed infant. *Clinics in Perinatology, 26*(2), 431–435.

Herman-Giddens, M. E., Brown, G., Verbiest, S., et al. (1999). Number of children killed by child abuse underreported. *Journal of the American Medical Association, 282*, 463–467.

Jeffery, H. E., and Megevand, A. (1999). Reduced airway protection in prone position may explain SIDS risk in prone position. *Pediatrics, 104*, 263–269.

Johnson, D. P., & Blasco, P. A. (1997). Infant growth and development. *Pediatrics in Review, 18*(7), 224–242.

Katcher, M. L. (1996). Cold, cough and allergy medications: Uses and abuses. *Pediatrics in Review, 17*(1), 12–17.

l'Hoir, M. P., Engelberts, A. C., van Well, G. T., et al. (1998). Case-control study of current validity of previously described risk factors for SIDS in the Netherlands. *Archives of Diseases in Children, 79*, 386–393.

Liptak, G. S., & Serletti, J. M. (1998). Pediatric approach to craniosynostosis. *Pediatrics in Review, 19*(10), 352–359.

Lucassen, P. L. Assendelft, W. J., Gubbels, J. W., et al: Effectiveness of treatments for infantile colic: Systematic review. *British Medical Journal, 316*, 1563–1569.

McCrindle, B. W., Shaffer, K. M., Kan, J. S., et al. (1996). Cardinal clinical signs in the differentiation of heart murmurs in children. *Archives of Pediatrics & Adolescent Medicine, 150*(2), 169–174.

National SAFE KIDS Campaign, December 1999.

Park, M. J., Namgung, R., Kim, D. H. et al. (1998). Bone mineral content is not reduced despite low vitamin D status in breast milk-fed infants versus cow's milk based formula-fed infants. *Journal of Pediatrics, 132*(4), 641–645.

Seidel, H. M., (Ed.) (1997). *Mosby's guide to physical examination* (4th ed.). St. Louis: Mosby Year Book.

Smith, G. A., Bowman, M. J., Luria, J. W., et al. (1997). Babywalker-related injuries continue despite warning labels and public education. *Pediatrics, 100*(2), E1.

Swenson, J. M., Fischer, D. R., Miller, S. A. et al. (1997). Are chest radiographs and electrocardiograms still valuable in evaluating new pediatric patients with heart murmurs or chest pain? *Pediatrics, 88*(1), 1–3.

Vaarala, O., Knip, M., Paronen, J., et al. (1999). Cow's milk formula feeding induces primary immunization to insulin in infants at genetic risk for type 1 diabetes. *Diabetes, 48*(7), 1389–1394.

Willinger, M., Hoffman, J. H., Wu, K. T. et al. (1998). Factors associated with the transition to nonprone sleep positions of infants in the United States. *Journal of the American Medical Association, 280*(4), 329–335.

Wright, C. M. (2000). Identification and management of failure to thrive: A community perspective. *Archives of Diseases in Children, 82* (1), 5–9.

Zitelli B. J., & Davis, H. W. (Eds.) (1997). *Atlas of pediatric physical diagnosis* (3rd ed.) (pp. 27–74). St. Louis: Mosby Year-Book.

Healthy Growth and Development of the Toddler

• SUSAN J. BRILLHART, MSN, RN, CS, PNP

INTRODUCTION

The toddler, ages 1 through 3, can be a delightful, engaging, and exasperating individual. Some toddlers are timid, some very spirited, and all will need to be very involved in the plan of care. Toddlers can be shy, inquisitive, and dependent, yet they enjoy asserting their opinions. One toddler has the ability to exhaust a whole group of adults. Toddlers will challenge adults with very definite needs and wants, yet they may lack the verbal skills to convey such wishes clearly. Their psychosocial growth is progressing rapidly, while their physical growth is slowing. Their health problems are, hopefully, few. Care of the toddler is true family-centered care, because few toddlers will cooperate in a primary care setting if their caregivers are not actively involved.

GROWTH AND DEVELOPMENT

A child's growth slows considerably after 12 months, with height and weight increasing in intermittent increments. Growth is about 3 in (7.7 cm) in length and 4 to 6 lb (1.8–2.7 kg) in weight per year, with most toddlers reaching an average height of 34 in (87 cm) and weight of 27 lb (12.3 kg) at 2 years. The toddler's height at 2 years is about half expected adult height. During the second year, head circumference normally increases about 1 in (2.6 cm). Between ages 2 and 5 years, growth continues at about ½ in (1.3 cm) per year.

The toddler generally begins to walk by age 12 to 15 months, displaying the classic protruding abdomen and bowleggedness. The abdomen will protrude less as the abdominal muscles develop, and the bowleggedness will disappear as the weight of the trunk becomes more proportional to the rest of the body. Other major milestones to be achieved are running, speaking a vocabulary of at least 200 words by age 2 years, walking backwards, and hopping on one foot by age 3 years. Toddlers generally do not alternate feet when climbing stairs.

Because the toddler's anatomy and physiology differ from those of the infant and adult, there are multiple normal variations of which the primary care provider should be aware for this age group. Some of these variations also require changes in examination technique.

Physical Development

Skin, Head, and Neck

There is a decrease in the proportion of subcutaneous fat during the second year. The posterior fontanelle should have closed at 2 months, with the anterior fontanelle closing by 2 years. Shoddy lymph nodes are normal, because they are more prominent than in adults.

Eyes

Permanent eye color usually is established by 1 year of age. A pink glow to the iris is indicative of albinism; black and white speckling is indicative of Down syndrome. Large spacing between the eyes may be normal but also may indicate a problem. Unfortunately, there is no accurate method to test visual acuity for the child younger than 3 years. The use of the red reflex and cover tests, however, may provide significant insights into possible visual deficits.

Ears

The auditory canal is directed upward, and the pinna should be pulled downward to aid visualization. The speculum should be inserted far enough so that the pneumatic otoscopy can be performed. After a child cries, a slight redness is normal as a result of increased vascularity. At a distance of 8 ft, the clinician should whisper a sound, command, or question appropriate to the child's developmental level. An adherent lobule of skin may be a normal variation on the external ear.

Nose

A nasal speculum usually is not necessary. The examination may be done by pushing the tip of the nose upward with the thumb and visualizing with a light. Watery discharge is normal if the child has been crying. When examining, the provider should remember that paranasal sinuses are not well developed until late childhood.

Mouth and Oropharynx

A toddler's crying is an opportunity to visualize the oral cavity. Tonsils are larger in children than adults, extending beyond the palatine arch until age 11 or 12 years. Foul odor in the mouth may indicate a foreign body in the nose. The tongue's mobility should be noted; protrusion may indicate mental retardation, while shortening affects speech. Timing and sequence of tooth eruption are noted by the following formula:

Child's age in months − 6 = number of teeth (up to age 2 years)

Thus, an 18-month-old toddler should have 12 teeth. By age 2½ years, 20 deciduous teeth should have erupted. If the child is cooperative, the examination may be done without a tongue blade.

Lungs

At this age, respiratory activity is abdominal; therefore, intercostal motion is abnormal. The toddler's chest normally is more resonant than that of the adult, and breath sounds are louder due to the thinness of the chest wall. The child's crying can be used as an opportunity to evaluate fremitus.

Heart

Up to age 7 years, the apical impulse often is visible and felt normally in the fourth intercostal space just to the left of the midclavicular line. Heart sounds are louder, with a higher pitch and shorter duration than adults. S_1 is louder than S_2 at the apex. Sinus arrhythmia occurs normally in many children, as do innocent murmurs, which must be distinguished from organic murmurs. More than 50% of children develop innocent murmurs during their childhood. Correct diagnosis of the murmur is important to rule out more serious heart disease. Innocent murmurs are usually systolic, of short duration, less than grade 3 intensity, and of a low-pitched, vibratory, musical quality. They often are poorly transmitted and are heard best with the bell along the left sternal border in the second or third interspaces, with the child lying supine (Bates, 1995). Murmurs vary in intensity and quality with position change. Innocent murmurs also are characterized by a physiologically split S_2 (the split between A_2 and P_2 varying with inspiration and expiration).

Abdomen

Up to age 4 years, the abdomen is larger than the chest, making the toddler appear "potbellied" both when sitting and standing. Abdominal respirations are normal up to age 7 years; lack of abdominal movement is indicative of a problem. Umbilical hernias are common in children younger than 2 years and in older children of some ethnic groups. Most resolve without intervention by age 5 years. The liver edge is palpable 1 to 2 cm below the right costal margin. Visible peristaltic waves and aortic beat in the epigastric region may be normal for thin children but always warrant further evaluation. Abdominal skin should be used to test skin mobility and turgor. Tenderness during examination may be determined by noting the child's expression or pitch of cry.

Rectum and Genitalia

Perianal skin tags are common in children. The clinician should observe for diaper rash. Forcible retraction of foreskin on an uncircumcised male should not be attempted. In females, vaginal and labial adhesions are noted, as is a pronounced clitoris. Parents should be reassured that such findings are normal and advised to diaper loosely to avoid irritation.

Musculoskeletal/Neurologic

Abduction of the forefoot distal to the metatarsal/tarsal line is common and usually corrects itself by 2 years. During infancy and young toddlerhood, many children appear "bowlegged." As toddlerhood progresses, they change to a "knock knees" appearance. In toddlers, thoracic convexity is decreased, and lumbar concavity is increased. Muscle strength, motor coordination, cognitive-perceptual development, and cranial nerve function are tested predominantly through observation and must be in relation to norms for growth and development.

Psychosocial Development

Psychosocial development is a major accomplishment during the toddler years, with Erikson describing the psychosocial crisis as *autonomy versus shame and doubt*. The general theme is that of holding on and letting go, with the significant person being the male caretaker. Ideally, the toddler has developed a sense of trust, has decreasing dependency needs, and is ready to begin to master six major areas: individuation (differentiation of self from others); separation from caregivers; control of body functions; communication with words; acquisition of socially acceptable behavior; and egocentric interactions with others. While accomplishing these goals, the toddler develops a sense of control, increasing independence, and autonomy. If the toddler is kept dependent in areas he or she has begun to master, or if the toddler is made to feel inadequate when attempting new skills, the child may develop a sense of shame and doubt. During this time of extensive psychosocial development, the continued need for a security object (eg, blanket) is expected, especially during times of stress.

Freud describes the toddler conflict of holding on and letting go as the *anal* stage (age 8 months–4 years). The focus shifts from the mouth to the anal area, with emphasis on bowel control. The child experiences both frustration and satisfaction as he or she attempts to gain control over withholding and expelling. The conflict between holding on and letting go gradually resolves as toilet training progresses.

Socially, toddlers play parallel, meaning beside rather than with other children. Play is the major socializing medium, and inexpensive toys found in the home are often the most popular—pots and pans, pencil and paper, "helping" the caretaker. Toddlers frequently engage in what is called "negativism" as a way of asserting their opinion. They are trying to convey that they have thought about what they want and have a reason for their decisions but are sometimes unable to convey the thought process due to limited vocabulary. For this reason, discipline can seem like a battle of wills at times. Caretakers need to be reasonable but consistent with discipline, offering the toddler appropriate choices whenever possible.

HISTORY AND PHYSICAL EXAMINATION

Table 9-1 presents critical foci for the toddler at different stages in the areas of history, physical examination, and health promotion. These guidelines can help providers as they conduct well child visits.

History

A caregiver with an ill toddler or multiple children in attendance may be unable to give a comprehensive history in the first visit. The history may be taken over several visits and entered together as a complete database, with the most important information pinpointed during the primary visit.

Topics

The following are topics to discuss during the history:

Informant: Who is giving the history?
Biographic data: Information should be briefly checked at every visit, especially when visits are 6 months apart. The child's current nickname and best way to reach the caregiver during office hours should be included.

Table 9-1.   CRITICAL FOCI IN THE HISTORY, PHYSICAL EXAMINATION, AND HEALTH PROMOTION ACTIVITIES DURING THE TODDLER PERIOD

	12–15 Mo	18 Mo	24 Mo	3 Y
History	Child "cruises." Child begins to stand alone. Child navigates stairs. Child points to/indicates wants. Child responds to music. Bowel movements are regular. Attention span increases. Vocabulary is three meaningful words.	Child walks without support. Child throws ball. Child turns book pages. Child uses spoon. Vocabulary is 10 words. Child follows directions. Child imitates adult behavior.	Child is aware of strangers. Child shows parallel play. Child has security object. Child opens doors. Child holds cup in one hand. Child scribbles. Child towers four to six blocks. Vocabulary is 200–300 words.	Child gives first and last names. Child asks "why?" Vocabulary is 900 words. Fantasy begins. Child takes turns. Child shows interest in colors. Child washes and dries hands. Child towers eight blocks. Child swings and climbs. Child drinks from straw.
Physical Examination	Birth weight has tripled. Two lower lateral incisors and four molars appear by 14 mo. Complete physical examination is conducted.	Anterior fontanelle closes by 19 mo in 90% of children. Abdomen protrudes. Fine motor coordination increases. Four cuspid teeth appear by 18 mo. Complete physical examination is conducted.	Height is about half adult height. Protruding abdomen disappears. Legs are slightly bowed. Handedness may appear. Complete physical examination is conducted.	Monitor blood pressure. Head circumference is no longer required at screening. Complete physical examination is conducted.
Health Promotion	Perform lead screening and PPD, based on risk factors. Parents should allow self-directed play. Encourage parents to show affection often. Promote safety. Encourage regular family reading. Encourage swim lessons. Discuss "terrible two's." Family should expose child to new foods.	Encourage tooth brushing. Promote safety. Set limits for sense of security, yet encourage exploring. Review common toddler behavior (eg, "no").	Remind parent that child does not know right from wrong. Child should start toileting. Encourage family meals. Promote safety. Perform lead screen. Perform cholesterol screen. Perform PPD, based on risk factors.	Child should have first dentist visit. Parents should provide color, blunt scissors, and paper for play. Encourage story-telling and dress-up play. Encourage consistent discipline. Help family handle tantrums. Teach traffic safety and importance of protective gear with activities (eg, helmets with bikes). Perform PPD based on risk factors; cholesterol screening as indicated.

Chief complaint/reason for visit: For a well child visit, an open-ended question, such as "How have things been going?" is often very productive.

Present health status: Current developmental status is addressed under this heading. Gross motor development (walks alone, skips, climbs), fine motor development (stacks blocks, draws with crayon, buttons, uses scissors), language skills (uses multiple words, speaks in sentences, uses baby talk, has speech problems), and cognitive development (remembers solutions to simple problems, understands different points of view for conflicting problems) should all be listed, with examples of the child's current level of mastery at home. Any such behaviors observed in the office setting also should be noted.

Family history: This section is important to update at every visit, because it may reveal stresses in the family/home and other issues that may affect the child and caregiver.

Past health status: Building on the data collected during the infant's first year, the clinician addresses the following at every visit:

Childhood illnesses: Include any recent exposures. What is the sickest the toddler has ever been? Include age and complications for chickenpox, rubella, measles, mumps, pertussis, strep throat, and frequent ear infections.

Serious or chronic illnesses: List age, when, and where treated and any complications for meningitis or encephalitis, seizure disorders, asthma, pneumonia or chronic lung problems, rheumatic fever, diabetes, kidney problems, sickle cell anemia, or allergies.

Serious accidents or injuries: Note age, extent of injury, when and how treated, and complications of head injuries, falls, auto accidents, burns, poisonings, fractures, traumas, and so forth.

Operations or hospitalizations: List what, where, when, why, by whom, complications, and the child's reaction. (A child who had a particularly frightening past experience may need special preparation for the examination to follow.)

Current medications: List what, why, when, how much, and any problems for prescriptions, over-the-counter drugs, vitamins, any home remedies, or complementary approaches.

Allergies: Include any reactions to drugs, foods, contact agents, and environmental factors (eg, lead, second-hand smoke, wood stoves).

Health maintenance: Include the last examination (when, where, why, by whom, and outcome). Also include dental examinations and all screening tests.

Immunizations: Note ages administered and any reactions.

Developmental history: The child's current developmental ability is recorded under "Present Health Status" (above). This section is a review of milestones and a general statement from the parents concerning this child's development compared with siblings and whether parents think the growth and development have been normal. List the age that the child achieved any milestones since the last visit.

Nutrition: Include food preferences or dislikes, overall appetite, vitamins, where child eats and with whom, whether child feeds self, whether caregivers feel there are feeding issues, and the amount and type of junk food consumption. Ask caregivers to provide a 24-hour diet recall, including the size of servings and frequency of meals and snacks. Inquire about bottles at night left in the crib.

Psychosocial history: How is the family unit? Has it changed since the last visit? What is the toddler's current security item (eg, toy, blanket)? Does the child display any repetitive behaviors? Who is the current primary caregiver? What are the current day care arrangements?

Activity: Describe the amount of active and quiet play, outdoor play, time spent watching television, and special hobbies or activities. List the amount of time spent reading per day. Is the child in day care or preschool? How many friends does the child have? Does the child show any problems with making friends?

Rest: List how long the child rests each day and night, where, and with whom. Note any nightmares or night terrors. Does the child sleep in a family bed? Does the child have any ritualistic nighttime behaviors? Is the child a sound sleeper, or does he or she awaken frequently?

Elimination: Include toilet teaching issues, ages of daytime bowel and bladder control, and nighttime bowel and bladder control. (Bowel and bladder control often are achieved separately, as are daytime and nighttime control.)

Stress management/coping skills: Have there been any recent changes or stresses? Has the child displayed recent changes in mood? Does the child have tantrums? If so, how often, and how does the caregiver respond?

Discipline: What method are caregivers currently using? Is it effective?

Environment: Are parents generally aware of the environment needed for a toddler to live safely? Include toys appropriate for age, car seats, stairs, yard equipment, protection from falling out of bed, poisons, description of neighborhood, and information on the family's residence (heat, ventilation, hot water, window gates). Asses for lead risk.

Review of Systems

The following is a general review of systems to be conducted during the history taking:

General: frequency of colds, infections, illnesses, fevers, or sweats; presence of edema; or changes in affect, behavior, or energy

Allergy: asthma, eczema, hay fever, hives, sinus disorders, food or drug allergies, sneezing, conjunctivitis

Skin: birthmarks, pigment or color changes, mottling, change in mole, rashes, lesions, easy bruising, easy bleeding, texture change, sweating or dryness, infection, hair growth, itching, change in nails

Head: headache, head injury, dizziness

Eyes: discharge, redness, itching, photophobia, visual acuity (where does the child sit to watch videos?), redness, pain, edema, strabismus

Ears: earaches, infection, drainage, auditory acuity, cleaning

Nose and sinuses: frequency of colds and runny noses, stuffiness, infection, drainage, nosebleeds

Mouth and throat: general condition of teeth, hygiene, dental visits, sores in mouth or tongue, sore throat, difficulty swallowing or chewing, mouth breathing

Speech: change in voice, hoarseness, clarity, articulation, vocabulary

Neck: swollen or tender glands, limitation of movement, stiffness

Respiratory: difficulty breathing, chronic cough, shortness of breath, wheezing or noisy breathing, croup history

Cardiovascular: cyanosis, fainting, exercise intolerance (can child keep up with peers?), murmurs

Hematologic: lymph node swelling, excessive bleeding or easy bruising, pallor, anemia, past exposure to lead/chelation

Gastrointestinal: abdominal pain, nausea and vomiting, history of ulcer, diarrhea, bowel habits/toilet training status, constipation or stool-holding problems, use of evacuation aids, rectal bleeding, stool color change, pinworms by history, perianal pruritus

Urinary: frequency of voiding, characteristics of urine, steadiness or force of stream, straining, unusual color or odor, previous urinary tract infection, urethral discharge

Genital: birth defects, discharges, odors, rashes, irritations, pruritus, screening for sexual abuse, note how sexuality is handled in the home, areas of parental concern

Musculoskeletal: sprains, fractures, joint pains or swelling, limitation of motion, twitching, cramping, pain, weakness, posture, gait ability

Neurologic: numbness and tingling, seizures (febrile versus afebrile), staring episodes, learning difficulties, coordination, balance, dominant hand, developmental problems, tic, tremors, tone changes

Endocrine: excessive hunger, thirst, or urination; abnormal hair distribution; intolerance to heat or cold; anorexia; sudden unexplained changes in weight

Physical Examination

Approach to Examination

The toddler is in Erikson's stage of developing autonomy. Basic dependency on the caregiver conflicts with the need to be independent and to explore the world. The results often are attempts to assert control and displays of frustration. Toddlers may be difficult to examine. They will be this way with almost everyone—their behavior should not be taken personally. The toddler has a heightened awareness of new environments, fears invasive procedures, and dislikes being restrained. This combination frequently will lead the child to be frightened and to cling to the caregiver.

Preparation

Advising the caregiver to bring along a favorite toy or security object (eg, blanket, stuffed animal) may be helpful. Because the 2-year-old does not like having clothing removed, clothes should be taken off one piece at a time during the examination. The provider begins by greeting the caregiver and child by name, but focuses mainly on the caregiver, giving the toddler room to adjust gradually and become familiar from a safe distance. The provider slowly gives attention to the child, focusing first on an object (dress, toy, bow in hair), then on how "big" the child is. A toddler will become engaged when ready—smiling, eye contact, talking, or accepting an object offered.

Toddlers like to have a sense of control and like to assert their opinion, often in the form of "no." Therefore, choices should be given, but only when any answer is acceptable. If asked, "May I listen to your tummy now?" the child may answer "No!" The clinician who does so anyway will lose the child's trust. The clinician should either instruct in a firm, caring voice that it is time to lay down so he or she can listen to the child's tummy, or ask "Would you like me to listen to your tummy first, or your heart?" Demonstrating all procedures on the caregiver may enhance cooperation. Praise should be repeated each time the child cooperates. Such an approach also provides role modeling for parents in how to engage their child's cooperation.

Positioning

If appropriate, toddlers should be offered the choice of being examined on their caregivers' laps or on the "special table." Young children are often most receptive to an examination while sitting on their caregiver's lap. During the part of the examination when they need to be supine, the provider should position the chair to be knee-to-knee with the caregiver. The child's head is then placed in the caregiver's lap, and the child's legs in the provider's lap. During parts of the examination where the child must be restrained for safety, the help of a cooperative parent may be vital.

Sequence

Gross and fine motor skills and gait should be observed during the history, when the toddler thinks the clinician is focusing on the caregiver. When finished with the history/observations, the clinician can begin with the "games." To evaluate the heart properly, the clinician listens through 10 noncrying heartbeats. This should be planned at an appropriate time for the child. "Game playing" continues during the examination (eg, "I'm going to listen to your belly. Can I guess what you had for breakfast this morning?"). The most invasive examinations—ear, nose, and throat—are left for last. Cold stethoscopes and new equipment can be frightening, so all equipment is warmed. Children should be allowed to handle the equipment, and all equipment should be tried out on the caregiver first. Finally, many toddlers like to listen to their own hearts and "blow out" the otoscope light.

General Appearance

Observations begin with the first contact. The provider should remember that there are at least two people to observe (child and caretaker). While taking the history, the provider observes for the child's race, sex, general physical development, nutritional state, mental alertness, evidence of pain, restlessness, body position, clothes, apparent age, hygiene, and grooming. The provider should remember that the level of care given to the child affects many of these particulars. Children's ability to amuse themselves while parents speak and their fine and gross motor skills as they play are observed. The provider gradually becomes involved with the child, to begin a "play" period with a Denver Developmental Assessment (Denver II). In this screening test, the provider examines gait, jumping, hopping, building a tower, and throwing a ball. Posture and alignment are evaluated while the child is sitting, standing, and walking. The child is observed as he or she rises from a supine position on the floor to gain good clues about balance, strength, and coordination and how the child uses the muscles of the neck, truck, arms, and legs (Fig. 9-1). Rolling a nickel under the chair or examination table will often easily get a child to lie down supine to reach for the nickel. The examination continues with evaluation of speech, hearing, and vision capabilities. Throughout, the child's social interaction is noted.

Measurement

Height, weight, head circumference, and vital signs normally are done first. In this age group, however, they may be deferred to a later part of the examination. The provider should proceed with chest, heart, and abdomen while the child is quietly sitting in the caretaker's lap. For this suggested sequence, all measurements except height, weight, and temperature are interspersed throughout the examination at the appropriate times.

Chest and Heart

After warming the stethoscope, the provider auscultates heart and breath sounds in all locations. If the child remains quiet, the clinician should pay particular attention to auscultating a normal physiologic split of S2 from a systolic or functional murmur. He or she should count heart rate and respiratory rate, proceeding to bowel sounds at this time. The chest is inspected for size, shape, configuration, symmetry, and respiratory effort. The precordium is inspected for pulsations. The point of maximal impulse (PMI) usually is seen in thin children, especially if one looks obliquely across the chest wall. Nipple and breast development is noted. The apical impulse is palpated, with location noted. The chest wall is palpated for thrills and any tactile fremitus. At this point, the child can lie down, either in the caretaker's lap or on the examination table.

Abdomen

The abdomen is inspected for contour and markings while the child sits, stands, and lies. After the child lies down, the

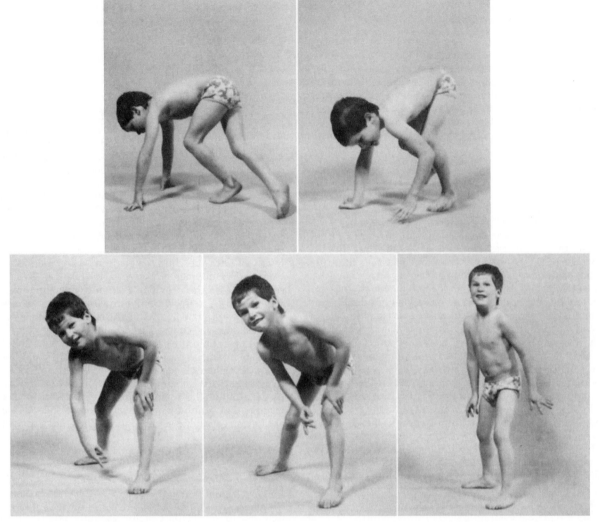

Figure 9–1 ■ Balance, strength, and coordination on rising from supine position on the floor. (Reprinted with permission from Swaiman, K. F., [1989] *Pediatric Neurology: Principles and practice.* St. Louis: C.V. Mosby.)

provider palpates for skin turgor, muscle tone, liver edge, spleen tip, kidneys, and any masses. The liver may be as low as 2 cm in this age group. It should be percussed to confirm findings. The kidneys and spleen are not normally palpable. The umbilicus and inguinal area are palpated for any sign of hernia. Inguinal lymph nodes are palpated, as are the femoral pulses, with their strength compared to the radial pulses.

Genitalia

The external genitalia should be examined with warm hands. For males, the clinician proceeds from the abdomen down, blocking the inguinal canals as he or she moves toward the scrotum. The provider should note if testes are not palpable and the scrotum does not have a "lived-in" look. Transillumination is needed if masses are present.

Lower Extremities

Alignment of legs and feet is noted. Toes, longitudinal arch, and skin condition are inspected. The dorsalis pedis is palpated. Hip stability is tested by checking gait, leg length, full abduction (to 180 degrees), and skin folds. The plantar,

Achilles', and patellar reflexes are elicited. The child should now return to a sitting position.

Upper Extremities

The arms, hands, and fingers are inspected for alignment and skin condition. The clinician should observe any palmar creases. The radial pulse is counted and palpated; blood pressure is measured. The biceps and triceps reflexes are tested.

Head and Neck

The head and facies are inspected for size, shape, and symmetry. The fontanelles, cranium, face, lymphatics, carotid pulses, trachea, thyroid gland, and sternocleidomastoids are palpated. The head circumference is measured.

Eyes

The external structures are inspected, with particular attention paid to the lacrimal duct and excessive tearing. The distance between the eyes is noted, as is any palpebral slant and distribution of the eyebrows. Corneal light and pupillary light reflexes are tested using a penlight, the focus of which should be moved to a favorite toy to elicit cardinal point of gaze. The thumb or a small index card is used for a cover/uncover test. Using an ophthalmoscope, the provider checks the red reflex and inspects the fundus as much as possible.

Nose

The external nose and skin condition are inspected. The nares are checked for mucosa, septum, turbinates, discharge, and foreign body (especially in a child with a "strange" odor) with a light.

Mouth and Throat

These may be done after the ears, because the child will frequently be crying, so the mouth will be wide open. Using a light, the clinician inspects the mouth, buccal mucosa, teeth, gums, tongue, frenulum, palate, and midline uvula. The tonsils, odor of the breath, and clarity/hoarseness of the voice are noted. A tongue blade should be used as a last resort.

Ears

The height of the ear is observed for proper position (in line with the midline of the eye). The auricle is inspected and palpated. Any discharge or foreign body is noted. An otoscope is used to examine the ear canal and tympanic membrane. Some children will enjoy playing with the light and cooperate, but most will need to be restrained even if they enjoyed playing with the light. Puppets or toys may be used as a distraction.

● **Clinical Pearl:** The key to a successful examination of the toddler is the caretaker's total involvement. The child must be given time to become familiar with the provider and the equipment, with as much "game playing" as possible. While they are acutely aware of new surroundings, toddlers' fears will be decreased if a calm, comfortable caregiver can appropriately distract them.

ASSESSMENT

A well child in this age group should meet several criteria:

Immunizations are up-to-date.
Physical examination is normal.
The child passes the Denver II (see screening section below).
No major child or caretaker social issues are present.
Caretaker is educated in the normal growth, development, and expectations of the toddler.
No other major outstanding issues are evident.

PLAN

For the well toddler in a healthy family and environment, the American Academy of Pediatrics (AAP) recommends visits at 12, 15, 18, and 24 months and 3 years. For children at risk due to adolescent parents, prematurity, inappropriate housing, medical conditions, or other factors, additional visits may be indicated.

The first toddler visit at 15 months provides an excellent chance to complete any health maintenance items that were unable to be completed at the 12-month visit (see Table 9-1). Any immunizations not previously given should be completed. A complete blood count with differential, sickledex, lead level, and purified protein derivative (PPD) should be done if not successfully completed at the 12-month visit. Hearing should be checked if there is any indication of a delay. Anticipatory guidance should be given, and referral to a social worker or health educator should be made if necessary. Brushing of teeth should have begun, and a dental referral might be necessary.

During the 18-month visit, any remaining vaccinations are completed. DDST evaluation continues, and the clinician follows up with any potential health issues. At this visit, the clinician can elect to adjust the visit schedule to every 6 months for low-risk children or every 4 months for moderate risk children. The schedule is maintained at every 3 months for higher risk children (those who have medical, social, or environmental concerns, whether acute or chronic). Premature infants, children of teenage parents, and chronically ill children should maintain accelerated visit schedules. Support and guidance are given to the caregiver as the toddler enters the "terrible two's," which begins during the second year, not at the second birthday.

The 24-month visit is sometimes the first visit where no immunizations need to be given. This visit is primarily for health maintenance, with assessments made of medical, social, developmental, and environmental health. Annual bloodwork and PPD should be done at this visit. Cholesterol screening should be initiated for children at high risk. All children should be up-to-date with their vaccinations and screened for hearing, vision (subjectively; objective screening begins at 36 months), lead, and developmental disabilities by this time. Once again, if all is well, the visit schedule may be adjusted. The well toddler may be seen at 36 months, while the child or family at risk may be seen at 3-, 4-, or 6-month intervals.

During the 36-month visit, many caregivers bring forms to be completed as the toddler enters a preschool/day care program. Annual bloodwork and PPD are done (based on the child's risk profile), as well as objective vision and hearing tests. Anticipatory guidance is given to parents about entering preschool/day care if the child has never been cared for outside the home.

SCREENING

The Denver II is the standard for developmental screening. It includes drawing simple lines, identifying pictures, building, and placing objects inside other objects. The "by report" of the Denver II should be done at every visit. If the child does not meet age-appropriate items, the full Denver II may be done or referral made for additional developmental assessment. When caring for a high-risk child, the provider should include many of the "by report" items into the routine history and let the child play with the test items during the interview to decrease the amount of actual testing time to under 5 minutes per visit.

ANTICIPATORY GUIDANCE

Anticipatory guidance is a critical component of the well child visit during the toddler years. Parents should be encouraged to write down the specifics of issues concerning them. Providers should be sure to reinforce safety.

Common Questions

The following are examples of common questions and ways to address them:

My child doesn't want to give up the bottle. Is there any nutritional reason to wean?

Answer: Yes. In some studies, persistence of bottle feeding after the second birthday (common to some ethnic groups) was highly associated with elevation of zinc protoporphyrin-to-heme ratio (ZPP/H). Education practices are important to prevent iron deficiency from overintake of cow's milk in the child who is still bottle feeding beyond the age of 2 years (Graham, Carlson, Sodergren, Detter, & Labbe, 1997).

My toddler is such a slow and picky eater. Is that normal?

Answer: Yes. On any given day, 52% of toddlers are not always hungry at mealtimes, 42% try to end meals after a few bites, 35% are picky eaters, and 33% have strong food preferences (Reau, Senturia, Lebailly, & Christoffel, 1996). Toddlers will switch between these trying characteristics from day to day.

What should I give my toddler to drink?

Answer: Plain water. Petter, Hourihane, and Rolles (1995) discovered that 72.5% of the preschool group studied and 50% of the infant group never drank plain water, an essential nutrient for the body. Baby fruits and vegetables (squash in this study) constitute a large portion of fluid and calorie intake. Attention needs to be given to children's daily intake of plain water. In fact, plain water should be promoted as a drink of choice over juices and sugared beverages.

My toddler had acute gastroenteritis last week but still has diarrhea. I'm really concerned. When will it stop?

Answer: Inquire about the child's current diet. Parents often continue the "clear fluids" portion of instructions longer than necessary and give more juice (high fructose/sorbitol) than the child's intestinal tract can absorb. Diarrhea thus results; moreover, such measures may actually provoke gastrointestinal symptoms of abdominal distention, flatulence, abdominal pain, and diarrhea (Hoekstra, 1998). Kneepkens and Hoekstra (1996) recommend a normalization of the toddler's feeding patterns according to the four "F's": fat, fiber, fluid, and fruit juices. Fat should be increased to 40% of the diet, fiber increased by increasing normal meal intake, fluids between meals decreased so that the child will be hungry for regular food at mealtime, and fruit juices eliminated as much as possible. In this age of specialty care, an explanation and dietary advice might not satisfy many parents, but they will notice that this simple advice is very effective within a few days.

I want my child to take a toddler swim class, but I am afraid of ear infections. Does swimming increase ear infections?

Answer: No, not even in the winter months. In fact, only 19% of toddler swimmers, compared to 43% of nonswimmers, had one or more ear infections (Robertson, Marino, & Namjoshi, 1997). All parents must be encouraged to "drown-proof" their toddlers with toddler swim/float classes.

I've carefully "toddler-proofed" my home—is there anything that many parents forget?

Answer: Parents sometimes forget to clean up after adult nighttime activities, and their toddler discovers these potential poisons first thing in the morning. An ashtray of cigarette butts has the potential for nicotine poisoning when a toddler chews on them. Not-completely-empty containers of alcohol increase the possibility of alcohol poisoning. Toddlers require very small amounts of ingested alcohol to reach toxic levels. Parents should be very diligent if little hands may reach these items before they do in the morning (Tovey, Rana, & Anderson, 1998).

I've tried EVERYTHING, and I can't get my toddler to sleep all night in her own bed.

Answer: If parents have tried the standard remedies, including Ferber's (1985) method, without success, they may need referral to the faded bedtime method (Ashbaugh & Peck, 1998).

My toddler keeps touching her genitals. What do I do?

Answer: Reassure the parent that this behavior is normal for toddlers and does not arouse the sexual feelings equivalent to those experienced by adults. The child should be taught that such behavior is unacceptable in public. Unreasonable restriction or punishment can lead to feelings of guilt or poor self-worth. Parents should use the proper terms for body parts at this time and should begin teaching about appropriate and inappropriate touch. Emphasize to parents that the way they express physical affection, wash their child's genitals, and respond to the child's genital exploration influences how the child begins to feel about his or her own sexuality (Finan, 1997).

Common Concerns

Nutrition

Nutrition is dramatically different during this period. Energy requirements are 100 kcal/kg/d. Fluid requirements are 115 to 125 mL/kg/d. Protein requirements are 1.8 g/kg/d. Growth slows at the end of the first year and is reflected in a decreased appetite. Because body tissues (especially muscles) continue to grow quite rapidly, however, protein needs are high. The toddler has 14 to 16 teeth, permitting easier chewing. The toddler's appetite is sporadic, and the child will intermittently favor or refuse specific foods. The average 2-year-old eats one-fourth the amount that he or she ate at age 1 year. This 75% decrease is compatible with the normal reduced growth velocity experienced in this age group. The average parent, however, may become concerned about this appetite decrease and may require reassurance.

Ritualistic toddler behavior is quite evident during meals and includes placement of tableware, seating preference, time of day, and specific foods. The child may display increasing independence by refusing certain foods or assistance from others when eating. The toddler's diet should consist of a wide range of nutritious foods from all food groups, in appropriately sized servings (two tablespoons of peas, a quarter cup of rice, or half an orange are all toddler-size servings). Iron-fortified dry cereals are excellent sources of iron during the second year. The AAP recommends that children drink whole milk from ages 12 months until 2 years. After 24 months, the toddler only needs 2 to 3 cups (16–24 oz) of 1% or skim milk per day.

Nutritious snacks become important to fulfill daily requirements. Fluids remain extremely important, with water being essential. Providers should encourage caregivers to assist the child in developing a taste for water. Juices should be diluted with water to half-strength or weaker to avoid empty calories; sodas and sports drinks are to be avoided. Most toddlers prefer to feed themselves and will typically master the ability to handle finger foods, drink from a cup held with both hands, and chew with their mouths closed. Toddlers need sufficient time to eat. Food should be removed when toddlers begin to play with it, because such behavior is a signal of fullness. Eating habits should be monitored, but mealtime struggles now may set negative patterns that prove difficult to break later.

Parents should be reminded that snacking two to three times a day helps toddlers to meet their nutritional needs, because they cannot eat very much at one time. If the child refuses vegetables, fruits can be substituted, because many of the nutrients in these food groups are the same. Most families also will experience a time when the toddler demands the same food repeatedly—a "food jag." Parents should serve the favorite food at one meal every day, giving small portions at the other meals. In this way, they provide both the favorite food (a control issue for the toddler) and a variety of other foods to preserve good nutrition. Nutrition-related safety issues at this age involve choking hazards. Foods such as nuts, grapes, raw carrots, popcorn, hard candy, hot dogs, chunks of meat, lumps of peanut butter, and raisins should be postponed until the child is older than 3 years. A young child should never eat unsupervised, nor should bowls of candies and nuts be left within reach.

Sleep

Sleep is an important adjunct to nutrition for proper growth in the toddler. Many autonomy issues are related to sleep at this age. Length and number of naps, bedtime, where to sleep, and where to fall asleep are all issues that caregivers have to address. Children in this age group also experience nightmares and night terrors. How the caregivers handle sleep issues may affect their children's lifelong sleep habits. The average toddler needs 11 to 12 hours of nighttime sleep. Average daytime sleep (naps) decreases from 2½ to 1 hour during the toddler period.

Nightmares are the most common reason that children over age 2 years awake in the middle of the night. Children should be comforted and made to know that they are safe and loved. ("Daddy's right here if you need him.") A frightened child should never be ignored.

Night terrors—a form of somnambulism—usually begin after age 3 years, although they can start as early as 6 to 8 months. They are terrifying for caregivers, but not for children, because they have no memory of the experience afterward. A terror can start with a hair-curling scream and include thrashing, yelling, profuse sweating, and even open eyes. The child may look wide awake but is not. The toddler will, however, be frightened if he or she awakens to see the caregiver standing over the bed, upset. Night terrors occur during the first few hours after the child falls asleep; they usually do not last for more than 10 minutes. The caregiver should stay with but not awaken the child.

The family bed is an issue with which each family deals differently. All children should, however, have their own bed, learn to go to sleep there, and be able to put themselves to sleep. If children are accustomed to sleeping in the family bed, moving them to their own bed as toddlers can be very difficult. Ferber (1985) describes a very successful method of addressing sleep issues in *Solve Your Child's Sleep Problems*.

Separation issues and fears at bedtime that seem irrational are common for toddlers. Caregivers should make responses as matter-of-fact as possible to avoid reinforcing the need to stay awake. Using a blanket, toy, or other security object is encouraged instead of picking the child up. Staying calm and reassuring and altering the sleep environment as needed (eg, keeping the door open, leaving the light on) should help the child through this developmental stage. See the Community Resources section for appropriate books, including *There's a Monster Under My Bed* (Howe, 1986).

Lack of sleep can be a major problem for both child and caregivers. Caregivers are strongly encouraged to address sleep issues early, consistently, and appropriately for developmental level, because sleep habits developed early can last for a lifetime. Rituals are important but should be limited to a reasonable time (eg, 10–20 minutes). Bedtime can be an excellent time for one-to-one caregiver–child bonding, review of the day, and some reading.

Elimination

Mastery of elimination and toileting issues is a major milestone for this age group. Most preschools do not accept children who are not reasonably continent, so lack of mastery could become an education or child care issue. Methods and philosophies of toilet training are numerous; some focus on the child's development and readiness, and some are more concerned with the caregiver's needs. The approach should be child oriented and directed. Most important is the readiness of the child. The four signals or requirements of readiness are that the child walks well (can get where he or she needs to go; poor muscle coordination also may indicate poor sphincter control); communicates well (can tell the caregiver he or she needs to go to the potty); can delay urination until getting to the potty (can sense the need to go before reflexive urination occurs); and is interested in pleasing caregivers. If the child is not ready to be continent, then the exercise will be frustrating and humiliating for both the child and caregiver.

Caregivers should provide positive reinforcement and should never shame the child when an accident occurs. Praise and rewards will reinforce the child's desire to please. Scolding, punishment, or yelling should not be part of the process. Saying "Next time I'm sure you'll remember" may work well after an accident. If accidents persist, the child may not have really been ready for toilet teaching. Complete regression could be a sign of illness or reaction to an event.

Learning daytime control can take 2 weeks to 2 months; learning nighttime control may take a year or longer. Bowel and bladder control often do not occur at the same time, with children differing as to what they master first. The toddler may wear underwear in the day but an underwear-type diaper at night until late into the third year.

Some basic hints for caregivers are to shop for the potty chair with the child, because different children like different chair styles. A child who doesn't like a type of potty chair will be reluctant to use it. The caregiver should be relaxed, supportive, able to give some guidance, and prepared to do a lot of laundry. Toilet teaching also is easier in the summer, if possible, when the child has fewer clothes to remove. Refer to Chapter 63 for more information on enuresis and encopresis.

Social

Toddlers are very social creatures, exploring themselves and their world constantly. Some caregivers dread the "terrible two's." The clinician should remind caregivers that their attitudes toward their child affect the child's behavior and self-esteem. Parents may negatively perceive a toddler as stubborn and demanding or positively as persistent and passionate—excellent traits to encourage as the child grows toward school-age. Instead of using negative terms like "difficult," "strong-willed," "obstinant," "bossy," or "defiant," positive terms to use include "spirited," "a sparkler," "zestful," "committed," and "tenacious." Caregivers will feel better about their children and their parenting if they use positive words and share this philosophy with family, friends, and day care providers. Negative behaviors should not be overlooked, but personality traits should be channeled positively.

Discipline

Tantrums are a common complaint of caregivers. Young children have neither the verbal skills to express what is wrong nor the emotional skills to deal with frustration. Caregivers should know that a child in the middle of a tantrum is clearly expressing that he or she cannot handle the frustration, fatigue, or hunger (or maybe all three) that has brought the toddler to the limit. The tantrum does not mean that the parent is a poor caregiver; it simply means that the child is overwhelmed. Frequent outbursts should be monitored, including how often, when, and what triggers them. If a child regularly has tantrums after a morning playgroup, then maybe an afternoon, postnap playgroup would be a better alternative.

The caregiver's reaction to a tantrum should be based on whether the child is having an involuntary overload reaction and really has lost control or is a calculated attempt to manipulate the caregiver. If it is a calculated attempt (usually older children), the caregiver should attempt to tune out the behavior. If the child is truly overloaded, hugging and talking with a calm voice often works. The caregiver should be aware that it often takes about 15 minutes to really calm an overloaded child.

The toddler's frequent use of the word "no" and bossy statements are really just symptoms of emotional growth exceeding verbal ability. Toddlers want to express what they think is correct and incorrect; caregivers should support this drive for independence as often as possible. Toddlers will often test limits, not usually just to test, but to be reassured that they are loved even when they behave badly. Stating that the behavior is bad, but not the child, will reassure the toddler of the caregiver's unconditional love. The toddler's insecurity will diminish with time.

Caregivers often struggle with the word "no" and how frequently they should use it to discipline their child. They can use other words that more accurately describe the circumstances instead—"hot," "yucky," "glass," and "danger" are excellent for appropriate situations. The child should then be removed and distracted. When caregivers use "no," they should state it in a gruff tone with a serious facial expression to avoid giving mixed messages. If the behavior persists, "time-out" should be used. Time-outs should last for approximately 1 minute per year of age. The high-chair turned into the corner can be a safe vehicle. Time-outs should be used only in dangerous or critical situations.

Inconsequential but extremely annoying behavior, such as whining, clinging, or screaming, should be ignored, as difficult as it may be. By ignoring the misbehavior, the caregiver is not rewarding the child for it. More importantly, the caregiver teaches the child that positive behavior will bring about the tender-loving attention the toddler craves. Often the parent needs to be creative with positive attention. On trying days, phrases such as, "I like the way you breathe," or "I like the way your heart beats" may be useful. In this fashion, when the toddler does something good, the child will begin to associate attention with his or her own positive behavior.

Sibling Rivalry

The toddler believes that he or she is the center of the world. That belief is crushed quickly when a new baby is born. Suddenly, the toddler is no longer the sole source of a caretaker's attention. It can be a trying time for all involved. About 1 month before the birth of a new baby, discussion is necessary regarding the new baby's feeding, diapering, and sleeping needs and how the toddler can help. It also is important to reassure the toddler that routines will stay the same and that the toddler's routines are as important as the baby's. After the birth, the toddler should be allowed and encouraged to help care for the new baby whenever possible so that the toddler feels included and important. The toddler should not be left alone, however, with the new sibling.

Safety

Childproofing the home is imperative. Breakables and small objects must be removed. Electric outlets and sharp corners must be covered. Parents must be aware of objects that the child can pull down, including tablecloths and cords. Poisons should be in closed, childproof containers kept out-of-reach in locked closets. Visiting relatives and friends are potentially dangerous if not watched closely. Falls can be prevented by using window guards and stair gates, with special care taken not to leave chairs near windows, stoves, and other hazardous places. Children should never be left alone near any water, especially in bathtubs. Toilets are potential hazards. Doors of potentially dangerous rooms should be locked. Properly installed car seats must be used when traveling any distance in a car. To avoid burns, hot water should be set to 120°F to eliminate the risk of scalding. Care is necessary when using heaters and hot irons, and parents should be aware of electrical cords and the handle position of pots on the stove. Plastic bags and balloons are suffocation hazards. All peeling paint must be cleaned up immediately. Remind parents to make the house child-safe before going to bed, including removing all ashtrays and almost-empty glasses of alcohol.

The child should never be left alone, and all play should be supervised. Safe play includes not throwing sharp objects or following a ball into the street. Toys should be checked to be sure that no parts are loose or can be bitten off. Sharp edges are another concern.

Common Conditions

Lead Poisoning

Lead poisoning is a toxic condition caused by the ingestion of lead-containing compounds. Deficient parental supervision and interaction is a major contributing factor, with the peak incidence at ages 1 to 5 years. It is significantly more prevalent in African Americans than in Caucasians. Findings may include behavioral changes, failure to gain weight, and serum lead levels above 19 μg/dL. Chelating medications are given, the child's environment must be cleaned, and the caretaker must be educated to understand the importance of age-appropriate interactions and supervision (Johnson and Oski, 1997).

Accidental Poisoning

Salicylate poisoning was common until the advent of childproof caps and the change from salicylate to acetaminophen and ibuprofen for children. Acetaminophen poisoning is a life-threatening overdose, possibly requiring emergency liver transplantation. Another increasing type of poisoning is "Grandma's bag"—overdoses of medications kept in the handbag of an individual whom a toddler is visiting. Sometimes elderly individuals, due to hand and finger mobility problems, do not have childproof caps on medication bottles that they carry with them or have at home. A toddler's natural curiosity is a potential source of trouble. It is very important that every parent knows the local Poison Control Center number and is aware of how to reach emergency services when away from home, because not all areas use 911. Families should keep syrup of ipecac in the home. "Mr. Yuck" should be taught to and used in the home of every toddler. Information may be obtained from the local Poison Control Center.

Child Abuse and Neglect

Abuse and neglect can be acts of omission or commission by any caregiver that prevent the child from reaching his or her potential for growth and development, whether emotional, intellectual, or physical. Providers are in a unique position to assess family interactions before any abuse takes place. Hopefully, they can intervene effectively when difficulties arise. Refer to Chapters 2 and 23 for more information.

Fractures

Several fractures fit under the category of "toddler fracture," all of which occur in the foot and tibia of young children. Any limping or leg pain should be investigated, especially if the child is unwilling to bear weight, even when distracted. The classic fracture is the nondisplaced spiral tibial fracture. Others include plastic bowing and buckle-type fractures, especially of the fibula; impaction, compression, or stress (fatigue) fractures of the tibia and fibula; and fractures of the metatarsal and tarsal bones. The fractures may be so subtle that they are very difficult to detect. Injuries of this kind are increasing as children enter sports (such as soccer) at increasingly younger ages (John, Moorthy, & Swischuk, 1997).

Communicable Diseases

Many common communicable diseases have been eliminated due to successful vaccination efforts. There are, however, diseases that are still common to this age group. For more information, see Unit Four: Primary Care of Episodic Illnesses.

COMMUNITY RESOURCES

Community resources to assist families with toddlers are listed in the following section:

American Red Cross: Tot Savers
Mothers of Preschool Children (MOPS) at local churches: support group for parents of young children.
Local Library, children's division: aware of many local services available to the toddler and the caretaker.
World Wide Web
  http://www.pedinfo.org: dedicated to the dissemination of on-line information for pediatricians and others interested in child health.
  http://www.aap.org: home page of the American Academy of Pediatrics.

http://www.nichd.nih.gov: home page of the National Institute of Child Health and Human Development (NICHD), a part of the National Institutes of Health.
http://PedsCCM.wustl.edu: a collection of resources for pediatric critical care professionals.
http://www.aspho.org: home page of the American Society of Pediatric Hematology/Oncology; has resources for both families of patients and professionals.
http://www.naspgn.org: home page for the North American Society for Pediatric Gastroenterology and Nutrition; for parents, patients, and professionals.
http://www.aacap.org: home page for the American Academy of Child and Adolescent Psychiatry. AACAP serves as a resource for members as well as for patients and their families; includes information on developmental, behavioral, emotional, and mental disorders affecting children and adolescents.

REFERENCES

Ashbaugh, R., & Peck, S. M. (1998). Treatment of sleep problems in a toddler: A replication of the faded bedtime with response cost protocol. *Journal of Applied Behavior Analysis, 31*(1), 127–129.

Bates, B. (1995). *A guide to physical examination and history taking* (pp. 609–610). Philadelphia: J.B. Lippincott.

Ferber, R. (1985). *Solve your child's sleep problems.* New York: Simon & Schuster.

Finan, S. L. (1997). Promoting healthy sexuality: Guidelines for infancy through preschool. *The Nurse Practitioner, 22*(10), 79–100.

Graham, E. A., Carlson, T. H., Sodergren, K. K., Detter, J. C., & Labbe, R. F. (1997). Delayed bottle weaning and iron deficiency in southeast Asian toddlers. *Western Journal of Medicine, 167*(1), 10–14.

Hoekstra, J. H. (1998). Toddler diarrhoea: More a nutritional disorder than a disease. *Archives of Disease in Childhood, 79*(1), 2–5.

Howe, J. (1986). *There's a monster under my bed.* New York: Simon & Schuster.

John, S. D., Moorthy, C. S., & Swischuk, L. E. (1997). Expanding the concept of the toddler's fracture. *Radiographics, 17*(2) 367–376.

Johnson, K. B., & Oski, F. A. (Eds.) (1997). *Oski's essential pediatrics.* Philadelphia: J.B. Lippincott.

Kneepkens, C. M. F., & Hoekstra, J. F. (1996). Chronic nonspecific diarrhea of childhood: pathophysiology and management. *Pediatric Clinics of North America, 43,* 375–390.

Petter, L. P., Hourihane, J. O., Rolles, C. J. (1995). Is water out of vogue? A survey of the drinking habits of 2–7 year olds. *Archives of Disease in Childhood 72*(2), 137–140.

Reau, N. R., Senturia, Y. D., Lebailly, S. A., & Christoffel, K. K. (1996). Infant and toddler feeding patterns and problems: Normative data and a new direction. Pediatric Practice Research Group. *Journal of Developmental and Behavioral Pediatrics, 17*(3), 149–153.

Robertson, L. M., Marino, R. V., & Namjoshi, S. (1997). Does swimming increase the incidence of otitis media? *Journal of American Osteopathy Association, 97*(3), 150–152.

Tovey, C., Rana, P. S., & Anderson, D. J. (1998). Alcohol ingestion in a toddler (letter). *Journal of Accident and Emergency Medicine, 15*(1), 69–70.

Healthy Growth and Development of the Preschool Child

• NOREEN MULVANERTY, MS, RN, CS, FNP, and DEE L'ARCHEVEQUE, MD

INTRODUCTION

The preschool child, ages 3 to 5, experiences a magical period of curiosity and activity. During these years, children require an enormous amount of attention; consequently, the primary care provider must be patient and innovative. He or she must fully assess the child during this period for changes in physical, psychosocial, cognitive, and emotional development. Identifying normal patterns of growth and development and detecting variations are important indicators as the preschooler progresses toward readiness for school. Parents and caregivers look to the clinician for advice about their child. Their concerns range from nutritional issues to nightmares and everything in between. A trusting relationship between provider, family members, and child is essential to provide quality patient care through health promotion, disease prevention, and anticipatory guidance.

GROWTH AND DEVELOPMENT

Developmental assessment is based on the conviction that patterns observed in the early years of life are sequential and predictable. Biologic maturation reflects developmental changes influenced by the environment. Individual variations from norms may be transient and simply need further evaluation. Assessment of development can be integrated in the pediatric examination. It involves a thorough history, familiarity with normal development, knowledge of familial and environmental influences, and awareness of developmental indicators.

Early clinical intervention in children with developmental problems is necessary for successful development. Such intervention only can occur by recognizing subtle variations in growth and development from the norm. Valid assessment requires both quantitative and qualitative measurements of the developmental process. A common clinical perspective is the identification of sequential milestones normally achieved at specific ages. Development also can be seen as a series of tasks to be mastered within certain stages. Other perspectives are derived from stage-based theories, such as Freud's theory of psychosexual stages or Piaget's stages of cognitive growth.

Physical Development

Gains in weight and stature usually are constant during the preschool years. Children ages 3 to 5 continue to grow at a much slower pace than they did in the first year of life. The average child gains 7 cm (2 in) in height and 2 kg (approximately 1 lb) in weight per year, with boys gaining slightly more than girls. As lordosis becomes less pronounced, the abdomen flattens and the body appears leaner. Head growth declines markedly, with head circumference increasing only 2 cm (1 in) each year; subsequently, the face becomes elongated. In comparison, the legs grow faster than the trunk, head, or upper extremities (Murphy, 1996).

Generally by age 3 years, visual acuity reaches 20/40; by age 4 to 5 years, it reaches 20/30; and by age 6 to 7 years, it reaches 20/20. By age 3 years, all 20 primary teeth have erupted. Muscle development and bone growth are still in the stages of maturation. Motor development increases in strength and refinement. Most children walk with a steady gait before the end of their third year. At age 3 years, the preschool child should be able to ride a tricycle, walk on tiptoe, and balance on one foot. By 4 years, the child can skip and hop on one foot and can catch a ball. By 5 years, the child can skip on alternate feet. Fine motor skills are evident in the abilities of drawing and dressing oneself. Table 10-1 outlines the age of presentation of physical and psychosocial developmental milestones (Levine, Carey, & Crocker, 1999).

● **Clinical Pearl:** As the child normally grows, the parents might mistake this for weight loss. Keeping clear records and growth charts can be reassuring to both the clinician and parents.

Understanding physical development is essential to understanding normal milestones attained during the preschool years. As external signs of change become evident, the internal organ infrastructure also undergoes growth, which allows the child to develop normally.

Neurologic Development

By age 2 years, significant brain maturation occurs, with myelinization finalized between the cortex and the thalamus and basal ganglia. All layers of the cortex reach a similar state of maturation between 15 and 24 months (Rabinowicz, 1986). The cognitive, emotional, and physical abilities of the preschooler are related to brain maturation. Sensory function becomes more developed, and the awareness of a full rectum or bladder accompanies the ability to control the rectal sphincter. As neural growth slowly continues, the child performs more complex tasks.

Cardiovascular Development

Growth of the cardiac structure continues through the preschool years. By the fifth year, the size of the heart has quadrupled since birth. The heart rate declines to 70 to 100 beats per minute as the myocardium grows and energy demands decrease. Adult levels of pulmonary vascular resistance and pulmonary arterial pressure are attained before reaching age 2 years; therefore, the physical exami-

Table 10–1. DEVELOPMENTAL MILESTONES IN PRESCHOOLERS

Milestone	Typical Age at Presentation	Age at Which Absence of Milestone Is Abnormal*
Gross motor		
Jumping and clearing ground	24 mo	30 mo
Doing a broad jump of 18 in	36 mo	48 mo
Alternating feet downstairs	36 mo	48 mo
Balancing on one foot for 2 s	36 mo	48 mo
Hopping on one foot	42 mo	60 mo
Fine motor		
Stacking five 1-in cubes	20 mo	27 mo
Stacking seven 1-in cubes	24 mo	36 mo
Copying a circle	36 mo	48 mo
Holding pencil with mature grasp	36 mo	48 mo
Copying a cross	40 mo	60 mo
Language		
Combining two ideas (eg, "Mommy, go!")	18 mo	24 mo
Naming one picture in a book	18 mo	27 mo
Following a two-step command	18 mo	27 mo
Using three- to four-word sentences	24 mo	36 mo
Using pronouns (I, you) appropriately	24 mo	30 mo
Identifying two colors	36 mo	42 mo
Naming the use of common objects	30 mo	36 mo
Speaking in a way understandable to a stranger	36 mo	48 mo
Social-adaptive		
Independent feeding with spoon and fork	24 mo	36 mo
Independent dressing without tying shoes	36 mo	48 mo
Independent toileting	36 mo	48 mo
Cognition		
Searching for lost object in several places other than place object was last seen	18 mo	24 mo
Playing with toys in functional way (eg, pushing a toy car around)	18 mo	24 mo
Reenacting familiar activities	18 mo	30 mo
Being able to imitate actions later	18 mo	30 mo
Using one object to stand for another object in play (a block for a telephone)	18 mo	30 mo
Using imaginary objects in play	36 mo	48 mo
Role playing several familiar people	36 mo	48 mo
Drawing face of a person with crude features	36 mo	48 mo
Planning out a story and assigning roles to self and others	48 mo	60 mo
Social-emotional		
Demonstrating shared attention: "Do you see what I see?"	18 mo	30 mo
Showing strong sense of self: using "No," "Mine"	18 mo	36 mo
Playing side by side with a single peer	24 mo	36 mo
Separating from parent without crying	36 mo	48 mo
Labeling feelings in self	36 mo	48 mo
Taking turns and sharing	36 mo	48 mo
Playing group games with simple rules	48 mo	60 mo

*The significance of an absent milestone must be assessed in the context of the child's complete physical and neurologic examination. Furthermore, the absence of a particular milestone may be "abnormal" earlier than indicated in the table in the context of a child's other accomplishments.

Data from Bayley Scales of Infant Development—II (N Bayley: Bayley Scales of Infant Development, 2nd ed. San Antonio, The Psychological Corporation, 1993); Denver II (Frankenburg WK, Dodds J, Archer P, et al: Denver II, Denver, Denver Developmental Materials, 1990; Frankenburg WK, Dodds J, Archer P, et al: The Denver II: A major revision and restandardization of the Denver Developmental Screening Test. Pediatrics 89:91, 1992); Developmental Rainbow: Early Childhood Development Profiles (Mahoney G, Mahoney F: Developmental Rainbow: Early Childhood Development Profiles. Tallmadge, OH, Family Child Learning Center, 1996); Early Language Milestone Scale (Coplan J: Early Language Milestone Scale, 1983. Modern Education Corp., P.O. Box 721, Tulsa, OK, 74101); The Revised Developmental Screening Inventory—1980 (Developmental Evaluation Materials, P.O. Box 27391, Houston, TX, 77277); Transdisciplinary Play-Based Assessment (Linder T: Transdisciplinary Play-Based Assessment. Baltimore, Paul H Brookes, 1990).

Valid screening for developmental delays should be done using a carefully developed or normed instrument/reference such as one of the preceding.

Reprinted with permission of Levine, M., Carey, W., & Crocker, A. (1999). *Developmental and Behavioral Pediatrics* (3rd ed.). Philadelphia: W.B. Saunders.

nation should reveal regular rate, with an innocent murmur possible as the heart gains size throughout this phase. See Chapter 37 for information on distinguishing heart murmurs.

Respiratory Tract Development

Growth and development of the respiratory system encompass changes in anatomy, mechanical properties, and metabolic and defense functions. The number of alveoli, the basic gas exchange unit, and its associated structures increase throughout childhood; conversely, the respiratory rate slows from infancy to approximately 20 to 30 breaths per minute. As the diaphragm matures, abdominal respiratory movement decreases. By the end of the fifth year, respiratory movement becomes more diaphragmatic.

Gastrointestinal Development

By age 5 years, the gastrointestinal (GI) tract is enzymatically mature, enabling the child to eat and digest a wide range of foods. Anatomically, the stomach is relatively small. Children who have anatomically intact GI tracts can enjoy many foods but need nutritional guidance to ensure normal growth. Healthy snacks should be encouraged between meals to support nutritional requirements (Murphy, 1996).

Psychosocial and Cognitive Development

As preschool children deal with the world around them, they use their developing language skills, knowledge of the environment, and play activities. Vocabulary increases during this period from 50 to 100 words to more than 2000. In turn, the use of language as an expressive tool increases. Language plays a critical role in the regulation of behavior. Children during these years understand the inhibitions that surround them and are able to express feelings, anger, and frustration without acting out.

● **Clinical Pearl:** Language-delayed children exhibit higher rates of tantrums and other externalizing behaviors (Behrman, Kilegman, Aruin, 1996).

The preschool period corresponds with Piaget's preoperational stage, which is characterized by magical thinking and egocentrism. The child uses magical thinking to explain the surrounding world; for example, "the sun goes down because it is tired and needs to sleep." Egocentrism is the inability to see another's point of view; however, this does not connote selfishness. The preschool child is developing hypotheses about the nature of the world as multiple aspects of a situation (Levine et al., 1999).

Play activities during the preschool years are increasingly complex and imaginative. This period also is marked by increased cooperative play and play that is increasingly governed by rules.

HISTORY AND PHYSICAL EXAMINATION

Primary care is delivered in myriad settings. Common to all settings is the consideration of privacy for the patient and family. The clinical setting should be a comfortable place for patients and family to sit and interact with the provider. A soothing environment with child-friendly artwork and furniture creates a pleasant atmosphere in which children feel relaxed, fostering better communication between the provider and family.

The examination room should be comfortable and safe for children of all ages. Providers should be mindful that wearing a white lab coat might evoke a fearful response from the pediatric patient. When interviewing the patient and family, the provider should sit, establishing and maintaining eye contact with the patient and family.

● **Clinical Pearl:** Friendly interaction with the patient's parents decreases the child's anxiety. Using a jovial and calming tone alleviates anxiety in both parent and patient.

History Taking

A thorough history is essential to a comprehensive well child visit (Display 10-1). Information related to the child's psychosocial environment is necessary for the provider to interpret information from the family during all subsequent visits and if problems arise in the child's growth and development.

● **Clinical Pearl:** Interest in the family is not only essential in treating the patient but also establishes good rapport with all family members that can assist in the development of a trusting relationship between provider and patient.

To satisfy the preschool child's need to know continually what is happening, the provider should explain each step of the examination. For example, "I'm going to talk to your caregiver(s) about how you are doing at home. If you have any questions or want to add anything, let us know." Treating the child as an active participant instead of a passive object will foster a positive relationship between the provider and the patient. Additionally, encouragement of verbal participation in the 3- to 5-year-old enhances the idea of active partnership in all aspects of their health care. The use of drawings to illustrate and explain parts of the anatomy and medical problems can be very helpful to the patient and the family.

Vague complaints or concerns voiced by parents present an opportunity for the provider to use anticipatory guidance about many psychosocial issues and to reassure the parent that the child is developing normally. The well child visit must allow adequate time to explore psychosocial aspects of the child's environment and to answer questions regarding

---

DISPLAY 10–1 • History Elements Reviewed During an Annual Preschool Child Visit

Family psychosocial status
Milestones
    Language
    Cognitive
    Emotional
    Spiritual
Elimination habits
Nutrition habits
Medication intake
Sleep habits
Television watching
Dental hygiene
Immunization status
Tuberculosis risk factors

Anticipatory guidelines are adapted from Murphy's 1996 section on the developmental management of toddlers and preschoolers in *Pediatric primary care: A handbook for nurse practitioners.*

topics such as eating and sleeping patterns, discipline issues, and television viewing.

During the preschool visit, it is important to elicit consistently the history of both physical and social development. During the initial well child visit, the provider should obtain additional historical information, including mother's prenatal history, pregnancy-related illness or medication or drug usage, birth information, neonatal history of growth and feeding, and significant familial genetic history. Understanding the child's environment is very important, and its importance should be clearly explained to the caregiver before asking questions regarding caregiver arrangements, home environment, people in the home, financial structure, occupation of caregivers, and marital status.

▲ **Clinical Warning:** The provider who is just focusing on the history and not observing the child is missing a key to the child's physical and psychosocial development.

Each primary care practice group should have a comprehensive format to follow to ensure everything from immunizations through anticipatory guidance are addressed during the initial and all subsequent patient visits. Each intake of information also should be tailored to the individual's needs and parental concerns. The provider should track intercurrent illnesses and major growth and developmental changes and have records available for parents to review. Educational materials and resources for reference also should be available.

Physical Examination

During the well child visit, most developmental testing should be completed (Display 10-2). The provider should use a standardized developmental tool, such as the Denver Developmental Screening Tool II. The child should be examined after the history and most developmental testing is completed. This helps to reduce the patient's anxiety toward

the provider, thereby increasing the caregiver's comfort when the provider examines the child.

Normal Versus Abnormal Variations

Growth can be measured within percentile ranges on standard growth charts for girls and boys, such as the classical National Center for Health Statistics (NCHS) growth charts from the 1960s and 1970s (Figs. 10-1 and 10-2). The following are four principles to assess normal growth:

- Accurate data
- Discontinuous growth
- Single value
- Time as a tool (Legler & Rose, 1998)

● **Clinical Pearl:** Crossing percentile lines on standardized growth charts between the ages of 3 to 12 for boys and 3 to 10 for girls is abnormal and requires further evaluation.

Height and weight should be measured appropriately and plotted on the child's NCHS growth chart at each annual well child visit and any interceding visits. Inaccurate or incorrectly plotted growth data may lead to an erroneous diagnosis of growth abnormality. For accuracy, the child should be weighed when he or she is not wearing clothes or shoes. After age 3 years, the child should be measured for height while he or she stands without shoes. Head circumference usually is not measured after 2 years unless there is a history or clinical reason to follow it. Staff should be educated about the importance of weight and height measurement accuracy, and if possible the same staff members should do the measurements.

The current guidelines create an impression that a child's growth occurs on a continuum; however, growth actually is a discontinuous process. Repeated observations of growth parameters determine if the child is exhibiting a discontinuous growth pattern. The deception of a single value measurement of growth is that it does not reflect a pattern of development. Time is a tool in assessment as both the age of the child and the presence or absence of significant clinical findings can be observed and evaluated over time.

▲ **Clinical Warning:** Abnormal growth patterns accompanied by abnormal findings necessitate immediate evaluation.

Growth curve variations can be below and above the normal standard of development. Table 10-2 shows some of the more common clinical reasons why differentiation from normal patterns of development may occur in the preschool child.

● **Clinical Pearl:** The standard growth curve was developed in the 1960s and 1970s, and deviation does occur depending on the child's ethnicity. Observation of Legler and Rose's (1998) principles is critical for accurate diagnosis of clinical problems.

The pediatric population is becoming more culturally diverse in the United States. Estimates are that by 2020, approximately 40% of school-age children will be from ethnic minority groups. The clinician must develop awareness through good history taking and observation of commonly held cultural beliefs and normal practices. Education and training to enhance the delivery of culturally effective health care must be integrated into provider practice (Fuentes & Afflick, 1999).

DISPLAY 10–2 • Physical Examination Elements During the Annual Preschool Child Visit

General physical appearance	Respiratory
Weight	Inspection
Height	Auscultation
Skin (take images)	Cardiology
Head	Auscultation
Size/shape	Gastrointestinal
Fontanelles closed	Hernias/organ size
Eyes	Rectum
Size/shape/equal	Genitourinary
Visual acuity	Females: Vagina
Red reflex	Males: Foreskin/testicles
Ears	Check for sexual abuse
Hearing	Neurologic
Internal canals	Motor
Nose/throat	Sensory
Teeth hygiene	Musculoskeletal
Nasal polyps	Exposure
Neck	Inspection
Lymph nodes	

Anticipatory guidelines are adapted from Murphy's 1996 section on the developmental management of toddlers and preschoolers in *Pediatric primary care: A handbook for nurse practitioners.*

GIRLS: 2 TO 18 YEARS
PHYSICAL GROWTH
NCHS PERCENTILES

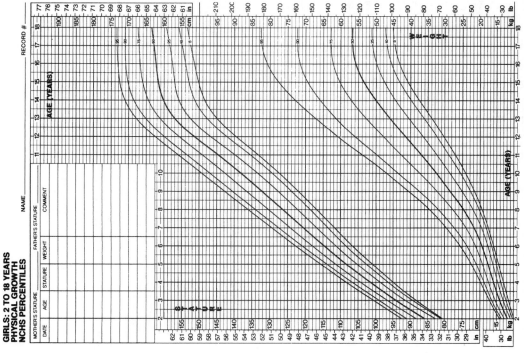

GIRLS: BIRTH TO 36 MONTHS
PHYSICAL GROWTH
NCHS PERCENTILES

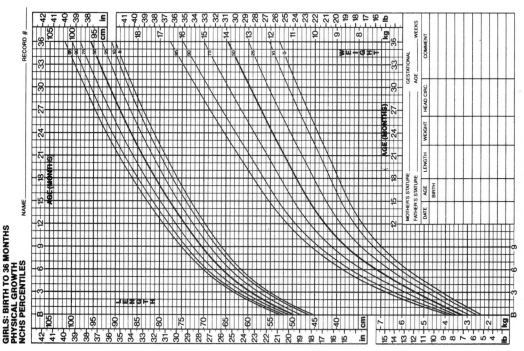

(Adapted from Hamill PVV, Drizd TA, Johnson CL, Reed RB, Roche AF, Moore AM: Physical growth: National Center for Health Statistics percentiles. Am J Clin Nutr 32:607–629, 1979. Data from the National Center for Health Statistics [NCHS], Hyattsville, MD. Figures provided through the courtesy of Ross Laboratories, Columbus, OH).

Figure 10–1 ■ Physical growth percentiles for girls up to 18 years. (Reprinted with permission from Bickley, L. S. [1999]. *Bates' guide to physical examination and history taking* [7th ed.]. Philadelphia: Lippincott Williams & Wilkins.)

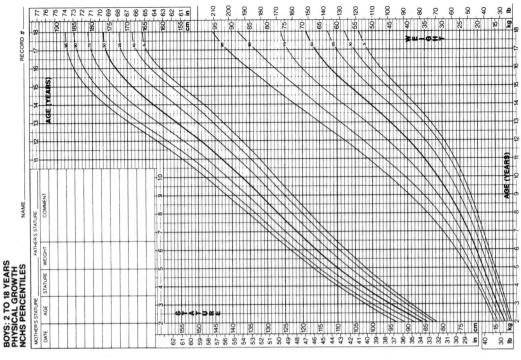

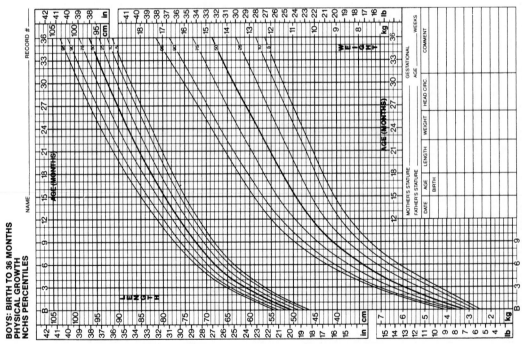

(Adapted from Hamill PVV, Drizd TA, Johnson CL, Reed RB, Roche AF, Moore AM: Physical growth: National Center for Health Statistics percentiles. Am J Clin Nutr 32:607–629, 1979. Data from the National Center for Health Statistics [NCHS], Hyattsville, MD. Figures provided through the courtesy of Ross Laboratories, Columbus, OH).

Figure 10–2 ■ Physical growth percentiles for boys up to 18 years. (Reprinted with permission from Bickley, L. S. [1999]. *Bates' guide to physical examination and history taking* [7th ed.]. Philadelphia: Lippincott Williams & Wilkins.)

Table 10–2. COMMON PATHOLOGIC ETIOLOGIES OF HEIGHT, WEIGHT, AND CRANIAL ABNORMALITIES IN THE NORMAL GROWTH PARAMETERS IN THE PRESCHOOL CHILD

Increased Height	Decreased Height
Endocrine	**Endocrine**
Excess production of growth	Growth hormone deficiency
Hyperthyroidism	Hypothyroidism
Metabolic	**Metabolic**
Homocystinuria	Chronic anemia
Genetic	Skeletal dysplasia/rickets
Klinefelter's syndrome	Major organ system failure
Marfan syndrome	**Genetic/psychosocial causes**
Increased Weight	**Decreased Weight**
Endocrine disorders	**Acquired immune and nutritional deficiencies**
Hypothyroidism	Iron deficiency
Excess production of cortisol (Cushing's disease)	Zinc deficiency
Thalamic or pituitary disorders	Major organ system failure
Genetic disorders	HIV infection and other cellular deficiencies
Down syndrome	Lead intoxication
Prader-Will syndrome	Psychosocial deprivation and malnutrition
Laurence-Moon syndrome	**Genetic/endocrine**
	Hypothyroidism
	Inborn errors of metabolism
Increased Head Size	**Decreased Head Size**
Hydrocephalus	Craniosynostosis
Primary	Prenatal insult
Secondary to associated disease of the central nervous system, such as Arnold-Chiari malformation	Maternal drug or alcohol abuse
	Maternal infection
Megalencephaly	Complications of pregnancy/birth
Primary	Chromosome defects
Secondary to associated disease of the central nervous system, such as neurofibromatosis or tuberous sclerosis	
Secondary to metabolic storage disease	

(Adapted from Legler, J. D., & Rose, L. C. [1998]. Assessment of abnormal growth curves. *American Family Physician, 58*[1], 153–158.)

As stated previously, growth curves are a tool, not an absolute predictor of normal growth and development; therefore, the provider must use comprehensive histories and physical examinations over time to ensure proper growth and development. Growth charts for children from some different cultures (eg, Asian heritage) and with various conditions (eg, Down syndrome) are available and should be used to evaluate the child when indicated.

● **Clinical Pearl:** The art of health care in the 21st century will be seen in how providers negotiate between the patient's cultural beliefs and the culture of health care. For a more comprehensive discussion of this topic, please refer to Chapter 1 of this book.

Sequence

Along with these objective data, vital signs, temperature (if indicated), pulse, respirations, and blood pressure with the proper size cuff (staring at the age of 3 years) are assessed.

Skin

The integument system, including the hair, should be both inspected and palpated for consistency and any abnormal growths or skin discolorations.

● **Clinical Pearl:** Taking a picture of skin abnormalities and following them with similar images is useful to the provider and allows the physical finding to be shared with other clinical specialists to provide greater diagnostic accuracy and comprehensive care.

Head and Neck

Examination of the head and neck should include inspection, palpation, percussion, and age-appropriate measurement of visual acuity and hearing. The head should be inspected for closure of the fontanelles, and size and symmetry should be assessed. Flexibility of the neck can be assessed by observation and through tests of active range of motion. The neck also is palpated to assess the carotid pulses and for significant lymphadenopathy.

● **Clinical Pearl:** Children who have recently recovered from head and neck infections have adenopathy of some of the head and neck lymph nodes. These nodes should be checked at another time, but the condition is not pathologic.

Eyes

The eyes are inspected, with the size and shape of the eyes noted. The pupils are checked for symmetry and red light reflex. The examiner looks for conjunctivae and color of the sclera. The muscles of the eyes are tested for extraocular movements to evaluate for any weakness, and visual acuity is assessed using an appropriate vision screen.

Ears, Nose, and Throat

The ears are inspected for size, shape, and symmetry. They are inspected internally for anomalies, discharge, and inflammation. Assessement includes the posterior ear to evaluate for skin infection and mastoid and postauricular node tenderness. Hearing should be tested using both gross and objective measures on well child visits throughout the preschool period.

● **Clinical Pearl:** The tympanic membrane is assessed using pneumatic otoscopy. Any abnormalities related to color, light reflex, bony landmarks, scars, and foreign bodies, especially when language development is delayed, should be further evaluated.

The nose should be inspected for size, shape, and patency. The mucosa is assessed for dryness and polyps. If there is a complaint of chronic nasal discharge, the nose should be inspected for foreign bodies.

When the child speaks, the mouth should be assessed for symmetry. The tongue is assessed for symmetry. The teeth are examined for caries, and the gums are checked for color and inflammation. The throat, palate, uvula, and tonsils are then inspected.

Chest and Lungs

Inspection of the respiratory system can uncover the common disorder pectus excavatum, in which there is sternal concavity of various degrees. Children with this deformity should be followed with other testing and more frequent visits. Physical activity should be encouraged.

● **Clinical Pearl:** Even though the pectus excavatum may be prominent visually, thoracic volume is less than 19% of the total lung capacity, and the child's ventilation is not limited.

Percussion and auscultation of the bony chest wall provide good indications of the health of the lung tissue underneath. Adventitious sounds, such as rales, rhonchi, wheezes, and rubs, should be followed up immediately with other diagnostic tests, such as pulse oximetry, chest x-ray, and pulmonary function testing.

Cardiovascular System

The cardiovascular system needs to be assessed next for proper growth and function. The provider should pay special attention to palpation of the point of maximum impact for thrills or heaves and to auscultation of heart sounds for murmurs and extra sounds. In children, it is necessary to distinguish innocent from organic murmurs, which may result from congenital defects or acquired diseases.

● **Clinical Pearl:** Because most congenital heart diseases are discovered before the preschool period, acquired heart diseases account for the greatest morbidity and mortality of conditions related to this system during this period.

Abdomen

After gaining the child's trust, the GI examination can be accomplished, followed by the genitourinary examination. The abdomen should be inspected for size, shape, and distension. As the diaphragm and chest structures mature, respiratory movements of the abdomen become normal. Inguinal, umbilical, and femoral hernias should be checked in all children.

● **Clinical Pearl:** Children as old as 4 years may have an umbilical hernia with no sequelae.

Auscultation of the abdomen for bowel sounds and palpation of organ size for abnormalities are advised in this age group. A liver edge may be palpated, which is normal. An enlarged spleen requires further investigation.

Genitalia and Rectum

The genitalia and rectum should be inspected together. The external female genitalia should be inspected for redness, swelling, lesions, and discharge. In males, the foreskin should be fully retractable by age 3 to 4 years. The position of the urethral meatus should be evaluated for hypospadias. The scrotal sac is evaluated for the presence of both testicles and hernias.

● **Clinical Pearl:** Persistent foul-smelling vaginal discharge needs gynecologic referral to rule out foreign body and chronic sexual abuse.

The rectum of both sexes needs to be inspected for fissures, tears, redness, and irritation.

● **Clinical Pearl:** Perineal irritation and lichenification may indicate the presence of worms and requires immediate treatment.

Musculoskeletal and Neurologic Systems

Throughout the examination, the child's musculoskeletal and neurologic development is assessed. The skeletal system can be observed by watching the patient's movements. Comprehensive neurologic checks include motor, language, and cognitive tasks that are assessed in developmental screening, along with tests of specific cranial nerve functions, such as vision and hearing.

● **Clinical Pearl:** The child's socks should be removed to check for malformations and hygiene of the feet. Problems could be preventing normal gait and posture (Boynton, Dunn, & Stephens, 1998).

SCREENING

During the yearly recommended examination, a language delay can be assessed using the Denver Developmental Screening Tool II. Underlying causes, such as mental retardation, child neglect or abuse, or physical limitations from ear infections, can be identified.

DISPLAY 10–3 • Health Promotion/Disease Prevention Elements Reviewed in an Annual Preschool Child Examination

Rhythmicity and daily patterns
  Child makes healthy food choices.
  Family shares meals.
  Family maintains nighttime rituals.
  Child regularly brushes teeth.
Emotional growth
  Family manages anger and resolves conflicts.
  Family shows affection.
  Child makes choices as appropriate.
  Parents praise good behavior and accomplishments.
  Family avoids power struggles.
  Parents set clear and consistent limits.
  Child has opportunities to play with other children of the same age.
  Child is provided with transitional objects.
  Family uses night-light (unless shadows increase a child's fears).
  Parents provide reassurance if nightmares occur.
Cognitive growth
  Parents limit television for child to 1 to 2 hours per day.
  Parents talk with child to develop vocabulary.
  Parents read to child to support language.
  Parents provide toys that child can use creatively.
  Parents listen with care and respond actively.
  Parents allow the child to explore.
Self-care
  Family encourages self-feeding.
  Parents anticipate child's interest in genital differences.
  Parents promote toilet training and hygienic habits.
  Parents promote physical activities in safe places.
  Family insists on use of a car seat.
Strength and coordination
  Child can exercise big muscles.
  Child sings and dances to music.
  Parents provide outdoor play opportunities in safe areas.

Anticipatory guidelines are adapted from Murphy's 1996 section on the developmental management of toddlers and preschoolers in *Pediatric primary care: A handbook for nurse practitioners.*

ANTICIPATORY GUIDANCE

A well child visit is incomplete without time allotted for anticipatory guidance. As discussed in the history-taking section, anticipatory guidance is interactive and occurs throughout the provider–patient interaction. The American Academy of Pediatrics (AAP) has issued two companion manuals to aid the provider in covering a variety of topics during each visit. Growth and development of a normal child are partly due to the environment, and health promotion and disease prevention assist in providing a safe and conducive environment for healthy development to occur.

Major goals involved in anticipatory guidance include gathering accurate information, establishing a therapeutic relationship, and providing education and guidance for the patient and family. During the preschool years, there are several areas of focus during the well child visit (Display 10-3). Anticipatory guidance should be reviewed at each visit with the parents and the child, with safety always a priority.

●**Clinical Pearl:** The AAP offers TIPP Age-related Safety Sheets on the Internet. These can be given to parents as reference materials after well child visits.

Common Questions

Anticipating common questions that parents have regarding growth and development assists providers in supporting parents in promoting healthy growth and development for their children.

- **My child is inventing imaginary friends and talking to them. Is this normal?**
  - **Yes.** Magical thinking accelerates during the preschool years, which allows the child to role play, develop sexual identity, and grow emotionally. Nightmares and fears of monsters are common. Calm reassurance that the monsters and dreams are not real usually is adequate to treat these sleep disturbances.
- **My child is "showing off" his or her genitalia and is curious about sex. Is this normal?**
  - **Yes.** The preschool child's mind is ablaze with thought and fantasy, and this is a normal manifestation. It should be observed carefully, however, to protect the child against individuals who might take advantage of the child's sexual curiosity. Examination of the child's genitalia at bath time or when a concern arises is appropriate. Children should be told that others are not to touch them in their private areas. See Chapter 23 for additional information on sexual abuse.
- **My child does not understand limits to activities. Does he or she overstep these limits just to anger me?**
  - Caregivers must agree and be united in decision making concerning their child. The rules must be consistently enforced. If expectations are made clear, the child will strive to achieve them. When reprimanding a child, it is most important that the parents criticize the deed, but never the child. The child is not trying to anger the parents; he or she is testing the parents' limits. Preschoolers are learning the boundaries of their new and challenging world. At the end of the preschool phase, the child will have learned how to temper fantasies of power and abide by rules for self-control.
- **When my child misbehaves, should I punish her?**
  - When dealing with preschoolers, it is especially important not to delay the consequences of inappropriate behavior. Punishment should be weighed carefully and within reason. A child should never be spanked or hit. Too often, a child is hit in anger when the parent or caretaker has lost control. Instead, restrictions on privileges often create positive effects. Encouraging and rewarding positive behavior can provide a mechanism for parents and children to communicate with love and care. Affection and praise can bring out beautiful qualities in all children. Principles of limit-setting should be elicited and reviewed to provide family members with a vehicle to verbalize thoughts and feelings related to this topic.

●**Clinical Pearl:** The action should be punished, not the child.

- **My child occasionally wets the bed after he witnesses a fight between my partner and me. Is this normal? Should I punish the child for these accidents?**

• Family counseling should be part of all plans for anticipatory guidance. Issues related to stress should be explored within the family unit, and counseling should be offered. Families need to be advised that children should never be punished for accidents. Rather, children should learn to understand the consequences of bed wetting by assisting parents with the removal of soiled bedding. Children should be rewarded for dry nights. See Chapter 63 on enuresis and encopresis for more information.

Common Concerns

Nutrition

The nutritional goal during the preschool years is the child's satisfactory growth. Energy expenditure for growth changes from infancy, when 40% of the total energy requirement was dedicated to growth. From age 2 through adolescence, only 2% is directed toward growth. Most energy is now expended on activity and basal metabolic maintenance (Smith, 1977). The calorie requirements for preschoolers are 70 to 90 calories/kg/d, including 1.5 to 2.5 g/kg/d of protein. Fluid requirements are about 100 mL/kg/d for average activity.

● **Clinical Pearl:** Remember these are guidelines. The child's activity level and the climate in which he or she lives determine the fluid requirements.

As part of neuronal development, preschoolers are learning mastery of their environment and are developing their own eating patterns. A good time to integrate mastery of the environment into meal preparation is by age 5, when the sense of self has developed. Children are more likely to eat foods they have helped to prepare (Levine et al., 1999). It is important to stress that healthy foods should be encouraged at this time.

● **Clinical Pearl:** A common concern regarding this age group is that children are not eating enough. If they are following a steady growth pattern and eating a healthy diet, they are doing well.

● **Clinical Pearl:** The gradual introduction of a wide variety of whole foods, including grains, fish, fruits, and vegetables, provides adequate nutrition and a strong foundation for growth, health promotion, and disease prevention.

Estimates are that 12 million Americans consider themselves vegetarians (Stevenson, 1998). All vegetarians do not practice the same eating habits. Lacto-ova vegetarians consume eggs and dairy products, while vegans exclude all animal food products. Because the average child in the United States has a diet based on meat, the protein intake of most children is double the necessary amount. This may raise concerns that the vegetarian child will lack the necessary protein for healthy growth and development. With proper anticipatory guidance, vegetarian children can meet their protein and nutritional needs. The provider should encourage vitamin B_{12} supplementation, because this vitamin is not found in plant foods. Calcium intake is important for growing bones and teeth. Vegetable sources of calcium, such as dark leafy greens, tofu, and beans, should be included in their diet. The family should be encouraged to seek out resources for assistance in menu planning and food preparation.

● **Clinical Pearl:** Good sources of protein for the vegetarian child are soybeans, fortified soymilk, tofu, legumes, nuts, seeds, and peanut butter.

▲ **Clinical Warning:** Discouraging a vegetarian diet in a child who is less than normal weight and height but is growing steadily and developing normally may be destructive to the patient–provider relationship and may isolate the child within a family that practices vegetarianism.

When serving a meal, the caregiver should be aware that the general consumption for preschoolers is about half an adult's portion. How a meal is presented often can entice a child to eat, but a child should never be forced to eat. Mealtime, including preparation and consumption, should be conducted in a relaxed and pleasant atmosphere. Food should be placed in front of the child and taken away when the child is finished. If the child eats, it is terrific; however, if the child does not eat, there should be no arguments or other disruptive behaviors.

● **Clinical Pearl:** Children will eat when they are hungry. The child should never be allowed to disrupt what should be a positive, happy, relaxed, mealtime atmosphere.

Sleep

Sleep contributes to the child's healthy growth and development and is essential for well-being. It should be discussed and assessed at every well child visit. As the brain undergoes myelinization and dramatically changes in the first 2 years of life, the child's sleep pattern will change to reflect this and other developments. The amount of overall sleep and rapid eye movement sleep decreases while quiet sleep increases (Lowery, 1986). By age 4 years, daytime sleep is no longer needed, and the child and family should have an established sleeping routine.

Sleep is not just a physiologic need, but an interactive activity between the family and child. The most frequent sleep disturbances during the preschool years are nightmares and night terrors that can be treated by reassuring the child. If other new sleep disturbances emerge, such as frequent night awakenings and bedtime difficulties, then causal exploration is warranted. Health conditions, such as pinworms, colic, hypothyroidism, or infections, can cause sleep problems. Additionally, parental mismanagement of sleep routines can impact the child's sleep habits. Preschoolers are developing a sense of self, so, as with mealtimes, bedtime should be a friendly and relaxed occasion. Having the child share a bed with a sibling or parent has been discouraged because co-sleeping children are two to three times more likely to have night awakenings than children who sleep alone. Before discouraging co-sleeping, the provider should explore the family's cultural practices and economic situation.

● **Clinical Pearl:** Sensitivity to the family's cultural and economic situation may help to ensure the child's continued growth and development.

▲ **Clinical Warning:** Persistent sleep disturbances in preschoolers should be evaluated for both physical and psychosocial causes. If the provider dismisses sleep disturbances, he or she may overlook physical ailments that can affect the child's long-term well-being.

Television and the Internet

Passive television viewing often takes the place of imaginative interactive play. Television and the Internet can positively influence a child's social behavior if he or she is exposed to prosocial programming. The amount of time a child views television peaks during the preschool years, with an average of 21 to 30 hours of viewing per week. A moderate amount of television viewing appropriate for age level can have a positive impact on development. Estimates are, however, that 80% of television viewing in today's children is developmentally inappropriate, containing five violent acts per hour of viewing (Hutson et al., 1992). Thus, an average 18-year-old has viewed about 200,000 acts of violence on television.

Shapiro (1999) synthesized the literature on the effects of children viewing violence from the 1960s through the 1990s. Findings were that children exhibited increased aggression after viewing violent television and experienced a greater sense of "arousal," which can lead to aggressive acts when the child is provoked or predisposed to aggression. Although the connection between viewing violence and the development of aggressive behavior continues to be debated, it has been identified that television viewing of more than 5 hours a day is associated with obesity and hypercholesterolemia (Wong, et al., 1992).

Electronic media are here to stay and have the potential to serve as educational tools that may escape cultural and language barriers. As with anything in the preschool child's life, unsupervised use of electronic media can have harmful effects. The AAP and the American Medical Association are lobbying for responsible programming and viewing.

Just as parents set limits regarding other activities of the child, they should set limits on television. Anticipatory guidance must be provided to families. In general, most experts believe that 2 hours or fewer a day of responsible television viewing is acceptable. The child's caregiver also must monitor use of the computer and Internet. Documentation of these behaviors also should be included as part of the ongoing well child assessment.

Common Conditions

Some of the most common conditions encountered from ages 3 to 5 years are febrile illness, vomiting and diarrhea, constipation, and upper respiratory tract infections. Detailed information on each of these topics can be found in Chapters 30, 31, 34, 36, and 38.

Acute viral infections cause most fevers. Unless extremely high (41.1°C [106°F]), fever does not specifically harm the patient and actually may help the immune system's response to the offending agents. Most fever treatment centers on providing adequate hydration and the use of antipyretics, acetaminophen, and nonsteroidal anti-inflammatory drugs. If the child does not have a history of febrile seizures and is not terribly uncomfortable, the child may not require pharmacologic treatment.

● **Clinical Pearl:** If the child has a history of febrile seizures, then the fever should be promptly treated.

▲ **Clinical Warning:** Alcohol or ice water baths should never be used to lower body temperature.

Constipation can be diagnosed many different ways (eg, rectal exam or stool on x-rays of the abdomen). Its cause in children usually is too little free water in the diet, inadequate intake of high-residue food, disruption of daily habits, or painful anal fissure. Treatment can include dietary counseling regarding natural dietary lubricants, such as prune and tomato juice, and high-residue foods, such as fruits and green vegetables. Pharmacologic therapy can be given for stool softening and anal fissure treatment. Medication dosage is based on weight.

Vomiting and diarrhea together usually are associated with a self-limiting viral gastroenteritis. Hydration status should be monitored. Clear fluids should be encouraged, and simple solid foods should be introduced slowly when the vomiting and diarrhea have subsided.

● **Clinical Pearl:** Intestinal obstruction, increased intracranial pressure, and accidental ingestion of theophylline and erythromycin can cause vomiting and should be suspected in cases of sudden vomiting without diarrhea.

Upper respiratory infection, or the common cold, is caused primarily by a respiratory virus. Viral infections that attack the mucous membranes can lower local resistance in the nose and throat, which can set the stage for secondary bacterial invasion. Treatment is symptomatic relief. If nasal discharge persists and becomes purulent, the provider should consider prescribing antibiotics.

COMMUNITY RESOURCES

Information available to the health care consumer has accelerated over the last 5 years through access to the Internet. Now patients and their families have other sources of information regarding anticipatory guidance other than their providers. The clinician should encourage families to use information that assists in a well child's growth and development.

A good recommendation is the AAP web site (*http://www.aap.org*), which not only offers TIPP Age-Related Safety Sheets, but also offers a wide variety of information, including immunization information and schedules, online Healthy Kids Magazine, provider referral services, and a provider-reviewed listing of the best pediatric web sites. Another helpful site for specific information is Healthfinder (*http://www.healthfinder.org*), offering high quality health information on a variety of topics. A good source of medication information for patients is Rx List (*http://www.rxlist.com*), which allows users to look up detailed information on specific drugs by their brand or generic names. Another good source of health information emphasizing alternative medicine is wellness web (*http://www.wellweb.com*). To verify the credibility of a website, one can search the medical watchdog site of Health on the Net Foundation (*http://www.hon.ch*). A prosocial site for the preschool child is the Public Broadcasting Station website (http://www.pbs.org.) and the Zoboomafoo website, the online companion to the daily children's show of the same name. The core activity of the television show—making friends with animals—is extended now to kids everywhere. There are three interactive games, a coloring book, and a who's who section. These activities are very interactive and test preschoolers' language, cognitive, and physical limits. Resources for vegetarian families include Vegetarian Journal: Vegetarian Resource Group, PO Box 1463, Baltimore, MD, 21203, phone: (410) 336-VEGE; Vegetarian Times, 4 High Ridge Park, Stamford, CT, 06905, phone: (800) 829-

3340; and Being Vegetarian: The Amercian Dietetic Association, Chronimed, 1996, phone: (800) 444-5951.

BIBLIOGRAPHY

Berkowitz, C. D. (1996). *Pediatrics: A primary care approach*. Philadelphia: W. B. Saunders.

Committee on Practice and Ambulatory Medicine, AAP. (1995). Recommendations for preventive pediatric health care. *Pediatrics, 96,* 373–374.

DuPont, H. L. (1999). Prevention of diarrhea by the probiotic, Lactobacillus GG. *Journal of Pediatrics,* 1–2.

Graef, J. (Ed.) (1997). *Manual of pediatric therapeutics* (6th ed.). Baltimore, MD: Williams & Wilkins.

Hamill P. V., Drizd, T., Johnson, C. L., Reed, R. B., Roche, A. F., Moore, W. M. (1979). Physical growth: National Center for Health Statistics percentiles. *American Journal of Clinical Nutrition, 32,* 607–629.

Heyman, M. A. (1986). Fetal and neonatal circulation. In F. H. Adams, G. C. Emmanouilides, & T. A. Riemenschneider (Eds.), *Heart disease in infants, children and adolescents* (5th ed.). Baltimore: Williams & Wilkins.

Hoekelman, R. A., Friedman, S. B., Nelson, N. M., & Seidel, H. M. (1992). *Primary pediatric care* (2nd ed.). St. Louis: C.V. Mosby.

Lampl, M., Veldhuis, J. D., & Johnson, M. L. (1992). Station and stasis: A model of human growth. *Science, 258,* 801–803.

Reiter, E. O., & Kaplan, S. L. (1996). Growth and disorders of growth. In A. M. Rudolph (Ed.), *Rudolph's pediatrics* (20th ed.) (pp. 1700–1702). Stamford, CT: Appleton & Lange.

Uphold, C. R., & Graham, M. V. (Eds.) (1998). *Clinical guidelines in family practice* (3rd ed.). Gainesville, FL: Barmarrae Books.

REFERENCES

Allen, A. (1999). The internet in medicine: An update. *Patient Care,* 30–54.

AAP Statement. (1993). "Lead Poisoning: From Screening to Primary Prevention." Elk Grove, IL: AAP.

AAP Statement. (1994). "Screening for Tuberculosis in Infants and Children." Elk Grove, IL: AAP.

American Academy of Pediatrics. (1996). Guidelines for health supervision and health supervision visit. Elk Grove, IL: AAP.

Behrman, R. E., Kliegman, R. M., & Arvin, A. M. (Eds.) (1996). *Nelson textbook of pediatrics* (15th ed.). Philadelphia: W.B. Saunders.

Boynton, R. W., Dunn, E. S., & Stephens, G. R. (1998). *Manual of ambulatory pediatrics* (4th ed.). Philadelphia: Lippincott Williams & Wilkins.

Fuentes, C. J., & Afflick, E. (1999). Culturally effective pediatric care: Education and training issues. *Pediatrics American Academy of Pediatrics,* 167–169.

Hutson, A. C., Donnerstein, E., Fairchild, H., et al. (1992). *Big world, small screen: The role of television in American society.* Lincoln, NE: University of Nebraska Press.

Legler, J. D., & Rose, L. C. (1998). Assessment of abnormal growth curves. *American Family Physician, 58*(1), 153–158.

Levine, M. D., Carey, W. B., & Crocker, A.C. (Eds.) (1999). *Developmental-behavioral pediatrics* (3rd ed.). Philadelphia, PA: WB Saunders.

Lowery, G. H. (1986). *Growth and development in children* (8th ed.). New York: Year Book.

Lustig, J. V. (1995). Approaching the pediatric patient. In W. W. Hay, J. R. Groothuis, A. R. Hayward, & M. J. Levin (Eds.), *Pediatric diagnosis and treatment* (pp. 1–8). Norwalk, CT: Appleton & Lange.

Murphy, M. A. (1996). Developmental management of toddlers and preschoolers. In C. E. Burns, N. Barber, M. A. Brady, & A. M. Dunn (Eds.), *Pediatric primary care* (pp. 101–121). Philadelphia: W.B. Saunders.

Nelson, W. E., Behrman, R. E., Kilegman, E. N., & Arvin, A. M. (Eds.), (1996). *Nelson textbook of pediatrics* (15th ed.). Philadelphia: W.B. Saunders.

Rabinowicz, T. (1986). The differential maturation of the cerebral cortex. In F. Falkner & J. M. Tanner (Eds.), *Human growth: A comprehensive treatise: Vol. 2. postnatal growth neurobiology* (2nd ed.). New York: Plenum Press.

Smith, D. W. (1977). *Growth and its disorders: Major problems in clinical pediatrics,* Vol 25. Philadelphia: W.B. Saunders.

Stevenson, S. S. (1998). Vegetarian children. *The Clinical Letter for Nurse Practitioners, 1*(2), 1–3.

Wong, N. D., Thomas, K. H., Qaqundah, P. Y., et al. (1992). Television viewing and pediatric hypercholesterolemia. *Pediatrics, 90,* 75–79.

Healthy Growth and Development of the School-Age Child

• ANDREA BERNE, RN, CPNP, MPH, and ELLEN FLYNN, RN, CPNP

INTRODUCTION

The school-age period (5–12 years of age) is a time of relatively slow but steady growth. It is a time of quiescence during which the primary care provider can rely on both the parent and child to give a history that directs the focus of the encounter. Excluding dentition and pubertal change, organs are developed and fully functioning. Major illness is not expected. Problems usually involve routine infection, known allergy, sports, and other injuries.

Many school-age children present with complaints of benign aches and pains of various body systems (eg, stomach ache, headache, and leg pain). The school-age child with a previously diagnosed chronic illness needs support to begin participating in the management of that illness. School entry and adjustment bring their own physical, developmental, psychological, and social challenges. During this period, learning difficulties, attention problems, and affective disorders surface.

The school-age child is on an early path toward independence. Successful academic achievement and acceptance from peers help in the development of initiative, competence, and confidence. Because school becomes the most important parameter of the child's cognitive development, providers must support the family with this transition.

GROWTH AND DEVELOPMENT

Physical Development

School-age children grow at a slow pace until they hit their "growth spurt." Expected growth is 2 in and 5 to 7 lb per year for both males and females. These parameters are particularly important in the identification of obesity for which today's school-age children are at high risk. In terms of stature, genetics play a role in normal variations, which may appear below the fifth or above the 95th percentile on standard growth charts. Abnormal etiologies may exist and include chronic illness, endocrine abnormalities, and neglect or abuse. The beginning of rapid adolescent growth for girls can be as early as 9 years of age and as late as 14 years, 6 months. Boys begin their growth spurt between 10 years, 6 months and 16 years. The median age for girls is 12 years; the median age for boys is 14 years (Bickley, Hoekleman, & Bates, 1999).

● **Clinical Pearl:** Growth charts should be graphed for height and weight at each visit. Significant crossing of percentiles is almost invariably abnormal in females between the ages of 3 and 10 and in males between the ages of 3 and 12.

Pubertal Development

Pubertal changes may begin in the school-age child. For girls, breast bud development is often the first sign of puberty and can appear as early as 7 years, 5 months and as late as 13 years. Normally, pubic hair follows 6 months later (Algranati, 1998). Each Tanner stage requires approximately 1 year, and menses usually begins sometime during breast Tanner stage IV (see Appendix XX) (Goldblum, 1997).

The first sign of puberty in boys is testicular enlargement and scrotal skin thinning, which can appear as early as 9 years and as late as 13 years, 6 months. The median age of occurrence is 11 years, 6 months. The onset of pubic hair growth occurs between 10 and 15 years. Normally, pubic hair appears 6 months after testicular enlargement begins. Penile enlargement occurs between ages 10 years, 6 months and 14 years, 6 months, 1 year after testicular enlargement (Algranati, 1998).

Motor Skills

Muscle bulk, coordination, and strength continue to develop throughout the school-age years. A 5-year-old child should be able to balance on one foot, walk on tiptoe, and tandem walk on a straight line. A 6-year-old child should be able to skip. An 8-year-old child should be able to hop twice on one foot and then on the other. Examples of appropriate fine motor abilities are the 6-year-old child who ties his or her own shoelaces and the 8-year-old child who performs rapid alternating movements of thumb to each finger of the same hand in succession (Algranati, 1998). Genetics help determine each child's unique skills and abilities. Normal variations include the clumsy child and the exceptionally athletic child.

Cognitive Development

Previously developed language skills become more fluid, resulting in advanced cognitive functioning in the school-age child. Vocabulary and understanding increase. Grammar and articulation are usually correct. Young school-age children ask many questions, solve simple problems, and use fantasy in their thinking processes. Fantasy thinking generates new fears. Between 6 and 11 years, the child further organizes thought and develops memory. He or she reads and reasons more completely.

Psychosocial Development

For the young school-age child, the family is the primary social group. Grade-school children usually have strong family ties and use their own parents or other adults close to the family as role models (ie, the child dresses up like mom). Relationships with parents and siblings are usually harmonious in younger years, becoming more challenging as puberty approaches. At this time, conflicts with parents regarding limit setting and expectations often arise. As they get older, school-age children begin to establish their independence, psychologically separate from their parents, and build their own identities. As they separate from parents, peers become increasingly important. Parents must recognize this as normal and allow children to separate.

The peer group provides an arena for older school-age children to establish independence and test out ideas. Friends are especially important during this time, and children begin to conform to a set of group standards. School-age children assume a sex role and engage energetically in group activities. How they view their competencies within these groups determines motivation, perseverance, and resilience. School-age children begin to incorporate values learned at home, in school, and from peers. The older school-age child begins to let go of fears, focusing more on reality. Approval, recognition, and enthusiasm are the hallmarks of the healthy child during this period. Role models shift to other adults outside the home. Normal variants describe personality differences that exist in children who are thought to be "different" but still function acceptably. Normal variants include shy, cautious, or contentious children. Parents need to seek help when a child fails to succeed at the tasks expected for his or her age because these personality differences are interfering with achievement.

HISTORY AND PHYSICAL EXAMINATION

The American Academy of Pediatrics (AAP) recommends that school-age children receive a complete history and physical examination at ages 5, 6, 8, 10, 11, and 12 years. Additional visits may be necessary for children who have some variations from normal (AAP, 1997). When the history and physical examination are complete, it is important to ask the child if he or she has any questions. Table 11-1 provides critical foci for history, physical examination, and health promotion.

History Topics

School-age children are valuable participants in providing the history. Providers should direct questions to both parent and child and ask both what their concerns are at each visit. In the late school-age years, it may be appropriate to take a history from the child privately as well as a history from the parent.

Physical Health

The following are questions to ask:

- What is the child's immunization status?
- Have there been any illnesses, accidents, injuries, or visits to emergency departments?
- Have you noticed any body changes? Has menses begun?
- Do you have any concerns about your body?
- Are you taking any medications?
- Can you see the blackboard, or do you have any trouble reading?
- Are there any problems with hearing?
- Do you brush your teeth and floss at least daily and have regular dental checkups? Do you have any cavities or dental problems? Do you have fluoride in your water? Is your water source municipal or well?

Mental Health

The following are questions to ask:

- Are you mostly happy or mostly sad?
- What things make you happy and sad?
- Are you worrying about anything?
- Are you angry with anyone or about anything?
- On a scale of 1 to 10, how do you get along with your parents and siblings?
- Are there any problems with peers?
- Do you ever think of hurting yourself or others?
- Have there been discussions between parent and child regarding sexuality?

Diet

The following are questions to ask:

- What do you eat during the course of the day? Give me an example of a typical meal.
- What are some of your snack foods?
- Do you eat between meals?
- Do you eat in front of the television?
- What do you drink?
- How much caffeine, sugar, or artificially colored or sweetened drinks do you consume?
- How much milk do you drink each day? What type of milk is it: whole, low fat, or skim?
- What are the healthy foods you eat?
- What are the "junk foods" you eat?
- What foods do you refuse to eat?
- Do you take any vitamins or other dietary supplements?
- How do you feel about your weight?
- Have you tried alcohol? Have you tried cigarettes?
- Do you eat in fast food restaurants?
- Are you a vegetarian or on any other special diet?

Habits and Physical Activity

The following are questions to ask:

- Do you have any habits (eg, nail biting, thumb sucking, tics, mannerisms, compulsions)?
- What physical activity do you get during the day?
- Do you play sports? If so, which ones, how many times a week, and what time of the year?

Sleep

The following are questions to ask:

- Are there any sleep problems (eg, difficulty getting to sleep, waking during the night, sleepwalking, nightmares, night terrors, late riser)?
- What time do you go to bed?
- What time do you get up?
- Are there battles about bedtime?
- Do you snore or have difficulty breathing during the night?

Elimination

The following are questions to ask:

- Is the child completely toilet trained? Are there any problems with accidents, enuresis, or encopresis?
- Do you have any problems with constipation or diarrhea? If so, are you using any medications or enemas?

TABLE 11-1. CRITICAL FOCI IN THE HISTORY, PHYSICAL EXAMINATION, AND HEALTH-PROMOTION ACTIVITIES DURING THE SCHOOL-AGE PERIOD

Age	History	Physical Examination (PE)	Health Promotion
5	Illness	Complete PE*	Explore and Support:
	Accidents	Immunizations	Healthy peer relationships
	Injuries	Vision	School adjustments
	Family changes	Hearing	Family relationships
	Eating problems	Mantoux	Discuss healthy diet and habits.
	Toileting problems		Encourage exercise.
	Sleep problems		Teach personal hygiene.
	ADL		Educate about injuries and accidents.
	Behavior problems		
	School adjustment		
	Activity/exercise		
	Habits		
	Dental hygiene		
	Fluoride supplement		
	Seat belts		
	Bicycle helmet		
	Sports safety		
	Stranger awareness		
	Gun awareness		
	Smokers in the home		
6	Nutrition	Complete PE*	Discuss dangers of cigarettes, alcohol, drugs.
	Exercise	Hgb	
7	Nutrition	Complete PE*	Discuss habit development.
	Exercise		
8	Sex education	Complete PE*	Discuss body changes.
		Cholesterol	
10	Body changes	Complete PE*	
	Special diet	Tanner stages	
	Supplements		
	Depression		
	Substance abuse		
11	Menses	Complete PE*	Discuss sexuality.
12	Sexual activity	Complete PE*	Discuss high-risk behaviors.

*Includes height; weight; vital signs, including BP; and scoliosis evaluation.

Social

The following are questions to ask:

- Who lives in the house?
- If parents are divorced or separated, what are the arrangements for visitation?
- Do both parents work? Are there any other caretakers?
- Do you have a best friend?
- What do you like best about school?
- Are there any specific difficulties?
- How many days have you missed from school this year?
- How did things go at the last parent–teacher conference?
- What do you do after school and on weekends?
- What do you read? What are your hobbies? Do you belong to any groups?
- Are there any behavior problems (eg, fighting, lying, stealing, sibling conflict, mood swings, aggression, defiance)?

● **Clinical Pearl:** The following are important questions to ask:

- How many hours are spent watching television or playing video games per day? What do you watch or play?
- How many hours are spent on the computer? What kind of computer use is usual?
- To what kind of music do you listen?
- Are there pets in the house?
- Are there smokers in the house?
- Are there guns in the house? If so, are guns and ammunition stored separately and in locked locations?

Safety

The following are questions to ask:

- Do you wear a seat belt at all times?
- Do you wear appropriate safety equipment for all sports (helmets and pads)?

- Do you know how to swim? Are you supervised when you swim?
- Do you know how to dial 911?
- Have there been family discussions about alcohol, smoking, and drug use?
- Do you know what to do if approached by a stranger?
- Do you know the difference between "good touch and bad touch?"

Physical Examination

School-age children should be "old hands" at visits to their providers. They understand the concrete operation of a physical examination and want to cooperate. The provider should praise children for their successful participation and reward them for cooperation. Each visit should be an opportunity to build the child's self-esteem.

Approach to Examination

Providers should speak to school-age children directly in a manner they comprehend and should listen to them when they speak. They are generally easier to engage when conversation begins with topics both familiar and important to them: best friends, sports, and school. They should be reassured regarding what to expect. Their major fears involve invasive procedures, especially "needles."

The child's emerging modesty should be protected during the physical examination. Children should be given the opportunity to cover themselves either with a gown or by removing and replacing articles of clothing one piece at a time. Allowing the school-age child some control reduces anxiety and improves cooperation. The clinician should be honest about discomfort and encourage the child to express feelings. He or she should praise healthy coping mechanisms for those things that the child fears. The provider should find something to praise in each child's performance.

Sequence

Measurements and Immunizations

To measure height and weight, the child should be without clothing or shoes and in the standing position. School-age children receive immunizations according to the AAP recommended schedule (see Chapter 13).

Skin

The skin is inspected and palpated for texture, color, and turgor. Lesions and rashes should be described. A normal variant for school-age children is superficial ecchymosis on the lower extremities. The fingernails and toenails are inspected for color and condition. The scalp is checked for inflammation, scaling, hair loss, and lesions. The eyebrows should be inspected as well. A common school-age problem for which the clinician must be alert is infestation with head lice.

Head, Neck, and Face

The head is assessed for general shape. The provider palpates for bony prominence, lymph nodes, and masses. The neck is inspected for bulges, head tilts, and an enlarged thyroid and palpated all over for any masses or enlarged or otherwise abnormal lymph nodes. The thyroid gland also is palpated. A normal variation in the preadolescent is a palpable thyroid even when not enlarged. Neck range of motion should be evaluated. The child's general mood and affect are noted. Any unusual facies (eg, open mouth, dry lips, allergic crease on nose, wide-set eyes, low-set ears) should be noted.

Eyes

Shape, size, and symmetry are inspected. Pupillary shape, reaction to light, and accommodation are evaluated. Ocular motion and corneal light reflex are assessed. The alternate cover test is used to assess muscle balance. Eye tests rule out strabismus and esotropia. The fundus is examined. Dark circles under the eyes (allergic shiners) may be a sign of allergies.

Ears, Nose, and Throat

The external ear is inspected and palpated. The pinna is pulled up and back and an insufflator is used to examine the ear canal and tympanic membrane for landmarks, color, translucency, and mobility. Traction applied to the pinna causes pain when a child has otitis externa (swimmer's ear).

The nose is inspected for patency and discharge. Flaring is noted. Turbinates, mucosa, and septum are examined. Nasal polyps can be mistaken for boggy, swollen, inflamed turbinates, which present with infection or allergy. Although nasal polyps are uncommon in children, they may be a presenting sign of cystic fibrosis. A ridge along the nasal bridge may represent an "allergic crease" due to frequent "allergic saluting" in a child with allergies.

The child's breath should be noted: Halitosis can be associated with pharyngitis, poor dental hygiene, sinusitis, and nasal foreign body. Lips should be examined for color, texture, lesions, and symmetry. At 6 years of age, children begin to lose their primary teeth; the permanent teeth erupt intermittently throughout the school-age years. Teeth are inspected for staining, caries, overcrowding, and malocclusion. Gums and mouth are checked for color, inflammation, and lesions. Common intraoral lesions include aphthous ulcers (chancre sores). A "strawberry" tongue is indicative of streptococcal infection. A "geographic tongue" (a tongue with areas of different coloration) is a benign normal variant.

The tonsils increase in size, with a peak between the ages of 3 and 8. Tonsils may appear large at this age due to physiologic lymphoid hyperplasia, which may be another common normal variant as long as the child has no problems with breathing, swallowing, or infection.

Chest and Cardiovascular System

The thorax is inspected for symmetry, excursion, and bulges. Scoliosis may produce an asymmetry of the chest. The heart and lungs are auscultated with the patient upright and recumbent. The precordium is palpated for the point of maximum impulse (PMI), thrills, heaves, and lifts. Rate, rhythm, and heart sounds are auscultated with the child upright and recumbent, because characteristics of a murmur may change when the child is in different positions. Innocent murmurs are a normal variant often first heard in the school-age child.

● **Clinical Pearl:** Assessment of physiologic splitting of the second heart sound is often critical in differentiating between innocent (functional) murmurs and their organic counterparts (see Chapter 37).

Respiratory rate is counted. All lung fields are auscultated for quality of breath sounds, with normal versus abnormal noted. The breasts, nipples, and axilla of males and females are inspected and palpated with the patient in the supine position. Tanner stage is noted. In females, breast budding may be asymmetrical and cause tenderness. Children with early, advancing adrenarche must be evaluated for precocious puberty. Premature thelarche defined alone, without any other evidence of puberty, is very common. The child and family should be assured that this is a normal variant and that an endocrinology work-up is rarely revealing. Such an examination should only be undertaken when other signs of precocious puberty are present.

Abdomen

The abdomen is inspected for asymmetry or bulges. Bowel sounds are auscultated before the abdomen is palpated. Because abdominal pain is a frequent complaint in school-age children, a helpful technique to determine true tenderness is for the provider to steadily increase pressure on the stethoscope as he or she listens to all four quadrants.

The four quadrants are palpated gently and more deeply (as the patient tolerates) for tenderness and masses. Constipation and a full bladder cause the most common benign masses found in this age group. Guarding and rebound tenderness are noted. The liver and spleen margins are palpated while the cooperative child takes and holds a deep breath. It is common to palpate a spleen tip in children who have had recent viral illness. While appendicitis is one cause, abdominal pain also is a presenting sign of group A *Streptococcus* infection and pneumonia. Often the child with an acute abdomen cannot tolerate jarring (eg, when jumping off the examining table, the child has difficulty standing straight).

Genitalia

Using correct terminology (vagina or penis), the clinician should explain to the child that every part of the body must be examined. This is a good opportunity to discuss who can and who cannot touch and look at "private parts." The inguinal lymph nodes and femoral pulses are palpated. The normal variant of shotty inguinal nodes should be expected. Inguinal hernias should be checked in both boys and girls.

For the female, the complete genitalia and anus are inspected with the child in the frog leg position. In the prepubertal girl, labial adhesions are a common variant.

● **Clinical Pearl:** Normal physiologic vaginal discharge is nonpurulent, watery, and not foul smelling. All other discharge must be evaluated for other etiologies (eg, foreign body, infection, abuse; see Chaps. 23, 41). Pubic hair development is inspected, with Tanner stage noted. Children with early, advancing adrenarche must be evaluated for precocious puberty (see Chap. 60).

For the male, the penis, urethra, scrotum, testes, and anus are inspected. Testicular size and scrotal skin thinning are noted. Pubic hair is inspected if present, with Tanner stage noted. Early, advancing testicular enlargement or adrenarche requires further evaluation. The scrotum and testes are palpated. It is normal for the left testicle to be slightly lower than the right, and for the right testicle to be slightly larger than the left. The child should bear down to enable the provider to examine for hernias. The penis and foreskin are examined. Ballooning of the foreskin with urination is a symptom of phimosis. Most school-age boys will have a fully retractable foreskin. Sometimes boys are concerned about penis size. The clinician can reassure the child by pushing down on the pubic fat pad to demonstrate actual penis size.

● **Clinical Pearl:** A useful technique for palpating testes in younger boys is to have the child sit "pretzel style" so that the provider can milk the testes into the scrotum.

Musculoskeletal System

Because of children's increased intense involvement with sports, a complete and thorough examination of the musculoskeletal system is necessary to check for both new and old injury. The head, neck, and extremities (including the hands and feet) are inspected for alignment, bulk, symmetry, and tone. Full range of motion is performed on all joints, with evaluation of muscle tone and strength. Gait is evaluated. Benign "growing pains" are a common complaint in the school-age child. Frequently, these complaints center on the thigh, calf, shin, or entire leg. They most commonly occur at night, and the physical examination is entirely normal. The most common cause of foot pain in children is poor-fitting shoes. Back pain, limp, and painful swollen joints should be taken seriously; they often are signs of pathology and must be fully evaluated. Children must be completely undressed when the spine is evaluated for curvature. The child should stand with feet together and arms at the sides. Unequal planes of shoulders and hips should be inspected. Bony prominences are noted, as is unequal length of the legs. The child should bend forward at the waist. Knees should be straight and arms dangling. The provider should check for asymmetry, curves, and unequal planes (Fig. 11-1). The spine is palpated. Symmetrical knock knees, bowing, and flat feet are common normal variants and require no intervention.

Neurologic System

Much of the neurologic history and examination has been conducted during the course of examining the previous sys-

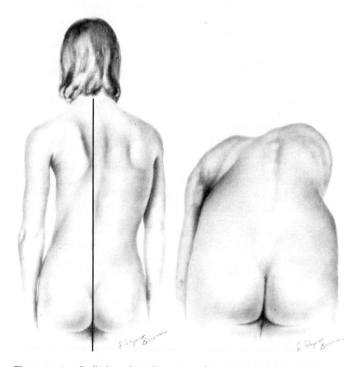

Figure 11–1 ■ Scoliosis—a lateral curvature of the spine—is shown here with a thoracic convexity to the right. The body has compensated for the curve and a plumb line from T1 drops through the gluteal cleft. Scoliosis may be structural, as illustrated, or functional. (Reprinted with permission from Bickley, L. S. [1999]. *Bates' guide to physical exam and history taking* [7th ed.]. Philadelphia: Lippincott Williams & Wilkins.)

tems. The child's general appearance, affect, and mood should be noted.

Cranial nerves II through XII are examined as follows:

- Nerve II (optic): The examination is based on the previously performed visual, optic fields, and fundoscopy tests.
- Nerves III (oculomotor), IV (trochlear), and VI (abducens): The examination is based on the previously performed ocular muscle balance test.
- Nerve V (trigeminal): The muscles of mastication are evaluated during the dental check when the child bites down to rule out malocclusion.
- Nerve VII (facial): Asymmetry and weakness of facial expressions (eg, crying and smiling) are evaluated.
- Nerve VIII (cochlea and vestibular): This is previously tested with an ideologic screen.
- Nerve IX (glossopharyngeal and vagus): This is previously examined during throat examination, with note made of palatal movement when the child says "Ah."
- Nerve XI (spinal accessory): This is previously examined when testing the strength of neck muscles during musculoskeletal examination.
- Nerve XII (hypoglossal): This is previously examined during mouth examination when tongue movements are assessed.

Coordination is observed in the waiting room and during the general examination. Tremors, tics, and other involuntary movements should be noted. Tics are common in the school-age child and are most likely to be benign, although they may be a sign of underlying pathology. Coordination is tested by having the child run the heel along the opposite shin. The child should perform rapid alternating movements by touching the thumb to successive fingers quickly. The child is asked to touch the finger to the nose. Normal variations found in young school-age children that may be signs of pathology in older school-age children are "soft signs." These include mirror movements of the opposite hand while the child performs rapid alternating movements of thumb and fingers and movements of the tongue while the child writes.

Most motor evaluation is completed through previous observation and palpation. The child's ability to walk, bend over, sit, run, and climb is evaluated. The child is asked to write, draw, and tie shoes to evaluate fine motor functioning.

Clonus at the ankles is tested; more than three beats of clonus is abnormal. Hypertonic, hypotonic, spastic, and ataxic tones are identified. Previously tested range of motion determines motor tone and strength. The fisted position with the thumb tucked under the fingers is a sign of increased tone.

Deep tendon reflexes should be elicited on the knees, brachioradialis, biceps, triceps, and Achilles' tendon. The child should lock and pull on opposite fingers to help facilitate this examination. A Babinski response should be absent.

The school-age child can cooperate in sensation detection. A nonthreatening tool is used to elicit sensation on different parts of the body.

ASSESSMENT

The well school-age child should follow the growth chart at a steady pace. A growth spurt is expected in the latter part of this period. Secondary sexual characteristics also should appear and progress sequentially by the middle to late part of the period.

The child demonstrates increasing skills and enthusiasm. Peers are becoming increasingly important, affecting feelings of competence and self-esteem and sometimes causing conflict. This is also a time of altered family dynamics, with interfamily tensions a possibility. The child now applies values learned at home to the enlarging social sphere. Most illness in this period is viral, with *Streptococcus* infections being the exception. Although this period is relatively harmonious, the child is at risk for injuries related to increasing independence and group activities like sports. Many complaints of benign body aches and pains are common; these must be differentiated from true pathology. Some children in this group will demonstrate the onset of chronic health problems like asthma, allergy, and obesity. These require intervention and education to ensure the child's eventual participation in management. Of course, school-age children are at risk for school problems with the increased physical, social, and cognitive demands placed on them at this time.

PLAN

The following are measures to plan for health promotion of the school-age child:

- Support healthy peer relationships and school adjustment.
- Support family relationships.
- Discuss healthy eating habits.
- Encourage exercise through sports and a less sedentary lifestyle.
- Discuss emerging sexual maturation, sexuality, and decision making regarding high-risk behaviors.
- Develop the child's self-management skills for health problems and chronic problems.
- Educate regarding injuries and accidents.
- Educate regarding high-risk behaviors associated with substance abuse.

SCREENING

The standard test for visual acuity in school-age children is the Snellen chart standardized at 20 ft. Children who do not recognize the letters of the alphabet can be tested with a tumbling E chart or HOTV letter chart. Visual acuity is expected to be 20/30 at 5 years of age. A two-line difference between eyes is considered a failed eye examination. Color vision should be tested at least once during the school-age years. Hearing is tested by pure tone audiometry in a sound-proof room. Vision and hearing screening should be evaluated once at 5 and again at 12 years of age (AAP, 1997).

Tuberculosis screening is done once on all children in the school-age years. Additionally, it is done whenever indicated for the child who presents with a history of exposure to tuberculosis or travel to a high-risk geographic area.

Hemoglobin and cholesterol are measured once between 5 and 12 years unless a child is high risk and requires more frequent assessment. Average hemoglobin for this age group is 12.5 g/dL. Cholesterol levels should be below 200 mg/dL; levels between 170 and 200 mg/dL should be considered borderline and followed up as needed.

● **Clinical Pearl:** A child with a high cholesterol should have a fasting lipid profile to assess cardiovascular risk and thyroid function tests because hypothyroidism can produce high cholesterol.

A urinalysis should be done once between 5 and 12 years. Blood pressure and vital signs are evaluated each year. The most common cause of an elevated blood pressure in a child is a blood pressure cuff that is too small. The second most common cause is anxiety.

ANTICIPATORY GUIDANCE

Common Questions

The following are common questions that parents of school-age children ask and that providers should be prepared to answer:

- Is my child overweight or underweight? How tall will he or she be?
- How many hours of sleep does my child need?
- Is my child's language age-appropriate?
- Is my child's activity level normal?
- Are these bruises on my child normal?
- My child fights with siblings and friends. Is this normal?
- How should I discipline my child?
- When should my child be able to read?
- In what activities should my child be involved now?
- When should I tell my child about body changes, menstruation, wet dreams, and puberty?
- Is my son's penis the normal size? Is my daughter's breast development normal?
- When and how should I warn my child about cigarettes, drugs, and sex?
- How do I introduce my date/significant other/partner?
- How do I handle my child's emerging assertiveness and rebellion?

Common Concerns

Nutrition

Nutritional requirements reflect the general steady state of physiology during this period. As children enter the school-age years, their energy requirements increase and vary based on level of activity, growth patterns, and size. On average, 5- to 7-year-olds require 90 calories/kg/d; 7- to 10-year-olds require 70 calories/kg/d; and children older than 10 years require 30 to 55 calories/kg/d.

Deficiencies of specific nutrients due to inadequate intake are relatively rare in North America. The one exception is iron deficiency. Boys' requirement for iron is less than prepubertal girls, whose bodies are preparing for menstruation. The school-age period is a time when dietary patterns and habits become set for life. Children who are spending more time away from the home assume more control over their daily intake. Their choices are influenced by their likes and dislikes, peer group, and newly found independence. The importance of appearance and body changes affects these choices. Therefore, it is important to ask questions about specific eating patterns, including any special diets and food supplements. Some children who choose special diets (ie, vegetarian) need to be counseled about certain additional vitamins and protein sources. There are different types of

vegetarian diets, so getting a detailed description of the child's diet is necessary. For example, a vegetarian diet that eliminates dairy products and eggs will generally not supply enough calcium, and children may need another source of calcium or a calcium supplement.

A scientific link between moderate sugar intake and behavior in children has yet to be made. Daily sugar intake, however, must be assessed because it contains empty calories and may predispose the child to obesity and dental caries. For this reason, sugar intake should be limited to 10% or less of daily intake to promote the consumption of nutrient-rich foods.

Fat intake recommendations for school-age children are the same as for adults. A 30% maximum of total fat calories, with less than 10% coming from saturated fats, and a 300-mg daily maximum of cholesterol continue to be the American Heart Association's recommendations. Parents should pay attention to ensuring that the child's regular diet does not drop below these guidelines. Less than a 20% daily fat intake may place the child at nutritional risk.

General health, height, weight, height–weight relationship, and hemoglobin remain the best parameters for assessing nutritional status. Fluoride supplements for dental health are recommended and can be supplied through the municipal water supply or by oral supplements.

Foods from the basic food groups need only be eaten every 2 to 3 days. These groups include dairy; meat, fish, poultry, eggs, nuts, legumes; vegetables; fruits; and cereal, rice, pasta, bread. Some helpful guidelines include two to three cups of low fat milk a day; breakfast cereals with a low sugar content; and vegetables and fruits as snacks. Children may need increased calories during growth spurts if they participate in competitive sports. Most school-age children who participate in competitive sports or intense physical activity do not need to increase any specific nutrients except water and calories to compensate for increased energy expenditure and water loss from exercise (Committee on Nutrition, AAP, 1993, and Barness, 1993).

In today's society, young school-age children are already obsessed with body image, weight, dieting, and special diets. This is a high-risk time for specific health problems related to nutrition. For example, it is often the school-age child who begins to put on excess weight, with obesity emerging as the result. In addition, eating disorder behaviors may appear. Providers need to improve parent and child awareness regarding these problems.

The following are measures to promote adequate nutrition and healthy diets:

- Eat some meals as a family; avoid eating in front of the television.
- Provide healthy choices for meals, school lunches, and snacks.
- Limit high-fat and high-sugar foods.
- Manage weight through diet *and* exercise.
- Recommend three glasses of skim milk (calcium) each day.

Sleep

It is important to establish a regular bedtime. By the age of 8, children typically sleep between 9 and 12 hours per night.

Health Promotion

The following are health-promotion measures to encourage for families of school-age children:

- Encourage physicals per the AAP guidelines and visits for health problems as necessary.
- Encourage flossing, brushing, regular dental visits, and adequate fluoride.
- Maintain a smoke-free environment.

Healthy Peer Relationships and School Adjustment

The following are measures to encourage healthy peer and school relationships for families of school-age children:

- Praise and encourage the child.
- Provide a safe after-school environment; oversee homework.
- Know the child's friends and their families.
- Teach the child how to resolve conflicts and handle anger.
- Discuss the transition to middle or high school.
- Discuss strategies for handling peer pressure.
- Encourage reading, hobbies, and talents.
- Create opportunities for peer group activities.
- Maintain open communication with teachers.

Family Relationships

The following are ways to strengthen family relationships:

- Create opportunities for family activities and responsibilities.
- Set reasonable expectations and limits.
- Teach the use of appropriate discipline to stop undesirable behaviors.
- Discuss appropriate discipline techniques (eg, loss of privileges, "grounding").
- Encourage good sibling relationships.
- Provide resources for family stress or alternative lifestyles (eg, adoption, separation/divorce, same-sex parents, interracial families, blended families).

Exercise

The following are ways for families to promote exercise:

- Encourage adequate sleep and physical activity.
- Limit television, video, and computer use.
- Discuss athletic conditioning and weight training

Sexual Maturation, Sexuality, and Decision Making Regarding High-Risk Behaviors

The following are ways for parents to handle issues related to sex:

- Teach personal hygiene and anticipated body changes.
- Use correct terms.
- Answer questions directly.
- Suggest age-appropriate books to be read together by parent and child.
- Initiate conversation regarding decision making, birth control, and safe sex.

Self-Management Skills

The following are ways for children to self-manage against health risks and chronic problems:

- Assign child-specific tasks that require age-appropriate decision making.
- Praise efforts *and* success.
- Provide literature and community support groups.

Injuries and Accidents

The following are measures to protect against injuries and accidents:

- Ensure adult supervision of activities with friends; discuss playground safety.
- Use seat belts, bike helmets, protective sports gear, and sun screen.
- Raise awareness and keep electrical tools, matches, poisons, and guns under lock and key.
- Perform tick checks where applicable.
- Teach stranger safety and the concept of "good touch/bad touch."
- Teach child how to dial 911; consider first aid and CPR classes.

High-Risk Behaviors Associated With Substance Abuse

The following are measures to educate children regarding substance abuse:

- Begin discussing dangers of tobacco, alcohol, and other drugs early.
- Encourage children to discuss what they and their friends hear or encounter in a nonthreatening manner.
- Identify and encourage intervention for the child who has begun experimenting with tobacco and drugs.

Common Conditions

During the school-age years, the following are the most common conditions encountered:

- Dental problems
- Unintentional injuries
- Allergies
- Increasing rates of homicide and suicide
- Behavior and emotional problems (eg, bullying)
- Learning problems
- Attention disorders
- Psychosomatic complaints
- Substance experimentation or abuse

COMMUNITY RESOURCES

Vast resources are available to the families of school-age children; these include churches and synagogues, schools and universities, gymnasiums, and community organizations like the YMCA, Big Brother/Big Sister, DARE, Scouts, and Little League. For children with special interests or talents, local museums and theaters often run educational programs centered on dance, drama, and music. Municipal police and fire departments also provide supervised activities for school-age children. All these resources provide role models, expanded peer groups, and opportunities for children to develop their social and physical skills. Primary care providers often act as liaisons between patient and community resources.

BIBLIOGRAPHY

Nader, P. R. (1997). School health and primary care: An idea whose time has come. *Pediatric Annals, 26,* 719–723.

Schor, E. L. (1998). Guiding the family of the school-age child. *Contemporary Pediatrics, 15,* 75–94.

REFERENCES

Algranati, P. S. (1998). Effect of developmental status on the approach to physical examination. *The Pediatric Clinics of North America, 45,* 1–22

American Academy of Pediatrics (1997). *Guidelines for health supervision III.* Elk Grove Village: Author.

Bickley, L. S., Hoekleman, R. A., & Bates, B. (1999). *Bates' guide to physical examination and history taking* (7th ed.). Philadelphia: Lippincott, Williams & Wilkins.

Goldblum, R. B. (1997). *Pediatric clinical skills.* New York: Churchill Livingstone.

Nelson, W. E. (1996). *Textbook of pediatrics.* Philadelphia: W.B. Saunders.

Healthy Growth and Development of the Adolescent

• PATRICIA A. BOLTIN, MSN, MPH, RN, CPNP

INTRODUCTION

Adolescents are human beings at crossroads. Their lives hang in the balance between childhood and adulthood. Myriad physical, psychosocial, and cognitive changes occur during adolescence. At the same time, adolescents live in a rapidly changing world that offers many challenges to their well-being. The primary care provider must appreciate the developmental changes that occur during adolescence to provide appropriate and timely advice regarding risky behaviors. The provider also must recognize and discuss the realities facing adolescents: early initiation of sexual activity; the commonness of sexually transmitted infections; the availability and addictiveness of cigarettes, drugs, and alcohol; and risks involved with motor vehicles, firearms, and other behaviors.

GROWTH AND DEVELOPMENT

Adolescence can be broken into three stages labeled early adolescence (typically ages 10–14), middle adolescence (ages 14–17), and late adolescence (ages 17–21). Physical, cognitive, and psychosocial changes define these stages. There is, of course, considerable variation, but using these stages as guidelines can aid in the approach to an adolescent patient.

Physical Development

Puberty is the term applied to the biologic processes that ultimately enable reproductive capacity. The changes of puberty can occur in as few as 2 to 3 years or may take as long as 6 to 7 years (Cronau & Brown, 1998). The physiologic changes of puberty are orchestrated by the hypothalamic-pituitary-gonadal axis. The hypothalamus releases gonadotropin-releasing hormone (GnRH) in a pulsatile fashion. GnRH stimulates the pituitary gland, nestled in the tella surca of the cranium, to release the gonadotropins: follicle-stimulating hormone and luteinizing hormone. These hormones signal the end organs, namely the ovaries, testicles, and adrenal glands, to release the hormones that foster secondary sexual characteristics. The hypothalamic-pituitary-gonadol axis is well developed at the time of birth. It is suppressed during most of early childhood, then is reactivated at the onset of puberty. The central nervous system controls the onset and progression of puberty.

Tanner, an English endocrinologist, described and outlined the usual sequence of physical changes in puberty. Most of these changes take place in early adolescence and are completed by middle adolescence. The defining sequence in girls is related to the breasts and pubic hair. In boys, the sequence is based on changes in the genitals and pubic hair. The Tanner stages, also known as sex-maturity ratings, help to predict other physical changes important to adolescents, such as the growth spurt, menarche, and spermarche. Tanner stage 1 is child-like, and Tanner stage 5 is adult-like.

In the female, the physical change that marks progression from Tanner stage 1 to stage 2 is the development of the breast bud or thelarche, which occurs on average at age 11. The growth spurt, defined by peak height velocity, occurs in girls between Tanner stages 2 and 3. Peak height velocity is recognized with the help of a growth chart. Menarche, or the beginning of menstruation, generally begins during Tanner stage 4 to 5. Thus, the clinician can reassure a 15-year-old girl at Tanner stage 3 who has not yet experienced menarche that there is no need for alarm.

In the male, the physical change heralding the onset of puberty is growth of the testicle. The immature testicle is less than 4 mL in volume, whereas the fully mature adult testis reaches a volume of approximately 20 to 25 mL. Testicle growth begins on average at age 12. The growth spurt in boys occurs between Tanner stages 3 and 4. Spermarche, or the first release of spermatozoa, does not occur before Tanner stage 3. Facial hair in males occurs only after Tanner stage 4 for pubic hair.

Cognitive Development

Cognitive development in the adolescent proceeds in halting steps. Jean Piaget had a strong influence on our understanding of adolescent thought processes. He used the terms concrete operational thinking and formal operational thinking to describe the transitions made in cognitive development from childhood to adolescence. Early to middle adolescents exhibit concrete thinking. Such thinking is oriented in the present. Concrete thinkers cannot think abstractly and have difficulty understanding the consequences of their behaviors. Formal operational thinking uses deductions, hypotheses, rules, and logic to solve problems. Middle to late adolescents are expected to exhibit operational thinking. Full abstract thought allows an individual to weigh the pros and cons of actions and to anticipate the future.

● **Clinical Pearl:** In times of stress, such as when dealing with a sexually transmitted infection (STI), the adolescent may regress in cognitive capacity. The safest course of action for the provider at such times is to be as concrete with an older adolescent as he or she would be with a younger one (Cronau & Brown, 1998).

Psychosocial Development

Sigmund Freud's general theory of psychosocial development provided Anna Freud, his daughter, with the framework upon which she built her theory of adolescent ego development. Anna Freud described puberty as the trigger for a sudden surge of strong erotic and aggressive impulses; this is the foundation for the traditional psychoanalytic conception of adolescence as one of stress and tumult. Other studies of adolescent development have found less tumultuousness and anxiety in the teenage years.

Erik Erikson described the adolescent struggle as identity formation versus identity diffusion. Identity formation describes the adolescent's attempts to answer the question "Who am I?" Identity diffusion is defined by an inadequate personal identity. Erikson's interpretation of adolescent psychosocial development sheds light on the teenage years as a necessary time of experimentation with alternative roles and value systems.

The three stages of adolescence (early, middle, and late) have characteristic findings in terms of psychosocial development. Early adolescents struggle to begin to separate from their parents. They are conflicted in their desire for separation, swaying between demands for independence and requests for their parents' assistance. In this struggle for independence, early adolescence is similar to toddlerhood. Early adolescents like to spend time alone. They are preoccupied with their rapidly changing bodies. A pimple may seem disastrous to the early adolescent, who feels "on-stage" and believes others to be just as preoccupied with his or her body. Early adolescents often spend time only with friends of the same sex. A common finding at school dances and parties is groups of boys and girls standing at opposite ends of the room.

Middle adolescents have begun to adjust to their external appearance. The peer group assumes importance as the adolescent further distinguishes the self from parents. Middle adolescents spend more time with their peers. They often dress and talk in ways that show the strong influence of the peer group. Conflicts with authority figures may occur. Dating can take place in groups, and romantic relationships have relatively short lives.

Late adolescents no longer have as strong a need for the peer group. They begin to form more adult-like relationships. They have adjusted to their body appearance and are less concerned about their peers' opinions regarding clothing and activities. This is a time when the adolescent assumes more adult responsibilities and begins working toward vocational goals.

▲ **Clinical Warning:** Risk-taking behavior tends to increase as adolescents get older.

HISTORY AND PHYSICAL EXAMINATION

Table 12-1 provides critical foci for the history, physical examination, and health promotion or disease prevention of the adolescent.

History

Adolescent history taking can involve the adolescent alone or together with parents. Parents should feel welcome in the clinical setting, but it should be clear to all that the adolescent is the priority person. The clinician can reinforce this idea from the outset by introducing oneself first to the adolescent and addressing most questions to him or her. If parents are present, all should meet together at the beginning of the adolescent history.

Confidentiality

At this time, the provider should explain the concept of confidentiality to the adolescent and caregiver, who need to understand that questions regarding high-risk behaviors, such as sexual activity, can be discussed by the patient and clinician in confidence. Communicating this concept clearly is important for all so that the adolescent will be willing to share information. Most adolescents will not share sensitive information unless they are assured that such information is held in strictest confidence (Ehrman & Matson, 1998). Adolescents may better understand the terms "privacy" or "just between you and me" than the word "confidentiality" (Ginsburg, Menapace, & Slap, 1997). The provider must inform the adolescent and parents that the provider is obligated to inform the parents if the adolescent tells the provider of an intention to hurt himself or herself or others. The provider may find it helpful to have written pamphlets that describe the concept of confidentiality available in the waiting room.

The parent may be asked to provide information on family medical history and parts of the teen's past medical history, of which the adolescent might not be aware. Parents also should be asked about any concerns they have regarding the adolescent's health. The clinician can address the remainder of the history taking directly to the adolescent. Some health care settings use a written questionnaire to assess risk behaviors in adolescent patients. All questionnaires should be marked as confidential; ideally, a quiet, private area away from parents should be available for the adolescent to complete the form.

TABLE 12–1.   CRITICAL FOCI: HISTORY, PHYSICAL EXAMINATION, AND HEALTH PROMOTION DURING ADOLESCENCE

Age	History	Physical Examination	Health Promotion and Disease Prevention
10–14	Concrete thinking	Tanner stage evaluation, scoliosis screen	Body changes, self-breast examinations, testicular self-examinations, abstinence, safer sex, pregnancy prevention, peer group influence, substance use prevention, bike safety, booster immunizations
14–17	Concrete thinking–formal operational thought	Tanner stage evaluation, scoliosis screen	Car safety, abstinence, safer sex, breast self-examinations, testicular self-examinations, pregnancy prevention, substance use
17–21	Formal operational thought	Growth generally complete	Car safety, safer sex, breast self-examinations, testicular self-examinations, pregnancy prevention, substance use, vocational goals

Parents who have difficulty separating from their offspring during the health visit may need to be reminded that individuation is a goal of adolescence. The health care visit is an opportunity for the teenager to practice independent interactions with an adult, whose goal is to guide the teen toward a healthy lifestyle. Most parents understand the teenager's need for privacy and appreciate the chance for the adolescent to discuss confidential health care issues with another adult.

Laws regarding minors' rights to confidentiality undergo continual modification. Medical conditions that may be treated without parental consent, depending on state law, include sexually transmitted diseases, human immunodeficiency virus (HIV) and acquired immunodeficiency syndrome (AIDS), contraception, pregnancy, abortion, sterilization, substance abuse, and mental health. Providers should become familiar with the statutes of their own state regarding confidential services for minors. One resource is a publication entitled State Minor Consent Statutes: A Summary, prepared by the National Center for Youth Law (English & Matthews, 1995).

The relationship between confidentiality and payment of services is an important consideration. A parent's discovery of an independent, confidential visit by means of a bill or insurance statement places both teenager and provider in very awkward positions. It may be impossible for the provider to promise full confidentiality unless services are provided for free or the adolescent can pay for the services. Referrals may be necessary if a payment issue precludes the clinician from providing confidential care. The clinician should be aware of area resources (such as federally funded family planning clinics) that base sliding fee scales on the adolescent's own income.

Review of Systems

The review of systems (ROS) can be asked in a head-to-toe manner. Early adolescents, who are very attuned to the changes occurring in their bodies, often provide detailed and seemingly superfluous answers to ROS questions. Patience and attentive listening help the adolescent feel that the provider cares about what is happening to the teen. Sometimes questioning the early adolescent can be improved by using explanatory adverbs and adjectives. Instead of asking the 13-year-old if he or she has stomach trouble, the provider might ask more specifically: "Do you get frequent stomach aches that bother you a lot?"

The female adolescent's ROS should include questions related to menstruation: age at menarche; frequency, length, and regularity of periods; and physical discomfort related to menstruation. An adolescent who reports dysmennorhea should be questioned as to what remedies she has tried, which remedies are beneficial, and if she misses school due to menstrual discomfort.

The ROS should include a general diet history and a review of sleep patterns. Growth requires energy and an adequate store of nutrients, yet adolescence is a time when diets are often irregular and loaded with "fast-foods" that have limited nutritional value. Screening for anorexia nervosa and bulimia nervosa also should occur at this time. The clinician should ask adolescents if they are happy with their body weight and if they have recently tried to lose weight. Females are at greater risk for eating disorders; however, some male athletes, such as wrestlers, may use drastic weight loss techniques to meet weight goals for their sport.

Adolescents also need to be screened for psychosocial problems in a standardized format. Studies have found such screening to be conducted sporadically for adolescent patients, with providers often avoiding emotionally sensitive issues (Elster, 1998). To address neglected areas, several different organizations have established guidelines for the adolescent visit. These include "Guide to Clinical Preventive Services" by the United States Preventive Services Task Force; "Guidelines for Adolescent Preventive Services" by the American Medical Association; "Age Charts for Periodic Health Examinations" by the American Academy of Family Physicians; "Bright Futures (BF): Guidelines for Health Care Supervision of Infants, Children, and Adolescents" by the Maternal and Child Health Bureau of the Health Resources and Service Administration; and "Recommendations for Pediatric Preventive Health Care" by the American Academy of Pediatrics. All these guidelines recommend screening regarding eating disorders, sexual activity, alcohol and other drug use, tobacco use, abuse, school performance, depression, and risk of suicide (Elster & Levenberg, 1997).

One method of organizing the adolescent interview to capture psychosocial data is to use the acronym HEADSSS (Reif & Elster, 1998). This is an adaptation of an acronym previously presented by Goldenring and Cohen (1988). The HEADSSS questionnaire encompasses all areas of screening recommended by the above organizations. It proceeds from less personal to more personal questions. Because many questions may be embarrassing to adolescents, it is often helpful to preface questions with a statement such as, "I know that some of these questions may be embarrassing, but I need to ask them to learn about your health." Another way to introduce topics that are possibly threatening to the adolescent is by first asking the adolescent about the habits of peers. For example, when asking about substance use, the provider may start by stating, "A lot of teenagers experiment with drinking alcohol. Do any of your friends drink beer, wine, or other types of liquor?" After talking about friends' habits, the adolescent may then feel more comfortable talking about himself or herself. The clinician should alter questions as necessary to obtain comfortably an accurate picture of how the adolescent is functioning within each of the psychosocial spheres designated by HEADSSS. Sample questions that could be used under each of the headings are as follows:

- H—Home and family: Who lives at home? Is anyone ill? How do you get along with your family members? Are any guns in your home?
- E—Education and school: Do you like school? What grade are you in? How were your grades on your last report card? How many days have you been absent so far this year? What are your plans after you finish high school?
- A—Activities and associates: What things do you do on an average day after school? Do you participate in any sports? Have you ever been injured playing sports? Do you work? How many hours a week do you work? Do you drive? Do you wear your seat belt in the car? Do you have close friends that you hang out with?
- D—Drugs, alcohol, and cigarettes: Do your friends or family members smoke? Some teenagers experiment with trying out different types of drugs. Have you tried smoking pot? Have you used inhalants, such as paint thinners and aerosol cans of whipped cream? Have you used crack or any other drug that could make you feel "high"? Have you tried using any kinds of drugs or dietary supplements to improve sports performance?

- S—Sexuality and sexual activity: Do you have a girl-friend or a boyfriend? Have you ever had sex with a girl, boy, or either? Has anyone ever forced you to have sex? How old were you the first time that you had sex? How many partners have you had in the last 6 months? Do you use condoms always, sometimes, or never? Have you ever had a sexually transmitted disease?
- S—Suicide and depression: Have you ever tried to hurt yourself? Do you often feel very sad? What do you do when you feel sad or very angry? Do you have someone that you can talk to when you are feeling down? A patient who reports any suicidal ideation needs to be asked specifics: Have you thought about how you would kill yourself? How easily could you accomplish this plan? Are you thinking about killing yourself in the near future? (Direct questions do not precipitate suicidal action and may allow the provider to intervene and save the life of a depressed adolescent.)
- S—Safety, violence, and abuse: Do you feel safe where you live? Have you ever had a relationship with someone who tried to hurt you? Have you ever been abused?

The provider must assess the developmental and social experience levels of the adolescent and gear questions to specific needs. For example, a 13-year-old who giggles, looks embarrassed, and responds negatively when asked about ever having dated probably will not need an in-depth sexual assessment that focuses on condom use and number of sexual partners in the last 6 months. The adolescent's negative response would, however, leave an opening for the clinician to assess the young adolescent's knowledge of pregnancy, to encourage abstinence, and to discuss briefly STIs and their prevention.

Important communication skills for providers to develop are the nonverbal techniques of recognizing and expressing emotions and the ability to express verbally sensitivity to the adolescent's feelings. Additionally, bidirectional communication, direct questions about psychosocial issues, and attentive listening to the patient's responses improve the diagnosis and management of health problems and the patient's satisfaction (Coupey, 1997).

Physical Examination

Approach to Examination

The adolescent physical examination can be approached in a head-to-toe manner with the exception of the genital examination, which is best left for last. Necessary tools for a complete examination include an ophthalmoscope, otoscope, blood-pressure cuff, and stethoscope. Other tools that may be needed include a scoliometer, magnifying glass, speculum, equipment for acquiring lab specimens, and a microscope. The examination is most easily accomplished with the adolescent undressed and wearing a gown. Some adolescents are very uncomfortable disrobing all at once. The clinician may allow the adolescent to stay dressed, removing one piece of clothing at a time as necessary for the examination to proceed.

Adolescents are concerned about disease transmission within the context of a physical examination. When ninth-grade students were interviewed concerning items that affected their decision to seek health care, the top two concerns were hand washing and the use of clean instruments. Students said that they wanted to see providers wash their hands and instruments removed from packaging (Ginsberg et al., 1997).

Sequence

Skin

The adolescent's skin should be carefully examined for bruises, tattoos, rashes, and lesions. Acne lesions are common concerns. Acne is commonly caused by the shift in hormones that occurs at puberty but also may be exacerbated by stress (Johnston & Saenz, 1997). The skin should be observed for open and closed comedones, cysts, and degree of oiliness.

Eyes

The eye examination should include assessment of eye movement and fundoscopy. Pupillary dilatation or constriction should not be ignored because either could indicate drug use. The provider should look for signs of conjunctivitis and possibly conduct a vision screen.

Ears, Nose, and Throat

The ear examination involves checking the tympanic membranes for appearance and movement. An auditory screen may be conducted. For the nose, the provider should look for a deviated septum, allergic rhinitis, or nasal irritation that could indicate a drug-sniffing habit. The clinician should check for dental caries, pharyngeal lesions, malformations of the uvula, and normal opening of the jaw.

Nodes

A thorough examination of nodes, including the cervical, occipital, supraclavicular, axillary, epitrochlear, and inguinal, is conducted. Any enlargement of supraclavicular nodes that would require a chest x-ray to rule out the possibility of infection or malignancy should be noted.

Thyroid

The thyroid should be observed for symmetry. It should be palpated while the adolescent swallows to check for nodules or masses.

Chest

Auscultation of all areas is necessary for wheezing, crackles, and proper aeration. Female patients need a breast examination, which involves palpation of both breasts in either a spiral or bicycle-spoke fashion. Teaching regarding breast self-examinations can be carried out at the same time as the breast examination (Fig. 12-1).

The male adolescent may exhibit firmness under the areola. Transient pubertal gynecomastia occurs in 65% to 70% of

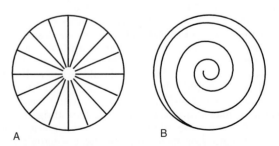

Figure 12–1 ■ Methods of performing a breast examination. **(A)** Bicycle spoke pattern. **(B)** Spiral pattern.

boys during Tanner stages 2 to 3, peaking around age 14. It may occur on one or both sides and generally resolves within 2 years. The most common type consists of a small, firm, tender, discoid subareolar mass measuring 2 to 3 cm in diameter (Hofmann & Greydanus, 1997). Idiopathic gynecomastia may be linked to transient imbalances in endogenous production of estrogen and testosterone with end-organ sensitivity. Organic causes that have been associated with gynecomastia include prescription drugs, such as tricyclic antidepressants and insulin; diseases, such as leukemia and hemophilia; and illicit drugs, such as marijuana and heroin (Hofmann & Greydanus, 1997).

Cardiac

The heart is examined for clicks, rubs, or murmurs. Both the femoral and radial pulses should be palpated.

Abdomen

The abdomen should be palpated for masses and signs of hepatosplenomegaly. A hard linear mass in the left lower quadrant may indicate constipation. Inguinal nodes and femoral pulses can easily be evaluated at this time.

Musculoskeletal System

The joints should be examined for range of motion. Extremities should exhibit equal strength, and musculature should exhibit bilateral symmetry. The back should be examined for signs of scoliosis. This is done by examining the adolescent's back as the teen leans forward with the knees straight, arms dangling, and palms of the hands facing each other. A scoliometer can be used to gauge roughly the degree of back curvature. This device looks like a wood-worker's level. The scoliometer should be placed over the adolescent's spine when the adolescent is bending forward. A curve of less than 7 degrees indicates that the actual curve is most likely less than 20 degrees and may not warrant radiographic evaluation (Skaggs & Bassett, 1996). Curves of 7 degrees or greater should be followed up radiologically with a scoliosis series. Curves that are progressive or are greater than 20 degrees measured by x-ray should be referred to an orthopedic surgeon for further evaluation.

Female Genitourinary System

All sexually active adolescent females or adolescents older than 18 should have a yearly pelvic examination that includes a Pap smear. Yearly or 6 month screening for STIs should be done for all sexually active adolescents. Non-sexually active, young adolescents, who are menstruating normally, generally just need to be examined for Tanner staging. The perineal area should be examined for lesions and discharge. The vaginal vault and cervix should be observed for lesions and type of discharge after insertion of the speculum. The estrogenized vaginal mucosa of the pubertal girl is dull, pink, moist, and thick, as opposed to the thin, red vaginal mucosa of the prepubertal girl. The external os usually is dark pink. A darker, erythematous area, indicating the squamous columnar junction, may surround the os. This condition, called cervical erosion or ectopy, is normal in adolescents.

The Pap smear generally consists of separate specimens obtained from the external cervix and the endocervix. The external cervix specimen for the Pap smear is obtained first. Testing for STIs should be done from the endocervix. Optimal sequencing for examining the cervix is Pap smear, gon-

orrhea testing, and *Chlamydia* testing (Emans, Laufer, & Goldstein, 1998). A sample of vaginal discharge for a wet preparation ("wet prep") and pH determination also can be obtained while the speculum is in place. Syphillis is detected by serum testing. As previously stated, serum testing for HIV should be offered to any sexually active adolescent.

● **Clinical Pearl:** Lubricant should not be used prior to endocervical testing.

After removal of the speculum, a bimanual examination should be performed. The examiner inserts one or two fingers into the vaginal vault and places the other hand onto the abdomen to palpate the uterus and adnexa. The cervix should be gently moved side to side to check for cervical motion tenderness.

Microscopic examination of the wet prep should be done using separate slides, with a drop of saline on one slide, and a drop of 10% KOH on the other. The saline slide may reveal clue cells indicating bacterial vaginosis or live trichomonads. The KOH slide may show the budding pseudohyphae from an infection with *Candida*. The KOH slide also may reveal a fishy odor. This is referred to as the "whiff" test that is often positive with bacterial vaginosis (Fig. 12-2).

Male Genitourinary System

The adolescent male should be examined for Tanner staging. The testicles should be palpated to make sure that there are two, with no testicular masses. The adolescent male can be taught at this time about the importance of regular testicular self-examination. The shaft of the penis should be examined for lesions. The urethral opening should be examined for hypospadias and lesions. The foreskin, if present, should be easily retractible. The clinician should check for inguinal her-

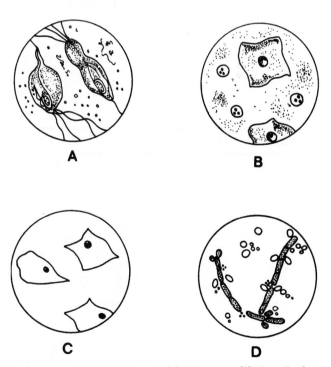

Figure 12–2 ■ Fresh vaginal smears. **(A)** *Trichomonas.* **(B)** Clue cells of bacterial vaginosis. **(C)** Leukorrhea. **(D)** *Candida.* A, B, and C are saline preparations; D is a KOH preparation. (Reprinted with permission of Emans, S. J., Laufer, M. R., & Goldstein, D. P. [eds.] [1998]. *Pediatric and adolescent gynecology* [4th ed.]. [p. 38]. Philadelphia: Lippincott Williams & Wilkins.]

nias by palpating the inguinal area while the patient turns his head to the side to cough. Sexually active males, if symptomatic, may be screened for STIs using a urethral swab. Alternatively, a urine test can now be used to screen for *Chlamydia* and gonorrhea. Serum testing can be performed for syphillis. HIV testing should be offered to all sexually active adolescents. Please refer to Chapter 41 for further discussion of STIs.

ASSESSMENT

The assessment of the adolescent should consider physical and psychosocial findings. Comments should be made in the assessment regarding positive findings of risk behaviors, such as smoking, frequent school absences, and unprotected sex. Specific physical findings that require treatment or follow-up need to be delineated. A comment also should be made regarding the adolescent's growth and development. A well teen with normal growth and development is an adolescent who is physically healthy, exhibits normal weight for height, and is dealing adequately with the developmental tasks of adolescence.

PLAN

Counseling and guidance of the adolescent must take into account developmental considerations. When teaching or counseling adolescents, providers should remember that teens are acutely self-conscious, have a short-term perspective, and may have a limited ability to understand abstract concepts (Coupey, 1997). Recommended health guidance for adolescents includes physical development; diet; exercise; tobacco, drug, and alcohol use; and pregnancy and injury prevention.

All adolescents at risk for HIV infection, including those who have had unprotected sex or admit to having used intravenous (IV) drugs, should be offered confidential HIV screening that includes pretest counseling. Pretest counseling is provided to ensure that the adolescent understands the difference between HIV and AIDS and the ramifications of a positive HIV test. Testing should be deferred in adolescents who report that they would harm themselves or others if their tests for HIV came back positive. Such teens should receive further psychological evaluation before HIV tests are performed (Sucich, 1999).

Immunizations should be updated as needed according to schedule (Table 12-2) (Committee on Infectious Diseases, 1997). Please refer to Chapter 13 for additional information.

Studies show that the estimated prevalence of mental health disorders in youths ranges from 14% to 25% (Stiffman, Chen, Elze, Dore, & Cheng, 1997). Despite the obvious need for adolescent mental health services, only a small proportion of youths receive needed care. This may be due partly to a lack of active seeking by teens or their families (Stiffman et al., 1997). Ideally, the clinician should have an established relationship with a child and adolescent clinical nurse specialist, social worker, or psychologist who is comfortable working with teenagers. The availability of one of these professionals during sessions when adolescent care is provided can assist in meeting significant psychosocial needs as they arise.

SCREENING

The following are screening recommendations for adolescents:

- Cholesterol screening is recommended if the adolescent has a positive family history for early cardiovascular disease or hyperlipidemia (Leverberg & Elser, 1995).
- Tuberculosis screening is recommended for adolescents at high risk (eg, adolescents recently immigrating from an endemic country or those living in homeless shelters). Otherwise, screening should be done every 5 years or more frequently if recommended by the local Department of Health.
- A hemoglobin or hematocrit level is an inexpensive way to assess an adolescent's physical and nutritional well-being. Interpretations of this screening test must consider the adolescent's age and sex.

TABLE 12–2.   IMMUNIZATION SCHEDULE FOR ADOLESCENTS

Td	Age 11–15 y or every 5 y for a puncture wound or other tetanus-prone injury.
MMR	A second MMR should be administered if the adolescent does not already have a history of two MMRs.
Hepatitis B	All adolescents should be offered the hepatitis B vaccine series. Hepatitis B is the only STI that currently can be prevented with a vaccine.
Varicella	Vaccine should be offered to all adolescents if they have not been vaccinated and do not have a reliable history of chickenpox. Adolescents younger than 13 y need a single dose. Adolescents older than 13 y need two doses separated by 4–8 wk.
Influenza	All adolescents with chronic illnesses, including asthma, cardiovascular disease, renal dysfunction, diabetes mellitus, hemoglobinopathy, or immunosuppression; adolescents residing in chronic care facilities; or receiving long-term aspirin therapy should be offered the influenza vaccine between September and December each year.
Pneumococcal	Adolescents who should be vaccinated include those who have anatomic or functional asplenia (including sickle cell disease), nephrotic syndrome, cerebrospinal fluid leaks, or conditions associated with immunosuppression, (including HIV).
Hepatitis A (HAV)	Administer to unvaccinated adolescents who plan to travel or work in a country that has a high endemicity of HAV infection, have chronic liver disease, are administered clotting factors, use illegal drugs, or are males who have sex with males.
Meningococcal	Vaccine should be administered to U.S. Military recruits, travelers to endemic countries, asplenic teenagers, and adolescents with terminal complement component deficiencies. The vaccine should be considered for college freshman, especially those who will be living in dormitories.

- Hepatitis B screening (surface antigen and antibody) should be offered to homosexual males and IV drug users if they have not received adequate immunization.
- All adolescents should be screened annually for hypertension.

ANTICIPATORY GUIDANCE

The following are some current statistics on adolescent behavior that have been compiled by the National Adolescent Health Information Center at the University of California, San Francisco:

- Twenty one percent of teenagers smoke their first cigarette by grade 6. An additional 22% do so by grade 8.
- By eighth grade, 22% of teenagers have drunk alcohol. By ninth grade, an additional 24% have had alcohol. By 10th grade another 19% have begun to use alcohol.
- Twenty percent of teenagers first experience getting drunk by grade 9. An additional 16% do so in grade 10 and another 12% by grade 11.
- Studies show that 40% of eighth graders and 66% of 12th graders report having had sexual intercourse (Lappa & Moscicki, 1997). There is an approximately 15% incremental increase per year in the number of adolescents who become sexually active. By age 19, more than 63% of females and 86% of males are sexually active.

Common Questions and Concerns

Parents may have questions regarding the adolescent's behavior or physical health. Care must be taken to ensure that the adolescent's needs remain the focus of the visit; however, parents must also feel welcome and appreciated. A wrap-up session with the parent, adolescent, and provider allows all participants to work as a team. Permission for immunizations, options for medical treatment, and any needs for referrals are items that may demand parental input. If the adolescent wishes, psychosocial issues, such as birth control or sexuality, can be discussed at this time. The presence of an objective third party like the provider sometimes can ease the trepidation adolescents and parents experience when discussing delicate issues.

If the parents want to speak to the provider alone, the provider should first assure the adolescent that he or she will not disclose any confidential issues discussed during the interview unless the teen would like the clinician to do so. Exceptions to this rule are disclosures that involve imminent harm to the teen or other (eg, an admission of suicidal ideation).

Parents may need reassurance regarding some of the seemingly outrageous behaviors and habits of their young son or daughter. The normalcy of an adolescent's struggle for individuation and independence may need to be clarified for parents. Adolescents need firm, fair, and explicit limits, but they should be involved in the limit-setting process as much as possible.

Neinstein (1984) has offered five suggestions that can improve parental–teen communication. These can be reviewed with parents who are struggling to relate to their teenage son or daughter:

- Empathize with the adolescent.
- Stress the adolescent's positive attributes.
- Deliver clear messages.

- Respect the adolescent's privacy.
- Involve the adolescent in the resolution of family conflicts.

Sex

The provider needs to provide counseling about sex that is relative to the adolescent's behaviors. Abstinence should be praised in non-sexually active teens. The clinician can provide pamphlets that encourage abstinence. Reasons to continue abstinence, including the risk of STIs and pregnancy, can be discussed.

Reality dictates that if an adolescent is already sexually active, he or she is likely to continue. One out of four adolescents report having four or more partners (Eng & Butler, 1997). Each year, approximately 3 million adolescents contract an STI, and 1 million teens become pregnant (Ryan & Futterman, 1997). Sexually active adolescents need tools to make sex safer, including discussion of STIs, the realities of parenting, condom usage, and birth control.

Approximately 1% to 2% of high school students view themselves as mostly or completely homosexual, while more than 10% are unsure of their sexual orientation (Brown & Cromer, 1997). Gay and lesbian youths are at increased risk for low self-esteem, depression, and suicide as they struggle to integrate a positive adult identity despite persistent negative stereotypes. Supportive relationships with peers and adults and the development of positive coping skills promote successful adapatation (Ryan & Futterman, 1997). The clinician should try to be objective when discussing sexuality with adolescents. Sexually active teens should be asked if they have had sex with males, females, or both. Such an approach demonstrates the provider's willingness to discuss homosexuality as a normal variation of sexual experience.

Pregnancy Prevention

Each year 1 million teens become pregnant (Ryan & Futterman, 1997). Birth control should be discussed with any adolescent who is sexually active or may become so. Methods of birth control, their benefits, and risks need to be described to the adolescent:

- Intrauterine devices (These are not commonly used in adolescents due to the increased risk of pelvic inflammatory disease [PID].)
- Diaphragm
- Spermacides
- Male and female condoms
- Oral contraceptive pills
- Depot medroxyprogesterone acetate (DMPA; Depo-Provera)
- Abstinence

Oral contraceptive pills and Depo-Provera are efficacious forms of birth control for many sexually active teenage girls. The adolescent provider needs to try to decrease external barriers to maintaining effective contraception, including cost, inadequate knowledge about methods, location and hours of adolescent services, and concerns about confidentiality (Brown & Cromer, 1997).

Tobacco Use

Tobacco use begins primarily during childhood and adolescence (Epps, Manley, & Glynn, 1995). A nationwide survey by the Centers for Disease Control and Prevention found that more than one third (36.4%) of students in the United States had smoked cigarettes more than once in the preceding month and that one fourth of the students had smoked a whole cigarette before age 13 (Kann et al., 1998). More than 9% of students reported the use of chewing tobacco or snuff. Adolescents need to be informed of the addictiveness and negative physical effects of tobacco use. Their providers can play a major role in decreasing tobacco use by discouraging its onset.

Substance Abuse

The following are some statistics regarding teens and substance abuse in the United States:

- Approximately 50% of students surveyed in 1997 reported at least one drink of alcohol within the last 30 days. One third of all students reported having had five or more drinks on at least one day during the preceding month (Kann et al., 1998).
- Forty seven percent of students had used marijuana at least once (Kann et al., 1998).
- Eight percent of students reported having used some form of cocaine, and 2% of students had injected illegal drugs during their lifetime (Kann et al., 1998).
- In a 1998 study by the University of Michigan, 20% of eighth graders reported having used an inhalant. Chemicals used as inhalants are found in hundreds of everyday products, from paint thinners and cleaning fluids to marking pens and aerosol cans of whipped cream (Janofsky, 1999).

Preventive counseling should address the real-life consequences of substance abuse, including drastic mandatory jail sentencing for use or possession of illegal substances.

Accidents and Injuries

In the United States, 73% of all deaths in individuals aged 10 to 24 years result from only four causes: motor vehicle incidents, other unintentional injuries, homicide, and suicide (Kann et al. 1998). Use of seat belts, not driving while intoxicated, gun safety, and use of bicycle helmets are preventive measures that merit discussion during the well-adolescent visit. Chapters 25 and 26 provide in-depth treatment of some of these issues.

Common Conditions

In this section, some of the more common adolescent medical conditions are discussed briefly. These include acne, dysmenorrhea, Osgood-Schlatter disease, mononucleosis, psychosomatic illness, STIs, and eating disorders.

Acne

Acne usually begins 1 or 2 years before puberty starts as a result of androgenic stimulation of the sebaceous glands. The blackhead, or open comedone, is more easily managed, because the contents of open comedones can easily escape, and inflammation does not occur. The whitehead, or closed comedone, is responsible for ongoing problems. The closed comedone does not allow for sebum to escape. The result is inflammatory changes that can include inflamed papules, pustules, and cysts. The bacterium *Propionibacterium acnes* acts to intensify the skin's inflammatory reactions. Therapy for acne depends on the type of lesions that are encountered. The severity of acne is graded from grade I to grade IV. Further information on the management of acne can be found in Chapter 58.

Dysmenorrhea

Dysmenorrhea is a frequent problem in adolescent girls after they have begun to ovulate. Ovulation typically starts approximately 24 months after menarche (Emans et al., 1998, p. 129). Primary dysmenorrhea refers to pain associated with menstrual flow that has no organic cause. Secondary dysmenorrhea is associated with organic disease, such as ovarian cysts, adhesions, or PID. Most cases of dysmenorrhea in adolescents are primary. A pelvic examination can rule out endometriosis or cervical abnormalities. A complete blood count (CBC) and erythrocyte sedimentation rate (ESR) can rule out PID. Cervical cultures and a pregnancy test also should be performed in the sexually active adolescent to rule out STIs and ectopic pregnancy. Absence of positive findings on pelvic examination, negative laboratory tests, and appropriate history indicate primary dysmenorrhea. Treatment consists of nonsteroidal anti-inflammatory agents or oral contraceptives.

Osgood-Schlatter Disease

Osgood-Schlatter disease is pain and enlargement over the tibial tubercle. Forceful and repetitive contractions of the quadriceps (such as those required in sprinting and jumping) transmit forces through the patellar tendon to the tibial tubercle. An ossification center over the proximal tibia is at risk for avulsion as a result of these stresses. Osgood-Schlatter disease typically presents during the growth spurt with an insidious onset of tenderness over the tibial tubercle. Treatment is symptomatic and consists of rest, stretching, and application of ice to the knee and ingestion of nonsteroidal anti-inflammatory agents. Refer to Chapter 44 for further discussion of Osgood-Schlatter disease and its management.

Mononucleosis

Infectious mononucleosis is commonly seen in adolescents. It is caused by the Epstein-Barr virus and is characterized by malaise, fever, sore throat, adenopathy, splenomegaly, headache, and nausea. Diagnosis is made by obtaining Epstein-Barr virus titers or by means of a Monospot test. A CBC will reveal lymphocytosis and the atypical monocytosis. Treatment consists of rest, analgesics (such as acetaminophen or ibuprofen), and avoidance of contact sports, especially in the presence of splenomegaly. Refer to Chapter 30 for more detail on the diagnosis and management of mononucleosis.

Psychosomatic Illness

Professionals who provide health care to adolescents will frequently encounter patients whose symptoms cannot be adequately explained by an organic cause. Stress can be defined as a demand for adaptation and coping, usually in response to life changes. Substantial evidence has linked stress to somatic symptoms in adolescents. Common psychosomatic symptoms include recurrent abdominal pain, headaches, chest pain, musculoskeletal pain, chronic fatigue, and other nonspecific symptoms, such as dizziness, hyperventilation, and syncope (Greene & Walker, 1997). Organic causes for these symptoms must be eliminated by a thorough history and physical examination and possibly laboratory testing.

Treatment consists of analgesics, antispasmodics, and dietary changes. The adolescent's pain should be acknowledged as real. The clinician should discuss the correlation between stress and physical symptoms and methods of stress reduction. A social worker may be of assistance in helping the adolescent to cope with the stressors in his or her life and with the physical symptoms.

Sexually Transmitted Infections

The reality of the existence of STIs and their possible negative effects need to be described to the adolescent. Abstinence or condom use needs to be encouraged as appropriate. Correct condom usage should be described. The female adolescent may need coaching about insisting on condom use. The following is an overview of some, but not all, of the STIs that can be encountered in the adolescent population. Comprehensive STI information is presented in Chapter 41.

- The most common STI is human papillomavirus (HPV). All sexually active adolescent females should have yearly Pap smears that test for cervical HPV. Condyloma acuminata and papular warts are external genital warts associated with HPV. Condyloma acuminata are typically soft and fleshy. Application of acetic acid can highlight genital warts by turning the lesions white. Most external HPV lesions are associated with benign HPV types, and many will spontaneously regress. Possible treatments for external genital warts include application of topical solutions and cryotherapy. Cervical HPV is associated with cervical cancer. All females with abnormal Pap smears need to be followed with repeat Pap smears and may need referral for colposcopy, depending on the grade of the lesion.
- *Chlamydia trachomatis* is considered the most common bacterial STI in the United States. *C. trachomatis* may cause urethritis in males, cervicitis in females, and proctitis. Infections may be asymptomatic in both sexes. Testing may be done with a urethral swab for males and a cervical swab for females. Urine testing for *C. trachomatis* using amplification techniques also is available but is costly. Symptomatic adolescents should be treated empirically, though testing should still be performed.
- *Neisseria gonorrhoeae* also is an important STI because of its high incidence. Clinical manifestations are similar to those for *C. trachomatis*, and testing is done at the same body sites. Urine testing for *N. gonorrhoeae* also is available but is costly.
- Herpes simplex virus (HSV) may cause urethritis. It often is associated with the presence of painful ulcers or blisters. In the United States, HSV-2 most commonly causes genital ulcers in adolescents. In the primary episode, herpes lesions can be extensive; systemic symptoms, including malaise and myalgia, occur in about half of patients. The herpes virus lays dormant in the sensory neurons of the involved area and is subject to reactivation. In recurrent episodes, lesions are usually smaller in size and number, and systemic symptoms are less frequent. Recurrent and primary herpes tend to be more severe in females.
- Syphilis is caused by the organism *Treponema pallidum*. Primary syphilis consists of painless papules or indurated ulcers called chancres that occur on the external genitalia, cervix, mouth, anus, lips, face, breast, and fingers. Nonpainful regional lymphadenopathy accompanies the lesion. Secondary syphilis begins on average about 3 weeks after the chancre develops. Symptoms consist of flulike discomforts, generalized lymphadenopathy, and a generally nonpruritic, bilateral body rash with a predilection for the palms of the hands

and soles of the feet. Latent syphilis is characterized by a positive serology (RPR, VDRL) for syphilis without any clinical signs and symptoms. Late syphilis may begin 2 to 10 years after exposure in inadequately treated patients. Late syphilis affects the nervous and cardiovascular systems.
- Inflammation of the upper genital tract in females as a result of a polymicrobial infection is called PID. Various organisms have been associated with PID, including *N. gonorrhea*, *C. trachomatis*, *Gardnerella vaginalis*, *Escherichia coli*, and group B streptococci. Symptoms of acute PID include lower abdominal pain, dyspareunia, right upper quadrant pain, increased vaginal discharge, fever, vomiting, and diarrhea. Abdominal pain tends to be constant and bilateral. On examination, the provider may find cervical motion tenderness, adnexal tenderness, and mucopurulent cervicitis. The differential diagnosis includes illnesses involving the gastrointestinal, reproductive, and urinary systems and reproductive illnesses, such as ectopic pregnancy and hemorrhagic ovarian cysts. Evaluation involves a pelvic examination with sexually transmitted disease testing. Other laboratory testing includes a CBC, ESR, or C-reactive protein and pregnancy testing. A gynecologist should be consulted for any unusual case or when treatment fails.
- Other STIs that occur in adolescents include hepatitis B, HIV, *Trichomonas vaginalis*, bacterial vaginosis, *Candida albicans*, *Hemophillus ducreyi*, and *Ureaplasma urealyticum*.

Eating Disorders

Caucasian female adolescents are the population at highest risk for eating disorders. Predisposing factors include an excessive concern with thinness, a perfectionistic temperament, difficulty communicating negative emotions and resolving conflict, and low self-esteem (Kreipe, 1995). Anorexia nervosa is a syndrome in which caloric intake is insufficient to maintain normal weight or growth. Affected individuals are under the delusion that they are fat and are obsessed with being thinner. Bulimia is an abnormal eating pattern that involves binge eating, followed by attempts to lose weight, most commonly through purging or by fasting and exercise. More than 80% of adolescents with bulimia engage in self-induced vomiting or laxative and diuretic abuse as methods to avoid weight gain.

Symptoms of malnutrition associated with eating disorders include amenorrhea, cold hands and feet, constipation, and dry skin and hair. Physical signs of malnutrition include hypothermia, acrocyanosis, hypotension, and loss of muscle mass. Physical signs of vomiting related to bulimia include salivary gland enlargement and dental enamel erosion.

Intervention is indicated for adolescents who have a distorted body image, weigh less than 90% of average for height, and use purging methods of weight control. Intervention is best accomplished with a therapeutic team that includes a psychologist, psychiatrist, nutritionist, and primary care provider. Refer to Chapter 22 for an in-depth examination of this issue.

COMMUNITY RESOURCES

Community resources that contain information related to adolescent health or adolescent services include the library, the Department of Health, school-based clinics, school psy-

WEB SITES

Web Site	Organization	Address
Adolescent Health on Line	American Medical Association	*www.ama-assn.org/adolhlth/adolhlth.htm*
Center for Disease Control	CDC	*www.cdc.gov/*
Adolescent Health Links	Health Care Information Resources	*www-hsl.mcmaster.ca/tomflem/teenhealth.html*
Morbidity and Mortality Weekly Report	CDC	*www.cdc.gov/epo/mmwr.html*
National Institute of Child Health and Human Development	National Institute of Health	*www.hih.gov/nichd/*

chologists, school nurses, school coaches, and the parks and recreation department. Community-based and school-based programs that focus on preventive measures are often best suited to address adolescent concerns. The adolescent provider should participate in these programs whenever possible. Possible activities include Junior ROTC, school-based clubs, YMCA programs, and parks and recreation programs.

REFERENCES

Brown, R. T., & Cromer, B. A. (1997). The pediatrician and the sexually active adolescent—sexual activity and contraception. *Pediatric Clinics of North America, 44*(6), 1379–1390.

Committee on Infectious Diseases. (1997). Immunization of adolescents: recommendations of the advisory committee on immunization practices, the American Academy of Pediatrics, the American Academy of Family Physicians, and the American Medical Association. *Pediatrics, 99*(3), 479–488.

Coupey, S. M. (1997). Interviewing adolescents. *Pediatric Clinics of North America, 44*(6), 1349–1364.

Cronau, H., & Brown, R. T. (1998). Growth and development: Physical, mental, and social aspects. *Primary Care, 25*(1), 23–45.

Elster, A. B., & Levenberg, P. (1997). Integrating comprehensive adolescent preventive services into routine medicine care: Rationale and approaches. *Pediatric Clinics of North America, 44*(6), 1365–1377.

Elster, A. B. (1998). Comparison of recommendations for adolescent clinical preventive services developed by national organizations. *Archives of Pediatric and Adolescent Medicine, 152,* 193–198.

Eng, T., & Butler, W. (Eds.) (1997). *The hidden epidemic: Confronting sexually transmitted diseases.* Institute of Medicine. Committee on Prevention and Control of STDs. Washington, DC: National Academy Press.

English, A., & Matthews, M. (1995). State Minor Consent Statutes: A Summary. Cincinnati, OH: Center for Continuing Education in Adolescent Health, Division of Adolescent Medicine, Children's Hospital Medical Center.

Emans, S. J., Laufer, M. R., & Goldstein, D. P. (Eds.) (1998). *Pediatric and adolescent gynecology* (4th ed.). Philadelphia: Lippincott-Raven.

Ehrman, W. G., & Matson, S. C. (1998). Approach to assessing adolescents on serious or sensitive issues. *Pediatric Clinics of North America, 45*(1), 189–204.

Goldenring, J. M., & Cohen, E. (1988). Getting into adolescents' heads. *Contemporary Pediatrics, 5*(7), 75–90.

Ginsburg, K. R., Menapace, A. S., & Slap, G. B. (1997). Factors affecting the decision to seek health care: The voice of adolescents. *Pediatrics, 100*(6), 922–930.

Greene, J. W., & Walker, L. S. (1997). Psychosomatic problems and stress in adolescence. *Pediatric Clinics of North America, 44*(6), 1557–1572.

Hofmann, A. D., & Greydanus, D. (Eds.) (1997). *Adolescent medicine* (3rd ed.). Connecticut: Appleton & Lange.

Janofsky, M. (1999, March 2). Fatal crash reveals inhalants as danger to youth. *The New York Times,* A12.

Kann, L., Kinchen, S. A., Williams, B. I., Ross, J. G., Lowry, R., Hill, C. V., Grunbaum, J. A., Blumson, P. S., Collins, J. L., & Kolbe, L. J. (1998). Youth risk behavior surveillance-United States, 1997. *In CDC Surveillance Summaries, MMWR, 47*(SS-3), 1–89.

Kreipe, R. E. (1995). Eating disorders among children and adolescents. *Pediatrics in Review, 16*(10), 370–379.

Lappa, S., & Moscicki, AB. (1997). The pediatrician and the sexually active adolescent-a primer for sexually transmitted diseases. *Pediatric Clinics of North America, 44*(6), 1405–1445.

Neinstein, L. S. (Ed.) (1991). *Adolescent health care—a practical guide* (2nd ed.). Baltimore: Williams & Wilkins.

Reif, C. J., & Elster, A. B. (1998). Adolescent preventive services. *Primary Care, 25*(1), 1–19.

Ryan, C., & Futterman, D. (1997). Lesbian and gay youth: Care and counseling. *Adolescent medicine-State of the art reviews, 8*(2), 207–374.

Skaggs, D. L., & Bassett, G. S. (1996). Adolescent idiopathic scoliosis: An update. *American Family Physician, 53*(7), 2327–2334.

Stiffman, A. R., Chen, Y., Elze, D., Dore, P., & Cheng, L. (1997). Adolescents' and providers' perspectives on the need for and use of mental health services. *Journal of Adolescent Health, 21*(5), 335–342.

Sucich, A. (July 20, 1999). Oral communication. Clinical Social Worker, Peekskill Area Health Center, Hudson Valley Health Care.

CHAPTER 13

Immunizations

- MARGARET F. CLAYTON RN, MS, CS, FNP

INTRODUCTION

According to Plotkin and Plotkin (1994), "The impact of vaccination on the health of the world's people is hard to exaggerate. With the exception of safe water, no other modality, not even antibiotics, has had such a major effect on mortality reduction and population growth" (p. 1). The immunization of children is the responsibility of each primary care provider. Barriers such as the lack of reliable tracking systems, missed opportunities, failure to provide simultaneous immunizations, and administrative or procedural policies against immunizations during certain types of visits still leave some children without adequate coverage. Using each patient encounter as an opportunity to assess immunization status and to administer all appropriate immunizations will continue to improve the rate of immunization coverage.

The recent focus on immunization practices stemmed from the measles outbreak of 1989 to 1991, which was responsible for more than 43,000 reported cases and over 130 deaths (The National Advisory Committee, 1991). Between 1985 and 1989, only 8% of children younger than 4 years had received the measles vaccine. Of these children, 40% were older than 15 months, the recommended age for measles vaccination, and thus should have been immunized. Measles, mumps, rubella (MMR) vaccine protects 95% of people who receive it; therefore, the 1989 measles epidemic resulted from a lack of immunization, not from poor efficacy of the vaccine itself (Orenstein, Atkinson, Mason, & Bernier, 1990; The National Advisory Committee, 1991). This outbreak led to an evaluation of general immunization policies for preschool children and ultimately to a reconsideration of the schedule for MMR administration and the development of the Standards for Pediatric Immunization Practices (Display 13-1). These standards reflect the immunization practice guidelines developed and recommended by the National Vaccine Advisory Committee, approved by the United States Public Health Service, and endorsed by the American Academy of Pediatrics (AAP). Unfortunately, not all providers are familiar with or adhere to these standards. A complete discussion of each standard can be found in the *Red Book: Report of the Committee on Infectious Diseases*, 24th edition (AAP, 1997).

DISEASES AND THEIR VACCINES

The goal of immunization is to prevent and ultimately to eradicate disease. This goal is slowly being achieved, as evidenced by the global eradication of smallpox in 1977 and the elimination of poliomyelitis in the Americas in 1991. The incidences of other diseases, such as tetanus, diphtheria, measles, mumps, pertussis, rubella, and *Haemophilus influenzae* type B (HiB), have been sharply reduced (AAP, 1997). In 1994, an international commission declared wild type polio to be eliminated from the western hemisphere, with the last reported case in 1991 (AAP, 1997; Rodewald, 1999).

These successes are partly due to the increasing adherence of pediatric providers to the Standards for Immunization and an increased focus on the benefits and cost effectiveness of immunizations, resulting in record high coverage levels. Currently, 30 vaccines are licensed in the United States (Table 13-1). Many more are in various stages of research and development, such as vaccines to protect against respiratory syncytial virus, Lyme disease, and herpes.

In 1996, the United States met the goal of 90% immunization coverage adopted by Healthy People 2000, using the 4:3:1 criteria (four or more doses of diphtheria, tetanus, and pertussis; three or more doses of polio; and one or more doses of measles vaccine). When three doses of HiB are added (4:3:1:3), the rate of coverage falls to 76% as estimated by the National Immunization Survey in conjunction with the Centers for Disease Control and Prevention (CDC) (Altemeier, 1998). These data contrast sharply with earlier literature showing the United States lagging behind many European and developing countries in rates of immunization coverage for preschool children (Guyer & Hughart, 1994; Altemeier, 1998). Varicella coverage in 1997 was estimated to be 25%, up from 19% in 1996.

ADMINISTRATION

Active immunization is defined as administration of all or part of a microorganism or modified product of that microorganism (such as a toxoid, purified antigen, or genetically engineered antigen) that invokes an immunologic response mimicking the natural infection (AAP, 1997). Usually this procedure poses little or no risk to the patient. Some vaccines provide complete protection throughout life with only one dose; others require multiple doses or boosters. Vaccines composed of an intact (whole) infectious agent are either live-attenuated or killed (inactivated). Many viral vaccines are live-attenuated preparations, where the infectious agent replicates but causes little or no adverse host reaction. Live-attenuated vaccines generally provide a wider range of immunologic response than killed preparations. Most bacterial and some viral vaccines are inactivated; therefore, the infectious agent does not replicate within the host. This type of vaccine often requires a booster. One advantage of this type of vaccine is that the infectious agent is not replicated and therefore not excreted by the patient. Thus, such a vaccine does not adversely affect immunocompromised patients or caregivers. Combination vaccines contain multiple killed or attenuated organisms and provide protection from disease with fewer injections. A well-known example is the diphtheria-tetanus-pertussis (DTP) vaccine.

Bacterial conjugate vaccines link a polysaccharide capsule to a carrier protein directly or using a spacer molecule. Pro-

DISPLAY 13–1 • Standards for Pediatric Immunization Practices

The Standards represent the consensus of the National Vaccine Advisory Committee (NVAC) and of a broad group of medical and public health experts about what constitute the most desirable immunization practices. It is recognized by the NVAC that not all of the current immunization practices of public and private providers are in compliance with the Standards. Nevertheless, the Standards are expected to be useful as a means of helping providers to identify needed changes, obtain resources if necessary, and implement the desirable immunization practices in the future.

Standard 1. Immunization services are readily available.

Standard 2. There are no barriers or unnecessary prerequisites to the receipt of vaccines.

Standard 3. Immunization services are available free or for a minimal fee.

Standard 4. Providers use all clinical encounters to screen and, when indicated, immunize children.

Standard 5. Providers educate parents and guardians about immunization in general terms.

Standard 6. Providers question parents or guardians about contraindications and, before immunizing a child, inform them in specific terms about the risks and benefits of the immunizations their child is to receive.

Standard 7. Providers follow only true contraindications.

Standard 8. Providers administer simultaneously all vaccine doses for which a child is eligible at the time of each visit.

Standard 9. Providers use accurate and complete recording procedures.

Standard 10. Providers co-schedule immunization appointments in conjunction with appointments for other child health services.

Standard 11. Providers report adverse events following immunization promptly, accurately, and completely.

Standard 12. Providers operate a tracking system to identify and notify patients due or overdue for immunization.

Standard 13. Providers adhere to appropriate procedures for vaccine management (storage and handling).

Standard 14. Providers conduct semiannual audits to assess immunization coverage levels and to review immunization records in the patient populations they serve.

Standard 15. Providers maintain up-to-date, easily retrievable medical protocols at all locations where vaccines are administered.

Standard 16. Providers operate with patient-oriented and community-based approaches.

Standard 17. Vaccines are administered by properly trained individuals.

Standard 18. Providers receive ongoing education and training on current immunization recommendations.

Used with permission.

tective antibody responses are directed against the specific polysaccharide capsule chosen, such as Hib. The goal of bacterial conjugate vaccines is to provoke a host antibody response to bacteria, such as gram-negative bacteria with polysaccharide capsules, which normally do not elicit a strong response in immunologically immature individuals (eg, those younger than 2 years). Obviously, these vaccines are targeted for this vulnerable age group; therefore, the use of a more immunogenic bacterial conjugate confers protection against these organisms even in very young children. Common examples are Hib and pneumococcal vaccines. Bacterial conjugate vaccines differ in composition and immunogenicity and therefore in recommendations for their use.

All vaccine preparations contain an active immunizing antigen and a fluid for the suspension of this antigen, such as sterile water, saline, or tissue culture fluids containing proteins such as eggs or gelatin. Vaccines also contain stabilizers or preservatives (including antibiotics) and occasionally adjuvants (most commonly an aluminum salt) to enhance immunogenicity. All the above may cause allergic responses in susceptible individuals.

▲ **Clinical Warning:** In all settings where vaccines are administered, facilities and personnel should be available for treating immediate allergic reactions (AAP, 1997).

Some vaccines require reconstitution. Reconstituting vaccines ahead of time should be discouraged, because doing so may alter their potency or effectiveness.

Vaccines can be administered orally or parenterally (intramuscularly or subcutaneously). The intramuscular site chosen depends on the volume of injected material and the size of the muscle. Generally, the anterolateral muscle of the thigh is chosen for the child younger than 1 year and the deltoid muscle for older children. Most parents feel that use of the deltoid muscle as opposed to the anterolateral thigh muscle reduces discomfort and distress in ambulatory children. Parents should be present to comfort the child during administration, and the child should be securely restrained during the actual delivery to avoid injury caused by grabbing at the needle or from a sudden unexpected movement.

Prior to administering any vaccine, the provider must inquire about adverse effects from previous immunizations. The provider also has a duty to warn the parent or guardian about the possible risks and benefits of vaccination. A duty is not the same as informed consent; rather, it is a federal requirement stemming from the National Childhood Vaccine Injury Act of 1986. This act requires health care providers to maintain permanent vaccination records and to report adverse events that follow immunization.

Since 1994, the federal government requires all health care providers who administer any vaccine containing diphtheria, tetanus, pertussis, measles, mumps, rubella, polio, varicella, hepatitis B, or Hib vaccine to provide a copy of the relevant vaccine information materials to the legal representative of any child prior to administration. These materials must be supplemented with visual presentations or oral explanations in appropriate cases. These vaccine information sheets are available through state health departments and the CDC as well as online at *http://www.cdc.gov/nip*. The provider's responsibility is to provide copies of informational material, discuss the information, answer questions, respond to concerns, and then document parental decisions. Some practices require a parent's or guardian's signature to refuse and to accept vaccinations because of lawsuits involving failure to vaccinate when a person acquires a disease preventable by vaccine (Rodewald, 1999).

The religious beliefs and philosophical practices of parents must be respected, but clinicians can assist parents to make informed decisions by providing information and allowing ample time to answer questions. The benefits of immunization to their child and any children who come in contact with that child should be strongly emphasized. Children who are unable to receive immunizations must rely on the immu-

Table 13-1.   VACCINES LICENSED IN THE UNITED STATES AND THEIR ROUTES OF ADMINISTRATION

Vaccine*	Type	Route†
Adenovirus‡	Live virus	Oral
Anthrax§	Inactivated bacteria	SC
BCG	Live bacteria	ID (preferred) or SC
Cholera	Inactivated bacteria	SC, IM, or ID
DTP	Toxoids and inactivated bacteria	IM
DTaP	Toxoids and inactivated bacterial components	IM
Hepatitis A	Inactivated virus	IM
Hepatitis B	Inactivated viral antigen	IM
Hib conjugates#	Polysaccharide-protein conjugate	IM
Hib conjugate-DTP (HbOC#-DTP and PRP-T# reconstituted with DTP)	Polysaccharide-protein conjugate with toxoids and inactivated bacteria	IM
Hib conjugate-DTaP (PRP-T# reconstituted with DTaP)	Polysaccharide-protein conjugate with toxoids and inactivated bacterial components	IM
Hib conjugate (PRP-OMP#)-hepatitis B	Polysaccharide-protein conjugate with inactivated virus	IM
Influenza	Inactivated virus (whole-virus), viral components	IM
Japanese encephalitis	Inactivated virus	SC
Measles	Live virus	SC
Meningococcal	Polysaccharide	SC
MMR	Live viruses	SC
Measles-rubella	Live viruses	SC
Mumps	Live virus	SC
Pertussis§	Inactivated bacteria	IM
Plague	Inactivated bacteria	IM
Pneumococcal	Polysaccharide	IM or SC
Poliovirus:		
OPV	Live virus	Oral
IPV	Inactivated virus	SC
Rabies	Inactivated virus	IM or ID¶
Rubella	Live virus	SC
Tetanus	Toxoid	IM
Tetanus-diphtheria (Td, DT)	Toxoids	IM
Typhoid		
Parenteral	Inactivated bacteria	SC
Parenteral	Capsular polysaccharide	SC (boosters may be ID)
Oral	Live bacteria	Oral
Varicella	Live virus	SC
Yellow fever	Live virus	SC

*Vaccine abbreviations: BCG indicates bacill Calmette-Guérin vaccine; DTP, diphtheria and tetanus toxoids and pertussis vaccine, adsorbed: DTaP, diphtheria and tetanus toxoids and acellular pertussis vaccine, adsorbed; Hib, *Haemophilus influenzae* type b vaccine; MMR, live measles-mumps-rubella viruses vaccine; OPV, oral poliovirus vaccine; IPV, inactivated poliovirus vaccine; Td, tetanus and diphtheria toxoid (for children ≥7 y and adults); and DT, diphtheria and tetanus toxoids (for children <7 y).

†Route abbreviations: SC indicates subcutaneous; ID, intradermal; and IM, intramuscular.

‡Available only to US Armed Forces.

§Distributed by the Division of Biologic Products, Michigan Department of Public Health, Lansing, Mich.

¶Human diploid cell rabies vaccine for intradermal use is different in constitution and potency from the intramuscular vaccine; it should be used for preexposure immunization only. Rabies vaccine adsorbed (RVA) should not be used intradermally.

Source: AAP. (1997). G. Peter (Ed.) *Red Book: Report of the Committee on infectious diseases* (24th ed.). Elk Grove Village, IL: Author. Used with permission.

nization status of others to prevent exposure to disease. This concept has been referred to as herd immunity. Ultimately, most states will allow exemptions from required school entry immunizations for religious or philosophical beliefs; however, each provider has the responsibility to ensure that parents receive all necessary information to make informed choices regarding immunizations for their children.

STORAGE

All vaccines are refrigerated or frozen. Storage procedures for vaccines vary but are extremely important to maintain the effectiveness of a product. Improper storage may render a vaccine ineffective. Providers should follow the manufacturer's guidelines closely regarding storage requirements for each vaccine.

▲ **Clinical Warning:** Varicella vaccine storage requirements are very specific, requiring a temperature of 5°F (−15°C). Refrigerators with open dormitory type freezers set within the refrigeration compartment are not suitable for the storage of varicella vaccine, because they are unable to achieve the required temperature for proper storage.

ROUTINE VACCINATIONS

Measles, Mumps, Rubella

The MMR vaccine is composed of three live attenuated vaccines. This highly effective vaccine is administered subcutaneously in two doses for those born on or after January 1, 1957. Those born before 1957 are assumed to have acquired immunity from having the actual disease. If a person's immunity is questioned, a titer can be drawn to verify antibody status. The first MMR dose is recommended at age 12 to 15 months and the second at the child's entry into school (age 4 to 6 years). Should an outbreak of disease occur in the community or if travel to an endemic area requires vaccination, the first MMR can be given as early as 6 months, and the second dose may be given before school entry. If the first dose is given before the first birthday due to disease outbreak, however, the recommended two doses on or after the first birthday must still be administered. For children already in school, the recommended age for the second dose is 11 to 12 years. The recommendation to administer a second dose was adopted in 1989 following recurrent outbreaks of measles in vaccinated children. Following one dose, given at age 15 months or later, 98% of immunized people demonstrate seroconversion. Following two doses given at least 1 month apart, on or after the first birthday, 99% of immunized people demonstrate seroconversion.

Because MMR is a live-attenuated vaccine, non–allergy-related side effects are noted 5 to 12 days following immunization. Fever and rash are relatively common, experienced by 5% to 15% of recipients. Transient arthritis has been reported. Very rarely, thrombocytopenia (less than 1 in 30,000) or encephalopathy (less than 1 in 1 million) occurs. A general rule of thumb is the "rule of 10"—about 10% of children get a rash approximately 10 days after vaccine administration. Immunization is not harmful to previously immune individuals. MMR vaccine should not be given 2 weeks before or 3 weeks after immunoglobulin administration or blood transfusion due to the possibility that antibodies will neutralize the vaccine virus, preventing seroconversion. Tuberculin skin testing should be done on the same day, or delayed for 4 to 6 weeks because the measles portion of this vaccine may suppress skin test reactivity. Human immunodeficiency virus (HIV)-positive individuals should be vaccinated, unless severely immunocompromised.

The purpose of the rubella portion of this vaccine is to protect against congenital rubella syndrome by preventing the occurrence of rubella, which, by itself, is a mild disease.

● **Clinical Pearl:** Pregnant women should not receive MMR due to theoretical risk to the fetus, although the presence of a pregnant woman in the household of a vaccinated child poses no risk. If a pregnant woman is inadvertently vaccinated or if pregnancy occurs within 3 months of immunization, the woman should be counseled about potential risks to the fetus, although receipt of this vaccine during pregnancy is not an indication for interruption of the pregnancy (AAP, 1997, p. 461).

History of anaphylactic response to neomycin is a contraindication to receiving MMR. (History of contact dermatitis to neomycin is not a contraindication to immunization with MMR [AAP, 1997]). Skin testing of egg-allergic children has not been predictive of those who will have an immediate hypersensitivity reaction (AAP, 1997).

● **Clinical Pearl:** MMR can and should be given to children who are allergic to eggs. The provider should ensure supervision during and after immunization until the child's response to MMR vaccine has been established.

Children who experience an anaphylactic response to vaccination should be tested for serum antibodies to determine the need for a second dose. If a second dose is needed, it should be administered only in a setting where life-threatening hypersensitivity reactions can be managed adequately. People with allergies to feathers or chickens are not at increased risk of allergic response to MMR vaccine.

The MMR vaccine is refrigerated. Shelf-life can extend to 2 years. After reconstitution, MMR must be protected from light and used within 8 hours.

Diphtheria, Tetanus, Acellular Pertussis

Diphtheria, tetanus, acellular pertussis (DTaP) is the currently recommended form of DTP, the first combination vaccine. Acellular pertussis, unlike whole-cell pertussis, contains few or no endotoxins. DPT or DTaP contains diphtheria toxoid, tetanus toxoid, and pertussis vaccine. As of 1996, two acellular preparations are licensed in the United States. When feasible, the same preparation should be used for the first three doses of vaccine. For the fourth and fifth doses, any licensed preparation is appropriate. When the preparation used for one or more of the first three doses is unknown, any licensed preparation may be used to complete the series (AAP, 1997). When compared to times before vaccines were available, the incidence of diphtheria and tetanus have decreased 99%. Pertussis incidence has decreased 98%. In 1995, 5000 cases of pertussis were reported in the United States (Rodewald, 1999). In 1996, there were no reported cases of tetanus and only four reported cases of diphtheria, none in children younger than 5 years (Rodewald, 1999).

The intramuscular route is used for DTaP (it is absorbed to aluminum salts). The three initial doses are given at ages 2, 4, and 6 months. The fourth dose is given 6 to 12 months after the third dose, usually at age 15 to 18 months. A fifth dose is given at age 4 to 6 years (school entry) unless the fourth dose was administered after the fourth birthday.

● **Clinical Pearl:** Split doses are not recommended and are not counted toward completion of the primary series by schools.

If DTP is used, acetaminophen is recommended for antipyretic prophylaxis (AAP, 1997). The use of DTaP reduces the incidence of pyretic responses. After age 7 years, adult-type tetanus and diphtheria toxoids (Td) are given. A Td booster is required every 10 years after completion of the primary series. For children in whom pertussis vaccine is contraindicated (eg, those with an immediate anaphylactic response or encephalopathy within 7 days not explained by other causes), the series may be completed using diphtheria, tetanus (DT) preparations.

Previously, the following circumstances were considered contraindications to receiving subsequent pertussis immunization: convulsions with or without fever occurring within 3 days of DTP or DTaP; persistent inconsolable screaming or crying for 3 or more hours within 48 hours of immunization; collapse or shock-like state within 48 hours; and temperature of 104.9°F or higher within 48 hours unexplained by other causes. Currently the AAP considers these situations as precautions because they have not been shown to cause permanent sequelae (AAP, 1997). Current contraindications to DTaP administration include an immediate anaphylactic response following vaccine administration and encephalopathy within 7 days of a previous dose unexplainable by other causes. In these cases, the series usually is completed with DT vaccine.

Before any subsequent vaccination with DTP or DTaP, the parent or guardian must be questioned regarding adverse events. The decision to administer or withhold immunizations should be evaluated on an individual basis based on the risks of disease exposure in the child's community and the risks and benefits of immunization (AAP, 1997). DTaP, DPT, and DPT/Hib vaccines should be stored refrigerated, not frozen. Shelf life may extend to 18 months.

▲ Clinical Warning: Children who have evolving neurologic conditions or an unevaluated seizure history should not be immunized with DTP or DTaP until evaluation and treatment have occurred and the child is stabilized.

Polio

In 1994, wild-type polio virus was considered interrupted in the western hemisphere (AAP, 1997). Poliomyelitis is still found in some underdeveloped countries, but the worldwide incidence has decreased 80% since 1988, due to the World Health Organization initiatives using oral poliovirus vaccine (OPV) (AAP, 1997). Since 1980, vaccine-associated paralytic poliomyelitis (VAPP) among recipients of OPV has accounted for eight to nine reported cases of polio per year in the United States. Trivalent OPV, also known as the Sabin vaccine, is a live-attenuated vaccine administered orally and stored frozen. Inactivated poliovirus vaccine (IPV), also known as the Salk vaccine, is a formaldehyde-killed preparation administered subcutaneously. It should be used for all immunocompromised people. IPV is refrigerated and may have a shelf life up to 18 months.

For either OPV or IPV, four doses are required prior to school entry (unless the third dose of the primary series occurs after the fourth birthday). The recommended series consists of two IPVs (to reduce the incidence of VAPP) at ages 2 months and 4 months, followed by two doses of OPV between ages 12 to 18 months and 4 to 6 years (school entry). The recommended interval between doses is 2 months. The minimum interval is 6 weeks, although if accelerated immunization is desired, this may be shortened to 4 weeks. All-OPV or all-IPV immunization schedules also are acceptable. As of January 1, 2000, the recommended polio sequence has changed to an all-IPV schedule (Advisory Committee for Immunization Practices [ACIP], 1999). The only adverse effects of polio immunization are related to VAPP occurring with the use of OPV. The incidence of VAPP from first-dose exposure is estimated at 1 per 1.5 million doses for a recipient case, and 1 per 2.2 million doses for a contact case (exposure to a first-dose recipient). For the subsequent doses, the risk is much lower for both recipient and contacts (AAP, 1997). The future IPV schedule has been recommended due to continuing progress toward eliminating poliomyelitis worldwide, coupled with the attendant risk of VAPP from

OPV. OPV will be acceptable under special circumstances, such as to control outbreaks, for imminent travel to polio-endemic countries (because it confers better gut immunity), and if parents refuse the number of injections required at the time of the third and fourth doses (ACIP, 1999).

No adverse effects have been reported due to IPV. Contraindications to IPV administration include allergic response to streptomycin or neomycin. OPV should not be given to children when close contacts include immunosuppressed individuals, due to the shedding of virus in the stool. Neither preparation should be given to pregnant women unless absolutely necessary; in such a case, OPV is recommended.

Varicella

Varicella is the newest recommended vaccine. Prior to its availability, approximately 4 million cases of varicella occurred each year, with 9000 hospitalizations and 100 deaths per year. Almost half these deaths were among previously healthy children and adolescents (Rodewald, 1999). Complications included secondary bacterial infections from scratching of lesions, including septicemia, cellulitis, erysipelas, toxic shock syndrome, and invasive "flesh-eating strep" primarily due to infection with Streptococcus pyogenes. Encephalitis usually is mild and self-limiting, often in the form of acute cerebellar ataxia. Additionally, the huge social cost of missed work time among those caring for ill children cannot be discounted. Varicella vaccine is a cell-free, live-attenuated vaccine. One dose is given subcutaneously at age 12 to 18 months or before age 13 years for individuals who lack a reliable history of varicella. Adolescents older than 13 years and young adults with no history of infection should receive two doses 4 to 8 weeks apart. Varicella can be administered concurrently with MMR vaccine (separate injections). If it is not administered on the same day as MMR, varicella immunization should be delayed until 30 days after the MMR immunization.

Precautions and contraindications include administration to immunocompromised children, including symptomatic and asymptomatic children with HIV. The presence of an immunocompromised household member is not a contraindication to vaccination, and no special precautions need to be taken unless the vaccinated child develops a rash. In this case, the child should avoid contact with the immunocompromised family member until the rash resolves. Other precautions and contraindications include administration to pregnant women (a pregnant woman in the household is not considered a contraindication) and to children receiving high doses of systemic corticosteroids (AAP, 1997). Children receiving more than 14 days of high-dose systemic corticosteroid therapy (2 mg/kg/d of prednisone or the equivalent or 20 mg of prednisone/d) should delay varicella immunization until 1 month after steroid therapy is completed. Inhaled corticosteroids are not considered a contraindication for immunization. Conception should be delayed 1 month following immunization. The effect of immune globulin on varicella vaccine is unknown. Based on its potentially inhibitory effect on passively transferred antibodies and its known effects on other live vaccines, varicella vaccination should be delayed 5 to 9 months following administration of immune globulins and blood products (except for washed red blood cells). The administration of salicylates should be avoided for 6 weeks after varicella immunization due to the potential association of Reye's syndrome with varicella and salicylates (although no cases of Reye's syndrome following immunization have been reported). Contraindications also include anaphylactic reactions to gelatin or neomycin (AAP, 1997; Rodewald, 1999).

Adverse effects include soreness, redness, and swelling at the injection site; a varicella-type rash at the injection site occurring within 2 weeks of immunization; and a varicella-type rash occurring elsewhere within 3 weeks of immunization. Varicella vaccine is stored frozen, at 5°F or −15°C, in a freezer that has a separate door from the refrigerator. With proper storage, shelf life is 18 months. After reconstitution, the vaccine must be administered within 30 minutes.

Hepatitis B

Hepatitis B is a viral infection transmitted through body fluids that are hepatitis B surface antigen (HBsAG) positive. Incubation periods may be 8 to 24 weeks. Onset may be acute, nonspecific, or asymptomatic and may progress to chronic infection. Young children are often asymptomatic. Chronic infection develops in 70% to 90% of infants born to HBsAG-positive mothers, as opposed to 30% who are infected at ages 1 to 5 years and 6% to 10% of those infected as adults (Fischbach, 1996; AAP, 1997). Vaccination prevents hepatitis B and its complications, namely chronic liver disease and hepatocellular carcinoma. Children infected at an early age are at greater risk of death due to liver complications than those infected at an older age (AAP, 1997). Infants born to hepatitis B-positive mothers should have their immunity status to hepatitis B evaluated at age 1 year.

Initially hepatitis B vaccine was targeted toward high-risk individuals, but due to the inability to control the spread of hepatitis B, this recommendation was revised in 1991 to include universal infant vaccination and in 1996 to include universal adolescent vaccination (Rodewald, 1999). Prenatal and neonatal testing to determine the need for prophylaxis or treatment also is recommended.

Hepatitis B vaccine is administered intramuscularly. Three doses induce seroconversion in 90% of healthy adults and 95% of infants, children, and adolescents. Initially, the first dose was given between birth and 2 months, the second dose at least 1 month after the first, and the third dose at least 2 months after the second. For infants who began the series at birth, the third dose was given after age 6 months. For those who began the series after age 2 months, the minimum recommended interval between the first and third doses was 4 months (AAP, 1997). In July 1999, the AAP modified its recommendations regarding infant hepatitis B vaccine because of a concern regarding thimerosal, a mercury-based preservative used in hepatitis B and other vaccines. Concerns revolved around the cumulative effect of thimerosal in the first 6 months of life (AAP, 1999b).

● **Clinical Pearl:** The new recommendations are to delay immunization until age 6 months for infants whose mothers are HepBSAg negative. Infants whose mothers are HepBSAg positive or whose status is unknown should receive hepatitis B vaccination at birth as per the January 1999 recommended childhood immunization schedule.

It is anticipated that the original immunization schedule will be readopted once thimerosal-free vaccines become more universally available. Should an individual fall behind in this schedule, it is not necessary to restart the series. Immunization can be completed regardless of the interval from the last dose of vaccine. Booster doses are not currently recommended, but detectable serum antibody levels have been demonstrated to decrease 13% to 60% after 10 years (AAP, 1997). A complete discussion of hepatitis B vaccine and its uses in special populations (such as the premature infant) can be found in the *Red Book* (AAP, 1997).

▲ **Clinical Warning:** Anti-HBs titers should be periodically assessed to ensure disease prophylaxis.

Adverse effects include local soreness at the injection site and low-grade temperature. Contraindications include serious allergic reactions to a previous dose and allergy to common baker's yeast. Anaphylactic response to hepatitis B vaccine is rare. Early data suggested a borderline significant association between Guillain-Barré syndrome and plasma-derived products. In 1993, the Vaccine Safety Committee of the Institute of Medicine concluded the evidence was inadequate to accept or reject a causal relationship between first-dose vaccination and Guillain-Barré syndrome. Plasma-prepared vaccine is no longer produced in the United States but is used in other countries. No association with Guillain-Barré syndrome has been reported with the currently licensed recombinant DNA preparations of hepatitis B vaccine (AAP, 1997). Immunization to hepatitis B that is started with vaccine prepared by one manufacturer may be completed with product from another. Hepatitis B vaccine is stored in the refrigerator, with a shelf life of up to 3 years.

Haemophilus influenzae Type b

The Hib vaccine has had a marked impact on the goal of disease prevention. Previous estimates were that 20,000 cases of invasive Hib disease occurred annually. The incidence of disease has been reduced 99% (Rodewald, 1999). Four preparations are licensed for administration in the United States. All are conjugated vaccines bound to a protein carrier. The difference between preparations is in the type of protein carrier used, which affects the schedule of administration. Notably, diphtheria toxoid carrier (PRP-D, trade name ProHIBIT) may only be used in children between ages 15 and 59 months. The other three preparations are PRP-T (tetanus toxoid carrier protein, trade name ActHIB or OmniHIB), HbOC (nontoxic mutant diphtheria toxin carrier protein, trade name HibTITER), and PRP-OMP (outer membrane protein complex of *Neisseria meningitidis*, trade name PedvaxHIB). Any of these three can be administered to infants age 2 months or older. Hib is available in combination products and alone. It is acceptable to complete the series with a preparation other than the original preparation used to start it. Number of doses and recommended schedule vary by age of the child and type of vaccine. The recommended schedule is two or three doses, based on manufacturer, given at 2 months, 4 months, and (for three-dose schedules) 6 months. A booster dose is given at age 12 to 15 months using any desired preparation, regardless of preparation used in the initial series (AAP, 1997). Providers are referred to specific product literature. Hib is not administered to infants younger than 6 weeks old. Hib may be administered simultaneously with any other vaccine. Adverse reactions include local swelling, redness, or pain. Serious systemic events are rare. Contraindications include anaphylactic response to prior Hib immunization. Hib vaccine is refrigerated and may be stored up to 2 years. Stability after reconstitution varies by manufacturer.

Other Licensed Vaccines: Influenza, Pneumococcal, Hepatitis A, Meningococcal

Influenza vaccine is available in the United States. This vaccine is grown in eggs. The composition is altered yearly depending on the expected viral strains for the coming winter. The vaccine is administered in the fall. Immunity lasts 1 year.

▲ **Clinical Warning:** Children younger than 13 years should receive only split-virus preparations. Split-virus or whole virus preparations may be administered to older children and adults. Children younger than 9 years receive two intramuscular doses of split-virus vaccine, 1 month apart, the first time they are immunized. Older children and adults receive one dose of split or whole virus preparation as appropriate.

Influenza vaccine is recommended yearly for children age 6 months or older and diagnosed with chronic pulmonary disease (including asthma), cardiac conditions, HIV, immunosuppressive conditions, sickle-cell disease, other hemoglobinopathies, diabetes, chronic renal or metabolic conditions, or on aspirin therapy. Immunization of the close contacts of such children also is recommended. Additionally, any healthy child may be immunized against influenza if parents request vaccination.

Adverse effects include local soreness, redness, and induration at the injection site. Immediate hypersensitivity reactions are rare. Contraindications include allergic responses to a previous influenza immunization and allergic responses to eggs or chickens. Influenza vaccine is refrigerated.

The current pneumococcal vaccine protects against invasive disease caused by *Streptococcus pneumoniae*. Because it is not immunogenic in infants, it is recommended for children older than 2 years who are at high risk for serious pneumococcal illness. Examples include children with chronic renal or liver disease, cardiovascular disease, pulmonary disease, sickle-cell disease, or immunosuppression, including HIV; those who have undergone a splenectomy; or those who experience cerebrospinal fluid leaks. Pneumococcal vaccine is administered intramuscularly or subcutaneously.

Adverse effects include mild local effects (experienced by approximately half of recipients) and fever or severe local reactions (experienced by less than 1% of recipients). Severe allergic reactions are rare, occurring in approximately 5 per 1 million doses. Contraindications include allergic response to a previous dose.

A new conjugated pneumococcal vaccine has recently received ACIP approval and is awaiting Food and Drug Administration (FDA) licensure for routine use in all children up to age 5 years. This vaccine targets the seven most prevalent pneumococcal serotypes in the United States and is immunogenic in children younger than 2 years. The ACIP recommendation is based on a phase III clinical trial that the Kaiser Permanente Vaccine Study Center conducted, involving 38,000 children. Results of the trial revealed no invasive pneumococcal disease (meningitis and bacteremia) in this study group, compared to 47 cases in the control group. There were also 8.9% fewer ill-child visits for otitis media and 20.3% fewer surgeries for tympanostomy tube placement. Given the increasing emergence of drug-resistant pneumococcal strains and the estimated $5 billion annual cost to society from otitis media, this vaccine will be medically and economically important (Black & Shinefield, 1999). The anticipated administration schedule is at 2, 4, and 6 months of age with a booster at 12 to 15 months. Observed side effects included injection site reactions, fever, irritability, drowsiness, and decreased appetite.

Immunization against hepatitis A is available using one of two licensed products. Hepatitis A vaccine is an inactivated viral vaccine made from human fibroblasts. It is adminis-

tered intramuscularly to children older than 2 years, using a two- or three-dose schedule. It is recommended for children who live in communities with increased risk of disease, homosexual males, intravenous drug users, and those with chronic liver disease or clotting factor disorders. Adverse effects include local soreness at the injection site. Serious adverse effects have not been reported (Rodewald, 1999). Contraindications are hypersensitivity reactions to vaccine components, including alum and phenoxyethanol. This vaccine is stored refrigerated.

Because of an increased incidence of fatal meningococcal infections in college students residing in dormatories (Harrison, Dwyer, Maples, & Billmann, 1999), the ACIP and AAP recently have recommended immunization for this at-risk population before they enter college. The current quadrivalent meningococcal vaccine is both safe and effective for serotypes A, C, Y, and W-135. It is not protective against type B strains, the most epidemic variety. Further, the current quadrivalent meningococcal vaccine is not immunogenic for children younger than 2 years.

ON THE HORIZON

New vaccines are under development. An oral vaccine to be given at ages 2, 4, and 6 months is newly licensed for rotavirus. It is not totally effective at this point, and not all insurance companies will pay for it. It can cost up to $50 per dose. At publication, preliminary evidence regarding an increased risk of intussusception in rotavirus vaccine recipients has led to an AAP policy statement recommending discretionary vaccine administration until more evidence is accumulated (AAP, 1999a). Two major studies involving 21,000 subjects, 45 sites, and 10 states are evaluating immunizations against Lyme disease. Results show the vaccine to be safe and effective (Sigal et al., 1998; Steere et al., 1998). A vaccine targeting respiratory syncytial virus will be important, because this disease is a leading cause of infant hospitalization. A trivalent live-attenuated intranasal pneumococcal vaccine for children younger than 2 years has been developed and is reported to be well tolerated, easily administered, and effective with no serious adverse effects (Belshe et al., 1998). New combination products will make administration of multiple vaccines more acceptable and available to patients and will further the goals of disease prevention and eradication.

MISSED OPPORTUNITIES

A missed opportunity is defined as lack of adherence to Standards 4 (administering all vaccines for which a child is eligible), 7 (failing to use only true contraindications to withhold immunizations), and 8 (withholding immunizations through failure to screen immunization status at each encounter). These missed opportunities contribute to less than desirable immunization levels and are costly to society.

In 1991 to 1992, the CDC awarded contracts to four major universities (in Philadelphia, Los Angeles, Baltimore, and Rochester, NY) to discover causes of underimmunization and to quantify missed opportunities. The report discovered that at least one missed opportunity occurred in 21% of the total 25,139 visits evaluated. Missed opportunities occurred during both sick and well visits but were more likely to occur during sick visits. Failure to administer all indicated vaccines simultaneously to an eligible child accounted for up to 15% of missed opportunities, depending on site (CDC, 1994). In this study, at least one missed opportunity to vaccinate occurred for approximately half of all children surveyed.

Many health maintenance organizations are auditing immunization records and requiring providers to comply with the Standards for Pediatric Immunization. Failure to immunize may be considered a liability issue (Lukes, 1995). The current use of combination vaccinations may improve parental and provider acceptance of immunizations and provider compliance with Standard 8 by reducing the number of injections given during a single office visit.

● **Clinical Pearl:** Many providers are reluctant to immunize children who have low-grade fever or mild acute illnesses, such as gastroenteritis, upper respiratory infection, and otitis media, despite recommendations that mild acute illness is not a true contraindication for withholding immunizations (AAP, 1997).

Misconceptions regarding true and false contraindications for immunization are common. They include redness or swelling or temperature below 105°F, exposure to an infectious disease, breastfeeding, a history of relatives with allergies or a history of nonspecific allergies, antibiotic allergies (except anaphylactic responses to streptomycin or neomycin), family history of seizures or sudden infant death syndrome, and malnutrition (AAP, 1997) (Table 13-2).

● **Clinical Pearl:** Barriers to receiving immunizations include practice policies. Identified practice policy barriers include requiring well checkups and appointments for administering immunizations, long waiting times, and limited office hours (AAP, 1997; Bates, Fitzgerald, Dittus, & Wolinsky, 1994; CDC, 1994; Fielding, Cumberland, & Pettitt, 1994; Szilagyi & Rodewald, 1994).

Since October 1, 1994, the U.S. Department of Health and Human Services has provided free vaccines through the Vaccines for Children (VFC) program at participating public and private sites. This program provides free immunizations to children with Medicaid, the uninsured child, Native Americans, and Alaskan Natives. Children whose health insurance does not cover the cost of immunizations also may use this program. Information on VFC is found at *http://www.cdc.gov/nip.*

Missed opportunities affect the U.S. workforce (Lukes, 1995). Children who are underimmunized are at risk for developing disease. If they become ill, employer-provided insurance pays the costs of their treatment, but parents incur expenses and lose wages while caring for ill children. If a child is not immunized during a minor illness, the parent may have to take additional time off work for another appointment to immunize this child, further increasing the likelihood of not returning for immunizations.

Debate continues among providers as to whether immunizations should be coupled with well child visits and whether immunizations should be given at sites other than primary practices, such as schools and day care centers. Some providers believe that a child immunized at episodic visits will not return for regular well child care. They therefore withhold vaccines for which children are eligible during visits for minor illness. This is not because providers believe immunization is harmful during acute illness, but because they think the child is already uncomfortable due to illness. It should be noted here that the *Red Book* (1997) still defines this type of encounter as a missed opportunity, regardless of the provider's future intentions.

Implementing tracking systems to identify children who are behind in their immunizations is universally recommended. The National Vaccine Advisory Committee has created a Workgroup on Immunization Registries. In 1998, in collaboration with the National Immunization Program, this workgroup launched the Immunization Registry Initiative and set the stage for implementing NIP's main strategies for increasing or maintaining immunization rates. These strategies involve using reminder or recall systems, assessment of provider immunization coverage rates with feedback and incentives, exchange of information between providers, and linkage with Women, Infants, and Children (WIC) immunization assessment and referral procedures (Linkins & Feikema, 1998).

Providers must assume responsibility for reducing missed opportunities for vaccination. Primary care practice must be better integrated with strong community-based public health delivery systems. The linkage with WIC supplemental nutrition program is especially effective. Nationally, more than 44% of infants have access to WIC programs. In 1997, approximately 5 to 7 million infants and preschoolers participated in WIC programs (Shefer & Mize, 1998). WIC eligibility is based partly on income. Many studies have shown the association between low income and underimmunization (Bates et al., 1994; Guyer & Hughart, 1994; Orenstein et al., 1990; Salsberry, Nickel, & Mitch, 1994). WIC's linkage with immunization efforts has been shown to increase immunization rates without harming WIC enrollment (Rodewald, 1999).

Administering OPV to a child with gastroenteritis elicits much debate among pediatric providers. Product literature for OPV lists gastroenteritis as a contraindication to administration. The AAP's *Red Book* (1997) acknowledges this and notes variations in product literature versus the recommendations regarding true contraindications for immunization by the ACIP and the Committee on Infectious Diseases (COID). The *Red Book* (1997) lists mild acute diarrhea as a false contraindication to the administration of OPV.

SPECIAL SITUATIONS

Special populations, such as premature children and children with neurologic diagnoses, present unique challenges to providers. A standard, up-to-date pediatric immunization schedule released each year by the AAP is used for premature and full-term infants. No schedules are specific for premature infants, and all childhood vaccines should be given to premature infants at the correct chronologic age using full-dose (not split-dose) preparations. The clinician should not use corrected gestational age. DTaP, Hib, and polio vaccines are given at the usual recommended ages of 2, 4, and 6 months. Hepatitis B vaccine should be deferred in the small and prematurely born infant whose mother is hepatitis B negative until the infant reaches the size and developmental level of a full-term 6 month old (AAP, 1999b). Varicella vaccination is given at 1 year, unless the infant has received blood products, immune serum globulin, or varicella zoster immune globulin. In any of these cases, the vaccine should be delayed for 5 months, because the antibodies present in these preparations may interfere with the ability to mount an immunogenic response (Arvin, 1997).

The *Red Book* advises that children who have proven or suspected neurologic diagnosis should be evaluated on an individual risk-benefit basis. Family history of neurologic

TABLE 13-2. CONTRAINDICATIONS FOR CHILDHOOD IMMUNIZATION

Symptom or Condition	Vaccinate?						
	HB	DTP/DTaP	Hib	OPV	IPV	MMR	Var
Allergies							
to baker's yeast (anaphylactic)	No	Yes	Yes	Yes	Yes	Yes	Yes
to duck meat or duck feathers	Yes	Yes	Yes	Yes	Yes	Yes	Yes
to eggs (anaphylactic)	Yes	Yes	Yes	Yes	Yes	Note 1	Yes
to gelatin (anaphylactic)	Yes	Yes	Yes	Yes	Yes	Yes	No
to neomycin (anaphylactic)	Yes	Yes	Yes	Yes	No	No	No
to penicillin	Yes	Yes	Yes	Yes	Yes	Yes	Yes
to streptomycin (anaphylactic)	Yes	Yes	Yes	Yes	No	Yes	Yes
nonspecific or nonanaphylactic	Yes	Yes	Yes	Yes	Yes	Yes	Yes
in relatives	Yes	Yes	Yes	Yes	Yes	Yes	Yes
Anaphylactic (life-threatening) reaction to previous dose of vaccine			See Note 2				
Antimicrobial therapy (current)	Yes	Yes	Yes	Yes	Yes	Yes	Yes
Breast-feeding	Yes	Yes	Yes	Yes	Yes	Yes	Yes
Convalescing from illness	Yes	Yes	Yes	Yes	Yes	Yes	Yes
Convulsions (fits, seizures)							
family history (including epilepsy)—See Note 3	Yes	Yes	Yes	Yes	Yes	Yes	Yes
within 3 d of previous dose of DTP or DTaP	Yes	Note 4	Yes	Yes	Yes	Yes	Yes
Diarrhea							
mild (with or without low-grade fever)	Yes	Yes	Yes	Yes	Yes	Yes	Yes
moderate to severe (with or without fever)	No	No	No	No	No	No	No
Exposure (recent) to infectious (contagious) disease	Yes	Yes	Yes	Yes	Yes	Yes	Yes
Fever							
low-grade fever with or without mild illness	Yes	Yes	Yes	Yes	Yes	Yes	Yes
fever with moderate-to-severe illness			See Note 5				

(continues)

N/A = Not Applicable

*See "HIV infection", recommendations differ slightly for that condition.

†An acute severe central nervous system disorder, generally consisting of major alterations in consciousness, unresponsiveness, or generalized or local seizures that persist more than few hours, with failure to recover within 24 h.

§Parent or household contact who has not been vaccinated with a vaccine the child is receiving.

Note 1: Children who are allergic to eggs may be vaccinated with caution. Consult the protocols for vaccinating such people (AAP, 1997).

Note 2: Contraindicates vaccination only with vaccine to which reaction occurred. (Also see "Allergies.")

Note 3: Consider giving acetaminophen before DTP or DTaP and every 4 h thereafter for 24 h to children who have a personal or a family history of convulsions. (If underlying neurologic disorder is involved, also see "Neurologic disorders.")

Note 4: Not a contraindication, but a precaution. Consider carefully the benefits and risks of this vaccine under these circumstances. If the risks are believed to outweigh the benefits, withhold the vaccination; if the benefits are believed to outweigh the risks (for example, during an outbreak or foreign travel), give the vaccine. (If convulsions are accompanied by encephalopathy, also see "Reactions to a previous dose of DTP/DTaP." If an underlying neurologic disorder is involved, also see "Neurologic disorders.")

Note 5: Children with moderate or severe febrile illnesses can be vaccinated as soon as they are recovering and no longer acutely ill.

Note 6: MMR should be considered for all symptomatic HIV-infected children, including children with AIDS, because measles disease in these children can be severe. Limited data on MMR vaccination among both asymptomatic and symptomatic HIV-infected children indicate that MMR has not been associated with severe or unusual adverse events, although antibody responses have been unpredictable.

Note 7: Do not give immune globulin products and MMR simultaneously. If unavoidable, give at different sites and revaccinate or test for seroconversion in 3 mo. If MMR is given first, do not give IG for 2 wk. If IG is given first, the interval between IG and measles vaccination depends on the product, the dose, and the indication. (See table).

Suggested Intervals

	Months before Measles Vaccination
TIG for tetanus prophylaxis	3
IG for hepatitis A contact prophylaxis of foreign travel	3
HBIG for hepatitis B prophylaxis	3
HRIG for rabies prophylaxis	4
VZIG for varicella prophylaxis	5
IG for measles prophylaxis (normal contact)	5
IG for measles prophylaxis (immunocompromised contact)	6
Blood transfusion (red blood cells [RBCs], washed)	0
Blood transfusion (RBCs, adenine-saline added)	3
Blood transfusion (packed RBCs [Hct 65%])	6
Blood transfusion (whole blood [Hct 35%–50%])	6
Blood transfusion (plasma/platelet products)	7
Replacement therapy for humoral immune deficiencies (given as IGIV)	8
Treatment of immune thrombocytopenic purpura (400 mg/kg IV)	8
Treatment of immune thrombocytopenic purpura (100 mg/kg IV)	10
Kawasaki disease	11

For guidelines, see *J Pediatr* 1993, 122:204–11. Also see *General Recommendations on immunization: Advisory Committee on Immunization Practices*, Jan. 18, 1994, for a more detailed version of this table.

TABLE 13-2.   CONTRAINDICATIONS FOR CHILDHOOD IMMUNIZATION (Continued)

Symptom or Condition	Vaccinate?						
	HB	DTP/DTaP	Hib	OPV	IPV	MMR	Var
HIV infection							
in household contact	Yes	Yes	Yes	No	Yes	Yes	Yes
in recipient (asymptomatic)	Yes	Yes	Yes	No	Yes	Yes	No
in recipient (symptomatic)	Yes	Yes	Yes	No	Yes	Note 6	No
IG administration (intramuscular or intravenous), recent or simultaneous (see suggested intervals in table)	Yes	Yes	Yes	Yes	Yes	Note 7	Note 8
Illness							
mild acute (with or without low-grade fever)	Yes	Yes	Yes	Yes	Yes	Yes	Yes
moderate-to-severe acute (with or without fever)	No	No	No	No	No	No	No
chronic			See Note 9				
Immunodeficiency*							
family history	Yes	Yes	Yes	Note 10	Yes	Yes	Note 10
in household contact	Yes	Yes	Yes	No	Yes	Yes	Yes
in recipient (hematologic and solid tumors, congenital immunodeficiency, long-term immunosuppressive therapy, including steroids) See Note 1	Yes	Yes	Yes	No	Yes	No	No
Neurologic disorders, underlying (including seizure disorders, cerebral palsy, and developmental delay)	Yes	Note 12	Yes	Yes	Yes	Yes	Yes
Otitis media							
mild (with or without low-grade fever)	Yes	Yes	Yes	Yes	Yes	Yes	Yes
moderate to severe (with or without fever)	No	No	No	No	No	No	No
resolving	Yes	Yes	Yes	Yes	Yes	Yes	Yes
Pregnancy, mother or household contact of recipient	Yes	Yes	Yes	Yes	Yes	Yes	Yes
Prematurity			See Notes 13 & 14				

(continues)

Note 8: Do not give varicella vaccine for at least 5 mo after administration of blood (except washed red blood cells) or after plasma transfusions, IG, or VZIG. Do not give IG or VZIG for 3 wk after vaccination unless the benefits exceed those of the vaccination. In such instances, either revaccinate 5 mo later or test for immunity 6 mo later and revaccinate if seronegative.

Note 9: The great majority of children with chronic illnesses should be appropriately vaccinated. The decision whether or not to vaccinate these children, and what vaccines to give, should be made on an individual basis.

Note 10: Do not give OPV or varicella vaccine to a member of a household with a family history of immunodeficiency until the immune status of the recipient and other children in the family is documented.

Note 11: A protocol exists for use of varicella vaccine in patients with acute lymphoblastic leukemia (ALL). See *Varicella Prevention: Recommendations of the Advisory Committee on Immunization Practices.*

Note 12: Whether and when to administer DTP or DTaP to children with proven or suspected underlying neurologic disorders should be decided individually. Generally, infants and children with stable neurologic conditions, including well-controlled seizures, may be vaccinated.

Note 13: The appropriate age for initiating vaccinations in the prematurely born infant is the usual chronologic age (same dosage and indications as for normal, full-term infants).

Note 14: For hepatitis B vaccine, if the mother is antigen positive, use the vaccine schedule in which the first dose is given at birth.

Note 15: Contraindicates vaccination only with vaccine to which reaction occurred. If tetanus toxoid is contraindicated for a child who has

not completed a primary series of tetanus toxoid immunization and that a child has a wound that is neither clean nor minor, give only passive vaccination, using tetanus immune globulin (TIG).

Note 16: Not a contraindication, but consider carefully the benefits and risks of this vaccine under these circumstances. If the risks are believed to outweigh the benefits, withhold the vaccination; if the benefits are believed to outweigh the risks (for example, during an outbreak or foreign travel), give the vaccine.

Note 17: Consider giving acetaminophen before DTP or DTaP and every 4 h thereafter for 24 h to children who have a personal or a family history of convulsions.

Note 18: The decision to give additional doses of DTP/DTaP should be based on consideration of the benefit of further vaccination versus the risk of recurrence of GBS. For example, completion of the primary series in children is justified.

Note 19: There is a theoretical risk that the administration of multiple live virus vaccines (OPV, MMR, and varicella) within 30 d of one another if not given on the same day will result in a suboptimal immune response. There are no data to substantiate this with current vaccines.

Note 20: Consider the benefits of immunity to measles, mumps, and rubella versus the risk of recurrence or exacerbation of thrombocytopenia after vaccination or risk from natural infections of measles or rubella. In most instances, the benefits of vaccination will be much greater than the potential risks and will justify giving MMR, particularly in view of the even greater risk of thrombocytopenia following measles or rubella disease. However, if a prior episode of thrombocytopenia occurred near the time of vaccination, it might be prudent to avoid a subsequent dose.

TABLE 13-2.   CONTRAINDICATIONS FOR CHILDHOOD IMMUNIZATION *(Continued)*

Symptom or Condition	Vaccinate?						
	HB	DTP/DTaP	Hib	OPV	IPV	MMR	Var
Reactions to a previous dose of any vaccine							
anaphylactic (life-threatening)—See Note 15	No	No	No	No	No	No	No
local (mild-to-moderate soreness, redness, swelling)	Yes	Yes	Yes	Yes	Yes	Yes	Yes
Reactions to previous dose of DTP/DTaP							
collapse or shocklike state within 48 h of dose	N/A	Note 16	N/A	N/A	N/A	N/A	N/A
persistent, inconsolable crying lasting for 3 or more h, occurring within 48 h of dose	N/A	Note 16	N/A	N/A	N/A	N/A	N/A
encephalopathy† within 7 d after dose	N/A	No	N/A	N/A	N/A	N/A	N/A
family history of any adverse event after dose	N/A	Note 17	N/A	N/A	N/A	N/A	N/A
fever of <40.5°C (105°F) within 48 h after a dose	N/A	Note 17	N/A	N/A	N/A	N/A	N/A
fever of ≥40.5°C (105°F) within 48 h after a dose	N/A	Notes 16 & 17	N/A	N/A	N/A	N/A	N/A
Guillain-Barré syndrome (GBS) within 6 wk after a dose	N/A	Note 18	N/A	N/A	N/A	N/A	N/A
seizures within 3 d after a dose	N/A	Notes 16 & 17	N/A	N/A	N/A	N/A	N/A
Simultaneous administration of vaccines See Note 19	Yes	Yes	Yes	Yes	Yes	Yes	Yes
Sudden infant death syndrome (SIDS), family history	Yes	Yes	Yes	Yes	Yes	Yes	Yes
Thrombocytopenia	Yes	Yes	Yes	Yes	Yes	Note 20	Yes
Thrombocytopenia purpura (history)	Yes	Yes	Yes	Yes	Yes	Note 20	Yes
Tuberculin skin testing, performed simultaneously with vaccination	Yes	Yes	Yes	Yes	Yes	Note 21	Yes
Tuberculosis (TB) or positive PPD	Yes	Yes	Yes	Yes	Yes	Yes	Yes
Unvaccinated household contact§—See Note 22	Yes	Yes	Yes	Yes	Yes	Yes	Yes
Vomiting							
mild (with or without low-grade fever) See Note 23	Yes	Yes	Yes	Yes	Yes	Yes	Yes
moderate to severe (with or without fever) See Note 23	No	No	No	No	No	No	No

Note 21: Measles vaccination may temporarily suppress tuberculin reactivity. MMR vaccine may be given after, or on the same day as, TB testing. If MMR has been given recently, postpone the TB test until 4–6 wk after administration of MMR. If giving MMR simultaneously with tuberculin skin test, use the Mantoux test, not multiple puncture tests, because the latter, if results are positive, require confirmation (and confirmation would then have to be postponed 4–6 wk).

Note 22: If the parent or other adult household contact of a child receiving OPV has never received polio vaccine, this person should consider being vaccinated with IPV before or at the same time as the child. Vaccination of the child should not be delayed.

Note 23: *Vomiting and OPV.* Infants sometimes do not swallow OPV. If, in the judgment of the vaccinator, a substantial amount of the vaccine is spit out or vomited within 5–10 min after administration, another dose can be given at the same visit. If this repeat dose is not retained, neither dose should be counted, and the vaccine should be readministered at the next visit.

Used with permission.

disease in itself is not a true contraindication to immunization.

▲ **Clinical Warning:** Infants with evolving neurologic disorders should not be given pertussis vaccine. Pediatric DT is given to these children until evaluation or treatment is completed.

Increasing parental participation in health care decision making can improve immunization goals. Additionally, providers must avoid assuming that a child is not at risk for underimmunization because of parental affluence or insurance coverage. Attitudes such as "trusting" the family to return for immunizations later need to be reexamined due to their potential to compound missed opportunities and impact financial resources.

The Clinical Assessment Software Application (CASA) developed by the CDC may assist providers with identifying the needs of their individual practices. Studies show providers consistently overestimate their patients' immunization levels (Bordley, Margolis, & Lannon, 1996; Bushnell, 1994; Szilagyi & Rodewald, et al., 1994). CASA is available through and administered by local health departments. This program takes approximately 4 hours to complete. Providers are given a report summarizing the immunization status of their patients based on random chart audits. A provider must participate in VFC to be eligible to use CASA software.

▲ **Clinical Warning:** Immunization coverage in the United States has improved dramatically in the 1990s. The job is not finished. Providers must continue to promote immunization for all children to ensure that epidemics of diseases such as polio, meningitis, and measles do not recur.

Primary care providers must take advantage of every opportunity to vaccinate children, coordinate efforts into integrated delivery systems, and reduce policy and procedural barriers to immunization. The availability of immunizations to every eligible child should be evident at each encounter with the health care system.

COMMUNITY AND PROFESSIONAL RESOURCES

The *Red Book* is updated approximately every 3 years. The journal *Pediatrics* publishes updated statements developed by the COID and approved by the AAP between editions of the *Red Book*, often in the January issue. The COID is composed of 12 pediatricians and liaisons from the CDC, the FDA, and the National Institutes of Health. This committee establishes vaccine recommendations, schedules, indications, and contraindications.

The other major influence regarding pediatric immunization comes from the ACIP, which advises the CDC. The ACIP consists of 10 experts in pediatrics, family medicine, infectious diseases, public health, vaccine research, and internal medicine, including representatives from the AAP and the American Academy of Family Physicians (AAFP). The ACIP also establishes preferred immunization schedules, indications and contraindications, and disease prevention strategies. Current ACIP guidelines can be found on the Internet at *http://www.cdc.gov/nip* or through the AAP at *http://www.AAP.org*. As they are updated, the ACIP guidelines are published periodically in the Morbidity and Mortality Weekly Report. Recently the ACIP, AAP (reflecting the recommendations of the COID), and the AAFP have coordinated recommended immunization schedules to minimize confusion and maximize the impact of new recommendations (Rodewald, 1999). This "harmonized" schedule reflects allowable differences regarding scheduling of immunizations, enabling offices to incorporate immunizations into individual office routines. It is necessary for each provider to check continually recommended delivery schedules because these are frequently changed and updated, reflecting new policies and recommendations. Up-to-date schedules can be found on the Internet at the AAP home page *http://www.AAP.org*.

The manufacturer and two federal agencies, the FDA's Center for Biologics Evaluation and Research and the CDC, assure safety of vaccines. Information can be obtained on the Internet at *http://www.fda.gov./cber*. This site also contains the appropriate forms for reporting adverse events through the Vaccine Adverse Event Reporting System, a surveillance system jointly administered by the FDA and the CDC. Events that providers are required to report are summarized in Table 13-3. Forms also are found at *http://www.cdc.gov/nip*; additionally, reports may be made by phone at 1-800-822-7967. Reporting an adverse event does not affect provider

Table 13-3.   REPORTABLE EVENTS FOLLOWING VACCINATION*

Vaccine/Toxoid	Event	Interval From Vaccination
Tetanus in any combination; DTaP, DTP, DTP-HiB, DT, Td, TT	A. Anaphylaxis or anaphylactic shock	7 d
	B. Brachial neuritis	28 d
	C. Any sequela (including death) of above	No limit
	D. Events described in manufacturer's package events insert as contraindications to additional doses of vaccine	See package insert
Pertussis in any combination; DTaP, DTP, DTP-HiB, P	A. Anaphylaxis or anaphylactic shock	7 d
	B. Encephalopathy (or encephalitis)	7 d
	C. Any sequela (including death) of above events	No limit
	D. Events described in manufacturer's package insert as contraindications to additional doses of vaccine	See package insert
Measles, mumps and rubella in any combination; MMR, MR, M, R	A. Anaphylaxis or anaphylactic shock	7 d
	B. Encephalopathy (or encephalitis)	15 d
	C. Any sequela (including death) of above events	No limit
	D. Events described in manufacturer's package insert as contraindications to additional doses of vaccine	See package insert
Rubella in any combination; MMR, MR, R	A. Chronic arthritis	42 d
	B. Any sequela (including death) of above events	No limit
	C. Events described in manufacturer's package insert as contraindications to additional doses of vaccine	See package insert
Measles in any combination; MMR, MR, M	A. Thrombocytopenic purpura	30 d
	B. Vaccine-strain measles viral infection in an immunodeficient recipient	6 mo
	C. Any sequela (including death) of above events	No limit
	D. Events described in manufacturer's package insert as contraindications to additional doses of vaccine	See package insert

*Effective March 24, 1997.
   These events are reportable by law to the Vaccine Adverse Event Reporting System (VAERS). In addition, individuals are encouraged to report any clinically significant or unexpected events (even if uncertain whether the vaccine caused the event) for any vaccine, whether or not it is listed in the table. Manufacturers also are required to report to the VAERS program all adverse events made known to them for any vaccine.
   Source: AAP American Academy of Pediatrics. (1997). G. Peter (Ed.). *Red book: Report of the committee on infectious diseases* (24th ed.). Elk Grove Village, IL: Author. Used with permission.

liability. Liability protection is provided by the National Childhood Vaccine Injury Act of 1986 through the Vaccine Injury Compensation Program.

Other sites of interest include information on recommended vaccines for travel, found at *http://www.cdc.gov/travel*, in the *Red Book* (1997), or through the CDC at 1-404-332-4559.

REFERENCES

Altemeier, W. A. (1998). Immunization rates: Where is the help when we need it? *Pediatric Annals, 27*(7), 325–327.

Advisory Committee for Immunization Practices (ACIP). (1999). Press release: ACIP votes for injected polio for all immunizations anticipated in 2000. *AAP News Release, June 17th.*

American Academy of Pediatrics. (1997). *Red book: Report of the committee on infectious diseases* (24th ed.). Elk Grove Village, IL: Author.

American Academy of Pediatrics. (1999a). Press Release: AAP issues public health advisory. *AAP News Release. July 15th.*

American Academy of Pediatrics. (1999b). Press release: AAP addresses FDA review of vaccines. Use of hepatitis B vaccines—Q & A. *AAP News Release, July 14th.*

Arvin, A. (1997). Live attenuated varicella vaccine. *Pediatric Annals, 26*, 384–388.

Bates, A. S., Fitzgerald, J. F., Dittus, R. S., & Wolinsky, F. D., (1994). Risk factors for underimmunization in poor urban infants. *Journal of the American Medical Association, 272*(14), 1105-1110.

Belshe, R. B., Mendelman, P. M., Treanor, J., King, J., Gruber, W. C., Piedra, P., Bernstein, D. I., Hayden, F. G., Kotloff, K., Zangwill, K., Iacuzio, D., & Wolff, M. (1998). The efficacy of live attenuated, cold-adapted, trivalent, intranasal influenzavirus vaccine in children. *New England Journal of Medicine, 338*(20), 1405–1412.

Black, S., & Shinefield, H. (1999). *A prospective study of conjugated pneumococcal vaccine in children.* Presentation at the Pediatric Academic Societies Meeting, San Francisco.

Bordley, W., Margolis, P., & Lannon, C. (1996). The delivery of immunizations and other preventive services in private practices. *Pediatrics, 97*, 467–473.

Bushnell, C. (1994). *The ABC's of practice-based immunization assessments. Proceedings of the 28th National Immunization Conference 1994* (pp. 207–209). Washington, DC: U.S. Department of Health and Human Services.

Centers for Disease Control and Prevention. (1994). Vaccines for children program, 1994, and impact of missed opportunities to vaccinate preschool-aged children on vaccination coverage levels-Selected U.S. sites 1991-1992. *Morbidity and Mortality Weekly Report, 43*(39), 705–718.

Fielding, J. E., Cumberland, W. G., & Pettitt, L., (1994). Immunization status of children of employees in a large corporation. *Journal of the American Medical Association, 271*(7), 525–530.

Fischbach, F. T. (1996). *A manual of laboratory and diagnostic tests* (5th ed.). Philadelphia: Lippincott-Raven.

Guyer, B., & Hughart, N. (1994). Increasing childhood immunization coverage by improving the effectiveness of primary health care systems for children. *Archives of Pediatric and Adolescent Medicine, 148*, 901–902.

Harrison, L. H., Dwyer, D. M., Maples, C. T., & Billmann, L. (1999). Risk of meningococcal infection in college students. *Journal of the American Medical Association, 281*(20), 1906–1909.

Linkins, R. W., & Feikema, S. M. (1998). Immunization registries: The cornerstone of childhood immunization in the 21st century. *Pediatric Annals, 27*(6), 349–354.

Lukes, E. (1995). Childhood immunizations: An update for occupational health nurses. *AAOHN Journal, 43*(12), 622–626.

Orenstein, W. A., Atkinson, W., Mason, D., & Bernier, R. H. (1990). Barriers to vaccinating preschool children. *Journal of Health Care for the Poor and Underserved, 1*(3), 315–330.

Plotkin, S. L., & Plotkin, S. A. (1994). A short history of vaccination. In S. A. Plotkin & E. A. Mortimer (Eds.), *Vaccines* (pp. 1–12). Philadelphia: W.B. Saunders.

Rodewald, L. E. (1999). Childhood immunizations. In R. A. Dershewitz (Ed.), *Ambulatory pediatric care* (3rd ed.). Philadelphia: Lippincott-Raven.

Salsberry, P. J., Nickel, J. T., & Mitch, R. (1994). Immunization status of 2 year-olds in middle/uppper and lower-income populations: A community survey. *Public Health Nursing, 11*(1), 17–23.

Shefer, A., & Mize, J. (1998). Primary care providers and WIC: Improving immunization coverage among high-risk children. *Pediatric Annals, 27*(7), 428–433.

Sigal, L. H., Zahradnik, J. M., Lavin, P., Patella, S. J., Bryant, G., Haselby, R., Hilton, E., Kunkel, M., Adler-Klein, D., Doherty, T., Evans, J., & Malawista, S. E. (1998). A vaccine consisting of recombinant *Borrelia burgdorferi* outer-surface protein A to prevent Lyme disease. *New England Journal of Medicine, 339*(4), 216–222.

Steere, A. C., Sikand, V. K., Meurice, F., Parenti, D. L., Fikrig, E., Schoen, R. T., Nowakowski, J., Schmid, C. H., Laukamp, S., Buscarino, C., & Krause, D. S. (1998). Vaccination against Lyme disease with recombinant *Borrelia burgdorferi* outer-surface lipoprotein A with adjuvant. *New England Journal of Medicine, 339*(4), 209–215.

Szilagyi, P. G., Rodewald, L. E., Humiston, S. G., Hager, J., Roghmann, K. J., Doane, C., Cove, L., Fleming, G. V., & Hall, C. B. (1994). Immunization practices of pediatricians and family physicians in the United States. *Pediatrics, 94*(4), 517–523.

Szilagyi, P. G., Roghmann, K., Campbell, J., Humiston, S., Winter, N., Raubetas, R., & Rodewald, L. (1994). Immunization practices of primary care practitioners and their relation to immunization levels. *Archives of Pediatric and Adolescent Medicine, 148*, 158–166.

The National Vaccine Advisory Committee. (1991). The measles epidemic: The problems, barriers, and recommendations. *Journal of the American Medical Association, 226*(11), 1547-1552.

CHAPTER 14

The Child Athlete: Preparticipation Screening and Common Issues

• KEITH REINSDORF, MD, and DENNIS CARDONE, DO

INTRODUCTION

The 21st century athlete encounters a vast array of options and information unavailable even a few short years ago. Knowledge in the areas of strength training, sports nutrition, and sports psychology is increasing. Common medical conditions, clearance issues, the use of anabolic steroids, the role of weather conditions in training, eating disorders, and problems unique to the female athlete are addressed in an effort to promote provider awareness and ultimately the healthy growth and development of the child athlete.

The child or adolescent intent on participating in athletics should undergo a preparticipation history and physical evaluation. This will enable the provider to determine the patient's general health status and to screen for any conditions that may limit participation or put the patient at risk for injury or sudden death. This encounter also establishes a relationship that will help address any problems should they arise over the course of athletic involvement. The examination of patients younger than 18 years should include parental input, because often children's versions of their history will differ from that provided by parents (Bratton & Agerter, 1995). Featured components of the preparticipation evaluation (PPE) include the patient's cardiopulmonary and injury histories in addition to a comprehensive orthopedic evaluation and assessment of the child's growth and development (Display 14-1) (Smith, Kovan, Rich, & Tanner, 1998). This evaluation is not a well child visit, nor is it meant to be exclusive of the components that constitute a general medical history and physical examination. The aim of providers is to assess a patient's ability to participate in a sport with only limited risk.

● **Clinical Pearl:** The ultimate goal is not to screen the patient with the idea of finding cause to exclude the individual from play, but rather to suggest more appropriate sports if indicated by the individual's presentation (Andrews, 1997).

Most patients will derive numerous benefits from athletics; thus, it is part of the provider's role to help the patient remain active. Table 14-1 provides a classification of sports according to their degree of contact and activity intensity. Fortunately, only about 1% of PPEs result in denied clearance. Roughly 10% of those visits require further evaluation (Bratton & Agerter, 1995).

EPIDEMIOLOGY

While many factors affect a patient's ability to participate in athletics, certain common conditions require familiarity

from primary care providers, because they often lead to questions regarding clearance to play. In addition, suggested guidelines exist for many conditions in terms of athletic participation (Appendix 14-1). Regardless of the illness, the provider must view each patient individually, including whenever possible parents, coaches, and athletic trainers who will be monitoring the child's well-being while he or she participates in the chosen sport.

An increase in physical activity leads to an increased demand on the cardiopulmonary system and can be associated with potential limitations. Hypertrophic cardiomyopathy, with a prevalence of 0.1% to 0.2%, is the leading cause of sudden cardiac death in athletes younger than 30 years and requires patients to restrict themselves to low-intensity athletics (Safran, McKeag, & Van Camp, 1998). Hypertension, as diagnosed by three separate elevated readings on separate occasions, varies according to criteria for each age group and is relatively uncommon in children. This condition generally results in limitation only if severe or associated with extensive secondary illness (Table 14-2).

Valvular disease and arrhythmias, while not uncommon, generally do not result in significant limitation unless they are seen together or cause symptoms. Mitral valve prolapse, present in about 5% of the population, can have associated exercise limitations, depending on family history, associated symptoms, and degree of regurgitation.

Individuals with Marfan syndrome should not participate in contact or collision sports but are otherwise cleared if they do not have aortic root dilation, mitral reguritation, or a family history of early sudden death. Monitoring of the aortic root dimensions every 6 months is recommended.

Patients with seizure disorders are allowed to participate in all sports as long as medication well controls their condition. High-risk sports, such as skiing, diving, swimming, auto racing, and high bar gymnastics, most likely should involve consultation with a neurologist. Athletes who suffer a concussion, a transient loss of consciousness with amnesia, are treated individually. Tables 14-3 and 14-4 discuss the initial management of concussion and guidelines for when to return to play (Quality Standards Subcommittee, 1997). Two certainties in concussion management are that patients with prolonged symptoms (ie, longer than 1 or 2 weeks) necessitate a workup and that all patients must be withheld from activity while they are symptomatic to prevent potentially fatal "second impact syndrome."

Exercise-induced bronchospasm, ranging in prevalence from 10% to 40% of the general population, is an extremely common problem. The use of peak flow meters and knowledge of exacerbating factors are critical to management. Diabetes mellitus, unless poorly controlled, is not a contraindication to exercise. Patients who have had the disease for at least 10 years, however, warrant close evaluation and follow-up, because they are more likely to experience complications (Fields & Fricker, 1997). Sickle

DISPLAY 14–1 • Standard Components of the Preparticipation Evaluation

Height
Weight
Eyes
   Visual acuity (Snellen chart)
   Differences in pupil size
Oral cavity
Ears
Nose
Lungs
Cardiovascular system
   Blood pressure
   Pulses (radial, femoral)
   Heart (rate, rhythm, murmurs)
Abdomen
   Masses
   Tenderness
   Organomegaly
Genitalia (males only)
   Single or undescended testicle
   Testicular mass
   Hernia
Skin
   Rashes
   Lesions
Musculoskeletal system
   Contour, range of motion, stability, and symmetry of neck, back, shoulder/arm, elbow/forearm, wrist/hand, hip/thigh, knee, leg/ankle, foot

Reprinted with permission from Smith, D. S., Kovan, J., Rich, B., & Tanner, S. (1998). *The physician and sports medicine* (2nd ed.). Minneapolis, MN: McGraw-Hill Healthcare.

cell trait, which has been associated with exertional rhabdomyolysis and heat illness, also is not a contraindication to athletic participation.

Acute viral illness of the upper respiratory tract is perhaps the most common condition seen by the primary care provider, with the average child affected as often as 10 to 12 times per year. Patients often are able to continue to participate unless fever, tachycardia, or other systemic signs are present. Patients with fever must be withheld from participation due to the increased likelihood of heat illness and the possibility of a potentially fatal myocarditis.

Infectious mononucleosis, with an attack rate of approximately 3% to 5% (Richmond & Shahady, 1996) of adolescents per year, requires that patients be restricted from activity for at least 3 weeks and 4 weeks if the patient is involved in a contact sport. This allows for resolution of any splenomegaly, which examination may not always detect. Patients with human immunodeficiency virus (HIV) must be viewed individually in terms of their general health and sport of interest. HIV alone is not a contraindication for any sport; however, sports such as boxing, football, soccer, wrestling, and rugby, where risk of exposure is high, should be viewed with more caution.

Common conditions in children and adolescents, such as Osgood-Schlatter disease and Sever's disease, are viewed in the same manner as acute sprains or strains. That is, clearance should be withheld if signs of inflammation, decreased range of motion, instability, or strength less than 85% relative to the unaffected side are present (Smith et al., 1998). Stress and avulsion fractures are more commonly seen in children than in adults. It is important to note that knee pain in children often is due to hip disease. A thorough examination can visually differentiate the etiology of symptoms.

Table 14-1. CLASSIFICATION OF SPORTS

Contact		Noncontact		
Contact/ Collision	Limited Contact/Impact	*Strenuous*	*Moderately Strenuous*	*Nonstrenuous*
Boxing	Baseball	Aerobic dancing	Badminton	Archery
Field hockey	Basketball	Crew	Curling	Golf
Football	Bicycling	Fencing	Table tennis	Riflery
Ice hockey	Diving	Field		
Lacrosse	Field	discus		
Martial arts	high jump	javelin		
Rodeo	pole vault	shot put		
Soccer	Gymnastics	Running		
Wrestling	Horseback riding	Swimming		
	Skating	Tennis		
	ice	Track		
	roller	Weight lifting		
	Skiing			
	cross-country			
	downhill			
	water			
	Softball			
	Squash, handball			
	Volleyball			

Reprinted with permission of Safron, M., McKeag, D., & Van Camp, S. (1998). *Manual of sports medicine.* Philadelphia: Lippincott-Raven.

TABLE 14-2.   CLASSIFICATION OF HYPERTENSION BY AGE

Age Group (y)	Significant Hypertension (mmHg)	Severe Hypertension (mmHg)
Children (6–9)	Systolic BP ≥122	Systolic BP ≥130
	Diastolic BP ≥78	Diastolic BP ≥86
Children (10–12)	Systolic BP ≥126	Systolic BP ≥134
	Diastolic BP ≥82	Diastolic BP ≥90
Adolescents (13–15)	Systolic BP ≥136	Systolic BP ≥144
	Diastolic BP ≥86	Diastolic BP ≥92
Adolescents (16–18)	Systolic BP ≥142	Systolic BP ≥150
	Diastolic BP ≥92	Diastolic BP ≥98

Reprinted with permission from Record of the Second Task Force on Blood Pressure Control in Children—*1987*: Task Force on Blood Pressure Control in Children; National Heart, Lung, and Blood Institute, Bethesda, Maryland; *Pediatrics* 1987:79(1):1–25.

HISTORY AND PHYSICAL EXAMINATION: THE PREPARTICIPATION EVALUATION

The primary goal of the PPE is to help promote safe participation in an activity that is enjoyable and suitable to the patient so that the patient can reap the many benefits that athletic involvement offers. The PPE should occur yearly in individuals younger than 18 years due to the relatively rapid and significant physical changes that occur during childhood and adolescence. Also, the evaluation should occur 1 month before the sport season starts so that any issues that arise can be addressed without the athlete having to miss much time from the sport. While one of the objectives is to determine general health, the PPE is not a substitute for a well child examination or vice versa. The PPE and the well child visit can be combined in one visit, however, if proper time is allotted.

The PPE is perhaps best completed in the primary care provider's office to foster confidentiality and disclosure of any private concerns. This can help maintain continuity of a therapeutic provider–patient relationship. Hopefully, the provider will be familiar with current PPE recommendations and clearance issues. In individuals younger than 18 years, parental input is encouraged regarding history taking, but certain sensitive issues may cause problems regarding confidentiality. Most states require that each child undergo a PPE

prior to each school year. This results in a large number of individuals needing to be evaluated at the same time. Station-based examinations are suitable for mass screening and often occur at local high schools and middle schools before the school year begins.

▲ **Clinical Warning:** One unfortunate disadvantage of station-based examinations is a relative loss of privacy and possible nondisclosure of more sensitive concerns.

States and governing bodies (the NCAA and United States Olympic Committee) have rules and regulations concerning the frequency of PPEs and allowable pharmaceuticals of which the provider needs to be aware to avoid inadvertently disqualifying an athlete. Please see Appendix 14-2, which has been endorsed by the American Academy of Family Physicians (AAFP), the American Academy of Pediatrics (AAP), the American Medical Society of Sports Medicine, the American Orthopedic Society for Sports Medicine, and the American Osteopathic Academy of Sports Medicine as a comprehensive preparticipation screening evaluation (Smith et al., 1998). Many major universities and athletic institutions also have adopted this sample for the screening of their athletes.

It is important to recognize that routine history and physical examination will never detect certain life-threatening conditions, such as idiopathic hypertrophic subaortic steno-

Table 14-3.   INITIAL MANAGEMENT FOLLOWING A FIRST CONCUSSION

Grade	On-Site Evaluation	Neurologic Evaluation	Same-Day Return to Play
Grade 1	Yes	Not required, but may be pursued depending on clinical evaluation	Yes, if normal sideline assessment while at rest and with exertion, including detailed mental status examination
Grade 2	Yes	Yes	No
Grade 3	Yes	Yes	No

(1997). Summary statement: Concussion in sports. *Neurology, 48*, 584.

TABLE 14-4.   WHEN TO RETURN TO PLAY AFTER CONCUSSION

Grade of Concussion	Time Until Return to Play*
Multiple grade 1 concussion	1 wk
Grade 2 concussion	1 wk
Multiple grade 2 concussions	2 wk
Grade 3—brief loss of consciousness (seconds)	1 wk
Grade 3—prolonged loss of consciousness (minutes)	2 wk
Multiple grade 3 concussions	1 mo or longer, based on clinical decision of evaluating physician

*Only after being asymptomatic with normal neurologic assessment at rest and with exercise.
(1997). Summary statement: Concussion in sports. *Neurology, 48*, 584.

sis, prolonged QT syndrome, or anomalous coronary artery syndrome. Only further investigation, such as with a 2-D echocardiogram or electrocardiogram (ECG), may identify these conditions.

History

At least 70% of potential problems are uncovered during the history, which is designed to screen for conditions that might lead to injury or death due to sports participation (Bratton & Agerter, 1995). The history must be reviewed with the child's parents to help prevent the omission of potentially significant information. The history consists mainly of questions pertaining to the cardiopulmonary, musculoskeletal, and neurologic systems. Also, questions regarding history of heat illness; drug, medication, or supplement usage; and chronic or congenital medical conditions are included. Appendix 14-2 provides a suggested history in further detail. This is adapted from the PPE monograph put forth by Smith et al. in 1998.

Physical Examination

The physical examination is similar to a general examination, with attention paid to blood pressure and the cardiopulmonary and musculoskeletal systems in particular. It is suggested that children with mild to moderate elevations of blood pressure be rechecked and, if cleared, followed up during the season. Elevations in blood pressure can be a sign of drug and supplement usage, especially with products that enhance the sympathic nervous system (weight loss products).

The cardiac examination focuses on the detection of murmurs and irregular rhythms. All diastolic murmurs are abnormal, and the systolic murmur of IHSS increases in intensity with maneuvers that decrease venous return (eg, standing, Valsalva's maneuver). Irregular heartbeats warrant ECG evaluation, and the provider must ask about recent viral infections due to the possibility of a potentially fatal myocarditis.

A thorough musculoskeletal examination involves the 14-step screening examination (Fig. 14-1), which takes no longer than 2 minutes to administer. It also should include sports-specific evaluations of the knee for football and soccer players, the shoulder for swimmers and baseball pitchers, and the ankle, which is heavily involved in almost all sports. Examining the ears of swimmers for chronic otitis externa and the skin of wrestlers for rashes (ie, herpes gladiatorum) is helpful not only to treat the patient, but also to promote disease prevention. No evidence supports obtaining routine blood or urine specimens for analysis during the PPE (Smith et al., 1998).

ANTICIPATORY GUIDANCE

Common Questions

The following are common questions asked of providers:

What aspect of participation should the coach emphasize?
- While teaching proper techniques and strategy is important, the coach should emphasize having fun and learning to function as a member of a team. Admittedly, winning does contribute to the enjoyment; however, it must remain a secondary goal for young athletes to foster an environment for children and their families to grow together and develop positive self-esteem. Table 14-5 and Display 14-2 refer to the behavioral goals of sports participation in childhood and adolescence (Mellion, 1999; Smith & Stanitski, 1987).

What is my role as a parent?
- The parent's role is to support and love the child both when he or she succeeds and stumbles. Parents should not be a source of stress but rather a source of comfort. The child, not the parent, should determine exactly how important it is to participate or succeed.

What if I am also the coach?
- The only thing different from above is that the coach is responsible for teaching the techniques and strategies. Blanket criticism can be very damaging to a child's self-esteem. Praise should be commensurate with the achievement and in the same nature as that given to the participants who are not the coach's child.

▲ **Clinical Warning:** Criticism should focus on the specific effort made or skill demonstrated.

How are youth sports organized into different levels of participation?
- Because individuals mature at different rates and girls generally enter puberty before boys, organization should be based on parameters such as weight and Tanner's stages rather than age (Mellion, 1999). Most sports involving contact use some combination of age and physical growth to determine which level of participation is appropriate for a child. It should be noted that there does not seem to be any evidence that shows organization based on age alone leads to higher injury rates among participants. However, there has been debate regarding boxing and trampoline usage (Mellion, 1999). The American Medical Association, AAFP, and AAP have all issued statements opposing boxing

Figure 14–1 ■ The general musculoskeletal screening examination consists of the following: (1) Inspection, athlete standing, facing toward examiner (symmetry of trunk, upper extremities); (2) Forward flexion, extension, rotation, lateral flexion of neck (range of motion, cervical spine); (3) Resisted shoulder shrug (strength, trapezius); (4) Resisted shoulder abduction (strength, deltoid); (5) Internal and external rotation of shoulder (range of motion, glomerular joint); (6) Extension and flexion of elbow (range of motion, elbow, and wrist); (7) Pronation and supination of elbow (range of motion, elbow and wrist); (8) Clench fist, then spread fingers (range of motion, hand and fingers); (9) Inspection, athlete facing away from examiner (symmetry of trunk, upper extremities); (10) Back extension, knees straight (spondylolysis/spondylolisthesis); (11) Back flexion with knees straight, facing toward and away from examiner (range of motion, thoracic, and lumbosacral spine; spine curvature; hamstring flexibility); (12) Inspection of lower extremities, contraction of quadriceps muscles (alignment, symmetry); (13) "Duck walk" four steps (motion of hip, knee, and ankle; strength; balance); (14) Standing on toes, then on heels (symmetry, calf; strength; balance). Adapted from Smith, D. S., Kovan, J., Rich, B., & Tanner, S. The Physician and Sports Medicine (2nd ed.). McGraw-Hill Healthcare, p. 22, figure 1.

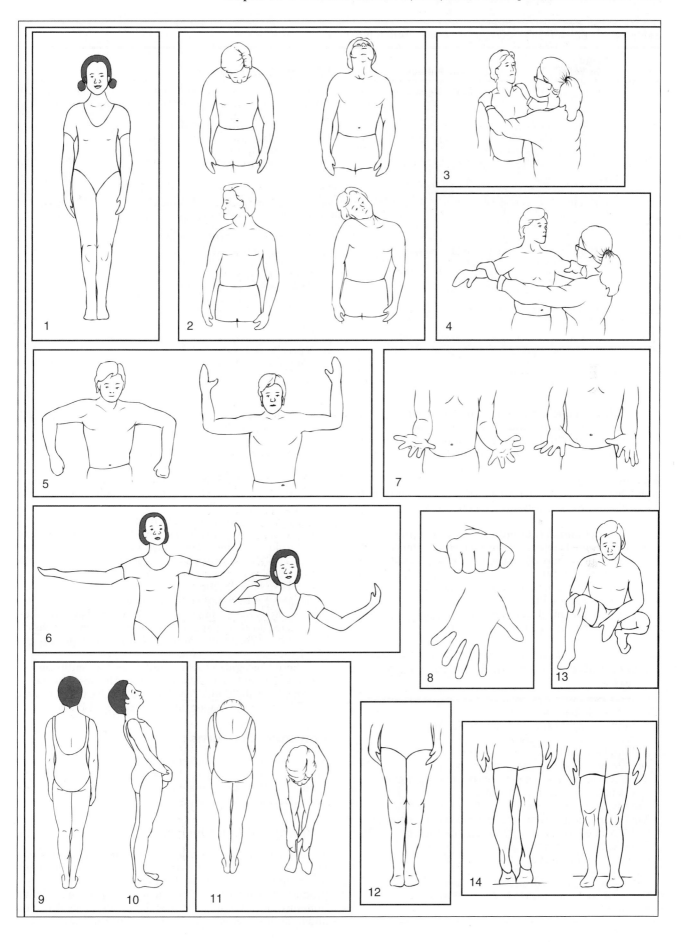

Table 14–5.   BEHAVIORAL GOALS OF SPORTS PARTICIPATION

	Age in Years	Characteristic Behavior	Behavior's Contribution
C H I L D H O O D	6–12	Age of social comparison	Fun, friends, skills; knowledge of sports, rules, and cooperation. Low-keyed introduction to competition: winning and losing avoided or minimized.
A D O L E S C E N C E	12–15	Stage of body awareness	Fun: Test new and changing physiques Confidence in new body
	15–18	Stage of sexual identity	Fun: Sexual identity enhanced Group identification Peer acceptance Enhanced self-image Pursuit of excellence
	18–21	Stage of separation	Fun: Experience separation from team and coach Limelight of sport Pursuit of excellence

for children due to a preserved high risk of head injury and chronic brain damage. The inconsistency in this argument is that the same position has not been taken on football, hockey, or the martial arts.

▲ **Clinical Warning:** Trampoline usage should occur only with trained instructors. The trampoline should be secured in a locked place when supervisors are not present.

Is strength training safe and productive for children?
- Yes, provided certain criteria are met, as outlined by the American Orthopedic Society for Sports Medicine and the National Strength Coaches Association. They include but are not limited to the following:
  - The need for a PPE
  - The requirement that the child have adequate emotional maturity to accept coaching
  - Supervision by competent coaches trained in strength training for the age group
  - Adequate warm up and cool down
  - No lifting to obtain the individual's maximum single repetition capacity ("maxing out")
  - Limiting strength training to three focused 30-minute sessions per week to help ensure adequate rest and recovery

Are young children more likely to get hurt?
- Actually younger children have far fewer injuries than do older children. The injury rate increases with age until high school. This is most likely due to older children being bigger, faster, stronger, and involved in more intense physical contact.

Do girls get hurt more often than boys?
- No. Boys have a higher total injury rate, believed to be related to their participation in more contact-collision sports. When boys and girls compete together, the injury rates are the same.

Is there a recognized set of guidelines for youth sports?
- Yes. The Bill of Rights for Young Athletes was developed by the American Alliance for Health, Physical Education, Recreation, and Dance (see Display 14-2).

Common Concerns

Some common issues in sports medicine include environmental effects on activity, performance-enchancing drugs, nutrition, eating disorders, menstrual disorders, and stress and performance anxiety.

Activity and Environment

Weather conditions play a large role in the individual's athletic performance. Heat illness, which ranges from relatively benign muscle cramps to heat stroke and possibly death, is a product of many factors. The ambient temperature, relative humidity, and the athlete's overall fitness, general health, and hydration status all play significant roles. The American

---

DISPLAY 14–2 • The Bill of Rights for Young Athletes

Right to participate in sports
Right to participate at a level commensurate with each child's maturity and ability
Right to have qualified adult leadership
Right to play as a child and not as an adult
Right of children to share in the leadership and decision making of their sport participation
Right to participate in safe and healthy environments
Right to proper preparation for participation in sports
Right to an equal opportunity to strive for success
Right to be treated with dignity
Right to have fun in sports

Reprinted with permission of the American Alliance, for Health, Physical Education, Recreation and Dance, 1990 Association Drive, Reston, VA 22091.

College of Sports Medicine (ACSM) recommends that runners participating in summer events replace their fluid loss with roughly 150 to 300 mL of both water and electrolyte-rich sport drinks every 15 minutes while competing (ACSM, 1996). It is recommended that summer events should occur in the morning or late afternoon to minimize heat exposure, while winter events are better scheduled for mid-day. Running in cooler, dryer air can exacerbate exercise-induced bronchospasm, and cold exposure also can lead to exacerbation of Raynaud's phenomenon, urticaria, frostbite, and hypothermia. Certainly, participants should be instructed to dress in removable layers of clothing and to remove any wet clothing. Rewarming is best accomplished in a controlled environment to prevent refreezing.

Performance-Enhancing Substances

The use of anabolic steroids, human growth hormone, erythropoietin, insulin growth factor-1, human chorionic gonadotropin, and amphetamines to enhance athletic performance is condemned for all individuals due to the various and significant adverse effects associated with them. Health care providers must emphasize that whatever apparent benefit may be gained by their use is far outweighed by the host of potential negative effects. This message should be conveyed whenever possible to parents, coaches, and athletes who, especially at the high school level, are exposed to significant rewards for "being the best." The use of creatine is widespread among athletes, even at the high school level and has been shown to enhance performance and recovery in high-intensity exercise. One limited study suggests that there are no adverse effects on kidney function in previously healthy individuals for up to 5 years (Poortmans & Francaux, 1999).

▲ **Clinical Warning:** There are no known adverse effects with short-term supplementation with creatine; little is known regarding the effects of long-term supplementation (Safran et al., 1998).

Nutrition

Various theories abound regarding optimum nutrition for both athletes and nonathletes. It clearly is best that all children have a balanced diet, (50% carbohydrate, 20% protein) and that children and their families should limit fat intake to no more than 30% of the daily caloric intake as recommended by the American Heart Association. Food rich in concentrated sweets and refined sugars also should be discouraged. It is recommended that for each hour of vigorous exercise (eg, jogging, running, jumping), the athlete should consume an additional 500 to 800 calories to prevent catabolism. The vast majority of these calories should come from carbohydrates, such as fresh vegetables and grains. If these parameters are met, additional supplementation is unnecessary. Optimally, individuals who consume five or six small snacks every 2 to 3 hours throughout the day rather than three large meals experience less fluctuation in hormonal response. Sports drinks are excellent in helping to replenish fluids and electrolytes both during and after exercise. Water and up to 16 oz/d of 1% low fat milk are still the best options when not exercising.

Eating Disorders

Anorexia and bulimia nervosa represent more extreme forms of distorted eating, and they affect roughly one third of all female athletes, as opposed to approximately 3% of the general population. Symptoms can begin as early as preado-lescence. Many athletes may not meet the strict *Diagnostic and Statistical Manual of Mental Disorders*, fourth edition, criteria for the disorders; however, some criteria often coexist in different forms of abnormal eating behaviors, which are associated with various medical problems. These include menstrual dysfunction; early osteoporosis; thyroid, gastrointestinal, and electrolyte abnormalities; anemia; and potentially fatal arrhythmias.

Screening for these disorders is essential and is best done in a private setting. Questions regarding the patient's menstrual history, recall of the patient's diet over the past 24 hours, exercise regimen, laxative and diet pill usage, vomiting, and overall sense of body satisfaction are all revealing indicators of disordered eating. The presence of lanugo, enlarged parotids, tooth enamel erosion, tachycardia, orthostatic hypotension, and low body weight are all revealing signs.

Treatment is multidisciplinary and should include a psychologist, nutritionist, nurses, and physicians who have experience in dealing with patients with eating disorders. Often, these patients need to be hospitalized. Patients who meet the criteria for anorexia or bulimia nervosa or have an associated condition that puts them at high risk need to be removed from athletic participation until they are in a better state of health. It is important to realize that eating disorders, while quite serious, almost always are a manifestation of the patient's difficulty in effectively dealing with underlying life stresses.

Menstrual Problems

Menstrual irregularity occurs in both adolescent and older female athletes with great frequency and thus is a common presenting complaint in primary care. Menstrual irregularity (oligomenorrhea or amenorrhea) has a higher prevalence in athletes, with as many as two thirds of women who routinely participate in intense athletics (see Table 14-1) affected (Safran et al., 1998). This refers to patients who do not suffer from primary amenorrhea but have had menarche and are experiencing missed menses or prolonged intervals (longer than 35 days) between menses. Exercise-induced menstrual dysfunction is a diagnosis of exclusion; hence, the provider must rule out causes such as pregnancy, polycystic ovary disease, and hypothyroidism. Potential complications of this condition include early osteoporosis and higher risk for both stress and pathologic fractures. The etiology of athletic amenorrhea is uncertain but may be related to inhibition of gonadotropin-releasing hormone and lutenizing hormone pulses. Treatment and prevention of this condition consist of maintaining adequate caloric intake and calcium supplementation of at least 1500 mg daily. Also, contraceptive pills or monthly progestin pulses may be used to protect the endometrium. Also, a reduction in the intensity of exercise should be recommended. The clinician should maintain a high index of suspicion for the presence of an eating disorder.

Stress and Performance Anxiety

Stress and performance anxiety are present to varying degrees in every athlete. Nobody wants to perform poorly, especially in front of friends, family, and teammates. Professional sport teams have sport psychologists who help the players cope with their stresses and maintain good mental health. Obviously, most adolescents do not have this luxury; thus, the burden falls on the children themselves and their supporters. This can be difficult, because children are still evolving physically and emotionally and have yet to establish a baseline for their behavior and athletic performance. An essential idea for parents and children to remember is that fun, and not winning, is the primary reason for participating.

Other things to know before participation include the time commitment and financial requirements of the sport. Are both parents and child mature enough to handle the prospect of losing and winning? One must realize that athletic stardom often is temporary. Academics must still be the first priority for children. These factors all can act as stressors on both the participant and the family and certainly can affect performance. The benefits of athletic participation and physical activity are well known and include enhancement of the child's self-esteem and social environment, in addition to helping shape the child's identity in a positive manner.

● **Clinical Pearl:** The child, and not the parent, must be the one who wants to play. Parents must learn and remain aware of the differences between supporting and pushing their child. While not every child is meant to be an athlete, all children can derive benefits from sports participation.

COMMUNITY RESOURCES

Sports and recreation are more popular than ever. People in general are more aware of their health; thus, the field of sports medicine is continually expanding in response to the numerous questions and issues that arise. Although there is no perfect resource for every question, the child athlete and family should feel comfortable in first turning to their provider with whom they have an established relationship to address their concerns. Ideally, the provider will have received added qualifications in sports medicine. The primary care provider is most capable of putting the patient in touch with the best available resources: other providers, qualified nutritionists, athletic trainers, or respected journals. Other good sources of information are certified athletic and personal trainers. In response to the veritable boom in exercise and nutrition that has occurred in recent decades, a variety of magazine and nutritional stores have an endless array of nutritional supplements and training techniques. The Food and Drug Administration does not regulate these supplements; therefore, they often have not been subjected to rigorous studies over time regarding their safety and efficacy. Before incorporating them into training, the patient should first check with his or her health care provider to eliminate any detrimental effect.

Journals and websites can serve as valuable resources to athletic patients. The list includes The Physician and Sports Medicine Journal and its web site *www.physsportsmed.com*; the American Journal of Sports Medicine; the Journal of Medicine and Science in Sports and Exercise; the web site of *www.acsm.org* for the ACSM; and the web site of the Gratorade Sports Science Institute, *www.gssiweb.com*.

REFERENCES

American College of Sports Medicine. (1996). ACSM position stand on exercise and fluid replacement. *Medicine and Science in Sports and Exercise, 28*(1), i–iv.

Andrews, J. S. (1997). Making the most of the sports physical. *Contemporary Pediatrics, March*, 185.

Bratton, R. L. D., & Agerter, D. C. (1995). Preparticipation sports examinations. *Postgraduate Medicine, 98*, 2, 123–123.

Fields, K. B., & Fricker, P. (1997). *Medical problems in athletes.* Boston: Blackwell Science LTD, XVI.

Mellion, M. B. (1999). *Sports medicine secrets* (pp. 28–32). St. Louis, MO; Mosby.

Poortmans, J. R., & Francaux, M. (1999). Long term oral creatine supplementation does not impair renal function in healthy athletes. *Medicine and Science in Sports Exercise*, 1108–1110.

Quality Standards Subcommittee. (1997). Practice parameter: The management of concussion in sports (summary statement). *Neurology, 48*, 581–585.

Richmond, J. C., & Shahady, E. J. (1996). *Sports medicine for primary care.* Boston: Blackwell Science LTD.

Safran, M., McKeag, D., & VanCamp, S. (1998). *Manual of sports medicine.* Philadelphia: Lippincott-Raven.

Smith, D. M., Kovan, J., Rich, B. S. E., & Tanner, S. M. (1998). *Preparticipation physical evaluation* (2nd ed.). Minneapolis, MN: McGraw-Hill Publishers.

Smith, N., & Stanitski, C. (1987). *Sports medicine: A practice guide.* Philadelphia: W.B. Saunders.

Medical Conditions in Sports Participation

This table is designed to be understood by medical and nonmedical personnel. In the "Explanation" section below, "needs evaluation" means that a primary care provider with appropriate knowledge and experience should assess the safety of a given sport for an athlete with the listed medical condition. Unless otherwise noted, this is because of the variability of the severity of the disease or of the risk of injury among the specific sports, or both.

Condition	May Participate
Atlantoaxial instability (instability of the joint between cervical vertebrae 1 and 2) Explanation: Athlete needs evaluation to assess risk of spinal cord injury during sports participation.	Qualified Yes
Bleeding disorder* Explanation: Athlete needs evaluation.	Qualified Yes
Cardiovascular diseases	
Carditis (inflammation of the heart) Explanation: Carditis may result in sudden death with exertion.	No

Hypertension (high blood pressure)
    Explanation: Those with significant essential (unexplained) hypertension should avoid weight
    and power lifting, body building, and strength training. Those with secondary hypertension
    (hypertension caused by a previously identified disease) or severe essential hypertension need evaluation.
	Qualified Yes

Congenital heart disease (structural heart defects present at birth)
    Explanation: Those with mild forms may participate fully; those with moderate or severe forms or
    who have undergone surgery need evaluation.
	Qualified Yes

Dysrhythmia (irregular heart rhythm)
    Explanation: Athlete needs evaluation because some types require therapy or make
    certain sports dangerous or both.
	Qualified Yes

Mitral valve prolapse (abnormal heart valve)
    Explanation: Those with symptoms (chest pain, symptoms of possible dysrhythmia) or evidence
    of mitral regurgitation (leaking) on physical examination need evaluation. All others may
    participate fully.
	Qualified Yes

Heart murmur
    Explanation: If the murmur is innocent (does not indicate heart disease), full participation is
    permitted. Otherwise, the athlete needs evaluation (see "Congenital heart disease" and
    "Mitral valve prolapse" above).
	Qualified Yes

Cerebral palsy Explanation: Athlete needs evaluation.	Qualified Yes

Diabetes mellitus
    Explanation: All sports can be played with proper attention to diet, hydration, and insulin therapy.
    Particular attention is needed for activities that last 30 min or more.
	Yes

Diarrhea
    Explanation: Unless disease is mild, no participation is permitted, because diarrhea may increase
    the risk of dehydration and heat illness. See "Fever" below.
	Qualified No

Eating disorders Anorexia nervosa, bulimia nervosa Explanation: These patients need both medical and psychiatric assessment before participation.	Qualified Yes

Eyes
Functionally one-eyed athlete, loss of an eye, detached retina, previous eye surgery, or serious eye injury
    Explanation: A functionally one-eyed athlete has a best corrected visual acuity of <20/40 in the
    worse eye. These athletes would suffer significant disability if the better eye was seriously injured
    as would those with loss of an eye. Some athletes who have previously undergone eye surgery
    or had a serious eye injury may have an increased risk of injury because of weakened eye tissue.
    Availability of eye guards approved by the American Society for Testing Materials (ASTM) and
    other protective equipment may allow participation in most sports, but this must be judged
    on an individual basis.
	Qualified Yes

Fever
    Explanation: Fever can increase cardiopulmonary effort, reduce maximum exercise capacity, make heat
    illness more likely, and increase orthostatic hypotension during exercise. Fever may rarely accompany
    myocarditis or other infections that may make exercise dangerous.
	No

Heat illness, history of
    Explanation: Because of the increased likelihood of recurrence, the athlete needs individual assessment
    to determine the presence of predisposing conditions and to arrange a prevention strategy.
	Qualified Yes

(continues)

Condition	May Participate

HIV infection
    Explanation: Because of the apparent minimal risk to others, all sports may be played that the
        state of health allows. In all athletes, skin lesions should be properly covered, and athletic personnel
        should use universal precautions when handling blood or body fluids with visible blood.
	Yes

Kidney: absence of one Explanation: Athlete needs individual assessment for contact/collision and limited contact sports.	Qualified Yes

Liver, enlarged
    Explanation: If the liver is acutely enlarged, participation should be avoided because of risk of rupture.
        If the liver is chronically enlarged, individual assessment is needed before contact/collision or limited
        contact sports are played.
	Qualified Yes

Malignancy Explanation: Athlete needs individual assessment.	Qualified Yes
Musculoskeletal disorders Explanation: Athlete needs individual assessment.	Qualified Yes

Neurologic
    History of serious head or spine trauma, severe or repeated concussions, or craniotomy
        Explanation: Athlete needs individual assessment for contact/collision or limited contact
            sports and for noncontact sports if there are deficits in judgment or cognition.
            Recent research supports a conservative approach to management of concussion.
	Qualified Yes

Convulsive disorder, well controlled Explanation: Risk of convulsion during participation is minimal.	Yes

Convulsive disorder, poorly controlled
        Explanation: Athlete needs individual assessment for contact/collision or limited contact
            sports. Avoid the following noncontact sports: archery, riflery, swimming, weight or
            power lifting, strength training, or sports involving heights. In these sports, occurrence
            of a convulsion may be a risk to self or others.
	Qualified Yes

Obesity Explanation: Because of the risk of heat illness, obese people need careful acclimatization and hydration.	Qualified Yes
Organ transplant recipient Explanation: Athlete needs individual assessment.	Qualified Yes
Ovary: absence of one Explanation: Risk of severe injury to the remaining ovary is minimal.	Yes

Respiratory
    Pulmonary compromise, including cystic fibrosis
        Explanation: Athlete needs individual assessment, but generally all sports may be played if
            oxygenation remains satisfactory during a graded exercise test. Patients with cystic
            fibrosis need acclimatization and good hydration to reduce the risk of heat illness.
	Qualified Yes

Asthma
        Explanation: With proper medication and education, only athletes with the most severe asthma
            will have to modify their participation.
	Yes

Acute upper respiratory infection
        Explanation: Upper respiratory obstruction may affect pulmonary function. Athlete needs
            individual assessment for all but mild disease. See "Fever" above.
	Qualified Yes

Sickle cell disease
    Explanation: Athlete needs individual assessment. In general, if status of the illness permits, all
        but high-exertion, contact/collision sports may be played. Overheating, dehydration, and
        chilling must be avoided.
	Qualified Yes

Sickle cell trait
    Explanation: It is unlikely that individuals with sickle cell trait (AS) have an increased risk of
        sudden death or other medical problems during athletic participation except under the most
        extreme conditions of heat, humidity, and possibly increased altitude. These individuals, like all
        athletes, should be carefully conditioned, acclimatized, and hydrated to reduce any possible risk.
	Yes

Skin: boils, herpes simplex, impetigo, scabies, molluscum contagiosum
    Explanation: While the patient is contagious, participation in gymnastics with mats, martial arts,
        wrestling, or other contact/collision or limited contact sports is not allowed. Herpes simplex
        virus probably is not transmitted via mats.
	Qualified Yes

Spleen, enlarged
    Explanation: Patients with acutely enlarged spleens should avoid all sports because of
        risk of rupture. Those with chronically enlarged spleens need individual assessment
        before playing contact/collision or limited contact sports.
	Qualified Yes

Testicle: absent or undescended Explanation: Certain sports may require a protective cup.	Yes

Reprinted with permission of American Academy of Pediatrics Committee on Sports Medicine and Fitness. (1994). Medical conditions affecting sports participation. *Pediatrics, 94*(5), 757–760.

Preparticipation Physical Evaluation

HISTORY   DATE OF EXAM _____

Name _____	Sex _____ Age _____ Date of birth
Grade _____	School _____ Sport(s)_____
Address _____	Phone _____
Personal primary care provider _____	

In case of emergency, contact
Name _____ Relationship _____ Phone (H) _____ (W) _____

Explain "Yes" answers below.   **Circle questions you don't know the answers to.**

	Yes	No
1. Have you had a medical illness or injury since your last checkup or sports physical?	☐	☐
Do you have an ongoing or chronic illness?	☐	☐
2. Have you ever been hospitalized overnight?	☐	☐
Have you ever had surgery?	☐	☐
3. Are you currently taking any prescription or non-prescription (over-the-counter) medications or pills or using an inhaler?	☐	☐
Have you ever taken any supplements or vitamins to help you gain or lose weight or improve your performance?	☐	☐
4. Do you have any allergies (for example, to pollen, medicine, food, or stinging insects)?	☐	☐
Have your ever had a rash or hives develop during or after exercise?	☐	☐
5. Have you ever passed out during or after exercise?	☐	☐
Have you ever been dizzy during or after exercise?	☐	☐
Have you ever had chest pain during or after exercise?	☐	☐
Do you get tired more quickly than your friends do during exercise?	☐	☐
Have you ever had racing of your heart or skipped heartbeats?	☐	☐
Have you had high blood pressure or high cholesterol?	☐	☐
Have you ever been told you have a heart murmur?	☐	☐
Has any family member or relative died of heart problems or of sudden death before age 50?	☐	☐
Have you had a severe viral infection (for example, myocarditis or mononucleosis) within the last month?	☐	☐
Has a physician ever denied or restricted your participation in sports for any heart problems?	☐	☐
6. Do you have any current skin problems (for example, itching, rashes, acne, warts, fungus, or blisters)?	☐	☐
7. Have you ever had a head injury or concussion?	☐	☐
Have you ever been knocked out, become unconscious, or lost your memory?	☐	☐
Have you ever had a seizure?	☐	☐
Do you have frequent or severe headaches?	☐	☐
Have you ever had numbness or tingling in your arms, hands, legs, or feet?	☐	☐
Have you ever had a stinger, burner, or pinched nerve?	☐	☐
8. Have you ever become ill from exercising in the heat?	☐	☐
9. Do you cough, wheeze, or have trouble breathing during or after activity?	☐	☐
Do you have asthma?	☐	☐
Do you have seasonal allergies that require medical treatment?	☐	☐

	Yes	No
10. Do you use any special protective or corrective equipment or devices that aren't usually used for your sport or position (for example, knee brace, special neck roll, foot orthotics, retainer on your teeth, hearing aid)?	☐	☐
11. Have you had any problems with your eyes or vision?	☐	☐
Do you wear glasses, contacts, or protective eyewear?	☐	☐
12. Have you ever had a sprain, strain, or swelling after injury?	☐	☐
Have you broken or fractured any bones or dislocated any joints?	☐	☐
Have you had any other problems with pain or swelling in muscles, tendons, bones, or joints?	☐	☐

If yes, check appropriate box and explain below.

☐ Head	☐ Elbow	☐ Hip
☐ Neck	☐ Forearm	☐ Thigh
☐ Back	☐ Wrist	☐ Knee
☐ Chest	☐ Hand	☐ Shin/calf
☐ Shoulder	☐ Finger	☐ Ankle
☐ Upper arm		☐ Foot

	Yes	No
13. Do you want to weigh more or less than you do now?	☐	☐
Do you lose weight regularly to meet weight requirements for your sport?	☐	☐
14. Do you feel stressed out?	☐	☐

15. Record the dates of your most recent immunizations (shots) for:

Tetanus _____   Measles_____

Hepatitis B _____   Chickenpox _____

FEMALES ONLY

16. When was your first menstrual period? _____
When was your most recent menstrual period? _____
How much time do you usually have from the start of one period to the start of another? _____
How many periods have you had in the last year? _____
What was the longest time between periods in the last year?_____

Explain "Yes" answers here: _____

_____

_____

_____

_____

I hereby state that, to the best of my knowledge, my answers to the above questions are complete and correct.

Signature of athlete _____ Signature of parent/guardian _____ Date _____

PREPARTICIPATION PHYSICAL EXAMINATION

Name _____ Date of birth_____ _____
Height _____ Weight _____ % Body fat (optional) _____ Pulse _____ BP ____/____ (____/____, ____/____)
Vision R 20/ _____ L 20/ _____   Corrected: Y   N   Pupils: Equal _____ Unequal _____

	NORMAL	ABNORMAL FINDINGS	INITIALS*
MEDICAL			
Appearance			
Eyes/Ears/Nose/Throat			
Lymph Nodes			
Heart			
Pulses			
Lungs			
Abdomen			
Genitalia (males only)			
Skin			
MUSCULOSKELETAL			
Neck			
Back			
Shoulder/arm			
Elbow/forearm			
Wrist/hand			
Hip/thigh			
Knee			
Leg/ankle			
Foot			

*Station-based examination only

Preparticipation Physical Evaluation
CLEARANCE FORM

□ Cleared

□ Cleared after completing evaluation/rehabilitation for: _____

□ Not cleared for: _____ Reason: _____

Recommendations: _____

_____

_____

_____

Name of provider (print/type) _____ Date _____

Address _____ Phone _____

Signature of provider _____

Pain and Children

• SUSAN J. BRILLHART, MSN, RN, CS, PNP

INTRODUCTION

Pain occurs in every child's life. The job of the primary care provider is to evaluate actual or anticipated pain, and to apply simple and appropriate pain measures that can help to make visits significantly less painful and frightening for children and their caregivers. This chapter explores recent research findings about pain in children and the broad recommendations for pain assessment, prevention, and management based on those findings. For specific doses and protocols, especially for pediatric conscious sedation, the reader is urged strongly to refer to the annually updated reference and protocol books.

PAIN MYTHS AND REALITIES

Until recently, pain in the pediatric population was neither recognized nor researched, even in the acute care setting. Professionals caring for children have long noted that the effects of pain on children have not been measured, explained, or described sufficiently (McGuire & Dizard, 1982; Richards, Bernal, & Brackbill, 1976; Schechter, 1985). For this reason, health care team members may misunderstand, minimize, or inadequately respond to the level or importance of a child's pain (Beyer & Byers, 1985; McCaffery, 1977; McGuire & Dizard, 1982). This problem is especially true for young children (Schechter & Allen, 1986). An examination of the literature of the 1970s, 1980s, and early 1990s reveals a frightening ignorance of the level of pain that children experience. Eland (1990) notes that before 1977, only one nursing article appeared in the pediatric pain literature (Schultz, 1971). This was a study describing pain perception in healthy 10- and 11-year-olds. Pediatric pain management was almost nonexistent in medical and nursing textbooks: Ten major pediatric texts totaling more than 12,000 pages contained less than one combined page on the topic (Rana, 1987). Fortunately, the situation has changed, and every current pediatric textbook addresses the issue of pain.

Past Research

Raising the critical question of whether children experience pain, Abu-Saad (1981) reminded readers of the belief, commonly held since the 1930s, that infants do not perceive pain to the same degree as adults because infants lack cortical pathways. Some practitioners still hold this belief; others believe that infants can feel pain but less strongly than adults. Actually, the opposite is true—infants are hypersensitive to pain because of incomplete physiologic development. Researching pain in adults, Melzack and Wall (1965) developed the revolutionary Gate Control Theory of Pain. Melzack (1975) proceeded to develop the widely used McGill Pain Questionnaire but did nothing to dispel long-standing pediatric pain myths or to address pain assessment

for children. Swafford and Allan (1968) reported only 2 out of 60 children (3%) on their surgical floor required pain medications. They anecdotally noted, "Pediatric patients seldom need medication for relief of pain. They tolerate discomfort well" (Swafford & Allan, 1968, p. 135). Other researchers reported repeatedly that children received fewer postoperative analgesics than adults (Beyer, DeGood, Ashley, & Russell, 1983; Eland & Anderson, 1977; Schechter & Allen, 1986).

Several comprehensive reviews of pain have appeared in both the earlier medical (Goldman & Lloyd-Thomas, 1991; McGrath, 1990; Schechter, 1984; 1985; 1989) and nursing (Abu-Saad, 1981; Eland, 1990; Ross & Ross, 1988) literature. The First International Symposium on Pediatric Pain was held in 1988. At the National Institute of Health Measurement of Pain Meeting in April 1988, however, the unique and complex problems of pediatric pain were not addressed at all, partially because of the problems of measurement (Loeser, 1990). This occurrence demonstrates that at that time, distinct knowledge about pediatric pain was lacking, especially the pain of children age 12 and younger.

Common Misconceptions

Many myths surround the topic of pediatric pain, most of which lead to inadequate treatment. The first and most serious is that infants do not feel pain. Research has proven that premature infants exposed to repeated heelsticks not only feel pain, but also develop an increased sensitivity to stimulation that outlasts the noxious stimulus by hours or days (Fitzgerald, Millard, & McIntosh, 1989). Because pain inhibitory systems are not fully developed, young infants actually may have an increased stress response to pain, compared with adults. These findings also refute the second serious myth: that children tolerate pain better than adults. Children actually tolerate pain better as they get older because their inhibitory systems become more developed.

The third myth is that infants and young children do not remember pain. Although this idea may be very soothing to the caregiver of a child in pain, it is untrue. Research of circumcised males during their 4- to 6-month vaccinations showed they had greater stress responses than uncircumcised males. In the same study, male infants who received a local anesthetic (EMLA in this case) for circumcision had a lower stress response than those who did not (Taddio, Katz, Ilerisich, & Koren, 1997). Although children may have no active memory of pain, a pain experience may have lasting effects on how individuals respond to future episodes throughout their childhood and possibly adulthood. Even the unremembered effects of pain should not be dismissed, as any family member of a person who has had surgery and sedation can attest. Disturbed sleep and behavior patterns are not uncommon in children and adults, even when surgical pain was "well controlled" (Orenstein, Manning, & Pelphrey, 1999).

Another myth is that children always tell the truth about pain. If they believe that admitting to pain will cause something more painful (especially an injection), children may be untruthful. For this reason, intramuscular (IM) injections should be a last resort for pain management in children. Children also may not really be aware of how much pain they have (slow-building chronic pain) or may assume that the provider knows how they feel. Physical indicators or mood changes may be the key to assessment in these children.

The fifth myth is that pain "builds character." It is not uncommon to hear caregivers make such comments to their children, especially older children and adolescents. The provider needs to remind parents that the pain *is* real. The clinician should tell all involved of the measures that he or she will use to decrease pain and measures that the family can continue at home to suppress pain. Adolescents may receive three to four booster vaccinations at once, some of which can be immediately extremely painful, with soreness lasting 7 to 10 days. Caregivers need to recognize this interruption in tissue integrity as an injury (even though a medical provider inflicted it) and treat the child's pain appropriately.

Another myth is that crying most often stems from fear rather than pain. While the older infant and toddler will greatly dislike being restrained, providers and parents should treat a procedure that is known to be painful as such. They should not lightly brush off a child's cries because the child is upset about being restrained. Children who have repeated painful procedures are not just fearful of being restrained; they have *increased* sensitivity to pain and should be assessed very carefully.

The seventh myth is that children cannot tell exactly where or how much they hurt. Children as young as 4 years can localize pain and can point to it on themselves or on drawings. Children as young as 3 years can effectively use the FACES rating scale (see discussion later in this chapter; Wong & Baker, 1988).

The eighth myth is that caregivers and health care providers can properly assess the child's pain. Children in chronic pain have different pain behaviors and may be in severe pain but may not "show" any pain response at all. Providers may then assume that the child has no pain and that pain reports are just attempts to gain attention. Multiple studies, recent and old, show that almost everyone, in every field of health care, underrates children's pain. Home caregivers also were found to underrate pain. Disappointingly, very little change has been made in this critical area of pain control. The message is to believe what the child says regarding the pain's severity, length, and so forth. Otherwise, chronic pain may lead to depression, anxiety, and low self-esteem (Zeltzer, Bush, Chen, & Riveral, 1997). The only way to treat pain appropriately is to listen to what children say about it.

The ninth myth is that all sedating or paralyzing drugs have an analgesic effect. In fact, many drugs used for sedation and paralyzation have no analgesic effect at all. The provider must remember to give analgesia, sedation, or a paralytic when needed, ensuring that each separate and necessary element is kept at the appropriate level. An active paralytic without sedation or analgesia can have disastrous psychological and physiologic effects. A sedated and paralyzed child in pain who does not receive analgesia will still display a change in vital signs and other physiologic effects, which can be potentially dangerous in the unstable patient.

The 10th myth, perpetuated by caregivers and health care professionals, is that children and adolescents will become addicted to narcotics if they are used. Providers should explain the difference between addiction (a *voluntary psychological or behavioral response* characterized by a compulsive drug-seeking behavior), tolerance (an *involuntary physiologic need* for larger doses to maintain the original analgesic effect),

and physical dependence (displayed by *involuntary physiologic* withdrawal symptoms when delivered narcotics are suddenly stopped or reversed). Everyone should understand that a child in pain does not become addicted when narcotics are used for pain control. Caregivers also should understand that a child who needs narcotics for weeks to months probably will develop tolerance or dependence. These children will be weaned slowly and successfully from those narcotics. Such weaning is a routine and expected part of discharge protocol in most major pediatric intensive care units.

The final myth is that children are more susceptible to opioid-induced respiratory depression than are adults. Multiple studies have shown narcotics to be as safe for children older than 3 months (and possibly younger) as they are for adults. As children increase their tolerance to the drug, they also increase their tolerance to respiratory depression. Pain is a natural antagonist to the action of opioids, so the more intense the pain, the more drug the child can receive safely. Respiratory depression also is rare in appropriate long-term opioid therapy, even if delivered in seemingly high doses (cancer pain).

Infant Pain Myths

The misperceptions about pain and infants are varied and far-reaching. This short section explores recent discoveries concerning the effects of pain on infants and potential long-term concerns.

Premature and full-term infants have a functional nervous system capable of perceiving pain and, when exposed to noxious stimuli, can experience changes in their physiologic status, biochemistry, behavioral state, cry features, and facial expression. Acute changes in physiologic status can be extremely dangerous for very premature or unstable infants. Increasing intracranial pressure can precipitate intraventricular hemorrhage (IVH). A state of hypermetabolism and catabolism ultimately may cause morbidity and mortality. In blinded, randomized trials (Anand, 1999), intravenous morphine reduced pain responses, stabilized vital signs, and decreased the incidence of poor neurologic outcomes (defined as death, grade III or IV IVH, or cystic periventricular leukomalacia). Treatment with the topical anesthetic EMLA (a eutectic mixture of 2.5% lidocaine and 2.5% prilocaine) has been found to reverse the hypersensitivity threshold for neonates with repeated heelsticks and to decrease the pain response for future vaccinations in circumcised male infants.

Individuals researching memory in very young infants have discovered interesting information. On their first breast-feeding, newborns chose the breast that was wiped with their own amniotic fluid over the breast that was wiped with a clean cloth. One-day-old infants respond differently to an odor once it has been paired with a reinforcing tactile stimulus. With these findings, it is no surprise that by age 6 months, infants show anticipatory fear when facing a previously painful stimulus (Porter, Grunau, & Anand, 1999).

● **Clinical Pearl:** The rule to follow for children of all ages is if the event would be painful for an adult, it will be as painful (or more so) to children.

PAIN ASSESSMENT

The assessment of pain in children is a much discussed and debated topic. The most important part of pain assessment in children is to *believe whatever the child is saying*. The World Health Organization has adopted McCaffery's (1977) definition of pain: *Pain is whatever the experiencing person says it is, existing whenever the person says it does.* Children "say" they have pain in different ways, verbal and nonverbal. The provider must understand what his or her beliefs are concerning pediatric pain and how those beliefs could influence practice.

Purpose and Goals of Assessment

Accepting that pain is multidimensional, the assessment of pain in children should accomplish several functions. Zeltzer et al. (1997) list multiple key functions for providers. All these suggestions should assist in developing pain management strategies optimally suited to each individual child.

First, determine how best to communicate with a child about pain, which may be a prerequisite to any other element of pain assessment. Evaluation of a child's developmental status and ability to understand pain, illness, and medical procedures is important.

Second, assess the intensity, quality, and characteristics of the child's pain experience; determine the child's pain management needs; and evaluate the effectiveness of ongoing pain-management strategies. Neglected or inexpert use of pain assessment is a major reason why children's pain often is undermanaged.

Third, review the psychosocial aspects of pain. Identifying the child's coping style, personality, and family factors will help target dysfunctional beliefs, attitudes, and coping skills. Then identify significant maladjustment or traumatic responses to pain (including depression and withdrawal) that may cause serious sequelae or encourage the development of dysfunctional attitudes and beliefs regarding pain, illness, and medical care.

Fourth, understand anxiety or behavioral stress in response to illness or procedures that may further exacerbate pain and make accurate estimation difficult.

Baker and Wong (1987) developed an overall approach called QUESTT that should be used for all pain assessments:

- **Q**uestion the child.
- **U**se pain rating scales.
- **E**valuate behavior and physiologic changes.
- **S**ecure parents' involvement.
- **T**ake cause of pain into account.
- **T**ake action, and evaluate results.

Questioning the child is the most important factor in pain assessment. The provider should ask the child questions using terminology familiar to that child. Hester and Barcus (1986) have developed an excellent pain experience history questionnaire that specifies questions for the child and for the caregiver. Their answers provide the basis for an effective plan of pain prevention. Caregiver involvement is crucial; children may deny pain to strangers yet admit it to a trusted caregiver. Children also may deny pain if they believe that admitting it will result in an injection or if they believe that they deserve the pain. Some children believe that they have been "bad" and are responsible for causing other negative events in their lives (eg, parents' divorce, illness of a sibling). This may lead them to believe they deserve any pain that they have.

Tools for Pain Assessment in Children

Multiple pain-assessment tools are available for children. All are effective for some children, though some are more effective for certain ages than are others. Tools should be used as part of a larger assessment that involves questioning the child and observing and evaluating behavioral and physiologic changes.

Some of the more common self-report pain assessment tools will be described. Whenever possible, the provider should present the same tool to the child at each pain-assessment session to avoid confusion between the different models. If one tool does not seem to work well, the provider should try another age-appropriate tool and record the name of the successful tool in a highly visible place.

The FACES Pain Rating Scale (Wong & Baker, 1988) can be used by children as young as 3 years. Several different scales use drawings or pictures of faces, but recent research (Chambers, Giesbrecht, Craig, Bennett, & Huntsman, 1999) has shown that subtle variations in format influence children's and parents' ratings of pain in clinical settings. The authors also found that the children and parents preferred scales that they perceived to be happy and cartoon-like (ie, the FACES scale). The FACES scale can be conveniently carried (Fig. 15-1).

The Adolescent Pediatric Pain Tool (Savendra, Tessler, Holzemer, & Ward, 1993) is a body outline that can be used by children other than adolescents. The provider asks the child to mark the outline wherever the pain is located and to make the mark as large or small as the painful area. Combined with a 1 to 100 analogue rating scale, this is an effective tool for expression of pain in mature children.

There are several numeric scales, ranging either from 1 to 10 or 1 to 100. The 1 to 10 scale is easily placed on the reverse side of the pocket-sized FACES scale for older children to use. The Word Graphic Rating Scale (Tessler et al., 1989) also uses a line but uses descriptive words instead of numbers. The provider may need to explain the words to younger children. To record a definitive score, the provider measures where the child placed the mark in millimeters, starting at the "no pain" end.

Special Assessment Considerations

The assessment of pain in preverbal, developmentally delayed, and neurologically impaired children is difficult and has been the topic of many recent studies. Assessment in young infants has focused on facial features, changes in auditory features of the cry, and changes in vital signs. Infants may attempt to change their body position in response to pain (eg, drawing up legs for abdominal pain, moving head side-to-side for ear pain, withdrawing foot for heelstick). Temperament is important to consider, even in very young children. A quiet child may be more passive but rate pain much higher than an actively fighting child. Providers should not be misled into thinking that the passive child is experiencing less pain; that child most likely is in greater need of pain-reduction skills.

Cultural differences may play a role in responses, although the differences are very slight at younger ages. One of the best assessment methods is observing for a change in behavior and vital signs after administering an analgesic. A return to normal often signifies appropriate pain relief, while persistent elevation can mean that relief is incomplete. A child who has been in pain for an extended period may appear to have depressed vital signs when pain relief finally is achieved. In actuality, the child has returned to normal sleeping vital signs.

PAIN PREVENTION AND MANAGEMENT

Pain is an individual's subjective response to noxious stimuli. Providers must view pain as a response of an intercon-

TRANSLATION OF FACES PAIN RATING SCALE

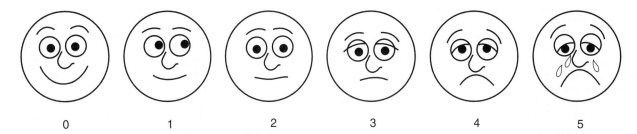

0	1	2	3	4	5

Explain to the person that each face is for a person who feels happy because he has no pain (hurt) or sad because he has some or a lot of pain. **Face 0** is very happy because he doesn't hurt at all. **Face 1** hurts just a little bit. **Face 2** hurts a little more. **Face 3** hurts even more. Face 4 hurts a whole lot. **Face 5** hurts as much as you can imagine, although you don't have to be crying to feel this bad. Ask the person to choose the face that best describes how he is feeling. Rating scale is recommended for persons 3 years and older.

Spanish. Epliquele a la persona que cada cara representa una persona que se siente feliz porque no tiene dolor o, triste porque siente un poco o mucho dolor. **Cara 0** se siente muy feliz porque no tiene dolor. **Cara 1** tiene un poco de dolor. **Cara 2** tiene un poquito más de dolor. **Cara 3** tiene todavia más dolor. **Cara 4** tiene mucho dolor. **Cara 5** tiene el dolor máximo aunque ni siempre causa el lloro. Pidale a la persona cual de las caras mejor describe su próprio dolor.

Esta escala se puede usar con personas de tres años de edad o más.

French. Expliquez à la personne que chaque visage repré-sent un personne qui est heureux parce qu'elle n'a pas point du mal ou triste parce qu'il a un peu ou beaucoup du mal. **Visage 0** est très heureux parce qu'elle n'a pas point du mal. **Visage 1** a un petit peu du mal. **Visage 2** a plus du mal. **Visage 3** a encore plus du mal. **Visage 4** a beaucoup du mal. **Visage 5** a autant mal que vous pouvez imaginer, bien que ces mauvais sentiments ne finissent pas nécessairement a vous faire pleurer. Demandez à la personne de choisir le

Japanese

　3歳以上の患者に望ましい。それぞれの顔は、患者の痛み (pain, hurt) がないのでご機嫌な感じ、または、ある程度の痛み・沢山の痛みがあるので悲しい感じを表現していることを説明して下さい。0＝痛みがまったくないから、とても幸せな顔をしている、1＝ほんの少し痛い、2＝もう少し痛い、3＝もっと痛い、4＝とっても痛い、5＝痛くて涙を流す必要はないけれども、これ以上の痛みは考えられないほど痛い。今、どのように感じているか最もよく表わしている顔を選ぶよう、患者に求めて下さい。

Chinese

　　解釋給人聽用每張臉譜來代表著一個人的感覺是因爲沒有疼痛〔傷痛〕而感快樂或是因爲些許疼痛或者是許多疼痛而感傷心。第零張臉是很快樂的因爲他一點也不覺得疼痛。第一張臉只痛一丁點兒。第二張臉又痛多了一些。第三張臉痛得更多了。第四張臉是非常痛了。第五張臉是爲人們所能想像到的劇痛既使感到這樣難過，卻不一定哭出來。請這人選擇出最能代表他現在感覺的一張臉譜。此量表適用於三歲以上的人。

Figure 15–1 ■ Translations of Faces Pain Rating Scale. [Reprinted with permission of Wong, D.L. (1995).*Whaley and Wong's Nursing Care of Infants and Children* (5th ed.). St. Louis, Mosby.]

nected mind–body system. Pain is real, whether its origin is physical (eg, knife wound) or psychological (eg, telling a test subject that you are about to repeat a painful procedure, when, in fact, you are not). Because of the physiologic changes that accompany it, pain from any source is real and must be taken seriously.

Developmental Considerations

The most effective approach toward preventing, assessing, and treating pediatric pain is developmental, as outlined by Wagner (1998). The developmental approach is especially

useful in children whose developmental age differs from their chronologic age. In pediatrics, there are at least two clients: the caregiver and the child. Pain management begins with creating a comfortable environment for both. Family-friendly waiting rooms and realistic scheduling are impor-tant. A caregiver with several young children will not be happy or calm after an extended wait, even if snacks and toys are provided. Clinicians also must remember the differ-ences in pain perception and response between adults and children. Adults can tell providers that they are in pain and understand reason, cause, and effect. They might not like what the provider is going to do but will (usually) cooperate.

Children scream and will do anything to get away. They are not rational about pain and cannot be coerced into cooperating by saying that the provider is hurting them to help them. A better way must be found.

Newborn to Six Months

Young infants generally have no fear of providers or procedures, but their caregivers do. Anxiety in an infant is usually a reflection of anxiety in the caregiver. The provider should gently take, swaddle, and rock the infant and use a gentle voice to calm the child and caregiver. These actions are instinctive to most pediatric primary care providers but may be new to parents who are watching an infant in pain for the first time from a procedure (eg, first immunization). During some procedures, caregivers may choose to leave the room, which providers should present as an acceptable option. The clinician should inform caregivers that swaddling, rocking, cooing, maintaining eye contact, speaking gently, and smiling are usually the most calming actions for the baby after a procedure. Caregivers also may want to distract the baby with a favorite toy, song, or bubbles. Providers should advise them to bring along such items. Pacifiers can be very helpful, possibly crucial, in calming infants who use them. If medically possible, the caregiver should feed the infant whatever fluids the baby is allowed to take immediately after the procedure. Feeding can be very reassuring to both the infant and the caregiver.

Six Months to Toddler

Most babies develop an inherent fear of strangers between 6 and 9 months of age, and the place they are most comfortable is on their caregivers' laps. If possible, any procedures should be done with the child held safely on the caregiver's lap. The caregiver should comfort the child immediately afterward. This method works especially well for immunizations.

Toddler to Six Years

Children of these ages can be delightfully challenging; they have appropriate pain control measures, but not all measures work for every child. The provider's task is to discover the measure that works best for each child (making sure to note on the chart successes and failures) and to modify that technique as the child grows.

These children are curious and willing to trust if adults give them a little time. Not wearing a white lab coat with these children is common practice, and some practitioners even remove examining tables from the room. Honesty, simple directions, and straightforward explanations of *everything* that will be done, how each step will feel, and what equipment will look like, at a level the child understands, is the best approach. The provider should never lie about pain. He or she should tell children how the procedure will feel without using the words "hurt" or "pain." The provider also should say exactly how long (or hopefully how short) the child will feel this way.

Children of these ages have imagination and believe in magical powers, which providers can use to their advantage. For example, the clinician can put "magic medicine" on children's skin so they will not feel anything. The provider can have them blow away the prick of a needle on a pinwheel (inserting the needle at the same time). He or she can encourage children to tell their parents a story involving such magical powers. Guided imagery works very effectively with these children. Actively doing something—whether in reality or a story—is as an effective distraction for both child and caregiver. Most caregivers know well what will distract their children and can either bring along items or advise providers of effective measures. Some practitioners have VCR monitors in procedure rooms with a variety of favorite shows. This might not work as well as active distraction but is certainly better than nothing.

During an examination, providers should be sure to maintain eye contact at the children's level at all times. Clinicians should keep their distance at first, letting children choose between their caregiver's lap or examining tables whenever possible. Caregivers should undress toddlers one area at a time. Preschoolers can undress themselves, showing how good they are at it. Watching their facial expressions is important, because expressions can alert providers to signs of increasing fear.

Once they gain children's trust, providers must keep it by explaining *exactly* what will happen and how it will feel. They also must explain what they expect—what behavior is allowed (eg, shouting, screaming, squeezing Mom's finger until Mom says "Ow!") and what is not (eg, moving, kicking, biting). Providers should keep children posted as they proceed. They should praise children for attempts at cooperation, even if unsuccessful. Children are afraid of disappointing their parents.

Praising a child for some positive behavior (eg, for not biting), especially when a child had difficulty cooperating, often will make both caregiver and child feel better. It also will set a positive tone for communication between caregiver and child about the behavior. Lack of cooperation is normal, not a flaw in the child.

After the painful procedure has ended, these children should be involved with a tangible task, such as putting on bandages or throwing away (clean) gauze. Rewards are important; providers can use stickers, pencils, or prescriptions to the local ice cream store after a particularly difficult or painful visit (a positive arrangement for the store, child, and provider). Providers and parents should reinforce rewards with reminders to be proud of bravery. Adults should not expect children to be perfect, just to try their best. They must help children to be proud of giving their best, even if it was not exactly perfect.

Seven Years to Adolescent

These children and adolescents usually are very willing to cooperate, provided they understand what will happen, know what is expected of them, and have some control. At these ages, adults and children are able to "make deals." Such deals, however, must be extremely concrete. Any deviation from the plan will be a deal breaker for the child; thus, providers must make sure it only takes 5 seconds to count to 5, not 15 seconds! If performing a procedure with postoperative involvement, the provider should make sure a child understands what behavior is expected after the procedure and the real ramifications of not following instructions (eg, infection, dehiscence, possible repeat of the procedure). Mature children who are older than 12 years should sign informed consent to show that they agree with the treatment plan and to display some sense of control.

Distraction is still key. Books, music, videos, and stories can be effective. If conducting an office procedure, the provider may suggest children bring whatever will give them comfort. Most children and adults are uncomfortable with needles and syringes. Preparing all syringes out of the client's site and making engaging conversation during needle insertion may decrease anxiety.

Nonpharmacologic Approaches

The most important nonpharmacologic measure is adequate preparation of the child. Using the developmental model, the provider should tell the child what will be happening and how it will feel, including the fact that it may not bother the child at all. Then, the provider should use as many pain-reduction techniques as possible for the procedure.

Cutaneous Stimulation

Cutaneous stimulation can include pinching, rubbing, applying ice (to the site or to the same site on the opposite extremity), applying an electric vibrator (electric tooth-brushes work well), massaging with lotion or powder, or applying a transcutaneous electrical nerve stimulation (TENS) unit to the skin. The TENS unit delivers low-voltage electricity to the skin through electrodes. It has been effective in relieving some chronic pain and may be an effective cutaneous distractor for the prevention of pain perception.

Relaxation, Positive Thoughts, and Distraction

Providers and caregivers alike can perform these unskilled techniques. During relaxation, the provider or caregiver can rock the infant, speaking softly. He or she can ask the older child to lay down and relax. Starting with the tips of the toes, the child should let each body part "go limp as a wet noodle," relaxing up to the head while exhaling.

Using positive thoughts, the provider or caregiver encourages the child to think only about positive aspects of the procedure. Having the child link short statements together and repeat them like a mantra ("short time, good veins, nice doctor, get stickers, go home") usually is effective. Children can close their eyes and concentrate only on the sound of their voice and the positive statements they are making. They can use this technique throughout their lives for painful, or just uncomfortable, procedures (eg, first pelvic examination).

Successful distraction techniques are very child specific, and caregivers should inform providers beforehand, if possible, what will be effective with their child. Hopefully, caregivers will bring some favorite items, including a pacifier if appropriate. Across different age groups, videos, music, puppets, game playing (eg, can you yell louder or whisper softer than I?), blowing bubbles or pinwheels, and looking though a moving kaleidoscope are usually somewhat effective. Kaleidoscopes have been studied specifically and shown to be effective because of their novelty and ability to change visual images constantly.

Guided Imagery

Guided imagery, a form of relaxation, uses the techniques of joining, leading, pacing, and choosing words. The child identifies a very pleasurable real or imagined experience that both adult and child describe in great detail during a procedure. This low-tech, cost-effective intervention can promote the child's personal coping abilities and sense of self-esteem. It also is very effective at an age when other techniques are less successful. Toddlers and preschoolers are master storytellers, and their desire to experience magical powers further enhances the possibilities of guided imagery. Ott (1996) discusses the experience of describing a tremendous snowball fight to a 3-year-old while a colleague started the child's IV, with the child so distracted that he did not know when the procedure was finished. Every provider is encouraged to acquire the basic skills of guided imagery and to use it with children whenever possible.

Behavioral Contracting

Behavioral contracting can be either informal or formal. In informal contracting, providers give tactile rewards (eg, stickers) for cooperative behavior and use actual timers to limit stalling in less cooperative children. Many providers believe that all children should receive a reward after a painful experience. The contracted reward may differ according to level of cooperation so that each child has something specific to work toward. During formal contracting (often used for the treatment of eating disorders), the provider and child develop a written contract that includes the realistic goal or desired behavior, a measurable behavior (eg, will not kick, bite, or move left arm during procedure), and the resultant rewards. All participants sign and date the contract.

Biofeedback

Very effective with some adults (especially for migraine headaches), biofeedback is being used increasingly and with some success for children (Hermann, Blanchard, & Flor, 1997). In biofeedback, the child learns how to control his or her physiologic responses. As a learned technique, biofeedback is used more in cases of chronic pain and its physiologic/psychological consequences.

Hypnosis

Medical practitioners have used hypnosis for decades but are rediscovering it for acute and chronic pain management in children. Iverson (1999) documents successful use in an emergency room of hypnosis for children with angulated forearm fractures and no possible access to analgesia during reduction. The children verbally protested during reduction, but no child had any painful memory of the procedure after the reduction was completed. The author describes a simple method of hypnotic induction. Steggles, Damore-Petingola, Maxwell, and Lightfoot (1997) completed an annotated bibliography of hypnosis for children and adolescents with cancer.

Pharmacologic Approaches

Significant strides in pediatric pain management have been made in the past 10 years because of a better understanding of the effects of pharmacologic agents on children. Proper analgesia for all situations should be available to every child. The job of the pediatric provider is to anticipate pain, prevent it as much as possible, and assess the effects of such efforts so that adequate analgesia can be delivered to every child at each intervention.

Morphine is still the "gold standard"—the best drug available for analgesia if medically indicated. Hydromorphone and fentanyl are effective substitutes. Demerol is discouraged due to the potential buildup of its toxic metabolite normeperidine. Diazapam and midazolam still are used frequently; they relieve anxiety, cause sedation, and provide amnesia but do *not* provide analgesia. In this current age of conscious sedation, providers must be mindful that they are providing analgesia, not just amnesia, during a painful procedure. Several articles provide excellent reviews of the basics of sedation and analgesia (Algren & Algren, 1996; Deady & Gorman, 1997). Along with the positive effects of conscious sedation come risks, and the provider must carefully evaluate and continuously monitor the sedated child. End-tidal CO_2 monitoring has been shown to provide an earlier indication of respiratory depression than pulse oximetry and respiratory rate alone (Hart, Berns, Houck, & Boenning, 1997). Providers should follow protocols carefully and review drug dosages annually with updated resource manuals.

Routes of administration include oral; sublingual, buccal, transmucosal; intravenous bolus; intravenous continuous; subcutaneous continuous; patient-controlled analgesia; epidural, intrathecal; IM; intranasal; intradermal; topical, transdermal; rectal; inhalation; and regional nerve block. With this vast array of routes and pharmaceuticals, providers should be able to provide children with effective analgesia.

Recent Research in Analgesia: Topical Anesthetics

A multitude of topical anesthetics is available. Different individuals prefer each type, and each has myths regarding its effectiveness. Roghani, Duperon, and Barcohana (1999) compared 5% EMLA cream, 10% cocaine, 10% lidocaine, 10% benzocaine, 1% dyclonine, and a placebo for effectiveness in the reduction of gingival pain. The authors found that 5% EMLA cream significantly reduced the pain threshold level, followed by 1% dyclonine and 10% benzocaine. Surprisingly, they also found *no significant difference* between the 10% cocaine, 10% lidocaine, and saline placebo. Statistically, except for EMLA cream, there was *no difference* in effectiveness between the placebo and all the drugs.

EMLA has been studied for effectiveness during dorsal penile nerve block (Serour, Mandelberg, Zabeeda, Mori, & Ezra, 1998) and was found to be very effective during needle penetration but to have no beneficial effect during infiltration. EMLA, however, was found to be an effective alternative to lidocaine infusion for analgesia during spinal needle insertion (Sharma, Gajraj, Sidawi, & Lowe, 1996). One of the most common uses for EMLA is as a topical anesthetic before office phlebotomy, and it has been proven very effective in that setting (Young, Schwartz, & Sheridan, 1996).

EMLA commonly is used on intact skin but is not available for laceration repair. Stewart, Simpson, and Rosenberg (1998) studied the effectiveness of soaking a simple laceration with 1% lidocaine and found that doing so did not decrease the pain for the subsequent lidocaine injection. Returning to the topic of dorsal penile nerve block, Serour, Mandelberg, and Mori (1998) found a significant difference in pain score between local anesthetic injected over a slow rate (10 mL over 100–150 seconds) versus a faster rate (10 mL over 40–80 seconds). The slower rate was found to reduce pain, a finding concurrent with other studies. The conclusion is that slow injection under the skin reduces pain.

Recent Research in Analgesia: Systemic Analgesia

Since its introduction into the pediatric population, ibuprofen has been recognized as a potent analgesic and antipyretic. In certain circumstances, however, it is less safe or effective than other measures. Harley and Dattolo (1998) discovered that for tonsillectomy pain, acetaminophen with codeine produced a lower hemorrhage rate (0% versus 12.5%), a decreased mean bleeding time, and a shorter time that medication was required compared with ibuprofen. This combination of factors is convincing evidence that sometimes acetaminophen with codeine is worth the additional effort of acquisition and administration.

Korpela, Korvenoja, and Meretoja (1999) studied postoperative pain and found that children given 40 to 60 mg/kg of rectal acetaminophen during induction of anesthesia had a significantly decreased need for morphine postoperatively. Moreover, these children also had less postoperative nausea and vomiting.

When looking for an ideal oral wound care analgesic (ie, one that is palatable and potent, has a rapid onset and short duration, and requires minimal monitoring), Sharar et al. (1998) found that oral transmucosal fentanyl citrate (OTFC) was safe and effective compared with hydromorphone. OTFC offers a palatable alternative route of administration without IV access for wound care procedures in children.

Common Conditions and Concerns Involving Pain

The pediatric provider will encounter a variety of situations and conditions that cause pain. Some of these are relatively common, recurrent, and usually relatively predictable. Schechter (1995) provides an excellent review of some of these topics for more information.

Injection Pain

Many painful office procedures involve injections, whether for vaccinations, sutures, or other procedures. The following is a short review of basic steps that providers can take to decrease injection pain. If providers use each measure with every child during every injection, starting with the first immunization (or earlier if necessary), children's perceptions of painful events may change significantly.

If time, money, and supply are available, every child with intact skin should receive topical anesthesia for all injections. EMLA is a very effective topical anesthetic at 3 to 5 mm of skin depth, but it must be acquired through a pharmaceutical supply house. It requires up to an hour's preparation time and can be relatively expensive. A relatively quick, easy, inexpensive, and accessible alternative to topical anesthesia is to place ice chips in the finger of a latex glove (or any other effective, convenient packaging) and apply the glove to the site before giving the injection. The child can put the ice back on the site once the injection is finished or actively dump it (and the pain) in the sink. Providers who choose to use a different application method can use ethyl chloride spray to achieve the same results.

Providers can incorporate several simple actions into their normal routine that will decrease injection pain. Beginning with preparation, the provider should choose the injection site carefully. The deltoid muscle is the appropriate site in children older than 12 months. Toddlers who received their immunizations in the anterior thigh had 250% more severe pain than those who received injections in the deltoid muscle. Once a child is walking, the anterior thigh should not be used. If a child must receive a large dose of medication and is older than 3 years, the ventrogluteal site is less painful than the thigh. If the provider must use the thigh, he or she should select the lateral thigh to minimize pain. To recap, the provider chooses the lateral thigh and ventrogluteal muscles over the anterior thigh and dorsogluteal muscles. Deltoid is preferable over all, if possible.

If possible, the clinician uses a 30-gauge needle, and if not, the smallest size allowable for the procedure. The liquid to be injected should be room temperature. If lidocaine is used, it should be buffered. Mixing 1 mEq sodium bicarbonate in 9 mL 1% lidocaine on the day of administration will increase the pH enough to decrease burning. The provider should pinch the child's skin just before injection (a distraction technique).

During the actual injection, several other techniques will continue to decrease the level of pain the child (and all others within hearing range) feels. Providers use the Z-track technique for IM injections. All injections are at a 90-degree angle and are swift and continuous until needle depth is achieved. The next step is to pause. Most people, including children, are most afraid of the actual needle insertion. Pausing gives them a moment to realize that the scariest action is over and that the provider did not lie about the level of needle pain. Children may not even have felt the needle and will actually look to confirm the skin puncture. Children should then take a breath and relax. An IM injection is easier and less painful if given into a relaxed muscle. The provider should tell the child how the actual medicine being injected may feel and remind the child not to move. The provider injects slowly, stopping and continuing at the child's request. Opening bandages beforehand and having the child hold them will give idle hands something to do. The child also will have control over an important step in the procedure. Engaging a child in conversation, distracting in other ways, and praising when finished are crucial.

Otitis Media

Otitis media is the most common reason for an unplanned office visit in children younger than 5 years. This common and painful condition often is undertreated from an analgesia standpoint. Surprisingly few analgesia studies have been published. There is a need to diminish antibiotic usage in otitis media with effusion, but no controversy should surround the need for analgesia. Children typically experience pain for at least 3 days; they should receive analgesia around-the-clock while awake. Acetaminophen provides an analgesic and antipyretic effect but no inflammatory action. Ibuprofen combines all three properties. It may be especially appropriate for acute otitis media in an effort to decrease confusion about treatment failures and the need to switch to a different antibiotic. If pain is severe and unresponsive, acetaminophen with codeine is appropriate. Topical solutions (Auralgan and Americaine are two brands) are marketed specifically to decrease the pain of otitis media, but they have no documented efficacy. Providers should not discontinue treatment with systemic analgesics in favor of other methods at this time.

Headaches

Results of a study drawn from pediatric primary care clinics of 100 consecutive children (ages 3–17 years) with headaches were startling (Lewis et al., 1996). The children wanted three things from their providers: the cause of the headache, what would make it better, and reassurance that they had no life-threatening illness. When asked to draw pictures of how they felt with a headache, 33% disclosed depressive features of helplessness, frustration, and anger. More than 20% of the adolescents depicted themselves as dead, dying, or about to be killed by their headache. Gladstein (1995) and Rothner (1995) wrote excellent articles identifying the most common causes of headaches in children, a methodology to identify them, and a treatment protocol. Gladstein maintains that primary care providers can evaluate and treat most children with headaches.

Analgesic rebound headache, a recognized phenomenon in adults, has just recently been studied in children (Vasconcellos, Pina-Garza, Millan, & Warner, 1998). With an increasing number of children using daily analgesics, this pain-management issue is becoming more common. Daily or near-daily analgesic rebound headaches can be stopped by discontinuing the daily analgesics and concurrently using amitriptyline.

Pharyngitis

Pharyngitis may be bacterial or viral. Children with strep throat consistently rate their pain as 4 or 5 on a scale of 5. For this reason, providing analgesic relief to all children with sore throat is important. Soreness of the throat can impede all other hydration, nutritional, and treatment efforts if it causes a child to refuse to swallow. Possibly because of its anti-inflammatory effect, ibuprofen has been shown to be slightly more effective than acetaminophen and much more effective than a placebo. The effectiveness of "home remedies" (eg, salt water gargles, lozenges, and local anesthetic sprays) is unproven, but such methods appear to be somewhat helpful.

Oral Viral Infection

The ulcers of herpetic gingivostomatitis and herpangina are often very painful, possibly interfering with eating and drinking. If pain persists unaddressed, the child is at risk for dehydration and possibly hospitalization. Drinking through a straw may help because it minimizes oral contact. "Magic mouthwashes" (1:1:1 combination of oral diphenhydramine, viscous lidocaine, and Maalox) seem to decrease discomfort when they are applied to the painful site. As with any product containing viscous lidocaine, such mouthwashes must be used with caution in younger children, who tend to swallow anything placed in their mouths. Swallowed lidocaine could diminish the gag reflex.

Urinary Tract Infections

Analgesia is underused in urinary tract infections across all ages of children. Phenazopyridine hydrochloride (Pyridium) is an effective local anesthetic now available over-the-counter. It is appropriate in children as young as 6 years (10 mg tablet of phenazopyridine hydrochloride). Phenazopyridine hydrochloride should not be used for more than 7 days and is contraindicated if glucose-6-phosphatase deficiencies are present. The tablet should not be crushed, because the dye will stain the mouth and tongue.

Cancer

Chronic cancer pain is the most difficult type of pain to relieve. The amount of medication (usually morphine) children with cancer require to achieve analgesia can be staggering to providers not accustomed to such doses. A constant concern is balancing the dose of morphine against the problems of respiratory depression. Most children who require oral or intravenous morphine for terminal cancer pain do not have problems with respiratory depression at doses that achieve adequate analgesia.

Currently, many of these children need regular pain medication and are effectively cared for at home, regardless of the route of administration. Pediatric hospice specializes in the care of terminal children with chronic pain. As experts in the field of chronic pain, hospice providers are often consulted for nonterminal children who have significant pain issues and are not responding well to standard measures. If a pediatric hospice is not found in the child's geographic area, many hospices are willing to provide guidance over the telephone for difficult issues. Pediatric narcotic analgesics are listed in Table 15-1.

TABLE 15–1.   PEDIATRIC NARCOTIC ANALGESICS

Drug	Dose	Dosage (mg/kg)	Onset (min)	Duration
Morphine sulphate	IM/IV/SC, children: 0.1–0.2 mg/kg/dose q2–4h p.r.n.	0.1 (IV, IM, SC)	5–10 (IV)	3–4 h
	PO: 0.2–0.5 mg/kg/dose (PO) q4–6h p.r.n. (immediate release)	0.2 (PO)	30–60 (PO)	4–6 h
	PO: 0.3–0.6 mg/kg/dose q8–12h p.r.n. (controlled release)	0.3 (PO)	30–60 (PO)	8–10 h
Hydromorphone	IV: 0.015 mg/kg/dose q4–6h p.r.n.	0.015 (IV-SC)	5–10 (IV)	3–4 h
	PO: 0.03–0.08 mg/kg/dose q4–6h p.r.n.	0.075 (PO)	30–60 (PO)	3–4 h
Fentanyl	1–2 μg/kg/dose q30–60 min p.r.n.	0.001 (IV)	3–8 (IV)	0.5–1h
Fentanyl oralet (Fentanyl lollipop)	10–15 μg/kg MAX 400 μg	0.010 (Transmucosal)	20–30 min	

COMMUNITY RESOURCES

Multiple resources are available to help those trying to decrease a child's pain. The American Pain Society (4700 W. Lake Avenue, Glenview, IL 60025-1485, 847-375-4715, http: *www.ampainsoc.org* or email *info@ampainsoc.org*) has a wealth of available resources. It is an excellent place to start looking for information and will be able to assist in a more intensive search.

REFERENCES

Abu-Saad, H. (1981). The assessment of pain in children. *Issues of Comprehensive Pediatric Nursing, 5*(5-6), 327–335.

Algren, J. T., & Algren, C. L. (1996). Sedation and analgesia for minor pediatric procedures. *Pediatric Emergency Care, 12*(6), 435–441.

Anand, K. J., McIntosh, N., Lagercrantz, H., Pelausa, E., Young, T. E., & Vasa, R. (1999). Analgesia and sedation in preterm neonates who require ventilatory support: Results from the NOPAIN trial. Neonatal Outcome and Prolonged Analgesia in Neonates. *Archives of Pediatric and Adolescent Medicine, 153,* 331–338.

Baker, C., & Wong, D. (1987). Q.U.E.S.T.: A process of pain assessment in children. *Orthopedic Nursing, 6*(1), 11–21.

Beyer, J., & Byers, M. L. (1985). Knowledge of pediatric pain: The state of the art. *Children's Health Care, 14,* 233–241.

Beyer, J., DeGood, D., Ashley, L., & Russell, G. (1983). Patterns of postoperative analgesic use with adults and children following cardiac surgery. *Pain, 17,* 71–81.

Chambers, C. T., Giesbrecht, K., Craig, K. D., Bennett, S. M., & Huntsman, E. (1999). A comparison of faces scales for the measurement of pediatric pain: Children's and parents' ratings. *Pain, 83*(1), 25–35.

Deady, A., & Gorman, D. (1997). Intravenous conscious sedation in children. *Journal of Intravenous Nursing, 20*(5), 245–252.

Eland, J. M. (1990). Pain in children. *Nursing Clinics in North America, 25*(4), 871–884.

Eland, J., & Anderson, J. (1977). The experience of pain in children. In A. Jacox (Ed.), *Pain: A sourcebook for nurses and other health professionals.* Boston: Little, Brown.

Fitzgerald, M., Millard, C., & McIntosh, N. (1989). Cutaneous hypersensitivity following peripheral tissue damage in newborn infants and its reversal with topical analgesia. *Pain, 39,* 31–36.

Goldman, A., & Lloyd-Thomas, A. R. (1991). Pain management in children. *British Medical Bulletin, 47*(3), 676–689.

Gladstein, J. (1995). Headaches: The pediatrician's perspective. *Seminars in Pediatric Neurology, 2*(2), 119–126.

Harley, E. H., & Dattolo, R. A. (1998). Ibuprofen for tonsillectomy pain in children: Efficacy and complications. *Otolaryngology-Head and Neck Surgery, 119*(5), 492–496.

Hart, L. S., Berns, S. D., Houck, C. S. & Boenning, D. A. (1997). The value of end-tidal CO_2 monitoring when comparing three methods of conscious sedation for children undergoing painful procedures in the emergency department. *Pediatric Emergency Care, 13*(3), 189–193.

Hermann, C., Blanchard, E. B., & Flor, H. (1997). Biofeedback treatment for pediatric migraine: prediction of treatment outcome. *Journal of Consultant Clinical Psychology, 65*(4), 611–616.

Hester, N. O., & Barcus, C. S. (1986). Assessment and management of pain in children. *Pediatric Nursing Update, 1,* 2–8.

Iverson, K. V. (1999). Hypnosis for pediatric fracture reduction. *Journal of Emergency Medicine, 17*(1), 53–56.

Korpela, R., Korvenoja, P., & Meretoja, O. A. (1999). Morphine-sparing effect of acetaminophen in pediatric day-case surgery. *Anesthesiology, 2,* 442–447.

Lewis, D. W., Middlebrook, M. T., Mehallick, L., Rauch, T. M., Deline, C., & Thomas, E. F. (1996). Pediatric headaches: What do the children want? *Headache, 36*(4), 224–230.

Loeser, J. D. (1990). Pain in children. *Advances in Pain Research Therapy, 15,* 1–4.

McCaffery, M. (1977). Pain relief for the child. *Pediatric Nursing, 3*(4), 7–8.

McGrath, P. A. (1990). Pain assessment in children: A practical approach. *Advances in Pain Research and Therapy, 15,* 6–30.

McGuire, L., & Dizard, S. (1982). Managing pain in the young patient. *Nursing '82, 12*(8), 52–55.

Melzack, R. (1975). The McGill Pain Questionnaire: Major properties and scoring methods. *Pain, 11*(3), 277–299.

Melzack, R., & Wall, P. (1965). Pain mechanisms: A new theory. *Science, 150*(3699), 971–979.

Orenstein, P. A., Manning, M. A., & Pelphrey, K. A. (1999). Children's memory for pain. *Developmental and Behavioral Pediatrics, 20*(4), 262–277.

Ott, M. J. (1996). Imagine the possibilities! Guided imagery with toddlers and preschoolers. *Pediatric Nursing, 22*(1), 34–38.

Porter, F. L., Grunau, R. E. & Anand, K. J. S. (1999). Long-term effects of pain in infants. *Developmental and Behavioral Pediatrics, 20*(4), 253–261.

Rana, S. (1987). Pain: A subject ignored. *Pediatrics, 79,* 309–310.

Richards, M., Bernal, J., & Brackbill, Y. (1976). Early behavioral differences: Gender and circumcision? *Developmental Psychobiology, 9,* 89–95.

Roghani, S., Duperon, D. F., & Barcohana, N. (1999). Evaluating the efficacy of commonly used topical anesthetics. *Pediatric Dentistry, 21*(3), 197–200.

Ross, D. M., & Ross, S. A. (1988). Assessment of pediatric pain: An overview. *Issues in Comprehensive Pediatric Nursing, 11*(2-3), 73–91.

Rothner, A. D. (1995). The evaluation of headaches in children and adolescents. *Seminars in Pediatric Neurology, 2*(2), 108–118.

Savendra, M. C., Tessler, M. D., Holzemer, W. L., & Ward, J. A. (1993). Assessment of postoperative pain in children and adolescents using the Adolescent pediatric pain tool. *Nursing Research, 42*(1), 5–9.

Schechter, N. L. (1984). Recurrent pains in children: An overview and approach. *Pediatric Clinics of North America, 31*(5), 949–968.

Schechter, N. L. (1985). Pain and pain control in children. *Current Problems in Pediatrics, 15*(5), 6–67.

Schechter, N. L. (1989). The undertreatment of pain in children: An overview and approach. *Pediatric Clinics of North America, 36*(4), 781–795.

Schechter, N. L. (1995). Common pain problem in the general pediatric setting. *Pediatric Annals, 24*(3), 139, 143–146.

Schechter, N. L., & Allen, D. (1986). Physicians' attitudes toward pain in children. *Developmental and Behavioral Pediatrics, 7,* 350–354.

Schultz, N. (1971). How children perceive pain. *Nursing Outlook, 19,* 670–673.

Serour, F., Mandelberg, A., Zabeeda, D., Mori, J., & Ezra, S. (1998). Efficacy of EMLA cream prior to penile nerve block for circumcision in children. *Acta Anesthesiology Scandinavia, 42*(2), 260–263.

Sharar, S. R., Bratton, S. L., Carrougher, G. J., Edwards, W. T., Summer, G., Levy, F. H., & Cortiella, J. (1998). A comparison of oral transmucosal fentanyl citrate and oral hydromorphone for inpatient pediatric burn wound care analgesia. *Journal of Burn Care Rehabilitation, 19*(6), 516–521.

Sharma, S. K., Gajraj, N. M., Sidawi, J. E., & Lowe, K. (1996). EMLA cream effectively reduces the pain of spinal needle insertion. *Regional Anesthesia, 21*(6), 561–564.

Steggles, S., Damore-Petingola, S., Maxwell, J., & Lightfoot, N. (1997). Hypnosis for children and adolescents with cancer: An annotated bibliography, 1985-1995. *Journal of Pediatric Oncology Nursing, 14*(1), 27–32.

Stewart, G. M., Simpson, P., & Rosenberg, N. M. (1998). Use of topical lidocaine in pediatric laceration repair: A review of topical anesthetics. *Pediatric Emergency Care, 14*(6), 419–423.

Swafford, L., & Allan, D. (1968). Pain relief for the pediatric patient. *Medical Clinics of North America, 52,* 131–136.

Taddio, A., Katz, J., Ilerisich, A. L. & Koren, G. (1997). Effect of neonatal circumcision on pain response during subsequent routine vaccination. *Lancet, 349,* 599–603.

Tessler, M. D., Savedra, M. C., Holzemer, W. L., & Ward, J. A. (1989). Children's words for pain. In S. G. Funk (Ed.), *Key aspects of comfort: Management of pain, fatigue and nausea.* New York: Springer Publishing.

Vasconcellos, E., Pina-Garza, J. E., Millan, E. J., & Warner, J. S. (1998). Analgesic rebound headache in children and adolescents. *Journal of Child Neurology, 13*(9), 443–447.

Wagner, A. M. (1998). Pain control in the pediatric patient. *Dermatological Clinics, 16*(3), 609–617.

Wong, D. L., & Baker, C. (1988). Pain in children: Comparison of assessment tools. *Pediatric Nursing, 14*(1), 9–17.

Young, S. S., Schwartz, R., & Sheridan, M. J. (1996). EMLA cream as a topical anesthetic before office phlebotomy in children. *Southern Medical Journal, 89*(12), 1184–1187.

Zeltzer, L. K., Bush, J. P., Chen, E., & Riveral, A. (1997). A psychobiologic approach to pediatric pain: Part I. History, physiology, and assessment strategies. *Current Problems in Pediatrics, 27,* 225–258.

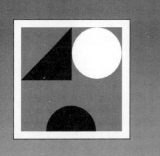

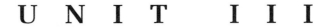
PRIMARY CARE OF CHILDREN WITH DEVELOPMENTAL AND ENVIRONMENTAL CHALLENGES

The Premature and Low–Birth-Weight Infant

- DAVID M. DEIULIO, MD, FAAP; STEVEN J. KOVACS, MD, FAAP; and WENDY MCKENNEY, MS, ARNP

INTRODUCTION

Since the advent of neonatology in the early 1960s, the management of premature and low–birth-weight newborns has undergone dramatic changes. Ever-smaller babies are surviving and as cost-containment efforts, which mandate the earliest possible discharges from neonatal intensive care units, (NICUs), increasing numbers of preterm babies are discharged home with unresolved health care needs and complex care issues. Graduates of NICUs experience a much higher rate of hospital readmissions during their first year than do their healthy full-term counterparts. This chapter reviews common and practical concerns for providers dealing with these infants before, during, and after NICU discharge. It is a basic guide to understanding the needs of such infants.

COMMON CONCERNS FOR PRETERM AND LOW–BIRTH-WEIGHT INFANTS

Primary care of preterm infants begins long before hospital discharge. The designated local primary care provider should communicate frequently with NICU staff from delivery to discharge to ensure that the provider is fully aware of the infant's clinical course and has a broad perspective of both baby and family. A discharge planning meeting may be necessary for some infants who have special needs (eg, oxygen therapy or monitoring equipment). The provider's participation in such a meeting is ideal but may be impractical. The American Academy of Pediatrics (AAP) (1998a) recently has published guidelines for predischarge collaboration between hospital staff and post-discharge provider, which should include arrangements for the following:

- Home nursing visits
- Any medical equipment going home with the baby
- Community referrals
- Specialist appointments, if indicated
- Plans for developmental follow-up
- Hearing and vision screening
- Immunization status
- Diet and medications
- Parental caregiving
- Education needs
- Questionable home environment or family issues

The NICU care provider should create a detailed discharge summary that includes ongoing problems and risk factors with recommendations for management.

▲ **Clinical Warning:** Providers who do not receive a discharge summary should contact the NICU to obtain one. It should contain recommendations specific to that infant's needs and should be a part of the clinician's office records.

The baby's first visit to the primary care provider should occur within a few days after discharge. The discharging neonatologist or neonatal nurse practitioner will recommend the timing of this initial visit according to the baby's specific needs. Some infants may need weekly or biweekly visits after discharge until adequate growth has been established, and the transition to the home environment is considered complete (Trachtenbarg & Miller, 1995).

Nutrition

At birth, premature infants are at a nutritional disadvantage, because they are born without the nutrient stores that the fetus normally accrues during the last trimester (Pursley & Cloherty, 1998). The nutrition goal for preterm infants is to approximate the rate of intrauterine growth (Nutrition Committee, Canadian Pediatric Society, 1995). Smaller (less than 1800 g) and younger (less than 34 weeks) premature infants require formula specifically designed to provide higher protein, mineral, and caloric contents. Human breast milk requires supplementation with special fortifiers to provide for those needs. Table 16-1 provides information about the vitamin and mineral supplementation needs of premature infants.

● **Clinical Pearl:** Poly-Vi-Sol with iron preparation contains sufficient amounts of vitamins A, D, C, E, B_1, B_2, B_6, B_{12}, niacin, and iron. It generally is given as 1 mL (1 dropperful) every 24 hours.

At discharge, preterm infants must be able to demonstrate competency with breastfeeding or bottle feeding. Providers can discontinue nutrient supplementation at a corrected age of 36 weeks in most infants or when exclusive breast-feeding has been established.

● **Clinical Pearl:** The primary care provider should follow infant and mother closely to ensure the baby's adequate growth and hydration. Obtaining a 24-hour diet history at the first office visit helps determine adequacy of feeding. The provider also should review stooling and voiding patterns to ensure that they are appropriate for the baby's chronologic age. The clinician should reinforce normal and expected patterns of feeding, including frequency of nursing. If the mother reports difficulty, she should feed the infant in the office so that the provider can assess the problem's origin. A referral to a lactation specialist may help the mother–infant dyad improve breast-feeding skills (Trachtenbarg & Golemon, 1998).

Table 16–1.   VITAMIN AND MINERAL SUPPLEMENTATION FOR THE PREMATURE INFANT

Vitamins and Minerals	Dose	Indication	Duration	Side Effects
Folate	50 mcg/d	Breast-fed premature infants	Until taking 150–200 mL/kg/d	Nontoxic
Iron	2–4 mg/kg/d	Breast-fed premature infants	From 2 mo of age through the first year of life	Generally minimal: GI upset, black stools, constipation, staining of teeth (liquid formulation)
Vitamin D	400 IU/d Daily multivitamin supplement provides an appropriate dose.	Premature infants	Formula fed: Until infant is taking in 1 L/d Breastfed: first 6 mo of life	Symptoms of toxic levels include nausea, vomiting, weakness, diarrhea, polyuria, failure to thrive
Fluoride	0.25 mg/d	Only in the absence of fluoridation of water source	6 mo through 12–14 y of age	Rare: rash, atopic dermatitis, urticaria, stomatitis, GI and respiratory allergic reactions
Vitamin E	5–25 IU/d Daily multivitamin supplement provides an appropriate dose.	Breast-fed premature infants	First 6 mo	Symptoms of toxic levels include GI upset, rash, headache, blurred vision

The AAP recommends exclusive formula feeding or breastfeedings for the first 5 to 6 months of life (Lucas, 1993), with caregivers postponing the introduction of solid foods until this time. Because this recommendation is based on the maturational status of the infant's nervous system, intestinal tract, and kidneys, premature infants need not necessarily wait until 5 to 6 months' corrected age. Some babies are indeed ready at 5 to 6 months' actual age, while others require more time. The primary care provider should be able to assess an infant's developmental progress and make an appropriate recommendation.

Breast-fed Infants

Many experts believe that human milk is the preferred diet for all infants. Breast milk benefits premature infants in many ways. Milk secreted the first 4 to 6 weeks after premature delivery differs in composition from milk secreted after term. Though the fat contents are similar in both, the fat in preterm milk is of a smaller globule size, enhancing its absorption. Absorption of fat from human milk is 95% compared with 85% in preterm formula. Many of the long-chain fatty acids necessary for brain growth also are higher in human preterm milk (Harnosh, 1994). Before 32 weeks' gestation, active transport of immunoglobulin G across the placenta does not begin in earnest and the immune system is immature. Thus, infants born before this time are immunologically disadvantaged (Goldman et al., 1994). The immunoglobulins present in human milk, however, offer protection to these vulnerable preterm babies. Studies have demonstrated fewer infections in breast-fed preterm infants (El-Mohandes et al., 1997; Goldman et al., 1994; Hylander, Strobino, & Dhanireddy, 1998). Moreover, all breastfed infants appear to have higher developmental and IQ scores (Tudehope & Steer, 1996; Horwood & Fergusson, 1998; Lucas, 1993) than do formula-fed babies.

Formula-Fed Infants

Preterm infants whose mothers do not plan to breast-feed require a formula designed to provide increased calories,

protein, and minerals. These infants generally are switched to a term formula at 36 weeks' corrected age. Wheeler and Hall (1996) concluded that infants who weighed less than 1800 g at birth and were kept on a preterm formula for 8 weeks after discharge were longer and had larger head circumferences 12 weeks after discharge than did preterm infants who received term formula. The short-term advantages are clear, but long-term benefits are less certain. Extremely premature (less than 28 weeks) babies often experience delays in reestablishing adequate growth after birth. Therefore, recommendations are to discharge these infants home for several months on an intermediate formula, such as Neocare, which has 22 kcal/oz. The long-term benefits of this approach have not been documented clearly.

Occasionally, an infant with high metabolic expenditures (eg, chronic lung disease, malabsorption, neurologic impairment, congenital heart disease) requires a higher kcal/oz formula after discharge as well. These babies are at slightly higher risk for hyperosmolar dehydration and may need monitoring of their electrolyte levels if they experience vomiting or diarrhea (Trachtenbarg & Golemon, 1998).

Growth

Adequate growth of premature babies should be documented using charts designed specifically for them, available through the AAP. Preterm infants experience catch-up growth that exceeds the rate of growth of term babies. Maximal catch-up growth occurs between 36 and 44 weeks' chronologic age. Babies who are small for gestational age experience the most rapid growth in the first 3 months of life, with catch-up growth continuing to school-age. A small percentage of infants never catch up to the term infant (Trachtenberg & Golemon, 1998a; Dusick, 1997).

▲ **Clinical Warning:** Poor growth and nutrition have major effects on developmental outcomes (Dusick, 1997). Providers must evaluate infants with poor growth for swallowing difficulties, gastroesophageal reflux, anemia, hypoxemia, or other factors (eg, feeding behaviors) that may be compromising ability to obtain sufficient nutrition. Providers can then initiate appropriate therapeutic interventions.

Immunizations

The AAP releases a standard, up-to-date pediatric immunization schedule each year, which is used for all babies, including premature infants. No schedules are specific for premature infants, who should receive all childhood vaccines at the correct chronologic age, not at corrected gestational age. Currently, the only exception is for the first hepatitis B vaccine, which should be administered when the baby weighs 2 kg if the mother is hepatitis B surface antigen-negative. Studies have demonstrated higher seroconversion in the group vaccinated at a weight greater than 2 kg (AAP, 1997). Refer to Chapter 13, Immunizations, for information concerning specific preparations and the timing of their administration.

▲ **Clinical Warning:** Infants with evolving neurologic disorders should not receive pertussis vaccine. They should receive pediatric Diptheria and Tetanus vaccine (without the pertussis component present in the DPT vaccine) instead.

Sleep

Prone sleeping has been associated with a higher incidence of sudden infant death syndrome (SIDS). In 1992, the AAP began recommending a supine or side-lying sleeping position for healthy term infants. Since then, the United States has experienced a 15% to 20% decrease in the incidence of SIDS (AAP, 1996). The risks and benefits of supine sleeping must be weighed individually for other than healthy term infants. If no contraindications to supine or side sleeping exist, the infant is switched to the supine position before discharge. Infants with neuromuscular disorders may need positioning that prevents secretions from pooling in the back of the throat. Babies with craniofacial abnormalities or evidence of upper airway obstruction require a prone sleeping position.

▲ **Clinical Warning:** To prevent smothering, parents must avoid using soft bedding and loose covers, including baby quilts. They must evaluate use of crib bumpers carefully, ensuring that the infant's head will not become lodged between bumper pad and crib rail (AAP, 1996).
In addition to sleep positioning, parents must be aware that premature infants sleep more hours total than term infants but experience more frequent awakenings. Transitioning the baby from the brightly lit and noisy nursery to the quieter home environment may take some time. Some parents have found that soft music or lighting helps soothe the baby during this time (Dusick, 1997).

COMMON CONDITIONS IN PREMATURE AND LOW–BIRTH-WEIGHT INFANTS

Cryptorchidism

Premature male infants are at risk for cryptorchidism (nondescended testes). Embryologically, the testes begin to descend from abdomen to scrotum between 28 to 30 weeks' gestation. By term, 95% of testes in infants are in the scrotum; most are fully descended by 6 to 9 months. At 1 year, testes remain undescended in only 0.7% of infants.

Cryptorchidism is associated with future development of testicular cancer. Surgical consultation will be necessary if the testes are not descended by 1 year, because it is unlikely for this condition to change after that time (Trachtenburg & Goleman, 1998; Kaplan, 1994).

Inguinal Hernias

Inguinal hernias are more common in premature males who have required prolonged mechanical ventilation. They may be repaired before discharge, because the risk for incarceration is high due to the small size of the inguinal ring. Infants with chronic lung disease may be discharged with plans for hernia repair when their respiratory status has improved. In any case, a hernia that is present at or discovered after discharge requires surgical intervention. These infants require close monitoring. Parents need to learn the signs of hernia incarceration and strangulation (Trachtenburg & Goleman, 1998; Ringer, 1998).

Bronchopulmonary Dysplasia

As technologic support for preterm infants has improved, the definition of bronchopulmonary dysplasia (BPD) has evolved (Bancalari et al., 1979; Northway, Rosan, & Porter, 1967). Shennan et al. (1988) define BPD as oxygen dependence at 36 weeks' postconceptional age, with radiologic abnormalities and a history of assisted ventilation. Infants with BPD have an increased risk for respiratory morbidity in the first few years of life. Studies have suggested using the term chronic lung disease (CLD) to describe these babies (Hack et al., 1991). Diagnosis of BPD at 28 days is still useful, however, because some who subsequently improve and are asymptomatic at discharge (and thus do not have CLD) still have abnormal pulmonary function tests (Abbasi & Bhutani, 1990; Myers et al., 1986).

▲ **Clinical Warning:** Infants with BPD are at greater risk of rehospitalization with concurrent respiratory infections. They have less pulmonary reserve than do babies without BPD.

Epidemiology

Incidence of BPD and CLD is inversely proportional to birth weight and gestational age. It is directly proportional to the presence and severity of respiratory distress syndrome (RDS), the absence of antenatal corticosteroid exposure, aggressive mechanical ventilation, high oxygen requirements, pneumothoraces, fluid overload, hemodynamically apparent patent ductus arteriosus (PDA), sepsis, Caucasian race, male sex, and low Apgar score. In addition, heredity seems to play a role, because incidence is associated with a strong family history of asthma and an HLA-A2 haplotype (Farrell & Fiascone, 1997; Abman & Groothius, 1994; Nickerson & Taussig, 1980).

Several advances in neonatal care responsible for the decreasing incidence of CLD may be responsible for the continued high incidence of BPD. These advances include the following:

- Maternal antenatal steroids. These decrease both the incidence of RDS and the need for mechanical ventilation and high oxygen supplementation. They also increase the concentration of antioxidants in premature lungs; these mitigate the toxic effects of supplemental oxygen.
- Surfactant therapy. This decreases mortality but has no real effect on incidence of BPD. This is probably because of the increasing survival of extremely premature babies, whose pulmonary anatomic immaturity compli-

cates their course and their response to surfactant, and increases the time they spend on a ventilator exposed to supplemental oxygen.

Etiology

The cause of BPD is multifactorial. Both ventilator-associated barotrauma and exposure to high oxygen concentrations are essential to survival in the treatment of RDS, to which premature babies are frequently exposed. Ventilator-associated barotrauma and exposure to high oxygen concentrations, however, are capable of initiating an inflammatory reaction in the lungs (Farrell & Fiascone, 1997). Each of these factors causes an influx of neutrophils into the lungs, damaging them by generating oxygen-free radicals that release inflammatory mediators. These mediators, in turn, attract more neutrophils, creating an ongoing cycle of damage (Frank, 1992; Groneck et al., 1994). Premature babies have underdeveloped pulmonary antioxidant systems, making them particularly susceptible to oxygen toxicity.

Infection and colonization of the airway with *Ureaplasma urealyticum* has been identified as a risk factor for BPD. Pneumonia of any viral or bacterial etiology also may contribute to the development and severity of BPD, because pneumonia leads to activation of the inflammatory cascade, prolonging the need for mechanical ventilation.

Management

Different neonatal units use different modalities, including the following:

- High-frequency ventilators
- Synchronized ventilation (reduces the incidence of pneumothoraces, thus decreasing incidence of BPD)
- Permissive hypercapnia (permits higher pCO_2 values [less barotrauma])
- Relative fluid restriction
- Postnatal steroid administration (equivocal effects on the incidence of BPD because of wide variation in its use [dosage, timing, length of treatment] as well as confounding variables, such as the diverse approaches to ventilator strategies, fluid management, between centers)

Primary care providers deal with a spectrum of patients with BPD after they graduate from the NICU. Their conditions range from apparently asymptomatic with normal growth, to mild CLD requiring diuretics and enhanced nutritional needs, to more severe CLD requiring supplemental oxygen and various medications.

● **Clinical Pearl:** Outpatient management for patients with BPD revolves around the use of supplemental oxygen, pharmacologic treatment (ie, inhaled bronchodilators, and diuretics, with occasional use of corticosteroids), and appropriate nutrition. In addition to well child care, the main focus should be on growth, monitoring respiratory symptoms, and appropriate use of and weaning from medications. The primary care provider can perform these functions in conjunction with a pediatric pulmonologist in more severe cases.

Assuming the provider participated in the baby's care prior to discharge, the initial outpatient visit should occur no longer than 2 weeks and ideally a few days after discharge. Follow-up visits may be necessary every few days to every few weeks until the infant has adjusted fully to home care

and is doing well clinically. The provider periodically should attempt to reduce or eliminate therapies when the patient is asymptomatic and growing well.

▲ **Clinical Warning:** Short-term oxygen saturation analysis in the office is not very predictive of long-term status and will fail to identify hypoxic episodes associated with stress, including sleeping, feeding, and crying. Episodic periods of desaturations can be measured and are not necessarily associated with apnea, bradycardia, or even cyanosis. They can therefore go undetected (Farrell & Fiascone, 1997; Garg et al., 1988).

As these patients grow, new lung tissue forms over a period of about 8 years, and pulmonary function improves. They may have abnormal pulmonary function for the rest of their lives, even if only noted in formal pulmonary function tests (Northway et al., 1990; Galdes-Sebaldt et al., 1989). They have experienced the double-edged sword of mechanical ventilation and supplemental oxygen during a critical period of lung development, ultimately leaving them with decreased numbers of larger-than-normal alveoli, gas exchange surface area, and pulmonary reserves.

Oxygen Therapy

Babies with BPD seem to require small amounts of oxygen for prolonged periods. Providers must avoid marginal oxygenation or hypoxia. The increased pulmonary vascular resistance that accompanies BPD improves with high-normal pO_2 levels and is worsened by low-normal levels or hypoxia. General recommendations are to maintain oxygen saturations above 92% (Rush & Hazinski, 1992; Koops, Abman, Accurso, 1984). Low-flow oxygen therapy by nasal cannula is preferred, because high flow use is associated with drying of the nasal mucosa. Adequate growth is a marker of adequate oxygenation (Moyer-Mileur et al., 1996).

The weaning process should begin when the baby has experienced no respiratory symptoms for weeks and has shown an increase in growth of 20 to 40 g/d. Providers should record oxygen saturations in all states. If a baby does well in some states but not others, support must increase during those times of stress. Feeding and deep sleep are examples of times when oxygen requirements increase; perhaps they should serve as the last frontier in the weaning process. Good growth is a very good indicator of the child's tolerance to the weaning process.

▲ **Clinical Warning:** Hypoxia can occur during different states (eg, activity, feeding, rest, deep sleep) (Dusick, 1997). Monitoring at different times is essential to knowing the patient's real oxygen requirements and to determining when weaning should begin. Oxygen therapy frequently is underused and stopped too quickly, resulting in alveolar hypoxia, poor growth, feeding difficulties, and pulmonary hypertension.

Pharmacologic Approaches

Airway hyper-reactivity frequently occurs in these patients, manifesting itself as increased work of breathing, inspiratory crackles, expiratory wheezing, and increased inability to handle concurrent viral illnesses. Bronchodilators are used widely for these problems and seem effective in decreasing the work of breathing, energy expenditure, and consequently caloric requirements. Of inhaled beta-mimetics, albuterol is most commonly used in NICUs.

Dosage starts at 1 mg in 2 to 3 mL of normal saline regardless of weight (0.2 mL of the 0.5% solution) and is adjusted either up or down, depending on its effects or the appearance of adverse reactions (eg, sustained tachycardia). Anticholinergic preparations like ipratropium bromide, especially in concert with beta-mimetics, also have been used successfully.

One difficulty concerns the method of administration (eg, nebulizer, metered-dose inhaler) and the variable delivery to the distal airways. In addition, controversy exists over chronic versus as-needed use, based on asthma literature suggesting that chronic therapy ultimately increases mortality and worsens control (Barrington & Finer Neil, 1998). Methylxanthines (aminophylline and caffeine) also can be used as bronchodilators but are more commonly used in the acute management of apnea. Few babies are discharged home on methylxanthines for CLD. These medications have a narrow safety margin (more true for aminophylline than caffeine). Many outside factors affect serum levels, side effects are common, and frequent levels are necessary. Their role as a major treatment modality even in asthma has fallen dramatically.

● **Clinical Pearl:** Frequent assessment for evidence of improvement is recommended with the use of inhaled bronchodilators. Providers should check breath sounds before and after administration. If no longer clinically useful, providers should discontinue and reuse them as needed. These concerns also are true for inhaled steroids.

At least early in its course, BPD is associated with interstitial pulmonary edema and responds to administration of diuretics. Additionally, diuretics seem to improve directly pulmonary function. Initial treatment is furosemide (Lasix), then combination therapy with spironolactone (Aldactone, 1–3 mg/kg per dose every 24 hours) and hydrochlorothiazide (1–2 mg/kg per dose every 12 hours) or chlorothiazide (10–20 mg/kg per dose every 12 hours) for their potassium and calcium-sparing properties. Most improvements are short term, and data are lacking on long-term benefits. These medications support improved nutrition through larger volume intake in addition to their beneficial effects on pulmonary function. Because chronic diuretic use is associated with electrolyte imbalance, providers must follow the infant's serum electrolyte levels, making adjustments to potassium and sodium chloride supplements that seem to be inevitably required. Caregivers can mix these supplements with feedings.

● **Clinical Pearl:** Providers should wean infants from diuretics gradually (or infants can "outgrow" the dose) but only after discontinuing supplemental oxygen. Subsequent deterioration (as with intercurrent viral illness) may warrant the reinstitution of oxygen therapy and short-term use of furosemide. Home equipment should remain available for an extended period after discontinuation for these likely events.

Administration of corticosteroids to premature babies with BPD modifies their clinical course and controls the pulmonary inflammatory process that treatment for RDS induces. Corticosteroids acutely reduce oxygen and ventilator pressure requirements, improve pulmonary function, and lead to earlier extubation. These effects, however, are short-lived. Once these drugs are discontinued, many affected infants gradually return to pretreatment requirements. Corticosteroids do not appear to increase significantly risk of infection, decrease length of hospitalization, improve mortality, or alter the incidence of BPD or CLD (Farrell & Fiascone, 1997; Barrington & Finer Neil, 1998; Van Schachyk et al., 1990). Data are lacking on their long-term pulmonary effects or potential effects on neurodevelopment. They impair short-term growth (although usually limited to the time of use) and cause hyperglycemia and hypertension (which are easily treated and self-limited) and biventricular myocardial hypertrophy (BMH) (Werner et al., 1992; Ohning, Fyfe, & Riedel, 1993). BMH is not associated with permanent changes and resolves over several weeks.

Intercurrent viral illnesses will likely require oxygen support, which providers should use liberally. Bronchodilators will also likely be needed if such infections are associated with worsening symptoms (eg, wheezing, increased work of breathing, tachypnea, cough). They may be accompanied by use of inhaled steroids (either by metered-dose inhaler with a spacer and face mask or nebulizer). Beclomethasone (Beconase AQ and Vancenase AQ) or flunisolide (Nasalide) are commonly used products. Providers should prescribe them in a few divided doses to reduce the incidence of oral candidiasis (Avent, Gal, & Ranson, 1994).

Inhaled steroids take longer than systemic steroids to work and should be used for several weeks before assessing their effectiveness. Cromolyn has been used but has not been shown to be of benefit to BPD. It has, however, been proven effective in asthma. It prevents mast cell degranulation and the subsequent release of inflammatory mediators and prevents bronchospasm (Frank, 1992). Cromolyn, a prophylactic medication to be used chronically, takes at least 2 weeks to produce an effect.

Nutrition

Nutrition is of paramount importance in patients with BPD. Poor nutrition can adversely affect host defenses and the ability of the lungs to undergo repair. Providing adequate nutrition for acutely ill, extremely premature babies with RDS is complicated. These babies never received the maternal transfer of many nutrients that normally occurs late in the third trimester (eg, trace elements and important cofactors for antioxidant enzyme production and function) (Frank, 1992). Growth failure, common in BPD, is associated with the increased oxygen consumption and work of breathing. These factors are further compounded by the relative fluid restriction used in treatment and the feeding difficulties these patients sometimes experience, including gastroesophageal reflux and aversion to oral feedings. Bronchodilators and methylxanthines commonly used in treatment also contribute to growth problems.

● **Clinical Pearl:** These babies require continued nutritional support after discharge. Enhanced support helps meet the increased requirements associated with pulmonary dysfunction and enhances adequate repair of damaged lung tissue and growth of new, normal lung tissue. Babies with BPD need formulas with increased caloric density (22–27 cal/oz) and additional support from carbohydrate and medium-chain triglyceride enhancers (eg, Polycose and MCT oil). Providers should decrease these formulas gradually and only after the baby is weaned successfully from oxygen and diuretic therapies.

● **Clinical Pearl:** Consultation before discharge with speech pathology or pediatric gastroenterology can help with feeding difficulties. If it does not occur before discharge, the primary care provider should arrange such consultation as soon as possible.

Complications

Patients with BPD have an increased risk for sudden death related to episodes of arterial oxygen desaturation that go undetected or to abnormal hypoxic arousal responses (Farrell & Fiascone, 1997). Cor pulmonale, rarely seen today, is associated with an increased risk for sudden death. It can be diagnosed and followed by echocardiograms and prevented or improved by resisting the urge to wean the patient off supplemental oxygen too soon.

Respiratory morbidity and rehospitalization from both upper and lower respiratory tract infections are high during the first 1 to 2 years after discharge (Dusick, 1997). Any common viral pathogen can cause serious infection with major deterioration in the patient's clinical state. The most common pathogens other than those associated with the common cold are respiratory syncytial virus (RSV), adenovirus, and influenza virus. Refer to the section on immunizations in this chapter for prevention and administration information and to Chapter 13.

The leading cause of lower respiratory tract infection in children is RSV, and risk of serious disease is high with prematurity and CLD. Currently, prophylaxis in these patients consists of monthly intravenous (IV) infusions of RSV-IVIG (Respigam) or monthly intramuscular (IM) injections of palivizumab (Synagis) during the RSV season, which varies across regions (Groothius et al., 1993; The PREVENT Study Group, 1997).

▲ **Clinical Warning:** Antibodies from RSV-IVIG interfere with immunity to measles vaccine. For this reason, the MMR vaccine should be held for 9 months after the last dose.

Guidelines for the use of Respigam are well established (AAP, 1997); it requires IV administration of a large volume of fluid (15 mL/kg) over several hours, which can compromise these volume-sensitive patients, who may require diuretic administration. In addition, Respigam generally is not administered in the office or home setting but is usually given in an outpatient facility.

Palivizumab solves many of the above problems in using Respigam. Palivizumab has been shown to be at least as effective as the IV preparation (the Impact-RSV Study Group, 1998). Advantages include its IM administration, lack of serious side effects, and efficacy at prevention of RSV that equals that of RSV-IVIG. Palivizumab can be given in the office or home setting, still as a monthly injection during the RSV season. In addition, it seems to show no interference with the measles vaccine. Indications for its use are now also available (AAP, 1998b). For premature infants being discharged who qualify for RSV prophylaxis, some neonatologists continue to give the first dose as Respigam, because this product also protects against other viruses. Palivizumab only protects against RSV. If Respigam was the initial predischarge formulation used, the primary care provider can safely and effectively continue monthly prophylaxis with palivizumab.

Hypertension of unknown etiology occurs with increased frequency in infants with CLD. It responds well to antihypertensives and resolves in essentially all these children over time. It remains important to follow blood pressures after discharge home (Farrell & Fiascone, 1997; Dusick, 1997). Some programs use home cardiorespiratory monitors for patients with CLD who require supplemental oxygen (Farrell & Fiascone, 1997; Abman & Groothius, 1994; Rush & Hazinski, 1992), but use of such monitors has not been shown to reduce mortality.

Apnea of Prematurity

Apnea of prematurity is a manifestation of immature central and peripheral respiratory control mechanisms, which can be affected adversely by the various metabolic, infectious, and environmental stresses to which premature babies are exposed. As these newborns mature, apnea generally resolves (Southall et al., 1983). Global maturation also must occur (ie, coordination of sucking, swallowing, and breathing), because this process will affect the presence and resolution of clinical apnea. Upper airway obstruction or gastroesophageal reflux also influence apnea.

For the purposes of this discussion, the following terms are defined:

- Apnea refers to the cessation of airflow and can be central, obstructive, or mixed in etiology.
- Short central apnea (less than 15 seconds) can be normal at all ages.
- Apnea of prematurity is apnea of longer than 20 seconds in a premature infant. It usually resolves by 37 weeks' postconceptional age, unless the infant is born prior to 28 weeks' gestation, in which case apnea of prematurity can persist beyond 40 weeks.
- Apnea of infancy refers to the cessation of airflow for longer than 20 seconds or shorter if associated with bradycardia, cyanosis, pallor, or marked hypotonia in patients whose onset of apnea appears later than 37 weeks' gestational age (Henderson Smart, 1981).

Apnea of prematurity frequently persists beyond term in infants delivered at 24 to 28 weeks' gestational age. Such apnea can therefore contribute to prolonged hospitalization (Malloy & Graubard, 1995) or to increased use of postdischarge monitoring.

Sudden Infant Death Syndrome and Acute Life-Threatening Events

Sudden infant death syndrome is the sudden death of a child younger than 1 year that remains unexplained after the performance of a complete postmortem investigation, including an autopsy, examination of the death scene, and review of the case history (Eichenwald, Aina, & Start, 1997). Its peak incidence is at age 2 to 4 months (95% of cases occur by 6 months of age).

● **Clinical Pearl:** All subsequent siblings of an infant who died from SIDS should be discharged home on a monitor.

An acute life-threatening event (ALTE) refers to an episode that is frightening to the observer and is characterized by some combination of apnea (central or obstructive), color change, marked change in muscle tone, choking, or gagging. In some cases the observer fears that the infant has died (Henderson Smart, 1981).

Pneumogram studies in the newborn period are not predictive of SIDS or ALTEs. Although premature babies are at increased risk of SIDS, apnea of prematurity itself does not seem to predispose to it. No evidence exists that apnea of prematurity predisposes to apnea of infancy (Henderson Smart, 1981).

● **Clinical Pearl:** There is no way to identify accurately which premature baby will ultimately die from SIDS. This fact has contributed to the confusion surrounding optimal management of these babies once discharged home.

Home Apnea Monitoring

No hard and fast rules govern which growing premature babies require home monitoring, how long to monitor them, and when to discontinue monitoring. Some things, however, have been generally agreed upon. Routine monitoring of asymptomatic preterm babies is not recommended, and the pneumogram should not be used as a screening tool (Henderson Smart, 1981). Most NICUs have a policy that requires some time during which the patient is apnea-free (between 5 and 10 days) before their discharge home without monitors. Only one study has examined how long the apnea-free period should be prior to discharge (Darnall et al., 1997). This study demonstrated that 36% of babies born before 28 weeks' gestation had apnea that persisted beyond 40 weeks. Infants who had been apnea-free for 8 days or more were unlikely to have another apnea episode, unless they had some other risk factor known to be associated with a resurgence of apnea of prematurity (eg, surgery, chronic lung disease, sepsis, RSV, immunizations). These findings support the notion of a waiting period before discharge, although more studies would be valuable. The increasing survival of extremely premature babies with known late resolution of apnea of prematurity speaks against setting fixed weight or postconceptional age as a criterion for discharge home. If a premature baby is not discharged home on a monitor, apnea of prematurity should have resolved and should not be an area of concern for the primary care provider.

▲ **Clinical Warning:** Shortening the apnea-free period before discharge to satisfy the push to decrease length of hospitalization is unwise.

Many centers use home monitors on premature babies who continue to have apnea or require methylxanthines to control apnea when they are otherwise ready for discharge home. Some facilities also monitor when gastroesophageal reflux has been shown to be the cause of documented apnea. Babies with CLD at discharge also are monitored frequently.

▲ **Clinical Warning:** Immunizations can be associated with resurgence of apnea for several days (Stefano et al., 1991), as can childhood illnesses, particularly respiratory tract infections (most notably RSV).

Given the foregoing, criteria are general and loose concerning the decision to send a baby home on a monitor. How well does monitoring work, and when is it discontinued? Again, reports, issues, and approaches are confusing and inconsistent. Cote et al. (1998) analyzed the frequency and timing of events in infants using home monitoring. They looked at former premature infants discharged on monitors for unresolved apnea of prematurity, infants with ALTE, siblings of babies with SIDS, and babies monitored for parental anxiety. Former premature infants were more likely to have events than all other groups. Most significant events began in the first month in all groups. Poor correlation existed between recorded events and clinically observed events.

Knowing which babies require home monitoring is difficult. Transient self-resolved bradycardia occurs in convalescent premature infants and even in healthy term infants up to 6 months of age. These babies look fine despite the alarm. In the NICU, clinical observers are trained to know that apnea or bradycardia alarms may go off for various reasons unrelated to apnea of prematurity, such as stretching or stooling. The cause impacts whether an alarm is recorded as an event.

▲ **Clinical Warning:** Families going home with a newborn on a monitor need to be well trained to make such judgments. Conversely, significant hypoxemia can occur without apnea or bradycardia in apparently well preterm infants. This factor influences the need to monitor oxygen saturation and heart and respiratory rates. These babies appear blue despite adequate heart and respiratory rates. Cause for concern may be warranted if these episodes occur repeatedly, because low saturations can adversely influence retinopathy, necrotizing enterocolitis, and periventricular leukomalacia. They also can play a role in the development of increasing pulmonary vascular resistance.

● **Clinical Pearl:** Monitors with capabilities of recording oxygen saturation and events are recommended. Providers should instruct parents to keep a log of all alarms, the clinical situation associated with each alarm, and their perception as to whether the event was real or false. Downloading the monitor's recording often can assist in documenting whether parents' perceptions of alarms are accurate.

At discharge home, alarm settings generally are established with the low heart rate limit at less than 80 beats per minute (bpm), the high heart rate limit at greater than 200 bpm, and the apnea limit at longer than 20 seconds. Oxygen saturation alarm, if available, should be set at less than 93%. If monitoring is used for many months, the provider may want to change the low heart rate limit to less than 70 bpm in the second and third months of life and to less than 60 bpm in the fourth through sixth months. Parents should only use the monitor when surveillance of the baby is not continuous. They need not use the monitor when they are holding, bathing, feeding, or constantly observing the infant.

The appropriate time at which to discontinue the monitor varies widely, but basically depends on the initial indication for its use. Most primary care providers require variable periods for no alarm episodes to pass before discontinuing the monitor. If a formal apnea center is not following the infant after discharge, probably the best criteria for discontinuing the use of home monitors comes from Cote et al. (1998):

- The monitor can be discontinued after 1 month without events unless events occurred after age 44 weeks' postconceptional age. In this case, the monitor is maintained for a minimum of 6 months, with discontinuation at that time after a 2-month apnea-free period (can discontinue at 6 months if 2 months have passed without apnea).
- If the baby is on methylxanthines (caffeine or theophylline), the monitor can be discontinued after 1 month without medications and events (again, unless event occurs after 44 weeks' postconceptional age).
- If parental anxiety was the initial indication, discontinuing the monitor when the parents no longer feel they need it is reasonable.

Anemia

Anemia is defined as a deficiency in circulating red cells and hemoglobin (Hgb) concentration that causes tissue hypoxia (U.S. Department of Health and Human Services, 1990). Multiple pathologic events cause anemia, including fetal-maternal hemorrhage, hemoglobinopathies, intracranial hemorrhage, and twin-to-twin transfusion syndrome. The focus of this discussion is on the expected postnatal course of events, which culminates in nonpathologic (or physiologic) anemia.

Physiology and Pathology

All infants normally experience anemia several weeks after birth; this is an expected consequence of the transition from a low-oxygen environment *in utero* to an oxygen-rich environment outside the womb. This phenomenon is called "anemia of infancy." Premature infants experience an exaggerated response that has been labeled "anemia of prematurity." To understand anemia of prematurity, a basic understanding of red cell physiology and the pathology of anemia is necessary.

The hormone erythropoietin (epo), which is manufactured in the fetal liver (Kannourakis, 1994), stimulates the production of red cells. In the presence of low partial pressure of oxygen, such as is the case *in utero*, epo levels are high, stimulating red cell production. Under normal circumstances, infants are born with relatively high hematocrit and Hgb levels. At birth, the infant moves to an oxygen-rich environment with adequate tissue oxygenation. The hypoxic stimulus to the bone marrow ceases, signaling the body to shut down production of red cells. Epo becomes virtually undetectable (Christou & Rowitch, 1998). Subsequently, both Hgb and hematocrit fall as senescent cells are removed from the circulation, giving rise to physiologic anemia.

Premature infants experience a more profound postnatal anemia when compared with term infants. Red cells in preterm infants are decreased in mass and have shorter lifespans. Rapid growth and expansion of intravascular volume in these babies result in hemodilution and decreased concentration of Hgb and red cells. These combined factors produce a significantly earlier and lower nadir of hematocrit and Hgb (Gladir & Naiman, 1991). Whereas term infants reach their nadir at 8 to 12 weeks, premature infants do so at 4 to 6 weeks, during which time Hgb levels may be as low as 6.5 to 7 g/dL. The low Hgb level decreases tissue oxygenation, which stimulates the kidneys to produce epo, initiating red cell production. During this production phase, the body rapidly uses its iron stores (Christou & Rowitch, 1998).

▲ Clinical Warnings:

- Preterm infants typically have iron stores to maintain Hgb synthesis for approximately 10 weeks. If they do not receive iron supplements, these babies will develop iron deficiency anemia (Gladir & Naiman, 1991).
- Infants who are symptomatic for anemia may display apnea, bradycardia, tachycardia, tachypnea, pallor, or poor weight gain. Infants on home oxygen therapy may have increased oxygen requirements. Oral feedings are difficult when the infant's respiratory rate exceeds 60 breaths per minute. All these factors lead to increased metabolic demands and caloric expenditures. A baby who feeds poorly does not grow.

Management

Recommendations are for iron supplementation to begin by 6 to 8 weeks after birth. The body does not use iron given before this time but actively stores it for later Hgb synthesis.

● **Clinical Pearl:** Iron supplementation should continue for 6 months in premature infants whose birth weights were more than 1500 g. Infants who weighed less than 1500 g at birth should receive iron supplements throughout the first year. Infants fed a formula supplemented with iron may not need additional supplementation. Infants fed human milk or a nonfortified formula must receive iron supplementation.

Iron dosages may be advanced to a maximum of 15 mg/kg/d (Ehrenkranz, 1993). The reticulocyte count and Hgb level can help in determining the infant's response to therapy and the need for dose adjustments. In general, the NICU graduate at discharge has a low but stable Hgb with a rising reticulocyte count and will probably not require further transfusions. The provider should check these every few weeks until sure that the reticulocyte count is rising.

Recombinant human erythropoietin (r-HuEPO) is a promising and controversial new treatment and prophylaxis for anemia of prematurity. Although not yet routine practice, preliminary studies have shown that administering r-HuEPO results in an increased hematocrit and number of reticulocytes and decreased frequency and volume of blood transfusions in large, healthy premature infants (Cohen & Marino, 1998). A U.S. multicenter trial demonstrated a mean age of 22 days for the first dose of r-HuEPO, with 600 mg divided into three weekly injections, continuing for 6 weeks (Miller & Martin, 1998). This trial demonstrated significant decreases in the number and volume of red cell transfusions in study infants. Administration of r-HuEPO without iron supplementation causes a rapid decline in serum iron and ferritin stores. It is recommended not to initiate r-HuEPO until iron supplementation can be given, generally once full enteral feeding has been established (Asch & Wedgewood, 1998).

The risks and side effects of r-HuEPO administration in adults include hypertension, bone pain, rashes, and, rarely, seizures. None have been reported in infant trials. Two studies reported a total of three infants who died from SIDS. Long-term studies are needed to determine if this rare adverse effect can be attributed to r-HuEPO administration (Ohis, 1998). R-HuEPO is administered subcutaneously. The clinician must balance benefits against the number of injections that will be required during treatment.

● **Clinical Pearl:** If anemia is suspected, the provider can check a reticulocyte count along with the hematocrit and Hgb levels. A general rule of thumb for deciding to transfuse is Hgb less than 6.5 g/dL or hematocrit less than 20% combined with a reticulocyte count of less than 3%. If the baby is symptomatic with higher values (poor weight gain, tachycardic, poor coloration, lethargic, and apneic), a transfusion also may be required (Kannourakis, 1994).

Hearing Impairment

Hearing is essential for the development of normal speech and language skills. Significant hearing impairment can affect these skills as early as the first 6 months of life. In the general population, estimates of the prevalence of newborn hearing loss are between 1.5 and 6 out of every 1000 live births (Parving, 1993). Prevalence of sensorineural hearing loss in NICU survivors is increased 10-fold, reported at 2% to 4% (Duara et al., 1986).

Hearing impairment is difficult to diagnose and many times is impossible to detect by physical examination alone. With technologic advances, screening for newborn hearing loss using auditory brainstem responses (ABRs) and otoacoustic emission (OAE) testing has become a practical modality. Current recommendations support screening for hearing loss in all newborns within the first 3 months and starting interventions by 6 months (Joint Committee on Infant Hearing, 1994; National Institute of Health, 1993; U.S. Department of Health and Human Services, 1990).

The ABR evaluates the hearing pathway from ear to brainstem. The automated model operates through disposable earphones and emits a 35-dB HL click at a rate of 37 pulses per second. Electrodes placed on the infant's forehead and nape of the neck detect brainstem responses and transmit them for computer-automated evaluation. The computer tabulates and prints the results as a "pass" or "refer." The advantage of ABR technology is its ability to screen with accuracy without requiring interpretation by a trained audiologist. Infants who register a "refer" unilaterally or bilaterally on repeat testing, however, require referral for further diagnostic evaluation to an audiologist with expertise in newborn hearing.

The OAEs are sounds that the cochlea creates as it processes noise. OAE testing identifies cochlear function. This technology measures cochlear sounds through a microphone placed in the clean ear canal (provided middle ear function is normal). It requires no electrodes and records OAEs in seconds under ideal conditions. The major advantage of OAE screening is its rapid testing time. Its disadvantage is that it requires a specialist with expertise for interpretation.

● **Clinical Pearl:** Ideally, screening for hearing will occur for all newborns, especially NICU graduates, before discharge.

Should an infant be discharged from an NICU in which universal hearing screening is unavailable, the AAP (1995) has made specific recommendations for infants with the following conditions:

- Family history of hereditary childhood sensorineural hearing loss
- *In utero* infection, such as cytomegalovirus, rubella, syphilis, herpes, and toxoplasmosis
- Craniofacial anomalies, including those with morphologic abnormalities of the pinna and ear canal
- Birth weight less than 1500 g (3.3 lb)
- Hyperbilirubinemia at a serum level requiring exchange transfusion
- Ototoxic medications, including but not limited to the aminoglycosides, used in multiple courses or in combination with loop diuretics
- Bacterial meningitis
- Apgar scores of 0 at 1 minute or 6 at 5 minutes
- Mechanical ventilation lasting 5 days or longer
- Stigmata or other findings associated with a syndrome known to include a sensorineural or conductive hearing loss

Once a significant hearing loss is identified, it is of utmost importance for the patient to be evaluated for sound augmentation. Small behind-the-ear hearing aids can assist even infants with very severe hearing loss. Babies should be fitted with two aids for binaural reception. Cochlear implants may be indicated for children who cannot benefit from conventional amplification. These patients should be enrolled in early intervention programs (EIPs) to assess for other developmental problems. Refer to Chapter 53 (Hearing Impairment and Disorders) for further discussion.

Retinopathy of Prematurity

Retinopathy of prematurity (ROP) is a recognized disorder of the retinal blood vessels in preterm infants. ROP is common in low–birth-weight infants and is responsible for total visual loss in as many as 2% to 4% of infants weighing less than 1000 g at birth (AAP, Section on Ophthalmology, 1997). Improved technologies and advances in neonatal care have helped to increase survival of small infants at earlier gestational ages; however, severe visual problems persist as long-term sequellae for these infants. The spectrum of ROP ranges from mild with complete resolution to severe with the potential for retinal detachment and blindness.

Pathology

Injury to the immature and delicate retinal capillary bed can cause ROP. Stresses such as hyperoxia, shock, sepsis, and asphyxia are all associated risk factors (Phelps, 1993). The healing process that follows often involves excessive regrowth of damaged retinal vessels at birth. This injury and its subsequent blood vessel maldevelopment are known as ROP.

In the past, theorists believed oxygen therapy to be the cause of ROP, related to the indiscriminate use of oxygen in the 1950s (Kinsey, Jacobus, & Hemophill, 1956). After severe restrictions were placed on the use of oxygen therapy, ROP virtually disappeared until the 1970s, when modern technologies emerged in intensive care nurseries, improving the survival of smaller and younger premature infants (Phelps, 1981). Today ROP is considered a nonpreventable disorder among infants whose retinal vasculature is extremely immature at birth (Gibson et al., 1990).

In 1984, investigators developed a nomenclature for categorizing ROP, which now is referred to as the International Classification of Retinopathy of Prematurity (ICROP, 1984). This classification, used throughout the world, describes the location, severity, and extent of ROP. It has enabled investigators to compare data from numerous centers meaningfully and accurately, which in turn has helped to launch multi-centered, prospective, and randomized trials evaluating various treatment modalities.

Three key criteria for classification are used by ICROP (Fig. 16-1):

- *Location* of the disease within the eye is described by the use of three zones. Zone I is the posterior portion of the eye near the optic disk, encompassing an area with a radius twice the distance from the macula. Zone II forms a region of the retina from zone I to the equator of the eye, involving the edge of the retina (ora serrata) on the nasal side. Zone III is the remaining retina outside zone II. Location of disease is critical to prognosis. For example, central vision is located in zone I. Severe ROP here bodes a much poorer prognosis than would ROP in zone 3, where peripheral vision is located.
- *Severity* of the vascular changes is indicated by stages. Stage I is the mildest detectable change. Stage II indicates moderate disease, but damage is still within the retinal substance. Stage III is of greatest concern because of the presence of intravitreal vessels. Stage IV is partial retinal detachment. Stage V is total retinal detachment.
- *Extent* of ROP is measured by viewing the retina as if it were the face of a clock, divided into 12 "hour" segments. The more "hours" that show damage, the worse is the case of ROP. In addition, the appearance of neovascularization (in which blood vessels become engorged and tortuous) is termed "plus disease" and is used as an additional descriptor.

▲ **Clinical Warning:** Some premature infants are ready for discharge at 35 to 36 weeks' postconceptional age. The potential exists for NICUs to discharge these infants before the incidence of ROP peaks. Very vigilant follow-up by an ophthalmologist with expertise in ROP and knowledge of ICROP is essential. A general ophthalmologist, pediatric ophthalmologist, or retinologist each may qualify, depending on experience. The primary care provider should inquire at the time of NICU discharge if the infant will require further

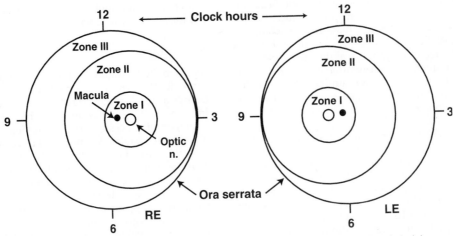

Figure 16–1 ■ Scheme of retina of right eye (RE) and left eye (LE) showing zone borders and clock hours employed to describe location and extent of retinopathy of prematurity. (Reprinted with permission of *Archives in Ophthalmology*, 1984, 102, 1130–1134.)

follow-up, which the neonatologist, primary care provider, and ophthalmologist should coordinate.

Management

Throughout the 1980s, cryotherapy (cryoablation) was the main treatment modality. It uses a special probe to freeze the avascular retina anterior to the region of active disease. Cryotherapy reduces the progression of ROP from 51% to 31% in the treated eye by preventing the development of retinal folds and detachment (Cryotherapy for Retinopathy of Prematurity Cooperative Group, 1988). The goal is to preserve the already vascularized retina by destroying the peripheral retina, in theory ablating the tissue yet to be vascularized and diminishing continued vessel growth. More recently, the indirect diode laser has replaced cryotherapy as the mainstay of treatment. Laser treatment is easier and reduces the side effects commonly observed with cryotherapy, such as swollen eyelids, apnea and bradycardia, and oxygen desaturations.

Sequellae of Regressed Retinopathy of Prematurity

Infants who have had ROP still may experience visual sequellae in spite of full regression of their disease. In particular, they may have myopia, strabismus, and amblyopia (Phelps, 1995). Myopia may be quite severe and require corrective lenses at an early age. Amblyopia may require patching of one eye.

▲ **Clinical Warning:** Aggressive therapy with glasses and patching should not be delayed, because it is necessary to salvage binocular vision. Patients require regular follow-up with a pediatric ophthalmologist or an informed general ophthalmologist.

WHAT TO TELL THE PARENTS

Parents need ongoing education and support to help them with the transition home. Anticipatory guidance will help families to make the experience positive. Providers should inform parents of common physical characteristics found in premature infants. These babies, particularly those with very low birth weights, frequently have a characteristic molding of the head as a consequence of gravity and positioning on a very malleable skull. The face appears long and narrow, with eyes close to the sides of the head. The skull looks flattened on both sides. These effects generally resolve by age 4 years (Trachtenberg & Golemon, 1998).

Developmental follow-up is very important. Many NICUs have developmental specialists who examine babies in clinics after discharge home. These specialists can ascertain early signs of developmental delay and can help families connect with community resources that will best meet their child's specific needs for EIPs. Depending on locale, such specialists also may coordinate follow-up with state or provincial health department support and staffing.

Primary care providers play a pivotal role in educating parents about the importance of accessing the services of child development clinics. They must emphasize to parents that their babies will meet critical milestones of growth and development at their corrected gestational, not chronologic, ages.

COMMUNITY RESOURCES

Because every community has different resources available, a good place to start when considering the need for external support is Appendix E, Community and Agency Resources, in Ballard, E. A. (1988). *Pediatric care of the ICN graduate* (pp. 329-330). Philadelphia: W.B. Saunders. No national or international umbrella organization exists for information on EIPs; providers can obtain local and regional information about this service from their own states or provinces. Providers also may want to use their referring NICUs as contact points for obtaining this information. Health department officials in children's services also may be of assistance.

Resources for parents include the following:

Harrison, H. (1983). *The premature baby book.* New York: St. Martin's Press. (Available through Amazon.com).
The Alexis Foundation (advocates for the rights of premature infants and their families)
PO Box 1126
Birmingham, MI 48012-1126
(248) 543-4169; Toll free (877) alexis-0

thealexisfoundation@prodigy.net,
http://pages.net/thealexisfoundation/THEALEXIS1.html.

**American Association of Premature Infants (AAPI)
(dedicated to improving health and service delivery)**
PO Box 6920
Cincinnati, OH 45206
(513) 956-4331
http://www.aapi-online.org

**Merter Hospital's Neonatology Unit (maintains a web site
for parents)**
Neonatology 6C
202 South Park St.
Madison, WI 53715
*http://www.medsch.wisc.edu/childrenshosp/parents of
preemies/index.html.*
Spanish version:
*http://www.medsch.wisc.edu/childrenshosp/Preemie Parent
Sp/spindex.html.*

**La Leche League (site on breast-feeding a premature
infant)**
http://lalecheleague.org/bfprem.html

**Preemie Parent Connection (contains a column co-
authored by Wendy McKenney, MS, ARNP)**
http://www.geocities.com/Heartland/Acres/1503/index.html

REFERENCES

Abbasi, S., & Bhutani, V. K. (1990). Pulmonary mechanics and energetics of normal, non-ventilated low birthweight infants. *Pediatric Pulmonology, 8,* 89.

Abman, S. H., & Groothius, J. R. (1994). Pathophysiology and treatment of bronchopulmonary dysplasia. *Pediatric Clinics of North America, 41,* 277–315.

American Academy of Pediatrics. (1998a). Committee of fetus and newborn: Hospital discharge of the high-risk neonate—proposed guidelines. *Pediatrics, 102,* 411–417.

American Academy of Pediatrics. (1998b). Policy statement. Prevention of respiratory syncytial virus infections: Indications for the use of palivizumab and update on the use of RSV-IVIG. *Pediatrics, 102,* 1211–1216.

American Academy of Pediatrics. (1997). *The red book* (pp. 247–260). Report of the committee on infectious diseases.

American Academy of Pediatrics. (1997). Committee of Infectious Diseases and Committee on Fetus and Newborn. Respiratory syncytial virus immune globulin, intravenous: Indications for use. *Pediatrics, 99,* 645–650.

American Academy of Pediatrics. (1996). *Positioning and sudden infant death syndrome: Update.* Policy statement.

Asch, J., & Wedgewood, J. (1998). Optimizing the approach to anemia in the preterm infant: Is there a role for erythropoietin therapy? *Journal of Perinatology, 17,* 276–282.

Avent, M. L., Gal, P., & Ranson, J. L. (1994). The role of inhaled steroids in the treatment of bronchopulmonary dysplasia. *Neonatal Network, 13,* 63–69.

Bancalari, E., Abdenour, G. E., Feller, R., et al. (1979). Bronchopulmonary dysplasia: Clinical presentation. *Journal of Pediatrics, 95,* 819–829.

Barrington, K. J., & Finer Neil, N. (1998). Treatment of bronchopulmonary dysplasia. *Clinics in Perinatology, 25,* 177–202.

Christou, H., & Rowitch, D. (1998). Hematologic problems. In J. Cloherty & A. Stark (Eds.), *Manual of neonatal care: Joint program in neonatology* (4th ed.) (pp. 453–460). Philadelphia: Lippincott-Raven.

Cohen, A., & Marino, C. (1998). Transfusion practices in infants receiving assisted ventilation. *Clinics in Perinatology, 25,* 97–111.

Cote, A., Hum, C., Brouillette, R., et al. (1998). Frequency and timing of recurrent events in infants using home cardiorespiratory monitors. *Journal of Pediatrics, 132,* 783–789.

Cryotherapy for Retinopathy of Prematurity Cooperative Group. (1988). Multicentered trial of cryotherapy for retinopathy of prematurity: Preliminary results. *Pediatrics, 81,* 697–706.

Darnall, R. A., Kattwinkel, J., Nattie, C., et al. (1997). Margin of safety for discharge after apnea in preterm infants. *Pediatrics, 100,* 795–801.

Duara, S., Suter, C. M., Bessard, K. K., et al. (1986). Neonatal screening with auditory Brainstem responses. Results of follow up audiometry and risk factors evaluation. *Journal of Pediatrics, 108,* 276–281.

Dusick, A. M. (1997). Medical outcomes in preterm infants. *Seminars in Perinatology, 21,* 164–177.

Eichenwald, E. C., Aina, A., & Start, A. R. (1997). Apnea frequently persists beyond term gestation in infants delivered at 24 to 28 weeks. *Pediatrics, 100,* 354–359.

Ehrenkranz, R. (1993). Iron, folic acid, and vitamin B12. In R. Tsang, A. Lucas, R. Uauy, & S. Zlotkin (Eds.), *Nutritional needs of the preterm infant* (pp 177–194). Baltimore: Williams & Wilkins.

El-Mohandes, A., Picard, M., Simmens, S.J., et al. (1997). Use of human milk in the intensive care nursery decreases the incidence of nosocomial sepsis. *Journal of Perinatology, 17,* 130–134.

Farrell, P. A., & Fiascone, J. M. (1997). Bronchopulmonary dysplasia in the 1990's: A review for the pediatrician. *Current Problems in Pediatrics,* April 1997.

Frank, L. (1992). Antioxidants, nutrition, and bronchopulmonary dysplasia. *Clinics in Perinatology, 19*(3), 541–562.

Galdes-Sebaldt, M., Sheller, J. R., Grogaard, J., et al. (1989). Prematurity is associated with abnormal airway function in childhood. *Pediatric Pulmonology, 7,* 259–264.

Garg, M., Kurzner, S. I., Bautista, D., et al. (1988). Hypoxic arousal responses in infants with bronchopulmonary dysplasia. *Pediatrics, 81,* 634–642.

Gibson, D. L., Sheps, S. B., Uh, S. H., et al. (1990). Retinopathy induced blindness: Birth weight specific survival and the new epidemic. *Pediatrics, 86,* 405.

Gladir, B., & Naiman, J. (1991). Erythrocyte disorders in infancy. In Shaffer & Avery (Eds.), *Diseases of the newborn* (pp. 798-827). Philadelphia: W.B. Saunders.

Goldman, A., Chheda, S., Keeney, S. et al. (1994). Immunologic protection of the premature newborn by human milk. *Seminars in Perinatology, 18,* 495–501.

Groneck, P., et al. (1994). Association of pulmonary inflammation and increased microvascular permeability during the development of bronchopulmonary dysplasia: A sequential analysis of inflammatory mediators in respiratory fluids of high-risk preterm neonates. *Pediatrics, 93,* 712–718.

Groothius, J. R., Simoes, E. A. F., Levin, M. J., et al. (1993). Prophylactic administration of respiratory syncytial virus immune globulin to high-risk infants and young children. *New England Journal of Medicine, 329,* 1524–1530.

Hack, M., Horbar, J. D., Malloy, M. H., et al. (1991). Very low birth weight outcomes of the National Institute of Child health and Human Development Neonatal Network. *Pediatrics, 87,* 587–597.

Harnosh, M. (1994). Digestion in the premature infant: The effects of human milk. *Seminars in Perinatology, 18,* 485–494.

Henderson Smart, D. J. (1981). The effect of gestational age on the incidence and duration of recurrent apnoea in newborn babies. *Australian Paediatric Journal, 17,* 273–276.

Horwood, L., & Fergusson, D. (1998). Breastfeeding and later cognitive and academic outcomes. *Pediatrics, 101,* 1–12.

Hylander, M., Strobino, D., & Dhanireddy, R. (1998). Human milk feedings and infection among very low birth weight infants. *Pediatrics, 102,* 38.

The Impact-RSV Study Group. (1998). Palivizumab, a humanized respiratory syncytial virus monoclonal antibody, reduces hospitalization from respiratory syncytial virus infection in high-risk infants. *Pediatrics, 102,* 531–537.

An international classification of retinopathy of prematurity. (1984). *Archives of Ophthalmology, 102,* 1130–1134.

Joint Committee on Infant Hearing. (1994). 1994 Position Statement. *ASHA, 36,* 38–41.

Kannourakis, G. (1994). The biology of erythropoietin and its role in the anemia of prematurity. *Journal of Pediatric Health, 30,* 293–295.

Kaplan, G. (1994). Structural abnormalities of the genitourinary system. In G. Avery, M. Fletcher, & M. MacDonald (Eds.), *Neonatology: Pathophysiology and management of the newborn* (4th ed.) (pp. 887–913). Philadelphia: J.B. Lippincott.

Kinsey, V. E., Jacobus, J. T., & Hemophill, F. M. (1956). Retrolental fibroplasia: Cooperative study of RF and use of oxygen. *Archives of Ophthalmology, 56,* 481.

Koops, B. L., Abman, S. H., & Accurso, F. J. (1984). Outpatient management and follow-up of bronchopulmonary dysplasia. *Clinical Perinatology, 11,* 101–122.

Lucas, A. (1993). Enteral nutrition. In R. Tsang, A. Lucas, R. Uauy, & S. Zlotkin (Eds.), *Nutritional needs of the preterm infant* (pp. 209–223). Pawling, NY: Caduceus Medical Publishers.

Malloy, M. H., & Graubard, B. (1995). Access to home apnea monitoring and its impact on rehospitalization among very-low-birth-weight infants. *Archives in Pediatric and Adolescent Medicine, 149,* 326–332.

Miller, H., & Martin, R. (1998). Pathophysiology of apnea of prematurity. In Polin & Fox (Eds.), *Fetal and neonatal physiology* (pp. 1129–1143). Philadelphia: W.B. Saunders.

Moyer-Mileur, J., Nielsen, D. W., Pfeffer, K. D., et al. (1996). Eliminating sleep-associated hypoxemia improves growth in infants with bronchoplmonary dysplasia. *Pediatrics, 98,* 779–783.

Myers, M. G., McGunness, G. A., Lachenbruch, P. A., et al. (1986). Respiratory illnesses in survivors of infant respiratory distress syndrome. *American Review in Respiratory Distress, 133,* 1011–1018.

National Institutes of Health. (1993). *Consensus statement: Early identification of hearing impairment in infants and young children, 11,* 1–24.

Nickerson, B. G., & Taussig, L. M. (1980). Family history of asthma in infants with bronchopulmonary dysplasia. *Pediatrics, 65,* 1140–1146.

Northway, W. H., Rosan, R. C., & Porter, D. Y. (1967). Pulmonary disease following respiratory therapy of hyaline-membrane disease. *New England Journal of Medicine, 276,* 357–368.

Northway, W. H., Jr., Moss, R. B., Carlisle, K. B., et al. (1990). Late pulmonary sequelae of bronchopulmonary dysplasia. *New England Journal of Medicine, 323,* 1793–1799.

Nutrition Committee, Canadian Paediatric Society. (1995). Position paper: nutrient needs and feeding of premature infants. *Canadian Medical Association Journal, 152,* 1765–1785.

Ohis, R. (1998). Developmental erythropoiesis. In Polin & Fox (Eds.), *Fetal and neonatal Physiology* (pp. 1071–1084). Philadelphia: W.B. Saunders.

Ohning, B. L., Fyfe, D. A., & Riedel, P. A. (1993). Reversible obstructive hypertrophic cardiomyopathy after dexamethasone therapy for bronchopulmonary dysplasia. *American Heart Journal, 125,* 253–256.

Parving, A. (1993). Congenital hearing disability epidemiology and identification: A comparison between two health authority districts. *International Journal of Pediatric Otolaryngology, 27,* 29–46.

Phelps, D. L. (1995). Retinopathy of prematurity. *Pediatrics in Review, 16,* 50–56.

Phelps, D. L. (1993). Retinopathy of prematurity. *Pediatric Clinics of North America, 4,* 705–714.

Phelps, D. L. (1981). Retinopathy of prematurity: An estimate of visual loss in the United States. *Pediatrics, 67,* 924.

The PREVENT Study Group. (1997). Reduction of respiratory syncytial virus hospitalization among premature infants and infants with bronchopulmonary dysplasia using respiratory syncytial virus immune globulin prophylaxis. *Pediatrics, 99,* 93–99.

Pursley, D., & Cloherty, J. (Eds.) (1998). *Manual of neonatal care.* Philadelphia: Lippincott Williams & Wilkins.

Ringer, S. (1998). Surgical emergencies in the newborn. In Cloherty, J. P., & Stark, A. R. (Eds.), *Manual of neonatal care: Joint program in neonatology* (4th ed.) (pp. 617–632). Philadelphia: Lippincott-Raven.

Rush M. G., & Hazinski, T. A. (1992). Current therapy of bronchopulmonary dysplasia. *Clinical Perinatology, 19,* 563–590.

Shennan, A. T., Dunn, M. S., Ohlsson, A., et al. (1988). Abnormal pulmonary outcomes in premature infants: Prediction from oxygen requirement in the neonatal period. *Pediatrics, 82,* 527–532.

Southall, D. P., Richards, J. M., de Swiet, M., et al. (1983). Identification of infants destined to die unexpectedly during infancy: Evaluation of predictive importance of prolonged apnea and disorders of cardiac rhythm or conductor. *British Medical Journal, 286,* 1092–1096.

Stefano, J. L., Anday, E. K., David, J. M., et al. (1991). Pneumograms in premature infants: A study of longitudinal data. *American Journal of Perinatology, 8,* 170–173.

Trachtenbarg, D., & Goleman, T. (1998a). Care of the premature infant: Part 1. Monitoring growth and development. *American Family Physicians, 57,* 2123–2130.

Trachtenbarg, D., & Goleman, T. (1998b). Office care of the premature infant: Part II: Common medical and surgical problems. *American Family Physicians, 57,* 2383–2390.

Trachtenbarg, D., & Miller, T. (1995). Office care of the small premature infant. *Primary Care, 22,* 1–20.

Tudehope, D., & Steer, P. (1996). Annotation: Which milk for the preterm infant? *Journal of Paediatrics and Child Health, 32,* 275–277.

U.S. Department of Health and Human Services. (1990). *Healthy People 2000.* Washington, DC, Public Health Services DHHS, PHS;91-5021.

Van Schachyk, C., Dompeling, D., van Herwaarden, H., et al. (1990). Bronchodilator treatment in moderate asthma or chronic bronchitis: Continuous or on demand? A randomized controlled study. *British Medical Journal, 303,* 1426–1431.

Werner, J., Sicard, R., Hansen, T. W. R., et al. (1992). Hypertrophic cardiomyopathy associated with dexamethasone therapy for bronchopulmonary dysplasia. *Journal of Pediatrics, 120,* 286–291.

Wheeler, R. E., & Hall, R. (1996). Feeding of premature infant formula after hospital discharge of infants weighing less than 1800 grams at birth. *Journal of Perinatology, 16,* 111–116.

The Challenged Family: Issues and Insights

• JANET BRANDT, RN, MS, FNP-C

INTRODUCTION

Childhood disability results in 26 million office visits and 5 million hospital days annually (Newacheck & Halfon, 1998). Childhood disability profoundly impacts the health care system, just as the health care system deeply affects family adaptation, functioning, and quality of life. Families with disabled children confront continual and daily stresses, many of which reflect the chronicity of care rather than the underlying disorder. These stresses may burden the family emotionally, socially, and financially. They also may necessitate dealing with complex and often bureaucratic systems to obtain health care, rehabilitation, education, and health insurance benefits.

The increased survival rate of low–birth-weight infants, children with spinal cord injuries and head trauma, and children with congenital disorders, such as heart disease and cystic fibrosis, has contributed significantly to the growing percentages of disabled children. The shift away from institutional care to care in the home environment requires exploration if new health care delivery models that focus on the family are to be developed. Creative, collaborative parent–provider approaches are necessary to meet the needs of these children. The clinician needs to be aware of critical issues that parents face when caring for a chronically ill or challenged child, while also recognizing the condition's potential impact on the family system itself. This chapter describes how a family might feel about and respond to the needs of their ill or developmentally challenged child, while underscoring the importance of the provider's role in helping that family manage the needs of all members.

THE ROLE OF THE PRIMARY CARE PROVIDER

Primary care providers are in the unique position of assisting disabled and ill children to reach their full potential. They can achieve this goal best by facilitating the integration of the child and family into the community, while minimizing the effects of the disability on the child's overall growth and development.

● **Clinical Pearl:** The Committee on Children With Disabilities suggests that the provider's role is to render a medical "home" that is responsive to the family's changing needs, working with other health care professionals, and responding to governmental agencies and third-party payers (American Academy of Pediatrics, 1997). Providers have a critical role in diagnosis, family adaptation, interdisciplinary coordination, acute care delivery, long-term treatment, and transition planning.

All the provisions of the Americans With Disabilities Act (ADA) apply to children and adolescents with disabilities (American Academy of Pediatrics, 1996). The provider who is familiar with these provisions can educate and counsel parents and patients about their rights, connecting them with appropriate resources. Furthermore, the practitioner can augment the intent of the ADA by increasing community sensitivity through advocacy: reducing barriers in and maximizing the child's interaction with the community. Chapter 18 may provide the reader with further insight.

The Message and the Messenger

From the moment parents suspect that something is not right with their child, they may seek answers in the hope of satisfying their angst with a reasonable explanation. Behind their questions may lie the fear that something is, in fact, seriously wrong. Worry and self-doubt prevail, part of the precariousness of parenthood. One parent described it in the following way:

> When your child has a problem it shakes the foundations of your relationships, your confidence in your own parenting, your faith in God, and your conviction that any problem is surmountable if only you work hard enough. The search for answers can be draining and frustrating as you slam against dead ends, and you may find yourself swinging between high motivation and inertia. Even when you are fortunate enough to find an answer, the journey has changed you forever. For better or worse, it has changed you (Unknown parent, Redbook Magazine, 1996, p.77).

Although parents may have had every indication that a problem existed and may have actively pursued the evaluation and diagnosis, hope protected them from their worst fears, which suddenly are made real in the conclusions rendered by the provider. In that moment, parents must begin to grieve the loss of their "perfect" child. Agitation, confusion, and repetitive questioning are part of the emotional response. The provider can and should acknowledge and validate feelings of shock, fear, sadness, and anger.

▲ **Clinical Warning:** Breaking bad news to a family about a child's condition is a challenging responsibility. The family will remember this news and its telling forever. They will painfully relive the memory of these few minutes again and again. The provider should not tell bad news to a parent who does not have a support system present or in an environment or manner unworthy of this solemn moment. This initial encounter will influence the parent's perception of health professionals, setting the tone for future trust and communication. Because much of this family's well-being hinges on the parents' ability to relate to and collaborate with needed professionals, a meaningful, positive connection is imperative.

Sad news is received initially in its emotional context. Expression of shock and distress is expected. Without explicit permission to be frightened and emotional, parents may conceal their feelings to maintain decorum and avoid embarrassment. The energy they direct toward suppressing these feelings distracts parents from attending to the information being communicated.

The provider can modify some of the suspense inherent in such a visit by encouraging the parents' involvement in the diagnosis throughout the appointment. The provider can ask parents to verbalize their observations about the child's condition, behavior, and development. Thus, the clinician confirms and further clarifies what the parents already know. This behavior also serves as a good first message to the parents, assuring them that they are knowledgeable about their child and that their instincts are correct and reliable.

Once the parents have reacted and described their feelings, they may be receptive to the basic information they need about the diagnosis. Only then can the provider begin to meet the present needs of the child and family. While the parents are likely to need a great deal of information, the presentation and timing of information are important considerations. The language used in this initial interaction is very meaningful.

● **Clinical Pearl:** The provider should avoid using specific diagnostic terms and euphemisms. Their use can increase parental anxiety.

As parents become accustomed to the medical terminology used in conjunction with describing their child, knowledge of specific diagnostic terminology may be empowering (Abrams & Goodman, 1998). Such knowledge helps them to speak openly with their provider about the diagnosis, the family's expectations, and their means of coping. Diagnostic terminology also facilitates access to educational materials and helps direct parents to the resources of specific support groups.

Abrams and Goodman (1998) analyzed how parents and professionals engaged in a process of negotiating what labels should be used and what developmental meaning should be ascribed in the diagnosis of disorders in young children. Their psycholinguistic analysis showed that professionals shied away from explicit use of labels, preferring to describe children's deficits with rate descriptors (eg, "slow"). Parties wavered between optimistic and pessimistic statements. When parents seemed despairing, professionals would try to offer hope; when parents were unrealistic, professionals gave more blunt statements. Parents who received the most ambiguous interpretations seemed left with diagnostic questions still unanswered. Those who received more forthright information appeared better able to move on to issues of prognosis.

The Value of Genetic Counseling

Recognized and commonly occurring syndromes have established networks of parent support with publications, treatment updates, conferences, and legislative and funding information. Knowing "what happened" can relieve some of the guilt, pain, and blame, as well as fear of outcomes for future children. Despite the fact that there are more than 1000 recognizable causes for mental retardation and developmental syndromes, in many instances the desired label is not currently ascertainable (Hirsch & Rader, 1998). Parents for whom no clear diagnosis can be offered report that they are driven to search for a conclusion (Redbook Magazine, 1996). They report that this is disturbing and distressful, distracting from the work of acceptance and adjustment.

● **Clinical Pearl:** The provider should identify the dominant features of the disorder and try to give it a name for parents. The clinician can then work with the family to find a support group that best fits the features of the named disorder.

The negative aspect of a definitive genetic diagnosis is the tendency to forget that the child is an individual whose presentation may not fit consistently with the syndrome. Hirsch and Rader (1998) describe the "syndrome, syndrome" in which parents and providers limit treatment, observation, and expectations based on anticipated outcomes. The reader is referred to Chapter 5 for more information on genetic counseling.

THE ROLE OF THE FAMILY

The diagnosis of a chronic illness or disability is just one point in the family's ongoing evolution. Over time, the family must learn a constellation of adaptive tasks to cope successfully and meet individual and family needs. Some tasks are practical, while others are emotional. Collectively, they represent a framework the provider can use in assessing the family and planning interventions. Display 17-1 identifies adaptive tasks that can assist parents to deal successfully with their child's disorder.

Coming to terms with their child's illness or disability is the initial difficult task. Shock and disbelief often are followed by a useful and purposeful period of denial in which the family masters the presenting threat. Prolonged denial impedes successful adaptation; a realistic view promotes it. Parents also need to become socialized into the health care system, because it is apt to become a major part of the family's environment. Its successful negotiation can reduce obstacles to care.

Cautious, subconscious grief begins the moment parents suspect a problem in their child's well-being or development. When suspicions are confirmed, the parents experience profound, often debilitating grief. This anguish is not linear, and parents must move through the stages of grief before they eventually accept their child's diagnosis.

● **Clinical Pearl:** For families with children who have chronic illness or physical or developmental disabilities, grief has no end point. The provider and parents should be aware of the cyclical nature of the grief process to understand better the family's needs over time.

In a cyclical model of grief, each new stressor, such as the need for surgery or the recognition that the child has not achieved a developmental milestone, can renew the grief

---

DISPLAY 17–1 • Parental Adaptive Tasks

1. Accept the child's disability.
2. Manage the child's condition on a day-to-day basis.
3. Meet the child's normal developmental needs.
4. Meet the developmental needs of other family members.
5. Cope with ongoing stress and periodic crises.
6. Assist family members to manage their feelings.
7. Educate others about the child's condition.
8. Establish a support system.

cycle. The disruptive effects of the cycle depend on the strength of the family and the severity of the stressor (Worthington, 1994). As the family meets the demands of the event, the grief resolves to a stable state. Benchmark events experienced by the siblings of a disabled child (eg, first slumber party, driver's license, graduation, wedding) can unexpectedly provoke renewed grief, as the family recognizes that the disabled child may never experience such an event.

Special consideration should be given to the dynamics of denial, an important defense mechanism that parents may use to cope with their grief and sadness. When the provider pushes harder to make a point a parent seems to deny, the parent's anxiety increases, amplifying the need for denial. The clinician may address the cause of the denial more effectively by acknowledging that the news is frightening and upsetting.

Anger is an expected emotion in the grief process. Without an opportunity for expression, a parent's anger can be turned inward and lead to clinical depression. Parents have described the intensity of emotions, including the feeling of "going crazy," as frightening in itself (Worthington, 1994). The provider should describe the grief process to prepare parents for this emotionality. Involvement in a support group can offer emotional validation and practical information, perhaps more effectively than that given by professionals. Providers may be expecting too much when they anticipate that the distraught parents of a newly diagnosed child will have the energy to seek out support opportunities. With the parents' permission, the clinician can arrange for a specific support group to reach out to them at the time of their child's diagnosis (Klein & Schive, 1996).

Meeting the child's developmental needs requires understanding the developmental tasks the child is facing and recognizing how the disability can interfere with mastery. A child's sense of self is constructed on accomplishments in psychosocial, developmental tasks. Normalization requires parents to engage in the same parenting activities they would perform for nondisabled family members. Parents need to focus on abilities, minimizing the limitations that their child's challenges impose.

Members of caregiving families are vulnerable to anxiety, guilt, fear, resentment, anger, and depression. Within the context of cultural variations, inhibition of emotional expression may be characteristic of maladaptive coping. Parents report difficulty handling their own emotions and difficulty helping their children to manage their feelings. Supportive family members, friends, and health professionals are important resources. Even more, support from parents in similar situations is highly successful (Canam, 1993). When parents have the resources to cope with their own feelings, they are more prepared to help their children cope as well.

Parents have reported difficulty talking about the child's illness to the child, to others within the family, and to people outside the family. Children who are included in the discussion and decision making recuperate faster and report greater satisfaction with health care (Canam, 1992). Ignorance of the disease and its ramifications by the ill child and others who have significant contact with the child interferes with the child's ability to cope effectively. Siblings must be prepared to answer questions that predictably arise. They should be able to explain the condition to their peers.

● **Clinical Pearl:** Social support has been identified as the single most powerful mediator of family adjustment (Canam, 1992).

The ability to share the responsibilities of care with extended family members and friends is associated with a significantly higher level of family functioning. Maintaining social relationships outside the home that are close and meaningful and that promote personal growth and satisfaction is important for all family members.

These adaptive tasks are related to the common issues that cross disease entities. Accomplishment of these tasks requires specific knowledge, skills, and resources. Parents who are unable to succeed at these tasks require specific intervention.

Stress, Coping, and Life Satisfaction

A significant amount of research indicates that families of handicapped children experience chronic stress. These potential stresses can threaten basic human needs (Tunali & Power, 1993):

- Financial resources
- Emotional relationships in the family
- Family activities and goals
- Family social life
- Family contact with large institutions
- Family grieving process

Ongoing stress related to the chronicity of care, periodic exacerbations and hospitalizations, and anxieties about their child's future can overwhelm the family's resources, leading to crisis. Primary care providers can mediate the stress of chronic illness by delivering care in a supportive environment. They can help parents to identify and problem-solve specific concerns, while also helping them predict and prepare for the future.

One psychological strategy that individuals may use when faced with an inescapable situation that threatens their needs is to redefine what constitutes the fulfillment of those needs. This redefinition plays a major role in the adaptation process. In managing the demands of life with a disabled child, parents may redefine what they see as ideal. In doing so, they may find alternatives. For example, the time needed to provide care may limit a mother's availability to pursue a career if she lacks available assistance. It is likely that this mother will redefine the way in which she will satisfy her achievement needs. She may fulfill them by emphasizing her parental role, stressing the importance of being a good mother, and placing a higher value on parenting than career development.

When parents feel rejected and isolated by their larger community, they are likely to satisfy their love and belongingness needs through the extended family. They may emphasize family-related values and activities, striving for a high level of family cohesiveness. These families often redefine parenting standards internally rather than externally. They may redefine a good marriage as one in which each partner is a good parent and provides emotional support, rather than one in which partners provide companionship and intimacy. When providers are aware of a family's recreated values, they can support the family's own means of coping.

Benevolent Overreaction

Benevolent overreaction is a cyclical, pathologic behavior exhibited by families of the chronically ill as a result of the natural, protective behaviors of parents (Murray & Hayes, 1996). It is characterized by a cluster of parental actions, including overprotection, overindulgence, and permissiveness. These actions are detrimental to the child's emotional welfare and contribute to low self-esteem, lack of initiative, and poor self-control. Parents caught in this cycle are unable to look beyond their child's challenges. They may be unable to imagine their child's potential for independence. Such a family's energy becomes focused on the illness itself and the need for caregiving. Psychosocial and developmental milestones are unmet. The result is that separation anxiety, usually common only in very young children, continues through the teen years and even into adulthood.

Murray and Hayes (1996) found that the incidence of social competency difficulties in chronically ill children is twice that of healthy children. Children with neurologic disorders (eg, epilepsy) or chronic disorders whose exacerbations and remissions lack predictability are at higher risk for adjustment problems.

The child's insecurity and focus on the handicap may elicit parental feelings of guilt, shame, and low self-esteem. These feelings drive the parents' overprotection, indulgence, and permissiveness. As a result, the child is deprived of new experiences, discipline, structure, and the frustration necessary to promote independence, self-control, and initiative. The child remains dependent on the parents, demanding of their attention, and developmentally immature. In turn, the parents feel frustration, resentment, ambivalence, anger, and, possibly, hostility. These emotions generally are expressed covertly. Passive-aggression and self-sacrifice are common in expressions of veiled feelings, but overt aggression also may be seen. Caught in this cycle, parents transfer these feelings to the child, who reacts with renewed insecurity and focus on the illness.

The child in this situation typically develops one of two maladaptive coping styles:

1. The child is so withdrawn and preoccupied with the health condition that he or she self-restricts activities, focusing on what he or she cannot do. Anxiety and vulnerability are characteristics of this coping style.
2. The child is irritable, acts out negative feelings, and is unable to manage emotions. This youngster appears unhappy and is uncooperative. The child has a poor self-concept, negative attitudes about the illness, and problems with following rules at home and at school (Murray & Hayes, 1996).

Common themes experienced by parents and child can include the following:

- Parents deny problems with behavior.
- Parents take little or no disciplinary action, apply discipline inconsistently, and set limits poorly.
- The child has few age-appropriate friends, with parents performing activities that the child is capable of performing. Examples include answering for the child or assisting with dressing, toileting, and feeding. The child seems immature for age. Even in older children, few demands are made.
- Parents routinely overlook many incidents of antisocial and hostile behavior, such as cursing, slapping, and spitting.

▲ **Clinical Warning:** Overprotection is a common parental reaction. All families should be assessed for this behavior. Providers who note this issue should refer the parents for counseling.

SUCCESSFUL COLLABORATION

Klein and Schive (1996) have written about the influence of the media and some professional literature in reinforcing a negative stereotype of parents with ill or disabled children. Though parents may present as nervous, guilty, anxious, depressed, or overprotective, the provider should remember that their observations of parents usually occur during times of significant stress. Sometimes, providers do not accept the concept of parents as experts and partners in care. They may misperceive a parent who speaks out for their child's needs as being aggressive or demanding. These negative stereotypes are detrimental obstacles to good communication and effective collaboration between parents and provider.

Confronting Obstacles

Hirsch and Rader (1998) outline specific problems in the parent–provider partnership, including the following:

- Improper focus on blame rather than partnership. Parents may blame providers for anything that does not go right, including missed opportunities, wrong treatments, overlooked clues, reluctance to get other opinions, lack of definitive answers, and failure to recognize the value of parental input. On the other hand, providers may blame parents for poor acceptance or participation in the plan, providing inaccurate information, having unrealistic expectations, not listening, and repeating already answered questions. These problems likely result from unclear guidelines about roles and responsibilities in the parent–provider partnership, as well as from basic misunderstandings of the nature of the child's condition.
- Provider intolerance for ambiguity. While the primary care provider functions in a scientific and orderly process, parental responses encompass emotional, cultural, and spiritual elements—all of which may seem to negate reason. Awareness and acceptance of this difference in perspective can lead to greater understanding, empathy, and effective collaboration.
- Lack of authenticity. Parental expertise often is not invited or valued. Parents are with their children over time and in a variety of settings. They coordinate input and recommendations from a variety of professionals. They are the experts. Helping parents report their information and experiences in a systematic, focused manner can help increase their credibility.
- Failure to address parental concerns. Parents often have difficulty expressing their concerns and formulating questions during hurried office visits. They are frustrated when providers fail to address their concerns and questions. Providers should invite parents to bring a list of questions, the most important of which providers should answer during the visit. They may defer other issues to a convenient later meeting, but within a reasonable time frame. Without spending time to listen to parental concerns, the provider cannot understand the parent's perspective.
- Frustration with their child's slow response to treatment. Treatment regimens may require time to demonstrate their effectiveness. Whenever a new treatment is introduced, parents have a tendency to hope for a miracle.

● **Clinical Pearl:** At the initiation of treatment, time lines should be discussed for evaluation of treatment effectiveness.

- Misunderstanding of the family's culture and ethnicity. Individual attitudes about health, disease, and disability, as well as the family's roles and dynamics, must be assessed in determining approaches to communication and treatment.
- Misunderstanding clinical limitations. Providers should constantly review the differing approaches to treating lifelong conditions versus curable disease states. Frequent acknowledgment of the overall picture can help keep both parent and provider appropriately focused on the capabilities and limitations of treatment.

To foster good communication, the provider should plan to meet with parents separately from the child. Meetings should be at convenient times for parents, considering the demands of child care, work, and so forth. Participants interact better when all are seated in equally comfortable chairs, at the same eye level, at a conversational distance, and in a position to take notes (Klein & Schive, 1996). A separate room or seating area other than an examining room is more appropriate for the uninterrupted privacy parents need and deserve.

Fathers should be included in meetings. Not doing so conveys an unspoken message that fathers need not attend because they are not necessary. A special invitation may be necessary. Such an invitation communicates the important role of the father in caregiving.

Meetings in which professionals outnumber the parents may overwhelm parents, discourage their participation, and lead to disorganization. More than three professionals is too many. It is also a good idea to follow up meetings with reports written in lay terms that summarize the collaborative treatment plans.

Another obstacle in the provider–family relationship includes frustration with long waiting times, which parents may see as a sign of disrespect. Long waiting times can be exceptionally challenging when parents must make several health care visits per week, necessitating child care for other siblings. Treatment plans need to be collaborative efforts with the family, realistically reflecting their goals and abilities.

Providing Hope

The line between honesty and pessimism can be very fine. Parents feel hurt and depressed when they leave a visit where the provider emphasizes the negative and offers little optimism. Careful language selection can influence a slight change in perspective. The provider can rephrase negative thoughts positively to inspire hope rather than despair. For example, informing parents that their child has a significant hearing loss is negative. Rephrasing the thought that their child has enough hearing to understand language and learn speech is positive. In this way, providers can help parents see possibilities rather than limitations (Weinhouse & Weinhouse, 1997).

The following statement is a plea from a parent. It dramatizes the need for families to hold hope for a positive future for them and for their children:

Provide Me with a Ray of Hope
Robbing me of hope is the worst thing you can do to me.
Remember that after I leave your office
I will create an atmosphere at home of hope or despair,
and surely one of hope is better for my child.
You can give me hope through your attitude
and through what you say.

Your belief that my child could defy the statistics
will soften the facts that you must tell me. (Alexander & Tompkins-McGill, 1987, p. 362)

Maintaining hopefulness can engender feelings of well-being and the belief that needs will be met. The provider can shape an optimistic perspective at every encounter. Sensitive interactions can strengthen families, expanding their resources and knowledge base, while acknowledging a child's positive possibilities.

COMMUNITY RESOURCES

The provider should know which community service programs are available for all children, including those offered by local and regional parks, recreation services, and libraries. Familiarity about where to obtain more information about public and private programs that support children with special health care needs is also important. Working with both the family and social services, the provider can help ensure that the family receives those services and information that voluntary agencies provide. Some of these include the following:

- ARC (formerly the Association for the help of Retarded Citizens)
- United Cerebral Palsy Association
- Cystic Fibrosis Foundation
- Crohn's and Colitis Foundation of America
- Alliance of Genetic Support Groups
- National Organization for Rare Diseases

The provider also should be aware of where to obtain information about publicly sponsored programs, such as early intervention, special education, Supplemental Security Income; mandated services of state/provincial health departments (in the United States, through Title V of the Social Security Act); and general patient information networks.

To maintain current knowledge about available services in the public and private sectors, providers can keep in contact with the local chapter of the national office of the American Academy of Pediatrics or their state Office of Services for Children With Special Health Care Needs. Alternatively, they may want to establish ties with a developmental pediatrics or chronic illness program at a local medical center (American Academy of Pediatrics, 1997).

The World Wide Web has proven to be a rich resource for parents and professionals. On-line support is available for every major disorder and disease and for many remote and rare disorders as well. Parents created many of these sites for mutual support and networking and can connect families to one another. These sites can offer much more than the health sections of on-line services or even on-line parent magazines (Koehl, 1997).

Parents Helping Parents (*http://www.php.com*) and others are creating a sense of community among families who would otherwise be isolated. Some of the best sites intend to link users to as many different childhood disability sites as possible. Examples include Internet resources for the following:

- Special Children (*http://www.irsc.org/*)
- Rare Genetic Diseases in Children (htt://mcrcr4.med. nyu.edu/~murphp01/homenew/htm)

- Wellness Web *(http://wellweb.com/index.htm)*
- The National Institute of Health home page *(http://www.nih.gov)* has dozens of links to highly specialized research studies. *http://www.familyvillage.wisc.edu* is a site for parents coping with childhood illness and disability.

Information related to health care policies is available through professional organizations, state advocacy organizations, and political organizations, such as Family Voices *(http:www.ichp.ufl.edu/MCH-NetLink/FamilyVoices)*. Family Voices is a national clearinghouse for information and education concerning the health care of children with special needs. The Children's Defense Fund is another such resource. Other resources include The National Parent to Parent Support and Information System (NPPSIS) (800-651-1151). This organization uses a database to match families nationally and internationally. It maintains local contact information for resources, services, and health care treatment. Parent Care, Inc. (317 872-9913) supports parents of critically ill children in neonatal intensive care units.

REFERENCES AND BIBLIOGRAPHY

Abrams, E. Z., & Goodman, J. F. (1998). Diagnosing developmental problems in children: Parents and professionals negotiate bad news. *Journal of Pediatric Psychology, 23*(2), 87–98.

Alexander, R., & Tompkins-McGill, P. (1987). Notes to the expert from the parent of a handicapped child. *Social Work, 32,* 361–362.

American Academy of Pediatrics. (1996). The role of the pediatrician in implementing the ADA. *Pediatrics, 98,* 146.

Brindle, S., & Boseley S. (1997, March). Parents' telling point on disability. *The Guardian, 1,* 11.

Canam, C. (1993). Common adaptive tasks facing parents of children with chronic conditions. *Journal of Advanced Nursing, 18*(1), 46–53.

Chedd, N. (1995, August). Genetic counseling: the science is the easy part. *The Exceptional Parent, 25*(8), 26(2).

Hirsch, D., & Rader, R. (1998). Questions parents ask. *Exceptional Parent, 28*(3), 14(2).

Janetti Publications, Inc. (1997). Family voices: Building voices for our children with special health care needs. *Pediatric Nursing, 23*(4), 400(3).

Klein, S., & Schive, K. (1996). Delivering difficult news. *The Exceptional Parent, 26,* 44–45.

Koehl, C. (1997). Finding a web of support/information for parents of children with defects and other health problems on the World Wide Web. Special education: Your child. *Newsweek, 129,* 50.

Malone, DM., Manders, J., Stewart, S. (1997). A rationale for family therapy specialization in early intervention. *Journal of Marital and Family Therapy, 23*(1), 65–79.

Murray, J., & Hayes, M. (1996). The benevolent overreaction: Nursing assessment and intervention in families coping with seizure disorder. *Journal of Neuroscience Nursing, 28*(4), 252(7).

Newacheck, P., & Halfon, N. (1998). Prevalence and impact of disabling chronic conditions in childhood. *The American Journal of Public Health, 88n4*(April 1998), 610.

Santelli, B., Turnbull, A., & Higgins, C. (1997). Parent to parent support and health care. *Pediatric Nursing, 23*(3), 303(4).

Tunali, B., & Power, T. (1993). Creating satisfaction: A psychological perspective on stress and coping in families of handicapped children. *The Journal of Child Psychology and Psychiatry, 34*(6), 945–957.

Unknown. (1996). Is my son normal? One mother's journey. *Redbook Magazine, 188,* 77.

Weinhouse, D., & Weinhouse, M. (1997). Parents' biggest needs from doctors: Honesty, sensitivity. *American Medical News, 40*(26) 15(2).

Worthington, R. (1994). Models of linear and cyclical grief: Different approaches to different experiences. *Clinical Pediatrics, 33*(5), 297(4).

The Physically Challenged Child

• ALEKSANDRA ALDERMAN, MD

INTRODUCTION

The term "physically challenged child" indicates that a child has a limitation in performance of motor function. This term encompasses a wide variety of diagnoses and affects all pediatric age groups. In the mildest expressions of these diagnostic entities, a child actually may overcome the condition. Most physical challenges, however, are chronic, persisting to varying degrees throughout childhood despite improvements achieved with intervention.

Physical medicine and rehabilitation is the medical specialty that deals with physically challenged children. A specifically trained physician (ie, the physiatrist), therapists, rehabilitation nurses, Clinical Nurse Specialists (CNSs), psychologists, and other support professionals manage interventions. These professionals focus on improving mobility, self-care, and quality of life.

Primary care providers can support the rehabilitation management of physically challenged children while integrating their families into this process. These children require extensive support. Functional limitations present major challenges to ego and personality development. Family members will need to work through their understanding of and feelings about the chronic limitations that their children will face. Participation in therapies and interventions inevitably alters family routines and time allotment.

● **Clinical Pearl:** Primary care providers often are the first health care professionals to whom parents turn when they suspect a developmental delay in their child. Clinicians must judge the seriousness of these concerns fairly and compassionately. Families will feel resentful when their providers tell them that their worries are unjustified, because their child "just needs to be observed for a while" or will "outgrow" the problem. Parents also will be angry if they do not receive any instructions for home programs and intervention. In retrospect, families report that such behaviors make them feel "put off" by their child's clinician. Chapter 36 provide suggestions for effective clinician behavior in such situations.

Certainly the initial recognition of a developmental delay, whether physical or neurointegrative, can be difficult. Observation may be appropriate, but during this period, clinicians should explain possible reasons for the problem. The family needs instruction in how to provide a home program of targeted exercises. Understanding and recognizing the functional dynamics involved in achieving developmental and physical milestones can provide the clinical foundation needed to determine the seriousness of the delay. This information also helps the provider to initiate rehabilitating therapies and to pursue additional workup for etiology.

● **Clinical Pearl:** For infants whose problems are not identified in the nursery, serial follow-up is the best method for detecting the onset of developmental or motor dysfunction. This is especially true during the first year of life, when most motor delays are diagnosed. Prematurity, low birth weight, neonatal complications, multiple birth, or lesions on cranial scans increase the risk of neuromotor dysfunction but are not predictive of it. The following discussion provides guidance for diagnosing and managing common motor limitations that require rehabilitative interventions.

HYPOTONIA

The infant with hypotonia (decreased muscle tone) exhibits motor limitations because of decreased strength aggravated by accompanying ligamentous laxity, especially if the hypotonia is neurologic in origin. The hypotonic infant exhibits decreased small excursion movements, weak sucking and crying, and decreased alertness. The most common clinical presentation is an infant who generally is delayed with decreased muscle tone of no obvious etiology. Identifiable causes of hypotonia include the following:

- Chromosomal aberrations (eg, Down syndrome), which are diagnosed in the nursery based on readily apparent physical features and confirming blood studies; may be present without obvious features as well, particularly in the newborn facies
- Many cerebral structural dysplasias
- Spastic cerebral palsy (CP; especially the dyskinetic types) in the first months of life
- Static brain lesions or encephalopathy
- A set level of spinal cord disruption
- Muscular dystrophies and myopathies
- Hypothyroidism
- Fetal alcohol syndrome
- Many hereditary metabolic states
- Toxin exposures
- Prader-Willi syndrome
- Autism

Epidemiology

Specific statistics on the incidence of hypotonia are unavailable, but the reader should be aware that hypotonia is a common newborn presentation. The epidemiologic literature has not described the relationship between the incidence of hypotonia and maternal behaviors. The reader is referred to the general epidemiologic information presented in Chapter 16 (The Premature and Low–Birth-Weight Infant).

History and Physical Examination

The following are indications of hypotonia:

- The infant has difficulty picking up the head, even to clear the nose when prone, with sagging, minimal, or no righting responses (head lag).

- The trunk exhibits no righting and tends to slip through the examiner's hands when he or she holds the baby up.
- The muscles have a softer feel when palpated, and the joints are less stable.

Diagnostic Criteria

When an infant is first noted to have diffuse hypotonia after discharge from the nursery, there are several diagnostic possibilities. Priorities are the infant's medical status, requirements, and maturational state.

● **Clinical Pearl:** Most developmental disabilities and psychomotor delays have varying degrees of associated hypotonia and ligamentous laxity, even if no etiology can be identified (as often is the case). Even if the underlying reason for hypotonia is unknown, intervention should begin as soon as the motor problem is noted. Rehabilitation is based on what the infant is doing and what movement difficulties are seen.

Diagnostic Studies

The infant with hypotonia who develops increased muscle tone after nursery discharge requires a diagnostic evaluation if earlier studies to provide a reasonable etiology were not done. For the infant whose cranial scans in the nursery showed lesions of cerebral insults (such as periventricular leukomalacia, porencephaly, and enlarged ventricles), hypotonia may be evident at first, even if spasticity emerges later.

● **Clinical Pearl:** If any doubt exists about the compatibility of previous findings with emerging signs, the infant should undergo a neurologic evaluation.

Management

After 9 months of age, manifestation of significant delays becomes increasingly unlikely if the infant has progressed normally through developmental stages. For example, infants who sit and crawl normally will be able to ambulate. By this age, the provider already should have identified any infant who is exhibiting gross motor delays or limitations, referring the child to an appropriate intervention program. The infant who exhibits deviations in normal motor function is likely to have alterations in pulling to stand and walking, unless interventions have minimized these problems. Some variations still may occur dynamically with pulling to stand or ambulating, even though previous patterns were normal. The reader who desires a review of normal motor development is referred to Chapter 8.

▲ **Clinical Warning:** Early recognition of manifestations of physical limitations, including relevant muscle tone deviations that may indicate a need for intervention, is crucial. Failure to meet a motor milestone is a strong sign that a child needs help. A delay in referring a child for intervention to see if he or she will "catch up" is not wise. Ignoring a motor delay can lead to extended follow-up.

If a pattern of development is deviated enough, intervention may need to begin before a delay actually appears. The provider must inform the family about which functional patterns may be inhibited, while giving them specific instructions for activities that will promote the infant's develop-

ment. With very mild deviations and borderline or no delays, this plan may be adequate in guiding the baby toward subsequent normal gross motor development. With early intervention, infants with mild delays and dynamic deviations may progress to normal functional levels and no longer be physically challenged. Depending on how a community manages their early intervention services, a provider may be able to follow the child and coordinate service delivery with the support of therapists until the child achieves functional mobility.

Several rehabilitative devices can assist the child with hypotonia to improve limb mobility and usefulness. In addition to standard devices, therapists can individualize rehabilitative equipment and regimens when specific needs exist. The provider should expect that therapists will recommend at least some of the following aids and activities for the child with hypotonia:

- Ankle level braces called supramalleolar orthoses (SMOs) to prevent deviations from worsening
- Articulating ankle foot orthoses (AFOs)
- Exercises to strengthen the quadricep and hamstring muscles, train the child to walk with a narrower base, and use more appropriate transitions. Such exercises require the family's intensive attention to help the child develop proper ambulation patterns so that they can become established habits.

HYPERTONIA

Hypertonia is a condition of increased muscle tone. Specific statistics on its incidence are unavailable. As with hypotonia, the reader should be aware that hypertonia is common in newborns. The epidemiologic literature has not described a relationship between the incidence of hypertonia and maternal substance abuse. The reader is referred to the general epidemiologic information that is presented in Chapter 16.

History and Physical Examination

To assess the infant appropriately, the provider needs adequate time to obtain a thorough history and to perform a complete examination of function and tone. The history should include the infant's feeding patterns, temperament, activity level, sociability, tolerance of handling, and any parental concerns.

● **Clinical Pearl:** Parental concerns are particularly valuable indicators for providers to consider when examining infants with hypertonia.

The examination requires placing the infant in the following positions: supine, prone, side-lying, and supported sitting on the examining table and parent's lap. The provider also should hold the child suspended in the air prone and sideways. The provider observes and handles the infant to assess quality of movements, tonal responses, primitive reflexes, quality of grasping, visual attending to hands and toys, social regard, and the ease with which crying can be calmed.

● **Clinical Pearl:** To identify hypertonicity early, the provider will need to conduct the examination serially over several visits.

Diagnostic Criteria

The earliest signs of hypertonia are reflected in the head, trunk, and extremities, with patterns often seen as precocious development. The following features identify hypertonia:

- In the first 2 months, maintenance of a fully elevated head while prone is sustained and excessive. Parents should monitor this behavior.
- The infant prefers the side-lying position, arching backward and possibly extending the legs, rather than lying in the normal flexed or curled position.
- Excessive hand-fisting is tighter and more sustained than the usual fisting prevalence seen in the first months. This sign is a possible indication of spasticity, as is the predisposition for extension in the lower extremities.
- The child exhibits an excessive support response, especially with the knees fixed in extension and with toed foot placement.
- The infant's body feels especially firm. Overall extremity movements are decreased both in frequency and range of excursions so that overall activity level is decreased. These findings may be seen in what otherwise is a more reactive system, with increased irritability, tremulous quality, inability to accept sudden changes, and overactive deep tendon, clonus, and primitive reflexes.
- The reflex grasp response is increased and sustained.
- The Moro reflex, the most familiar of the postural primitive reflexes, is excessive and prolonged in expression, lasting beyond the expected age.
- Sustained tonic neck reflex, obligatory or expressed with increased intensity, lasts beyond the expected age.

● **Clinical Pearl:** These extension patterns are seen as transient hypertonic patterns in many premature infants. Subsequent normalized development may follow, especially when flexion is facilitated. These signs, however, also may be the first manifestations of spasticity that will continue to increase as the nervous system matures.

Management

The foregoing manifestations of hypertonia are key to detecting significant motor problems. They also are the focus of intervention programming, with therapies directed at inhibiting these signs to facilitate more volitional control. Hypertonic patterns and reflexes can predict pending delays even when actual milestones are still normal. Not all these signs and reflexes will be present, and they may appear at different times. While continuing to support the family, the provider should refer the infant with hypertonia to a pediatric neurologist for a more focused evaluation and to devise appropriate management strategies.

Feeding difficulties that may occur in the infant with hypotonia or hypertonia can be dealt with by improving positioning. A specially trained speech therapist can work with the baby to enhance oromotor responses.

CEREBRAL PALSY

Cerebral palsy is the most frequently seen disorder of major hypertonic motor limitation. Most sources quote an incidence of between 2 and 5 out of 1000 births (Braddom, 1996; Nelson, Behrman, Kliegman, & Arvin, 1996; Nelson, 1998). CP is defined as a nonprogressing encephalopathic injury or lesion to the developing brain. The affected child presents with abnormal muscle tone and varying movement disorders.

Pathology

Causes of CP vary; it may be congenital or result from an insult prenatally, at birth, or during early infancy. Manifestations of CP may be delayed.

● **Clinical Pearl:** The most prevalent risk factors for CP are marked prematurity (younger than 32 weeks) and very low birth weight (less than 1500 g) (Braddom, 1996).

In premature infants, the less-developed vascular beds are particularly prone to hemorrhage in the germinal matrix, with involvement in the intraventricular or periventricular areas. The latter problem leads to periventricular leukomalacia, one of the most frequently seen predisposing cerebral insults among premature infants who develop CP. Many factors can establish an environment for cerebral injury, however, and prenatal factors are increasingly being considered more relevant. Infections are emerging as an important cause. Most premature infants do not go on to have CP.

Nearly half the children who have CP were not premature (Nelson, 1998). Causes of CP in term infants vary. The cerebrum is more mature and less vulnerable in term infants than in premature infants, especially because its vascularity is improved. The mechanics of the delivery process and all the etiologies that can lead to malformation or brain injury prenatally, during birth, or in the neonatal period, however, still can occur. For many children, a cause is never identified. The reader should refer to a current pediatric neurology text for further information on the causes of CP.

History and Physical Examination

Infants with CP present with different categories of muscle tone and movement disorders. A spastic muscle tone pattern is most common, occurring in approximately 75% of cases (Nelson, 1998). Spasticity is a specific form of hypertonicity, resulting from injury to the pyramidal part of the nervous system. Spasticity manifests as abnormal upper motor neuron reflexes, persistent primitive reflexes, increased muscle tone, and increased resistance to muscle stretch or elongation. The latter condition is known as a clasp knife phenomenon, with distinct release of resistance during stretching that is reproducible. Spasticity usually occurs in a diplegic, hemiparetic, or quadriparetic pattern, reflecting the location of cerebral motor involvement. Diplegia affects primarily the lower extremities. Hemiparesis affects the upper and lower extremity on the same side. Quadriparesis affects the bilateral upper and lower extremities. The hemiparetic form is slightly less frequent than the other variants, while the diplegic pattern is particularly likely with prematurity. Triplegic presentations are rare, usually with relative sparing of an upper extremity.

Dyskinetic Cerebral Palsy

Dyskinetic CP reflects injury to the extrapyramidal system. This form usually has a quadriparetic involvement manifested by involuntary, irregular movements. Hypotonia and developmental delays are the initial features seen in early infancy with dyskinetic CP.

Athetosis is the most frequent form. Fluctuating muscle tone is the basic feature, ranging from flaccidity to rigid posturing. The intensity of irregular writhing movements varies and will be increased by stress or activity. These movements may be absent or mild at rest but may involve the entire limb when the child tries to reach. Speech may be blocked or very dysarthric. Swallowing may be difficult, leading to drooling and feeding problems. Another prominent feature of athetosis is persistent and exaggerated primitive reflexes, which are present in the initial hypotonic phase that precedes other findings. The most likely cause of athetosis is diffuse prenatal brain insults. Thus, athetosis is more likely to be seen in the premature infant who is susceptible to this damage at lower bilirubin levels. It may present during infancy, with tonal fluctuations commonly seen first about the mouth and face.

Ataxic CP, quite rare, is considered a dyskinetic type of CP, because fine and gross motor incoordination have the quality of a movement disorder generated by the nervous system that is not based primarily on a tonal state. The major feature is hypotonia of trunk and extremities, with unsteady postural patterns resulting from decreased equilibrium and titubation. The child's extremities exhibit jerky, coarse tremors, dysmetria, and past pointing. Dysarthria and nystagmus also are common. The dynamics described with ataxia suggest cerebellar damage. When it is present, the provider must consider cerebellar tumors, vascular and metabolic pathology, and many genetic syndromes. A careful diagnostic evaluation should be done, with referral to a geneticist and a pediatric neurologist. Ataxia appears earlier than athetosis, with unsteady reaching, difficulty in propping on upper extremities, and unsteadiness with sitting that may be titubating or with irregular jerky shifts. The child with ataxia usually will gain skills, although delays depend on the degree of ataxia and hypotonia.

Mixed-Type Cerebral Palsy

A frequent presentation is mixed-type CP. Most children with spasticity also have underlying hypotonia noted with head and trunk control. A common combination is a mix of athetosis with spasticity and underlying hypotonia. Other less frequent combinations include ataxia or dystonia. Management is based on controlling the primary deviating clinical patterns to facilitate development. Hypotonic CP is another rare form, presenting with severe, diffuse hypotonia. A pediatric neurologist will need to do the workup for this child (as described under hypotonia). Only when a more specific diagnosis is not possible will the diagnosis be made of hypotonic CP (Nelson, 1998).

Management

The provider should initiate intervention with physical, occupational, and speech therapies as soon as functionally limiting signs appear. Therapists should instruct family members about their role in carry over of therapy. Rehabilitative activities require comanagement by therapist and family so that interventions occur daily or more frequently. The provider's role as coordinator of services is key to successful intervention, because he or she can support the family through the stresses and demands of carrying out a therapeutic regimen several times every day.

The therapy team teaches the family how to carry out proper stretching methods at home, where the child is most comfortable and relaxed. The family can establish a routine that works best and allows adequate time for the activity. Diversion of the stretching regimen to home means that therapists can use their sessions to concentrate on helping the child develop more varied mobility and postural control skills.

Family and therapists must incorporate supportive seating early for proper postural symmetry and trunk alignment that will prevent spastic trunk hyperextension or underlying hypotonic sagging. They must facilitate rolling, crawling, sitting, and eventually, assisted standing. These children usually require AFOs to control toeing and to maintain proper alignment with standing. They may need AFOs very soon if sustained plantar flexion posturing is of a degree that would lead to range loss. Children progress to gait training when they have achieved adequate postural control. Children who are able to override their primitive reflexes by 18 months and sit independently with control by 2 years are likely eventually to walk at a functional level, although usually with braces (Nelson, 1998).

● **Clinical Pearl:** Whether the child is ambulatory or not, the goal is to work with the child at regular therapy intervention levels until he or she has achieved a functional plateau and quality of movement dynamics. At that point, therapies are reduced gradually to monitoring frequency. The amount of function the child achieves depends not only on the type and degree of neurologic disability, but also on the child's intelligence, temperament for working with the rehabilitation process, and degree of carry over by family and, when applicable, school.

Complications

Spasticity

Even though the primary management of spasticity is through mobilization, stretching, relaxation techniques, positioning, and bracing (Glenn & Whyle, 1990; Molnar, 1991), medications also may cause some mild decreases. Because the effects achieved with medications are mild and not striking, they are not used widely with severely spastic children (Nelson, 1998). Table 18-1 provides information for clinicians about medications that may be used by the pediatric physiatrist or neurologist to manage spasticity. The provider should not prescribe these agents, but rather, should refer the patient for subspecialist management.

Two neurosurgical procedures are available to reduce spasticity. These procedures are selective posterior rhizotomy and intrathecal baclofen administration. They require very careful patient selection by a physiatrist, pediatric neurologist, pediatric neurosurgeon, and often a medical social worker or CNS working in concert with the rehabilitation team. The appropriate procedure is selected in tertiary medical centers.

Selective posterior rhizotomy is contraindicated for dyskinesias. This procedure is performed at the lumbar level, usually with a laminectomy to expose nerve roots that are selectively stimulated at multiple spinal nerve levels to ascertain response. Extensive experience with the procedure is necessary to judge the degree of sectioning of the posterior nerve that will best diminish spasticity while preserving sensation and sphincter function. Optimally, this surgery improves the quality of gait and functional mobility in patients older than 2 years. Selective posterior rhizotomy requires very intensive rehabilitation, including committed family involvement.

Intrathecal baclofen was approved in 1996 for children at least 4 years old. In this alternative procedure, a very small catheter is inserted into the spinal canal and connected to a computerized delivery pump placed in the subcutaneous abdomen. The pump dispenses baclofen in precise amounts

Table 18-1.   MEDICATIONS USED BY THE PEDIATRIC SUBSPECIALIST TO TREAT SPASTICITY

Drug	Dosage/Frequency	Route	Indications	Contraindications	Side Effects	Clinical Advice
Dantrolene	0.5 mg/kg b.i.d.; titrate by 0.5 up to 3 mg/kg b.i.d. to q.i.d. p.r.n. Do not exceed 100 mg q.i.d. Half-life 9 h.	PO	Spasticity from upper motor neuron disorders	Hypersensitivity, active hepatic disease, when child uses spasticity to maintain upright posture/balance	Drowsiness, dizziness, diarrhea, tachycardia, weakness, general malaise, fatigue, liver dysfunction	Safety has not been established in those younger than 5 y. Avoid using with CNS depressants and alcohol. Must monitor liver function studies.
Diazepam	1–2.5 mg t.i.d. to q.i.d. Half-life 20–80 h	PO	As an adjunct to rest, physical therapy, and other measures for the relief of discomfort associated with acute, painful, musculoskeletal disorders	Hypersensitivity, psychoses, acute narrow angle glaucoma	Drowsiness, ataxia, confusion	Increases levels of cimetidine, BZ, disulfiram, fluoxetine, isoniazid, ketoconazole, metoprolol, propoxyphene, propranolol, and valproic acid.
Baclofen	5 mg t.i.d. for 3 d, 10 mg t.i.d. for 3 d, 15 mg t.i.d. for 3 d, 20 mg t.i.d. for 3 d. Do not exceed 80 mg/d. NOTE: NO pediatric dose provided. Half-life 3–4 h	PO	Spasticity	Hypersensitivity, skeletal muscle spasm resulting from rheumatic disorders, stroke, CP, or Parkinson's	Drowsiness, depression, excitement, euphoria, hallucinations, tinnitus, ataxia, nystagmus, diplopia, dry mouth, anorexia, taste disorder, diarrhea, urinary retention, dysuria, impotence, rash, edema, weight gain, increased perspiration, elevated blood sugar, elevated AST	Taper drug to avoid psychoses and hallucinations. Use with caution in those with seizure disorders.
Clonidine	5–25 mcg/kg/d, divided q6h	PO	Spasticity	Hypersensitivity	Dry mouth, dizziness, sedation, constipation, impotence	Abrupt discontinuance may result in rebound hypertension. Safety and efficacy have not been established in children. It may induce bradycardia.
Botulinum Toxin (Botox)	Depends on the muscle being injected	Inject	Unlabeled uses: spasms, dystonias, head and neck tremor unresponsive to other therapies; has been designated an orphan drug for the treatment of dynamic muscle contracture in pediatric patients with cerebral palsy.	Hypersensitivity to any ingredient in the formulation	Paralysis	It must be stored and reconstituted properly. Patient may create antibodies to the drug, reducing effectiveness. Botox injection is considered more of a procedure than a medication.

Note: The information provided on this table is meant for reference *only*. Prescription and/or administration of these agents is reserved for the pediatric subspecialist.

and sustained fashion. The initial titration is done in the hospital. The advantage for the very severe patient is that baclofen can be delivered to its functional location without systemic side effects, which would otherwise be very likely with muscle-relaxing doses. Unlike selective posterior rhizotomy, baclofen therapy is reversible and removable (Brin, 1997).

Contractures

Providers must monitor joint ranges in children with CP for the development of contractures. In the child who is spastic, contractures will occur for ranges that are sustained with synergistic posturing. If stretching approaches to treat contractures are too tight for management with manual stretches and splinting, then Botox injection can be used by the specialist for selected muscles. If these approaches do not achieve adequate range improvement and positioning or function is significantly limited, then an additional referral to a pediatric orthopedist is indicated for evaluation for surgical tendon lengthening or release with muscle transfer (Brin, 1997).

The provider must observe hip integrity very closely. Abnormal muscle tone patterns cause muscular forces to be unbalanced, leading to structural straightening of the femoral neck. Synergistic posturing favors shifting the femoral head to a more shallow position in the hip joint, which can lead to hip subluxation, one of the most common secondary complications of CP. Providers need to monitor the clinical findings for hip dislocation carefully. Often the first sign is increased tightening of hip adductors, followed by a decrease in hip abduction. These findings warrant obtaining hip x-rays, which are likely to show early partial subluxing with partial femoral head unroofing. The provider needs to refer the child to a pediatric orthopedist for possible surgical release of hip adductors. More severe hip pain sublaxation will require femoral osteotomy as well.

BRACHIAL PLEXUS INJURY

The provider must prescribe an initial rest period for the newborn diagnosed with a brachial plexus injury to allow edema and any hemorrhaging to clear. Following resolution of these problems, the provider should refer the infant to therapy so that the family can learn how to provide gentle ranging. This therapy usually begins in approximately 1 week for the absent active ranges.

If the infant does not demonstrate rapid recovery within the first weeks of gentle ranging, the provider will need to arrange for motor training to be incorporated with the mobilization. Motor training requires the skills of an experienced pediatric occupational therapist, who will establish a specific exercise regimen of functional movements for compromised muscles. The therapist should teach the exercises to family members so that they can do them daily and incorporate them into the handling of the child. Nerve regeneration occurs slowly, usually at 1 mm/d. Thus, upper arm lesions can recover in 4 to 5 months, while distal arm recovery may take 7 to 9 months. Recoveries taking 2 years and, less frequently, 6 to 8 years also have been reported (Campbell, 1991; 1994).

One of the greatest challenges of brachial plexus injuries is preventing the development of substitution patterns. Because other muscle groups work more easily than those in the affected area, the infant is strongly predisposed to avoid using the compromised muscles. For example, the child may learn that tilting the trunk and using other shoulder girdle muscles to elevate the arm is easier than using the deltoid muscle and will lean the trunk in the direction of the reach instead of extending the elbow. The results are trunk asymmetry and disuse atrophy of avoided muscles. Hand manipulations done in deviated wrist positions that favor the stronger muscles strengthen them further, thus increasing the deviations. Once the use of substitution dynamics becomes habituated, avoiding their perpetuation becomes very difficult.

● **Clinical Pearl:** Continuing therapy input for many years is advisable to ensure that the child has achieved optimal muscle recovery for normalized dynamics, rather than substituted patterns.

Diagnostic Studies

Any infant who does not respond to initial gentle ranging activity requires referral to a pediatric neurologist or physiatrist who can assist the provider in interpreting electrodiagnostic studies. Either the clinician or the specialist can perform such studies, which will delineate the lesion more objectively. Electrodiagnostic studies should be done in the first months and repeated several months later to follow up on nerve regeneration.

Management

The provider should support the family's participation in any prescribed exercise regimen and in orthotic and splinting use to optimize nerve regeneration and subsequent muscle function. The success of the use of therapeutic electrical stimulation has not been established, with no consensus on intensity or endurance of nerve stimulation. Providers should consider neurosurgical intervention with neuroplasty when the child exhibits little recovery of antigravity strength for functionally crucial ranges. Specialists with extensive experience in this procedure should perform such surgery.

BRACHIAL PLEXUS PALSY

When a brachial plexus injury involves the entire upper extremity, the condition is designated as brachial plexus palsy. Infants usually sustain such injuries from traction or compression during delivery. Brachial plexus palsy, however, also has been seen with cesarean deliveries. It has been reported to be 14 times more likely in subsequent births.

Upper extremity palsies present variably. Erb's palsy involves injury primarily to C-5 and C-6. Upper arm paresis or paralysis is present, and the child is unable to abduct and externally rotate the shoulder, supinate the forearm, and extend the wrist. The results are shoulder adduction and internal rotation, forearm pronation, and flexed wrist positioning. The affected child can extend the elbow, and the hand is functional. Klumpke's palsy involves the distal arm with injury primarily to C-8 and T-1. It occurs much less frequently than Erb's palsy. The affected child presents with a paretic or flaccid limb and usually some degree of wrist weakness (Abbot, 1998).

▲ **Clinical Warnings:**

- Erb's palsy occasionally is associated with ipsilateral phrenic nerve involvement, compromising diaphragmatic movement.
- In infants with Klumpke's palsy, providers must look for Horner's syndrome with ipsilateral ptosis and decreased pupillary dilation with reduced light. These findings may

overlap if nerve involvement extends beyond C-8 and T-1 roots.

When an extremity is hypotonic or flaccid but structurally normal (as in upper extremity palsies and many cases of spina bifida), then positioning with soft supports is sufficient. Initial management consists of partial immobilization and rest of the arm for approximately 1 week. After this phase, gentle passive ranging and massage should begin to maintain ranges and to stimulate muscular activation. Prognosis depends on the degree of nerve injury and is best when findings are due to edema or hemorrhage and not nerve disruption. Management usually does not progress beyond this point during the nursery stay.

SPINA BIFIDA AND MYELOMENINGOCELE

Pathology

Spina bifida is the most frequently encountered serious congenital malformation with complex associated problems. It results from abnormal embryonic neural tube development and closure that occurred before or at 26 to 30 days postconception, when the caudal portion closes. Folic acid supplementation before and during pregnancy has a protective role in the prevention of spina bifida. Myelomeningocele indicates the inclusion of spinal neural tissue along with the meninges through the unfused vertebral arches.

The level of lesion in spinal cord involvement determines the child's potential for mobility. Seventy-five percent of lesions occur in the lumbosacral area, causing various levels of flaccid paralysis or other mixed paraplegia (Nelson, Behrman, Kliegman, et al., 1996). This problem is further compounded in children born with orthopedic conditions originating from in utero positioning that resulted from the lesion level.

Children with L1 to L3 level lesions have marked muscular imbalance because of hip flexion and adduction, which is present with little opposition and tends to cause contractures and hip dislocation. Imbalance in knee flexors also will result in deviations. Scoliosis will develop with higher level lesions but can be managed with thoracolumbosacral orthosis (TLSO) and surgery. Children with L4 to L5 level lesions have some hip abduction and extension, although not sufficient to prevent imbalance about the hip. Flexion contractures and hip dislocation may emerge slowly, often in late childhood or adolescence. Foot deformities occur early because of innervation of ankle dorsiflexors and weak plantar flexors. An S1 to S2 lesion is associated primarily with foot deformity resulting from imbalanced innervation of intrinsic foot muscles. The child usually presents with cavus foot deformity and possible valgus or varus deviations.

Management

The infant with spina bifida or myelomeningocele requires management in a setting with multidisciplinary pediatric specialists, including a neurosurgeon, urologist, orthopedist, and physiatrist. The initial priority is to close the myelomeningocele in the first days and to assess the status of the cerebrum and spinal cord for anomalies. Daily joint ranging should be done gently to support any existing active mobility. Ninety percent of patients with spina bifida are reported to have hydrocephalus (Braddom, 1996), which may be present at birth or may develop in the first week of life. Hydrocephalus requires cerebral scanning, monitoring of head circumference, and placing of shunts when indicated.

A renal system evaluation is required. Neurogenic bladder sphincter dysfunction has to be addressed early to ensure bladder emptying and avoidance of urinary infections that can damage the kidneys. The urologist will set up management if evidence exists of urine reflux or residual bladder urine. If residual bladder urine exceeds 10 to 20 mL after voiding, intermittent catheterization should be initiated. The family needs to learn how to manage this procedure.

The provider typically performs subsequent continuous monitoring of hydrocephalus and neurogenic bladder. Careful and frequent monitoring of head circumference is necessary to ensure adequate shunt function and to monitor for delayed hydrocephalus, which can develop months or years later. Monitoring of urine also is done at the primary level, with the goal of preventing infection. Should infection occur, the provider must treat it promptly to protect renal status. Providers prescribe prophylactic antibiotics when necessary to prevent frequent infections.

▲ **Clinical Warning:** All children with myelomeningocele require physical therapy, the intensity of which depends on the lesion level and associated complications. The therapist should be experienced in pediatric rehabilitation and focus on stretching limited ranges, strengthening weak muscle groups, and facilitating optimal positioning and mobility. The family requires extensive instruction to perform carry over for these activities.

Children with lumbosacral lesions, hip dislocation, knee contractures, and talipes equinovarus (clubfoot) are seen often and require the attention of a pediatric orthopedist. Contractures and dislocations that interfere with symmetric and functional positioning require correction even when ambulation is not a goal, as with high lesions. Positioning bracing is key to maintaining ranges in flaccid, mobile joints and to prevent gravity-accommodating contractures. Assisted standing is introduced after the child is 1 year. The goal is eventually to progress to swing-through ambulation using a walker or possibly even crutches.

The rehabilitative goal for children with L1 to L3 lesions is household level ambulation using crutches and a special brace. The child may use a wheelchair for functional mobility. These children will be functional ambulators with AFO level bracing. Typically they eventually will not require crutches but will still need a wheelchair for very long distances, when braces require repair or adjustment, or if skin breakdown occurs to ankles or feet. The patient with a level S1 to S2 lesion will have completely functional ambulation. Shoe inserts or low-level SMOs are likely to be sufficient bracing. Refer to Chapter 59 (Chronic Orthopedic Problems) for more information.

Because of the lack of sensation associated with the spinal level lesion, skin breakdown can be a major problem, requiring the family to learn how to pay careful attention to the child's positioning with sleep and sitting, while also monitoring brace use and fit. Skin breakdown can create major obstructions to the child's rehabilitation, quickly leading to contractures. In such cases, maintenance activities have to be curtailed to remove all pressure while ulcerations heal.

▲ **Clinical Warning:** Because the child lacks sensation, pathologic fractures can occur readily and may not be easily detected. The provider and family should maintain a high level of suspicion for swollen sites.

Long-term management requires the clinician to monitor the child's progress continually. In addition to observing for signs of shunt dysfunction, changes in neurologic examination can indicate a tethered cord resulting from traction and canal deformity. This situation requires immediate neurosurgical intervention. The practitioner must monitor renal status as needed in comanagement with the pediatric urologist. The provider is often in the best position to support the family in its management of their child's need for intermittent catheterization. Bowel continence is usually more achievable than urinary continence. The provider can establish a regular bowel program using stool softeners, suppositories, digital anorectal stimulation, or manual removal as needed.

As the child ages, obesity becomes a major nutritional concern and can limit mobility. The provider helps the family to manage diet and activity before obesity occurs. Finally, the practitioner can be a powerful advocate for the child's learning, ensuring that he or she receives adequate educational support. Occupational therapy may help improve aspects of organizational skills needed for learning and provide assistive equipment that can expand self-care and educational independence.

Scoliosis and Kyphosis

Scoliosis can be seen as an orthopedic complication of CP, but also can occur in the idiopathic variety in normal children. Untreated scoliosis can evolve into a serious motor limitation. The disorder results from muscular asymmetry in the trunk that directly affects the spine, an uneven sitting base set up by pelvic obliquity, or hip subluxation. In turn, scoliosis increases the likelihood of hip subluxation, leading to aggravation of the spinal curve. Prevention includes a great deal of rehabilitative management directed at establishing postural symmetry to the degree that is possible, while also facilitating symmetric movement patterns. Scoliosis is particularly likely to develop in nonambulatory children with CP, because their muscular limitations are greater and more sustained.

● **Clinical Pearl:** Surgical correction is considered at approximately 40 degrees and should be done by a pediatric orthopedist or spinal orthopedic specialist. Refer to Chapter 59 (Chronic Orthopedic Problems) for further information on the diagnosis and management of scoliosis.

Kyphosis also can develop as a spinal deformity when children have poor underlying muscle tone and sit with a sagged posture for a prolonged duration. Tight hamstrings also will pull the pelvis forward in sitting, causing a slouched position with kyphotic spinal curve. If the child spends a great deal of time in this position, the spine can become fixed. As with scoliosis, kyphosis prevention is based on erect postural patterns and sitting position and diligent hamstring stretching.

As the spinal curve increases and becomes more fixed, bracing is initiated, usually with a TLSO. With the asymmetric muscular tone that is seen with CP, TLSO use can be considered earlier than with the more commonly seen idiopathic scoliosis that is usually braced at 20 degrees. The judgment for timing TLSO initiation is based on the degree of asymmetric forces exerted on the spine, the degrees of the curve, and the degree of stiffness in the curve when reduction and counter-rotation are attempted.

Scoliosis occurs more frequently than kyphosis. It is possible to have both deformities, known as kyphoscoliosis.

Associated Conditions

The primary care provider following the child with CP should be aware of certain comorbid conditions. Learning disabilities, attention deficit hyperactivity disorder (ADHD), language dysfunction, and processing disorders for functions like motor planning and sensory integration are much more likely to occur with CP than in the general population. Incidences of hearing and visual impairment and strabismus are increased (Nelson, 1998). An increased incidence in seizures, reported to be as high as 30% to 50%, is most frequently seen in children with spastic quadriplegic and hemiparetic CP (Braddom, 1996; Alexander & Molmar, 2000). Table 18-2 presents conditions associated with CP and their common manifestations. The reader is referred to Chapters 21, 46, 52, 53, 57, and 44 for more specific information.

Mental retardation is not part of CP but is reported in approximately two thirds of patients with CP. Retardation is mild in half these children and severe in the other half (Alexander, 1998). Because the spastic diplegic and hemiparetic types of CP represent more focal cerebral insults, normal intelligence is most likely to be seen in this group. Retardation is most likely to be seen with spastic quadriparetic CP. The likelihood of severe retardation is increased if microcephaly, severe spasticity, or seizures are present.

Hydrocephalus usually will appear early but not always. Compensated hydrocephalus has been reported to become progressive. Thus, providers must continue to measure head circumference beyond the usual infancy period. This is also a valuable measure for brain growth.

Table 18–2 CONDITIONS ASSOCIATED WITH CEREBRAL PALSY

Condition	Common Manifestation
Seizures	Refer to Chapter 46 for more information.
School problems	Communication, behavior, learning disabilities, ADHD
Visual impairment	Nystagmus, strabismus, optic atrophy
Hearing impairment	Hearing deficit
Auditory processing disorder	Child hears communication as something other than what it is; refer to Chapter 53 for more information.
Respiratory infections	Aspiration pneumonia (due to supranuclear bulbar palsies)
Nutritional problems	Swallowing difficulties
Gastroesophageal reflux disease	Refer to Chapter 16 for more information.
Fractures	

▲ **Clinical Warning:** When symptoms of increasing head circumference raise concern, the provider should refer the child for further evaluation, optimally by a pediatric neurosurgeon or neurologist. Continued family support and coordination of rehabilitative services underscore provider management. Because of the complexity of such coordination, the provider should use the services of a social worker or CNS with skills in this area. Their functions and roles are discussed in more detail at the end of this chapter.

PROGRESSIVE NEUROMUSCULAR DISEASES

Anatomy, Physiology, and Pathology

A variety of diseases with different etiologies share the common symptom of hypotonia in infancy or childhood that progresses throughout life. These diseases occur primarily at the level of the muscle cell or its directly innervating nerve cell or motor unit. Many are genetic, rare, and difficult to diagnose. It is not within the scope of this chapter to discuss the different diseases beyond mentioning some representative examples. If desired, current neurology texts can provide more in-depth information, including incidence, diagnosis, and management.

The spinal muscular atrophies are primarily genetically recessive, with progressing degeneration of the anterior horn cells in the spinal cord. These cells innervate voluntary or striated muscles. Disease progression, therefore, does not affect intellect. The several subtypes of spinal muscular atrophies vary in severity and rate of progression. Some children become totally incapacitated, dying in infancy. Other children experience gradual, progressive weakness and may survive into middle adulthood. Other hereditary progressive peripheral neuropathies exist that are less severe, such as Charcot-Marie-Tooth disease or peroneal muscular atrophy. These are managed as weakness states.

The muscular dystrophies are manifested by genetic, progressive degeneration at the muscle fiber level. Duchenne muscular dystrophy is the best known and most common, although other unrelated dystrophies exist of greater or lesser severity. Some patients have more focal presentations, such as limb girdle dystrophy. Duchenne muscular dystrophy is genetically transmitted as an X-linked recessive disease in boys. Some hypotonia is evident in infancy but usually does not cause gross motor delay until the onset of walking. In some patients, walking is not delayed. These children do not begin to exhibit hypotonia until they transition to standing. At this point, the well-described Gower's sign is evident, with the boy needing to push his arms against his thighs to stand because of early hip extensor weakness. The posture becomes lordotic and the gait pattern deviated, with lateral shifting from gluteus medius weakness and toe walking. These changes are compensations in the center of gravity with associated gastrocsoleus contractures.

Wheelchair dependence with ambulatory loss usually occurs between ages 7 to 10 years. Extremity contractures and scoliosis progress quickly because of the inability to move. Fortunately, the muscular fibrosis usually is not painful. Often obesity emerges, aggravating the progressive cardiomyopathy and respiratory failure characteristic of muscle fiber degeneration. These problems are the usual causes of the patient's death by early adulthood. Even though the primary disease is at the muscular level, mild mental retardation has been noted as part of the complex of symptoms in some boys with Duchenne muscular dystrophy.

Myotonic muscular dystrophy is the next most common muscular dystrophy. The term myotonia refers to the unique slow relaxation phase after the muscle contracts. Incoordination, caused by muscle weakness and slowed relaxation, is characteristic, resulting in slurred speech and swallowing irregularity. Myotonic muscular dystrophy has a more complex, genetically based presentation that affects not only voluntary striated muscles, but also the smooth muscles of many organs. It often is associated with intellectual impairment. Unlike the other dystrophies with more proximal involvement initially, weakness usually is mild in the early years, with a subsequent decrease in muscle mass seen distally at the face and neck. Progression usually is slow so that the child can ambulate into adulthood, although bracing is often necessary.

Numerous rare metabolic myopathies exist, with muscle dysfunctions based on structural abnormalities within a cell or enzymatic defects that weaken the muscle cell's function. These changes also may affect other organ functions, with varying degrees of progressive weakness.

History and Physical Examination

The provider must be suspicious for these muscular dystrophies when evaluating an infant or child with hypotonia, if any progression in hypotonia is evident, or if a family history of muscle weakness exists.

Diagnostic Studies

If the history and physical examination suggest Duchenne muscular dystrophy, the clinician needs to obtain a serum creatine phosphokinase level. An extremely elevated level is suggestive and needs to be confirmed by muscle biopsy, unless the disease already has been confirmed by family history.

● **Clinical Pearl:** The other disorders are much harder to diagnose specifically. The provider should refer any child with uncertain progressive neuromuscular disease to a pediatric neurologist with access to a laboratory that can do the necessary assays on blood and muscle biopsies. Muscle biopsy usually is required for diagnosing most of these disorders.

A neurologist also may order electrodiagnostic studies. These can contribute to diagnosis when patterns of slowed nerve conduction, denervation, or myopathic electromyographic discharges are demonstrated.

Management

Accurate diagnosis is important for guiding prognosis and decisions about therapeutic approaches and possible surgical interventions. Following diagnosis, the provider should refer parents and patients who reach reproductive age to a geneticist for genetic counseling.

The approach to rehabilitation for progressive neuromuscular disease incorporates the interventions described for hypotonia. Providers should note that the severity of muscle weakness and functional limitations will increase to varying degrees, depending on the disorder; therefore, they must adjust therapy, bracing, and equipment accordingly. The clinician will coordinate care with intensive support from occupational and physical therapies to maintain function as long as possible, including flexibilitiy and ambulatory ability. Monitoring of the progression of dysfunctions, such as hip dislocation and scoliosis, is important. Rehabilitative professionals can provide ongoing support, monitoring guidance, and therapeutic assistance in these efforts.

The provider needs to carry out periodic review with the family to determine the need for assistive equipment like motorized wheelchairs, voice-activated computer software (especially helpful for the child in carrying out school assignments), bath chairs, commodes, transfer lifts, and hospital beds. The family will require a great deal of support as their child's physical abilities wane. They have the very difficult circumstance of knowing that in spite of their efforts with exercises, ranging, and positioning, their child's condition will progress relentlessly in many cases, leading to an early demise. Refer to Chapter 49 (The Child With Chronic Illness) for more information about how to support the family dealing with their child's chronic disease.

ARTHROGRYPOSIS

Anatomy, Physiology, and Pathology

Arthrogryposis is a nonprogressing neuromuscular deformity primarily affecting the extremities. The disorder is thought to result from events in the first trimester. Arthrogryposis is characterized by nerve and muscle involvement that causes weakness, immobilization, joint contractures, and eventually fibrosis. Children with arthrogryposis usually have normal intelligence.

History and Physical Examination

Etiology is not known, but viral infection with fever is considered a possible cause, as are circulatory compromises and maternal uterine septum defect. Lower extremities are more frequently and diffusely involved than are upper extremities. Hips are usually flexed or abducted and often dislocated. Feet are clubbed, and knees, elbows, and wrists are deformed in flexion or extension. Muscles opposing the contracted positions are often very weak.

Management

Providers should refer any patient they suspect of having arthrogryposis to a pediatric neurologist for a more complete evaluation. The child will require referral for ongoing rehabilitative support. Physical therapy is an important part of the management plan for contractures, scoliosis if it occurs, and ambulation support. Providers also will need to refer the patient for pediatric orthopedic intervention to reduce deformities, release contractures and fibrotic joint capsules, and transfer muscles to increase mobility.

Despite the foregoing efforts, significant mobility and functional limitations will remain. The provider's ongoing role is one of supporting the family, while coordinating rehabilitative interventions that optimize development and function.

RHEUMATOID ARTHRITIS

The pediatric rheumatologist and primary care provider usually manage rheumatologic conditions with medications. Rehabilitation support is dictated by the inflammatory state. When acute inflammation is present in a joint, the joint is rested in a functional position and supported with a splint if necessary. When the inflammation lessens, more active mobilization with stretching and progressive strengthening is done. More than with the other conditions discussed, family involvement forms the basis of rehabilitative management.

The family learns to rest acutely involved joints and to mobilize and strengthen them when the process has quieted. They learn exercises along with joint-conserving functional dynamics. Assistance can be provided for pacing the day's activities to avoid fatigue. Children may require rest periods built into the school day. Physical education is adapted to provide activity for endurance, while avoiding stressful joint impact and wear. Mobilization of the spine and neck for range maintenance is also useful. Walking, biking, and swimming are particularly good endurance activities. Crafts can make hand mobility fun. For tightened ranges that tend to be less responsive to stretching, night splinting can be used without interfering with day activities. In home-based programming, the family can respond to the changing course of inflammation. They can adjust resting and mobilization activities to family schedules, causing the least interruption of family life while still sparing joints and maintaining as much strength as possible.

SUPPORTING THE FAMILY

Families of children with physical challenges face psychological challenges. The child's physical condition alters the family's experience in many ways. Initially, parents experience an emotional adjustment when they learn that projected aspirations for their child may be impossible and that demands on them will be great. They will need to expend significant energy and time on therapies and their carry over, placing parents in the position of having to perform additional activities that their child may not favor. Many activities that parents normally teach their children will be more difficult or will need to be repeated patiently many times. Children may be less motivated to do tasks because they are difficult. Through it all, these children still share the desires, needs for play, and issues involving attachment and separation that all children face.

Parents of children with physical challenges have less time to socialize or pursue entertainment interests. Their social experiences may be shifted to other families with challenged children and the agencies that serve them, which can be positive. Socialization for these children is more difficult than for nonchallenged youngsters, often because of language limitations, decreased ability to participate fully in peer activities, and inability to process social cues. Unfortunately, even though families and educational laws bring children together in mainstreamed situations, nothing can guarantee acceptance or positive engagement.

Primary care providers can help these families to focus on the fact that everybody in the family is important. Each family needs to set common goals and decide how individual members should interact to maintain a functional and supportive unit. Even though the child who is challenged has more obstacles to overcome and may face more disappointments than other children, the family should view all activities as socialization experiences. They should not accept maladaptive responses. Children should feel loved and nurtured for who they are, and family members should recognize their accomplishments. Parents should not sacrifice other siblings to the needs of the physically challenged child.

Referral to appropriate rehabilitative and mental health professionals is key to family success. Effective clinicians encourage families to seek out and become a part of a peer group of families facing similar challenges. The Community

Resources section at the end of this chapter can guide such efforts. Chapter 27 (Grief, Loss, and Coping With Change) may support the provider who is working with a patient dealing with a progressive disease. Chapter 50 (Multidisciplinary Support of the Chronically Ill Child and Family) should guide the clinician in how to integrate professional suggestions into an effective, family-focused management plan.

Children who exhibit neurologically based motor problems are more likely to experience behavioral maladjustments with neurologic processing dysfunctions, such as ADHD, poor frustration tolerance with antisocial reactions, impulsivity, decreased transitioning skills, perseveration, and general emotional immaturity. Providers should suggest and coordinate behavior modification approaches for the child to enact in family and educational settings. Refer to Chapter 21 (School Problems) for ideas on dealing with these problems.

A child's additional therapeutic, rehabilitative, cognitive, behavioral, and social needs may be so complex that they exceed available coordination time. In such an instance, the clinician may be well supported by referring the patient and family to a CNS or social worker who can spend time with the family, explaining the child's condition and needs sensitively. This professional should remain available as an ongoing resource for follow-up of the child and family. The provider, CNS, or social worker should recommend physical, occupational, and speech therapies and equipment as needed. He or she should arrange these services so parents can understand treatment goals, participate in the process, and provide carry over with implementation. Because of the complexity that many of these cases present, this professional can serve as a family coordinator, providing support while ensuring comprehensive integration of any intervention.

The family coordinator also should be able to seek out funding available to the child and additional support services. These intentions are encompassed in the Early Intervention Program (EIP), established with PL 99-457 as an optional program with federal and state funding for children up to age 3 years. The level of disability that is eligible for EIP service varies among states. Intensity of services is also very inconsistent. Individual states implement EIPs differently (Wallace, Biehl, MacQueen, & Blackman, 1997). Usually a comprehensive pediatric rehabilitation agency will be the best source in a community or region, employing professionals with experience in working as part of interdisciplinary teams.

Although individually contracted therapists and case coordinators may be very qualified, integration among services is difficult. Comprehensive rehabilitation programs usually provide additional activities for families, such as play groups for parents and children, parent peer groups, and other community resource connections. Primary care providers must recognize any emerging problem(s), setting up the referrals for EIPs. A major problem exists for the child who does not meet the eligibility criteria. Children who receive Medicaid can receive care at rehabilitation centers as outpatients. They will receive available comprehensive programming. The child in managed care or a system that requires referral, however, may not be approved for what are deemed to be developmental services. Even if evaluations are done, longer duration interventions usually are not covered.

Providers must encourage the family to review and remain active participants in their child's activities and programs. Parents should stay closely engaged with therapists and teachers so that home carry over continues.

● **Clinical Pearl:** The primary care provider should be aware of the presence of these programs, be able to identify children who need them, and support families in their involvement with their children's interventions.

COMMUNITY RESOURCES

Providers should encourage families to be active in advocating in their community for their children. Parents should establish contact groups within a school district, a broader locality, or as an extension of a rehabilitation agency. Because so many of the discussed programs vary in service delivery, contact groups enable families to compare program effectiveness to advocate for change or other needed actions.

Families can approach various organizations to support children's special equipment needs when insurance will not provide for them. Communities may establish volunteer or organization services for respite or family assistance. Parent groups can exert political influence, lobbying their legislators for improved insurance coverage. They also can recruit political officials to support their concerns. Parent contact groups have been effective in influencing legislators for money allocations that improve the availability and effectiveness of programs.

A number of national organizations are particularly supportive of advocacy and providing information for families. The following sources list some organizations for conditions discussed in this chapter.

The Association for Persons With Severe Handicaps
7010 Roosevelt Way, N.E.
Seattle, WA 98115
(206) 361-8870

Muscular Dystrophy Association
3300 East Sunrise Drive
Tucson, AZ 85718
(602) 529-2000

National Council on Disability
800 Independence Ave., S.W. Suite 814
Washington, DC 20591
(202) 267-3846

National Down Syndrome Society
666 Broadway
New York, NY 10012
(800) 221-4602

National Organization for Rare Disorders
P.O. Box 8923
New Fairfield, CT 06812
(203) 746-6518

National Organization on Disability
910 16th St., N.W., Suite 600
Washington, DC 20006
(202) 293-5960

National Rehabilitation Information Center
(800) 346-2742

Spina Bifida Association of America
4590 MacArthur Blvd., N.W., Suite 250
Washington, DC 20007
(800) 621-3141

United Cerebral Palsy Association
1522 K Street, N.W., Suite 1112
Washington, DC 20005
(800) USA-5UCP

REFERENCES

Abbot, R. (1998). *Brachial plexus palsy* (seminar). Institute for Neurology and Neurosurgery at Beth Israel Medical Center, New York, NY, Nov. 16, 1998.

Alexander, M. (1998). *The spectrum of medical problems in children with cerebral palsy, and nonsurgical management of spasticity: What works, what doesn't* (seminar). Cerebral Palsy, New Insights, New Interventions. Schneider Children's Hospital, New Hyde Park, NY, Nov. 3.

Alexander, M. A., & Molmer, G. E. (2000). *Physical medicine and rehabilitation.* Philadelphia: Hanley and Balfus, Inc.

Braddom, R. L. (1996). *Physical medicine and rehabilitation.* Philadelphia: W.B. Saunders.

Brin, M. (Ed.) (1997). *Spasticity, etiology, evaluation, management and the role of botulinum toxin type A. Muscle and nerve, supplement 6.* New York: John Wiley & Sons.

Campbell, S. K. (Ed.) (1991). *Pediatric neurologic physical therapy, clinics in physical therapy* (2nd ed.). New York: Churchill Livingstone.

Campbell, S. K. (Ed.) (1994). *Physical therapy for children.* Philadelphia: W.B. Saunders.

Glenn, M. B., & Whyle, J. (1990). *The practical management of spasticity in children and adults.* Philadelphia: Lea & Febiger.

Molnar, G. E. (Ed.) (1991). The child with physical disability. *Physical Medicine and Rehabilitation State of the Art Reviews, 5,* 2.

Nelson, K. B. (1998). *The causes of cerebral palsy: New insights* (seminar). Cerebral palsy: New insights, new interventions, by Schneider Children's Hospital, New Hyde Park, NY, Nov. 3, 1998.

Nelson, W. E., Behrman, R. E., Kliegman, R. M., & Arvin, A. M. (1996). *Nelson's textbook of pediatrics.* Philadelphia: W.B. Saunders.

Wallace, H. M., Biehl, R. F., MacQueen, J., & Blackman, J. A. (1997). *Mosby resource guide to children with disabilities and chronic illness.* St. Louis: C.V. Mosby.

Asperger's Syndrome and Pervasive Developmental Disorders

• JOSEPH P. DAMORE, JR., MD

INTRODUCTION

Pediatric primary care providers are in the enviable position of watching children grow and develop from infancy through childhood, adolescence, and often beyond. Perhaps no other specialty affords clinicians with the opportunity to witness such unparalleled change. Those who work in pediatric primary care also observe many children of various ages and developmental stages. As a result, they become acquainted early on with the broad range of normal variations that characterize such development.

Often in such practice, providers will encounter a child who presents with behavioral or emotional symptoms that are outside the range of normal development. It is not uncommon for the pediatric practitioner to be the first to diagnose children with attentional deficits, hyperactivity, or other difficulties, such as mood disorders and anxiety. Less frequently, providers may encounter and appropriately diagnose a child with autism. Usually, such diagnoses are made in the presence of clear-cut symptoms or during particularly severe decompensations in behavior. Often, however, children with less profound behavioral disorders "fall through the cracks" of pediatric watchfulness. Busy primary care providers may overlook these children, who often present with odd mannerisms, deficits in social skills, or remarkable facility with language or memory. This is particularly common when such characteristics do not create problems at home or school. Even when problems occur, these children are often misdiagnosed and treated for the component parts of their syndrome (Perry, 1998).

Though the category of pervasive developmental disorders includes such problems as autism, Rett's disorder, and childhood disintegrative disorder, this chapter focuses specifically on the presentation, diagnostic criteria, and treatment of children with Asperger's syndrome and pervasive developmental disorder not otherwise specified (PDD NOS). The reasons for this are twofold. First, discussion of all the pervasive developmental disorders is beyond the scope of this text. Secondly, the sequellae of disorders such as autism and Rett's disorder are so profound that they usually are easily identified at an early age and thus referred early for treatment. Cases of Asperger's syndrome and PDD NOS, however, are often misdiagnosed or undiagnosed. Though rare, they are more likely to be seen in pediatric primary care practice. This chapter is not an exhaustive discussion of these syndromes; rather, it will enable readers to become familiar with the presentation and treatment of these disorders.

PATHOLOGY

Asperger's Syndrome

In 1944, the Viennese child psychiatrist Hans Asperger, while studying the capacity for group formation in children, first described a cohort of children who demonstrated social isolation coupled with odd and unusual behavior (Szatmari, Tuff, Finlayson, & Bartolucci, 1990). This condition was first described as autistic psychopathy, terminology that led to misunderstanding because of the similarity of the term psychopathy to sociopathy. For this reason, the disorder became known as Asperger's syndrome. This disorder describes children with eccentricities of speech, nonverbal communication, social interaction, motor coordination, and skills and interests. Most of these children demonstrate a strong interest in repetitive activities and a strong desire to avoid changes in their environment. Children with Asperger's syndrome usually acquire the capacity for language at the same age as unaffected children, though the content of the speech tends to be repetitive, pedantic, and loquacious (Wing, 1981). Similarly, they demonstrate difficulty in initiating and maintaining two-way conversation. Children with Asperger's syndrome exhibit a paucity of emotional expression and facial gestures. Quite commonly, these youngsters become intensely interested in unusual subjects, such as floor plans for buildings, fish, or machinery (Szatmari et al., 1990; Howlin & Asgharian, 1999).

They also tend to excel at board games. These children are reported to be clumsy and uncoordinated and often demonstrate problems with drawing and writing. Their posture and gait may be described as odd (Wing, 1981).

● **Clinical Pearl:** Often, stereotyped interests may resemble other interests found in unaffected children of the same age, such as astronomy, geology, or dinosaurs. What distinguishes the child with Asperger's syndrome is the intensity and circumscribed nature of his or her interest. Children with Asperger's syndrome have excellent rote memories and may obtain every fact available about their chosen interest.

Wing (1981) suggested that Asperger's syndrome should be considered part of an autistic continuum (ie, a mild variant of autism in relatively intelligent children). Though in agreement with the notion that Asperger's syndrome and autism share features, other authors later proposed that those with Asperger's syndrome demonstrate no cognitive or language delays (Tantum, 1988). Baron-Cohen and Wheelwright (1999) examined the behavior of children with Asperger's syndrome. In surveying 92 parents of such children, they found that the obsessive behaviors of Asperger's syndrome are not in fact random acts but are organized around the notion of what they term "folk physics," meaning a fascination with how things work. This finding is in contrast with what the authors term "folk psychology," which means a curiosity about how people work.

Few studies have been able to demonstrate a link between Asperger's syndrome and pathologic conditions, though associations with neurologic disorders and amino-aciduria have been reported (Tantum, 1988). Sobanski, Marcus, Hennighausen, Hebebrand, and Schmidt (1999) describe disturbed eating behavior and, hence, significantly decreased body mass index (BMI) in male children with Asperger's syndrome compared with healthy control children. Of 36 subjects, 13 children had BMIs below the 10th percentile, while three had BMIs under the third percentile. Their findings suggest that providers should evaluate any child with Asperger's syndrome for eating problems as well.

Some studies suggest an association between Asperger's syndrome and lesions of the right cerebral hemisphere (Tantum, 1988). Interestingly, Wing (1981) observed that approximately half of children affected with this disorder had a history of prenatal, postnatal, or perinatal complications, though other investigators did not observe such findings in other samples (Szatmari, Bremner, & Nagy, 1989). Though several studies suggest a genetic etiology to the disorder, no firm genetic relationship has been established (Gillberg, 1989).

Pervasive Developmental Disorder Not Otherwise Specified

Unlike Asperger's Syndrome, little is known about PDD NOS as a distinct clinical entity. Various euphemisms for the disorder include atypical autism and high functioning autism, because most children with PDD NOS demonstrate some or most characteristics seen in children with autism (Howlin & Asgharian, 1999).

In a study of 390 children younger than 5 years conducted by Dahl, Cohen, and Provence (1986), 24 children demonstrated odd behavior, eccentric thinking, and impairments in social interaction. In a similar study, Levine and Demb (1987) reported that of 18 preschool children diagnosed with PDD NOS, only about one third had an IQ in the normal or borderline range. More than two thirds of the children in Levine's sample had a history of abnormal speech acquisition. More than 90% of these children had abnormal speech characterized by echolalia, abnormalities of prosody, and pronoun reversal. In addition, Levine and Demb noted these children to be markedly provocative or clinging with their parents, and almost all demonstrated ritualistic behaviors. Other authors have described the consistency of these findings over time as well (Baron-Cohen & Wheelwright, 1999; Berument, Rutter, Lord, Pickles, & Bailey, 1999; Coplan, 2000).

● **Clinical Pearl:** In general, the social, intellectual, and language impairments of children with PDD NOS are considerably more profound in presentation than those seen in Asperger's syndrome. When taking a developmental history, a child with Asperger's syndrome should not have demonstrated a delay in either language acquisition or cognitive milestones (Howlin & Asgharian, 1999). Such delays are common in children with PDD NOS.

EPIDEMIOLOGY

Asperger's Syndrome

In a study examining the prevalence of Asperger's syndrome, Wing (1981) determined that 0.6 per 10,000 children met criteria for the syndrome and for mild mental retardation; 1.1 per 10,000 met criteria for autism in early life, though these children later developed features more consistent with Asperger's syndrome. Gillberg and Gillberg (1989) examined children of normal intelligence, with criteria somewhat different from those listed in the *Diagnostic and Statistical Manual of Mental Disorders,* fourth edition (DSM-IV). They reported a prevalence rate of 10 to 26 per 10,000 for Asperger's syndrome. Similarly, Ehlers and Gillberg (1993) reported a total population prevalence of 71 per 10,000, though again they used less stringent criteria for this study than those found in the DSM-IV. In all studies of Asperger's syndrome, the disorder was found to be more common in boys than in girls, with a ratio of 3.8 to 10.5 to 1 (Szatmari et al., 1990; Wing, 1981; Baron-Cohen & Wheelwright, 1999; Filipek et al., 1999; Howlin & Asgharian, 1999).

Pervasive Developmental Disorder Not Otherwise Specified

Because of the lack of a precise definition of PDD NOS, prevalence rates of the disorder vary. Steffenburg and Gillberg (1986) reported a prevalence of 2.2 per 10,000 in a population of Swedish children. Burd, Fisher, and Kerbeshian (1987) reported a prevalence of 1.99 per 10,000 in a population of children from North Dakota. Like Asperger's syndrome, the disorder appears significantly more common in boys (Volkmar, Cohen, Hoshino, Rende, & Paul, 1988; Filipek et al., 1999; Sobanski et al., 1999). A genetic basis is emerging as a factor in the epidemiology of the PDDs (Barrett et al., 1999; Mbarek et al., 1999).

No epidemiologic evidence exists that supports the notion that measles, rubella, or mumps vaccines can precipitate PDD NOS (DeStefano & Chen, 2000). Furthermore, seasonal variability has not proven to be a precipitating factor in incidence of autism or PDD (Landau, Cicchetti, Klin, & Volkmar, 1999).

DIAGNOSTIC CRITERIA

Asperger's Syndrome

The diagnostic criteria for Asperger's syndrome according to the DSM-IV (1994) are as follows:

- Qualitative impairment in social interaction, as manifested by at least two of the following:
  - Marked impairment in the use of multiple nonverbal behaviors, such as eye-to-eye gaze, facial expression, body postures, and gestures to regulate social interaction
  - Failure to develop peer relationships appropriate to developmental level
  - A lack of spontaneous seeking to share enjoyment, interest, or achievements with other people (eg, by a lack of showing, bringing, or pointing out objects of interest to others)
  - Lack of social or emotional reciprocity

- Restricted repetitive and stereotyped patterns of behavior, interests, and activities, as manifested by at least one of the following:
  - Encompassing preoccupation with one or more stereotyped and restricted patterns of interest that is abnormal either in intensity or focus
  - Apparently inflexible adherence to specific, nonfunctional routines or rituals
  - Stereotyped and repetitive motor mannerisms (eg, hand or finger flapping or twisting or complex whole-body movements)
  - Persistent preoccupation with parts of objects
- The disturbance causes clinically significant impairment in social, occupational, or other important areas of functioning.
- There is no clinically significant general delay in language (eg, child uses single words by age 2 years, uses communicative phrases by age 3 years).
- There is no clinically significant delay in cognitive development or in development of age-appropriate self-help skills, adaptive behavior (other than in social interaction), and curiosity about the environment in childhood.
- Child does not meet criteria for another specific PDD or schizophrenia (American Psychiatric Association, 1994).

Pervasive Developmental Disorder Not Otherwise Specified

The DSM-IV (1994) states that the diagnosis of PDD NOS is appropriate if impairment in reciprocal social interaction or verbal and nonverbal communication skills is clear or when stereotyped behavior, interests, or activities are present; however, the child does not meet the criteria for a specific pervasive developmental disorder, schizophrenia, or personality disorder (American Psychiatric Association, 1994). When evaluating a child who seems particularly odd with regard to mannerisms, areas of interest, or behavior, providers should have a high degree of suspicion that these findings could represent Asperger's syndrome. A high degree of suspicion greatly reduces the probability of tunnel vision in seeing only the problematic behavior, such as hyperactivity or distractibility, and thus misdiagnosing the disorder.

MANAGEMENT

The management of Asperger's syndrome and PDD NOS is both challenging and complex. Treatment is always multimodal, involving individual and family psychotherapy, parent training, social skills training, educational counseling, special education, behavior modification, and pharmacotherapy. Optimal outcomes involve early recognition of the syndrome and appropriate timely referral to a specialist familiar with it (Volkmar, Cook, Jr., Pomeroy, Realmuto, & Tanguay, 1999). Usually, such specialists work in child study centers, which are specialized neuropsychiatric institutes associated with major medical universities. Once diagnosed, a therapist skilled in working with such children and their families is critical. Ideally, this therapist will coordinate parent training, individual skills training, group work, and educational needs required in the treatment of such children. The evaluating clinician may be able recommend a qualified therapist.

Some children, particularly those who demonstrate poor coordination, can benefit from physical and occupational therapy. Such therapy needs to target better gross and fine motor control. Most large communities have individuals skilled in doing this work.

Medications have been used with varying degrees of success to control the obsessive and repetitive behaviors often observed in Asperger's syndrome and the sometimes oppositional and irritable behaviors that such children occasionally display. A child psychiatrist who is experienced in working with these patients is usually the most familiar with medications used to treat these features.

▲ **Clinical Warning:** Children with Asperger's syndrome and PDD NOS can often have paradoxical reactions to some medications and preferential responses to others (Perry, 1998). Damore, Stine, and Brody (1998) were first to report an exacerbation of impulsivity and behavioral disregulation in children with Asperger's syndrome who were taking fluoxetine (Prozac) and resolution of these behaviors when these children were switched to divalproex sodium (Depakote).

From an educational perspective, working closely with the school staff and the child's committee on special education is a vital component of treatment. These children demonstrate unusual learning disabilities, especially in the areas of social skills. Neuropsychological testing is helpful in diagnosing learning disabilities (Szatmari et al., 1989; Filipek et al., 1999; Bristol-Power & Spinella, 1999). The reader is referred to Chapter 21, which provides a more in-depth discussion of the diagnosis and management of conduct disorder.

Finally, the diagnosis of Asperger's syndrome or PDD NOS requires that parents receive a thoughtful and cogent explanation of the disorder and its relationship to other similar disorders, such as autism. Parents need to know that the behavior and social interaction of children with Asperger's syndrome, and to some extent PDD NOS, improve with age. They need to know that the day-to-day care of these children can be both enriching and exhausting (Szatmari et al., 1989; Volkmar et al., 1999; Coplan, 2000). Primary care providers can help these children and their families by coordinating the unique and varied multimodal care that these disorders require.

COMMUNITY RESOURCES

The following sources can provide support and information for both the clinician and families:

Yale Child Study Center
Yale University School of Medicine
New Haven, CT

New York University Child Study Center
New York University School of Medicine/Bellevue Medical Center
550 First Avenue
New York, NY 10016
(212) 263-6205

REFERENCES

American Psychiatric Association. (1994). *Diagnostic and statistical manual of mental disorders* (4th ed.). Washington, DC: Author.
Baron-Cohen, S., & Wheelwright, S. (1999). "Obsessions" in children with autism or Asperger syndrome. Content analysis in terms

of core domains of cognition. *British Journal of Psychiatry, 175,* 484–490.

Barrett, S., Beck, J. C., Bernier, R., Bisson, E., Braun, T. A., Casavant, T. L., Childress, D., et al. (1999). An autosomal genomic screen for autism. Collaborative linkage study of autism. *American Journal of Medical Genetics, 88*(6), 609–615.

Berument, S. K., Rutter, M., Lord, C., Pickles, A., & Bailey, A. (1999). Autism screening questionnaire: Diagnostic validity. *British Journal of Psychiatry, 175,* 444-51.

Bristol-Power, M. M., & Spinella, G. (1999). Research on screening and diagnosis in autism: A work in progress. *Journal of Autism and Developmental Disorders, 29*(6), 435–438.

Burd, L., Fisher, W., & Kerbeshian, J. (1987). A prevalence study of pervasive developmental disorders in North Dakota. *Journal of the American Academy of Child and Adolescent Psychiatry, 26,* 700–703.

Coplan, J. (2000). Counseling parents regarding prognosis in autistic spectrum disorder. *Pediatrics, 105*(5), E65.

Dahl, E., Cohen, D., & Provence, S. (1986). Clinical and multivariate approaches to the nosology of Pervasive Developmental Disorders. *Journal of the American Academy of Child and Adolescent Psychiatry, 25,* 170–180.

Damore, J., Stine, J., & Brody, L. (1998). Medication induced hypomania in Asperger's Disorder. *Journal of the American Academy of Child and Adolescent Psychiatry, 37,* 248-49.

DeStefano, F., & Chen, R. T. (2000). Autism and measles, mumps, and rubella vaccine: No epidemiological evidence for a causal association. *Journal of Pediatrics, 136*(1), 125–126.

Ehlers, S., & Gillberg, C. (1993). The epidemiology of Asperger syndrome: A total population study. *Journal of Child Psychology and Psychiatry, 34,* 1327–1350.

Filipek, P. A., Accardo, P. J., Baranek, G. T., Cook, E. H., Jr., Dawson, G., Gordon, B., Gravel, J. S., et al. (1999). The screening and diagnosis of autistic spectrum disorders. *Journal of Autism and Developmental Disorders, 29*(6), 439–484.

Gillberg, C. (1989). Asperger syndrome in 23 Swedish children. *Developmental Medicine and Child Neurology, 31,* 520–531.

Gillberg, I. C., & Gillberg, C. (1989). Asperger syndrome—some epidemiological considerations: A research note. *Journal of Child Psychology and Psychiatry, 30,* 631–638.

Howlin, P., & Asgharian, A. (1999). The diagnosis of autism and Asperger syndrome: Findings from a survey of 770 families. *Developmental Medicine and Child Neurology, 41*(12), 834–839.

Landau, E. C., Cicchetti, D. V., Klin, A., & Volkmar, F. R. (1999). Season of birth in autism: A fiction revisited. *Journal of Autism and Developmental Disorders, 29*(5), 385–393.

Levine, J., & Demb, H. (1987). Characteristics of preschool children diagnosed as having an atypical pervasive developmental disorder. *Journal of Developmental and Behavioral Pediatrics, 8,* 77–82.

Mbarek, O., Marouillat, S., Martineau, J., Barthelemy, C., Muh, J. P., & Andres, C. (1999). Association study of the NF1 gene and autistic disorder. *American Journal of Medical Genetics, 88*(6), 729–732.

Perry, R. (1998). Misdiagnosed ADD/ADHD; Rediagnosed PDD. *Journal of the American Academy of Child and Adolescent Psychiatry, 37,* 113–114.

Sobanski, E., Marcus, A., Hennighausen, K., Hebebrand, J., & Schmidt, M. H. (1999). Further evidence for a low body weight in male children and adolescents with Asperger's disorder. *European Child and Adolescent Psychiatry, 8*(4), 312–314.

Steffenburg, S., & Gillberg, C. (1986). Autism and autistic-like conditions in Swedish rural and urban area: A population study. *British Journal of Psychiatry, 149,* 81–87.

Szatmari, P., Bremner, R., & Nagy, J. (1989). Asperger's Syndrome—a review of clinical features. *Canadian Journal of Psychiatry, 34,* 554–560.

Szatmari, P., Tuff, L., Finlayson, M. A., & Bartolucci, G. (1990). Asperger's Syndrome and autism: Neurocognitive aspects. *Journal of the American Academy of Child and Adolescent Psychiatry, 29,* 130–136.

Tantum, D. (1988). Asperger's syndrome. *Journal of Child Psychology and Psychiatry, 29,* 245–255.

Volkmar, F., Cohen, D., Hoshino, Y., Rende, R., & Paul, R. (1988). Phenomenology and classification of the childhood psychoses. *Psychological Medicine, 18,* 191–201.

Volkmar, F., Cook, E., Jr., Pomeroy, J., Realmuto, G., & Tanguay, P. (1999). Summary of the practice parameters for the assessment and treatment of children, adolescents, and adults with autism and other Pervasive Developmental Disorders. *Journal of the American Academy of Child and Adolescent Psychiatry, 38*(12), 1611–1616.

Wing, L. (1981). Asperger's syndrome: A clinical account. *Psychological Medicine, 11,* 115–129.

The Intellectually Gifted Child

• PHYLLIS ALDRICH, AB, MA, SDA

INTRODUCTION

The phenomenon of a "gifted child" is one of the most misunderstood and underdiagnosed conditions throughout the western world. Claims of "giftedness" arouse strong (and mostly negative) reactions in many adults, including educators. These feelings seem more a product of adults' own personal experiences than objective analysis, impeding the identification and nurturing of these children's gifts. Attitudes toward giftedness reflect a deep paradox in western culture. While society may value outstanding intellectual achievement, such as breaking the genetic code or inventing the microchip, a deep abiding distrust of precocity in children prevails. Society often perceives gifted children as "misfits" whose intellectual power develops in direct proportion to diminished attractiveness.

Primary care providers can play a vital role in correcting this situation. If providers become more aware of some of the presenting signs of intellectual giftedness, then they can be persuasive advocates for these children, both with parents and teachers. Consequently, these children will be able to realize more of their promise. This chapter provides the reader with an understanding of some of the observable behaviors and varieties of intellectually gifted children. It also gives suggestions for supporting gifted youngsters and their parents.

ANATOMY, PHYSIOLOGY, AND PATHOLOGY

Ever since the Terman (1905) studies began and the Stanford-Binet intelligence test was designed to sort out unsuitable soldiers from service in World War I, psychologists have defined giftedness as a kind of unitary hereditary factor. They assumed intelligence to be a general kind of special prowess present from birth and waiting for the right conditions to appear. The Marland Report (1972) proposed a more encompassing description of giftedness that included at least six domains, describing children who demonstrate outstanding potential or performance in any one of these areas:

- General intellectual ability
- Specific academic ability
- Creative or productive thinking
- Leadership ability
- Visual and performing arts ability
- Psychomotor ability

Howard Gardner (1993) examined the effects of trauma on differing sites in the brain. He posits eight separate kinds of intelligence, including the following:

- Linguistic
- Music
- Logical/mathematical reasoning
- Spatial
- Bodily/kinesthetic
- Interpersonal
- Intrapersonal
- Naturalist

In 1995, The World Council on Gifted and Talented Children adopted this definition of giftedness:

> "Giftedness is asynchronous development in which advanced cognitive abilities and heightened intensity combine to create inner experiences and awareness that are qualitatively different from the norm. This asynchrony increases with higher intellectual capacity. The uniqueness of the gifted renders them particularly vulnerable, requiring modifications in parenting, teaching, and counseling if such children are to develop optimally" (Tolan, p. 172, 1998).

● **Clinical Pearl:** There is no typical gifted child. Each is unique and displays special abilities in highly personal ways. Recognition of giftedness is contextual in nature and demands astute observation from medical and education professionals to analyze the extent and exact nature of the ability.

Are emotional problems the cause or result of giftedness? Until the 1920s, psychologists, physicians, and teachers believed that most highly gifted children were emotionally disturbed. Some early studies linked giftedness with madness (Lombroso, 1891). Seminal work by Hollingsworth (1926, 1931, 1942), however, showed that the social isolation felt by many highly gifted students did not result from emotional instability, but from the absence of a compatible peer group. The more extreme the child's gift, the more acute the discomfort he or she experienced in a traditional school setting. Hollingsworth found that between the ages of 4 and 9, highly gifted children were particularly vulnerable to this isolation. Twenty-five years of work at the Johns Hopkins Center for Talented Youth shows that when young, precocious students (as identified on off-level tests, such as the SAT-M and SAT-V) study advanced material with intellectual peers, their social development flourishes (Benbow & Stanley, 1997). Association with intellectual peers in play and study often eliminates social isolation and concomitant loneliness.

EPIDEMIOLOGY

In studies of extraordinary talent development, both Bloom (1985) and Csikszentmihalyi, Rathunde, and Whalen (1993) found that children best actualize their potential when parents and teachers recognize their specific gifts and when positive school experiences and challenging mentor relationships in their areas of talent are available during the teen years. Adults should not view gifted children as a homogeneous group. Giftedness varies by domain and degree of variation from the normal population. Generally, the estimate of intellectually gifted children ranges from 2% to 3% of the population, with some educators including as many as 15% of children (Marland, 1972). Different levels of intellectual ability are associated with attendant differences in cognitive and emotional functioning. Differences in high performance can be seen in Table 20-1.

The potential for unusual intellectual ability is present in all ethnic, racial, and cultural groups and in both sexes. One example of stereotypical thinking is the designation of Asian children as mathematically or musically gifted. It is true that early training in music is widespread for some Asian children. It also is true that the mathematics curricula in most Asian countries are much more demanding than those in U.S. schools (Peak, 1996; Stevenson & Stigler, 1998). For these reasons, a logical consequence is that more Asian children display accomplishment in music and math. But Asians also excel in other ways. Asians with writing talent often are neglected because of the prevalence of the math myth. Another similar display of stereotypical thinking is the belief that native Americans and other aboriginal peoples (including those of Australia, the Pacific Rim, and Central and South America) display giftedness in the specific areas of spatial and natural arts.

Providers should recall that manifestations of giftedness differ according to what opportunities a culture presents. Wayne Gretzky would not have achieved his level of hockey playing without someone introducing him to ice and skates. Mozart required the musical culture of the 18th century, early immersion in music, and constant practice on the piano to develop his composing genius. Booker T. Washington needed someone to teach him to read before he could go on to create a new intellectual institution at Tuskegee.

Socioeconomic factors influence the identification of intellectual giftedness. More middle class parents are aware of the significant precursors for potential giftedness in linguistics or numeracy than are poor families.

▲ **Clinical Warning:** Economically disadvantaged families with limited educational backgrounds may have so many survival issues that they have a special need for help to identify intellectual potential early. Some ethnic groups may require encouragement to elicit reports of advanced behaviors because of different cultural attitudes about giftedness.

Both extreme deficit and high ability can coexist. Providers should assess closely various apparently handicapping conditions for evidence of possible high ability. Certain challenges, such as dyslexia, learning disability, Asperger's syndrome, and extreme emotional impulsivity mask high potential for skill. Emotional immaturity may disguise extreme intellectual capacity in one or more domains.

Conversely, discriminating between giftedness and Asperger's syndrome is important (Neihart, 1998). Children with Asperger's need proper diagnosis so that they receive essential services. Developmental history is critical to distinguish between the gift and the deficit (Klin & Volkmar, 1995). For instance, misbehavior can stem from boredom in a routine classroom that offers only tasks the student has already mastered (Guevremont, 1990). Without knowledge of these factors, such behavior may lead to an improper diagnosis of attention deficit hyperactivity disorder (ADHD). Refer to Chapters 19 (Asperger's Syndrome and Pervasive Developmental Disorders: The Different Child) and 21 (School Problems) for a more in-depth examination of these topics.

HISTORY AND PHYSICAL EXAMINATION

Intellectual giftedness presents independent of any specific physical characteristics. Direct evidence of giftedness in the provider's office usually is limited to observation of a child's verbal skills, but other factors may inhibit even these. Parental reports have been determined to be quite accurate (Silverman, 1993). Taking a careful developmental history is very important. The provider should listen when parents report any of the following presenting characteristics about their child:

- Child has acute awareness of physical surroundings.
- Child has acute awareness of emotional surroundings.
- Child uses advanced vocabulary, sentence structure, or loves to play with words. For example, a grandmother reported overhearing her 4-year-old grandson telling his mother, "Oh Mom, I love you so. In fact it's not just that I love you, I adore you!"
- Child asks questions about abstract ideas like love, feelings, relationships, or justice. He or she insists that people be "fair" and complains when things are "unfair."
- Child gives complex answers to questions. For example, a 5-year-old child coughing at a birthday party responded to his hostess's concern with, "Don't worry, Mrs. Jones. I am not choking. It's just that the birthday cake was stuck for a moment on my epiglottis."
- Child explains ideas in complex and unusual ways.
- Child is very interested in clocks, calendars, maps, or structures.
- Child has a long attention span for activities of interest. For example, a 4-year old spent 8 hours a day for 1 week playing with a new Capsela construction set, only to discard it when he had explored all the adaptations.
- Child moves around a lot, is very active, sometimes seems hyperactive, craves stimulation and activity, and rarely is content to sit idly.
- Child reacts intensely to noise, light, smells, or touch but is able to function in a social setting.
- Child is extremely curious, asking why, how, and what if.
- Child becomes so involved that he or she is not aware of anything else ("lost in own world").
- Child has vivid imagination and may have trouble separating the real from the unreal.
- Child has an advanced sense of humor.
- Child prefers playing with older children or being with adults. (The provider must discern this preference from behavior often exhibited by the only child of urban professional parents. Such a youngster might not be so much "gifted" as privileged.)

Table 20-1. RANGE OF LEVELS OF INTELLECTUAL GIFTEDNESS (GROSS, 1993)

Level	IQ Range	Distribution (Stanford-Binet Revised Form IV)
Mild giftedness	115–129	1:6–1:44
Moderately	130–144	1:44–1:1000
Highly gifted	145–159	1:1000–1:10,000
Exceptionally	160–179	1:10,000–1:1 million
Profoundly	180+	fewer than 1:1 million

- Child becomes extremely frustrated when the body cannot do what the mind wants it to.

DIAGNOSTIC CRITERIA

Because of the lack of agreement on precise definitions, no uniform diagnostic categories of giftedness have been established. For this reason, prevalence rates usually are arbitrary. While disagreement exists about the limitations of IQ testing, individual IQ tests remain the best way to pinpoint some degrees of advanced ability. Although the use of standardized IQ tests has been criticized for cultural bias, Ehrlich (1986) concludes that often the test itself is not a source of bias. Rather, the person administering the test may not have ensured that the test used is appropriate to the child's age.

Language and cultural issues can make it challenging to identify the gifted child who is economically disadvantaged or ethnically or culturally different from other students (Ford, 1996). Providers should encourage parents and day care providers to maintain a portfolio of a child's strengths observed in the home, school, and community. Anecdotes, observations, and records of achievement can validate hunches about a child. These can assist teachers in adjusting the pace and depth of the learning experience, enabling schools to develop these exceptional talents in children.

While no definitive criteria guarantee a diagnosis of intellectual giftedness, the following can serve as useful guidelines for a multifaceted collection of data in determining level of giftedness:

- Formal IQ tests individually administered by a psychologist, such as the WISC or Stanford Binet, can give some indication of intellectual strengths for students older than 6 years. They are not very accurate when used with younger students (Silverman & Kearney, 1992).
- Informal inventories and checklists gathered from multiple sources also can be useful (DeLisle, 1984).
- Self-referrals are important.
- Student products and performance data from class, church, synagogue, or day care are informative.

DIAGNOSTIC STUDIES

Intellectual precocity may be detectable as early as 12 months, but most current diagnostic tools have limited predictive ability. While studies do pinpoint some behavioral markers, they are not definitive.

In comparing children of ages 12 and 24 months, the Bayley Scales of Infant Development had weak predictive value for high IQ. Performance on the Fagan Test of Infant Intelligence and later scores on the Stanford-Binet at 36 months have found moderate correlations (Fagan & Detterman, 1992). A significant factor seems to be performance on visual recognition memory tasks. While infant intelligence tests have limited value in predicting later high IQ scores, they do seem to predict some developmental abnormalities in at-risk children (Siegel, 1981).

Although studies are not yet definitive, some strong evidence indicates that early intervention factors may be significant in the development of intelligence. These factors include the following:

- The quality of maternal care; interactive behaviors between mother and infant
- Maternal talk
- Focused gaze

Tactile intervention and music may increase measured intelligence. These findings seem to be particularly true for infants in sparse home environments; however, more research is needed. Diagnostic studies of the intellectual development of children ages 3 to 6 years are complex, because their physical, social, and cognitive development is so rapid and variable. Some tests ordered by a child psychologist at this age include the following:

- The Peabody Picture Vocabulary Test (emphasizes language)
- The Columbia Mental Maturity Scale (measures abstract reasoning with minimal emphasis on language)
- The Draw-A-Person (gives information about perception, recall, basic knowledge using a minimum of expressive language, and culture dependence)

One of the best ways for a primary care provider or preschool teacher to learn about a child's abilities and interests is to interview the child. Some suggested interview questions include the following:

- What are some of the things that you do best?
- What are some of the things that you like to do?
- What are some of things that are hard for you?
- What don't you like in school? Why?
- What are some things that might make school (or preschool) better for you?
- What are some things you might like to be and do when you are grown?
- If you had three wishes that could come true, what would they be (Smutny, Walker, & Meckstroth, 1998)?

MANAGEMENT

Primary care providers can do several things to support the gifted child and family. Some efforts include the following:

- Take careful developmental histories. Look at many areas for evidence of accelerated language or motor, interpersonal, or academic development (Osborn, 1996).
- Expect complexity in the cognitive and emotional experiences of gifted children.
- Respect parental reports; they are usually accurate.
- Encourage parents to turn off the television, seek out enrichment opportunities, and read to their children daily.
- For in-depth assessment, refer parents to a psychologist with experience in gifted children.

What to Tell Parents

The following are common questions that cover many behavior problems, parenting issues, and educational decisions:

- **How long will the condition last (ie, will children grow out of their giftedness)?**
  Most likely, gifted children will continue to need more stimulation than their agemates. Without intervention

and appropriate stimulation in school, emotional and behavioral problems may develop. Unless parents ensure a proper educational match, a gifted child may develop poor self-esteem, patterns of underachievement, or poor study skills, subsequently appearing less gifted.

- **What is the best kind of school program for the gifted child?**

Because so many different school settings and local varieties of curricula are available, there is no easy answer. Parents can use as a template a principle defined by Robinson (1993) as optimal match: Is the child engaged in learning at a level appropriate to ability and skills? Is the child being stretched a little but not overwhelmed? All children learn best when they are challenged moderately. If schoolwork is too easy, they get bored, tune out, underachieve, and do not develop intellectual muscle. If the work is too hard, they also tune out.

- **What about grade skipping? Is that the only choice for a gifted child?**

Grade skipping may be a good choice if a child is socially mature and comfortable with older friends. This decision is best made by a child study team of teachers, school psychologist, and parents (Southern & Jones, 1991). Other learning options include cluster grouping in the classroom or placement in a multiage class, such as a Montessori group where students work at their own paces and in fluid cohorts. Advanced curricula in a special, full-day, intensive, self-contained classroom also can be advantageous. Mentors who share a child's interest, such as an architect or biologist, often can successfully motivate gifted students. Many configurations are possible. In all cases, the key starting point is to diagnose the extent of the specific gift so that a proper match can be made.

▲ **Clinical Warning:** Grade skipping may not be a solution because the child may overtake older classmates quickly. Therefore, an analysis of the curriculum over several years is important when parents request skipping. Grade skipping for an intellectually gifted but socially or physically immature child may lead to a totally new variety of problems.

- **What can the family provide to nurture the young child's intelligence?**

Parents should seek out as many different exploratory experiences as possible. These can include visits to museums and parks, walks in city neighborhoods, access to open space for running around or moving to music, listening to classical music, and reading stories, nursery rhymes, and poetry. Manipulative toys that allow the imagination to flourish (eg, wooden blocks, tinker toys, Lego or Capsela) are helpful. Children should have easy access to crayons, colored pencils, newsprint, old clothes for dress up, puppets, and simple tools (eg, hammers, screwdrivers, nuts, and bolts). Also important is an area for quiet and calm reflection. Such a place should have clean pillows for snuggling, picture books, and some prints or photos (Smutny, Veenker, & Veenker, 1989).

- **Can parents overstimulate the child? What about the "hurried child" syndrome?**

Providers should reassure those who fear that acknowledging children's giftedness will place too much pressure on them that most gifted children have an insatiable desire to learn. Winner (1996) has called this phenomenon a "rage to learn." To ignore the signifi-

cance of this drive could lead to a child being punished for restlessness, poor attention to the teacher, sloppy work, or diverting creative urges into destructive mischief.

Without space and time for quiet reflection, overstimulation could become a problem. Elkind (1981) has recommended, however, that children of very high intelligence may have a greater need for information and movement than normal.

▲ **Clinical Warning:** Playful exploration is preferable until a child demands formal lessons. Parents should wait for signals from the child before presenting any direct academic instruction at home.

- **Is there any connection between ADHD and the high energy level of gifted children?**

The high intensity and curiosity of gifted children may present as some of the same behaviors exhibited by children with ADHD. These conditions are not incompatible. Diagnosis is difficult in the primary care provider's office because of the unnatural setting. Office visits also may be tinged with anxiety. To determine the presence of ADHD, providers should collect detailed data from parents and teachers. School psychologists often are helpful. For instance, gifted children may lack the persistence for tasks that seem irrelevant to them. They may question rules and authority. Conversely, children with ADHD need a low-stimulus environment for concentration and have trouble processing directions (Brody & Mills, 1997; Vail, 1987). Refer to Chapter 21 (School Problems) for more information on ADHD.

- **What kind of education intervention should parents request from their child's school?**

Parents should ask the school to conduct an in-depth assessment of their child's strengths in specific areas. Proper diagnosis of actual skills can help a family decide how best to accommodate the gift. Out-of-level testing may be necessary for a school to learn the true "ceiling" of a child's learning.

● **Clinical Pearl:** Because treating the needs of gifted children is not federally mandated, schools are not required to make any curricular adjustments. Consequently, nurturing must be initiated by parents and sustained by informed child advocates, such as school nurses, guidance counselors, and primary care providers. A provider's carefully written recommendation can serve as a powerful impetus to service provision by the school, especially in adjusting a child's curriculum to achieve a more optimal match.

Once a diagnosis of giftedness is made, a school may suggest a variety of accommodations, ranging from in-class enrichment to grade acceleration. Many schools have enrichment consultant specialists who are helpful in guiding the decision of the child study team. Unfortunately, such specialists are too rarely available to poorer or rural schools.

- **How should a primary care provider follow up?**

Annual well child visits can be very important to monitoring. Primary care providers should be alert for symptoms of depression or underachievement. They should encourage parents to call the child's school if they notice negative changes in their child's behavior. Parents can gain more information through reading lists and joining parent groups. Some problem areas to watch out for include the following:

- Depression in adolescent girls. To fit in with their peers, young girls may try to hide their capacities and purposely underachieve (Pipher, 1994). Depression and poor self-esteem may result. Refer to Chapter 28 (Depression) for more information.
- Socioeconomic disadvantage or non-Caucasian status. Gifted students who are economically or socially disadvantaged or who are non-Caucasian are also vulnerable to pressures not to "sell out" to the dominant culture. If children are economically disadvantaged, their access to resources for talent development can be limited significantly. Emotional support from the primary care provider for such children and their families can be very important. The clinician should learn what resources and service scholarship opportunities are available locally, referring the family to affordable options that can support the child's giftedness.
- ADHD. Families or schools may confuse a child's low attention span of ADHD with boredom (Brody, 1997). The primary care provider should write up the symptoms observed, referring parents to the school or school district specialist in gifted child education. Refer to Chapter 21 (School Problems) for further discussion of this topic.

Why Bother?

Primary care providers usually do not consider giftedness to be a disorder, but manifestations of giftedness may evoke negative reactions from teachers, school administrators, and the child's own peers and their parents. Such reactions may range from peers feeling uneasy around the child to dread in school administrators who view giftedness as causing disorder in their institutions. Giftedness can present significant challenges to all involved because it means that these children, who prefer to "march to their own drummers," really have a "rage to learn" (Winner, 1996). They are precocious. They may be out of step with regular school curricula designed to fit the norm.

● **Clinical Pearl:** Giftedness means that children will challenge the system. Many schools do not heed the observations of parents alone. Armed with objective, corroborating observations from primary care providers, parents will have a better chance of being persuasive when requesting an appropriate curriculum match.

Studies have shown that unrecognized intellectual strength may lead to many problems, even emotional disorders that include depression, behavior problems, and inappropriate aggressiveness. Uninformed people, including professional educators, often assume that the development of "gifted" children will take care of itself—that somehow talent usually finds a way. This is not true. In fact, the most recent national study concluded that the United States is wasting the precious assets gifted children have to offer (Office of Education Research and Improvement, 1993).

Primary care providers see children regularly over time. They are in the unique position of observing developmental milestones. In taking patient histories and carefully listening to parents, providers can detect important patterns for potential. A proactive stance in educating parents about their important role in this talent development is critical, especially for those who are not confident members of the dominant, middle class culture. Bloom (1981) warned not to underestimate the role of parents. The provider's observations and carefully written recommendations to the school are very powerful supports for parental requests for

an appropriate "optimal learning match" for their gifted child (Hoelscher, 1998; Robinson & Olszewski-Kubilius, 1996).

Boredom and repeated experiences with assignments well below their level of mastery can erode children's passion. They may even turn to socially and personally destructive channels. Early intervention supported by advice from primary care providers can prevent such undesirable outcomes.

COMMUNITY RESOURCES

Webb, J. T., Meckstroth, E. A., & Tolan, S. S. (1994). *Guiding the gifted.* Scottsdale, AZ: Gifted Psychology Press.
Winebrenner, S. (1992). *Teaching gifted kids in the regular classroom.* Minneapolis: Free Spirit Publishing.
Understanding our gifted. Boulder, CO: Open Space Communications. (800) 494-6178. *Gifted Child Today.* Waco, TX. (800) 998-2208; *www.prufrock.com.*
Free Spirit Press (publisher of parent-friendly materials). (800) 735-7323; *www.freespirit.com.*

Many websites are available as well. Hoagies Gifted Education Page has many annotated links to related programs and resources for gifted education at *http://www.ocsc.com/hoagies/gift.htm.* The Center for Talented Youth in the Institute for the Academic Advancement of Youth at the Johns Hopkins University has one of the most respected research centers for gifted children. They offer reading lists, diagnostic help, and special academic experiences at *www.jhu.edu/gifted.* The National Association for Gifted Children (*www.nagc.org*) has a wealth of information for each state's regulations. Membership includes excellent journals for parents and teachers. The National Research Center on the Gifted and Talented (*www.gifted.uconn.edu*) is a consortium of Universities (University of Connecticut, Yale, University of Virginia, Stanford University) supported by a grant from the U.S. Office of Education Research and Instruction. They publish a newsletter and sponsor research that parents can translate into practical use.

REFERENCES

Benbow, C. P., & Stanley, J. C. (1997). Inequity in equity: How "equity" can lead to inequity for high potential students. *Psychology, Public Policy, and Law, 2*(2), 249–292.
Bloom, B. S. (1981). *All our children learning: A primer for parents, teachers, and other educators.* New York: McGraw-Hill.
Bloom, B. S. (Ed.) (1985). *Developing talent in young people.* New York: Ballantine.
Brody, L. E., & Mills, C. J. (1997). Gifted children with learning disabilities: A review of the issues. *Journal of Learning Disabilities, 30,* 282–297.
Csikszentmihalyi, M., Rathunde, K., & Whalen, S. (1993). *Talented teenagers.* New York: Cambridge University Press.
Delisle, J. R. (1984). *Gifted children speak out.* New York: Walker.
Ehrlich, V., (1986). *Gifted children: A guide to parents and teachers.* Englewood Cliffs, NJ: Prentice-Hall.
Elkind, D. (1981). *The hurried child: Growing up too fast too soon.* Reading, MA: Addison-Wesley.
Fagan, J. F., & Detterman, D. K. (1992). The Fagan test of infant intelligence: A technical summary. *Journal of Applied Developmental Psychology, 13,* 173–193.
Ford, D. Y. (1996). *Reversing underachievement among gifted black students: Promising practices and programs.* New York: Teachers College Press.
Gardner, H. (1993). *Multiple intelligences: The theory in practice.* New York: Basic Books.
Gross, M. U. M. (1993). *Exceptionally gifted children.* New York: Routledge.

Guevremont, D. (1990). Social skills and peer relationship training. In R. Barkley (Ed.), *Attention deficit hyperactivity disorder: A handbook for diagnosis and treatment.* New York: The Guilford Press.

Hoelscher, P. D. (1998). The role of the pediatrician. In J. F. Smutny (Ed.), *The young gifted child* (pp. 347–352). New York: Hampton Press.

Hollingsworth, L. (1926). *Gifted children: Their nature and nurture.* New York: Macmillan.

Hollingworth, L. (1931). The child of very superior intelligence as a special problem in social adjustment. *Mental Hygiene, 15*(1), 3–16.

Hollingworth, L. (1942). *Children above 180 IQ.* Yonkers, NY: World Book.

Klin, A., & Volkmar, F. R. (1995). *Guidelines for parents: Assessment, diagnosis and intervention of Asperger syndrome.* Pittsburgh: Learning Disabilities Association of America.

Lombroso, C. (1891). *The man of genius.* London: Walter Scott.

Marland, S. Jr. (1972). *Education of the gifted and talented.* Report to the Congress of the United States by the Commissioner of Education. Washington, DC: US Government Printing Office.

Neihart, M. (1998). *Gifted children with Asperger's syndrome.* Unpublished Paper presented at the Annual Convention of the National Association of Gifted Children. 11/14/98. Louisville, KY.

Office of Education Research and Improvement. (1993). *National excellence: A case for developing America's talent.* Washington, DC: U.S. Government Printing Office.

Osborn, J. (1996). Gifted children. *Youth mental health update.* NY: Division of Child and Adolescent Psychiatry, Schneider Children's Hospital and Hillside Hospital of Long Island Jewish Medical Center, the Long Island Campus for the Albert Einstein College of Medicine May-June, 1–4.

Peak, L. (1996). *Third International Math and Science Study: Pursuing excellence.* Washington, DC: US Dept of Education, National Center for Education Statistics.

Pipher, M. (1994). *Reviving Ophelia.* New York: Ballantine.

Robinson, N. M. (1993). Identifying and nurturing gifted very young children. In K. A. Heller, F. J. Monks, & A. H. Passow (Eds.), *International handbook of research and development of giftedness and talent* (pp. 507–524). Oxford, UK: Pergamon.

Robinson, N. M., & Olszewski-Kubilius, P. M. (1996). Gifted and talented children: Issues for Pediatricians. *Pediatrics in Review, 17*(12), 427–434.

Siegel, L. (1981). Infant tests as predictors of cognitive and language development at two years. *Child development, 52,* 545–557.

Silverman, L. K., & Kearney, K. (1992). The case for the Stanford-Binet L-M as a supplemental test. *Roeper Review, 15,* 34–37.

Silverman, L. K. (1993). *Counseling the gifted and talented.* Denver: Love.

Smutny, J. F., Veenker, K., & Veenker, S. (1989). *Your gifted child: How to recognize and develop the special talents in your special child from birth to age seven.* New York: Ballantine Books.

Smutny, J. F., Walker, S. Y., & Meckstroth, B. A. (1998). *Teaching young gifted children in the regular classroom.* Minneapolis, MN: Free Spirit Publishing.

Southern, W. T., & Jones, E. D. (Eds.) (1991). *The academic acceleration of gifted children.* New York: Teachers College Press.

Stevenson, H. W., & Stigler, J. W. (1998). *The learning gap: Why our schools are failing and what we can learn from Japanese and Chinese education.* New York: Summit Books.

Terman, L. M. (1905). A study in precocity and prematuration. *American Journal of Psychology, 16*(2), 139–144.

Tolan, S. S. (1998). Beginning brilliance. In J. F. Smutny (Ed.), *The young gifted child: Potential and promise, an anthology* (pp. 165–180). Cresskill, NJ: Hampton Press.

Vail, P. (1987). *Smart kids with school problems.* New York: E. P. Dutton.

Winner, E. (1996). *Gifted children.* New York: Basic Books.

School Problems

• HERSCHEL R. LESSIN, MD

INTRODUCTION

It is an all too common scenario: The primary care provider is conducting an annual health maintenance examination on a school-age child. As the clinician is about to leave the examining room, the parent says, "Oh, by the way, my child is having trouble in school. The teacher thinks he might be hyper. I don't know what to do." School problem is a very broad term than can include almost any reason that a child does poorly in school. Whether in learning, behavior, or both, school problems are among the most common complaints that parents bring to the provider, who often is the first professional they contact for help. School problems can be broadly divided into three categories:

• Cognitive (learning disability, central auditory processing defect, attention deficit hyperactivity disorder [ADHD])
• Psychological (school avoidance, separation anxiety, shyness)
• Physical

Considerable overlap exists within these categories and with other mental health disorders. This chapter provides a brief overview of school problems, with special emphasis on ADHD. Other problems, such as anxiety, depression, oppositional and conduct disorders, and major psychiatric problems (such as bipolar disorder and psychosis), are discussed as comorbidities under the diagnosis section of ADHD.

● **Clinical Pearl:** The provider's role is to identify that a problem exists, make a diagnosis if possible, use appropriate pharmacologic therapy, make the proper referral for further care with mental health or educational professionals, and work closely with the family and school to provide support and counseling as needed.

COGNITIVE PROBLEMS

Several cognitive problems manifest as school problems, the most dominant of which is ADHD. The following discussion provides a brief synopsis of learning disability and central auditory processing defect, with a more detailed examination of ADHD. More significant mental health diagnoses usually require a referral to an experienced mental health professional. These are discussed under the section on diagnosis of ADHD.

Learning Disability

Learning disability, a general term that encompasses many disorders of varying severity, is the most common cognitive disorder, occurring in 5% to 17.5% of children (Shaywitz,

1998). The Diagnostic and Statistical Manual-IV (DSM-IV) defines learning disability as individual achievement that is substantially below that expected for age, schooling, and level of intelligence. It represents a difference in how the brain processes information that it receives, not in the actual reception of the information (eg, visual or auditory impairment). It only is noted to be a problem when the disability causes functional impairment to the patient. Dyslexia, the most commonly used term, has no solid definition, although it usually refers to a problem with reading.

Learning disability should be suspected if a child of average or better intelligence has difficulty learning basic educational skills (eg, math or reading), and the skills in certain areas fall below performance in other areas. Learning disability is both familial and heritable (Shaywitz, 1998); thus, a thorough family history is extremely important for the child who presents with signs of learning disability. If the history suggests a learning disability, the provider must refer the patient to a child psychologist or other pediatric mental health professional who is able to perform psychoeducational testing. Learning disability is diagnosed when a discrepancy is found in performance or achievement and intelligence, as measured by standardized testing. Once diagnosed, specific educational remediation must be initiated based on the child's individual needs.

▲ **Clinical Warning:** Learning disability must be differentiated from true diminished mental capacity. True diminished mental capacity can be due to neurologic damage, genetic disorders and syndromes, trauma, central nervous system infection, and nonspecific causes of mental retardation. A child with true diminished mental capacity is limited in learning in any realm, as opposed to a child with learning disability, who has specific problem areas. Depending on the severity of the problem, the child with learning disability requires a specific educational program (mainstreaming or separate special education classes). A whole array of specific learning disabilities can be found in DSM-IV (1994).

Central Auditory Processing Defect

Although an exact figure is unavailable, a defect in central auditory processing is a cognitive problem seen fairly often in pediatric practice. The child with a disorder of central auditory processing has normal hearing but is unable to process the information heard and so does not understand it. Clinically, the youngster is suspected to have hearing loss, but repeated hearing tests are normal. A defect in central auditory processing thus sometimes is confused with ADHD.

● **Clinical Pearl:** If a child's history suggests that attention problems may be linked to failure to understand directions, the provider should refer the patient for audiologic evaluation. Specific central auditory processing tests by an audiologist can diagnose a defect in central auditory processing. Refer to Chapter 53 for a more in-depth discussion.

Attention Deficit Hyperactivity Disorder

The DSM-IV (1994) defines ADHD as only one of a spectrum of attention deficit disorders. The syndrome has been known by many names over the years, including minimal brain damage, minimal brain dysfunction, hyperkinesis, attention deficit disorder, and ADHD. The various revisions of DSM have reflected these name changes by emphasizing different parts of the symptom complex in its classification and description, with DSM-IV (1994) dividing ADHD into various subtypes.

Clinicians often find themselves inundated with requests from schools and parents to evaluate large numbers of children for this problem. Depending on their level of interest and commitment, providers can effectively evaluate children with uncomplicated ADHD, but it takes substantial time and effort to do so properly. The use of pharmacologic therapy, particularly stimulant medications, has been the subject of longstanding and ongoing controversy in the media. The fact that medications used for ADHD are controlled substances in the amphetamine group also has troubled many providers and parents alike. There remains the undercurrent of whether any child who acts up in class should be medicated. Is this therapy prescribed for the patient's benefit or for the teacher and parents? What has become clear over the past few years is that ADHD is a real disorder with a real physiologic defect and a real and effective treatment.

Pathology

Although the symptoms of ADHD have been recognized for more than 50 years, no theory has been universally accepted to explain the pathophysiology of the underlying defects. Rapid advances in neurobiology and noninvasive imaging, however, have lent support to the theory that ADHD is due to disregulation of neurotransmitters in the frontal lobes of the brain. Structural neuroimaging of the brain with magnetic resonance imaging (MRI) has shown abnormalities in the caudate nucleus and corpus callosum (Castellanos et al., 1996; Semrud-Clikeman et al., 1994). Functional brain imaging with MRI and positron emission tomography (PET) scanning has demonstrated diminished frontal lobe activity (Bush et al., 1998; Zametkin et al., 1990). All these studies, however, suffer from some methodologic flaws and other limitations.

While it is clear that ADHD is highly heritable, the actual genetic defect has yet to be determined. Molecular genetics studies suggest defects in the dopamine receptor and the dopamine transporter genes, giving support to the theory that defects in either gene result in diminished dopamine entry in frontal lobe synapses (LaHoste et al., 1996). This could explain why stimulants, which increase dopamine at the synapse, are helpful in children with ADHD. However, how do stimulants, such as amphetamines, paradoxically result in decreased motor activity? Barkley (1997) proposes that ADHD is a motor disinhibition syndrome. The frontal lobes are responsible for the regulation of motor activity. The neurons responsible for inhibiting such activity are underactive, due to a defect in dopamine transport. According to Barkley, by increasing available dopamine, stimulants allow the normal amount of inhibition to take place, thereby accounting for their paradoxical effects. The frontal lobes also are responsible for a wide range of high-level executive reasoning functions that are compromised in patients with ADHD. For a full discussion of this theory, the reader is

referred to Barkley's publications and books, several of which are annotated at the end of this chapter.

Other factors that may be implicated in the pathogenesis of ADHD include a history of the following:

- Birth trauma
- Head trauma
- Prenatal teratogenic exposure, including maternal smoking (Millberger, Biederman, Faraone, Chen, & Jones, 1996) and drugs association with other syndromes, such as Gilles de la Tourette's

● **Clinical Pearl:** Despite numerous studies clearly demonstrating the contrary, the idea that diet causes ADHD persists in the public mind. Diets such as that proposed by Feingold (1975) have been shown to have no significant beneficial effects (National Advisory Committee on Hyperkinesis and Food Additives, 1980). Studies conducted in intervening years have not altered this fact. Sugar ingestion is not correlated with hyperactivity (Woolraich, Wilson, & White, 1995).

Epidemiology

The prevalence of ADHD has been reported as between 2% and 9% of all school-age children, making it one of the most common disorders of childhood (Bauermeister, Canino, & Bird, 1994). The DSM-IV (1994) reports ADHD prevalence as being 3% to 5%. The male-to-female ratio is between 3:1 and 8:1. ADHD occurs across all socioeconomic strata. It clearly runs in families (Faraone & Biederman, 1994), with 80% of its variance explainable by family history (Barkley, 1998). Most children with ADHD have some other comorbidity, including one or more of the following:

- Oppositional defiant disorder (ODD) (65%)
- Learning disability (30%–40%)
- Depression (30%)
- Anxiety disorder (10%–20%)
- Conduct disorder (20%)
- Tic disorders (10%) (Biederman, Newcorn, & Sprich, 1991)

History and Physical Examination

A good history must include a general discussion of the following:

- Behavior, including discerning whether there are problems at home or school, or discipline problems, including issues with aggression and anger
- Performance in varied areas, including school work, homework, and household tasks, as well as organizational skills, staying with tasks, and overall learning difficulties
- Social skills and behavior, including interaction with parents, teachers, and peers
- Emotional responses to stressful situations, as well as frustration tolerance

The provider should ask a series of specific questions that are targeted to the diagnostic criteria discussed in the next section. In addition, the clinician must ask questions that can lead to diagnosis of the many comorbidities discussed previously, particularly ODD and depression. The age of onset of all symptoms and the realm in which they occur should be noted. The reader is referred to Chapters 19 and 28 for further discussion of relevant comorbid conditions. A workbook with lists of questions based on DSM-IV (1994) criteria is annotated at the end of this chapter. This resource can serve as a template for the interview (Barkley & Murphy, 1998). The following suggestions also can be used to frame this interview:

- The clinician should obtain a complete past medical history, with emphasis on possible central nervous system trauma.
- The clinician also must obtain a thorough developmental history, with particular emphasis on birth history, temperament, and developmental milestones.
- If any outside psychoeducational testing has been performed, the provider should review it.
- Given the high incidence of heritability, the provider should elicit a careful family history, with emphasis on the parents' own home and school histories.
- The clinician also may explore symptoms of adult ADHD and, finally, discuss whether there is a family history of mental health problems, especially depression, bipolar disorder, anxiety disorder, and psychosis. This latter information is critical to making an informed determination.

In addition, the provider should ask whether there is a history of primary nocturnal enuresis (PNE). Special needs children have higher rates of PNE. This is especially true for youngsters diagnosed with ADHD. PNE in such children may be partly related to a "hyperactive" bladder or to behavioral problems encountered in toilet training. These problems may have emerged because of attentional impediments to efficient learning. Pervasive and chronic hyperactivity of the parasympathetic nervous system also may play a role in uninhibited bladder contractions (Yakinci, Mungen, Durmaz, Balbay, & Karabiber, 1997). Refer to Chapter 63 for more information about the diagnosis and management of PNE.

As with any patient contact, a thorough physical must be performed with special attention to the neurologic examination. The examination should focus on finding any signs of other neurologic disorder, metabolic problem (eg, hyperthyroidism), genetic disorder (eg, fragile X syndrome), hearing or visual impairment, or other developmental syndrome (eg, autism or pervasive developmental disorder). Refer to Chapters 19, 32, 46, 52, 53, and 60 for further information.

Diagnostic Criteria

Diagnosis of ADHD is primarily based on history. Symptoms often present around the age of 3 years, but diagnosis usually is delayed until around age 7 years. With the recent publicity about ADHD, diagnosis is suspected much earlier than in the past. The presentation in very young children is not the same as in older children. ADHD in very young patients is characterized by temperamental problems, such as high activity level, low adaptability, high approach to novel stimuli, emotional intensity, negative persistence, and fearfulness with anxiety.

The DSM-IV (1994) diagnostic criteria for ADHD are listed in Table 21-1, demonstrating that the history must be taken to elicit the appropriate answers to all the criteria outlined. Key points in meeting the DSM-IV criteria include the following:

- Symptoms have persisted for more than 6 months.
- Symptoms are maladaptive (ie, the child is impaired).
- Symptoms are inappropriate for the child's developmental level.
- Symptoms must have had their onset before age 7 years.

- The impairment must be noted in at least two settings (eg, home and school).
- Another disorder cannot explain symptoms.

The diagnosis is then made as one of three diagnoses:

- ADHD: Primarily inattentive type
- ADHD: Primarily hyperactive-impulsive type
- ADHD: Combined type

● **Clinical Pearl:** Most children seen in a primary care setting will present with the combined type of ADHD. Some controversy exists as to whether the primarily inattentive type is actually a subtype of ADHD or a completely different illness. Resolution of this issue is yet to be determined.

Although the diagnostic criteria are well described, a diagnosis of ADHD is not an all-or-none phenomenon. It is not like a diagnosis of type 1 diabetes, in which the patient is either insulinopenic or not. ADHD is more like a trait, such as intelligence or height (Barkley, 1998). It is distributed along a normal curve. Those with ADHD symptoms to the far right of the curve (greater than 1 standard deviation) probably show some symptoms and may be impaired. The further the child's symptoms are on this curve, the more likely the child is to be impaired and to have an actual diagnosis of ADHD.

● **Clinical Pearl:** In evaluating diagnostic criteria, the provider also must consider the patient's intelligence and ability to cope. Those with superior intelligence will take longer to come to diagnosis, especially if the hyperactive component is not prominent, because they are better equipped to develop their own compensatory mechanisms. Even with superior intelligence and coping skills, however, severely affected children will eventually become impaired, even if it is not noted until high school or college.

Diagnostic Studies

No true studies can help the provider in making the diagnosis of ADHD; it is a clinical judgment based on history. A number of standardized questionnaires, however, can be useful in not only helping reach a diagnosis, but also in monitoring the patient's progress and response to therapy. These can provide some objective evidence of change in symptoms over time and with treatment.

The most common tools used in a primary care setting are the Revised Connors Scales and the ACTERS scales. They are short, easy to score, and convenient to use. They are available for parents and teachers and, in the case of the Connors scale, adolescent self-evaluation. Somewhat more complex instruments, such as the Child Behavior Checklist (CBCL) and the Behavioral Assessment Scales for Children (BASC), are also available but are more difficult to interpret. They usually are used by those with more psychological training or interest, such as child or behavioral psychologists. Sources for obtaining these scales are provided at the end of this chapter.

▲ **Clinical Warning:** The clinician should note that the diagnosis of ADHD cannot be made simply by using standardized questionnaires. They are helpful adjuncts but not substitutes for a complete evaluation.

Management

Comprehensive treatment of ADHD encompasses much more than handing a parent a prescription for stimulant

Table 21–1.   DSM-IV CRITERIA FOR ADHD

A. Either (1) or (2):

  (1) six (or more) of the following symptoms of **inattention** have persisted for at least 6 months to a degree that is maladaptive and inconsistent with developmental level:

  Inattention

    (a) often fails to give attention to details or makes careless mistakes in schoolwork, work, or other activities

    (b) often has difficulty sustaining attention in tasks or play activities

    (c) often does not seem to listen when spoken to directly

    (d) often does not follow through on instructions and fails to finish schoolwork, chores, or duties in the workplace (not due to oppositional behavior or failure to understand instructions)

    (e) often has difficulty organizing tasks and activities

    (f) often avoids, dislikes, or is reluctant to engage in tasks that require sustained mental effort (such as school work or homework)

    (g) often loses things necessary for tasks or activities (eg, toys, school assignments, pencils, books, or tools)

    (h) is often easily distracted by extraneous stimuli

    (i) is often forgetful in daily activities

  (2) six (or more) of the following symptoms of **hyperactivity-impulsivity** have persisted for at least 6 months to a degree that is maladaptive and inconsistent with developmental level:

  Hyperactivity

    (a) often fidgets with hands or feet or squirms in seat

    (b) often leaves seat in classroom or in other situations in which remaining seated is expected

    (c) often runs about or climbs excessively in situations in which it is inappropriate (in adolescents or adults, may be limited to subjective feelings of restlessness)

    (d) often has difficulty playing or engaging in leisure activities quietly

    (e) is often "on the go" or often acts as if "driven by a motor"

    (f) often talks excessively

  Impulsivity

    (g) often blurts out answers before the questions have been completed

    (h) often has difficulty awaiting turn

    (i) often interrupts or intrudes on others (eg, butts into conversations or games)

B. Some hyperactive–impulsive or inattentive symptoms that caused impairment were present before age 7 years.

C. Some impairment from the symptoms is present in two or more settings (eg, at school [or work] and at home).

D. There must be clear evidence of clinically significant impairment in social, academic, or occupational functioning.

E. The symptoms do not occur exclusively during the course of a Pervasive Developmental Disorder, Schizophrenia, or other Psychotic Disorder, and are not better accounted for by another mental disorder (eg, Mood Disorder, Anxiety Disorder, Dissociative Disorder, or a Personality Disorder).

Code based on type:

314.01 Attention-Deficit/Hyperactivity Disorder, Combined Type: if both Criteria A1 and A2 are met for the past 6 months.

314.00 Attention-Deficit/Hyperactivity Disorder, Predominantly Inattentive Type: if Criterion A1 is met but Criterion A2 is not met for the past 6 months

314.01 Attention-Deficit/Hyperactivity Disorder, Predominantly Hyperactive-Impulsive Type: if Criterion A2 is met but Criterion A1 is not met for the past 6 months.

Coding note: For individuals (especially adolescents and adults) who currently have symptoms that no longer meet full criteria, "In Partial Remission" should be specified.

Note. From American Psychiatric Association (1994). Copyright 1994 by American Psychiatric Association. Reprinted by permission.

medications. While in many cases stimulant and other pharmacologic interventions are helpful and needed, they are not enough. A comprehensive treatment plan must include a program to help the following:

- The family deal with the child's behavior and any physical, mental, and other challenges
- The school deal with the child's behavior and any physical, mental, and other challenges
- Pharmacotherapy tailored to the child's individual needs and comorbidities

The first order of business is to be sure that all comorbidities have been properly identified. If the clinician is not con-

fident in this ability, he or she should make a referral for diagnostic evaluation to a mental health professional who is skilled in testing for ADHD.

▲ **Clinical Warnings:**

- Unless comorbidities are treated properly first, treatment of ADHD will fail. For example, children with ODD or conduct disorder require some sort of family systems intervention. This work should be referred to an experienced therapist.
- Children with depression, bipolar disorder, anxiety disorders, or psychosis may need complex pharmacologic intervention with or without therapy. This usually is

beyond the scope of a provider and should be referred to a child psychiatrist. Children with tic disorders, seizures, or other neurologic illness also may have complex treatment needs. Consultation should be sought with a pediatric neurologist or at least a general neurologist with experience in this area.

Pharmacotherapy

Three classes of drugs are used in the treatment of ADHD:

- Stimulants, including methylphenidate, dextroamphetamine, mixed salts of dextroamphetamine (Adderall), and pemoline (Cylert)
- Antidepressants, including tricyclics (desipramine and nortriptyline), and bupropion
- Antihypertensives, including clonidine and guanfacine.

Of these, the stimulant class is the most studied and so most likely to be used by clinicians.

● **Clinical Pearl:** Stimulants are the first line of drug therapy for ADHD. The general consensus is that the stimulants work by different actions at the synapse so that if one type does not work and the diagnosis is sure, then another stimulant can be tried.

STIMULANTS

Stimulant drugs have been used for more than 70 years and have been examined in several hundred controlled studies. Overall, about 70% of children with ADHD have a positive response to stimulant pharmacotherapy. Children with hyperactive symptoms have a 90% response rate, while only 50% of primarily inattentive children respond positively. Overall, the safety record of stimulants is excellent. There is a clear linear dose response to increasing dosages of stimulant medications.

● **Clinical Pearl:** If mild improvement occurs, it is reasonable to push the stimulant dose a bit higher to get maximal benefit.

All stimulants have similar side effects, which are usually minor, with the exception of the hepatotoxicity associated with pemoline (see below). The most common side effects are anorexia, insomnia, headache, dizziness, rebound as doses wear off, and mood disturbance (either from peak dose or from rebound). Most side effects are easily managed by changing the timing of medication, overlapping doses, giving medication with meals, or changing the stimulant used. Some concern has arisen over impairment of linear growth, but this has not been fully documented and may not be significant. Risk of substance abuse always is mentioned when discussing stimulants. Certainly all of these drugs have abuse potential.

▲ Clinical Warnings:

- Patients and their parents should be strongly warned not to share their medications with others. Studies have shown that medicating children with ADHD actually lowers their own risk of developing substance abuse disorders (Biederman, Wilens, Mick, Faraone, & Spencer, 1999).
- Stimulant medications can unmask an underlying tic disorder, particularly Gilles de la Tourette's syndrome. While tics are not an absolute contraindication to stimulants, serious consideration must be given to alternative choices of medications for treating ADHD, including antidepressants and antihypertensives.

The choice of which stimulant to prescribe is up to the clinician. Each drug has certain advantages and problems. The choice of short- or long-acting forms also depends on the clinical situation. The following discussion and Table 21-2 provide a framework for drug choice:

- *Methylphenidate:* Onset of action is 20 to 30 minutes, with a duration of 3 to 4 hours. It should be dosed at least b.i.d. Every 4 hours is an acceptable dosing regimen. It is strongly recommended that at least t.i.d. dosing be used during the school year to cover homework and late afternoon hours. The dose range is 0.3 to 2.0 mg/kg/d (0.3–10.6 mg/kg/dose). Dosing should start at 2.5 to 5 mg/dose and can be increased every 1 to 2 days until an acceptable response is reached. Methylphenidate does not accumulate, and results can be quickly assessed without long periods of observa-

Table 21–2. MEDICATIONS FOR ADHD

Name	Dosage Range	Frequency	Chewable	Onset	Duration	Side Effects
Methylphenidate	0.3–2.0 mg/kg/d 0.3–0.6 mg/kg/dose	q4h b.i.d. t.i.d. (preferred)	Yes	20–30 min	3–4 h	Anorexia, insomnia, headache, dizzyness, tics, rebound effect, mood disturbance (peak/trough), growth disturbance
D-amphetamine	0.1–1.0 mg/kg/d 0.1–0.3 mg/kg/dose	q4h b.i.d. t.i.d. (preferred)	Yes	30 min	3–4 h	Same as methylphenidate
D-amphetamine spansules	0.1–1.0 mg/kg/d 0.1–0.5 mg/kg/dose	q6h b.i.d.	No	1 h	6 h	Same as methylphenidate (less mood disturbance and rebound)
Dextroamphetamine (mixed salt) (Adderall)	0.1–1.0 mg/kg/d 0.1–0.5 mg/kg/dose	q6–8h b.i.d	Yes	1 h	6–8 h	Same as methylphenidate (less mood disturbance and rebound)
Pemoline	0.5–3.0 mg/kg/d	q.d.	Yes	gradual over days	24 h	Same as methylphenidate Hepatoxicity

tion. The maximum single dose is 40 mg. Dosing forms are 5-, 10-, and 20-mg tablets, which can be chewed but are meant to be swallowed. Methylphenidate also comes in a sustained-release preparation (SR formulation). Standard sustained release tablet is 20 mg, although a 10 mg preparation has recently been released. These tablets cannot be cut in half. The SR is supposed to have an onset of action of 1 hour and a duration of 6 hours, but many clinicians report that its absorption is irregular, not lasting much longer than the short-acting preparation. It is acceptable to combine both short and SR preparations to titrate to an effective dose.

● **Clinical Pearls:**

- One SR tablet of 20 mg is equivalent to 10 mg of the short-acting form. Therefore, when switching from regular to SR formulations, the single dose mg dosage should be doubled.
- The SR formulation cannot be chewed; it must be swallowed. Only thus will its prolonged length of action be preserved.

Dextroamphetamine: It comes in both long- and short-acting forms. Short-acting tablets have an onset of about 30 minutes and last 3 to 4 hours. Dosing is b.i.d. or t.i.d., as with methylphenidate. Total daily dose range is 0.1 to 1.0 mg/kg/d. Dextroamphetamine is available only in 5-mg strength and can be chewed or swallowed. Dextroamphetamine is about twice as potent as methylphenidate, with 10 mg of dextroamphetamine equivalent to 20 mg of methylphenidate. Long-acting spansules in 5-, 10-, and 15-mg strengths are available. Onset is about 1 hour, and duration is about 6 hours. Spansules should be dosed b.i.d. As with methylphenidate, it should be started with a low dose and increased every few days until effects are noted.

Mixed salts of dextroamphetamine (Adderall): This relatively new product is longer acting than the others mentioned. It seems to have a more favorable side-effect profile. To date, mixed salts of dextroamphetamine is not as well studied as the others but appears to be similarly effective. Dose range is 0.1 to 1.0 mg/kg/d. Mixed salts of dextroamphetamine is dosed b.i.d. at 6- to 8-hour intervals. There is some evidence that a single larger morning dose can be used on a once-a-day basis. More research is needed to document the efficacy of using this method. This drug comes in 5-, 10-, 20-, and 30-mg tablets, which are scored and can be chewed or swallowed. Titration of dose is as with the others. Dosage equivalence of 15 mg of mixed salts of dextroamphetamine is comparable to 20 mg of methylphenidate.

Pemoline: Pemoline is very long acting and is usually dosed once daily, but it can be used b.i.d. It can be chewed. The dosage range is 0.5 to 3.0 mg/kg/d. Tablets come in 18.75-, 37.5-, and 75-mg strengths.

▲ **Clinical Warning:** Cases of serious hepatotoxicity with pemoline have been reported; thus, frequent liver function tests are recommended. This risk should be assessed against the potential benefit before prescribing. Many providers have abandoned this drug because of associated risks.

ANTIDEPRESSANTS

The tricyclic category has been more extensively studied than most other drug groups, with dozens of published trials. Newer drugs like bupropion are just beginning to be examined in clinical trials and used clinically. The tricyclics are useful in children who do not respond to stimulants and youngsters with comorbid depression. Advantages include once-a-day dosing without rebound or insomnia, increased dosing flexibility, and little abuse potential. These medications, however, are more complicated to use.

▲ **Clinical Warning:** Tricyclics have been associated with serious cardiac arrhythmias. Electrocardiograms must be followed. Tricyclics are very dangerous when taken in overdose. Drug levels of tricyclics should be monitored.

Side effects of tricyclics include dry mouth, constipation, headache, gain and loss of weight, drowsiness, and irritability. While some clinicians have experience in using these medications for this purpose, often referral to a child psychiatrist is indicated, at least for initiation of pharmacotherapy and recommendations for treatment planning.

ANTIHYPERTENSIVES

Antihypertensives, such as clonidine and the newer guanfacine, are used primarily as mood modulators. They are particularly useful in children who have significant problems with aggression and hyperactivity. Antihypertensives also are useful in patients with tic disorders. They are much less effective for ADHD than the other two classes of drugs. Guanfacine has the advantage of producing much less sedation, which is a major problem with clonidine. Side effects include sedation, depression, hypotension, and rebound hypertension.

▲ **Clinical Warnings:**

- Four cases of sudden death have been reported in children taking clonidine. As of this writing, no causal link has been established.
- As with the tricyclics, only a few providers feel comfortable with the use of these drugs without some consultative support. The clinician is advised to consult with a child psychiatrist or neurologist before undertaking management of ADHD with antihypertensive therapy.

What to Tell the Family

A complete discussion of family and school interventions is beyond the scope of this chapter. Several references and resources listed at the end of this chapter can be consulted for more information. Important measures for the clinician include the following:

- Educate parents as to the nature of the problem, reinforcing that ADHD is not a personal failure on their or the child's part.
- Emphasize the need for consistency. The chronicity of ADHD means that parents must be consistent in their approach to the child and in every aspect of the child's life.
- Teach parents to identify situations and settings in which their child will have difficulty. Parents should avoid such occurrences if possible and manage them when they happen. The goal is to improve the child's environment, making it easier for the child to succeed, not to try to punish away their child's behavior.
- Encourage parents to accept their child, celebrating strengths while working within their youngster's limitations.
- Teach parents to apply behavioral techniques, such as using time out, remaining calm, and setting limits. Again, the key to success is consistency.

- Make parents aware that long-term damage to self-esteem can occur if reactions to the child are constantly negative. They need to minimize negativity.

● **Clinical Pearl:** The primary care provider should teach parents to pay positive attention to their child. Positive attention means "catching" their child engaged in positive behavior. It is not false praise, nor does it remove the need for consequences in the case of negative behavior.

- Remind parents that feedback—whether positive or negative—must be immediate and more powerful than used for other children.
- Emphasize that caregivers should act, not talk.

● **Clinical Pearl:** The child with ADHD does not respond well to lectures about behavior, whether good or bad. If an action is to be taken, whether punishment or reward, the parent needs to do it, not talk about doing it.

- Inform parents that the home setting should be as structured and organized as possible. This task may be difficult if the clinician is relying on parents who have problems similar to those of their child.
- Parents should mean what they say and be careful how they say it. Explain that parents should not ask the child if he or she would like to do something. Rather, they should simply tell the child what he or she needs to do. Parents then should have the child repeat to the parent what he or she just heard.

● **Clinical Pearl:** Parents need to understand that what they say and what the child hears may not be the same.

These youngsters need more rewards than punishments. They also will need rewards for behaviors that other children will do without recompense. For many, particularly younger children, parents should develop some sort of concrete and formal reward system. This may involve tokens like poker chips or some other objects the child can value. Chore cards and posted rules are also helpful. The provider may want to duplicate Display 21-1, which summarizes the

---

DISPLAY 21–1 • Hints for Parents of the Child With ADHD

ADHD is a real disease with a real treatment. It is not a personal failure!
Consistency is one of the keys to effective treatment.
Make it easier for your child to succeed rather than punish failure.
Celebrate your child's strengths. Work with your child's weaknesses.
Use behavior techniques, such as enforcing time out, setting limits, and remaining calm.
Minimize negativity. It will destroy your child's self-esteem.
Pay positive attention.
Feedback must be *immediate* and more *powerful* with ADHD children.
Do it–don't talk about doing it.
Home environments should be as structured and orderly as possible.
Give clear, powerful instructions, and ask your child to repeat them to you.
Concrete reward systems are helpful, particularly with younger children.

DISPLAY 21–2 • Hints for Teachers Working With the Student With ADHD

Children with ADHD need rewards for doing things that other kids do not need rewards to do.
Rewards and consequences must be more frequent than with other kids.
Rewards and consequences must be more immediate than with other kids.
Use a daily assignment book that both parents and teachers must check and sign.
Break down long-term projects into small pieces, each with its own deadline for completion.
Smaller, more structured settings are helpful.
Use behavior techniques, such as enforcing time out, setting limits, and remaining calm.

---

preceding points, and give it to parents as part of their anticipatory guidance.

▲ **Clinical Warning:** Adolescents with ADHD are much harder to manage than are younger children. Behavioral programs are far less effective with this age group. The provider should consider referring such adolescents to a mental health professional skilled in dealing with ADHD in teenagers.

What to Tell the School

School systems today are overwhelmed with special education mandates and costs. Nevertheless, all publicly funded schools are legally obligated to provide an adequate education to children with disabilities such as ADHD. Most school systems are willing to work with parents to maximize the child's classroom performance. Too often, however, parent and school get into a cycle of blame for the child's behavior, and little gets accomplished.

The clinician should work hard to facilitate collaboration between parents and school. Contact with the child's teachers or principal is helpful and can educate them about the needs of children with ADHD. Teachers must recognize that students with ADHD need rewards for things that other children do not. They also must understand that both rewards and consequences need to happen more frequently and with greater speed than with other children. Feedback between parent and teacher must be constant, particularly regarding homework and assignments. An assignment book that must be filled out and signed daily is useful. Long-term projects should be broken down into small components, each with its own deadline for completion. If available, small, highly structured classes are best. School personnel easily can use many of the behavioral techniques discussed for parents. Display 21-2 provides a synopsis of these points, which the provider may want to duplicate and distribute to the teacher or school administrator on behalf of the patient with ADHD.

Some Final Strategies

In working with the child who has ADHD, the provider should remember the following:

- Close monitoring and support improve results. The patient should be seen at least quarterly and far more often when dosing changes are made. Height, weight, and blood pressure should be recorded at these visits. A careful interval history should be taken that covers home, and school, performance, social issues, and medication side effects. An evaluation of the dose of medications should be performed. The frequent use of monitoring scales, such as Connors or ACTERS, should be encouraged.

- Higher doses and more frequent dosing of stimulant medications should be used. The dose response is linear; thus, a higher dose may result in a large clinical improvement.
- ADHD does not disappear in the afternoon or on weekends. Use of medication at these times can lessen the condition's constant assault on the child's self-esteem and can provide the cushion needed for the patient to perform best. Drug holidays may not be in the child's interest.
- Adolescents of driving age should *never* drive without being medicated. Risks associated with adolescent driving are much higher in teens with ADHD than in their peers. This fact is not surprising, given the disorder's characteristic impulsivity.
- Comorbidity must be diagnosed and treated before ADHD. Comorbidity should be assessed in siblings and parents as well.
- The clinician should treat and monitor patients frequently. They should not wait for crises to happen. They should not write prescriptions without following up to assess the medication's effects.
- The provider should be conscientious in educating the family, working with parents, children, and school.

Making outcome statements about ADHD is difficult because of the high rate of comorbidity that complicates the disorder and, if present, certainly affects outcome. One question that all parents ask is, "Will my child grow out of it?" It was believed in the past that nearly all children outgrew ADHD. Especially in light of increasing evidence of a neurobiologic basis for ADHD, the general consensus is that it is a disorder with lifelong sequellae. Estimates are that there is at least 70% persistence into adolescence. Persistence into adulthood is variable, estimated at 10% to 60% (Spencer, 1998). The actual rate of persistence depends on how it is defined. If it is depicted as meeting the full DSM-IV (1994) criteria, persistence is at the low end of that range. When defined as meeting half the criteria, persistence is higher. If one describes persistence on a functional basis, asking whether the patient is functioning well, even fewer children outgrow ADHD.

Factors that correlate with remission rates include a strong family history of ADHD, level of psychiatric comorbidity, and level of psychosocial stress in the family. What is clear is that a syndrome of Adult ADHD definitely exists. Adult ADHD may need modified diagnostic criteria from the childhood syndrome of ADHD. Many adults are now being treated in similar ways as children, with interventions at home, at work, and with pharmacotherapy.

Patients should be referred to a pediatric neurologist, psychiatrist, or other mental health provider for any of the following:

- The clinician does not have the time, interest, or experience to evaluate properly the child with school problems.
- The child has a complicated presentation or symptomatology.
- Significant comorbidity is suspected or diagnosed.
- Significant or dangerous side effects from pharmacotherapy develop.

- Complex polypharmacy appears to be necessary.
- At any time, the clinician feels uncomfortable with the diagnosis or the patient's clinical course.

The main clinical warnings are to be aware of and not fail to diagnose serious comorbidity. In addition, the clinician needs to be aware of the rare dangerous side effects of some of the medications used to treat ADHD.

PSYCHOLOGICAL PROBLEMS

Psychological problems related to school can run the gamut from mild adjustment problems to severe mental illness. Discussion here is limited to the milder end of the spectrum. This section addresses school avoidance, separation anxiety, and shyness.

School Avoidance

School avoidance is one of the most common emotional problems encountered in pediatric primary care. To avoid attending school, the child may complain of a variety of often vague somatic complaints, such headache, dizziness, nausea, or abdominal pain. The youngster may have specific complaints, such as sore throat and earache. Typically, the complaints miraculously resolve after school and on weekends, but sometimes they persist. The child may miss significant school time before parents seek medical attention. The challenge for the provider is to take a very careful history as to the timing, severity, and frequency of symptoms and noting family and school dynamics. A careful physical examination should be performed, but the provider who suspects school avoidance should avoid feeding into the situation by ordering laboratory or imaging studies. If secure with the diagnosis, the provider should emphasize that the problem is behavioral, not physical. Parents should tell the child firmly that he or she must attend school. They should prevent or limit absences as much as possible. If the child stays home and gets better, he or she should return to school, even for part of the day. If the child stays home, he or she should not be allowed to participate in fun activities. If such intervention is not successful, a mental health referral should be made.

Separation Anxiety

Separation anxiety usually is a problem among day care and preschool populations, but may persist into kindergarten and first grade. In younger children, separation anxiety often is related to a developmental or attention-getting stage and is dealt with best by advising the parent to be matter-of-fact when dropping off the child. In older children, separation anxiety often is indicative of a more significant disorder in the parent–child relationship.

● **Clinical Pearl:** If separation anxiety significantly affects school attendance or performance, a counseling referral should be considered.

Shyness

Excessive shyness is a problem in the pediatric population that, if not acknowledged and handled, can persist into adulthood. Excessive shyness may reflect the child's inborn temperament and may resolve over time. At its extreme, excessive shyness may progress to point where the child refuses to speak while in school. This problem, known as mutism, is potentially serious.

▲ **Clinical Warning:** The provider must refer the child with mutism to a pediatric mental health specialist who can provide needed intervention.

PHYSICAL PROBLEMS

Difficulty in school can be due primarily to physical problems or disabilities. Obvious disabilities, such as cerebral palsy, neuromuscular disorders, visual impairment (including blindness), and auditory impairment (including deafness), can significantly compromise school performance, even if the child's intellectual capacity is intact or superior. Such students need multidisciplinary support and special education plans to maximize their achievement. In the United States, state and federal laws mandate the provision of services for disabled students, and the same is true to varying degrees for other Westernized nations. In the United States, referral to appropriate specialists and therapists, as well as contact with the school, is mandatory. The provider should strive to understand appropriate laws, because correct information helps in obtaining services for the child and family.

In addition to obvious motor and perceptual disabilities, children with chronic medical problems, such as asthma, diabetes, seizure disorder, sickle cell anemia, cystic fibrosis, and even recurrent otitis media, can face school problems due to repeated absences and diminished ability to pay attention to school work. The emotional toll also should be considered, because ongoing illness may compromise the child's self-esteem and ability to fit in with peers. The provider can work closely with the family and school to bring the illness under control and to handle the child's real and perceived disabilities. For more information, refer to Units III and V, which deal with psychosocial challenges and chronic disease in pediatric primary care.

COMMUNITY RESOURCES

Resources for Providers

- *Attention Deficit Hyperactivity Disorder: A Handbook for Diagnosis and Treatment*, by Russell Barkley, 1998, is a comprehensive text on theory, diagnosis, and treatment.
- *Attention Deficit Disorder: A Clinical Workbook*, by Russell Barkley and Kevin Murphy, 1998, is a manual of templates and forms that can be used for history-taking and monitoring.
- *Connors Rating Scales*, published by Multi-Health Systems, Inc. (800) 456-3003. This is a multitude of standardized ratings scales for parents, teachers, and adolescents. Workbooks that discuss scoring and interpretation of the scales are also available from this resource.
- *ACTERS Rating Scales* is published by Metritech, Inc. (217) 398-4868.
- DSM-IV, *Diagnostic and Statistical Manual of Mental Disorders*, 4th ed., 1994, is published by the American Psychiatric Association.
- *Pharmacotherapy of ADHD Across the Lifecycle*, by Thomas Spencer and Joseph Biederman, et al., is published in *Journal of the American Academy of Child and Adolescent Psychology*, 35(4), 409–1432, 1996.

Resources for Parents

- Children and Adults with ADD (CHADD). A National support group with extensive information services, a national magazine, newsletters, national meetings, and many local chapters. They can be reached at 499 Northwest 70th Ave, Suite 109, Plantation, FL 33317. (800) 233-4050. They are on the web at *www.chadd.org*.
- *Taking Charge of ADHD*, by Russell Barkley, 1995, is one of the best of the many books available. It has the benefit of an extensive discussion of home and school management, as well as theory and drug treatment.
- ADD Warehouse. This is a catalog of books, videos, and products for children with ADHD. (800) 233-9273.
- *The Difficult Child*, by Stanley Turecki and Leslie Tonner, is a wonderful book about the inborn temperament of children and how to manage it.

REFERENCES

American Psychiatric Association. (1994). *Diagnostic and statistical manual of mental disorders* (4th ed.). Washington, D.C.: Author.

Barkley, R. (1998). *ADHD: A handbook for diagnosis and treatment*. New York: The Guildford Press.

Barkley, R. (1997). Behavioral inhibition, sustained attention, and executive functions: Constructing a unifying theory of ADHD. *Psych Bulletin, 121*, 65–194.

Barkley, R., & Murphy, K. (1998). *ADHD: A clinical workbook*. New York: The Guildford Press.

Bauermeister, J. J., Canino, G., & Bird, H. (1994). Epidemiology of disruptive behavior disorders. *Child and Adolescent Psychological Clinics of North America*, 177–194.

Biederman, J., Newcorn, J., & Sprich, S. E. (1991). Comorbidity of ADHD. *American Journal of Psychiatry, 148*, 564–1577.

Biederman, J., Wilens, T., Mick, E., Spencer, T., & Faraone, S. V. (1999). Pharmacotherapy of attention-deficit/hyperactivity disorder reduces risk for substance use disorder. *Pediatrics, 104*(2):e20.

Bush, G., Frazier, J. A., Rauch, S. L., Seidman, L. J., Whalen, P. J., Jenike, M. A., Rosen, B. R., & Biederman, J. Anterior Cingulate Cortex Dysfunction in Adults with ADHD Revealed by MRI and the counting stroop. *Biological Psychiatry, 45*,(12): 1542–1552.

Castellanos, F., Giedd, J., Eckburg, P., Marsh, W., Hamburger, S., Vaituzis, A., Dickstein, D., Sargatti, S., Vauss, Y., Snell, J., Rajapakse, J., & Rapoport, J. (1996). Quantitative brain MRI in ADHD. *Arch Gen Psych, 53*, 607–1616.

Faraone, S., & Biederman, J. (1994). Genetics of ADHD. *Child and Adolescent Psychological Clinics of North America, 3*(2), 285–1301.

Feingold, B. (1975). *Why your child is hyperactive*. New York: Random House.

Lahoste, G. J., Swanson, J. M., Wigal, S. B., Glabe, C., Wigal, T., King, N., & Kennedy, J. L., (1996). Dopamine D4 Receptor Gen Polymorphism is Associated with ADHD. *Molecular Psychiatry, 1*.

Millberger, S., Biederman, J., Faraone, S. V., Chen, L., & Jones, J. (1996). Is maternal smoking during pregnancy a risk factor for ADHD in Children? *American Journal of Psychiatry, 153*(9), 1138–11142.

National Advisory Committee on Hyperkinesis and Food Additives. (1980). New York: Nutritional Foundation.

Semrud-Clikeman, M. S., Filipek, P. A., Biederman, J., Steingard, R., Kennedy, D., Renshaw, P., & Bekken, K. (1994). ADHD: MRI morphometric analysis of the corpus callosum. *Journal of the American Academy of Child and Adolescent Psychiatry, 33*, 875–1881.

Shaywitz, S. E. (1998). Dyslexia. *New England Journal of Medicine, 338*, 307–1312.

Spencer, T., Biederman, J., Wilens, T. E., & Faraone, S. (1998). Adults with ADHD: A controversial diagnosis. *Journal of Clinical Psychiatry, 59*(suppl 7), 59–168.

Woolraich, M. L., Wilson, D. B., & White, J. W. (1995). The effect of sugar on behavior or cognition in children: A meta analysis. *Journal of the American Medical Association, 274,* 1617–1621.

Yakinci, C., Mungen, B., Durmaz, Y., Balbay, D., & Karabiber, H. (1997). Autonomic nervous system functions in children with nocturnal enuresis. *Brain and Development, 19*(7), 485–1487.

Zametkin, A. J., Nordahl, T. E., Gross, M., King, C., Semple, W. E., Rumsey, J., Hamburger, S., & Cohen, R. M. (1990). Cerebral glucose metabolism in adults with hyperactivity of childhood onset. *New England Journal of Medicine, 323,* 1361–11366.

Eating Disorders

• ENITZA D. GEORGE, MD

INTRODUCTION

Eating disorders are those in which an individual is preoccupied excessively with body weight or shape or in which food intake is grossly inadequate, irregular, or chaotic. Such disorders are not uncommon among children and adolescents. In 1997, the Centers for Disease Control and Prevention (CDC) found that 30.4% of students diet, 4.9% use diet pills, and 4.5% induce vomiting or use laxatives after meals to lose weight (CDC, 1998).

The most commonly diagnosed eating disorders in pediatric populations are anorexia nervosa (AN), bulimia nervosa (BN), and obesity. Other disordered eating patterns observed among children are selective eating, food avoidance, emotional disorder, binge eating, and pervasive refusal syndrome. These latter patterns of disordered eating do not fulfill the strict criteria for eating disorders but may cause diagnostic confusion.

Eating disorders have numerous damaging effects. Poorly nourished children attain low scores on standardized achievement tests (especially tests of language ability) and have difficulty resisting infection. They are more likely than other children to become sick, miss school, and fall behind in class. Restricting meals can delay growth and sexual development. Obesity, which results from overeating and physical inactivity, affects 25% to 30% of children and adolescents in the United States (Keller & Stevens, 1996). In adults, obesity causes at least 300,000 deaths yearly. In later adolescence, eating disorders are associated with psychosomatic disorders and risk-taking behaviors, including the use of tobacco, alcohol, and marijuana; suicidal ideation and attempts; and unprotected sexual activity (Neumarker et al., 1997).

Because these conditions have immediate and long-term deleterious consequences on health, growth, and intellectual and social development, early recognition and treatment of eating disorders are paramount. This chapter discusses the most salient clinical features of AN, BN, and obesity in children and adolescents. It also presents prevention and treatment for these disorders and ways for providers to help affected children and their families.

ANOREXIA NERVOSA

A multidetermined syndrome, AN has various biologic, psychological, and social components. Children with AN are very hungry but choose to starve themselves because they have an irrational aversion to food. Affected individuals believe they are fat no matter how much they actually weigh.

Pathology

Heritability is high among patients with AN. The concordance rate for AN in dizygotic twins is 5% compared with 56% for monozygotic twins. The frequency of the disorder in female relatives of patients with AN is 8 to 20 times higher than in the general population (Gorwood, et al., 1998). The exact mode of inheritance and the specific genes that influence risk are not yet known. Some evidence has supported a disordered hypothalamic-pituitary-adrenal axis as a cause. Hypercortisolemia, nonsuppressive dexamethasone suppressive tests, and increased central nervous system fluid levels of corticotropin-releasing hormone have all been demonstrated in AN (Kaye, 1998). Recent studies show increased levels of cerebral serotonin in patients with AN, leading theorists to believe that high levels of serotonin may lead to reduced food intake (Walsh & Devlin, 1998). Research also has suggested that a high level of cholecystokinin, a gastric peptide, is associated with delayed gastric emptying, causing a constant sense of satiety in patients with AN (Fujimoto et al., 1997).

The psychosocial profile of children with AN demonstrates a premorbid history of high achievement and perfectionism. These children often come from families with rigid homeostatic systems. Parents of children with AN may be overinvolved or overprotective, avoid conflict, or have high and unrealistic expectations. As a result, these children struggle for autonomy, identity, and self-respect, gaining a sense of control by restricting severely the amount of food they eat. Thus, the ability to do without food becomes a way to cope with stress.

Psychological trauma, especially sexual abuse, may contribute to AN. Between 34% and 83% of children with AN report some form of sexual trauma (Schmidt et al., 1997). Children and adolescents with AN often have other associated psychological disorders, including major depression (50%–75%), bipolar disorders, obsessive-compulsive disorder (10%–13%), substance abuse, and borderline personality disorder (Halmi et al., 1993). Refer to Chapters 23, 25, and 28 for more information on these comorbidities.

The relationship between social influences and AN is worth exploring. For example, the use of tall and emaciated teen fashion models in the mass media conveys an unrealistic, unhealthy, and dangerous standard of beauty for very receptive children and adolescents. More information is needed to understand how such images may contribute to AN and other eating disorders.

Epidemiology

Prevalence of AN in the United States is 0.5% to 1% among adolescents, and the incidence is rising (Pawluck & Gorey, 1998). Incidence almost certainly is lower in young children, but the exact numbers are not known. Pattern of onset is bimodal, with peaks at ages 13 to 14 years and later at ages 17 to 18 years. In adolescents, AN is observed overwhelmingly among females (90%–95% of cases). In children with AN, 19% to 30% of cases are observed in boys (Bryant-Waugh & Lask, 1995).

History and Physical Examination

Patients with full-blown AN often wear several layers of clothing to keep warm and to hide their thinness. During examination, patients must disrobe completely for providers to determine their weight accurately.

Untreated patients with AN will show obvious signs of emaciation. Several physical signs of AN include the following:

- Body weight less than 85% of expected
- Bradyarrhythmia
- Bradypnea (respiratory compensation for alkalosis)
- Hypotension (systolic blood pressure below 90 mmHg)
- Hypothermia (rectal temperature below 96.6°F)
- Lanugo (fine, downy hair) on the arms and face with loss of scalp and pubic hair
- Lower extremity edema
- Muscle atrophy and emaciation
- Carotenemia (yellowish hue of the skin), especially of the palms and soles
- Dry skin with desquamation
- Small uterus and cervix
- Pink and dry vaginal mucosa

Diagnostic Criteria

The criteria of the *Diagnostic and Statistical Manual of Mental Disorders*, fourth edition (DSM IV), for diagnosis of AN include the following:

- Body weight less than 85% of that expected or failure to grow, resulting in body weight that remains less than 85% of expected
- Fear of gaining weight
- Body weight disturbance or denial of the seriousness of low body weight
- Absence of three consecutive menstrual cycles in postmenarcheal females

Timely diagnosis is crucial but can be difficult. Patients often are secretive about their problem; many of them deny they have AN. Early "red flags" in a child or adolescent include the following:

- Practicing ritualistic eating habits, such as cutting up meat in very small bites
- Hoarding food
- Refusing to eat in front of others
- Suddenly deciding to become a vegetarian or choosing low- or no-fat and low-calorie foods
- Continuously exercising
- Insisting that he or she is very fat when he or she obviously is not
- Displaying highly self-controlled behavior
- Showing a depressed mood and social isolation
- Being hypersensitive to cold

Diagnostic Studies

Diagnosis of AN usually is obvious and based on the patient's history, attitude toward food, associated symptoms, and physical examination. No specific biologic test is used to diagnose this disorder. Early in the diagnosis, the only abnormality providers may observe is an elevated blood urea nitrogen that results from dehydration. Later, providers may note iron deficiency anemia with microcytosis, hypocalcemia, hypoglycemia, hypomagnesemia, and hypophosphatemia, all due to starvation. Patients with AN have severe but reversible hypercholesterolemia (Stone, 1994). Later, serum aminotransferase may be elevated.

▲ **Clinical Warning:** Elevation of serum aminotransferase signals a critical, life-threatening condition associated with multiorgan failure. The patient requires urgent calorie repletion (Ozawa et al., 1998).

Providers must perform an electrocardiogram and echocardiography on patients with AN to evaluate for cardiac muscle damage. Patients may develop decreased left ventricular wall thickness, reduced heart size, bradycardia, and nonspecific ST-T wave changes. They may have a low-voltage ECG. Echocardiography may reveal mitral valve prolapse (Cheng, 1997). These alterations make patients with AN prone to sudden death (Neumarker et al., 1997).

Anorexia nervosa severely alters the endocrine system; therefore, measurements of leuteinizing hormone (LH), follicle-stimulating hormone (FSH), and estradiol are necessary, as are thyroid function tests. The starvation that accompanies AN disrupts the hypothalmic-pituitary-adrenal axis, resulting in low levels of LH and FSH. For this reason, adolescents with AN who previously have experienced menarche become amenorrheic with anovulation. Because they are estrogen deficient, these patients do not experience withdrawal bleeding after progestin challenge. Between 30% and 50% of patients with AN become amenorrheic even before they experience significant weight loss. Resumption of menses often is delayed until some time after they regain weight, perhaps because the body produces high cortisol levels as a response to the stress of starvation (Kaye, 1998). In males with AN, hypogonadism with low levels of testosterone, LH, and FSH may be seen. In either sex, thyroid function tests are abnormal with elevated reverse T_3, reduced total T_3, low normal T_4, and normal TSH. Reduced metabolic rate accounts for the hypothyroid-like presentations of bradycardia, cold intolerance, constipation, and dry skin.

One of the most important complications of AN is osteoporosis resulting from estrogen deficiency. Photon absorptiometry will assist in evaluating fracture risk. When amenorrhea is prolonged, sustained bone loss may not be reversible even once menses resume. Therefore, these patients are at an increased risk for fractures throughout their lives (Hotta et al., 1998).

Management

Several complications are associated with refeeding patients with AN:

- Self-limited edema. Providers should treat this condition with a salt-restricted diet, leg elevation, and support stockings.
- Abdominal bloating. Providers should consider giving metoclopramide if bloating is severe.
- Constipation. Providers should prescribe a high-fiber diet, stool softeners, and hydration.
- Congestive heart failure. Providers should hospitalize and treat patients with digoxin and diuretics.
- Hypophosphatemia. Providers should give oral phosphate and monitor serum phosphate every other day.

Providers must conduct refeeding carefully to prevent complications and progression to bulimia. The goal for the female patient is to gain 2 lb per week until she reaches the weight at which she previously menstruated and is within 15% of her ideal weight. The goal for the male patient is to achieve a weight within that same ideal range. Providers prescribe a diet that provides 2000 to 4000 calories each day (Walsh & Devlin, 1998). Open trial studies have shown zinc supplementation (100 mg/d) to double the rate of increase in the body mass index (BMI) of patients with AN (Birmingham et al., 1994). Patients require calcium supplements of at least 1 g/d and need multivitamins as well. Because refeeding may cause severe hypophosphatemia, recommendations are for patients to be started on oral phosphate when feeding is initiated. Providers need to monitor serum phosphate every 1 to 2 days for at least the first week of refeeding.

More research is needed regarding the use of force-feeding, which may be necessary in life-threatening cases that are refractory to treatment (Mehler & Weiner, 1995). Force-feeding may be performed by nasogastric tube or through total parenteral nutrition. Generally, force-feeding is used only with extreme cases of AN, including patients who may lose weight again, necessitating repeated treatments. When force-feeding is conducted, the patient should be detained in a hospital that also provides psychotherapy. Other medical therapies will not be possible until the patient has steadily gained some weight. Some experts disagree with force-feeding, suggesting that repeated episodes of it can adversely affect ultimate success (Draper, 1998). To resolve this controversy in the United Kingdom, the Mental Health Commission issued guidelines about when patients with AN can be detained, treated, and fed without consent (Mental Health Commission, 1997).

Providers must decide on the need for hospitalization versus the appropriateness of treating individuals as outpatients. Indications for the hospitalization of patients with AN are as follows:

- Severe malnutrition: Weight loss is more than 30% of ideal weight for height.
- Rapidly losing weight: Weight loss is more than 30% in less than 3 months.
- Medical complications: Cardiac arrhythmia, intractable hypokalemia, hypothermia, and altered mental status occur.
- Suicidal ideation or acute psychotic reaction exists.
- Attempts to treat as outpatient have failed.

● **Clinical Pearl:** The goal of hospitalization is to stabilize the patient medically and nutritionally and to help the patient attain as close to a healthy weight as possible.

While the patient is in the hospital, providers must maintain a caring, highly structured, nonpunitive environment. Often, health care professionals will present a written contract to the patient and family on admission (Robin et al., 1998). The contract must describe the goals of hospitalization, criteria for discharge, a nutritional rehabilitation plan, and rules regarding exercise, visitation, and system of rewards. Display 22-1 presents a sample contract. Generally, achievement of these goals takes about 4 to 6 weeks; however, in today's era of managed care, most hospitals discharge patients within 2 weeks. Criteria for discharge from the hospital include the following:

- Patient has reached 85% to 90% of ideal body weight.
- Patient is eating and gaining weight regularly.
- Parents have learned how to work with their child in taking care of the eating disorder.
- Providers have treated all secondary medical complications.
- Patient has received psychological evaluation, and therapeutic plan has begun.

DISPLAY 22-1 • Sample Contract to Present When Admitting Patients With Anorexia Nervosa

1. You will be given three meals and several snacks each day.
2. We expect you to eat 100% of your food.
3. You will be given the opportunity to exclude three aversive foods. We expect you to eat all other foods that are on your tray.
4. You will have 30 minutes to eat everything on your tray. You will eat in the playroom with a nurse present to encourage and monitor you.
5. You cannot have food brought in from outside the hospital.
6. If you are unable to eat all your food within 30 minutes, you will be given 15 additional minutes to drink a nutritious milkshake equal to the amount of food remaining on your tray. If you cannot drink the milkshake, we will ask you to preserve your energy by staying on bed rest until the next meal. During bed rest, there are no activities or TV.
7. You will remain in the playroom with the nurse for 30 minutes following each meal.
8. If you eat breakfast completely, you have earned telephone privileges.
9. If you eat all three meals completely, you have earned 1 hour of visitation in the evening.

Adapted with permission from Robin, A. L., et al. (1998). Treatment of eating disorders in children and adolescents. *Clinical Psychology Review, 18*(4), 421–446.

An alternative to full hospitalization for refeeding is to discharge patients as they approach their target weight and admit them into a parital pediatric day treatment program from 8:00 AM to 10:00 PM. Robin et al. (1998) report success using this method, with 84% of patients reaching and retaining their ideal weight after 9 months of follow-up treatment.

Psychotherapy is fundamental to the treatment of AN. Ego-oriented individual therapy (EOIT) and cognitive-behavioral treatment (CBT) have both proven useful. EOIT combines weekly individual sessions for the patient with collateral sessions twice a month for the parents. Individual sessions focus primarily on the youngster's ego strength, coping skills, individuation from the nuclear family, confusion about identity, and other interpersonal issues related to physical, social, and emotional growth. In these sessions, therapists examine the connection between such issues and eating, weight expectations, and body image. Conversely, CBT uses cognitive restructuring to modify distorted beliefs and attitudes about the "meaning" of weight gain. Compared with CBT, restoration of weight is slower with EOIT, but changes in eating, attitudes, depression, ego-functioning, and family interactions are comparable (Robin et al., 1998). Providers should refer patients whose families are interested in pursuing either EOIT or CBT to mental health professionals skilled in their application with adolescents.

Family therapy and parental counseling are essential. Parents need treatment to relieve them of guilt. Providers must educate parents about the medical, nutritional, and psychological aspects of the eating disorder. They should ask family members to work with the affected child by taking charge of the eating disorder. Providers ask parents to take a proactive supportive role in their child's eating by planning menus, supervising meal intake, providing snacks, and monitoring progress without being controlling or judgmental.

▲ **Clinical Warnings:**

- Medications have no clear role in the treatment of AN during the weight-gain phase (Attia, 1998). Research on the use of fluoxetine after weight restoration has rendered mixed results (Kaye, 1998; Strober, 1997).
- Current adjunctive treatment of AN with fluoxetine only is recommended when evidence of a significant mood disturbance or obsessive compulsive disorder (OCD) persists or emerges after weight is restored (Mayer & Walsh, 1998). Fluoxetine can be administered in doses of 10 to 20 mg/d. Close monitoring of side effects is recommended because of the physiologic disturbances associated with AN.

Many individuals recover fully from AN; however, 50% of patients have a poor long-term outcome, remaining irrationally concerned about weight gain and thus never achieving a normal body weight. Fatality from AN is 25%. Complications of starvation or from suicide are approximately 5% per decade of follow-up (Walsh & Devlin, 1998).

BULIMIA NERVOSA

Bulimia nervosa is characterized by repeated bouts of overeating and excessive preoccupation with controlling body weight. Patients adopt extreme measures to mitigate the "fattening" effects of ingested food, including vomiting, fasting, excessively exercising, and misusing diuretics, laxatives, or enemas. During the course of their illness, 30% to 80% of patients alternate between BN and AN. This bimodal pattern of disease is known as bulimarexia.

Pathology

Patients with BN generally are perfectionists. They have an impaired self-concept, affective instability, poor impulse control, and a lack of adaptive functioning for maturational tasks and developmental stresses (eg, puberty, peer and parental relationships, sexuality). Substance abuse is observed in 33% of patients. Overall, between 2% and 50% of adolescents with BN have some type of personality disorder, most commonly borderline, antisocial, histrionic, or narcissistic personality disorder (Mcgilley & Pryor, 1998). Presence of these additional comorbidities in adolescents may pose extra challenges for providers.

Epidemiology

Incidence of BN is about 3% among adolescent girls (Mcgilley & Pryor, 1998) and about 0.2% in adolescent boys (Andersen & Holman, 1997). The disorder typically begins in adolescence or early adulthood, with peak age of onset between 13 and 20 years. There are no reports of prepubertal BN.

As with AN, BN has multiple biologic and psychosocial etiologies, and a genetic predisposition for BN may exist (Allison & Faith, 1997). Researchers have found that first- and second-degree relatives of patients with BN have increased incidences of depression and manic-depressive illness, eating disorders, and substance abuse (Lilenfeld, et al., 1998). In contrast with AN, individuals with BN have poor serotonergic function, contributing to their persistent binge eating

(Jimeson, 1997). In some patients, the capacity of the stomach is enlarged, and the release of the satiety hormone cholecystokinin after a meal is blunted (Walsh & Devlin, 1998).

History and Physical Examination

Early in the disease, no physical signs of BN are apparent. Later, three signs unmistakably suggest self-induced vomiting that has continued for years:

- Erosion of dental enamel
- Russell's sign
- Bilateral hypertrophy of the parotid glands

Gastric acid erodes the tooth enamel, most commonly over the lingual surfaces of the upper teeth. Patients with BN have an increased rate of caries, pyorrhea, and other gum disorders. They may complain of increased temperature sensitivity in the teeth and gums. Mouth lesions, which are mostly irreversible, require regular dental care (Rytomaa et al., 1998). Self-induced vomiting also may damage the upper gastrointestinal tract by causing oral lesions, sore throat, esophagitis, and esophageal tears. Most damage is benign and can be treated with antacids and throat lozenges. Esophageal or gastric ruptures are rare but lethal complications.

Russell's sign presents as bleeding, scarred, or callused knuckles. It develops because the hand is in repeated contact with the front teeth in the patient's effort to induce vomiting (Daluiski, 1997). Russell's sign is not observed in all patients with BN, because individuals often use toothbrushes or other objects to induce vomiting. Also, some patients are able to vomit by placing pressure on or contracting the abdominal muscles.

Eight percent of patients with BN develop parotid hypertrophy, the exact etiology of which is unknown. It is painless and occurs within days of vomiting. Although cosmetically distressing, it is medically benign. No treatment is needed, as parotid hypertrophy disappears once vomiting stops (Andersen & Holman, 1997).

Diagnostic Criteria

Bulimia nervosa can be very difficult to diagnose. The median duration of symptoms before diagnosis is 6 years. The DSM IV (1994) diagnostic criteria for BN include the following:

- The individual has recurrent episodes of binge eating:
  1. The patient eats an amount of food within 2 hours that is definitely larger than most people would eat.
  2. The patient senses a lack of control over his or her eating during the episode.
- The individual displays recurrent inappropriate compensatory behaviors to prevent weight gain, such as self-induced vomiting; misuse of laxatives, diuretics, enemas, or other medications; fasting; or excessive exercising.
- Binge eating and compensatory behaviors occur at least twice a week for 3 months.
- Body shape and weight unduly influence self-evaluation.
- The disturbance does not occur exclusively during episodes of AN.

There are two specific types of BN:

- Purging type: The individual regularly engages in self-induced vomiting or misuses laxatives, diuretics, or enemas.

- Nonpurging type: The individual uses other inappropriate compensatory behaviors, such as fasting or excessive exercise.

Early "red flags" of BN in a normal-weight adolescent include the following:

- Making frequent excuses to go to the bathroom after meals
- Showing mood swings
- Buying large amounts of food that suddenly disappear
- Having unusual swelling around the jaw (parotid gland hypertrophy from repeated self-induced vomiting)
- Eating large amounts of food on the spur of the moment

● **Clinical Pearl:** In addition to the above signs, family members or friends may frequently find laxative or diuretic wrappers in the trash that they share with adolescents who have BN.

Diagnostic Studies

History, physical examination, and serum electrolyte disturbance prove diagnostic in 80% of patients with longstanding BN. About 50% of patients have serum abnormalities resulting from vomiting, most commonly hypochloremic metabolic alkalosis and hypokalemia (Crow, 1997). The electrolyte disturbances caused by vomiting can have serious consequences. Initially, the patient may complain of fatigue, fainting, abdominal distension, shortness of breath, muscle spasms, paresthesias, and heart palpitations, which are caused by intermittent hypokalemia.

▲ **Clinical Warning:** Left undiagnosed and untreated, hypokalemia will lead to tetany, seizures, or lethal cardiac arrhythmia.

Management

Substantial evidence exists that pharmacotherapy is effective as adjunctive treatment of BN. Multiple medications have been studied, including tricyclic antidepressants, selective serotonin reuptake inhibitors, monoamine oxidase inhibitors, and trazodone. The Food and Drug Administration has approved fluoxetine for the treatment of BN and considers it the drug of choice because it has been extensively studied, and information regarding the effective dose is available. Patients who receive 60 mg/d of fluoxetine have a 67% reduction in binge eating and a 56% reduction in vomiting (McGilley & Pryor, 1998).

▲ **Clinical Warning:** Because of its side-effect profile and because it can exacerbate the physiologic side effects associated with BN, fluoxetine use should be monitored closely.

The best psychotherapeutic approach for patients with BN is CBT. Patients treated with CBT are directed to monitor the thoughts, feelings, and circumstances that surround binge-purge episodes, to cease dieting and begin regular eating, and to systematically challenge their assumptions linking weight with self-esteem. Patients receiving medications in combination with CBT experience greater improvement in binge eating and depression than do patients who receive other psychotherapeutic approaches (Walsh & Devlin, 1997). Providers should refer patients whose families are interested in pursuing CBT or other psychotherapeutic approaches to mental health professionals skilled in their application with adolescent patients.

The long-term outcome of BN is unknown. With treatment, 60% to 80% of patients achieve remission within 3 months. Most patients have an episodic course. Research shows that 30% of patients rapidly relapse, and up to 40% remain chronically symptomatic (McGilley & Pryor, 1998).

CHILDHOOD-ONSET OBESITY

Traditionally, obesity was defined as a weight above the 90th percentile for height on the growth charts from the National Center of Health Statistics or weight in excess of 120% of the median for a given height. More recently, the Expert Committee on Clinical Guidelines for Overweight in Adolescent Preventive Services has recommended the use of the BMI to help define childhood (6–10 years), adolescent (11–21 years), and adult obesity (Lazarus et al., 1996). A child or adolescent with a BMI greater than the 95th percentiles for age and sex should be considered obese. A recommended BMI upper limit of normal values has not been developed for children younger than 6 years.

Pathology

The exact etiology of obesity is unknown. In children, prenatal, genetic, behavioral, and familial factors may contribute. Two and, possibly, three critical periods exist for the development of obesity in children:

- Gestation and early infancy
- The period of adiposity rebound that occurs between ages 5 and 7 years
- Adolescence

Theorists have suggested that *in utero* nutritional exposure influences the risk of later obesity, possibly by altering the transfer of metabolic substrates between mother and fetus (Whitaker & Dietz, 1998). The discovery and cloning of five mutations that cause spontaneous obesity in mice has led to a search for a genetic etiology of obesity, with multiple genes being implicated (Chagnon et al., 1998). The role of these genes in humans is still unclear.

Depression and low self-esteem have been associated with obesity in children (Pierce & Wardle, 1997). In today's image-conscious society, even children associate overweight drawings with poor social functioning (Schonfeld-Warden & Warden, 1997). Children as young as 5 years have expressed such negative stereotypes.

Epidemiology

Obesity affects approximately 25% of all children and adolescents (Schonfeld-Warden & Warden, 1997). More Hispanic (56%) and African American children (46%) are obese than are Caucasian children (28%) (Keller & Stevens, 1996). Controversy exists regarding the role of dietary fat in the rising prevalence of childhood obesity, particularly because of the increased frequency of children eating in fast food restaurants. Most studies agree, however, that energy expenditure is lower in obese children. A strong association exists between the prevalence of obesity and inactivity, especially related to the extent of television viewing (Bar-Or et al., 1998).

History and Physical Examination

Most obese children have no underlying or secondary etiology for their obesity, making their condition idiopathic.

Rarely, it may be important to exclude possible endogenous causes of obesity in children, which occur in conjunction with hormonal diseases (eg, hypothyroidism, hypercortisolism, primary hyperinsulinism). Endogenous obesity also is observed in children who are suffering from rare genetic syndromes like Prader-Willi, Laurence-Moon, Cohen, or Weaver's syndrome (Moran, 1999). In most instances, clinicians can distinguish between idiopathic and endogenous obesity based on the child's history and a detailed physical examination. An expensive laboratory workup rarely is needed. Table 22-1 presents some characteristics that will assist providers to make this distinction.

Obese children and adolescents commonly have hyperlipidemia, increased heart rate and cardiac output, hepatic steatosis with elevated transaminases, and abnormal glucose metabolism. Obese girls have an earlier menarche. Obese boys may have either delayed or early sexual maturation. Gynecomastia is a common problem in obese adolescent boys. Refer to Chapters 56, 60, and 61 for more in-depth discussion.

Because of the excess weight that obese children carry, they are at increased risk for orthopedic problems like slipped capital femoral epiphysis, tibial torsion, bowed legs, and symptoms of weight stress in the joints of the lower extremities (Moran, 1999). Pediatric studies suggest that obstructive sleep apnea occurs in approximately 17% of obese children and adolescents. Obstructive sleep apnea may be an important contributing factor to learning disability and school failure (Slyper, 1998). It is well recognized that atherosclerosis begins in childhood. Obesity in childhood or adolescence increases the likelihood of adult morbidity and mortality from atherosclerotic disease (Dietz, 1998).

Diagnostic Criteria

Schonfeld-Warden and Warden (1997) have found that primary care providers recognize and initiate treatment in less than 20% of obese children. The most commonly used anthropometric indexes for assessing the degree of overweight in children is weight-for-height. After weighing and measuring the child, the provider plots the measurements on a growth chart from the National Center for Health Statistics for comparison with the "standard."

▲ **Clinical Warning:** If the child's weight for height is above the 90th percentile on the growth chart, the child is considered obese.

● **Clinical Pearl:** The weight-for-height method does not consider that some children may be overweight because of increased lean body mass. Measuring skinfold thickness can help make this distinction. Skinfold thickness can be performed at the triceps, biceps, axilla, midabdomen, subscapular, and suprailiac areas. Thickness above the 85th percentile for age and sex suggests obesity.

Assessing the child for central body fat also is important, because fat in this area is associated with a greater risk for developing hypertension, dyslipidemia, hyperinsulinemia (and subsequent type 2 diabetes), and cardiovascular disease. There are no reliable means of assessing childhood and adolescent visceral fat other than radiologically using magnetic resonance imaging. Waist circumference and trunk skinfold measurements, however, are suitable indicators of abdominal adipose tissue in children (Schonfeld-Warden & Warden, 1997).

Management

Despite the prevalence of obesity in children, relatively few treatment programs are available. The primary goal of treatment is for the child to achieve a weight closer to ideal without impairing growth. Other important goals in treating obese children include preventing the development of obesity comorbidities in adulthood, promoting long-lasting lifestyle modifications, and involving the entire family in healthy eating and physical activity (Williams, et al. 1997).

Diet

The use of weight maintenance versus weight loss to achieve weight goals depends on each patient's age, baseline BMI percentile, and presence of medical complications (Barlow & Dietz, 1998). In moderately obese children, a weight-maintenance program will normalize body weight because of future growth. This can be achieved by simply eliminating "junk food," including sugared sodas, juices, and excess milk in the diet. Milk products should be low- or non-fat. A weight-loss program is necessary for markedly obese children.

Depending on the child's age and medical condition, a balanced hypocaloric diet restricts the child's usual intake by 30% to 40%. The caloric distribution of the diet is as follows:

- 25% to 30% fat
- 50% to 55% complex carbohydrates
- 20% to 25% protein

This diet supports growth with slow reduction in weight and can be used in children as young as 5 years (Schonfeld-Warden & Warden, 1997).

Table 22–1.   CHARACTERISTICS OF IDIOPATHIC AND ENDOGENOUS OBESITY

Idiopathic Obesity	Endogenous Obesity
>90% of cases	<10% of cases
Tall stature (usually 50th percentile)	Short stature (usually fifth percentile)
Family history of obesity	Family history of obesity uncommon
Mental function normal	Mental impairment common
Normal or advanced bone age	Delayed bone age
Physical examination otherwise normal	Associated stigmata on physical examination

Adapted with permission from Williams, C. L., et al. (1997). Management of childhood obesity in pediatric practice. *Annals of the New York Academy of Science, 817,* 225–240.

▲ **Clinical Warning:** A safe rate of weight loss is 1 to 2 lb per week. Further restricting caloric intake in a child can be dangerous.

Exercise

Exercise is an essential component of the treatment of obesity in children. A realistic goal is for the child to decrease inactivity rather than to begin vigorous exercise routines. To achieve this goal, parents should provide rewards when the child decreases the time they spend watching television and playing computer games. Providers should suggest regular physical activity that is fun for the child and encourage family involvement. Families can experience good fun while walking, biking, or playing team games. When the family is involved in the weight-loss program, the efforts are more effective and last longer (Noonan, 1997).

Behavior modification is another very important component of the treatment of obesity in children. Self-monitoring increases children's awareness of when, where, why, what, and how much they eat. Even if self-report of food intake and activity is quantitatively inaccurate, it helps children learn how they may be using food to pacify inner feelings or to kill boredom. CBT alerts children to these triggers. CBT is effective for treating obese children, even without a strict dietary prescription (Braet, 1997). Providers should refer the child whose family is interested in pursuing CBT to a mental health professional skilled in its application with children and adolescents.

▲ **Clinical Warning:** The use of drug therapies for the treatment of obesity in children is limited and experimental. Surgical procedures should be avoided in children.

PREVENTION OF EATING DISORDERS IN CHILDREN AND ADOLESCENTS

Most weight-loss programs can produce short-term benefits. Attempts to treat obesity in children are of limited efficiency in the long run, except in specialized centers with highly competent workers with unusual dedication and tenacity. Despite national efforts to promote weight reduction, pediatric obesity is increasing. Eighty percent of obese adolescents become obese adults (Schonfeld-Warden & Warden, 1997).

Parents control most food choices available in the home. They also are role models for physical activity or its lack. Changing poor eating and exercise behaviors in parents may be one of the most effective ways to prevent eating disorders in children. Clinicians can provide parents with educational materials on nutrition and exercise, reminding them to send children to school with healthy lunches and snacks. They should counsel parents to avoid packing convenience foods, including sugary sodas and juices. Convenience foods are notoriously devoid of nutritional value, while being high in fat and empty calories. If feasible, a referral to a nutritionist may assist parents in understanding appropriate food choices for their growing child, while also helping them to determine normal portion sizes. Parental involvement in school policy-making about offerings in cafeterias and vending machines is also important.

Parents should avoid focusing on their child's looks. Providers should caution parents to avoid comments such as, "You are too fat," or "You are too thin," or even "You look great." Such remarks can encourage obsessions with body image. Instead, parents should redirect their focus toward their child's health and behavior. Comments such as, "I've noticed that you are skipping meals" or "I'm concerned for your health" can be helpful.

To prevent obesity, parents should avoid insisting that children finish every bottle or meal. Rather, they should respect their children's appetites. They should not use food for non-nutritive purposes, such as comfort or reward.

Schools are ideal settings for nutrition education. More than 50% of youths in the United States eat one of their three daily meals in school (MMWR, 1996). Schools should provide appealing, low-fat, low-sodium foods in vending machines. They should make an effort to serve healthy, well-balanced meals in the cafeteria. The school curriculum should include nutrition education from preschool through secondary school. Such education must be culturally relevant and fun. It should include participatory activities that involve social learning strategies and teach students how to use nutrition labels to make healthy food choices.

Coaches must de-emphasize weight. In working with coaches, providers can encourage them to avoid constantly weighing athletes. Coaches should not make comments about weight and should focus instead on areas such as strength and mental conditioning. Coaches, parents, and providers alike can all point to athletes who are models of fitness and wellness. Caring providers also stress to children, parents, coaches, and others never to ridicule children with eating disorders but to encourage their participation in team sports.

REFERRAL POINTS AND CLINICAL WARNINGS

Anorexia Nervosa

- Current adjunctive treatment of AN with fluoxetine is only recommended when evidence of a significant mood disturbance or OCD persists or emerges after weight restoration (Mayer & Walsh, 1998). Fluoxetine at 10 to 20 mg/d can be used. Close monitoring of side effects is recommended because of the physiologic disturbances associated with AN.
- Elevation of serum aminotransferase signals a critical, life-threatening condition associated with multiorgan failure and requires urgent calorie repletion.

Anorexia Nervosa and Bulimia Nervosa

- Providers should monitor use of fluoxetine for AN or BN closely, because of its side-effect profile and because it can exacerbate the physiologic side effects associated with BN.

Bulimia Nervosa

- Left undiagnosed and untreated, hypokalemia will lead to tetany, seizures, or lethal cardiac arrhythmia.

Obesity

- If the child's weight for height is above the 90th percentile on the growth chart, the child is considered obese.
- A safe rate of weight loss is 1 to 2 lb per week. Further restricting caloric intake in a child can be dangerous.
- Referral to a nutritionist may assist the parents in understanding appropriate food choices for their growing child, while also helping them to determine normal portion sizes.

- The use of drug therapies for the treatment of obesity in children is limited and experimental.
- Surgical procedures should be avoided in children.
- The provider should refer the child whose family is interested in pursuing CBT to a mental health professional who is skilled in its application with children and adolescents.

COMMUNITY RESOURCES

Providers should encourage the parents of children with eating disorders to contact appropriate local agencies that deal with the specific illness. These agencies assist with education, research, cure, and prevention efforts related to these illnesses. They provide free self-help group meetings for children, parents, and siblings and send newsletters to members. For nationwide referrals for children who have anorexia, bulimia, or obesity, contact the following:

The American Anorexia/Bulimia Association, Inc.
165 W. 46th Street #1108
New York, NY 10036
(212) 575-6200
http://www.aabainc.org

The American Obesity Association
1250 24th Street N.W., Suite 300
Washington, DC 20037
(800) 98-OBESE
http://www.obesity.org/who.html

Many print resources are available for children from preschool to junior high regarding body awareness and prevention of eating disorders. The following is a sample:

Preschool Age

- *Fat, Fat Rose Marie,* by Lisa Passen, New York, Henry Holt and Company 1991.

Young Readers through Junior High

- *Am I Fat? Helping Young Children Accept Differences in Body Size,* by Joanne Ikeda, MA RD, and Priscilla Naworski, MS CHES. ETR Associates, (800)-321-4407, PO Box 1830, Santa Cruz, CA 950619.
- *Nell's Quilt,* by Susan Terris, New York, Farrar, Straus, and Giroux, 1987.
- *The Pig-Out Blues,* by Jan Greenberg, New York, Farrar, Straus, and Giroux, 1982.
- *Good Answers to Tough Questions About Weight Problems and Eating Disorders,* by Joy Berry, Chicago, Children's Press, 1990.

REFERENCES

Allison, D. B., & Faith, M. S. (1997). Issues in mapping for eating disorders. *Psychopharmacology Bulletin, 33*(3), 359–368.

Andersen, A. E., & Holman, J. E. (1997). Males with eating disorders: Challenges for treatment and research. *Psychopharmacology Bulletin, 33,* 391–397.

Attia, E., Haiman, C., Walsh, B.T., & Flater, S.R. (1998). Does fluoxetine augment the inpatient treatment of anorexia nervosa? *American Journal of Psychiatry, 155*(4), 548–551.

Bar-Or, O., Foreyt, J., Borechard, C., et al. (1998). Physical activity, genetic, and nutritional considerations in childhood weight management. *Medic Sci Sports Exerc, 30*(1), 2–10.

Barlow, S. E., & Dietz, W. H. (1998). Obesity evaluation and treatment: Expert committee recommendations. The Maternal and Child Health Bureau, Health Resources and Services Administration and the Department of Health and Human Services. *Pediatrics, 102*(3), e29.

Birmingham, C. L., Golder, E. N., & Bakon, R. (1994). Controlled trial of Zinc supplementation in anorexia nervosa. *International Journal of Eating Disorders, 15*(3), 251–255.

Braet, C., Van Winkle, M., Van Leeuwen, K., (1997). Follow-up results of different programs for obese children. *Acta Peaediatrica, 86*(4), 397–402.

Bryant-Waugh, R., & Lask, B. (1995). Annotation: Eating disorders In children. *Journal of Child Psychology, 36*(2), 191–202.

Centers for Disease Control and Prevention. (1998). Youth risk behavior surveillance B US 1997. *Morbidity and Mortality Weekly Report, August 14,* 47(SS-3).

Chagnon, Y. C., Perusse, L., & Weisnagel, S. J., et al. (1998). The human obesity gene map: The 1997 update. *Obesity Research, 6*(1), 76–92.

Cheng, T. O. (1997). Mitral valve prolapse in patients with anorexia nervosa. *American Family Physician, 56*(1), 52, 55.

Crow, S. J., Salisbury, J. J., Crosby, R. D., et al. (1997). Serum electrolytes as markers of vomiting in bulimia nervosa. *International Journal Eating Disorders, 21*(1), 95–98.

Daluiski, A., Rahbar, B., & Meals, R. A., (1997). Russell's Sign. Subtle hand changes in patients with bulimia nervosa. *Clinical Orthopedics, 343,* 107–109.

Dietz, W. H. (1998). Childhood weight affects adult morbidity and mortality. *Journal of Nutrition, 128*(2 Suppl), 411S–414S.

Draper, H. (1998). Treating anorexics without consent: Some reservations. *Journal of Medical Ethics, 24*(1), 5–7.

Fujimoto, S., Invi, A., Kiyoto, N., et al. (1997). Increased cholecystokinin and pancreatic polypeptide responses to a fat-rich meal in patients with restrictive but not bulimic anorexia nervosa. *Biological Psychiatry, 41*(10), 1068–1070.

Gorwood, P., Bouvard, H., Moren-Simeon, M. C., et al. (1998). Genetics and anorexia nervosa: A review of candidate genes. *Psychiatric Genetics, 8*(1), 1–12.

(1996). Guidelines for school health programs to promote lifelong healthy eating. *Morbidity and Mortality Weekly Report, 45*(RR-9), 1-33.

Halmi, K., et al. (1993). Anorexia and bulimia: You can help. *Patient Care, 27*(6), 24–52.

Hotta, M., Shibasaki, T. Sato, K., & Denura, H., (1998). The importance of body weight history in the occurrence and recovery of osteoporosis in patients with anorexia nervosa. *European Journal of Endocrinology, 139*(3), 276–283.

Jimeson, D. C., Wolfe, B. E., Metzger, E. D., et al. (1997). Decreased serotonin function in bulimia nervosa. *Archives of General Psychiatry, 54*(6), 529–534.

Kaye, W. H. (1998). The role of the central nervous system in the psychoneuroendocrine disturbance of anorexia and bulimia nervosa. *Psychiatric Clinics of North America, 21*(2), 381–396.

Keller, C., & Stevens, K. (1996). Assessment, etiology, and intervention in obesity in children. *Nurse Practitioner, 21*(9), 31–42.

Lazarus, R., Baur, L., Webb, K., et al. (1996). Body mass index in screening for adiposity in children and adolescents: Systematic evaluation using receiver operating characteristic curves. *American Journal of Clinical Nutrition, 63,* 500.

Lilenfeld, L. R., Kaye, W. H., Greeno, C. G. et al. (1998). A controlled family study of anorexia nervosa and bulimia nervosa: Psychiatric disorders in first degree relatives and effects of proband comorbidity. *Archives of General Psychiatry, 55*(7), 603–610.

Mayer, L. E., & Walsh, B. T. (1998). The use of selective serotonin reuptake inhibitors in eating disorders. *Journal of Clinical Psychiatry, 59*(Suppl 15), 28–34.

Mcgilley, B. M., & Pryor, T. L. (1998). Assessment and treatment of bulimia nervosa. *American Family Physician, 57*(11), 2743–2750.

Mehler, P. S., & Weiner, K. A. (1995). Treatment of anorexia nervosa with total parenteral nutrition. *Nutrition Clinical Practice, 10*(5), 183–187.

Mental Health Commission. (1997). *Guidance on the treatment of anorexia under the Mental Health Act 1983.* London: HMSO.

Moran, R. (1999). Evaluation and treatment of childhood obesity.

American Family Physician, 59(4), 861–868.

Neumarker, K. J., et. al. (1997). Mortality and sudden death in anorexia nervosa. *International Journal of Eating Disorders, 21*(3), 205–212.

Noonan, S. S. (1997). Children and obesity: Flunking the fat test. *New Jersey Medicine, 94*(6), 49–51.

Ozawa, Y., Shimizu, T., & Shishiba, Y. (1998). Elevation of serum aminotransferase as a sign of multiorgan disorders in severely emaciated anorexia nervosa. *Internal Medicine, 37*(1), 32–39.

Pawluck, D. E., & Gorey, K. M. (1998). Secular trends in the incidence of anorexia nervosa: Integrative review of population-based studies. *International Journal of Eating Disorders, 23,* 347–352.

Pierce, J. W., & Wardle, J. (1997). Cause and effect beliefs and self-esteem of overweight children. *Journal of Child Psychology and Psychiatry, 38*(6), 645–650.

Robin, A. L., Gilroy, M., & Dennis, A. B., et al. (1998). Treatment of eating disorders in children and adolescents. *Clinical Psychology Review, 18*(4), 421–446.

Rytomaa, I., Jarvinen, V., Kanerva, R., & Heinomen, O. P., (1998). Bulimia and tooth erosion. *Acta Odontologica Sandinavica, 56*(1), 36–40.

Schmidt, U., Tiller, J., , Blanchard, M., et al. (1997). Is there a specific trauma precipitating anorexia nervosa? *Psychology and Medicine, 27*(3), 523–30.

Schonfeld-Warden, N., & Warden, C. H. (1997). Pediatric obesity. An overview of etiology and treatment. *Pediatric Clinics of North America, 44*(2), 339–361.

Slyper, A. H. (1998). Childhood obesity, adipose tissue distribution, and the pediatric practitioner. *Pediatrics, 102*(1), e4.

Stone, N. J. (1994). Secondary causes of hyperlipidemia. *Medical Clinics of North America, 78*(1), 117–141.

Strober, M., Freeman, R., DeAntonio, M., et al. (1997). Does adjunctive fluoxetine influence the post-hospital course of restrictor-type anorexia nervosa? *Psychopharmacology Bulletin, 33*(3), 425–431.

Walsh, B. T., & Devlin, M. J. (1998). Eating disorders: Progress and problems. *Science, 280*(5368), 1387–1390.

Whitaker, R. C., & Dietz, W. H. (1998). Role of the prenatal environment in the development of obesity. *Journal of Pediatrics, 132*(5), 768–776.

Williams, C. L., Campanero, L.A., Squillace, M., & Bollella, M., (1997). Management of childhood obesity in pediatric practice. *Annals of the New York Academy of Science, 817,* 225–240.

C H A P T E R 23

Abuse

- PHILIP W. HYDEN, MD, JD; JAMIE HOFFMAN-ROSENFELD, MD; CATHERINE KOVEROLA, PhD;
  MARY MORAHAN, LCSW, MSW; and LEAH HARRISON, MS, C-PNP

P A R T 1 ▲

Maltreatment and Failure-to-Thrive

- PHILIP W. HYDEN, MD, JD

INTRODUCTION

The field of child abuse investigation is of growing importance for pediatric primary care providers, with clinicians treating an overwhelming number of cases in the past decade. Primary care providers increasingly are being acknowledged as indispensable components of child advocacy teams and recognized experts in the field. This chapter provides a foundation for understanding what is meant by child maltreatment, which includes physical abuse. Bruises, burns, fractures, head trauma, and abdominal trauma are the most common types of injuries involved in physical abuse. The material discusses the criteria that constitute neglect. It also presents information about failure-to-thrive (the result of intentional nutritional deprivation) and statutory mandates for provider reporting. The chapter also provides content meant to assist clinicians in discerning potential or actual abuse from clinical presentations that are not related to abuse.

▲ Clinical Warning: As generalists, primary care providers need awareness of the basic principles for recognizing and reporting child abuse. All 50 U.S. states and many westernized countries consider providers to be mandated reporters. Aside from ethical considerations, providers outside the United States should acquaint themselves with their national or regional statutory regulations. Cultural conflicts can arise when parents of a different culture relocate to a country that considers their ethnic childrearing practices abusive. Providers should endeavor to acquaint such parents with accepted disciplinary norms in the adopted country to avoid possible charges of child abuse.

Identification criteria demand that within their professional scope, providers report child abuse or maltreatment immediately if they suspect that either has occurred or if a child would be in imminent danger were reporting delayed. Statutory requirements subject providers who violate their mandated responsibility to specific penalties,

both civil and criminal. The law also protects them with tort immunity if they make a report in good faith, even if incorrect. Primary care providers must be able to recognize the signs and symptoms of child maltreatment, even if children do not make up the majority of patients they see in their practice. In addition to clinical practice, providers may come into contact with children in waiting areas or examining rooms.

CHILD MALTREATMENT

Child maltreatment encompasses several categories of abuse and neglect. The child abuse statutes of some jurisdictions combine excessive corporal punishment and neglect under the heading of maltreatment, distinguishing these acts from physical or sexual abuse. Other jurisdictions combine all actions or omissions against children as either abuse or maltreatment, including failure-to-thrive.

The primary care provider may be the first individual to recognize a child in distress, especially when triage is in the emergency department (ED) rather than the private office or general clinic. Providers need to understand and anticipate warning signs and behaviors that may warrant intervention.

Maltreatment involves neglect of a child's medical, nutritional, educational, or emotional needs. Behaviors of the child that may indicate but are not diagnostic of abuse or neglect include sudden behavioral changes, sleep or eating disorders, recent onset of bed wetting or thumb sucking, and school-related problems. Long-term effects of maltreatment can lead to low self-esteem, depression, and suicide. Many older children and adolescents will exhibit runaway behavior, promiscuity, or substance abuse.

Abuse

Reports of child abuse are very high, with some statistics showing approximately 4 million cases per year. Recently, the U.S. Department of Health and Human Services (1999) estimated that out of 3.2 million reported cases in 1997, substantiated cases decreased to fewer than 1 million. Possible explanations for the decrease include an improved economy and a decline in the use of crack and cocaine, but no clear reasoning for this change has emerged. A recent study suggests, however, that death from child abuse may be under-reported by as much as 60%. These findings were based on a retrospective review of medical examiner data, wherein the state vital records system under-recorded children who died from battering or abuse (Herman-Giddens et al., 1999). Worldwide, child abuse numbers are staggering. Recent estimates show that 40 million children from ages newborn to 14 years are abused or neglected (McMenemy, 1999).

For severe physical abuse, children younger than 2 years are most likely to suffer major trauma. Child abuse is a leading cause of death in infants. In a study linking birth and death certificates of all U.S. births between 1983 and 1991, half the homicides occurred by the fourth month of life. Perpetrator risk factors included the following:

- Maternal age younger than 15 years for a first birth or younger than 17 years for a subsequent birth
- No prenatal care
- Mother who had fewer than 12 years of education

Mothers were more likely to be abuse perpetrators in children who died within the first week of life. Fathers or stepfathers were more likely to be abuse perpetrators in children who died after the first week until age 3 years. After age 3 years, children were more likely to be victims of an unrelated perpetrator. Risk factors for infant victims included low birth weight, low gestational age, male sex, and low Apgar scores (Overpeck, Brenner, Trumble, Trifiletti, & Berendes, 1998).

Diagnostic Criteria

The differential diagnosis for bruising should include the presence of birth-related cutaneous manifestations, such as mongolian spots. In this case, the provider should question the historian in a non-leading manner. (ie, "How long has the mark been present?"). In cases of significant unexplained bruising, the clinician may need to rule out a bleeding disorder, such as idiopathic thrombocytopenic purpura, Henoch-Schönlein purpura, hemolytic-uremic syndrome, von Willebrand's disease, or classic hemophilia.

History and Physical Examination

Whether in the ED or pediatric clinic, the primary care provider may observe behavioral indicators that can help to identify abuse. If the child's caregiver is the suspected perpetrator, the clinician should observe the interaction carefully between the child and the adult. Even though nonspecific, a child's fear or a caregiver's hostility may be subtle clues to an underlying problem.

Any part of the child's body can be an abuse target, so the provider needs to complete a thorough physical examination before determining if a child has been injured. In some cases, internal organs may be affected without any evidence of superficial injury, so more invasive studies may need to be performed to rule out abuse.

● **Clinical Pearl:** Symptoms are important in cases of child abuse, because overt clues may not be readily apparent.

Fantuzzo, Weiss, et al. (1998) assessed maltreated children attending Head Start. They found that children with a history of maltreatment had decreased peer play interaction. The researchers interpreted this finding to indicate a decreased ability to respond positively to others. These children also did not show empathy in response to peer distress, were unable to solve social problems, and avoided conflicts. Teachers observed maltreated children to show decreased self-control in social interactions and to display fewer interpersonal skills than their nonmaltreated peers. The maltreated children were identified negatively more often than their peers, and they exhibited more internalizing adjustment problems, such as withdrawal and sadness. Abused children appeared to use approach-avoidance conflicts nondiscriminantly, preventing potentially ameliorative relationships from forming and thus increasing the risk for social isolation and further withdrawal (Fantuzzo, Weiss, et al., 1998).

▲ **Clinical Warning:** These behavioral indicators also may suggest sexual abuse. Any of these indicators, however, may be nonspecific and are not diagnostic of maltreatment. Refer to Part 2 for more information.

History taking is essential in determining what may have happened to a child. Beyond the actual event described as the cause of injury, the interviewer needs to assess possible risk factors through general questioning. Topics should include the following:

- Familial history of abuse or excessive corporal punishment
- Cultural or familial practices (eg, some parents use corporal punishment to enforce discipline)
- Teen parenthood
- Drug misuse
- Socioeconomic data, including lack of economic or emotional support or unemployment

▲ **Clinical Warnings:**

- The provider should evaluate the age-appropriateness of the child's behaviors carefully, because the child's developmental capabilities may not fit the scenario the family presents as the cause of the injury. Additionally, in many cases of child abuse, parents may blame a sibling for serious injury to another child. This should raise suspicion that the actual perpetrator is attempting to avoid or is being shielded from discovery.
- Interviewing the child separately from the caregiver or other individual who brings in the child for evaluation is essential. Discrepant or inconsistent histories are suspicious. Delay in seeking health care also may be an indicator that a caregiver deliberately injured a child, in that the caregiver prevented treatment to obscure possible disclosure or discovery of an intentional injury. Previous visits to other hospitals or clinics for similar problems also should increase a provider's suspicion that a caregiver prevented a case from being reported or that the caregiver may have Munchausen syndrome by proxy. Though relatively rare, this latter scenario arises when a caregiver attempts to gain attention by harming his or her child (ie, the caregiver's proxy).
- Providers should remind all parents, including immigrants whose discipline practices may be seen as excessive by the host country, that where their family now lives determines the appropriateness of the punishment, not their cultural heritage or country of origin. It is imperative that clinicians be culturally sensitive to differences, discussing appropriate discipline practices in the host country without denigrating the parents' ethnic practices. Practitioners must reinforce the need for safe and child-centered discipline that is neither excessive nor abusive by the host country's standards.

● **Clinical Pearl:** Optimally, the provider should interview the child alone. He or she should ask both caregivers and child open-ended, nonjudgmental, and objective questions. He or she also should contact the referring hospital, law enforcement agency, or social worker to learn about any other history. This information may be helpful both in gaining additional information and also uncovering possible discrepancies.

The diagnosis of physical abuse frequently is based on the presence of injuries to the child, which are apparent through physical examination or radiographs. The provider who encounters a child dressed in inappropriate clothing for the season should investigate the youngster's physical status thoroughly. An example is a child wearing long sleeves on a hot summer day. The child or family may be using such a shirt to hide a bruise on the arm. Conversely, a child dressed in a snowsuit during the winter should occasion no initial suspicion. When the child is sitting in a warm waiting room still dressed for outdoors, however, the provider needs to be especially vigilant in assessing the child's status, even if the child is not the patient he or she is treating.

▲ **Clinical Warning:** If assessment reveals that a child's well-being or safety is threatened, the provider needs to ensure placement of the child in protective custody. The steps to follow for initiating protective custody vary among jurisdictions. Providers should acquaint themselves with statutory and institutional policies. In the extreme case in which a clinician believes a child's life to be in danger, he or she must take steps to remove the child from the environment immediately and, if necessary, admit the child to the hospital.

The following discussion describes specific injuries that providers may observe while examining a child who may have been abused.

Bruises

Most injuries involve the skin, with bruises being the most frequent finding. The following are sites where bruises may be inflicted rather than accidental:

- Buttocks and lower back
- Genitals and inner thighs
- Cheeks, ear lobes, upper lip, and frenulum
- Neck

When clinicians note bruises, they should measure them and document findings on the appropriate clinic sheet, with any accompanying "fill-in" anatomic diagrams. Several types of bruises may have a certain configuration or pattern. Human hands can leave a variety of markings, such as oval grab marks from fingertip compression, trunk encirclement marks from the hand grasping the pelvic girdle and abdomen tightly, linear marks on the face from slapping, resulting in the appearance of individual finger marks, and hand prints or pinch marks.

▲ **Clinical Warning:** Bite marks are sometimes visible and are of serious concern if an adult inflicted them. To distinguish a bite injury caused by an adult rather than a child, the provider must be able to delineate the intercanine distance of the maxillary bite impression. The primary maxillary canines of children are normally less than 3 cm apart; the upper central incisors of adults are much wider. The measurement alone is not sufficient to identify a possible perpetrator, however. Clinicians need to evaluate the location, shapes, and size of individual teeth and the configuration of the entire bite impression (Feldman, 1997). Bites by dogs and other carnivorous animals usually tear through skin, whereas human bites compress the tissue, causing abrasions, contusions, and lacerations but rarely avulsions of flesh (Committee on Child Abuse and Neglect, 1999)

Strap marks may appear as linear bruises from belts or whips or as loop marks from electrical cords. Sometimes the marks may be rather bizarre and in a pattern, as from a blunt instrument, a homemade tattoo, circumferential tie marks, or gag marks.

An indicator of chronic abuse is the presence of multiple bruises at different stages of resolution. Bruises may resolve at different times based on severity, location, and depth of hemorrhage. Classically, bruises are tender, swollen, and purple, red, or blue when they are new, changing from green to yellow to brown as they resolve. Wide variations and differences exist, however, in interpretation of color and age. The provider must differentiate between an old and a more acute injury (Stephenson & Bialas, 1996).

Accidental bruises often occur over bony prominences, such as the forehead, knees, and shins. Children also can scratch themselves and, in rare cases, self-mutilate. Cultural markings may result from folk medical practices or rites of developmental passage. Depending on the mechanism of injury, some of these markings are relatively benign, but clinicians need to evaluate each case individually to determine if the family is neglecting health care or subjecting the child to a harmful practice. An example is cao gio, an Asian remedy for pulmonary illness that involves rubbing a coin on the child's body, creating a linear, petechial rash. Cupping, a remedy that uses an inverted hot cup to apply suction to the chest and back, produces lesions similar to those of coin rubbing. Providers should instruct parents how to render safe and effective health care, while informing them of possible consequences if they continue these practices.

● **Clinical Pearl:** Phytophotodermatitis is an anecdotal skin finding sometimes mistaken for child abuse. This cutaneous manifestation is the result of activation of a chemical compound in plant substances exposed to ultraviolet light, which creates a pattern on the skin. Providers can mistakenly diagnose both burns and bruises in a child who presents with this phenomenon. The plants most likely to cause this reaction are lemons, limes, celery, and parsnips. One scenario involved a father making Margaritas with fresh squeezed lime juice while simultaneously attempting to keep his young toddler away from the swimming pool during a barbecue. Brown lines resembling handprints under the axillae and around the waist of the child were evident a day later, following sun exposure. Because a detailed history was obtained, the family was spared a lengthy investigation.

If clinicians suspect a medical cause for bruising, they should order coagulation studies, such as prothrombin time, partial thromboplastin time, fibrinogen, fibrin-split products, bleeding time, and platelet count. Refer to Chapter 42 for more information on diagnosis and management of these common problems.

▲ **Clinical Warning:** An important concept to remember is that child abuse can exist concurrently with a coagulopathy.

Burns

The primary care provider may observe burns in the ED, burn unit, or clinic. In addition to accidental burns caused by scalding, contact, chemical, electrical, and fire sources, burns also may be intentional. Burns comprise 10% to 25% of all cases of child abuse, with scalds from tap water being the most common intentional burn injury (Feldman, 1997). In determining a burn's etiology, it is important to identify the following:

- Configuration
- Location
- Distribution
- Severity
- Uniformity

Whether a burn is circumferential or linear helps to distinguish an immersion burn from a contact burn. Immersion burns usually result from a triggering event that somehow offended, frustrated, or angered the perpetrator. Either because of malicious intent or neglect, the perpetrator places the child in a tub or sink with hot water directly from the faucet. Many adults and most children do not realize the danger of hot water. Stocking-feet and gloved-hand burn configurations are observed in this type of inflicted injury, as are circumferential trunk burns and "doughnut-shaped" burns on the buttocks from contact with the cool porcelain tub surface. A burn located exclusively on the buttocks implies an injury resulting from discipline after a toileting accident. Deeply excavated circular burns on the feet render the image of an angry caregiver repeatedly applying a cigarette to the child's feet. A pour burn with an arrowhead or triangular configuration will be that shape because, as liquid cools, it does so from the outside to the center. Gravity forces the liquid to move downward, creating the pattern.

● **Clinical Pearls:**

- Whether a child could have self-inflicted a burn depends on the child's length, not height. The provider must ascertain the maximum length a child can attain to reach an object—his or her arm span and leg length with foot flexed (tiptoe).
- If the burn is anterior on the lower face and chest in the arrowhead configuration, the child may have pulled hot liquid directly onto himself or herself. If the back is burned, however, it is unlikely that the child was able to self-inflict this injury.

In 1997, 24,000 children were seen in EDs for scalds. Hot water directly from the tap accounts for nearly 25% of all scald burns among children (U.S. Health and Human Services, 1999). Children younger than 5 years and adults older than 65 years are at highest risk for scalds because of their age-related inability to make a swift decision about the water's temperature, decreased ability to ambulate, developmental limitations in the elderly, and decreased sensation.

▲ **Clinical Warning:** Most infants are comfortable bathing in water that is 101°F. Hot tubs are usually between 104°F and 108°F. Adults perceive water greater than 109°F as painfully hot but will not sustain severe burns at temperatures below 120°F. At 114°F, it takes approximately 6 hours to sustain a split thickness burn. The rate of burns increases rapidly after 130°F, in which it takes 35 seconds to cause a deep second-degree burn in an adult's skin. It takes only 10 seconds to cause the same severity of burn in a preschooler. At 140°F, it takes 5 seconds for an adult and 1 second for a child to sustain the same degree of burn (Feldman, 1997).

About 30 years ago, the U.S. Consumer Products Safety Commission and hot water heater manufacturers reached a voluntary agreement to have a normal setting of 120°F. Once out of the factory, however, appliance temperature easily can be increased. Few municipalities enforce 120°F as the safest maximum temperature. Solutions to this problem are obvious. Recently, ordinances have established maximum temperature settings in designated housing, for example, by installing expensive pressure-valve components. These devices prevent sudden bursts of scalding water from diverted flow. More practically, inexpensive heat-sensitive metal alloy fixtures are available, which stop water flow if the temperature exceeds 119°F. Although not directly addressing the housing most in need, including older and poorly maintained units, this type of governmental intervention recognizes the need for child safety and has effectively reduced the incidence of scald-related injuries and deaths secondary to hot tap water (U.S. Health and Human Services, 1999).

Fractures

Fractures are important components of abuse. Certain types of skeletal injury are of increased concern because they do not occur commonly by simple, short falls. Spiral fractures, although not pathognomonic of abusive injury, are worrisome. These injuries result from a twisting mechanism, leaving a corkscrew configuration of fracture on an anteroposterior and lateral radiograph. This injury can occur when an ambulating child falls because of planted foot, which then twists and breaks or when the child is running and suddenly slips, twisting the leg. In nonambulating infants, this type of injury can occur by a perpetrator grasping and wrenching the femur forcibly during a diaper change (Kleinman, 1998).

▲ **Clinical Warning:** Spiral fractures are of concern in a child younger than 3 years because of the amount of force required for their occurrence.

Metaphyseal avulsion fractures are of great concern because of the physical mechanism involved in their origin. The lack of mineralization weakens the bone's integrity at this location, making it very susceptible to shearing forces. The torsion and whiplash effect of a child being vigorously shaken and the isolated twisting above and below a joint cause this type of injury. Metaphyseal avulsion fractures are a highly specific result of maltreatment (Spivak, 1992).

Rib fractures in children most commonly result from child abuse. Sustained, intense compression directed toward the chest, not blunt trauma, causes rib fractures. The mechanism of these fractures is consistent with a young infant being grasped compressively around the chest and then shaken or thrown (Spivak, 1992).

Most rib fractures are not detected acutely and are only visualized on plain radiographs after callus formation. When force is applied to the posterior ribs, the bending is against the transverse process, which protects the side of the applied force. Such force causes tensile failure on the rib's opposite side. The intact posterior cortex prevents displacement and decreases the visibility of an acute fracture, especially on frontal radiographs. In these cases, a bone scan may reveal an otherwise hidden injury (Spivak, 1992).

● **Clinical Pearl:** CPR is not considered the cause of rib fractures in infants, regardless of the resuscitative provider's experience. The mechanism of rib fractures is one of sustained intense compression around the chest rather than anterior pressure on the sternum.

Skull fractures can be either accidental or abuse-related, but certain features help to delineate the etiology. These features include the velocity or acceleration of impact, height of a fall, presence of any forces other than gravity that increased the velocity or acceleration, and any pathology that may decrease bone strength.

▲ **Clinical Warning:** Although no minimum height has been adequately established that would cause a linear skull fracture, falls less than 30 in do not appear to do so. Initial velocity before the fall increases the force of impact, suggesting the likelihood of high-energy pathology.

Head Trauma

Intracranial injury, the source of the most severe sequellae of abuse, generally is accepted as responsible for at least 50% of deaths in children caused by nonaccidental trauma. Children are anatomically at risk until age 4 years, with most injuries occurring in infants. Severe shaking of an infant has been coined "shaken baby syndrome." This injury causes sudden accelerative-decelerative forces to shear internal vessels, leading to subdural hematomas and retinal hemorrhages. Duhaime et al. (1992) postulated that blunt head trauma also was required to produce the severe forces needed to cause significant injury, leading to the term "shaken-impact syndrome."

Important mechanisms that can help the provider to ascertain the presence of subdural hematomas include computed tomography (CT) scan, which can delineate acute hemorrhage. Magnetic resonance imagery (MRI) can be used to discern acute, subacute, and chronic hemorrhage. MRI detects blood breakdown components and, based on particular weighted images, may be able to differentiate blood from cerebrospinal fluid and possibly determine the age of hemorrhage. Ophthalmoscopy can reveal the presence of retinal hemorrhages. If suspicions of abuse are present in a child younger than 2 years, both a skeletal survey and an ophthalmoscopic examination are important tools to help rule out nonaccidental trauma.

A rare but important disease entity that can predispose a patient to having subdural hematomas and retinal hemorrhages with minimal trauma is glutaric aciduria type 1 (GA1). This autosomal recessive, inborn error of metabolism is caused by deficiency of the enzyme glutaryl-CoA dehydrogenase. Macrocephaly, bilateral frontotemporal atrophy or widening of the Sylvian fissure, and subdural effusions are the clinical manifestations of GA1. No skeletal abnormalities have been reported, so GA1 does not predispose a child to fractures. Additionally, if a subdural hematoma is present without coexistent frontotemporal atrophy, GA1 is probably not present. This information is important to consider when confronted with the multiple clinical symptoms of the disease so that in an investigation of suspected child abuse, clinicians can appropriately exclude GA1 (Morris et al., 1999).

Abdominal Injury

Generally abdominal injuries are accepted as the second most common cause of death in physically abused children, with greatest risk between ages 2 and 4 years (Canty & Brown, 1999). Symptoms include abdominal pain, nausea, recurrent vomiting, abdominal distention, absent bowel sounds, and localized tenderness. More severe symptoms on presentation may include ileus, hematemesis, hematochezia, hematuria, peritonitis, and hemorrhagic shock. Because the abdominal wall is flexible, the internal organs usually absorb the force of the blow, so overlying skin typically may be free of bruises. Specific injuries include ruptured liver or spleen, the most common organs injured secondary to blunt trauma. Less common are tears or hematomas of the small intestine at sites of ligamental support, such as the duodenum and proximal jejunum, which can lead to perforation or possible obstruction. Pancreatic chylous ascites and pseudocysts

have been reported, and hematuria may occur as a result of blunt trauma to the kidney (Johnson, 2000).

Typically, the caregiver postpones seeking medical attention. Thus, the child presents in an advanced stage of illness. Because the perpetrator denies the event that precipitated the injury, accurate clinical history data are lacking. Frequently, associated central nervous system injury further contributes to the difficulty and delay in diagnosis.

The most practical evaluation of this type of injury is first to obtain a detailed history of any possible blunt injury to the abdomen. The provider should then perform a careful physical examination, noting the presence or absence of skin bruising. A flat plate of the abdomen and a film in the lateral decubitus position may help to show ileus or peritoneal free air but may not reveal a significant acute injury. Better imaging modalities include both ultrasound and abdominal CT. A stool guaiac will reveal occult blood, and helpful laboratory tests include a complete blood count (CBC), amylase, lipase, and liver functions.

Neglect

The primary care provider often must determine if a child is obtaining adequate nurturing and support from parents or other caregivers. Families must meet minimum standards for health, education, shelter, and clothing. Sometimes families are not financially capable of offering certain elements to their child. Often, parents lack education or knowledge of available resources.

▲ **Clinical Warning:** If families refuse resources or intentionally deprive children of minimum standards, providers must notify child protection authorities. Religious motivation sometimes creates conflicts with health care intervention, yet most U.S. and Canadian laws protect children who require life-saving treatment.

Obtaining appropriate intervention for children who do not receive immunizations is difficult until they reach school age. At that time, the state may be able to intervene, because schools require immunizations before children may enter. If the parent does not permit immunizations, the school may not be able to admit the child, depending on individual state laws. In this instance, the parent will be neglecting the child proximally, depriving him or her of education.

The provider also must consider cases in which a child is injured accidentally but while left unsupervised or in which a child suffers an unintentional injury at a caregiver's hands. If these injuries were foreseeable, avoidable, and unreasonable, they would be classified as neglect resulting from inadequate supervision or lack of parenting.

Deaths secondary to motor vehicle accidents also may involve neglect for infants and toddlers who are not adequately restrained in appropriate seating. According to 1996 U.S. Vital Statistics Data, the largest accident subgroup in children ages 1 to 4 years were victims of motor vehicle accidents. More than 50% of these children were passengers at the time of death, and many were not properly restrained in a car seat (Spivak, 1998).

FAILURE-TO-THRIVE

Failure-to-thrive (FTT) traditionally has been divided into two realms—organic and nonorganic. This nomenclature is expanding into a more complex diagnostic system. The definition of nonorganic FTT originated from observations of inadequate maternal–child interaction. Outcomes were seen to include possible emotional deprivation, infant behavior abnormalities, and chronic undernutrition. This definition has evolved to possibly renaming FTT as growth failure secondary to a feeding skills disorder. The trend is to use the terminology "the syndrome formerly known as failure-to-thrive."

Three criteria describing FTT use traditional standard growth charts from the National Center of Health Statistics (Hamill et al., 1979):

- A child younger than 2 years whose weight is below 3% to 5% for age on more than one occasion
- A child younger than 2 years whose weight is less than 80% of ideal for age
- A child younger than 2 years whose weight crosses two major percentiles downward on a standardized growth grid, using 90%, 75%, 50%, 25%, 10%, and 5% as major percentiles

Note that exceptions to the above criteria exist:

- Children of genetic short stature
- Small-for-gestational age infants
- Preterm infants
- "Overweight" infants whose rate of height gain increases while rate of weight gain decreases
- Infants who are normally lean (Zenel, 1997)

Failure-to-thrive encompasses more than mere malnourishment. The provider needs to assess the overall home environment, because factors other than nutrition may be affected, including language development, reading, social maturity, behavior, and intelligence. To diagnose and differentiate FTT as related to malnutrition from other factors, several traditional methods are used that involve hospital admission to evaluate weight gain, laboratory testing, and separating etiology of FTT into organic or inorganic types (Zenel, 1997).

▲ **Clinical Warning:** In infants, daily weight gain of 15 to 30 g is considered adequate growth. Failure to achieve this change is an early indicator of malnutrition. By establishing this baseline at the first 2-week clinic visit and then following the child closely, the provider may be able to intervene earlier than the ordinary 2-month well-baby checkup (Gahagan & Holmes, 1998).

History and Physical Examination

Usually FTT occurs for several reasons. Most cases result from the caregiver's psychosocial problems involving child care, parent and child interactions, and mental health. As in every case involving abuse or neglect, the history is the most important tool available to assist in evaluating for FTT.

▲ **Clinical Warning:** Clinicians should investigate all possible causes of FTT, including an acute or chronic illness, feeding problems, and the child's behavior. He or she should distinguish between bottle feeding and breast-feeding. After obtaining the parent's impression of the child's intake and ability to feed, the provider should explain what the child requires.

● **Clinical Pearls:**

- Approximately eight feedings a day provide adequate nutrition for a breast-fed infant. The infant's suck and energy level during feedings are important clues to underlying disease or illness. If the child is bottle fed, type of formula, preparation, and amount are important to note. The provider should identify who feeds the child and the feeding schedule. For toddlers, the provider should ask about the frequency of feeding. Small children should eat six small meals a day and not sit for long periods at the table. Parents should restrict juices, sport and soft drinks, and "junk" foods, because they may cause appetite suppression or obesity.
- Taking a diet history depends on the caregiver's accuracy and integrity. Providing a narrative probably is not adequate, because faulty memory may cause a parent to overestimate the amount of foods a child ingested or to omit certain items. The best and preferred method for obtaining a dietary history is in writing. The parent writes down the child's food intake over 2 or 3 days, with one day being on a weekend. Rather than stating amounts in servings, the parent should record the number of tablespoons or slices of food placed on the plate and how much the child ate. Many parents will find it difficult to measure portions in ounces or cups; using an eating utensil as a measuring device will be easier (Gahagan & Holmes, 1998).

Providers must complete growth charts, including height, weight, and head circumference. They also should plot the parents' heights if possible. If head circumference, weight, and height are proportionately reduced, the child actually may have hereditary or congenital defects. Infants and children with normal head circumference and weight that is slightly reduced or proportionate to height may have an endocrine abnormality, genetic dwarfism, or constitutional growth delay (Marcovitch, 1994). Refer to Chapter 60 for further discussion.

● **Clinical Pearl:** Most infants with FTT have normal head circumference. Weight is reduced out of proportion to height because of malnutrition, malabsorption, or altered metabolism.

Diagnostic Studies

Laboratory testing is seldom needed when inadequate food intake is the most likely etiology, but in certain instances, such testing may be helpful. Examination of the stool, both macroscopically and microscopically, may reveal possible parasites, inflammatory bowel disease with presence of blood, diarrhea, sugar malabsorption, or colonic inflammation or infection by presence of leukocytes. A CBC will detect iron deficiency anemia. Urinalysis and urine cultures may assist in recognizing renal tubular acidosis and possible infection. The child may require hospitalization if he or she is considerably undernourished, abused, or has a specific medical condition requiring immediate intervention. If the admitted child begins to thrive with weight gain and favorable personality changes, a psychosocial rather than an underlying organic etiology may be present.

▲ **Clinical Warning:** If a youngster is admitted because of inadequate nutrition, the provider should document close monitoring of the family's interactions with the child during feedings. Philosophies about hospitalization are mixed. Many providers believe that the mother should be actively involved in the child's care and feeding while the child is in the hospital; others fear obfuscation of data if the mother, instead of nursing staff, feeds the child. Case-by-case management may be the best approach in guidelines regarding maternal participation in feeding.

In rare cases, a mother will intentionally deprive a child of food so that the infant will require medical attention. This scenario is an example of Munchausen syndrome by proxy, wherein a perpetrator, usually a mother, feigns or induces an illness in a child. She subsequently seeks medical attention, vicariously receiving gratification for the attention given to the child and herself.

● **Clinical Pearls:**

- Diagnosis of FTT is strongly supported if a child begins to thrive in the hospital, as evidenced by weight gain and favorable personality changes.
- Daily visits rather than hospitalization for investigation and observation of mother–child interaction may be more valuable, because the stigma to the parent may be decreased; the child will be less likely to contract an iatrogenic or nosocomial infection; and the parent will be actively involved with the ongoing evaluation. These factors possibly may contribute to a more positive outcome for the entire family.

Management

Whatever the plan, the primary care provider should remain active in the management process, even if intentional deprivation or neglect is considered the cause for malnutrition. Because of the problem's complexity, the provider is important in assisting the family with frequent follow-up visits, careful documentation of weight gain, and ongoing observation of parent–child interaction, noting improvements and success (Gahagan & Holmes, 1999).

ANTICIPATORY GUIDANCE

Providers must remember that anticipatory guidance is a mandatory component of a health visit. Besides offering preventive mechanisms, such as how to make a home or car safe, clinicians may ask questions about and identify certain stressful factors that a family should address. They can discuss with parents the use of corporal punishment versus other forms of discipline, offering resources to those who may need economic or therapeutic support.

If a child presents with signs or symptoms of abuse, neglect, or FTT, the provider must be aware of the mandated reporting laws in the state where he or she is treating the child and intervene immediately. Although the provider legally does not have to inform the family that he or she may file a report, he or she ethically is obligated to alert the family that a report is being made as part of his or her legal responsibility as a health provider.

● **Clinical Pearl:** An important message to deliver to the family is that the practitioner is acting on the child's behalf, not as an adversary to the family.

After the case is reported and the department of social services or law enforcement has initiated intervention, the provider may want to continue the child's health management and offer services to the family. In this way, the family may realize that the practitioner is attempting to preserve rather than dissolve the family's integrity. These visits may involve both primary care and psychosocial interventions. Scheduled visits should occur frequently and consistently. The Department of Social Services should know about these appointments and perhaps assign them as a component of the family's rehabilitation plan:

- For cases of abuse, providers can monitor resolution of injuries.
- For cases of neglect, providers can visualize improvement and progress.
- For cases of FTT, frequent visits can help providers evaluate growth, assist parents with improving their skills, and recognize the child's needs.

Hopefully, return clinic visits can provide a mechanism for positive reinforcement that will alter a parent's attitudes about the child, while rewarding parents for active efforts in improving relationships within the family. These efforts can help ensure that the child has a much safer and more caring home.

COMMUNITY RESOURCES

Provider Resources

American Academy of Pediatrics Task Force on Abuse and Neglect

National SAFE KIDS Campaign
1301 Pennsylvania Avenue
Suite 1000
Washington, DC 20004-1707
(202) 662-0600 voice
(202) 393-2072 fax
http://www.safekids.org

Other Resources

The following resources can assist both provider and family:

- Childhelp, U.S.A. 1 (800) 4-A-CHILD
- American Professional Society on Abuse of Children
- National Association of Child Abuse
- Parents Anonymous

REFERENCES

American Academy of Pediatric Dentistry, Committee on Child Abuse and Neglect, (1999). Oral and dental aspects of child abuse and neglect. *Pediatrics*, 104:348–350.

Canty, T. G., Sr., Canty, T. G., Jr., & Brown, C. (1999). Injuries of the gastrointestinal tract from blunt trauma in children: A 12-year experience at a designated pediatric trauma center. *Journal of Trauma-Injury Infection & Critical Care, 46*(2), 234–240.

Duhaime, A., Alario, A.J., Lewander, W.J., et al. (1992). Head injury in very young children: Mechanisms, injury types, and ophthalmologic findings in 100 hospitalized patients younger than 2 years of age. *Pediatrics, 90*(2).

Fantuzzo, J. W., Weiss, A. D., et al. (1998). A contextually relevant assessment of the impact of child maltreatment on the social competencies of low-income urban children. *Journal of the American Academy of Child and Adolescent Psychiatry, 37*(11), 1201–1208.

Feldman, K. W. (1997). Evaluation of physical abuse. In M. E. Helfer, R. S. Kempe, & R. D. Krugman (Eds.), *The battered child* (5th ed.). (pp. 175–220).

Gahagan, S., & Holmes, R., (1998). A stepwise approach to evaluation of undernutrition and failure to thrive. *Pediatric Clinics of North America, 45*(1). Chicago: University of Chicago Press.

Hamill, P. V., Drizd, T. A., Johnson, C. L., et al. (1979). Physical growth: National Center for Health Statistics percentiles. *American Journal of Clinical Nutrition, 32*, 607–629.

Herman-Giddens, M. E., Brown, G., et al. (1999). Underascertainment of child abuse mortality in the United States. *Journal of the American Medical Association, 282*(5), 463–467.

Johnson, C. F. (2000). *Abuse and neglect of children* (pp. 110-119). In Behrman, R. E., Lkiegman, R. M., & Jenseon, H. B. (eds). Nelson's textbook of pediatrics (16th ed.). Philadelphia: W. B. Saunders.

Kleinman, P. K. (1998). *Diagnostic imaging of child abuse* (2nd ed.) St. Louis: Mosby.

Marcovitch, H. (1994). Fortnightly review: Failure to thrive. *British Medical Journal*, 35–38.

McMenemy, M. C. (1999). WHO recognises child abuse as a major problem. *The Lancet, 353*(9161), 1340.

Morris, A. A., Hoffman, G. F., Naughton, E. R., et al. (1999). Glutaric aciduria and suspected child abuse. *Archives of Disease in Childhood, 80*(5), 404–405.

U.S. Health and Human Services. (1999). *National Safe Kids Campaign*. Washington, D.C.: Author.

Overpeck, M. D., Brenner, R. A., Trumble, A. C., Trifiletti, L. B., Berendes, H. W. (1998). Risk factors for infant homicide in the United States. *New England Journal of Medicine, 339,* 1222–1226.

Spivak, B. S. (1992). The biomechanics of nonaccidental injury. In S. L. Ludwig & A. E. Kornberg (Eds.), *Child abuse: A medical reference* (2nd ed.) New York: Churchill Livingston.

Stephenson, T., & Bialas, Y. (1996). Estimation of the age of bruising. *Archives of Disease in Childhood. 74*(1), 53–55.

Zenel, J. A. (1997). Failure to thrive: A general pediatricians' perspective. *Pediatrics in Review, 18*(11), 371–378.

P A R T   2   ▲

Sexual Abuse

- JAMIE HOFFMAN-ROSENFELD, MD, and
  LEAH HARRISON, MS, C-PNP

INTRODUCTION

Sexual abuse of girls and boys has occurred across time and in all races, cultures, societies, and socioeconomic backgrounds. Many misinformed people believe that sexual abuse of children is rare. It actually is a major health problem that often is unrecognized because children are unable to disclose that it happened or are not believed when they do tell. Often, primary care providers fail to recognize the signs and symptoms of sexual abuse in children.

PATHOLOGY

In 1977, C. Henry Kempe said that child sexual abuse is a hidden pediatric problem (1978). Though no longer "hidden," sexual abuse remains a significant issue. Providers need time, knowledge, experience, and understanding of the diagnosis to provide appropriate in-depth assessment of both girls and boys.

No definition of child sexual abuse has been universally accepted. Depending on the professional perspective (eg, legal, child protective) and the geographic region, the definition varies, compounding the problem of determining whether a child has been abused. The provider must be familiar with the definition of child abuse in his or her state or province, as well as the definitions of legal and child protection systems. In the United States, some states follow their social service laws, while others follow their penal laws. Laws may differ in their language and with respect to the ages of the victim and perpetrator, which are used to define their relationship.

Kempe (1978) defines child sexual abuse as "engaging a child in sexual activities that the child cannot comprehend, for which the child is developmentally unprepared and cannot give informed consent, and/or that violate the social and legal taboos of society" (p. 382). In a 1977 article, Brandt and Tisza describe sexual abuse as "exposure of a child to sexual stimulation inappropriate for the child's age, the level of psychosexual development, and the role in the family" (p. 80).

Frequently, families will verbalize their fears that their children are being or will be sexually abused at school or by a stranger. Parents will tell their children not to talk to strangers, warning them about being "snatched." Although these fears can be well grounded, primary care providers must teach parents to be more aware of the risk of sexual abuse by people who have easy access to their children. In most instances, perpetrators of sexual abuse are individuals known to children. The latest National Incidence Study (NIS) report states that a parent or parent-substitute is the perpertrator in approximately 50% of cases of sexual abuse (Sedlak & Broadhurst, 1996). In contrast, Elliott and Briere (1994) report that the perpetrator is a parent figure in only 25% of cases, while family members overall are guilty in about 50% of cases. They state that a stranger is responsible in only a very small percentage of cases.

In a 1980 study, approximately 22% of perpetrators were younger than 26 years at the time of the abuse and were predominately male (Finkelhor, 1980). This figure has not altered appreciably in intervening years (Sedlak & Broadhurst, 1996). Providers should note that even though females are not usually perpetrators, a small percentage of women sexually abuse children. Identifying perpetrators is difficult because they typically do not fit a uniform character profile. Siblings who abuse siblings often are unrecognized, even though reports have shown that sibling abuse is prevalent (Caffaro & Caffaro, 1998). Parents may not realize or may deny the possibility that one of their own children might be sexually abusing another child in the family. Refer to Part 3 for further discussion.

EPIDEMIOLOGY

The third NIS of Child Abuse and Neglect, based on a national sample of professionals and agencies serving 42 U.S. counties, cites that the annual incidence of sexual abuse doubled from 1986 to 1996 (Sedlak & Broadhurst, 1996). In the United States, 217,000 children were victims of sexual abuse, representing an 86% increase from the 1993 NIS report (Sedlak & Broadhurst, 1996). Providers should remember that this number represents only children who have disclosed sexual abuse or sought assistance. Thus, this statistic does not represent the true number of children who have been sexual abuse victims.

Many children never tell that they have been abused. NIS III reported that girls have been sexually abused three times more often than boys. The report found the age of abuse to be very broad, representing all age groups. Children younger than 3 years, however, comprised the smallest category (Sedlak & Broadhurst, 1996). Added to this alarming information is the finding that 6% to 62% of women and 3% to 30% of men were sexually abused as children (Finkerhor, 1994). The wide range can be explained partially by the varying definitions of sexual abuse used. A final, chilling fact is that a child who is disabled is at 1.75 times greater risk of being a victim of sex abuse (National Center on Child Abuse and Neglect, 1993).

The NIS III did not find race to be a significant determining factor for sexual abuse (Sedlak & Broadhurst, 1996). Sexual abuse occurs in all racial, ethnic, and cultural groups, though the recognition of abuse may differ in various groups. Sexual abuse is still a taboo diagnosis in most cultures. Children typically cannot disclose their abuse because they fear being ostracized by their family or society, and they fear retaliation. Finally, child sexual abuse occurs irrespective of income, although NIS III reported that children were 18 times more likely to be sexually abused when their family's annual income was less than $30,000.

HISTORY AND PHYSICAL EXAMINATION

A child victim may present for examination immediately after an acute sexual assault or may come to medical attention after disclosing sexual abuse later. A child also may present to a primary care provider for evaluation if a parent or other individual becomes concerned that the youngster has been abused. The local Department of Social Services, law enforcement, or the school system also may refer children for evaluation.

History

Primary care providers may not feel adequately prepared to perform a medical evaluation for sexual abuse; therefore, they need to be familiar with local community resources. The United States, Canada, and most westernized countries have child abuse laws mandating that clinicians concerned about or suspicious of sexual abuse in a child make a report to the appropriate authorities. All providers must be familiar with the laws in their own states and countries and the guidelines that determine how and when to make a report. Both law enforcement and local child protective agencies may need to be involved, depending on the details of the particular case. Different parts of the United States, Canada, and other countries have different guidelines as to who will interview the child. This does not preclude the practitioner from taking a standard pediatric history or from performing a routine physical examination.

As described in Part 3, many municipalities are developing multidisciplinary teams to provide a coordinated response to abuse, including child sexual abuse. Increasingly, the interview is conducted in a "joint interview" format that allows a "lead interviewer" to question the child while other professional team members observe, preferably from the other side of an observational mirror. By reducing the number of interviews to which they subject a child victim, professionals can minimize the trauma for the child of recounting painful events.

▲ Clinical Warning: When a child's initial disclosure of sexual abuse is to a primary care provider, the clinician should do a "minimal facts" medical interview so that the child receives necessary and appropriate health care. The practitioner should refrain from asking for details with only forensic value. Law enforcement, child protective services, or both inevitably will interview the child for forensic data at a later time.

A body of literature is growing on suggestibility in children and its implications for conducting "forensically sound" interviews. Not surprisingly, the younger the child, the more likely he or she is to acquiesce to false suggestions of sexual abuse. By the time children reach 10 or 11 years, they are no more suggestible than are adults. Display 23-1 provides interview suggestions and strategies based on the literature about interviewing children for a sexual abuse evaluation. The provider should conduct an age-appropriate interview without asking leading questions. Table 23-1 illustrates leading questions for examiners to avoid and open-ended questions for examiners to use when conducting this sensitive interview.

Physical Examination

The physical examination for sexual abuse has several goals:

- Identifying injuries that require treatment
- Targeting medical conditions (eg, sexually transmitted infections [STIs] and pregnancy) that require health care attention
- Gathering medical–legal evidence when present
- Preserving an unbroken chain of evidence
- Noting other signs of abuse and neglect

DISPLAY 23–1 • Strategies for Conducting an Interview When Evaluating for Sexual Abuse

- The interview setting should be one in which the child is comfortable.
- Interviewers should be friendly and approach the interview with an open mind.
- Interviewers should orient the child to the interview process, tell about other observers when appropriate, and question the child alone whenever possible.
- They should encourage the child to be truthful and not to pretend.
- They should explain to the child that they are uninformed and need the child to explain and clarify the facts.
- They should encourage the child to admit confusion or ignorance rather than guessing the answers to questions.
- They should tell the child that when a question is repeated, it does not mean that the answer was wrong the first time.
- They should give the child permission not to answer questions that are too difficult to discuss at the moment.
- They should encourage the child to correct interviewers if they misstate the facts.
- Questions should be developmentally appropriate for the child.
- Interviewers should avoid leading and coercive questions and repetitive questions.
- The interview should start with open-ended questions and proceed to more focused questions if necessary.
- Interviewers should document relevant questions and responses verbatim in the record.
- Interviewers should not display shock, disbelief, or surprise.
- Interview adjuncts, such as anatomically correct dolls, should be used only by professionals specifically trained in their use.

Adapted from Morgan, M. (1995). *How to interview sexual abuse victims.* (pp. 47–48). Thousand Oaks, CA: Sage Publications, and Reed, L. D. (1996). Findings from research on children's suggestibility and implications for conducting interviews. *Child Maltreatment, 1*(2), 105–120.

Table 23–1.   Examples of Leading Questions Versus Open-Ended Questions When Conducting the Evaluation Interview for Child Sexual Abuse

Leading Questions to Avoid	Open-Ended Questions to Use
"Don't you have a problem with Daddy?"	"Can you tell me more?"
(Or "Uncle," or "Your mother's boyfriend?")	
"Doesn't he touch you down there?"	"What happened next?"
"Did your Dad say that?"	"When did that happen?"
"Was it hard or soft?"	"Who said that?"
	"What did it feel like?"

● **Clinical Pearl:** The provider *must* reassure both child and caregiver that the victim is not "damaged," and physical injuries will heal.

The examination should not be traumatic. If the child is uncooperative, whenever feasible, the clinician should allow more time for preparing the child for the examination and helping the child to relax. If necessary, the child can return later for a second visit. In some circumstances (eg, active genital bleeding secondary to trauma), the clinician cannot delay a physical examination and thus may need to arrange for sedation or anesthesia.

The child should have the company of a supportive adult, although depending on the abuse circumstances, this person may not always be the parent. Often adolescents will choose to be examined alone, and providers should respect this request. The examination time also may offer the provider the opportunity to ask questions about consensual sexual relations and cigarette, alcohol, and other drug use.

The clinician should explain the examination to the child beforehand. He or she should familiarize the patient with any tools that may be used, such as swabs for obtaining culture specimens, vaginal speculum (post-puberty), and the colposcope.

The timing of the examination depends on the history of the abuse. If the alleged abuse has occurred within the past 72 hours, the evaluation may include using a forensic evidence collection kit. If signs and symptoms are acute, the provider should expedite the examination. If the incident occurred more than 3 days before and no acute symptoms are present, the clinician should schedule the evaluation for the earliest possible time.

● **Clinical Pearl:** Whenever possible, the provider should avoid sending the child to an ED for sexual abuse evaluation. Professionals who are neither skilled nor comfortable with performing this type of evaluation usually are on the staff of EDs, which may not have pediatric providers available. When an inexperienced provider performs the evaluation, the chances are increased that a more skilled clinician will need to repeat it, adding to the child's discomfort and anxiety. In many communities, police and child protective workers have protocols that serve as guidelines to help triage children away from EDs and into specialized programs, such as child protection centers or Advocacy Centers.

The provider should conduct a thorough examination, paying particular attention to the child's physical develop-

ment, stage of sexual maturation, and emotional status. The clinician may use instruments that enhance lighting and provide magnification, such as a hand-held otoscope, to examine the child's genitalia. Specialized programs have begun to rely on a photocolposcope, an instrument originally designed for cervical examination during gynecologic examinations, to provide magnification and a bright light source for performance of the ano-genital examination. This instrument is able to document the examination with either 35-mm photos, video, or digital photography. Photo documentation of the examination findings allows for teaching, second opinions, and case conferencing, which may serve as important evidence in a trial. When the results of an evaluation are inconclusive, photos may serve as important documentation of a "baseline."

The clinician should describe carefully any signs of trauma, including extragenital trauma. If possible, the provider should sketch these signs on a standardized form designed for this purpose. Health care providers who conduct sexual abuse examinations should familiarize themselves with the nomenclature standardized by the American Professional Society on the Abuse of Children (1995a). Using uniform terminology is important so that other professionals who read the chart or testify as to its contents will have an accurate idea of what has been documented.

Considerations for Female Patients

The provider may examine the female child in several positions, including the supine frog-leg position, with the soles of the feet together and the knees abducted toward the table; the supine lithotomy position; or prone, with the chest pressed toward the examination table and the buttocks raised in the air. The clinician first must separate the labia and then apply outward and downward traction to allow for adequate examination of the hymen, vaginal opening, fossa navicularis, and posterior fourchette.

● **Clinical Pearl:** The clinician should document the examination position in the medical record.

Many things can influence the appearance of the genitalia and the size of the vaginal opening: the degree of the child's relaxation, the degree of traction applied to the labia majora, the child's position, and the presence of secretions, which may cause tissue to adhere to itself or surrounding tissues. At times, the clinician may need to gently manipulate the child's hymen with a small swab (eg, Calgi) to examine its architecture adequately. He or she may use a syringe to squirt water or saline at the tissues to wash away any agglutinating secretions. The examiner should become acquainted with the variety of normal hymenal configurations (eg, crescentic, annular), which can change over time. The annular configuration is most common in infancy, while the crescentic configuration is most common in girls older than 3 years (Berenson, 1998).

The clinician should examine the anus for scars, bruises, tears, or abnormalities of tone. Some anal sphincter dilatation may be normal, particularly when stool is in the rectal vault.

▲ **Clinical Warning:** Examiners should never use a speculum or perform internal examinations in prepubertal girls. They should inspect the external genitalia for discharge, acute abrasions, tears, ecchymosis, or alterations in color or architecture, which might indicate a scar from old injury.

Considerations for Male Patients

In males, the provider should examine the penis and scrotum for urethral discharge, discrete lesions (eg, vesicles), bruises, scars, or bite marks. The clinician should check the anus for scars, bruises, tears, or abnormalities of tone. Some anal sphincter dilatation may be normal, particularly when stool is in the rectal vault.

Interpreting Examination Results

Because of the forensic importance of an abnormal physical examination, multidisciplinary teams often wait anxiously for the results to decide how to proceed in investigating the case.

▲ **Clinical Warning:** Providers should realize that a normal physical examination is common even when sexual abuse has occurred. Multiple studies have reviewed the incidence of abnormal physical examination findings in children who were allegedly sexually abused. Normal examinations were reported in 26% to 73% of girls (mean 50%) and in 17% to 82% of boys (mean 53%). Even when physical examination helped to detect some abnormality, most reports have shown that the abnormality was nonspecific and therefore not diagnostic of sexual abuse. Diagnostic findings have been reported in only 3% to 16% of cases (Bays & Chadwick 1993).

There are multiple reasons for a normal physical examination in sexually abused children:

- Because of the hidden nature of the problem, discovery or disclosure of abuse may be delayed significantly, leading to a delay in seeking a health evaluation.

- Many types of sexual abuse, such as fondling and oral sodomy, do not leave any traumatic findings. The younger the victim, the less likely that sexual molestation included genital-genital contact or penetration.
- Hymenal tissue is elastic and can stretch to allow for full penetration by a finger or penis without causing visible trauma. Even when tissue has been damaged, healing may be rapid and complete. Once a female has reached puberty, estrogen changes of the genital mucosa may obliterate any evidence of prior injury.
- The anus can stretch to allow for passage of large-caliber stools without injury. Thus, it also can accommodate large, penetrating objects.

Because of delays in seeking evaluation, retrieval of forensic evidence (eg, semen, pubic hair) is rarely successful (Bays & Chadwick, 1993).

Many factors affect the likelihood of finding signs of traumatic injury after sexual abuse. These include the type of molestation, degree of force used, age of the child, chronicity of the abuse, and use of lubricants (Bays & Chadwick, 1993).

There have been multiple attempts to classify examination findings into levels of certainty for a diagnosis of sexual abuse. Some findings are specific, while others are nonspecific and may be attributable to other causes. Nonspecific findings become more important in the face of a clear history of molestation and so may serve to corroborate that history. Display 23-2 presents a framework for interpreting physical findings of the sexual abuse examination.

● **Clinical Pearl:** Because anogenital anatomy varies, the most experienced provider available must conduct sexual abuse examinations. He or she is less likely to miss subtle traumatic injury or to mistakenly attribute normal

---

DISPLAY 23–2 • Evaluating the Physical Findings of the Examination for Sexual Abuse

Diagnostic for Sexual Abuse
Presence of semen, sperm, or acid phosphatase
Pregnancy
Fresh genital or anal injuries in the absence of an adequate accidental explanation
Positive test or culture for syphilis, gonorrhea, or HIV (not perinatal or IV acquired)
An enlarged hymenal opening for age with findings of hymen disruption (absent hymen, healed transections, hymenal remnants) in the absence of an accidental or surgical explanation

Consistent With Sexual Abuse
Genital or anal *Trichomonas*, *Chlamydia*, human papillomavirus, herpes II (not perinatal)
Disruptions of hymen tissue, posterior or lateral angular concavities (clefts or notches), transections, absence or decrease in amount of hymen, and scars
Anal scars or skin tags outside the midline, dilation 13–20 mm without stool in the ampulla
Marked dilation of the hymenal opening, persisting in different examination positions

Sometimes Seen Following Sexual Abuse
Bacterial vaginosis
Extensive labial adhesions in girls several years out of diapers
Posterior fourchette friability

Repeated anal dilation of less than 15 mm
Edema of the perianal tissues, shortening or eversion of the anal canal, perianal fissures, thickened perianal skin, and reduction of rugae
Penile erection maintained during examination in prepubertal boys

Unlikely to be Due to Abuse
Labial adhesions in girls still in diapers
Erythema of the vestibule, perianal erythema
Midline avascular areas of the fossa navicularis or posterior fourchette
Urethral dilation with labial traction
Concavities of the hymen that are anterior or smooth, curved, and shallow
Intravaginal ridges and rugae behind a normal hymen
Perianal erythema, increased pigmentation, or venous engorgement after 2 minutes in the knee–chest position
Smooth areas or skin tags in the midline anterior and posterior to the anus
Single episode of anal dilation 15–20 mm or anal dilation with stool in the ampulla

Adapted from Bays, J. & Chadwick, D. (1993). The medical diagnosis of the sexually abused child. *Child Abuse and Neglect, 17*, 91, with kind permission from Pergamon Press Ltd., Headington Hill Hall Oxford OX30BW, UK.

variations as injuries from sexual abuse. For example, indentations or notches of the hymenal membrane have different significance, depending on their depth and location.

▲ **Clinical Warning:** Notches that extend the depth of the hymen to the vestibule have not been documented in girls who have not been sexually abused. In particular, notches in the posterior portion of the hymen (between 5 and 7 o'clock) are believed to be especially significant and consistent with abuse (Berenson, 1998). Many perianal findings once believed to suggest abuse have since been shown to occur in nonabused children. Fissures and tags in other than a midline location, however, are seen infrequently in nonabused children, as is anal sphincter dilatation in the absence of stool in the rectum. Acute findings, such as lacerations, abrasions, and hematomas, are seen primarily only in abused populations (Berenson, 1998).

DIAGNOSTIC CRITERIA

A sexually abused child may come to the primary care provider under various circumstances. Because careful inspection of the genitalia should be part of the routine examination of every child, providers may detect traumatic genital injury or other physical findings suggestive of sexual abuse (eg, grab marks on the inner thighs) during any physical examination. Examination of the genitalia in a child without specific symptoms is no less important than is looking in the ears or listening to the chest of an asymptomatic child. Providers should never defer such examination. Most parents will be pleased by the thorough nature of the examination and may even welcome the opportunity to address concerns that they may have been avoiding.

A sexually abused child may present with physical complaints, such as genital or anal bleeding, vaginal discharge or pain, or pain with urination. While each symptom may be present in a child whose diagnosis does not point to sexual abuse, clinicians must always at least consider sexual abuse in the differential diagnosis.

▲ **Clinical Warning:** If the differential diagnosis of sexual abuse is not made in cases of genital or anal bleeding, vaginal discharge or pain, or pain with urination, instances of child sexual abuse will be missed.

Sexualized behavior inappropriate for the child's developmental level, enuresis, encopresis, and a variety of other behavioral problems have been identified in sexually abused children. A number of studies comparing behaviors in sexually abused and non-sexually abused children have found behavioral symptoms to be more common in sexually abused children. No single symptom, however, has been described in the majority of victims of sexual abuse (Kendall-Tacket, Meyer-Williams, & Finkelhor, 1993).

Many behaviors that seem suspicious of sexual abuse, such as masturbation, can be normal developmental variants or nonspecific manifestations of emotional stress. While behavioral complaints may support a diagnosis of sexual abuse, they should not by themselves constitute that diagnosis. Sexual abuse should be one of many possible etiologies in the differential. The primary care provider should become familiar with the broad range of developmentally normal sexual behaviors in children (Friedrich, 1998). Display 23-3 outlines these behaviors as well as suspicious physical findings.

DISPLAY 23–3 • Possible Indicators of Sexual Abuse

Behavioral
- Sexualized behavior that is inappropriate for developmental level, including excessive masturbation or forcing sexual acts on other children
- Sleep disorders, nightmares
- Phobias, extreme fear of the physical examination
- Clinging, low self-esteem, and general anxiety
- Aggression, social problems among peers
- Abrupt behavioral change, withdrawal, fantasy, or regression
- School problems, delinquency, or runaway behavior
- Depression, self-injurious behaviors (suicide attempts), substance abuse, prostitution

Physical
- Vaginal discharge, STIs, bleeding, itching, possible pregnancy
- Encopresis, constipation, painful defecation
- Enuresis, dysuria
- Grasp marks
- Foreign body in the vagina or rectum
- Abdominal pain, headaches, or other genitourinary complaints
- Bruises to the hard or soft palate

Source: Botash, A. (1994). What office-based pediatricians need to know about child sexual abuse. *Contemporary Pediatrics, 11,* 83–100. Used with Permission.

Child sexual abuse is unique from other medical entities because of its secretive nature. A myriad of motivational issues may cause a child not to reveal the abuse. For this reason, primary care providers must be willing to entertain the diagnosis of sexual abuse. Because most often the perpetrator is in the child's family or at least well known to the child, disclosure of victimization is frequently accidental and tentative and often follows initial denial. Recantation or withdrawal of an allegation sometimes occurs during the process of disclosure, at rates ranging from 12% to 33%. In 93% of instances, the child reaffirms the original complaint. Factors that may compel children not to tell include being threatened with harm or punishment, being afraid of removal from or the dissolution of their family, and fearing that a loved one may go to jail (Sorenson & Snow, 1991).

DIAGNOSTIC STUDIES

In the United States, many states have kits that include all necessary specimen collectors and detailed instructions for obtaining forensic evidence. In the setting of child sexual abuse, the yield of these kits has not been well established. Most sexual offense medical protocols advise completing a forensic evidence examination if the child is seen within 72 hours of the abusive incident. Maintaining an unbroken chain of evidence is important so that collected specimens can be accounted for from the moment of collection until they are introduced into court as evidence. Each health care facility must establish a procedure for the transfer of the specimen kit by a law enforcement official to the crime lab. The health record must document the names of all individuals who handle the kit and dates of its transfer.

Though the detection of forensic evidence or a positive culture for STIs may be the only "evidence" that a child has been sexually abused, this diagnostic testing is most often negative for many reasons. Most child sexual abuse does not come to medical attention within 72 hours of the abuse; therefore, successfully detecting sperm or semen is uncommon. In addition, the prevalence of STIs in sexually abused children is low.

Photography

Many U.S. state laws allow for photographic documentation of injuries in child abuse evaluations, without a parent's or guardian's consent. The American Professional Society on the Abuse of Children has developed guidelines for the photography of visible lesions on a child (1995b).

● **Clinical Pearl:** In child sexual abuse evaluations, photography may be useful in documenting bite marks or suction marks (hickeys), as well as marks on the buttocks or lower extremities consistent with grabs.

The colposcope is a noninvasive magnifying instrument with an excellent built-in light source and camera attachment. First used by Teixeira in 1981 to study the external female genitalia of possible child abuse victims, the colposcope is very important in advancing the medical diagnosis of child sexual abuse. Its benefits include the following:

- Enhanced visualization with magnification up to 25 times
- Filters to improve visualization of subtle changes in vascularity
- Photographic preservation of examination findings as evidence in a criminal proceeding
- Documentation of a "baseline" in a child whose abuse cannot be proven and who may continue to live in a high-risk situation
- Provision for a second opinion and peer review
- Avoidance of the need to repeat examinations at the request of defense counsel. The slides can be made available to a defense expert.

Testing for Sexually Transmitted Infections

The transmission of STIs to sexually abused or assaulted children is possible. The determination that a child has an STI may be the first or only indication that he or she has been sexually abused. Multiple factors have thwarted the determination of the risk of transmission of STIs to children and STI prevalence in sexually abused children. Some infections that are clearly sexually transmitted in adults may be transmitted from mother to child at the time of delivery. These infections may be asymptomatic for long periods, making the determination of route of transmission very difficult. The incubation period of STIs varies from several days (eg, gonorrhea) to months (eg, human papillomavirus), making it difficult to determine the time during which sexual contact took place. In addition, many STIs in children are asymptomatic and therefore may not come to prompt medical attention (Hammerschlag, 1998).

Strong indications for testing for STIs include the following:

- The child has genital or anal symptoms including pain, dysuria, or discharge.
- The alleged perpetrator is known to have an STI or to engage in high-risk behaviors (eg, intravenous drug use).

- A history of oral, anal, or genital contact is evident.
- Contact history includes pain, bleeding, or contact with the perpetrator's blood or semen.
- Prevalence of STIs in the child's local community is high.
- Physical examination reveals findings consistent with anogenital trauma.
- The child is too young to give a clear history, or the family is very anxious about STIs.

The American Academy of Pediatrics, Committee on Child Abuse and Neglect (1999) has published implications of various STIs for detecting and reporting child abuse. Because the prevalence of STIs varies regionally and from across countries, precise recommendations for STI testing are beyond the scope of this chapter. Primary care providers should be familiar with the appropriate specimen collection technique for each of the STIs. For example, standard culture is the gold standard for the detection of both Chlamydia and gonorrhea in prepubertal girls. DNA probes and enzyme-linked immunoassays have not been approved for use in this age group and should not be used (Hammerschlag, 1998). Table 23-2 describes the implications for the diagnosis and reporting of STIs in children. Refer to the Chapter 41 for more information on their diagnosis and management.

● **Clinical Pearl:** Because the prevalence of STIs is low in child victims of sexual abuse, antibiotic prophylaxis is not routinely recommended for prepubertal children. It should be offered to adolescents, however, after sexual assault.

▲ **Clinical Warning:** Pubertal girls should have a pregnancy test, which may need to be repeated depending on the timing of the sexual abuse relative to the evaluation. Providers need to consider postexposure prophylaxis against human immunodeficiency virus (HIV), which depends on the circumstances of the abuse, the perpetrator's HIV status (if

---

TABLE 23–2. IMPLICATIONS OF COMMONLY ENCOUNTERED SEXUALLY TRANSMITTED DISEASES (STDs) FOR THE DIAGNOSIS AND REPORTING OF SEXUAL ABUSE OF INFANTS AND PREPUBERTAL CHILDREN

STD Confirmed	Sexual Abuse	Suggested Action
Gonorrhea*	Diagnostic[†]	Report[‡]
Syphilis*	Diagnostic	Report
HIV[§]	Diagnostic	Report
*Chlamydia**	Diagnostic[†]	Report
Trichomonas vaginalis	Highly suspicious	Report
Condylomata acuminata* (anogenital warts)	Suspicious	Report
Herpes (genital location)	Suspicious	Report[‖]
Bacterial vaginosis	Inconclusive	Medical follow-up

*If not perinatally acquired.
[†]Use definitive diagnostic methods, such as culture or DNA probes.
[‡]To agency mandated in community to receive reports of suspected sexual abuse.
[§]If not perinatally or transfusion acquired.
[‖]Unless there is a clear history of autoinoculation. Herpes 1 and 2 are difficult to differentiate by current techniques.
From: American Academy of Pediatrics, Committee on Child Abuse and Neglect. (1999). Guidelines for the evaluation of sexual abuse of children: Subject review. *Pediatrics, 103* (1), 186–191. Used with permission.

known), and the local epidemiology of HIV. The provider needs to be familiar with local/regional guidelines. He or she should consider testing for syphilis and hepatitis B. For more complete information on STI testing, the reader is referred to the guidelines published by the Centers for Disease Control and Prevention in January 1998.

MANAGEMENT

When the primary care provider suspects that a child has been a victim of abuse, he or she must sit down with the (nonoffending) parent(s) alone to outline concerns and discuss a plan of action. The clinician also should discuss what steps the parents will need to take to protect the child from further abuse. Many parents will be shocked—even incredulous—that their child has been victimized. Still others may disclose that they also had similar concerns. When discussing the results of the history, physical examination, and reasons for suspicion, providers need to realize that parents will not always fully comprehend what they have been told. If the physical examination is within normal limits, the parents may erroneously believe that abuse has been eliminated as a possibility.

The most important information that providers should relay to parents is the need for them to be supportive throughout the initial evaluation, treatment, and any future proceedings. Despite therapy, children who do not have supportive parents will have poor long-term mental health outcomes (Berliner & Elliott, 1996). If the parent is unable to be supportive or believe what the child has disclosed, the youngster may need to be placed in a protective, nurturing environment.

▲ **Clinical Warning:** Not infrequently, a nonoffending parent may have had reason to believe or may even have been told that the child was being abused. The nonoffending parent is culpable in this circumstance for failing to protect the child.

Pediatric providers are in a unique position of dispelling many myths about child sexual abuse in their dealings with families, teachers, child protective services, law enforcement officers, attorneys, and judges. The following discussion highlights some of these myths, as identified by Bays and Chadwick (1993):

- **Myth 1:** If physical evidence of sexual abuse cannot be found, then it did not occur.
  - **Fact:** Definitive physical evidence of sexual abuse is rare. Documentation of a normal physical examination should avoid phrases such as "exam negative for sexual abuse" and "hymen intact" because they falsely suggest that sexual abuse was disproved.
- **Myth 2:** Boys are rarely sexually abused.
  - Fact: Studies of pedophiles indicate that more than two thirds of their victims are male. Sexual abuse of males remains extremely underdetected and underreported.
- **Myth 3:** STIs are frequently the result of nonsexual transmission.
  - **Fact:** While some infectious organisms have been found to survive on inanimate objects, actual transmission by fomites has not been clearly documented.
- **Myth 4:** Injuries to the hymen can be accidental (eg, the result of straddle injuries, tampon insertion, or masturbation).

- **Fact:** Most straddle injuries involve bruises to the overlying protective structures of the labia majora and minora. Even a penetrating injury caused by a fall on a sharp object would be more likely to penetrate through the lateral vaginal wall, injuring surrounding structures, than to injure only the hymen while sparing the surrounding soft tissue. No data have supported either tampon insertion or masturbation as causes of genital injury. Masturbation usually involves touching anteriorly over the sensitive clitoral tissue and would not, in normal children, be expected to be traumatic in nature.
- **Myth 5:** A girl can be born without a hymen.
  - **Fact:** No cases of congenitally absent hymen have been documented. Even in cases of congenital genital abnormality, hymenal tissue can be found.

What to Do After a Child Discloses

The provider must prepare a child for what will happen after that youngster discloses. The clinician should give positive feedback to the child, acknowledging the courage that it takes to tell, while reassuring the patient that he or she has not done anything wrong. The provider needs to explain that other professionals will also have to be told to protect the child. Nonoffending parent(s) will need support as well. In explaining the "next steps" to the child and parent(s), the provider should be supportive and encouraging but should not make promises, offer false hopes, or be unrealistic.

● **Clinical Pearl:** The primary care provider cannot be sure of what might happen over the ensuing weeks and months as the legal and child protective investigation takes place. Therefore, the prudent clinician will avoid going into too much detail about precisely what will happen following disclosure.

Reporting Sexual Abuse

In 1963, just 1 year after Dr. C. Henry Kemp published the landmark article describing the "battered child syndrome," state legislatures began enacting child abuse reporting laws. In addition to their most immediate function of protecting children, these laws have allowed for the systematic collection of data about the prevalence of child abuse, both sexual and physical.

Professionals who work with children are required to report any suspicion of child abuse to appropriate legal or child protection authorities. The list of "mandated reporters" includes, among others, teachers, health care providers, and social workers. While state reporting laws may differ slightly, the basic concepts are the same. The law mandates a professional to make a report when he or she only suspects abuse. Professionals are not in violation if they report a suspicion of abuse that turns out to be unfounded. As long as the report is made in good faith and uses reasonable professional judgment, the mandated reporter is immune from civil and criminal liability. This does not mean that a professional cannot be sued but, rather, that such suit is unlikely to be successful. All U.S. states have mechanisms that allow for children to be taken into temporary protective custody by police officers, child protective service workers, or health care professionals if a child is believed to be in imminent danger (Myers, 1992). Readers in other countries are advised to learn whether similar statutory measures hold true. Table 23-3 provides guidelines meant to assist in making the decision to report sexual abuse.

TABLE 23–3. GUIDELINES FOR MAKING THE DECISION TO REPORT SEXUAL ABUSE OF CHILDREN

Data Available			Response	
History	Physical Examination	Laboratory Findings	Level of Concern About Sexual Abuse	Report Decision
None	Normal	None	None	No report
Behavioral changes[†]	Normal	None	Variable depending on behavior	Possible report;* follow closely (possible mental health referral)
None	Nonspecific findings	None	Low (worry)	Possible report;* follow closely
Nonspecific history by child or history by parent only	Nonspecific findings	None	Intermediate	Possible report;* follow closely
None	Specific findings[‡]	None	High	Report
Clear statement	Normal	None	High	Report
Clear statement	Specific findings	None	High	Report
None	Normal, nonspecific or specific findings	Positive culture for gonorrhea; positive serologic test for HIV; syphilis; presence of semen, sperm acid phosphatase	Very high	Report
Behavior changes	Nonspecific findings	Other sexually transmitted diseases	High	Report

*A report may or may not be indicated. The decision to report should be based on discussion with local or regional experts or child protective services agencies.

[†]Some behavioral changes are nonspecific and others are more worrisome.[7]

[‡]Other reasons for findings ruled out.[13]

From: American Academy of Pediatrics, Committee on Child Abuse (1999). Used with permission.

What to Tell Parents

Children who are maltreated often experience adverse affects in their cognitive, physical, emotional, and social development. The emotional, psychological, and physical effects of child maltreatment depend on many variables, including the type and extent of the abuse and the child's stage of development. A child's personal characteristics, such as self-esteem and cognitive ability, may buffer the experience of sexual abuse. The presence of a supportive adult who believes the child and gives a sense of protection also may serve to limit the damaging effects of victimization (The David and Lucille Packard Foundation, The Center for the Future of Children, 1998).

When a child's sexual abuse comes to light, the primary care provider must be aware of not only the importance of the physical examination and the collection of forensic evidence, but also the necessity for a thorough psychosocial assessment and evaluation of the patient's ongoing mental health needs. The clinician needs to be familiar with local resources for referring the child for psychological assessment and treatment.

Prevention

The three types of prevention are primary, secondary, and tertiary. Primary prevention is targeted to the general population to increase the awareness of a specific topic. This is often seen through the media as a public service announcement. Elementary schools have initiated many programs to increase children's awareness of "good touch, bad touch, and secret touch." Through educational programs starting in preschool and continuing through the sixth grade, children enrolled in such programming learn what abuse is and how

to protect themselves (The David and Lucille Packard Foundation, The Center for the Future of Children, 1998).

Providers can use educational materials, available to complement any discussions that might be conducted during a scheduled pediatric health care appointment, as an integral part of anticipatory guidance. The use of written educational materials is a practical adjunct to addressing the topic of child sexual abuse during the health care appointment. The clinician should introduce and discuss the topic with both the child and parent(s). Their responses will help determine the advice needed to help prevent abuse. If the provider is concerned that a patient's or parent's responses signal that the child is at risk or might be a victim of abuse, then he or she will need further time to explore concerns.

During the physical examination, asking the child about what he or she calls body parts allows for the patient to be more aware of body parts and for the provider to teach that no one should touch them. Traditionally, children are told to listen to adults. The provider must teach children that it is ok to say "No" if someone tries to touch them and that they should run and tell someone. While conducting the physical examination, the practitioner should explain to the child that it is ok if a parent helps him or her go to the bathroom or cleans him or her in the bath. The provider should also explain that it is appropriate for the provider to touch the child, as long as the parent is there and says that it is ok.

Secondary prevention targets a specific high-risk group that has demonstrated behaviors that put their children's safety at risk. Knowing which specific children are at increased risk of abuse is difficult. The provider must take the time to discuss family relationships, communication between all family members, caretaking arrangements, school performance, behavior problems of concern, and resistance of the child to spending time with specific people. Whenever interview responses or reactions to anticipatory guidance alert the provider, then a referral for further evaluation and treatment is warranted.

Tertiary prevention occurs following abuse, when protection and treatment are indicated. Though the extent to which the primary provider can be involved in the management of the sexually abused child may vary considerably, it is incumbent on all clinicians to be familiar with the signs and symptoms of sexual abuse.

▲ **Clinical Warning:** Child sexual abuse often happens to vulnerable children. Whenever a history of abuse is positive, treatment is imperative. Children who have been victimized are at increased risk for aggressive behavior, trouble with peers, depression, poor self-esteem, and difficulties in school performance. Children who have been victims of abuse are at increased risk for being the victim of adult abuse or of perpetrating abuse on others.

COMMUNITY RESOURCES

Several available websites offer valid resources for providers, educators, and families. One such site follows:

- Sexual Assault Information Page
  Child Sexual Abuse
  http://www.cs.utk.edu/~bartley/index/childSexualAbuse/
  (many good links and resources)
- Stop it Now (A resource for adults who are interested in prevention activities)
  PO Box 495
  Haydenville, MA 01039
  (413) 268-3096
  (413) 268-3098 (fax)
  Stop it Now HELPLINE
  (888) PREVENT
  (888) 773-8368

REFERENCES

American Academy of Pediatrics, Committee on Child Abuse and Neglect. (1999). Guidelines for the evaluation of sexual abuse of children: Subject review. *Pediatrics, 103*(1), 186–191.

American Professional Society on the Abuse of Children. (1995a). *Descriptive terminology in child sexual abuse medical evaluations.* Chicago, IL: Author.

American Professional Society on the Abuse of Children. (1995a). *Practice guidelines: Photographic documentation of child abuse.* Chicago, IL: Author.

Bays, J., & Chadwick, D. (1993). The medical diagnosis of the sexually abused child. *Child Abuse and Neglect, 17,* 91–110.

Berenson, A. (1998). Normal anogenital anatomy. *Child Abuse and Neglect, 22*(6), 589–596.

Berliner, L., & Elliot, D. M. (1996). Sexual abuse of children. American Professional Society on the abuse of children. In J. Briere (Ed.), *The handbook on child maltreatment* (p. 961). Thousand Oaks, CA: Sage Publications.

Botash, A. (1994). What office-based pediatricians need to know about child sexual abuse. Contemporary Pediatrics, 11, 83-100.

Brandt, R. S. T., & Tisza, V. (1997). The sexually misused child. *American Journal of Orthopsychiatry, 47,* 80–90.

Centers for Disease Control and Prevention. (1998). 1998 sexually transmitted diseases treatment guidelines. *Morbidity and Mortality Weekly Report, 47*(RR-1), 1–116.

The David and Lucille Packard Foundation, The Center for the Future of Children. (1998). *The future of children: Protection of children from abuse and neglect, 18*(1), 47–48.

Elliot, D., & Briere, J. (1994). Forensic sexual abuse evaluations: Disclosure and symptomotolgy. *Behavior Sciences and the Law, 12,* 261–277.

Finkerhor, D. (1994). Current information of the scope and nature of childhood sexual abuse. *Future of Children, 4,* 31–53.

Finkerhor, D. (1980). Sex among siblings: A survey of prevalence, variety, and effects. *Archives of Sexual Behavior,* 171–193.

Friedrich, W. N., Fisher, J., Broughton, D., et al. (1998). Normative sexual behavior in children: A contemporary sample. *Pediatrics (electronic pages), 101*(4), E9.

Hammerschlag, M. (1998). The transmissibility of sexually transmitted diseases is sexually abused children. *Child Abuse and Neglect, 22*(6), 623–635.

Kempe, C. H. (1978). Sexual abuse: Another hidden pediatric problem. The 1977 C. Anderson Aldrich Lecture. *Pediatrics, 62,* 382–389.

Kendall-Tacket, K., Meyer-Williams, L., & Finkelhor, D. (1993). Impact of sexual abuse on children: A review and synthesis of recent empirical studies. *Psychological Bulletin, 113*(1), 164–180.

Morgan, M. (1995). *How to interview sexual abuse victims.* Thousand Oaks, CA: Sage Publications.

Myers, J. E. B. (1992). *Legal issues in child abuse and neglect.* Thousand Oaks, CA: Sage Publications.

National Center on Child Abuse and Neglect. (1993). *A report on the maltreatment of children with disabilities.* Washington, DC: U.S. Department of Health and Human Services.

Reed, L. D. (1996). Findings from research on children's suggestibility and implications for conducting interviews. Child Maltreatment, 1(2), 105-120.

Sedlak, A. J., & Broadhurst, D. D. (1996). *Executive summary of the Third National Incidence Study of Child Abuse and Neglect.* Washington, DC: U. S. Department of Health and Human Services.

Sorenson, T., & Snow, B. (1991). How children tell: The process of disclosure in child sexual abuse. *Child Welfare, LXX*(1), 3–15.

Teixeira, W. (1981). Hymenal colposcopic examination in sexual offenses. *American Journal of Forensic Medical Pathology, 2,* 209–215.

PART 3 ▲

Children Exposed to Domestic Violence

- CATHERINE KOVEROLA, PhD, and
  MARY MORAHAN, LCSW, MSW

INTRODUCTION

During the course of practice, every primary care provider will work with numerous families who present with a history of children who have been affected by violence in the home. Pediatric practitioners are in a unique position to intervene. The most typical dynamics of domestic violence are that the child and mother are isolated with few outside contacts. While significantly more rare, fathers, too, can be victims of domestic violence. Urging a woman to leave a domestic violence situation prematurely is misguided and often can lead to deadly consequences, unless a well thought-out plan of action with supports has been developed. The practitioner's primary role needs to be the identification, assessment, and referral of the family. A team of professionals who can ensure that the mother and children have access to all needed resources must do the actual intervention and follow-up. Some families will require shelter; it is strongly recommended that clinicians have liaisons with local shelters. Similarly, some families will require specialized legal counsel.

Exposure to domestic violence represents a significant physical and mental health problem for millions of children in all countries. Research has documented that by "asking the questions," that is, by screening for domestic violence, children and their abused parents will talk about their situation, and providers can refer them appropriately (Siegel, Hill, Henderson, Ernst, & Boat, 1999). The purpose of this chapter is to furnish critical information on how to assess these situations and, most importantly, how to effectively intervene in the complex and intricate web of domestic violence.

▲ **Clinical Warning:** Each provider is ethically responsible to screen and provide referrals for appropriate interventions on behalf of their pediatric patients.

PATHOLOGY

Historically, practitioners have been reticent to address the issues of domestic violence, believing it to be a private family matter. Compounding this misconception is that actually addressing the problem and reporting its existence to legal authorities may jeopardize the victim's safety (Rodriguez, Craig, Mooney, & Bauer, 1998). Furthermore, patients may perceive a clinician who reports domestic violence as a threat to their family. Of course, cultural values play a role in the pathology of domestic abuse, especially when these values encourage women to "keep silent," to maintain family unity, and avoid embarrassment (Leung, Leung, Lam, & Ho, 1999;

Bhatt, 1998). The result may be that the victim is unwilling to disclose abuse, preferring to keep it private.

Domestic violence is not a private matter. The World Health Organization (WHO) recognizes domestic violence as a worldwide public health issue. WHO reports that domestic violence is the leading cause of death and injury to women of childbearing age (Naumann, Langford, Torres, Campbell, & Glass, 1999). Generally these women are, like other mothers, the primary caregivers of the provider's pediatric patients. Mothers who live in constant fear of physical violence and are subjected to psychological and emotional intimidation and control by their perpetrators are unable to care adequately for their children. Similarly, the partners who perpetrate violence against mothers are equally unavailable in their parental role.

Children exposed to domestic violence not only are deprived of adequate parenting, but also are traumatized. Research over the past 15 years has documented the devastating impact of domestic violence on development, particularly in the areas of emotional and behavioral development, interpersonal skills, and academic achievement (Kolbo, Blakely, & Engleman, 1996). Children exposed to violence within their homes are at increased risk for developing a wide range of serious initial and long-term adjustment difficulties (Edleson, 1999; Stephens, 1999). Table 23-4 describes the signs and symptoms of domestic violence at different ages and stages of development. Display 23-4 provides emotional and behavioral indicators of exposure to domestic violence, categorized by age.

Increasingly, clinicians, researchers, and policy makers are beginning to define exposure to domestic violence as a form of emotional/psychological child abuse. In some jurisdictions, exposure to domestic violence serves as grounds for reporting to child protection services and, in some cases, apprehension of the child. Regardless of whether the expo-

TABLE 23–4. DEVELOPMENTAL STAGES AND BEHAVIOR PATTERNS SEEN IN CHILDREN EXPOSED TO DOMESTIC VIOLENCE

Stage/Age	Victim Behaviors
Infant/toddler	Diminished curiosity about the world
	Insecure relationships
	Impaired sense of self-development
	No autonomy development
	Confused sense of right and wrong
Preschool	Poor interpersonal boundaries, either withdrawn or intrusive
	Sense of self damaged and diminished
	Belief that domestic violence is their fault
	Delayed cognitive development
Childhood	Sense of self damaged
	Interpersonal relationship capacity inhibited
	Rationalizing/blaming overdeveloped
	Extremes on continuum (ie, selfless or demanding of others)
Adolescence	Rejection of sexuality or oversexualized/violent
	Rejection of true intimacy
	Delayed development of abstract thinking
	Overly self-reliant or compulsive relationships without boundaries

---

DISPLAY 23–4 • Behavioral and Emotional Indicators of Domestic Violence Exposure

---

Infants/Toddlers

- Excessive crying
- Clingyness
- Difficult to soothe
- Lethargic and fatigued
- Nonresponsive
- Developmental delays

Preschoolers

Externalizing

- Aggression
- Noncompliant, oppositional, overactive
- Destructive
- Cruel to animals
- Excessive neediness
- Enuresis and encopresis

Internalizing

- Excessive neediness
- Withdrawal, shyness
- Sadness
- Anxiety, separation anxiety
- Nightmares

Social Competence

- Delayed peer relationship capacity
- Intrusive inappropriate boundaries
- Delays in speech and communication

School-Age Child

Externalizing

- Aggression
- Noncompliant, oppositional, overactive
- Destructive to property
- Cruel to animals
- Excessive neediness
- Enuresis and encopresis
- Fire-setting
- Early substance abuse
- Truancy
- Penis displacement disorder
- Low empathy

Internalizing

- Excessive neediness
- Withdrawal, shyness
- Sadness
- Anxiety, separation anxiety
- Nightmares
- Overachieving/highly compliant

Social Competence

- Lack of peer relationships
- Intrusive inappropriate boundaries
- Delays in speech and communication
- Poor problem-solving skills
- School avoidance

Adolescence

Externalizing Symptoms

- Aggression/rage, destructive behaviors
- Precocious sexuality
- Cruelty to animals
- Gang affiliation
- Alcohol and drug use
- Suicidal attempts

Internalizing Symptoms

- Depression
- Anxiety
- Self-blame
- Withdrawal

Social Competency

- Social isolation and peer rejection

Post-Traumatic Stress Disorder Symptoms (applicable to ALL ages)

- Symptoms of intrusion
- Nightmares, flashbacks, repetitive play with themes or aspects of the trauma
- Acting or feeling as if the traumatic event were recurring
- Trauma specific re-enactment
- Distress at exposure to cues that symbolize or resemble the traumatic event
- Behavior problems reported at school
- Efforts to avoid thoughts, feelings, or conversations associated with the trauma
- Efforts to avoid activities, places, or people that cause recollections of the trauma
- Numbing of general responsiveness, restricted range of affect
- Feeling detached from others
- May have parentified role in family
- Symptoms of physiologic arousal
- Difficulty falling or staying asleep
- Difficulty concentrating
- Hypervigilant or exaggerated startle response

---

sure to domestic violence is legally defined as child abuse in the provider's jurisdiction, witnessing violence within the family home has devastating emotional and psychological sequellae for the child. This warrants thorough assessment and appropriate referral and intervention.

Historic Perspective

Societal views on domestic violence continue to evolve. Similarly, the response of providers, social welfare authorities, and mental health and law enforcement professionals continues to improve. The change in response to domestic violence has arisen primarily from the feminist movement. Early feminists were the first to define domestic violence as a social problem derived from a male-dominated oligarchy (Gordon, 1988). Early feminists linked a woman's right to divorce with male drunkenness and the right not to be hit. This link was important because, traditionally, society viewed women and children as property. Society saw it as the husband's right to beat his wife and children as he deemed necessary. While the westernized world no longer considers this view "politically correct" or legal, some societies and even some health care professionals continue to hold these sentiments and values.

The child protection movement initially was resistant to responding to domestic violence. It has since developed a significantly more sympathetic attitude toward children and women in these situations. A more proactive, appropriate response is now in place in some jurisdictions.

Somewhat surprisingly, the women's and child protection movements have a history of being in conflict, and in many places ideologic disputes persist, compromising care for mothers and their children. All too often, child protective services remove children from their mother's care because of her "failure to protect" while the father is victimizing the family. Rather than providing the mother with appropriate supports to maintain her children with her in a safe home, "the system" further victimizes her. Children who have been traumatized by domestic violence then enter the bewildering child welfare system, often separated from both siblings and parents.

● **Clinical Pearl:** The systems that are involved in the intervention and resolution of issues of domestic violence are parts of massive bureaucracies. Children's needs are all too often lost in the shuffle of papers. While progress has been made, these systems are far from perfect. Practitioners can be critical advocates for children in the midst of this complexity.

The Dynamics of Domestic Violence

Domestic violence is a process rather than a single event. It is defined as a documented set of behaviors that forms a pattern over time, involving the progressive, insidious domination of one intimate partner over another. In addition to physical abuse, this domination usually includes psychological abuse, intimidation, economic control, and isolation (Campbell, 1998; Levendosky & Graham-Bermann, 1998). These factors lead to a typical set of family dynamics in which the child is psychologically orphaned or at a minimum, deprived of adequate parenting by both caregivers.

Most often, the perpetrator is a male partner. In only 4% of cases of violence perpetrated against men, the aggressor was an intimate female partner. Only a small percentage of these male victims were fathers (National Center for Juvenile Justice, 1997). Children come to view the male perpetrator as destructive, abusive, controlling, and emotionally unavailable as a parent. In contrast, the child comes to see the victimized mother as ineffective, powerless, and, many times, in need of caretaking herself. Unless she can leave her abuser, she may be incapable of addressing the child's needs. Thus, the child has no adequate, stable, caring parent figure. The youngster waffles between allegiance to the destructive but powerful perpetrator figure and to the weaker, but at times potentially nurturing, mother figure.

The issues are more complex for children of gay or lesbian parents. Research has documented that intimate partner violence in gay and lesbian couples is as high as 33%. The dynamics of the violence mirror that of heterosexual couples. Of great concern is that these families may be more isolated and have access to fewer services, such as protective orders, shelters, and legal protection, than do heterosexual families (Barnes, 1998; Burke & Follingstad, 1999). No known studies on the effects of same-sex domestic violence on children have been done. In the clinical experience of the authors, the effects of domestic violence are even more detrimental on these children.

An important and particularly difficult factor in domestic violence is its intergenerational nature, which makes intervention by primary care providers and others challenging.

The intergenerational nature of domestic violence means that the child tend to emulate either the mother or father. Children who identify with their fathers are at risk for becoming perpetrators, while children who identify with their mothers are at risk for choosing future relationships with individuals who victimize them.

● **Clinical Pearl:** Intervention is critical to break the cycle of domestic violence. Initial research on effectiveness of intervention points to its efficacy with children (Miller, 1999; Kot, Landreth, & Giordano, 1998). Interventions for batterers hold much less promise.

Psychological Abuse: Intimidation, Economic Control, and Isolation of the Victim

Psychological abuse of the mother results in the destruction of her self-esteem and self-worth. Most mothers in domestic violence situations present with chronic post-traumatic stress disorder (PTSD). PTSD has three major categories of symptoms: intrusive symptoms related to the trauma itself, avoidance symptoms related to the trauma, and physiologic reactivity. Key symptoms that may be noted in a mother who has PTSD include the following:

* Sleep problems, often due to persistent intrusive symptoms (eg, flashbacks, nightmares)
* Irritability
* Anger
* Lack of patience
* Hopelessness
* Flat affect
* Powerlessness
* Confusion
* Fears
* Sense of a foreshortened future
* Difficulty concentrating
* Heightened startle reflex

Psychological abuse also often results in the development of depressive symptoms and generalized anxiety. Psychological abuse clearly diminishes a person's ability to parent and to make appropriate healthy decisions for herself and her children (Wilson, 1998).

The perpetrator intimidates the mother by making threats that typically include harm to the children, pets, and her immediate family members. Perpetrators often carry out these threats to some degree. In 50% of domestic violence cases, the perpetrator also abuses the children, regardless of whether they are his biologic offspring (Edleson, 1999). Thus, intimidation of the mother has a reverberating and negative impact on her children's sense of safety and ability to seek help and refuge.

In westernized societies, in which economic independence is critical for survival, a perpetrator's deliberate destruction of the victim's independent economic viability often is a primary factor in preventing the woman from leaving the home. Economic control is particularly intertwined in families with children, because the person exerting authority provides shelter, food, clothing, and in some families, opportunities, such as private education. It is well documented that in divorced families, the mother's and children's quality of life is diminished. This issue is heightened in situations of domestic violence because the perpetrator has systematically ensured that the mother cannot be financially viable without him (Campbell, 1998).

Isolation is the culmination of psychological abuse, intimidation, and economic control. The perpetrator systematically isolates the family from outside influences that could intervene positively, including health care, education, social welfare, the legal system, and extended family and friends. Not only is the mother often isolated, but so, too, are the children. This deprives the child of other healthier role models who could ameliorate the impact of exposure to domestic violence, while also solidifying the perpetrator's power. This scenario ensures dependence of both mother and child on the perpetrator (Kilpatrick & Williams, 1998).

EPIDEMIOLOGY

Domestic violence is woven into the very fabric of all societies, regardless of race or ethnicity (Hedin, Grimstad, Moller, Schei, & Janson, 1999; Leung et al., 1999; Marais, de Villiers, Moller, & Stein, 1999; Miller, 1999; Bhatt, 1998; Campbell, 1998; Sheridan, 1998). Millions of children each year suffer a multiplicity of problems following exposure to violence. The complex dynamics create barriers for normal development (Kolbo et al., 1996). In the United States alone, the severity of domestic abuse as a significant public health issue is exemplified by the statistic that 2 to 4 million women are severely physically abused each year by their partners (Wilson & Daly, 1993). Campbell (1998) states the following:

- The United States spends $5 to $10 billion per year on health care, criminal justice, and other social service costs of domestic violence.
- One million women seek medical treatment for domestic violence injuries each year.
- Of women seen in EDs, 22% to 35% are seen for injuries inflicted by their husbands or boyfriends.
- Medical expenses arising from domestic violence assaults in the United States cost more than $44 million per year.
- One in six adult pregnant women and one in five pregnant teenagers are abused by their partners.
- Domestic violence has been documented to occur with a number of other conditions within the family, further jeopardizing the children's well-being.
- In approximately 50% of domestic violence cases, alcohol or drug abuse is ongoing.
- In approximately 50% of domestic violence cases, children also suffer direct physical abuse by the perpetrator.
- Among women of childbearing age infected with HIV, approximately 50% also experience domestic violence.
- Of boys aged 12 to 20 who were incarcerated for murder, 63% had killed their mother's abusers.

Of further concern is the fact that 87% of children in homes with domestic violence witness the actual physical act of abuse. These children know what happened. They are able to provide detailed descriptions about the violence and its incidence in their home (Edleson, 1999). Beyond direct witnessing, they see their parents' faces, lie in bed listening, hear the tone of voices, and see the injuries and bruises the next day. Providers should be especially concerned that children are present 25% of the time when abusers kill their mothers (Miller, 1999).

Overwhelming consensus in the international literature has shown that the incidence of domestic violence is significantly increased in homes where one or both adult partners is depressed, abuses substances, or both. Perception of increased life stress is also a commonly reported factor.

O'Farrell, Van Hutton, and Murphy (1999) found that domestic violence decreased significantly in the year following a behavioral marital therapy alcoholism treatment program for 88 alcoholics and their wives. They also reported that domestic violence rates returned to their previous levels in participants who resumed drinking.

In a large, diverse South African sample, Marais et al. (1999) described a significant association, ranging from 35% to 48%, between domestic violence and either major depression or PTSD in racially diverse female patients who were victims of abuse. These women also were more likely to report suicidal ideation or attempts, compared with women who had not experienced domestic abuse.

A recent survey of Alaskan native youth revealed that 45% of participants saw drug and alcohol abuse as problems for their rural communities. The respondents also reported that domestic abuse was an associated phenomenon (Seyfrit, Crossland, & Hamilton, 1998).

The interplay of domestic violence and chemical dependency increases the risk factors for children. Substance abuse presents another layer of health concerns through which practitioners must sort to best help the child. When both parents are addicted, no adults are able to focus on the child's health and emotional needs. Boundaries within the family are weak, often leading to one child becoming parentified. The isolation experienced by children in domestic violence families is heightened when substance abuse is also a factor.

The dynamics of secrecy typified by substance abusing families is extremely powerful, with detrimental effects for children. These youngsters have fewer social, physical, emotional, and mental resources than do children who are not exposed to parental substance abuse. In half of spousal homicide cases, alcohol was considered a factor, especially since 25% to 50% of violent men also have chemical dependency issues (Rodriguez et al., 1998).

HISTORY

The assessment of domestic violence should be a component of each history taking. Many providers have historically been reluctant to ask about domestic violence. Because domestic violence is a health issue, it is not a private matter. The practitioner needs to conceptualize the assessment of domestic violence as a routine procedure to be implemented with every patient.

When assessing for issues of family violence and addiction, the provider also should include questions about the extent of chemical dependency, how often the violent behavior occurs while the batterer is drinking or on drugs, and whether anyone in the family uses alcohol and drugs to recover from the violence. Some victims will use alcohol and drugs to self-medicate against the physical and emotional pain of the violence. One dynamic to which the practitioner should be alert is the tendency for both victim and perpetrator to "blame the substances" or to excuse violence committed under the influence. When assessing the role of substance abuse in violent relationships, the practitioner should not join in the very destructive dynamics that justify and condone the violence.

● **Clinical Pearl:** It is strongly recommended that each mother or primary female caregiver be screened privately for domestic violence. This will require the clinic to make provisions for the mother to have at least part of the history taking completed separate from the child. If the interview reveals domestic violence or behavioral or emotional indicators in the child point to its possibility, the child also needs to be interviewed privately.

Questions for the Parent

What follows is a list of questions to include in each clinical history taking of a child's mother or primary caregiver. The male partner (or perpetrator) should not be present for this component of history taking. The provider should preface with the comment, "These are questions that I ask all the mothers of my patients." Then the clinician should ask the following:

- "Has anyone hit you, hurt you, or threatened you within the past year? If so, whom?"
- "Are you afraid of your current or previous partner? Has he ever threatened you or hurt your children?"

If the mother responds affirmatively to either of these questions, the provider must activate the institution or clinic's domestic violence protocol. In addition, the provider must ask the following questions:

- "Are there any children involved who are in danger?" If yes, the provider must make a child abuse report.
- "Is it safe for the patient to go home?" If the mother answers "no," the clinician should ask whether she and her child can stay with family or friends or if the provider should arrange for a shelter. If she answers "yes," the provider must ask whether she has a safety plan for getting out of the house, with the children, if violence recurs.

● **Clinical Pearl:** The provider must give the patient a list of shelters, resources, and hotline numbers that can be accessed locally.

Questions to Ask the Pediatric Patient

Preschoolers

The primary care provider should begin the interview with a preliminary discussion about feelings: happy, sad, angry, and scared. He or she can use face charts as a prompt. The clinician should include questions about how people show feelings at their house, including asking whether they hug, hit, break things, and so forth.

The practitioner should then shift the discussion to asking about adult conflict, stating, "All grown ups get mad at each other sometimes. At your house when they get mad, what do they do? Do they use their voice? Do they yell? Do they throw things? Do they hit each other? Do they wave knives?" It is important that the provider then ask, "Are there guns at your house?" and "Has anyone ever made a bang or a loud noise with a gun?" Start with open-ended questions, and then move to specific questions if the child does not respond.

If the child discloses exposure to domestic violence, the clinician must remain very calm and unperturbed, regardless of how distressed he or she feels. The practitioner should tell the child that he or she is very glad the child told about these feelings. The provider must reassure the child that he or she and all the people with whom the clinician works want to be sure that the child is safe. The provider should tell the child that he or she will talk to some social workers and other people who will help Mommy and the child to be safe so that no one gets hurt

anymore. The practitoner must then immediately activate a domestic violence protocol, following the reporting guidelines of their jurisdiction.

School-Age Children

The provider can use the same question format as with the preschool child, using age-appropriate language and props. Sometimes school-age children prefer to answer questions by engaging in a written dialogue. Should the child be somewhat resistant or hesitant, the practitioner should ask if the child would like to draw pictures as answers. Alternatively, the clinician can write a question, with the child then writing the answer. Some children enjoy writing, especially if they can use a computer. This format is particularly useful because it provides an immediate, written document of the child's responses. This provider should keep this document with the patient's chart.

Should the provider identify that the child has been exposed to domestic violence, he or she again must reassure the patient of concern for the child's safety and that of the youngster's mother, and the practitioner will work with the child on this concern. The clinician must then immediately activate the domestic violence protocol.

Adolescents

Depending on their level of maturity, questions asked of adolescents will be more similar to those asked of adults; for example, "Do you feel safe at home?" and "Are other family members safe?" Adolescents who are in families with domestic violence are extremely vulnerable to victimization because of their efforts to seek help and gain acceptance from people outside of the family. They may have a history of having been sexually victimized or be at risk for dating violence. The provider appropriately should ask adolescents whether they think it is acceptable for individuals to hit, slap, shove, or push each other. The reader is referred to Part 1 and Part 2 for further discussion.

DIAGNOSTIC CRITERIA

As seen in Table 23-4 and Display 23-4, children and adolescents exposed to domestic violence can present with many different symptoms, ranging from almost none to severe disturbance. A number of psychological and psychiatric disorders are common to children who are exposed to domestic violence:

- PTSD
- Oppositional defiant disorder
- Conduct disorder
- Learning disabilities
- Separation anxiety disorder
- Depression
- Encopresis
- Enuresis

Physical symptoms can include the following:

- Chronic headache
- Abdominal pain
- Sleep disorders
- Speech disorders

▲ **Clinical Warning:** Clinicians should be aware that they may see atypical presentations of symptoms. Furthermore, behavioral or psychogenic problems do not necessarily indicate abuse. Providers should have a high index of suspicion when a constellation of symptoms is present or when they occur in a child for whom no other reasonable explanation can be found. As such, symptomatology should simply serve as part of the differential diagnosis.

● **Clinical Pearl:** It would be extremely unusual for a child or adolescent to report exposure to domestic violence that was not occurring or did not happen. In these rare situations, such disclosure would indicate a very unusual and disturbed child. Immediate referral to a psychologist will help to clarify the situation.

MANAGEMENT

Domestic Violence Intervention Protocol

Providers must ensure that their service delivery unit has access to multidisciplinary wrap-around services for victims of domestic violence. In many centers, these programs are already in place. In those hospitals and clinics with established programs, practitioners will be able to refer immediately and activate a well-developed response. In contrast, many practitioners will need to develop their own network within their own geographic region. Regardless of size and geographic isolation, setting up a well-coordinated, multidisciplinary response is not only possible, but imperative.

● **Clinical Pearl:** Every program that now exists was initiated by a small group of individuals who wanted to make life safe for children.

Wrap-around services for victims of domestic violence and their children require at minimum the following interdisciplinary components:

- Medical
- Mental health
- Social services
- Law enforcement and prosecution

Additional professionals and organizations whose services can strengthen the interdisciplinary model for violence intervention include the following:

- Visiting/public health nurses
- Pastoral care
- School personnel
- Community groups
- Shelters
- Civic groups
- Legal clinics

▲ **Clinical Warning:** Situations that require that the provider report to child protection or law enforcement include suspicion of child abuse, neglect, or failure-to-thrive; weapons; or a mother who presents with injuries from domestic violence

The provider's response to domestic violence needs to include the following:

- Identification of the domestic violence
- Treatment of injuries as needed

- Reporting to child protection/law enforcement, depending on laws in the jurisdiction
- Mental health assessment of the mother
- Mental health assessment of each child
- Legal advocacy for the mother (eg, assistance in obtaining restraining orders)
- Information about community resources available to the family
- Ongoing mental health and advocacy resources

● **Clinical Pearl:** The provider must have resources available that address chemical dependency treatment conjointly with domestic violence. With respect to treatment, consensus in the literature is that chemical dependency issues must be addressed first.

More specifically, in the case of an addicted victim, she must obtain treatment for chemical dependency and become sober before being able to address the dynamics of violence. For children, treatment issues should be dealt with concurrently.

Special Considerations

Undocumented Women (Immigrants)

Depending on location, some providers deliver health care to children whose mothers are undocumented. These mothers live in considerable fear of deportation and separation from their children, particularly if their partner is a legal resident or citizen. Perpetrators often use immigration status as a component of threat, intimidation, and isolation. They often tell mothers that if they ever disclose the domestic violence, they will be deported and lose their children. In the United States, the practitioner can tell the woman that she can apply for amnesty under the Violence Against Women Act (VOWA) if the batterer is a legal resident and she is legally married to him (Goldman, 1999). VOWA is a federal act, applicable in all jurisdictions of the United States. Most communities have legal counsel for women in this situation, and the multidisciplinary team typically will provide these resources to them. Providers in other countries need to acquaint themselves with their own federal laws regarding protection against deportation for their undocumented patients.

● **Clinical Pearl:** Sharing information related to VOWA with a mother who is particularly fearful can support her increased willingness to talk. She may be less fearful of reporting the abuse.

Women Infected With Human Immunodeficiency Virus

The overlap between domestic violence and infection with HIV is very high. Studies indicate that in approximately 50% of cases of HIV-positive mothers, a history of domestic violence also is present, with HIV infection caused by their batterers (Degani, Ferris, & Norton, 1997; Kalichman, Williams, Cherry, Belcher, & Nachimson, 1998; Molina & Basinait-Smith, 1998; Stevens & Richards, 1998).

▲ **Clinical Warning:** Clinicians providing services to children who are HIV positive, whose mothers are HIV positive, or both should be aware that HIV is an additional high-risk indicator for domestic violence.

Abused Children

Research literature extensively documents the overlap between domestic violence and child abuse. In at least 50% of homes with domestic violence, children are physically abused as well as adults (Edleson, 1999; Reams, 1999; Kolbo et al., 1996). The provider must be alert to issues involved in reporting child abuse and adhere to the relevant protocols. In a small percentage of domestic violence cases, the perpetrator also sexually abuses the children. Usually, these victims are nonbiologic children (Koverola & Morahan, 2000).

Children Abused by Siblings

A disturbing trend that clinicians and researchers have reported is sibling-on-sibling violence (Caffaro & Caffaro, 1998). The issues involved are particularly complex in terms of both assessment and treatment of the family. Child protection plays an important role in these cases. Mothers are often extremely resistant, particularly when it results in the removal of an older child. Older children are often the only support available to the mother. The mother then is conflicted in her needs to protect children against the need for someone to help manage her workload.

▲ **Clinical Warning:** It is a mistake to conceive of an aggressive older sibling as a perpetrator. The nature of the older child's behavior must be identified and acknowledged as serious. Without swift and intensive intervention, this older sibling is well on the road to becoming an adult perpetrator.

Primary Prevention

Providers should have posters displayed and pamphlets available in the clinic area. A number of short educational videos can be played in waiting areas. Children exposed to domestic violence need and deserve intervention, which begins with screening. Pediatric practitioners can play a vital role in identifying and referring these children for appropriate intervention services. Regardless of jurisdictional differences across regions and countries, multidisciplinary wraparound services are essential if these children are to be effectively reached and the cycle of intergenerational domestic violence broken.

● **Clinical Pearl:** The provider and clinic can join other members of the multidisciplinary team to heighten awareness. Schools are an excellent place to provide workshops and seminars to personnel, parents, and students.

COMMUNITY RESOURCES

Resources and Websites for Providers, Families, and Victims

- National Domestic Violence Hotline
  (800) 799-SAFE (7233); (800) 787-3224
- (TDD) RAINN: Rape Abuse Incest National Network
  (800) 656-HOPE (4673)
- Domestic Violence Information
  http://www.feminist.org/911/crisis
- U.S. Department of Justice
  http://www.orp.usdoj.gov/vawo/

Books

The provider may want to suggest any of the following texts to adult survivors of domestic violence:

- Betancourt, M. (1997). *What to do when love turns violent: A practical resource for women in abusive relationships.*

- Ferrara, F. F. (1999). *Conquered legacy: A healing journey.*
- Landes, A. (1997). *Violent relationships: Battering and abuse among adults.*

REFERENCES

Barnes, P. G. (1998). *Domestic violence: From a private matter to a federal offense.* New York: Garland.

Bhatt, R. V. (1998). Domestic violence and substance abuse. *International Journal of Gynaecology and Obstetrics, 63*(Suppl 1), S25–31.

Burke, L. K., & Follingstad, D. R. (1999). Violence in lesbian and gay relationships: Theory, prevalence, and correlational factors. *Clinical Psychology Review, 19*(5), 487–512.

Caffaro, J. V., & Caffaro, A. (1998). *Sibling abuse trauma: Assessment and intervention strategies for children, families, and adults.* Binghamton, NY: Haworth.

Campbell, J. C. (Ed.). (1998). *Empowering survivors of abuse: Health care for battered women and their children.* Thousand Oaks, CA: Sage.

Degani, N., Ferris, L. E., & Norton, P. G. (1997). Are wife abuse and HIV transmission connected? *Canadian Family Physician, 43*(1), 13–15, 20–23.

Edleson, J. L. (1999). Children's witnessing of adult domestic violence. *Journal of Interpersonal Violence, 14*(8), 839–870.

Goldman, M. (1999). The Violence Against Women Act: Meeting its goals in protecting battered immigrant women? *Family and Conciliation Courts Review, 37*(3), 375–392.

Gordon, L. (1988). *Heroes of their own lives: The politics and history of family violence.* Boston: Penguin.

Hedin, L. W., Grimstad, H., Moller, A., Schei, B., & Janson, P. O. (1999). Prevalence of physical and sexual abuse before and during pregnancy among Swedish couples. *Acta in Obstetrics and Gynecology, 78*(4), 310–315.

Kilpatrick, K. L., & Williams, L. M. (1998). Potential mediators of post-traumatic stress disorder in child witnesses to domestic violence. *Child Abuse and Neglect, 22*(4), 319–330.

Kalichman, S. C., Williams, E. A., Cherry, C., Belcher, L., & Nachimson, D. (1998). Sexual coercion, domestic violence, and negotiating condom use among low-income African American women. *Journal of Women's Health, 7*(3), 371–378.

Kolbo, J. R., Blakely, E. H., & Engleman, D. (1996). Children who witness domestic violence: A review of the empirical literature. *Journal of Interpersonal Violence, 11*(2), 281–293.

Koverola, K., & Morahan, M. (June, 2000). Differential impact of exposure to domestic violence and child sexual abuse: Maternal functioning as a mediating variable. Presented at the Victimization of Children and Youth: An International Research Conference , Durham, New Hampshire.

Kot, S., Landreth, G. L., & Giordano, M. (1998). Intensive child-centered play therapy with child witnesses of domestic violence. *International Journal of Play Therapy, 7*(2), 17–36.

Leung, W. C., Leung, T. W., Lam, Y. Y., & Ho, P. C. (1999). The prevalence of domestic violence against pregnant women in a Chinese community. *International Journal of Gynaecology and Obstetrics, 66*(1), 23–30.

Levendosky, A. A., & Graham-Bermann, S. A. (1998). The moderating effects of parenting stress on children's adjustment in women-abusing families. *Journal of Interpersonal Violence, 13*(3), 383–397.

Marais, A., de Villiers, P. J., Moller, A. T., & Stein, D. J. (1999). Domestic violence in patients visiting general practitioners—prevalence, phenomenology, and association with psychopathology. *South African Medical Journal, 89*(6), 635–640.

Miller, L. (1999). Treating posttraumatic stress disorder in children and families: Basic principles and clinical applications. *American Journal of Family Therapy, 27*(1), 21–34.

Molina, L. D., & Basinait-Smith, C. (1998). Revisiting the intersection between domestic abuse and HIV risk. *American Journal of Public Health, 88*(8), 1267–1268.

Naumann, P., Langford, D., Torres, S., Campbell, J., & Glass, N. (1999). Women battering in primary care practice. *Family Practice, 16*(4), 343-352.

National Center for Juvenile Justice. (1997). *Justice for children and families (annual report).* Pittsburgh: Author.

O'Farrell, T. J., Van Hutton, V., & Murphy, C. M. (1999). Domestic violence before and after alcoholism treatment: A two-year longitudinal study. *Studies in Alcoholism, 60*(3), 317–321.

Reams, R. (1999). Children birth to three entering the state's custody. *Infant Mental Health Journal, 20*(2), 166–174.

Rodriguez, M. A., Craig, A. M., Mooney, D. R., & Bauer, H. M. (1998). Patient attitudes about mandatory reporting of domestic violence. Implications for health care professionals. *Western Journal of Medicine, 169*(6), 337–341.

Seyfrit, C. L., Crossland, C. R., & Hamilton, L. C. (1998). Alcohol, drugs, and family violence: Perceptions of high school students in southwest Alaska. *International Journal of Circumpolar Health, 57*(Suppl 1), 459–466.

Siegel, R. M., Hill, T. D., Henderson, V. A., Ernst, H. M., & Boat, B. W. (1999). Screening for domestic violence in the community pediatric setting. *Pediatrics, 104,* 874–877.

Sheridan, D. J. (1998). Health care-based programs for domestic violence survivors. In J. C. Campbell (Ed.), *Empowering survivors of abuse: Health care for battered women and their children* (pp. 23–31). Thousand Oaks, CA: Sage.

Stephens, D. L. (1999). Battered women's views of their children. *Journal of Interpersonal Violence, 14*(7), 731–746.

Stevens, P. E., & Richards, D. J. (1998). Narrative case analysis of HIV infection in a battered woman. *Health Care of Women International, 19*(1), 9–22.

Wilson, C. (1998). Are battered women responsible for protection of their children in domestic violence cases? *Journal of Interpersonal Violence, 13*(2), 289–293.

Wilson, M., & Daly, M. (1993). Spousal homicide risk and estrangement. *Violence and Victims, 8,* 3–16.

The Addicted Newborn

• DANIEL RAUCH, MD

INTRODUCTION

Drug abuse, a well-documented problem found in all socioeconomic groups, knows no cultural boundaries. It does not spare pregnant women; in fact, pregnancy magnifies drug problems because both mother and child experience the consequences. Pregnant women are vulnerable physiologically and psychologically, while the fetus suffers both directly from the drug and indirectly from comorbid effects of the mother's drug use. The long-term outcomes are just now coming to light, and effects on the infant clearly can be lifelong. Identifying those at risk is not easy, and options that are available once identification has been made are not ideal.

The "addicted newborn" is not an agreed-upon clinical term. It is used to refer to infants who exhibit some behavioral changes during the newborn period and who test positive for drugs of abuse. The term's true meaning is that providers are able to recognize some infants who have been exposed to drugs of abuse. It does not include exposed infants who are not detected in the newborn period or whose mothers, for medical reasons, used prescription drugs, the effects of which may not be known. A useful reference about the safety and potential effects of most prescription drugs in pregnancy and breastfeeding is *Drugs in Pregnancy and Lactation* (Briggs, Freeman, & Yaffe, 1998).

ANATOMY, PHYSIOLOGY, AND PATHOLOGY

Although not all primary care providers are involved in obstetric care, an understanding of pregnancy can help them to comprehend the effects of drug abuse on the mother and unborn child. Intoxication, a well-described risk factor for unprotected sex and therefore pregnancy, may affect the woman's response to a resulting pregnancy for which she was unprepared. While the psychological effects on the woman cannot be underestimated, the conceptus is spared any direct physiologic effects because no transfer of toxins occurs before implantation in the uterus. Once the conceptus has implanted in the uterus, all subsequent nourishment comes from the placenta. The growing fetus then is exposed to the same things as the mother. The degree of exposure depends highly on the substance. The mother rapidly metabolizes some drugs, so the fetus is relatively spared. The placenta may easily transfer drugs with a longer half-life, with effects concentrating in the fetus. The fetus has certain capabilities, which vary according to fetal age and level of exposure, to metabolize and clear drugs. Pregnancy is a huge metabolic demand on the mother; when combined with drug use and poverty, it often results in poor maternal nutrition. Further, maternal drug use clearly is associated with sexually transmitted infections (STIs), many of which can infect and damage the fetus.

Physiologic Effects of Teratogens

The effects of any teratogen, including drugs of abuse, are more pronounced in the early stages of pregnancy when the vital organs are developing. Understanding the critical role of timing is essential, because the fetus is most at risk during the time when many women are still unaware that they are pregnant. Therefore, even "recreational" drug use can profoundly affect the fetus.

Cigarette and marijuana use creates an abnormally high carboxyhemoglobin level in the mother, which can induce a chronic mild fetal hypoxia. The most visible outcome is the small-for-gestational age baby born secondary to placental insufficiency. Less obvious effects are late cognitive deficits as a result of hypoxia in the developing central nervous system (CNS). Cocaine also may produce hypoxic damage by causing vasospasm with resultant decrease in blood flow to the affected area. These infarctions can happen in the brain or any other end organ. Placental infarctions can cause premature labor, exposing the infant to the additional risks of prematurity. Infants of opiate-using mothers have earlier lung maturation, possibly secondary to chronic fetal distress.

Jones and Smith (1973) coined the term fetal alcohol syndrome (FAS) to describe a constellation of signs and symptoms seen in children born to alcohol-abusing mothers:

- Growth retardation
- Dysfunction of the CNS, most often mental retardation, but also learning disabilities, attention deficit, hyperactivity, poor impulse control, and others
- Facial anomalies, including short palpebral fissure, flat midface, short nose, indistinct philtrum, and thin upper lip

The child with full FAS exhibits symptoms of all three categories. Less affected children are described as having fetal alcohol effect. Estimates are that 5000 cases of FAS (1 in 750 births) occur each year. According to the most recent data, FAS is the leading known etiology of mental retardation (Abel & Sokol, 1987; Barone, 1996).

Neurobehavioral and Cognitive Effects of Teratogens

Subtler neurobehavioral or cognitive effects may take much longer to reveal themselves. Clearly, gross mental retardation and developmental delay become apparent within the first year of life; less profound effects may take longer to appear. Significant controversy exists over the long-term effects of drug exposure. During the crack cocaine epidemic in the early 1990s, many studies of "crack" babies described infants with much the same CNS involvement as children with FAS. Anonymous screening of pregnant mothers at delivery, however, indicates that incidence of maternal exposure to crack was much higher than was the number of "crack" babies. Thus, some babies were not exhibiting this "crack syndrome." Later studies have not found any consistent deficits in these babies as they grow up, after confounding for effects such as poverty and prematurity. Other studies have demonstrated a relationship with the amount of exposure. This is only to say that the effects are not predictable at birth (Datta-Bhutada et al., 1998; Richardson & Day, 1994). Recent studies on children of smoking mothers have demonstrated lasting behavioral consequences (Williams et al., 1998).

Economic Impact of Drug Addiction in Newborns

The cost to society of maternal drug abuse is staggering. Increased length of stay and additional tests for these babies increase medical costs. Added to these costs are the need for social work and other services. If the child is removed from the mother, foster care and associated legal and bureaucratic expenses are incurred. When the mother is allowed to keep the baby, it is usually with the aid of additional services, such as a visiting nurse to check on the child. Later costs include long-term management and treatment of children who have behavioral or cognitive deficits. Lifelong costs can be tremendous, with estimates of an annual expenditure of over $300 million for children with FAS alone (Abel & Sokol, 1987; Streissguth et al., 1991).

EPIDEMIOLOGY

Estimates of the numbers of pregnant women who abuse drugs are unclear and vary according to the study method used. Self-reported use during prenatal care is considered accurate for those who report drug abuse. Self-reporting measures do not provide data about pregnant women who choose not to report or deny drug use or who are lost to reporting measures because they do not receive prenatal care. Other reports represent results of toxicology screening at delivery, which is an accurate indicator of drug use immediately preceding delivery but is inaccurate about drug use that may have occurred earlier in the pregnancy. Data from the most recent national survey of pregnancy and health (National Institutes of Health, 1992) suggest that 10% of pregnant women smoke cigarettes, 10% drink alcohol, and 5% use illegal drugs. Rates of illegal drug use were higher among unmarried, uneducated, and unemployed women and among women on public assistance. The problem exists, however, in all socioeconomic, ethnic, and geographic groups. The most common illegal drug used was marijuana, followed by cocaine (National Institutes of Health, 1996). At least 12% of babies born in the United States are exposed perinatally to drugs of abuse. Even if one added up the frequency of all the different diseases routinely screened for in the newborn period, from metabolic diseases to hearing loss, the total would not come close to the incidence of perinatal drug exposure.

DIAGNOSTIC CRITERIA

Detection of at-risk mothers and infants can be difficult. Clearly, providers should take seriously any woman self-reporting drug use and test the woman for all the drugs of abuse because of the possibility of multidrug use. The clinician should obtain a careful history of the prepartum mother whenever possible and screen the mother as appropriate. Routine screening based on epidemiologic risk factors without clear cause is a potentially difficult practice that varies based on each state's laws.

Often, suspicious behavior in the newborn is the first clue that the mother has abused drugs. The "jittery" or "irritable" baby is the classic description of the addicted newborn. Jitteriness is described as coarse, tremulous movements of the face and extremities. The term "irritable" is used to describe the infant who is hypersensitive to all environmental stimuli. Vomiting, diarrhea, or both usually accompany irritability.

● **Clinical Pearl:** Published behavioral scales have rated objectively an infant's behavior. Examples of tools used frequently are cited at the end of this chapter. The clinician should consult with a child psychiatrist, child behaviorist, or other pediatric mental health professional who is skilled in assessment and testing of the drug-addicted infant.

▲ **Clinical Warning:** The provider should always keep in mind that there are other causes for these behaviors, including hypoglycemia, electrolyte abnormalities, and infection. All these other organic reasons can represent neonatal emergencies that providers must address rapidly and appropriately. This sometimes makes drug testing more difficult.

Jitteriness is associated with maternal perinatal cocaine use, although methamphetamines probably produce a similar effect, as can nicotine. Cocaine is commonly used "recreationally" and may go undetected in the newborn period if the mother used it early in the pregnancy. On the other hand, crack is well known for its ability to induce labor, and the pregnant woman may use it when she wants to deliver. Irritable babies with vomiting, diarrhea, or both may be exhibiting neonatal abstinence syndrome, which is consistent with exposure to a depressant, such as an opiate (eg, heroin) or alcohol. Even when these babies are found to have another etiology for their behavior, providers should not forget drug effects because maternal drug abuse is associated with prematurity and low birth weight, putting the infant at higher risk for infection.

▲ **Clinical Warning:** The provider must be aware that withdrawal may not occur in the newborn nursery. Withdrawal can occur days to even a few weeks after discharge home. Providers should follow the infants of all mothers identified as drug abusers closely after discharge.

DIAGNOSTIC STUDIES

Newborn behavior that is suspicious for addiction or maternal report of drug use in pregnancy should provoke a confirmatory drug test. Three major options are available for providers to use in newborn testing:

- Urine
- Meconium
- Hair

Each has advantages and disadvantages. Urine toxicology screens are probably the most widely used and available tests. Optimally, the provider should send the infant's very first void for testing, although this specimen may be lost in the delivery room. Advantages are that renally excreted products are concentrated in the urine, and urine is usually easily obtained. Disadvantages are that many drugs are rapidly metabolized so that any delay in obtaining urine means a significant decrease in the ability to detect the substance. It also means that urine testing indicates peripartum use, which may not reflect any long-term habits. The provider should be aware of how urine screens are done and exactly which drugs are routinely tested versus those that must be requested specifically. Some laboratories initially test urine for broad classes of substances, such as opiates or barbiturates. If the overall level is high enough, then the laboratory will test for specific substances, such as morphine or heroin. It is possible to be positive for a drug class but have low enough levels of the individual substance and its metabolites that the final report is negative.

Positive drug findings in meconium and hair reflect a longer history of maternal use than does a positive urine test. The fetus starts to produce meconium in the second trimester, so meconium can reflect exposure over a much longer period than can urine. Additionally, meconium is rather easy to obtain and is rarely used for any other testing relative to the infant's well-being. Many laboratories can now test meconium, although not as many as can test urine. Hair testing is not currently a standardized test (Marques, 1996).

MANAGEMENT

Addiction in a newborn is often the signal that brings the drug-using mother to attention. Clearly, it is too late to prevent any damage that has already been done to the newborn. Therefore, the most effective treatment is to counsel women of childbearing age and treat them before they become pregnant. Chapter 5 provides more information on this topic. With the cost of dealing with addicted children so high, the cost effectiveness of treatment before pregnancy is self-evident.

For the pregnant mother identified as a drug user, treatment during pregnancy depends on the drug of abuse. Clearly, abstinence is a goal, but the psychological and physiologic toll of eliminating an addiction must be considered. Providers also should remember that women who use drugs during pregnancy may be held legally accountable for their behavior. In the United States, some states have prosecuted drug-using pregnant women for child abuse.

Treatment of the drug-addicted infant is usually symptomatic. Most infants literally can be nursed through any symptoms with careful attention. Swaddling the child to provide comfort and limiting extrasensory stimulation are effective. Vomiting and diarrhea usually are not severe enough to affect the infant's electrolyte balance, although providers should monitor both electrolyte and calorie intake. Occasionally, additional medical management is necessary for serious symptoms, such as seizures, severe vomiting and diarrhea, and poor weight gain.

▲ **Clinical Warning:** Medications should be used with consultation from a pediatrician or neonatologist who is experienced in treating addicted newborns. Paregoric commonly is used for severe diarrhea. The starting dose is 0.2 to 0.3 mL/dose every 3 to 4 hours, which can be increased by 0.05 mL/dose until symptoms abate. Alternatively, a 25-fold dilution of opium tincture may be used in an equal dose. Phenobarbital is effective as an antiepileptic. It is given as a loading dose of 15 to 20 mg/kg at a rate not greater than

1 mg/kg/min. Opiate withdrawal may be treated with a methadone taper, with actual methadone withdrawal usually requiring a longer taper than heroin withdrawal.

● **Clinical Pearl:** The provider must thoroughly evaluate any addicted newborn for associated illnesses. Drug-using mothers have a much higher incidence of STIs. Evaluating and treating the infant for congenital infections, including human immunodeficiency virus (HIV), is appropriate.

The discharge disposition of the child is clearly an issue. Most providers have serious misgivings sending a newborn home with a documented drug-using mother. Drug use alone may not be sufficient for invoking the local version of child protective services, although the provider must treat each case individually and with some knowledge of prevailing local standards. Visiting nurse services are an excellent way to monitor the infant for late-onset withdrawal and the quality of the home environment. The provider may want to see these infants within the first week and even weekly after that for a month or two to carefully monitor the child's progress.

Long-term treatment of addicted newborns remains controversial. Most experts recommend referral to early intervention services, although the outcomes of such programs are unclear. Reports on the efficacy of occupational and physical therapy in premature infants suggest that the major effect is to produce stronger mother–child bonding without any significant developmental benefits. Bonding should not be underestimated, however, because attachment to the child has been associated with better maternal outcome in terms of drug abstinence. Clearly, some of these infants have neurobehavioral deficits that will be lifelong. Such children require special education, therapy, and even ongoing management for these problems. Refer to Chapters 21 and 24 for further discussion of these problems. These chapters also examine expected outcomes of treatment beyond the newborn stage.

Ethical Concerns

Identification of an addicted infant and his or her drug-abusing mother raises issues beyond primary care management fix double break. A multidisciplinary team approach, including providers, social workers, and counselors, is necessary. A social context in which drug use occurs is clear, and the possibility for an individual provider to affect that context may seem minimal. The provider must be familiar, however, with potential means for social intervention.

▲ **Clinical Warning:** The child's protection should be paramount at all times. Involvement of child protection services may be warranted, although other means of invoking services are often preferable. Right-to-privacy issues are involved with testing infants and mothers; the provider should be aware of state and local regulations.

Supporting the Family

In addition to referring the family of the addicted newborn to appropriate professionals, such as addiction treatment and mental health, the primary care provider also may need to refer them for visiting nurse/public health nurse support. Nurses and other professionals associated with their agencies, including social workers and physical therapists, can provide a fragile family with the physical and emotional support they need to accomplish activities of daily living.

Nurses especially can assist the family in learning how to be safe and effective parents. Most municipalities also provide social workers as family support resources. No one needs such support more than the family struggling with addiction. Should a provider in the United States be concerned about a child's safety, federal and state statutes require the provider to report such beliefs to child protection authorities. Providers in other national jurisdictions need to abide by legal, professional, and ethical standards.

It is not uncommon for the addicted newborn to be parented, temporarily if not permanently, by a grandparent. Most often this individual is the grandmother. She may be filled with love for her grandchild, may resent the intrusion in her life, or may be conflicted about her feelings. She also may be dealing with unresolved issues about the child's parents, especially the mother. Finally, if she herself is an older individual, she may be struggling with the physical effects of her own aging. Income may be limited. These and other issues can quickly lead to caregiver burnout and, perhaps, lay the foundation for child abuse. The provider is ethically bound to seek out referral services to assist this individual in her task. In some larger municipalities, local senior services include support group activities for grandparents who are raising their children's children. The provider should be acquainted with any and all services, both municipal and church or service related, which might be available to help the multigenerational family. Refer to the Chapter 23 for more information and ideas about supporting the family.

REFERRAL POINTS AND CLINICAL WARNINGS

Withdrawal can occur days to even a few weeks after discharge home. The infant of any mother identified as a drug abuser should be closely followed after discharge.

- Newborn behavior that is suspicious for addiction or maternal report of drug use in pregnancy should provoke a confirmatory drug test.
- If unfamiliar with drug withdrawal therapies, the provider should consult with a pediatrician or neonatologist experienced in treating addicted newborns before initiating treatment for withdrawal.
- Evaluating and treating the infant for congenital infections, including HIV, is prudent.
- Referral to early intervention services may be warranted in some instances. Periodic developmental testing to provide tracking and occupational and physical therapy services are available at no charge through state children's services.
- Involvement of child protection services may be warranted, although other means of invoking services are often preferable.

COMMUNITY RESOURCES

Resources for Provider and Family

Many resources for dealing with addiction are available to both provider and family. A selection of these include the following:

- Child Welfare League of America (This is a resource for printed materials and information on current child advocacy needs.)
  1st Street, 3rd Floor
  Washington, DC, 20001-2085
  (202) 638-2952; Fax (202) 638-4004
  http://www.cwla.org
- Children's Aid Society (This society provides emergent and long-term child and family counseling services for its clients in northern New England, Connecticut, and New York. Phone consultation services are available, as are referral services.)
- Alcoholics Anonymous (AA); Narcotics Anonymous (NA); Al-Anon; AL-A-Teen (These provide intensive support services in most localities. AA and NA target the abuser. Al-Anon and Al-A-Teen provide group support for family members.)

Additional Resources for Providers

Briggs, G. G., Freeman, R. K., & Yaffe, S. J. (1998). *Drugs in pregnancy and lactation: A reference guide to fetal and neonatal risk* (5th ed.). Baltimore, MD: Williams & Wilkins.
Brazelton, T. B. *The neonatal behavior assessment scale* (3rd ed.). Clinic in Developmental Medicine, 88.
Korner, A. F., & Thom, V. A. (1990). *The neurobehavioral assessment of preterm infant.* New York: The Psychological Corporation.
Finnegan, L. P. (1986). Neonatal abstinence syndrome: Assessment and pharmacology. In F. F. Rubatelli & B. Granati (Eds.), *Neonatal therapy: An update.* New York: Excerpta Medica.
Lester, B. M., & Tronick, E. Z. The NICU Network Neurobehavioral Scale. National Institute of Child Health and Human Development contract N01-HD-2-3159.

REFERENCES

Abel, E. L., & Sokol, R. J. (1987). Incidence of fetal alcohol syndrome and economic impact of FAS-related mental retardation. *Drug and Alcohol Dependence, 19,* 51–70.
Barone, M. A. (ed.). (1996). *The Harriet Lane Handbook* (14th ed.). St. Louis: Mosby.
Datta-Bhutada, S., Johnson, H. L., & Rosen, T. S. (1998). Intrauterine cocaine and crack exposure: Neonatal outcome. *Journal of Perinatology, 18*(3), 183–188.
Jones, K. L., & Smith, D. W. (1973). Recognition of the fetal alcohol syndrome in early infancy. *Lancet, 2,* 999–1001.
Marques, P. R. (1996). Factors to consider when using hair as a cocaine-exposure measure for mothers or newborns. *NIDA Research Monograph, 166,* 183-97.
National Institutes of Health. (1996). *National Pregnancy and Health Survey Drug use among women delivering livebirths: 1992,* National Institute on Drug Abuse, NIH publication #96-3819.
Richardson, G. A., & Day, N. L. (1994). Detrimental effects of prenatal cocaine exposure: Illusion or reality? *Journal of the American Academy of Child and Adolescent Psychiatry, 33*(1), 28–34.
Streissguth, A., et al. (1991). Fetal alcohol syndrome in adolescents and adults. *Journal of the American Medical Association, 265*(15), 1961–1967.
Williams, G. M., et al. (1998). Maternal smoking and child psychiatric morbidity: A longitudinal study. *Pediatrics, 102*(1).

Adolescent Substance Experimentation and Abuse

• RICHARD HEYMAN, MD, FAAP

INTRODUCTION

The use of mind-altering substances is arguably the most significant and dangerous risk behavior that adolescents exhibit. While the use of tobacco, alcohol, and other drugs (TAOD) is just one of many problems today's teens are facing, the distorted thinking that accompanies such use puts children at greater risk than does any other behavioral health problem (American Academy of Pediatrics, 1997). The pediatric primary care provider must play an important part in prevention, identification, and assessment of substance use. This chapter discusses this role in the context of the primary care practice setting.

PATHOLOGY

A variety of factors influence a young person's decision to experiment with TAOD. Family factors, including tolerance of aberrant behavior and parental role modeling, are certainly critical. Acceptance of use in the community and at school and the degree to which authorities curtail such behavior affect availability and use patterns. Some teens feel compelled to announce their independence through rebelliousness and antisocial behavior. Some teens experiment with mind-altering drugs simply to feel better and obliterate underlying feelings, such as depression, alienation, anger, and anxiety.

▲ **Clinical Warning:** Teens who are not activity oriented and have no commonly identified peer group (eg, teammates, Scouts, fellow musicians) may spend inordinate time "hanging out." When mixed with self-esteem issues and poor motivation, a lack of positive interests is an additional risk factor.

As they consider these risk factors, providers must recognize that substance use is, in fact, a continuum. Many individuals will experiment with mind-altering substances only to abandon use or use infrequently and only under controlled circumstances. Others will develop the pattern of high-reward compulsive use and experience adverse consequences in life, work, relationships, and health. Individual risk and protective factors will play an important role in determining these issues. Display 25-1 provides information that the primary care provider can use when assessing adolescent risk for TAOD use.

Putting a young person's choice to use mind-altering substances into the context of other risk behaviors may help to explain the phenomenon further. Jessor (1991) has defined such behaviors as those that jeopardize the individual's physical, emotional, or psychological health. Examples include truancy, delinquency, inappropriate sexual behavior,

TAOD use, membership in gangs, carrying weapons, and even athletic activities pursued in an unsafe manner. Such risk behaviors tend to cluster (because the risk factors for such activities are similar). Thus, the provider identifying one risk behavior should be vigilant about looking for others. Furthermore, for the various kinds of risk factors there are antidotes, or "protective factors." The net influence of such risk and protective factors helps to determine the behaviors of young people. Jessor (1991) has defined five "domains" of risk and protective factors, presented in Table 25-1. Identification of risk and protective factors in an individual patient is an excellent way to initiate a discussion of risk behaviors and lifestyle. It may furthermore represent an important method of helping to build self-esteem and encourage family activities.

EPIDEMIOLOGY

Use of TAOD among adolescents increased significantly throughout the last decades of the 20th century. The "Monitoring the Future" (MTF) study (Johnston, O'Malley, & Bachman, 1999), conducted annually by the University of Michigan on behalf of the National Institute on Drug Abuse, samples more than 50,000 students in grades 8, 10, and 12 and is generally regarded as a benchmark in assessing usage patterns. Among its 1999 findings was the continued widespread use of alcohol among teenagers. Among eighth graders, 10% admitted to having gotten drunk within the 30 days immediately preceding the survey. Nearly one in four 10th graders had done so, and a third of high school seniors reported so-called "binge drinking" (defined as having had at least four [for women] or five [for men] drinks in a row).

Ninety percent of those people who will ever smoke begin before their 19th birthday. In fact, of adults who are regular smokers, the average age at which they began was 12½ years. Most had progressed to regular use within 2 years (Centers for Disease Control and Prevention, 1994).

Some 37% of eighth graders admit to having used an illegal drug at some point in their lifetime. That number rises to 50% by 10th grade but goes up only an additional 2% by high school graduation, suggesting that generally, teens make the decision to experiment by age 15. Marijuana is the most commonly used illegal substance (though of course purchase of alcohol and tobacco products is also illegal for the students surveyed). The MTF study consistently shows that 50% of high school seniors have tried marijuana, as have 40% of 10th graders and 22% of eighth graders. While there is slight male predominance and a geographic skew toward the coasts, the numbers have remained remarkably steady throughout the 1990s (Johnston et al., 1999).

Inhalant abuse, the deliberate inhalation of volatile substances, frequently constitutes a young teen's first exposure to mind-altering drugs. Among eighth graders, 12% admit-

DISPLAY 25–1 • Why Young People Start Using Drugs

Family
- Lack of supervision
- General parental permissiveness
- General parental rigidity
- Parental role modeling
- Biogenetic factors

Community/School
- Ready availability and perception of normativeness
- Tolerance and acceptance of drugs
- Neighborhoods with high crime/use patterns
- Lack of commitment to school and future
- Absence of attachment to social institutions

Peer Factors
- Desire to belong
- Peer pressure and acceptance
- Lack of attachment
- Boredom/group antisocial behavior
- Sense of affinity and common interest with group that uses

Self Factors
- Sense of rebelliousness
- Need for independence
- Tendency toward reckless, risk-taking behavior
- Acquisition of desired image (usually as portrayed by advertising and media)
- Need for increased self-esteem
- Desire to look older
- Curiosity
- Desire to feel better

Source: Heyman, B. B., & Adger, H. (1997). Office approach to drug abuse prevention. *Pediatric Clinics of North America, 44*(6), 1447–1455.

("ecstasy") and methamphetamine have become increasingly available and are current drugs of choice for young people exploring the world of mind-altering drugs. Use of narcotics and cocaine also has shown steady upward trends, as purer forms have made alternate routes of administration, such as smoking and nasal inhalation ("snorting"), available.

▲ **Clinical Warning:** Most people usually make the decision to use TAOD during the second decade of life. Thus, providers caring for children and teenagers have a major responsibility to identify those at risk and convey the prevention message at every available opportunity.

HISTORY

As one concerned with the total welfare of the individual and family, the primary care provider is perfectly situated to take an active role in the prevention and identification of substance abuse. Ideally, the provider should address this issue throughout his or her relationship with the family.

Age-Appropriate Strategies

During a prenatal visit, issues related to TAOD use should be at the forefront of discussion. The effects on the fetus when a pregnant woman consumes alcohol are well defined and span the gamut from full-blown fetal alcohol syndrome (which includes specific facial defects and cognitive and social problems) to the milder forms of alcohol-related brain damage and neurodevelopmental disorders (see Chap. 24). Pregnant women should not drink: no dosage is safe for a fetus. The provider should emphasize this point repeatedly.

Smoking is hazardous as well. Infants born to mothers who smoke during pregnancy may have underdeveloped lungs and low birth weight. They are at increased risk for sudden infant death syndrome (Schoendorf & Kiely, 1992). Pregnant women should quit smoking, and those caring for them should offer cessation assistance (including nicotine replacement therapy if indicated) (Fiore et al., 2000). Infants and children exposed to environmental tobacco smoke have an increased incidence of upper respiratory and middle ear infections. They tend to experience more episodes of bronchitis and pneumonia and are more likely to have asthma (Etzel, Pattishall, Haley, Fletcher, & Henderson, 1992).

Finally, illegal drugs, including cocaine, narcotics, and even marijuana, may have adverse fetal effects. Decreased placental circulation resulting in low birth weight and devel-

ted to having used inhalants in the previous year; that number tapers to 9% for 10th graders and 7% for high school seniors. These findings suggest that inhalants are a "starter" drug, with teens moving to other substances as they get more sophisticated (Johnston et al., 1999).

Teens use other illegal drugs commonly as well. Hallucinogens such as LSD showed a pattern of steadily increasing use throughout the 1990s. Chemicals such as MDMA

Table 25–1.   FIVE DOMAINS WITH RISK AND PROTECTIVE FACTORS

Domain	Risk Factors	Protective Factors
Biology/genetics	Family history of alcohol abuse or mental health disorder	High intelligence; good health
Social environment	Poverty; easy access to TAOD in community or school	Quality schools; intact family; sense of belonging and responsibility
Perceived environment	Peer substance abuse; use by adults; lack of positive adult role models; media and advertising imagery depicting use as positive	Productive peers with conventional values; family attachment and supervision; positive role models
Personality	Low self-esteem; lack of attachment; enjoyment of thrill seeking; sense of limited options for future	Desire to achieve success in a somewhat conventional way
Behavior	Low aspirations, expectations, motivation	Participation in social activities; sense of purpose, with goals and aspirations

opmental disorders, as well as an infant who is drug-addicted, are sad consequences of maternal use. Providers should advise pregnant women who are using drugs to seek treatment. They always should offer treatment in lieu of taking legal action. Refer to Chapter 24 for more information.

Children growing up in homes where alcohol and drug abuse are problems may display a wide range of psychosocial problems as well. Neglect and abuse are certainly more common in such families. Extensive research on children of alcoholics reveals that more subtle problems, such as low self-esteem, anxiety and other mental health disorders, decreased school achievement and learning ability, problems with social relationships, and the child's use of alcohol and drugs, are often seen as well (Zucker & Fitzgerald, 1991).

As children grow, their exposure to the media becomes a major factor in introducing them to TAOD. Advertising (Evans, Farkas, Gilpin, Berry, & Pierce, 1995) is a major force in promoting substance abuse as it creates the imagery, for example, that smoking makes one cool, sexy, popular, rich, successful, and thin. Beer is promoted as the normal reward for all successes, the necessary accompaniment of good times, and the natural key to popularity and social prowess. Unfortunately the media rarely show negative consequences. Advertisements depict smokers as suave, not emphysematous. Drinkers are sophisticated, never drunks. Even the "moderation" commercials some brewers have produced depict partying as fun, with drinking as an integral element.

Movie and television scripts and commercials portray tobacco and alcohol use as universal. Many films and programs associate cigars, fine wines, and liqueurs with sophistication and financial success. Teens who see their favorite actresses and actors using alcohol and tobacco perceive the behavior as "normal." Again, the entertainment industry rarely shows the consequences of substance abuse, and often the characters are young and especially appealing to adolescents.

Children are keen observers of parental use as well. Parents who model appropriate use of alcohol as a beverage, not a chemical to consume to get drunk, actually may promote their children's subsequent use of alcohol in an equally appropriate fashion. Those who serve alcohol every time a guest is in the house, who convey that good times always entail drinking, and who overuse the substance themselves are providing a dysfunctional role model.

Most young people experiment with tobacco and alcohol in middle school and junior high school. Statistics repeatedly show that of those who smoke regularly as adults, 15 is the mean age at which most had become regular smokers. Studies show that those who start using tobacco early are at increased risk of progressing to other drugs (Center on Addiction and Substance Abuse at Columbia University, 1995). The topic of TAOD use should occupy a prominent place in the anticipatory guidance menu of the care provider seeing this age group. Useful lines of discussion include "deconstructing" tobacco and beer ads to show how they manipulate young people through imagery and asking why the patient thinks tobacco and beer use are so prevalent. Answers to these kinds of questions may shed some insight into how young people see themselves and their peer group and may provide parents and care providers with information as to how best to promote non-use.

Finally, all adolescents will be exposed to TAOD use. They all will know people who use; most will have tried tobacco and alcohol. As formal operational thinking develops toward college age, young people may be better able to understand the concept of "responsible use." While drinking and drug use are rampant in society, not everyone partakes. A reasonable approach might be to discuss drinking, tobacco, and marijuana use on college campuses from the standpoint of "harm reduction." That is to say, drinking and smoking are inherently dangerous activities. Individuals can minimize risks in a number of ways, including abstaining from tobacco, limiting alcohol consumption, not driving while intoxicated, not riding with intoxicated drivers, avoiding drinking games, not using illegal drugs, and being careful about activities pursued while drinking.

Interviewing Children and Adolescents in the Office Setting

When interviewing young people, providers must establish from the outset the principle of confidentiality. They can do so by discussing the provider's policy of confidentiality with both parent and child at age 11 or 12, before most sensitive adolescent issues are likely to arise. Most parents are, in fact, pleased that the provider will address these topics. Providers can reassure the occasional parent who is anxious about such issues that they will discuss them carefully and that they will involve the parent if significant problems become evident.

Discussing sensitive issues requires asking the parent to leave the room and interviewing the young person alone. The care provider's opening remarks should discuss the concept of confidentiality, the limits of such confidentiality, and how he or she will handle an issue that requires parental involvement. Defining these ground rules is essential for trust to be established, yet it helps the provider pursue critical issues, such as suicide or sexual abuse, appropriately. Refer to Chapter 12 for specific information on the adolescent interview. Chapter 26 also provides interview ideas and red flag information.

The care provider addressing sensitive issues must be comfortable with the concept of "open-ended questioning." Asking "yes" or "no" questions frequently leads to one-word answers or nondescript grunts. Starting with nonthreatening inquiries, such as how things are going at home and school, is useful and can lead logically to discussions of friends and pastimes. To ask about TAOD use, for example, one might start by asking if the teen has friends who use TAOD or knows people who do. The clinician might continue this line of questioning by asking if the patient has ever been offered TAOD or been at a party where others were using TAOD. This leads logically to the provider's inquiring if the patient has ever tried cigarettes, beer, or other substances and if so, what it was like. If the patient has not used, the provider should commend the decision and reinforce reasons for abstaining.

The provider should assess in a casual and nonthreatening way the teen who admits to having experimented with TAOD. What experience has the teen had with such substances? Has the teen ever been "drunk" or "stoned?" Has he or she experienced any adverse consequences in the areas of personal or family relationships, school, work, or recreational activities? Providers may find the CAGE assessment presented in Display 25-2 useful.

▲ **Clinical Warning:** While not statistically validated for adolescents, a positive answer to any of the four CAGE questions suggests a problem with alcohol or drugs.

If a provider suspects that a young person has problems with TAOD, a comprehensive assessment is the proper approach. Urine screens for drugs of abuse have limited accuracy and may fail to detect alcohol. They furthermore reflect the patient's status at one isolated point in time and may be

---

DISPLAY 25–2 • The CAGE Assessment

- Have you ever felt the need to **C**ut down on your use of alcohol or drugs?
- Have you ever felt **A**ngry because someone suggested you use too much?
- Have you ever felt **G**uilty about your alcohol or drug use?
- Have you ever felt the need for an "**E**ye-opener" to get your day going?

---

subject to adulteration if the patient is able to do so. A much more appropriate approach is to obtain a professional consultation with someone skilled in performing such assessments, using one of the variety of instruments available to screen for problem drug behavior. Only in this way can a valid diagnosis be made and a treatment plan developed.

Stages of Substance Abuse

All substance abuse begins with the decision to try a drug for the first time. This choice can have devastating consequences if a young person decides he or she likes the feeling and begins to use the drug regularly or has a serious adverse consequence. In assessing young people in the office, determining the "stage" of substance abuse is useful. The *Diagnostic and Statistical Manual,* fourth edition (1994) and the *Diagnostic and Statistical Manual for Primary Care* (1996) provide useful definitions of "substance abuse" and "substance dependence." For teenagers using alcohol and other drugs, providers should define stages of use, as outlined in Display 25-3.

DISPLAY 25–3 • Stages of Substance Abuse

- Potential for abuse: need for excitement and peer acceptance; decreased impulse control; lack of long-term goal orientation; availability of alcohol and other drugs
- I. Experimentation: learning the mood swing (usually with alcohol, nicotine, and marijuana); learning how to use the drug under controlled circumstances with few consequences and maintenance of normal lifestyle
- II. Regular use: enjoying the mood swing and seeking it; advance to additional drugs, including prescription stimulants, sedatives, and hallucinogens; more regular use eventually leading to gradual deterioration in life functions, including hygiene and appearance, school, work, activities, sports, with early involvement of discipline administered by family, school, or courts.
- III. Preoccupation: needing drugs to get through the day; use of additional drugs more frequently and in greater amounts, with concomitant deterioration in life functions; association mainly with drug-using peers; major consequences of use imposed by family, school, judicial system.
- IV. Addiction: needing drugs to feel normal; heavy use of multiple substances; marked physical, social, and mental deterioration; physical symptoms of withdrawal when drugs not available.

Source: MacDonald, D. I. (1984). *Drugs, drinking and adolescents.* Chicago: Year Book Medical Publishers.

● **Clinical Pearls:**

- "Abuse" implies significant impairment and failure to fulfill obligations in the domains of work, family, or school; frequent use associated with hazardous situations; problems with the law; and use despite consequences.
- "Dependence" implies symptoms, including tolerance (increased amounts needed for the same clinical effect), withdrawal, use that is out of control, and the desire to decrease such use; the consumption of great time and effort to obtain the drug; abandonment of other responsibilities in pursuit of the drug; and use despite major life consequences.

● **Clinical Pearl:** Perhaps the most important aspect for primary care providers to understand is that, unfortunately, some use of TAOD is "normal." Most teenagers try a cigarette or two, experiment with alcohol and even marijuana, and suffer no consequences. Staying in stage I or early stage II is the rule: most adolescents who try TAOD will experiment, use occasionally, and do well. The provider's goal is to identify those who are at risk of progressing or are already having symptoms (late stage II and stages III and IV). These young people need referral and assessment.

DIAGNOSTIC CRITERIA

Adolescent drug users can be great "con artists" and even better liars. They can look their parents directly in the eyes and sheepishly protest their innocence without a twinge of conscience or guilt. Eventually, though, the constellation of signs and symptoms becomes too obvious for parents, teachers, and the primary care provider to ignore.

Changes in personal appearance and hygiene may be the first clue. Slovenliness, "hippie"-type dress, clothing with prodrug messages, body piercing, and tattoos may become the teen's new uniform as he or she becomes part of the drug-using community.

Physical symptoms may include red eyes, chronic cough, excessive sleeping, or periods of prolonged waking and activity. Changes in appetite with resultant weight loss or gain are common as teens use drugs that alter the way their minds and bodies work. Moodiness and abrupt changes in attitude are a hallmark of the drug-using teen. Lack of motivation, failure to complete assignments or chores, and generalized truculence and noncommunicativeness are all part of the biochemical changes the drug use is inducing. Secretive behavior, lying, spending excessive time alone and away from the family, strange phone calls, new "friends," and unknown visitors may represent the teen's gathering and using time.

School performance usually declines, and dropping out of former activities, such as sports, Scouts, church, or anything that requires association with straight, nonusing peers, follows. The teen appears chronically bored, as drug using becomes the only real outlet and sole activity that sparks any interest.

Finally, of course, parents may find paraphernalia suggestive of drug use in the home or car. Fake identification cards; matches; pipes; rolling papers; stashes of seeds and herb-like material; odor cover-ups, such as incense or breath spray; and missing alcohol and prescription drugs all point to the teen's drug use. "I'm just holding it for a friend" is the usual response to being discovered; parents should not be fooled by such an excuse.

MANAGEMENT

The decision to intervene in the life of a young person using alcohol and other drugs requires confidence and commitment on the part of the primary care provider. Clinicians may find it an ongoing challenge to work with teens whose thinking has been distorted by drugs and alcohol and to convince them that a problem exists. Most providers believe that further assessment is necessary when substance abuse has begun to interfere with life functions, including job, school, activities, personal relationships, safety, or health.

▲ Clinical Warning: Untreated substance abuse is a fatal disease. In every sense, it is a family disease as well. Because insurance, consent, and transportation issues usually are involved, obtaining treatment means breaking confidentiality with the teenager. How this is done can be critical in helping young people to break through the denial of the effects their substance abuse is having on them and their family.

One useful model involves the process of "intervention," which is done by arranging a meeting between the provider, the teen, and people who care about the teen's well-being. Such people might include the family, one or more peers (preferably abandoned "straight" friends), a concerned adult (eg, teacher, guidance counselor, religious leader, coach), and even a trusted relative. One at a time, each person speaks to the teen and explains how the substance abuse is affecting the patient's life as well as the relationship with the speaker. When an intervention goes well, the teen may respond with a willingness to accept the diagnosis and to acknowledge the need for treatment. When intervention fails, at least those involved know that they have made a concerted attempt to break through the denial, opening the issue for discussion. This may lead to progress at a later date.

▲ Clinical Warning: The individual conducting an intervention must be knowledgeable about counseling techniques, crisis intervention, treatment facilities, and grief management. The primary care provider who does not feel capable of running such a conference should identify a provider in the community who can assist. The provider should identify community resources in the area and have knowledge of those that are appropriate and available to the patient, based on insurance considerations.

Arranging treatment for the teen who is abusing substances requires knowledge of available treatment facilities, indications for different levels of care, information as to what services are covered under a patient's insurance, and personal experience as to which programs are comprehensive and effective. Limitations on available programs, the family's insurance coverage or ability to pay privately, and the teen's willingness to enter treatment will all significantly impact the provider's recommendations. The clinician should be aware of available options, acting as an advocate with insurance companies and health maintenance organizations for the most appropriate care available.

Comorbidity of Substance Abuse and Mental Health Disorders

Providers must recognize the frequent coexistence of substance abuse and mental health disorders in children and adolescents. Depression occurs more often in girls, whereas conduct disorder occurs more often in boys. These disorders represent major risk factors for the use of mind-altering drugs. While both may be primary diagnoses, a comprehensive psychiatric assessment should be performed once the patient has stopped using TAOD for at least 1 month (American Academy of Pediatrics, Committee on Substance Abuse, 2000). Suspicion of mental health problems may be heightened when they exist elsewhere in the family, when the condition predated the onset of drug use, or when the patient does not seem to improve when not using drugs (Grilo et al., 1995). Refer to Chapters 21 and 28 for more information about the diagnosis and management of behavioral and mental health needs.

What to Tell Parents

Substance abuse represents a major health threat to children and adolescents. Chemicals may have severe effects on growing and developing tissues, including the brain. While some degree of experimentation with tobacco, alcohol, and even marijuana may be normal for today's adolescents, the primary care provider must not only watch vigilantly for signs and symptoms that such use is occurring, but also to give prevention messages and anticipatory guidance to all young patients.

Convincing a family to obtain treatment for a child's substance abuse may at first be difficult. Issues of denial, time constraints, and finances may pose barriers to treatment. Providers should remind parents that substance abuse and dependence is a disease—one that is progressive and fatal if not treated. Treatment for substance abuse works. Statistics suggest that success rates are as good for substance abuse as for other conditions, such as cancer and obesity. The primary care provider's firm but gentle advice may be the motivating factor that persuades the family to seek treatment.

COMMUNITY RESOURCES

The American Society of Addiction Medicine (1996) has created its "Adolescent Crosswalk," a graphic representation of treatment options that outlines criteria for selecting a substance abuse treatment facility. The Adolescent Crosswalk recognizes five levels of treatment, starting with early intervention for those who have some insight into their problem, a solid family support system, and no underlying medical or psychosocial problems. Level I outpatient treatment is indicated for those who need a bit more structure and support, while more intensive level II outpatient treatment may be indicated for those who have underlying emotional concerns, are in denial, and have a less than ideal home situation. Levels III (medically monitored inpatient treatment) and IV (medically managed inpatient treatment) are reserved for those who have more severe symptomatology, including withdrawal symptoms, severe emotional problems, high resistance to treatment, and likelihood of subsequent relapse, as well as an unsupportive or even dangerous home environment.

REFERENCES/BIBLIOGRAPHY

Rockville, MD: U. S. Department of Health and Human Services, Public Health Service.
American Academy of Pediatrics, Committee on Substance Abuse. (1997). Tobacco, alcohol and other drugs: The role of the pediatrician in the prevention and management of substance abuse. *Pediatrics, 101,* 125–128.
American Academy of Pediatrics, Committee on Substance Abuse. (1996). *The classification of child and adolescent mental diagnosis in primary care.* Elk Grove Village, IL: Author.

American Academy of Pediatrics, Committee on Substance ABuse. (2000). Indications for management and referral of patients involved in substance abuse. *Pediatrics, 106,* 143–148.

American Psychiatric Association. (1994). *Diagnostic and statistical manual of mental disorders* (4th ed.). Washington, DC: Author.

American Society of Addiction Medicine. (1996). *ASAM patient placement criteria for the treatment of substance-related disorders* (2nd ed.). Chevy Chase, MD: Author.

Center on Addiction and Substance Abuse at Columbia University. (1995). *National Survey of American Attitudes on Substance Abuse.* New York: Author.

Centers for Disease Control and Prevention. (1994). *Preventing tobacco use among young people: A report of the Surgeon General.* Atlanta, GA: US Department of Health and Human Services, Public Health Service, 66-67.

Etzel, R. A., Pattishall, E. N., Haley, N. J., Fletcher, R. H., & Henderson, F. W. (1992). Passive smoking and middle ear effusion among children in day care. *Pediatrics, 90,* 228–232.

Evans, N., Farkas, A., Gilpin, E., Berry, C., & Pierce, J. (1995). Influence of tobacco marketing and exposure to smokers on adolescent susceptibility to smoking. *Journal of the National Cancer Institute, 87,* 1538–1545.

Fiore, M. C., Bailey, W. C., Cohen, S. J., et al. (2000). Treating tobacco use and dependence. *Clinical Practice Guidelines.* Rockville, MD: U.S. Department of Health and Human Services. AHRO Publication #00-0032.

Grilo, C. M., Becker, D. F., Walker, M. L., Levy, K. N., Edell, W. S., & McGlashan, T. H. (1995). Psychiatric comorbidity in adolescent inpatients with substance use disorders. *Journal of the American Academy of Child and Adolescent Psychiatry, 34*(8), 1085–1091.

Heyman, R. B., & Adger, H. (1997). Office approach to drug abuse prevention. *Pediatric Clinics of North America, 44*(6), 1447–1455.

Jessor, R. (1991). Risk behavior in adolescence: A psychosocial framework for understanding and action. *Journal of Adolescent Health, 12,* 597–605.

Johnston, L. D., O'Malley, P. M., & Bachman, J. G. (1997). *Monitoring the future: Questionnaire responses from the nation's students 1997.* Ann Arbor, MI: Institute for Social Research, University of Michigan.

MacDonald, D. I. (1984). *Drugs, drinking and adolescents.* Chicago: Year Book Medical Publishers.

Schoendorf, K. C., & Kiely, J. L. (1992). Relationship of sudden infant death syndrome to maternal smoking during and after pregnancy. *Pediatrics, 90,* 905–908.

Zucker, R. A., & Fitzgerald, H. E. (1991). Early developmental factors and risk for alcohol problems. *Alcohol, Health and Research World, 15*(2).

Self-Destructive Behavior

• ROGER NUÑEZ, MD; MIRIAM T. VINCENT, MS, MD; and DAISY ARCE, MD

INTRODUCTION

Children and adolescents who display self-destructive attitudes most likely are involved in several risk behaviors that may result in injury or even death (Jessor, 1991). One common risk behavior among adolescents is unsafe and premature sexual activity, which contributes to unintended pregnancies and the spread of sexually transmitted infections (STIs), including human immunodeficiency virus (HIV). Other self-destructive behaviors include smoking, drinking alcohol, using drugs, missing school, carrying weapons, participating in potentially violent groups, contributing to unintentional and intentional injuries, eating poorly, and self-mutilating.

Primary care providers are in an ideal position to address the needs of children who are or may be at risk for self-destructive behavior. They have the advantage of knowing children and their families for many years and thus can anticipate the development of self-destructive behavior. The following chapter provides a framework for the identification of and intervention in the cycle of self-destructive behavior.

PATHOLOGY OF SELF-DESTRUCTIVE BEHAVIOR: CAUSES AND DETERMINANTS

Examining any self-destructive behavior in isolation is difficult because all such behaviors can be antecedents to or consequences of any of the others. Many biologic, genetic, environmental, and psychological factors have been proposed to explain the general development of self-destructive behaviors; however, no single theory or combination of different theories has been able to do so fully. One well-known theory is the primary socialization theory, which asserts that all human social behaviors are learned or at least have major components that are learned. The theory's core is that adolescents are enmeshed in a social network consisting of primary socialization sources, including the family, school, peer clusters, and media (Oetting & Donnermeyer, 1998; Strasburger, 1997). Any interference with bonding or communication of norms through primary socialization sources will become a risk factor for the development of self-destructive behavior. Table 26-1 presents primary socialization sources and risk factors for self-destructive behavior.

The Role of the Family

Family factors can contribute significantly to the onset of self-destructive behavior in children and teens. Lack of supervision, general parental permissiveness, and, conversely, parental rigidity, are all problems. The absence of appropriate adult role models (including parents themselves), family history of substance abuse or alcoholism, biogenetic predisposition, history of mental health disorder, parental rejection, physical or sexual abuse, history of domestic violence, poor financial and housing status, and unemployment are all familial risk factors for self-destructive attitudes.

Parental use, patterns, and opinions about tobacco, alcohol, and other drugs range from permissiveness to rigid condemnation. Children of alcoholics and substance abusers are at tremendously increased risk for use (Heyman & Adger, 1997). Survivors of childhood sexual abuse have higher rates of self-harm, eating disorders, sexual dysfunction, and teen pregnancy than do others (Romans, 1996; Jarvis, 1997; Elders, 1998). Primary care providers must be prepared to identify all these risk factors associated with the family to design management and monitoring strategies for troubled adolescents and their families.

The Role of Schools

Schools are primary sources for acquiring and testing prosocial norms. Reiff (1998) reports that better students do poorly when moved into worse schools, while poorer students often improve when placed in better schools. Better schools are best characterized as those that emphasize academics, allow teachers autonomy to meet the education needs of individual students, and have programmatic flexibility systems of incentives and rewards that allow students to assume responsibility for their own behaviors.

Epidemiologic studies support the premise that children who fail to form appropriate bonds in school are at increased risk for drug use, early pregnancy, and other deviant behaviors. Adolescent school failure, a powerful indicator of self-destructive behavior, results from an array of forces, many of which are outside the adolescent's control (Reiff, 1998). School failure is the result of a long process. Because schools frequently measure progress through grades and group achievement testing, many opportunities are available for preventing school failure.

Low self-esteem is a significant predictor of school failure (Reiff, 1998). Because strong family relationships and success in school contribute so greatly to it, self-esteem in a teen likely signifies good bonding with these primary socialization sources, which in turn are likely to discourage self-destructive behavior (Oetting, Deffenbacher, & Donnermyer, 1998). Both children and adolescents who have low self-esteem about their academic ability require individualized opportunities for successful academic experiences.

One disorder likely to result in self-destructive behavior is attention deficit hyperactivity disorder (ADHD). The symptomatic inattention, forgetfulness, and inability to stay focused on a task are likely to create bonding problems both at home and in school. ADHD is associated with anger and aggression, which are likely to disrupt further the child's bonding with family, school, and prosocial peers (Barkley, 1997). If parents and teachers are able to deal effectively with

Table 26–1. PERCENTAGE OF HIGH SCHOOL STUDENTS WHO ENGAGE IN SELECTED HEALTH-RISK BEHAVIORS, BY GRADE GROUP

Behavior	High School Grade				
	9	10	11	12	Total
Rarely used safety belts[+']	21.2	16.6	19.5	19.7	19.3
Rarely used motorcycle helmets[¶][0]	41.5	33.3	35.0	34.9	36.2
Rode with a drinking driver**	9.7	11.5	19.9	25.3	16.9
Participated in physical fight[+'+]	44.8	40.2	34.2	28.8	36.6
Carried a weapon[§–§]	22.6	17.4	18.2	15.4	18.3
Lifetime cigarette use[¶][0]¶	66.7	70.0	68.8	73.7	70.2
Current cigarette use***	33.4	35.3	36.6	39.6	36.4
Current smokeless tobacco use[+'++]	9.7	6.8	10.0	10.5	9.3
Lifetime alcohol use[§–§§]	72.0	77.4	81.9	84.0	79.1
Current episodic heavy drinking[¶][0]¶¶	25.7	29.9	37.5	39.3	33.4
Lifetime marijuana use****	38.8	45.9	50.3	52.4	47.1
Current marijuana use	23.6	25.0	29.3	26.6	26.2
Lifetime cocaine use[+'+++]	6.7	7.5	9.1	9.2	8.2
Ever injected drugs	3.0	2.5	1.6	1.5	2.1
Ever had sexual intercourse	38.0	42.5	49.7	60.9	48.4
Sexual intercourse with more than three sex partners	12.2	13.8	16.7	20.6	16.0
Used condom during most recent sexual intercourse	58.8	58.9	60.1	52.4	56.8
Used birth controls during most recent sexual intercourse	7.8	12.0	15.6	24.0	16.6
Reported having been taught about HIV in school	89.8	91.6	92.4	92.2	91.5
Reported having been taught about HIV by guardian	61.6	62.1	62.2	65.6	62.8
Ate fruits and vegetables[v]	31.3	31.7	27.2	27.2	29.3
Ate foods typically high in fat[ð@]	43.0	39.4	35.0	33.1	37.7
Thought they were overweight	27.1	26.0	28.1	27.9	27.3
Engaged in moderate physical activity[f–]	28.1	22.3	17.4	14.8	20.4

'+Safety belts used "always" when riding in a car or truck as a passenger.
[0]¶Helmets used "always" among respondents who rode motorcycles.
***Role at least once during the 30 days preceding the survey in a car or other vehicle driven by someone who had been drinking alcohol.
'+Fought at least once during the 12 months preceding the survey.
-§§Carried a gun, knife, or club at least 1 day during the 30 days preceding the survey.
[0]¶¶Ever tried cigarette smoking, even one or two puffs.
****Smoked cigarettes on 1 or more of the 30 days preceding the survey.
'+++Used chewing tobacco or snuff on 1 or more of the 30 days preceding the survey.
-§§§Ever drank alcohol.
[0]¶¶¶Drank five or more drinks of alcohol on at least one occasion during the 30 days preceding the survey.
*****Ever used marijuana.
*++++Ever used cocaine.
'oAmong the respondents who had who had sexual intercourse during the 3 months preceding the survey.
vvAte five or more servings of fruit and vegetables the day preceding the survey.
@ðAte more than two servings of foods typically high in fat the day preceding the survey.
-f Walked or rode a bicycle at least 30 minutes at a time on 5 or more of the 7 days preceding the survey.
Adapted from Centers for Disease Control and Prevention. (1998). Youth Risk Behavior Surveillance-United States, 1997. *MMWR, 47,* SS3.

a child who has ADHD, bonding with the family or school will not suffer. The probability of substance use and other self-destructive behavior will not be increased (Oetting et al., 1998). Successful management of conduct disorder (CD), an externalized behavioral/emotional disorder, is the same as for ADHD: behavioral techniques, cognitive-behavioral training, and possibly stimulant medication (Reiff, 1998). ADHD and CD are easily recognizable in the classroom. Early intervention can support the formation of prosocial bonds. Refer to Chapter 21 for more information.

Teachers, coaches, and peers are less likely to identify internalized behavioral and emotional disorders, depression, or anxiety. Primary care providers must inquire about and identify any internalizing behavior problems in children who are performing poorly in school. Clinicians may be the only professionals outside school who are prepared to diagnose and

treat these children. Chapter 28 provides more information on internalized behavioral and emotional disorders.

The Role of Peers

Literature spanning the last 5 decades strongly supports the influence of peers on self-destructive behavior (Oetting & Donnermeyer, 1998). Strong selection factors in the formation of peer clusters, some of which are external to the individual and imposed by culture, the environment, or chance, include age differences, gender, ethnicity, living in the same neighborhood, and classroom seating. Although superficially it may appear paradoxical, weak bonds with healthy peers can lead ultimately to strong bonds with deviant peers. Healthy peers often reject younger children who express deviant attitudes.

● **Clinical Pearl:** When child–family and child–school bonds are weak, peers may dominate the youngster's primary socialization. Children with weak bonds to family and school will seek out or be attracted to other youth with similar problems. The resulting peer clusters transmit norms through discussion and shared experiences and directly monitor and reinforce the attitudes and self-destructive behaviors of their members.

The Role of Personal Traits

Personality theory views behavior as emerging from and explained by personality traits. This approach has a fundamental problem. Personality traits rarely account for more than a small proportion of the variance in behavior, particularly self-destructive behavior. In contrast, socialization links, such as schools, families, and peers, can account for a large proportion of variance in behavior. Traits are likely to lead to self-destructive behaviors when they interfere with bonding with family, school, or peers or if personal traits interfere with the transmission of prosocial norms (Oetting et al., 1998). Children with underlying issues, such as obsessive-compulsive disorder (OCD), CD, or ADHD, may find the comfort with deviant peers that they cannot attain with family or normal children (Kaplan, 1996).

Even in the presence of a genetic predisposition to anger and aggression, behaviors are learned traits. Anger and aggression appear early in a child's development. Early problems in family–child bonding can lead the child to act out and use anger as a means of expression. This is particularly true when parents model anger or when their discipline is inconsistent or overly harsh. Such modeled behaviors exacerbate the child's anger and stimulate further problematic parent–child interactions, reinforcing anger and aggression. A child with high levels of anger and aggression may affect others in a peer cluster. When children of similar traits interact, their anger and aggression can become normalized within that peer cluster. Thus, anger and aggression become part of the group's subculture. The result is a peer cluster with poor bonds to prosocial influences and a high potential for self-destructive behavior (Oetting et al., 1998).

Low self-esteem results from being unable to conform to conventional standards of family, school, and peer groups. Children with low self-esteem then form links with deviant peers to reduce self-derogation. Low self-esteem seems to occur only at specific times, after failure with prosocial primary socialization sources and before bonding with deviant peers.

Although not directly related to low self-esteem, evidence suggests that sensation seeking may have at least a partial genetic basis (Benjamin et al., 1996). Members of a sensation-seeking cluster may encourage one another to perform risky, deviant behaviors, including excessive drinking, high-speed driving, and using drugs.

The Role of Media and Advertising

Television and other media represent one of the most important and least recognized influences on the health and behavior of children and adolescents. Objections to various programming and advertising practices have come from common sense, philosophical, aesthetic, humanistic, and public health perspectives. An increasing number of studies document the existence of serious problems (Strasburger, 1997; Strasburger & Donnerstein, 1999).

Children and adolescents are a captive audience for entertainment producers. On average, young people watch 16 to 17 hours of television weekly, beginning as early as age 2

years (Nielsen Media Research, 1998). Video games and video cassettes comprise an additional 2 to 4 hours of viewing per week. Some teenagers spend as many as 35 to 55 hours each week in front of the television set. Regardless of all other issues, the viewing of television, video cassettes, and video games exerts a significant displacement effect of 2 to 3 hours per day, meaning that children and adolescents spend less time engaged in physical activity, reading, or interacting with friends. Many adolescents also spend many hours listening to the radio, although they generally use music to accompany other activities. Few data currently are available about young people's use of the Internet, but past evidence suggests that "surfing the Net" will prove as popular as television, videos, video games, and music (William, Montgomery, & Pasnik, 1997).

● **Clinical Pearl:** Self-destructive behavior is learned. Such learning occurs in social groups—families, peer groups, and gangs. Television and other media may function as a "super peer" in this respect.

Whether at the movies, on videos or television, or in music, young people view an estimated 10,000 acts of violence each year. The National Television Violence Study examined 10,000 hours of television programming for 3 years and found that 61% of programming contains violence. Children's programming is the most violent, and 26% of violent interactions on these programs involve the use of guns (Federman, 1998). Researchers have concluded that children learn their attitudes about violence at a very young age; once learned, these attitudes tend to be lifelong (Eron, 1995).

A comprehensive analysis of music videos demonstrated that 22.4% of all videos played on Music Television (MTV) portrayed overt violence. Heavy metal music, which is more rebellious than other types of rock music, abounds with lyrics that glorify hatred and abuse (Shank & Gabel, 1996; DuRant et al., 1997; Christenson & Roberts, 1998). Caucasian male teens who engaged in five or more risky behaviors were most likely to name a heavy metal music group as their preferred music choice.

▲ **Clinical Warning:** Research on the relationship between media violence and real-life aggression is voluminous and clear: A cause-and-effect relationship exists. High levels of television viewing are causally related to aggressive behavior and acceptance of aggressive attitudes. This correlation is stable over time, place, and demographics (Donnerstein, Slaby, & Eron, 1995; Smith & Donnerstein, 1998).

Although more than 1000 studies have linked media violence to real life violence, only five studies have demonstrated any connection between media with high sexual content and changes in the sexual behavior or attitudes of teens. Thus, for sexual activity, inferences must be drawn from the violence literature. The Internet offers unparalleled access to hard core pornography with just a few keystrokes (Log-On Data Corporation, 1996). *Playboy* or *Playgirl* has been read by 92% of males and 84% of females by age 15 (Strasburger & Donnerstein, 1999). Data suggest that the media (television, movies, and magazines) account for 39% of teenagers' sexual information (Kaiser Family Foundation, 1997). The glut of inappropriate sexual messages in the mainstream media, coupled with the absence of appropriate messages about abstinence and the use of birth control, may partially account for the United States continuing to have the highest teenage pregnancy rate in the western world (Alan Guttmacher Institute, 1996).

● **Clinical Pearl:** Each year teenagers view nearly 15,000 sexual references. Fewer than 170 deal with abstinence, birth control, STIs, or pregnancy. Family hour on prime time television contains more than eight sexual incidents per hour (Strasburger & Donnerstein, 1999).

Correlation studies indicate a positive relationship between alcohol and tobacco advertisement and exposure and consumption (Schooler, Feighery, & Flora, 1996; Strasburger & Donnerstein, 1999). Commercials involving cartoon characters, such as the Budweiser frogs (promoting an alcoholic product), had a 73% recall by children 9 to 11 years old (Leiber, 1996). In one well-publicized study, children as young as 6 years old were likely to mistake Old Joe Camel as being the Mouseketeer logo for the Disney channel or to associate him directly with cigarette smoking (Fischer, Schwart, Richards, Goldstein, & Rojas, 1991). One third of teenagers own cigarette promotional items, and these adolescents are four times more likely to be smokers (Sargent et al., 1997). One third of all adolescent smoking is causally related to tobacco promotional activities (Pierce, Chol, Gilpin, Farkas, & Berry, 1998).

Few studies have examined the factors that may lead susceptible individuals to undertake acts of sefl-mutilation. Showcasing criminal acts in the mainstream media has likely influenced susceptible individuals to undertake self-mutilating acts (Catalano, Morejon, Alberts, & Catalano, 1996). The mainstream media has taken notice (Egan, 1997). Just as anorexia nervosa and bulimia nervosa did several

years ago, self-mutilation is making its way into public consciousness. If predictions are correct, a large number of self-mutilators, especially repetitive cutters and burners, can be expected to seek treatment, and pressure will be exerted to develop innovative, effective therapy (Kehrberg, 1997).

The Role of the Community

The community in which a child lives and grows exerts tremendous influence. Neighborhoods with high crime rates and tolerance or acceptance of drug use create an environment of normalized deviance. The likelihood of an individual associating with deviant peer clusters increases when a child lives within or near these clusters. Conversely, healthy family–child and school–child bonding greatly reduces an individual's deviance, notwithstanding deviant influences in the child's community (Oetting & Donnermeyer, 1998).

EPIDEMIOLOGY

The Centers for Disease Control and Prevention (CDC) conduct Youth Risk Behavior Surveys every 2 years to examine the relationship between self-destructive behavior and subgroups, such as age, gender, and ethnicity. Subgroup findings from the national 1997 Youth Risk Behavior Surveillance System (YRBSS) are shown in Tables 26-2, 26-3, 26-4, and 26-5. These data can assist primary care providers in identifying

Table 26–2.   COMPARISON OF HEALTH RISK BEHAVIORS OF HIGH SCHOOL STUDENTS BY GENDER

Male Students Were More Likely Than Female Students to Report:	**Female Students Were More Likely Than Male Students to Report:**
Rarely or never wearing seat belts	Engaging in suicide-related behaviors
Driving after drinking alcohol	Not using a condom
Carrying weapons	Not eating fruits and vegetables daily
Carrying guns	Using laxatives or vomiting and taking diet pills either to lose weight or to keep from gaining weight
Participating and being injured in a physical fight	Not participating in vigorous physical activity
Carrying a weapon on school property	Not participating in strengthening exercises
Being threatened or injured with a weapon on school property	Exercising for less than 20 min during PE class
Being in a physical fight on school property	Not participating in sports teams
Having property stolen or deliberately damaged on school property	
Using smokeless tobacco	
Engaging in episodic heavy drinking	
Using marijuana (lifetime and current)	
Using cocaine (current)	
Using illegal steroids and inhalants (lifetime)	
Initiating cigarette, alcohol, and marijuana use before 13 y of age	
Using smokeless tobacco, alcohol, and marijuana on school property	
Being offered, sold, or given an illegal drug on school property	
Not talking with parents or older adult family members about AIDS or HIV infection	
Initiating sexual intercourse before age 13 y	
Their partner not using birth control pills	
Using alcohol or drugs at last sexual intercourse	
Eating more than two servings of foods typically high in fat content daily	

Adapted from Centers for Disease Control and Prevention. (1998). Youth Risk Behavior Surveillance-United States, 1997. *MMWR, 47,* SS-3.

Table 26–3. COMPARISON OF HEALTH RISK BEHAVIORS OF HIGH SCHOOL STUDENTS BY ETHNICITY

Caucasian Students Were More Likely Than African American or Hispanic Students to Report:	African American Students Were More Likely Than Caucasian or Hispanic Students to Report:	Hispanic Students Were More Likely Than Caucasian or African American Students to Report:
Driving after drinking alcohol	Rarely or never wearing seat belts or bicycle helmets	Rarely or never wearing motorcycle helmets
Currently and frequently using cigarettes	Carrying a gun	Riding with a driver who had been drinking alcohol
Initiating cigarette use before 13 y of age	Participating and being injured in a physical fight	Carrying weapons and guns
Using cigarettes on school property	Being in a physical fight on school property	Being threatened or injured with a weapon on school property
Using smokeless tobacco	Being threatened or injured with a weapon on school property	Feeling too unsafe to go to school
Using smokeless tobacco on school property	Feeling too unsafe to go to school	Engaging in suicide-related behaviors
Using alcohol (current and lifetime)	Not being taught about AIDS or HIV infection in school	Currently using cigarettes
Episodic heavy drinking	Having had sexual intercourse during their lifetime	Using alcohol (lifetime and current)
Not talking with parents or other adult family members about AIDS or HIV infection	Being currently sexually active	Episodic heavy drinking
Not using condoms	Initiating sexual intercourse before 13 y of age	Using cocaine (lifetime and current)
Using alcohol or drugs at last sexual intercourse	Having had four or more sex partners during their lifetime	Using lifetime "crack" steroid, inhalant, and other illegal drugs
Not participating in moderate physical activity	Not using birth control pills	Initiating cigarette, alcohol, marijuana, and cocaine use before 13 y of age
Not attending PE class daily	Ever being pregnant or getting someone else pregnant	Using alcohol and marijuana on school property
	Eating more than two servings of foods typically high in fat content daily	Being offered, sold, or given an illegal drug on school property
	Not participating in vigorous physical activity	Not being taught about AIDS or HIV infection in school
	Not participating in strengthening exercises	Not talking with parents or other adult family members about AIDS or HIV infection
	Not participating in school-sponsored sports teams	Having had sexual intercourse during their lifetime
		Initiating sexual intercourse before 13 y of age
		Not using condoms or birth control pills
		Using laxatives or vomiting
		Not participating in vigorous physical activity
		Not participating on sports teams

Adapted from Centers for Disease Control and Prevention. (1998). Youth Risk Behavior Surveillance-United States, 1997. *MMWR, 47,* SS-3.

the need for education and services based on a higher prevalence of risk behavior in identified subgroups. For example, findings have shown that African American and Hispanic children (57% and 45%, respectively) are significantly more likely than Caucasian non-Hispanic children (17%) to engage in high or very high-risk behaviors. Children who are 1 year older than their classmates (behind one modal grade) have a 20% to 30% greater chance of dropping out of school, even when controlled for achievement, social status, and gender. Race and ethnicity cease to become factors in school dropout when control for social status is exerted (Reiff, 1998). Because the biannual YRBSS surveys are conducted among high school students, results do not include adolescents who have dropped out of school. It is likely that

the risk behavior indices are much higher in the drop-out population.

● **Clinical Pearl:** Both academic and social success in school are excellent markers for general adolescent well-being. School failure and low grades are powerful predictors of high-risk behaviors, including delinquency, substance abuse, and pregnancy (Reiff, 1998).

In the United States, 43% of children 1 to 4 years, 51% of children 5 to 14 years, and 75% of adolescents and young adults 15 to 24 years died from four major causes in 1997: motor vehicle crashes, other unintentional injuries, homicide, and suicide (CDC, 1997). For every death from injury

Table 26–4.   COMPARISON OF HEALTH RISK BEHAVIORS OF HIGH SCHOOL STUDENTS BY GRADE

Students in Grades 9 and 10 Were More Likely Than Students in Grades 11 and 12 to Report:	Students in Grades 11 and 12 Were More Likely Than Students in Grades 9 and 10 to Report:
Carrying weapons	Driving after drinking alcohol
Being threatened or injured with a weapon on school property	Using alcohol (lifetime and current)
Participating in a physical fight	Episodic heavy drinking
Being in a physical fight on school property	Using marijuana (lifetime)
Having property stolen or deliberately damaged on school property	Having had sexual intercourse during their lifetime
Feeling too unsafe to go to school	Having had four or more sex partners during their lifetime
Engaging in suicide-related behaviors	Being currently sexually active
Using inhalants (lifetime)	Ever being pregnant or getting someone else pregnant
Initiating cigarette, alcohol, and marijuana use before 13 y of age	Not participating in stretching and strengthening exercises
Initiating sexual intercourse before 13 y of age	Not being enrolled in a PE class
Not using birth control pills	Not attending PE class daily
Eating more than two servings of foods typically high in fat content daily	Not participating in non–school-sponsored sports teams

Adapted from Centers for Disease Control and Prevention. (1998). Youth Risk Behavior Surveillance-United States, 1997. *MMWR, 47,* SS-3.

Table 26–5.   PRIMARY SOCIALIZATION SOURCES AND RISK FACTORS FOR SELF-DESTRUCTIVE BEHAVIOR

Family	**School**
Lack of supervision	Behind one modal grade
General parental permissiveness	Lack of individualized successful academic experiences
General parenting rigidity	Lack of mentored learning experiences
Lack of appropriate adult role models	Lack of a focus on basic academic skills
History of mental health disorder	Lack of teacher's autonomy to meet individual student needs
Physical or sexual abuse	Inflexible school programs
Parental rejection	Not allowing students to take responsibility for their own behavior
Minimal parental warmth	Lack of system of incentives and rewards for students
Parental criminality/deviance	Raising school standards without raising school quality
Unemployment	Grouping classes by ability (psychological cost for low achievers)
Poor financial and housing status	Lack of school-based mental health teams
Family composition/absence of parents	Lack of follow-up of early intervention programs
Marital discord	
Substance abuse by parents	
Peers	**Youth (Personal Traits)**
Desire to belong to a contemporary group	Sense of rebellion
Failure to form prosocial bonds	Need for independence
Contagion effect of deviant peers	Anger and aggression
Self-esteem derived from peers versus school or family	Need for increased self-esteem
Normalized deviant subculture	Sensation seeking
Lack of attachment	Tendency toward reckless behavior
Media	**Community**
Displacement effect	Tolerance and acceptance of drugs
Media and advertising portrayal that use is normative	High crime
Stylized violence	Absence of attachment to social institutions
Glut of violence and inappropriate sexual behavior	Lack of community support for school programs
Lack of appropriate education on violence and sex	Lack of prenatal drug and alcohol counseling
Child-friendly promotion of alcohol and cigarettes	
Easy access to pornography through internet and cable television	
Musical lyrics glorifying hatred and abuse	

that occurs among adolescents, an estimated 41 hospitalizations and 1100 emergency department visits also occur (Kelton & Shank, 1998). The leading causes of mortality and morbidity among youth also are implicated for adults, meaning that the self-destructive behavior of youth can continue into adulthood.

Results from the 1997 YRBSS demonstrate that many high school students engage in behaviors that increase their likelihood of death from those four main causes. Nationally, about 60% of all adolescent accidental fatalities are from motor vehicle crashes. In the United States, more than 50% of the adolescents who died from motor vehicle crashes were found to have a blood alcohol level of 0.1 mg/dL or greater (Kelton & Shank, 1998). According to the 1997 YRBSS, 19.3% of high school students rarely wore a seat belt. During the 30 days before the survey, 16.9% of high school students had driven a vehicle on one or more occasions after drinking alcohol, and 36.6% had been passengers in a vehicle with a driver who had been drinking alcohol. Nationwide, nearly one third (31%) of students reported their first drink of alcohol (more than a few sips) occurred before age 13 years. More than half (50.8%) of all students had at least one drink of alcohol within the 30 days before the survey. Approximately 10% of students nationwide had tried marijuana before age 13 years. One fourth (26.2%) of all students used marijuana on one or more occasions during the 30 days before the survey (ie, current marijuana use), and 1.1% had tried cocaine before age 13 years. Overall, 3.3% of students had used some form of cocaine at least once during the 30 days preceding the survey. Two percent of students reported illegal drug use, and 17% stated that they had used other illegal drugs during their lifetime. Across the United States, 18.3% of students carried a weapon on one or more occasions within 30 days preceding the 1997 survey. Perhaps related to this phenomenon, 7.7% of students attempted suicide during the 12 months before the survey.

Significant morbidity and social problems also result from approximately 1 million pregnancies and the estimated 3 million cases of STIs that occur each year among adolescents. Results of the 1997 YRBSS indicate that 48.4% of all high school students had sexual intercourse and that 16% of students already had four or more sexual partners. Nearly one half of students (43.2%) did not use condoms, and one fourth (24.7%) of students used alcohol or other drugs during their last sexual intercourse. Overall, 6.5% of students had been pregnant or gotten someone pregnant (CDC, 1998).

Of all the deaths among adults older than age 25 years 67% resulted from two causes: cardiovascular disease and cancer. Most risk behaviors associated with these causes of death develop during childhood and adolescence. In 1997, 36.4% of high school students had smoked cigarettes during the 30 days preceding the survey; 70.7% had not eaten five or more servings of fruits or vegetables during the day preceding the survey; and 72.6% had not attended physical education classes daily as assigned (CDC, 1998).

Self-mutilation, a form of self-directed violence, is more common among female than male adolescents. Determining the precise incidence of self-mutilating behavior is difficult, because it has been shown to be seriously underreported (Dallam, 1997). In the primary care setting, most self-mutilators appear as normal, nonpsychotic individuals who do not have mental or developmental disabilities. These individuals are classified as superficial/moderate self-mutilators, based on the degree of tissue destruction and the rate and pattern of behavior. Superficial/moderate self-mutilation is the most common form of self-mutilation, with prevalence in the general population of at least 1000 per 100,000 population per year (Favazza, 1998). Superficial/moderate self-mutilation refers to acts such as trichotillomania, nail biting, skin pricking, and persistent scratching, any of which can be seen in the individual with OCD.

Skin cutting, carving, burning, piercing, bone breaking, and interference with wound healing all characterize the episodic and repetitive type of self-mutilating personality. Most individuals who exhibit superficial/moderate self-mutilation are females, but many males are diagnosed as "accidents," thus skewing the overall picture (Frost, 1995). A few small-scale studies have recorded the prevalence of self-harm in specific populations. Self-injury in the form of head banging, self-biting, burning, and cutting has been found in 41% of physically and sexually abused children.

Self-cutting has been reported in 83% of psychiatrically hospitalized adolescents who reported being sexually abused. Self-mutilation has been reported in 48% of inpatient female adolescent drug and alcohol abusers, 40% of patients with bulimia, and 35% of those with anorexia (Dallam, 1997). Studies have shown that individuals with elaborate tattoos and piercings exhibit more psychopathology than do control groups (Favazza, 1998).

Stereotypic self-mutilation refers to acts such as head banging and hitting, orifice digging, arm hitting, throat and eye gouging, self-biting, tooth extraction, and joint dislocation. These acts tend to be monotonously repetitive and occasionally rhythmic. Stereotypic self-mutilating behaviors are highly prevalent in 21% of mentally or developmentally retarded children who are institutionalized (Briere, 1998). Stereotypic self-mutilation may be present as a symptom or associated feature in cases of acute psychosis, schizophrenia, autism, Lesch-Nyhan syndrome, de Lange's syndrome, and Gilles de la Tourette's syndrome (Favazza, 1998).

Major self-mutilation refers to infrequent acts, such as eye enucleation, castration, and limb amputation. Acts of major self-mutilation are not essential symptoms of any disorder but may appear most commonly as associated features of psychosis, including acute psychotic episodes, schizophrenia, mania, severe depression, and acute intoxication (Favazza, 1998).

CONSEQUENCES OF SELF-DESTRUCTIVE BEHAVIOR

Teen Pregnancy

Each year, approximately 1 million teenagers become pregnant in the United States. Approximately 51% of teenage pregnancies end in live birth, 35% end in induced abortion, and 14% end in miscarriage or stillbirth. The teenage birth rate in the United States (54.7 live births out of 1000) was higher in 1996 than in 1980. Of adolescents who give birth, 83% are from poor or low-income families, as are 61% of those who have abortions. One third of adolescents who become parents (both males and females) are themselves the products of teenage pregnancies. Approximately 50% to 60% of adolescents who have become parents have a history of childhood sexual or physical abuse.

Among all developed countries, the United States has the highest adolescent birth rate, despite sexual activity rates that are similar to or lower than those of western European teenagers (The Alan Guttmacher Institute, 1996). The discrepancy may be related to the universal sexual education that exists in some European countries. Another contributing factor may be the differences in the values of some American subcultures that accept pregnancy as a norm.

Adolescents with self-destructive behavior often engage in sexual activity primarily to express their frustration, anger, nonconformity, or defiance. Sexual acting out increases the incidence of STIs and teen pregnancy. The family environment and dynamics, including financial and housing status, unemployment, family composition, substance abuse by parents, and parental history of neglect, physical and sexual abuse, are all thought to be predisposing factors for the adolescent to engage in early sexual promiscuity. Such behavior carries with it the higher risk of teen pregnancy. Women who were sexually abused as children are at higher risk for early pregnancy, self-harm, eating disorders, and sexual dysfunction (Jarvis, 1997).

Female youth with self-destructive attitudes are at considerable risk for pregnancy and should be provided with effective family planning methods of their choosing. Adolescent mothers are in special need of effective contraception after the birth of their child. The pregnant adolescent must have a comprehensive program that addresses her many nutritional, medical, psychological, and other needs. Refer to Chapter 26 for more information.

Sexually Transmitted Infection and Human Immunodeficiency Virus Risk

Sexual activity and associated risks are common among adolescents and preadolescents. According to the 1997 Youth Health Risk Survey, 48.4% of high school students reported sexual intercourse. Seven percent of these students reported initiation of sexual activity before age 13. Sixteen percent reported having intercourse with four or more partners, and 6.5% of students reported getting pregnant or getting someone pregnant. Most, 91.5%, had received HIV education, but only 56.8% reported using condoms during their last sexual intercourse. Only 16.6% of students reported birth control use for themselves or their partner at the time of their last sexual intercourse (CDC, 1998).

Studies of juvenile prostitutes report that 50% to 65% had a prior history of physical and sexual abuse (including incest), rape, sexual molestation, and pregnancy. These adolescents often have low self-esteem and may believe their body image is defined only in sexual terms. A minority are diagnosed with borderline personality disorder, mental retardation, and certain psychiatric disorders. Sequelae of juvenile sexual promiscuity are many, including continued sexual abuse, STIs, pregnancy, physical assaults, depression, various other psychiatric disorders, adult prostitution, and even death (Greydanus, Pratt, Patel, & Sloane, 1997; Bardone, 1998).

Alcohol Use and Binge Drinking

According to the 1997 U.S. YRBSS, 79.1% of adolescents have had at least one drink of alcohol; 50.8% of adolescents report current alcohol use; and 33.4% report episodic heavy drinking (CDC, 1998). Family violence targeted against adolescent members has been associated with increased use of alcohol in the adolescent victim. There is a 30% chance of alcohol use among men who had been corporally punished during adolescence. Children of alcoholics and substance abusers are at tremendously increased risk for use. General availability in the school and the community and a child's perception that drug use is pervasive and even normative influence the choice.

● **Clinical Pearl:** Violent behavior, carrying a weapon, and engaging in physical fighting have been linked with alcohol use, binge drinking, and drinking while driving. Abuse of alcohol also has been reported more commonly in patients with underlying psychiatric pathology (Melzer-Lange, 1998).

Tobacco and alcohol are the most common drugs used by young people, and invariably the drugs are used first. Children understand that those who choose to use tobacco and alcohol are more likely to go on to use other drugs (Heyman & Adger, 1997). The distilled spirits industry is making a comeback in the world of advertising, from Europe to North America. In both Britain and the United States, for example, major wine cooler manufacturers and brewers continue to find increasingly clever ways to use cartoons and other child-friendly images to sell their products. Their use of media influences children in their product choices and in beginning to drink.

● **Clinical Pearl:** All substances of abuse except tobacco are associated with one fundamental characteristic: They produce some degree of euphoria and change the user's perception of reality. Once the process begins, substance abuse develops its own energy and may become habitual simply because it relieves stress and unhappiness and allows the young person to escape their environment (Heyman & Adger, 1997; Kessler, Nelson, et al., 1996)).

Tobacco Use

Adolescents frequently try cigarettes before their 13th birthday. Teenagers smoke 1.1 billion packs of cigarettes yearly and account for more than $200 billion in future health costs (Woolf, 1997). Tobacco use in adolescents represents another health risk behavior that is dependent on adolescent risk-taking behavior. Family tobacco use, peer pressure, educational level, and cultural factors all play a part in a teen's decision to smoke or chew tobacco. Tobacco also is strongly related to alcohol and illicit drug use and to violent behavior (Melzer-Lange, 1998; Escobedo, Reddy, & Durant, 1997).

Drug Abuse

The use of illegal drugs continues to climb steadily among school children and youth. Among eighth-graders, 24% admit to having used an illegal drug in the preceding year. By the 10th grade, 38% admit to having used illegal drugs. An additional 2% of children state that they have used illegal drugs such as cocaine, heroin, LSD, phencyclidine (PCP), amphetamine, or marijuana by the time they reach 12th grade (Johnston, O'Malley, & Bachman, 1996; CDC, 1997). These data suggest that people make the decision to begin using drugs at an early age. It is well known that tobacco use is comorbid with other risk-taking and self-destructive behaviors (Kessler, Nelson, et al., 1996). Regardless of ethnicity, boys who report drug activities are more likely to smoke cigarettes, drink alcohol, carry a gun, engage in sexual intercourse, and experience school failure or expulsion than are those boys not involved in drug activities (Black & Ricardo, 1994).

Primary care providers must discuss risk behavior, paying particular attention to problems associated with driving or having sexual relationships while under the influence of mind-altering drugs. Refer to Chapter XX for help in identifying which teens need intervention and which can be managed expectantly with counseling and education.

Self-Mutilation

Children who have experienced incest, rape, abuse, or neglect often are evasive or deceptive when others ask about their injuries. Family members naively accept fabricated stories when they accidentally discover wounds, because they are eager to deny the truth about the child's self-harm and its implications. Children who self-mutilate often dress to camouflage their injuries. Because of the secrecy involved, primary care providers may only become aware of injuries if they require medical intervention or are discovered during an unrelated physical examination.

The initial step is to ask the child about self-injurious practices and closely inspect the skin, hair, teeth, mouth, and eyes. Genitalia also may warrant close examination. Body piercings can appear on external and internal structures. Physical indicators of self-inflicted abuse include numerous unexplained scars, burns, or superficial cuts (Dallam, 1997). Areas that children most often select for self-mutilation are the arms and frontal body from the shoulder to the knees (Favazza, 1998). Barstow (1995) recommends asking the following questions:

- "Have you had accidents like this before?"
- "What were you thinking and feeling prior to the accident?"
- "Have you found a pattern to these accidents?"
- "How did you feel after the accident?"

Primary care providers must have a high index of awareness when an adolescent presents with elaborate tattoos and body piercings. From a psychological perspective, if this behavior fails to provide a cathartic challenge to feelings of oppression or social isolation, then further injury is likely (Clarke & Whittaker, 1998). Once self-harm is established or even just suspected, the assessment should involve a thorough evaluation of the child's medical, psychiatric, and family history, as well as previous injuries, self-destructive behaviors, interaction patterns and relationships, current stressors, and coping style (Dallam, 1997). Display 26-1 presents areas for provider assessment when self-mutilation is suspected.

Establishing a trusting relationship appears to be the most critical and perhaps difficult component in treating adolescents who self-mutilate. Because the physical and sexual abuse of a child is based on an abuse of power and disregard for the child's needs, survivors of abuse have difficulty trusting others (Dallam, 1997).

Cutting behavior should be treated with minimal attention. The patient is given a tetanus shot if necessary and counseled never to share razor blades with other people because of the potential for HIV transmission. After medical stabilization, the most critical task is to determine the risk of escalating self-mutilation and to provide appropriate psychological or psychiatric referrals. Hospitalization is warranted only if the individual is judged to be at risk for suicide or serious injury. Psychotic and intoxicated individuals require hospitalization.

▲ **Clinical Warning:** OCD should be part of the differential diagnosis for an adolescent exhibiting self-cutting behavior. A referral to a child psychiatrist or psychologist for further evaluation and follow-up management is warranted.

If management for an actively mutilating individual is to be outpatient, the provider must obtain a no-suicide contract. In this written statement, the patient promises not to

---

DISPLAY 26-1 • Assessment of Self-Mutilators

- Rule out biobehavioral disorders associated with self-mutilating behavior:
  Mental retardation (particularly after institutionalization)
  Stereotypic self-mutilation, such as head banging, self-biting, orifice digging, and scratching. Self-injury occurs without shame or guile, even in the presence of on-lookers.
  These behaviors may be present as a symptom or associated feature in cases of acute psychosis, schizophrenia, autism, Lesch-Nyhan syndrome (self-injury usually takes the form of unremitting finger chewing), Gilles de la Tourette's syndrome (self-injury usually takes the form of head banging), de Lange's syndrome (self-injury often takes the form of face slapping).
- Rule out other psychiatric conditions, such as acute psychotic episodes, schizophrenia, and mania.
  Acts of major self-mutilation are uncommon and difficult to prevent.
  Major self-mutilation refers to acts such as eye enucleation, castration, and limb amputation.
  A drastic change in appearance in psychotic or intoxicated adolescents, such as severe hair plucking, may be a harbinger of major self-mutilation.
  Self-injurious behavior often occurs in response to command hallucinations or persecuting delusion and preoccupations with sexuality or religion, especially when the adolescent is involuntarily confined.

- Obsessive compulsive disorder (OCD): Patients with OCD who have compulsions with few or no obsessions.
  Self-injury often takes the form of trichotillomania, skin picking and nail biting.
- Gender identity disorder:
  Self-harm may take the form of a carefully planned transsexual self-castration.
- Munchausen syndrome:
  Self-mutilation is done to simulate a disease or illness.
- Assess for depression and anxiety. These are often concurrent disorders.
- Explore the family history for trauma, sexual or physical abuses, alcoholism, neglect, abandonment or violence.
- Assess sociocultural variables to determine if the self-mutilating behavior has any special meaning within the adolescent's religion, ritual, and healing traditions.
- Assess current stressors and losses.
- Determine the motives, methods, and process of self-injury. Establish the frequency and type of self-harm. Assess the risk for suicide. Acts of self-mutilation escalating in frequency and intensity may lead to demoralization and bona fide suicide attempts.
- Inquire about other self-damaging and addictive behaviors, such as anorexia, bulimia, substance abuse, gambling, kleptomania, abusive relationships, and dangerous sexual practices.

Adapted from Dallam, S. J. (1997). The identification and management of self-mutilating patients in primary care. *Nurse Practitioner, 22*(5), 151–165.

do anything self-destructive, accidentally or on purpose, without calling the primary care provider or therapist. The primary care provider informs the individual that, if needed, a 24-hour-a-day number is available for help. The clinician needs to assure the adolescent that the teen does not have to self-hurt to see either the primary provider or a therapist again.

MANAGEMENT

Prevention

Adolescent self-destructive behavior is a predictor of more serious medical problems, poorer self-reported overall health, lower body mass index, alcohol and marijuana dependence, tobacco dependence, more lifetime sexual partners, STIs, and early pregnancy. Primary care providers must identify risky behaviors to intervene quickly and effectively. Clinicians see adolescents in a variety of settings, including primary care, sports, reproductive health, school-based, and subspecialty clinics, as well as in emergency departments, hospitals, and detention centers. Primary care providers must take the opportunity in these settings to screen adolescents for drug, alcohol, and tobacco use and sexual activity and violent behavior. Providers should develop acute interviewing skills for teenagers that will enable them to assess adolescents adequately for potential and actual risk factors (Melzer-Lange, 1998; Fuller & Cavanaugh, 1995). Refer to Chapter 12 (Adolescent) for further information on interviewing techniques and Heads approach.

● **Clinical Pearl:** Acceptance from a specific, healthy peer group and attachment to productive activities, including school-based clubs and teams, jobs, or church activities, may help create an atmosphere in which the adolescent is less likely to choose drugs and other self-destructive behaviors.

Intervention

Once identified, adolescents whose behavior is self-destructive need their providers to show understanding and refer them to appropriate treatment resources. Youth-centered community services also can assist. Other family members also may need help. Psychosocial treatment of adolescents with self-destructive behavior involves therapy directed at adolescents themselves, parental figures, and other family members. Individual therapy is directed toward improving the adolescent's prosocial skills regarding interpersonal issues, communication, relationship building and maintenance, problem solving, conflict resolution, negotiation, and avoiding problem situations. The most effective family interventions aim at building skills in communication, behavior monitoring, and effective discipline. Parents can learn how to alter interactions with their adolescents to promote prosocial behavior, thereby decreasing deviant behavior. In this regard, family therapy can be helpful. Family therapy focuses on building cohesion and emotional warmth, strengthening adaptive behavior in the adolescent, and minimizing marital problems that can interfere with effective parental functioning (Greydanus et al., 1997).

Family intervention also may be required to build communication skills and the parenting skills needed to monitor behavior, provide effective discipline, and promote prosocial behavior. These skills can help the family and the adolescent in decreasing self-destructive attitudes. Youth-centered programs use individual psychotherapy, group psychotherapy, behavior therapy, cognitive therapy, pharmacotherapy, and residential treatment (Greydanus et al., 1997). Although expensive, most programs are eligible for coverage by private health insurance. Some programs accept Medicaid payment.

COMMUNITY RESOURCES

Many community-based programs and resources address youths at risk for self-destructive behavior. Such programs, many of which have been used effectively for many years, involve a variety of treatments. Examples of community resources valuable to primary care providers include the following:

AIDS and Adolescents Network
666 Broadway, Suite 520
New York, NY 10012

Teens and AIDS Hotline
(800) 440-TEEN

National Runaway Switchboard
(800) 621-4000

National Campaign to Prevent Teen Pregnancy
2100 M Street NW
Suite 300
Washington, DC 20037
(202) 261-5655

Campaign for Our Children
120 West Fayette Street
Suite 1200
Baltimore, MD 21201
(410) 576-9015
http://www.cfoc.org

National Parenting Center
(800) 753-6667
http://www.tnpc.com

How to Help Self Injury
http://www.palace.net/~llama/psych/self injury.html

Big Brothers Big Sisters of America
230 North 13th Street
Philadelphia, PA 19107
(215) 567-7000
http://www.national@BBBSA.org

Al-Anon/Alateen
Family Group Headquarters, Inc.
1600 Corporate Landing Parkway
Virginia Beach, VA 23454-5617
(800) 344-2666

REFERENCES

Bardone, A. M. (1998). Adult physical health outcomes of adolescent girls with conduct disorders, depression, and anxiety. *Journal of the American Academy of Child and Adolescent Psychiatry, 37*(6), 594–601.

Barkley, R. A. (1997). Behavioral inhibition, sustained attention, and executive functions: Constructing a unifying theory of ADHD. *Psychology Bulletin, 121*(1), 65–94.

Barstow, D. G. (1995). Self-injury and self-mutilation: Nursing approaches. *Journal of Psychosocial Nursing and Mental Health Services, 33*(2), 19–22.

Benjamin, J., Li, L., Patterson, C., Greenberg, B. D., Murphy, D. L., & Hamer, D. H. (1996). Population and familial association between the D4 dopamine receptor gene and measures of novelty seeking. *Nature Genetics, 12*(1), 81–84.

Black, M. M., & Ricardo, I. B. (1994). Drug use, drug trafficking, and weapon carrying among low-income African-American, early adolescent boys. *Pediatrics 93*, 1065–1072.

Briere, J. (1998). Self-mutilation in clinical and general population samples: Prevalence, correlates and functions. *American Journal of Orthopsychiatry, 68*(4), 609–620.

Shapiro, J., & Balka, E. R. (1995). Longitudinally predicting late adolescent and young adult drug use: Antecedent and intervening process. *Journal of the American Academy of Child and Adolescent Psychiatry, 34*(8), 1076–1083.

Brown, J. D., & Sheele, J. R. (1995). *Sex and the mass media.* Menlo Park, CA: Kaiser Family Foundation.

Catalano, G., Morejon, M., Alberts, V. A., & Catalano, M. C. (1996). Report of a case of male genital self-mutilation and review of the literature, with special emphasis on the effects of the media. *Journal of Sex and Marital Therapy, 22*(1), 35–46.

Centers for Disease Control and Prevention. (1998). CDC surveillance summaries, August 14, 1998. *Morbidity and Mortality Weekly Report, 47* (No. SS-3).

Centers for Disease Control and Prevention. (1997). Deaths and death rates for the 10 leading causes of death in specified age groups: United States, preliminary data for 12 months ending June 1996. *Monthly Vital Statistics report, April 30*, 45 No. (S) 2.

Christenson, P. G., & Robert, D. F. (1998). *It's not only Rock "N" Roll: Popular music in the lives of adolescents.* Cresskill, NJ: Hampton Press.

Clarke, L., & Whittaker, M. (1998). Self-mutilation: Culture, contexts and nursing responses. *Journal of Clinical Nursing, 7*(2), 129–137.

Dallam, S. J. (1997). The identification and management of self-mutilating patients in primary care. *Nurse Practitioner, 22*(5), 151–165.

Donnerstein, E., Slaby, R., & Eron, L. (1995). The mass media and youth aggression. In L. Eron, J. Gentry, & P. Schlegal (Eds.), *Reasons to hope: A psychological perspective on violence and youth.* Washington, DC: American Psychological Association.

DuRant, R. H., Rich, M., Emans, S. J., Romes, E. S., Allred, E., & Woods E. (1997). Violence and weapon carrying in music videos: A content analysis. *Archives in Pediatric and Adolescent Medicine, 151*, 443–448.

Egan, J. (1997). The thin red line. *New York Times Magazine, July*, 21–35, 43–48.

Elders, M. J. (1998). Adolescent pregnancy and sexual abuse. *Journal of the American Medical Association, 280*(7), 648–649.

Eron, L. R. (1995). Media violence. *Pediatric Annual, 24*, 84–87.

Escobedo, L. G., Reddy, M., & Durant, R. H. (1997). Relationship between cigarette smoking and health risk and problem behaviors among US adolescents. *Archives in Pediatric and Adolescent Medicine, 151*, 66–77.

Favazza, A. R. (1998). The coming of age of self-mutilation. *Journal of Nervous and Mental Disorders, 186*(5), 259–268.

Federman, J. (1998). *National television violence study III.* Thousand Oaks, CA: Sage.

Fischer, P. M., Schwart, M. P., Richards, J. W., Goldstein, A. O., & Rojas, T. H. (1991). Brand logo recognition by children aged 3 to 6 years: Mickey Mouse and Old Joe the Camel. *Journal of the American Medical Association, 266*, 3145–3153.

Frost, M. (1995). Self-harm and the social work relationship. *Social Work Monographs*, Norwich NR4 7 TJ. Monograph 134.

Fuller, P. J., & Cavanaugh, R. M. (1995). Basic assessment and screening for substance abuse in the pediatrician's office. *Pediatric Clinics of North America, 42*, 295–315.

Greydanus, D., Pratt, H., Patel, D., & Sloane, M. (1997). The rebellious adolescent: Evaluation and management of oppositional and conduct disorders. *Pediatric Clinics of North America, 44*(6), 1457–1485.

Heyman, R., & Adger, H. (1997). Office approach to drug abuse prevention. *Pediatric Clinics of North America, 44*(6), 1447–1455.

Jarvis, T. S. (1997). Child sexual abuse as a predictor of psychological co-morbidity and its implications for drug and alcohol treatment. *Drug and Alcohol Dependence, 49*(1), 61–69.

Jessor, R. (1991). Risk behavior in adolescence: A psychosocial framework for understanding and action. *Journal of Adolescent Health, 12*, 597–605.

Johnston, L. D., O'Malley, P. M., & Bachman, J. G. (1996). *Monitoring the future: Questionnaire responses from the nation's students.* Ann Arbor, MI: Institute for Social Research, University of Michigan.

Kaiser Family Foundation. (1997). *Sexual content in the media: The future of effects research.* Menlo Park, CA: Author.

Kaplan, H. B. (1996). Empirical validation of the applicability of an integrative theory of deviant behavior to the study of drug use. *Journal of Drug Issues, 26*(2), 345–377.

Kehrberg, C. (1997). Self-mutilating behavior. *Journal of Child and Adolescent Psychiatric Nursing, 10*(3), 35–40.

Kelton, G. M., & Shank, J. C. (1998). Adolescent injury and death: The plagues of accident, self-infliction and violence. *Primary Care Clinic in Office Practice, 25*(1), 163–179.

Kessler, R. C., Nelson, C. B., McGonagle, K. A., Edlund, M. J., Frank, R. G., & Leaf, P. J. (1996). The epidemiology of co-occurring addictive and mental disorders in the National Comorbidity Survey: Implication for prevention and service utilization. *American Journal of Orthopsychiatry, 66*(1), 17–31.

Leiber, L. (1996). *Commercial and character slogan recall by children aged 9 to 11 years: Budweiser Frogs versus Bugs Bunny.* Berkeley, CA: Centers on Alcohol Advertising.

Log-On Data Corporation. (1996). *White paper on issues to consider.* Anaheim, CA: Author.

Lowry, R., Kann, L., Collins, J. L., & Kolbe, L. J. (1996). The effect of socioeconomic status on chronic disease behavior among US adolescents. *Journal of the American Medical Association, 276*, 792–797.

Melzer-Lange, M. (1998). Violence and associated high risk health behaviors in adolescents: Substance abuse, sexually transmitted diseases, and pregnancy of adolescents. *Pediatric Clinics of North America, 45*(2), 307–317.

Nielsen Media Research. New York, 1998. Report on TV viewing time for children: United States, Canada, and Britain. http://www.reseau-medias.ca/enhg/issues/stats/usetv.htm.

Oetting, E. R., & Donnermeyer, J. F. (1998). Primary socialization theory: The etiology of drug use and deviance I. *Substance Use and Misuse, 33*(4), 995–1026.

Oetting, E. R., Deffenbacher, J. L., & Donnermyer, J. F. (1998). Primary socialization theory. The role played by personal traits in the etiology of drug use and deviance II. *Substance Use and Misuse, 33*, 1337–66.

Pierce, J. P., Chol, W. S., Gilpin, E. A., Farkas, A. J., & Berry, C. C. (1998). Tobacco industry promotion of cigarettes and adolescent smoking. *Journal of the American Medical Association, 279*, 511–515.

Reiff, M. I. (1998). Adolescent school failure: Failure to thrive in adolescence. *Pediatrics in Review, 19*(6), 199–207.

Romans, S. E. (1995). Sexual abuse in childhood and deliberate self-harm. *American Journal of Psychiatry, 152*(9), 1336–1342.

Sargent, J. D., Dalton, M. A., Beach, M., Bernhardt, A., Pullin, D., & Steven, M. (1997). Cigarette promotional items in public schools. *Archives in Pediatric and Adolescent Medicine, 151*, 1189–1196.

Schooler, C., Feighery, E., & Flora, J. A. (1996). Seventh graders self-reported exposure to cigarette marketing and its relationship to their smoking behavior. *American Journal of Public Health, 86*, 1216–1221.

Shank, J. C., & Gabel, L. L. (1996). The adolescent plague of injury, violence, and death. *Family Practice Recertification, 18*, 31–48.

Smith, S. L., & Donnerstein, D. (1998). The harmful effects of exposure to media violence: Learning of aggression, emotional desensitization, and fear. In R. Geen & E. Donnerstein (Eds.), *Human aggression: Theory, research and policy.* San Diego, CA: Academic Press.

Strasburger, V. C. (1995). *Adolescents and the media: Medical and psychological impact.* Thousand Oaks, CA: Sage.

Strasburger, V. C. (1997). "Sex, drugs, rock 'n' roll" and the media: Are the media responsible for adolescent behavior? *Adolescent Medicine State of the Art Review, 8*, 403–414.

Strasburger, V. C., & Donnerstein, E. (1999). Children, adolescents, and the media: Issues and solutions. *Pediatrics, 103*, 129–138.

The Alan Guttmacher Institute. (1996). *Facts in brief: Teen sex and pregnancy.* New York: Author.

William, W. S., Montgomery, K., & Pasnik, S. (1997). *Alcohol and tobacco on the web.* Washington, DC: Center for Media Education.

Woolf, A. D. (1997). Smoking and nicotine addiction: A pediatric epidemic with sequelae in adulthood. *Current Opinion in Pediatrics, 9*(5), 470–477.

Grief, Loss, and Coping With Change

• BARBARA PISICK, MED, RN, CS

INTRODUCTION

The cycle of birth, life, and death is ongoing and ever changing. Buddhist philosophy, which emphasizes rebirth and evolution of the soul over time, exemplifies the process of transformation. The death of old ideas that no longer serve current purposes gives birth to new concepts and technologies that alter the process of living. Often, fearful people respond to new information with a more rigid defense of their old beliefs. The ability to cope effectively with change, however, is a critical component of successful living.

This chapter discusses grief, loss, and change from a developmental perspective. It provides content meant to assist primary care providers in identifying children who are struggling with these basic life concepts. It also presents intervention strategies for such children.

CHANGE IN FAMILIES

Change in families occurs through new experiences as different family members grow, marry, have children, age, and die. These experiences continuously transform the family system. The role of parents is to help children develop age-appropriate coping skills and to assist with the process of change as children gain independence.

Primary care providers have a unique opportunity to assess and target interventions for at-risk children. Clinicians can provide an environment for helping to transform dysfunctional communication patterns within the family, in addition to teaching parenting and coping skills. Parents who are unable to help and nurture their children appropriately often lack such abilities not because of disinterest, but because their own parents lacked such skills. Every parent's style of childrearing reflects his or her own experiences of being parented. Providers must perform all interventions without judgment to enhance relationships among all family members. Providers can be role models for clear communication, teaching children how to be accepted, respected, and understood.

Influence of Birth Order Position

Birth order position is a significant variable that influences a child's growth and development. The way a child views the world usually is established by age 6 years. Children's perceptions of the world tend to serve as a filter for them throughout life. Awareness of a child's perceptions is essential to understanding the factors that motivate him or her.

The first-born child usually provides parents with their first parental experience. Parents often give this child some measure of power over younger siblings. The trauma of dethronement usually occurs for the first-born child at the birth of the second child. The intensity of that experience depends on the number of years between the two siblings

and other variables. Parents can help older children accept new siblings by giving all family members sufficient attention and affection.

Clinicians may be able to understand parents better by considering the framework of the parents' experience as well. Often parents treat children differently according to their own birth order placement and childhood relationships with siblings.

Loss Through Moving

When families move frequently, children lose connections with their schools and communities. The disruption they experience with a move heightens the loss of friends and familiarity. During this process, children may have difficulty making new friends and, consequently, feel isolated. Parents should consider the child's level of psychosocial development and the concurrent adjustment to the new situation to respond appropriately to their child's behavior. From ages 10 to 12 years, girls value intimacy and exclusiveness in friendships. They usually play in small groups. Boys generally play in large groups, and recreation often involves sports. As both groups move into adolescence, cliques and friends become extremely important.

Parents need to follow through with children after a move, exploring whether children are adjusting to the new school and environment. Parents must actively pursue information. Children may feel shame, guilt, and discomfort when entering a new social milieu. Developing new friendships can be quite difficult if a child is shy or if groups and cliques at the new school already are established. Many children suffer in silence rather than face humiliation. Table 27-1 provides developmentally appropriate suggestions for parents to help children deal with the loss of beloved friends or pets through moving.

Loss Through Divorce

Approximately 1.25 million children live in divorced families. When families divorce, many children feel like they are losing one parent. They may have to share parents because of remarriage and blending of families. Children of divorce often feel left out and isolated. Children experiencing parental divorce find it very stressful. They may feel emotionally distraught, afraid, guilty, and angry. These feelings can disrupt school performance and peer relationships.

Children younger than 3 years usually demonstrate regressive behavior. Children between ages 3 and 6 years can experience a more concrete realization of the meaning of divorce, which may be manifested through shock and depression. Children ages 4 to 6 years often use fantasy and self-blame as a way of coping with their stress. They may regress, withdraw, and have tantrums. Through the normal developmental process, the school environment often serves as an alternative "home," dedicated to children's development and social well-being. School-age children coping with parental divorce often experience somatic symptoms and

Table 27–1. DEVELOPMENTALLY APPROPRIATE INTERVENTIONS FOR CHILDREN WHO LOSE A FRIEND OR PET THROUGH MOVING

Developmental Stage	Special Considerations	Interventions
Toddler and preschooler (2–6 y)	• Children lack ego skills to handle feelings.	• Evaluate the relationship the child had with the friend or pet. • If an animal dies, plan a family ritual for burial with family members talking about the pet, which helps the child mourn within the family context. • Parents should not buy replacement pets until the child has grieved the loss.
School-age (6–12 y)	• Child socializes and learns about loyalty, justice, and leadership. • Child may belong or be excluded from from cliques or gangs at school. • This age group is very vulnerable.	• At the loss of a friend, children may feel devastated. Lack of acceptance from new peers can compound a sense of isolation. • Child may be shy and lack the social skills to make new friends.
Adolescent (12–18 y)	• Friends play an important role. • Friendships usually are very close.	• Teens should be included in parental discussions regarding moving and loss of friendships. • They can understand separation from friends but emotionally may feel a tremendous loss of their special friends and may withdraw.

deteriorating school performance. Peer relationships may suffer, and children may isolate themselves from peers and adults. Adolescents are often very aware of difficulty between their parents. They may look to other family members and peers for support. They may side with one or the other parent.

Long-term effects of divorce depend on the child's age when it happens. Usually young children and adolescents have the best outcomes, while preadolescent children in middle school suffer the worst long-term effects. The findings of a 15-year study of 100 children from divorced families found children had the best outcomes when they had contact with both parents and were able to maintain their relationships (Wallerstein & Blakeslee, 1989).

Children of any age who have good relationships with parents and can talk about the effects of divorce will handle the situation more effectively. Providers can help families address post-divorce issues by helping them identify parenting resources, values, and visitation arrangements. Table 27-2 highlights developmentally appropriate interventions for providers to use to help patients whose parents are divorcing.

Loss Through Other Circumstances

Children are at tremendous risk if they grow up in abusive homes, including those with alcohol, drug, sexual, or physical abuse; live in homes where parents are teenagers or the family experiences poverty; or attend schools in which violence occurs. Children in these circumstances usually do not complain. They may either withdraw out of fear or act out their aggression.

Loss Through Abuse

Families coping with substance addiction are found at all socioeconomic levels. These families often experience role confusion, with the oldest children being forced into a parental role. Arguments, illogical thinking, and denial are paramount characteristics of these families. Children are

often fearful when parents are out of control. In these families, children do not learn the healthy coping skills they need for adaptation in society. These youngsters are often withdrawn, aggressive, angry, and anxious. They experience developmental problems and difficulties discerning between fantasy and reality.

Early childhood neglect or abuse causes anxiety and insecure attachment in children. These children may become severely upset when separated from their parents, which can lead to subsequent problems in forming and maintaining intimate relationships (Schneider-Rosen & Cicchetti, 1984). Beck (1976) asserts that parental abuse is an antecedent to depression. Adult women whose parents were addicted to alcohol score high for depression (Benson & Heller, 1987). Depression is common in adults and adolescents who were molested as children (Browne & Finkelhor, 1986; Jehu, Gazan, & Klassen, 1984–1985).

Many adults who abuse children are themselves victims of childhood abuse, demonstrating multigenerational patterns of abuse. Chapters 22, 23, and 28 offer content that can give the reader further insight into the causes and consequences of childhood abuse.

Providers should know that when parents have such problems, their children often suffer in silence. Children depend on their parents to protect them, even when parents are abusive. Often, these children believe they have nowhere to turn. Through sharp awareness, practitioners can evaluate situations to protect children involved. For example, a practitioner who worked in a pregnancy clinic was treating an underage adolescent and called in the parents for discussion. The clinician noticed an abnormal interaction between the daughter and father and suspected that the patient was pregnant with her father's child. The provider then met with the girl separately, confirming this fact. The child subsequently was taken out of the home. This situation highlights the importance of keen observation on the part of the primary care provider (Scipio-Bannerman, 1999). Refer to Chapter 23 for additional discussion of the causes and outcomes of abuse.

Table 27-2. DEVELOPMENTALLY APPROPRIATE INTERVENTIONS FOR CHILDREN WHOSE PARENTS ARE DIVORCING

Developmental Stage	Special Considerations	Interventions
Toddler and preschooler (2–6 y)	• Child does not understand that parents have a different relationship than they have with the parents. • They start to understand things can exist when not visible. • They are very vulnerable to parental separation and divorce and experience anger, fear, rejection, and guilt. • They may feel they are responsible for the divorce because they were angry at one of the parents or were bad. • Loss incurred through divorce can be as devastating as death. • Children can begin to understand the separated parent is in their lives even if not there physically. • Loss of the intact family often results in feelings of guilt, self-blame, anger, and fantasy of a parental reunion. • Children can understand parental interactions more clearly. • They may have difficulty resolving the loss that occurs with parental separation.	• Children need to know parents love them and that they are not the cause of separation. Both parents should explain that they will always be a part of children's lives. • Providers can assist parents to deal with the child and handle life situations in a healthy way. • Parents must learn how to cooperate in plans for the child. • The child should have a bed and space in each home. • Parents should not use child as a messenger. They should not tell children about problems within the relationship.
School-age (6–12 y)	• The ability for limited logical process of understanding a relationship develops.	
Adolescent (12–18 y)	• Teen may experience mood swings, rebellion, and confusion. • They have better problem-solving skills and increased ability to cope. • Teens may turn to friends and siblings for social support. • They may also turn to nicotine, drugs, or alcohol to handle the chaos and stress in the family. • They may socially withdraw or develop suicidal thoughts	• Observe this group for social isolation; divorce may affect a teen's ability to strive for autonomy from parents.

● **Clinical Pearl:** Providers must intervene as often as possible before children are affected, thereby breaking the multigenerational cycle of abuse. Doing so can help prevent children from carrying their emotional burdens into adulthood.

Loss Through Poverty

Children born to teenage parents often suffer because their parents are not developmentally ready to assume parenting skills. Many of these children grow up in poverty. Approximately 13.5 million children in the United States, 4.9 million of whom are younger than age 6 years, live below the poverty line (National Center for Children in Poverty, 1999). Many of these children live in less than adequate environments and lack a basic standard of living. Parents may be focused on providing a home under severe stress. Often, they cope with stress by using drugs or alcohol, isolating the child even more.

Loss Through Trauma and Violence

Decades ago, Levy (1945) found that after surgery, children experienced nightmares. He equated this observation with the trauma experienced by soldiers who fought on the battle-fields of Europe in World War II. Trauma in children, however, was not studied extensively until the 1970s and 1980s. Terr (1990) followed children ages 1, 4, and 5 years after a kidnapping in California. Her study was the first to document the effects of childhood trauma and the enduring patterns of emotional scarring after the event. She found that children may appear outwardly unaffected, but the terror of such an event results in post-traumatic stress. Her work highlights the need for parents, teachers, and providers to be aware of what to look for in children who are experiencing psychological trauma and ensure that they receive treatment.

Symptoms of post-traumatic stress include changes in the child's personality, from easy-going to angry, moody, and mistrustful. The youngster may have a moody outlook, a sense of lost invincibility, perpetual mourning, and day-dreams about death and disfigurement. These children may intensify fears and displace anger by incorporating their negative feelings into themselves. Normal development means that a child begins to achieve autonomy. When safe movement toward autonomy is taken from a child, the powerful result usually is shame and guilt. Children must learn how to master their trauma in order for the bereavement process to occur (Pynoos & Nader, 1991).

What is most obvious is that there are so many ways in which practitioners can be observant early. Their assessments can help in developing a plan of action. When adult victims of childhood trauma learn positive life skills, including how to parent, they can move in the direction of healthy family building.

Loss Through Death

When a family member dies, each family member experiences the loss differently. The complexities of the impact of that loss within a family system are so profound that clinicians must address each situation as they find it.

● **Clinical Pearl:** Practitioners cannot impose their own values or belief systems on families. Rather, they must create opportunities for family members to grieve and mourn in their own way, giving support and understanding.

For those who are confused about death, allowing exploration is a healthy goal. Children feel guilty when they are unable to resolve their anger at a deceased family member about things that happened in the past or if the person died before they could right the wrong. Providers should understand the dynamics of the parent–child and deceased individual–child relationships so they can help conflicted individuals to heal.

Children are often left "in the dark" about death in the family. Adults may not allow them to attend funerals or to grieve appropriately. Adults may preclude them from the family grieving process, leaving children isolated while adults progress through distress and mourning. Grieving adults may think that children are fine and should be spared from knowing anything about death. Unfortunately, these children miss the chance to mourn the loss fully within a protective family network.

Young children's underdeveloped verbal skills may mask their turmoil in response to loss. Parents who experience extreme emotionality, loss of control, or both may be rendered unable to care for their children.

● **Clinical Pearl:** Children should be part of the family grieving process. They should discuss their feelings about death and loss. If a family has difficulty talking about these issues, the provider should refer the family to a mental health professional for assistance.

A child's awareness of death is a developmental process that evolves toward an increasingly more mature understanding. As children age, they are better able to distinguish between thoughts and deeds. Children must attain a certain level of cognition before they can fully integrate the concept of death. Providers need to be aware of children's reactions. Table 27-3 highlights the knowledge of death and the fear it can cause among preschoolers, school-age children, and adolescents.

Loss Through Chronic Illness

When a parent is chronically ill and facing death, family members often have high expectations of the children. They often require the children to be quiet and not to make demands. Because they are focusing on the ill parent, adults have less attention to give to the children. An impending death of a parent may cause children to feel guilty or abandoned. Protracted terminal illness causes prolonged stress and suffering that may prove harder to deal with than handling the death itself. Acknowledging the family's feelings and supporting them through the process of loss can help them deal with the situation (Barakat, Sills, & Bagnara, 1995).

Parental death in early childhood can increase an individual's risk for depression by a factor of two or three. For example, Siegel, Karus, and Raveis (1996) found that children facing the death of a parent from cancer had elevated levels of depression and anxiety prior to that death. Seven to 12 months after the parent's death, children's depression and anxiety diminished to the levels of peers who had not experienced such losses.

In families with a chronically sick child, siblings often do not receive sufficient attention. Because parents must give so much attention to the sick child, siblings may feel isolated and left to fend for themselves. They are losing a sibling, but they also lose the experience of a "normal childhood," because the whole family is steeped in ongoing grief about the sick child. The child's illness so overwhelms the parents that they are unable to cope with the problems of other family members.

When a child dies, parents may be so consumed by their own overwhelming grief (and perhaps guilt) that they become unable to care for their other children. Brent, Moritz, Bridge, Perper, and Canobbio (1996) found that siblings experience prolonged grief symptoms for up to 3 years. Surviving children may feel guilty or ambivalent because of unresolved sibling rivalry, depending on the relationship. Parents and provider must consider the child's level of psychosocial development.

Loss Through Sudden Death

In the case of sudden death, children naturally are shocked. When a parent dies from trauma, the surviving parent usually experiences surprise and disbelief. Often he or she is so consumed with grief that care for children suffers. In such cases, children suffer not only the actual physical loss of a parent, but also the psychological loss of the surviving parent who cannot respond adequately. If the surviving parent cannot deal with the situation, family members and providers must take an active role.

A parent's suicide can be similarly traumatic. How a child handles a parent's suicide greatly depends on the remaining parent's reaction and emotional availability. Usually, the entire family experiences shock, anger, and shame. Both clinician and parent should consider the child's developmental stage. Preschool and school-age children will have difficulty understanding what is happening, and psychological intervention is necessary.

Furman (1984) describes the child's process of mourning. The youngster must understand the reality of the death, mourn the loss, and, after approximately 6 to 18 months, be able to choose a parent substitute or to redefine the relationship with the remaining parent.

Providers need to identify any patient at risk and plan accordingly for necessary interventions, referring the child to a therapist who specializes in child bereavement. This professional should be an integral part of planning and implementing care for the youngster and family. Play therapy, which encourages children to express their emotions, can be helpful. Many localities have formalized grief programs for children and families. Providers should seek out such programming to refer families to a sound and valuable support service.

Bereavement: Loss of a Relationship, Now and Forever

Many people carry their childhood losses of a sibling, parent, friend, or grandparent into adulthood. This finding is especially true if individuals never dealt properly with the

Table 27–3. KNOWLEDGE OF DEATH AND ATTENDANT FEAR BY AGE GROUP

Developmental Stage	Special Considerations	Interventions
Preoperational: ages 2–6 y	• Two-year-olds understand more than they say. • They learn about death from their environment, relative, friend, or pet. • They are egocentric and cannot distinguish between thoughts and actions (Piaget, 1965). • Their understanding of death is incomplete; they have fears of death and about body intactness (Erikson, 1968). • They are concerned with how the body is treated after death. • For 4- to 5-year-olds, death is temporary: If someone is shot, he or she is still alive. Death is short-term and reversible. • Death may upset them, and they may think they are responsible because they were bad. • If they were angry at the person who died, they may think their thoughts caused the person's death. • They associate events that occurred before the death as significant or magical. • They fear a similar illness will affect them. • They worry about death in relation to their family. • A 5- to 7-year-old has a better understanding of death's permanence (Palombo, 1981). • They lack ego skills necessary to handle intense feelings. • Development to this point does not allow for understanding the concepts of death as inevitable and irreversible.	• Children this age do not have ego controls and need parents to handle their environment for them. • The loss of a central person in the child's life is devastating. • These children are vulnerable, as manifested by irrational fears. • If a child asks, "When are you going to die?" the parent should reply, "Mommy will be there to take care of you." • Do not tell a child that death is like going to sleep; the concreteness of the child's thinking may lead them to fear sleep. • When a relative dies, parents should not tell children that the person "went on a trip." Children are sensitive to adult behavior and are often upset at not being told the truth. • Explanations about death should be made according to the family's religious belief; for example, some may explain that the person is in heaven with God.
Concrete operations: 6–12 y	• Between 7 and 11 y, the ability to reason and decreased egocentricity allow children to recognize death's irreversibility. • Before age 10 y, children do not have the ability to resolve and understand loss. They may not think death will happen to them. • Between ages 9–12, the child's thinking becomes logical and able to deal with abstractions. • Children focus on post-death decay. • Sibling rivalries can be very intense; death of a sibling may cause guilt because of anger and hostile thoughts.	• This age group is very vulnerable. Cognitive skills help child understand some of the ramifications of death, but ego skills for coping are lacking. • Children can understand the biologic concept of death and that death is irreversible but not why. • Children ages 7–8 y may have sleep disturbances and concerns for others' safety. • Practitioners can recommend that children be told to focus on memories of the loved one so they will remain in their hearts.
Formal operations: 12–18 y	• The individual can reason logically and deal with abstract thoughts (Piaget, 1965). • They have the ego skills that allow them to cope. • They experiment with different roles and are working on issues of intimacy and isolation (Erikson, 1968). • Increased emotion and impulse control are issues (Carter, 1998). • These children understand death is universal, irreversible, and natural. • At older ages, they often understand death in an abstract, religious/spiritual context. • When a sibling dies, they may feel guilty that they survived.	• At this age, a parental death can have a profound effect. Providers should assist the surviving parent and family members. • Adult support for the adolescent is critical; while teens may appear to cope, they may feel emotionally incapacitated. The overwhelming pressures may result in identity confusion. • Teens may experience an anniversary reaction a year after the death.

(Adapted from Piaget, 1965)

loss when it occurred. Some people may carry forever within their psyches the loss of significant unresolved relationships. Grief is a natural reaction to any type of loss. Mourning or bereavement means the way an individual resolves grief.

During bereavement, the grieving individual becomes preoccupied with the image of the deceased, has guilty feelings, feels hostile, and deviates from usual behavioral patterns. The individual must work through grief to achieve separation from the deceased and eventually return to normal patterns of functioning. The closeness of the relationship between the child and deceased determines the level of loss. The child's level of psychosocial development will help the clinician assess the type of intervention he or she requires. Younger children do not experience phases of grief as do adults because their psychosocial and intellectual development is less advanced. The adolescent's mourning process is similar to that of the adult.

Children who experience inadequate mourning after a parent's death may have difficulty forming relationships in later years. Inadequate mourning also can lead to depression. These problems result from a disruption in the normal developmental process (Worden, 1991). Children at risk for suicide are those who experienced the loss of a loved one before age 12 years. Other risk factors include family history of depression and suicide, violence, and severe family pressures (Workman & Prior, 1997).

COMMUNITY RESOURCES

Community-based suicide prevention programs should be available to help children. Bereavement support groups for children can reduce anxiety and decrease isolation caused by the loss of a loved one (Mulcahey & Young, 1995). Schools can be excellent resources for providing mental health services (Van Epps, Opie, & Goodwin, 1997).

Local schools, religious organizations, and hospitals often have bereavement programs.

The following are sources for films, books, and tapes related to bereavement focusing on children:

The Rainbow Coalition Catalog
471 Hannah Branch Road
Burnsville, NC 28714

The Good Grief Program
Judge Baker's Children's Center
295 Longwood Avenue
Boston, MA 02115

National Center for Death Education Library
Mt. Ida College
777 Dedham Street
Newton Centre, MA 02159

REFERENCES

Barakat, L. P., Sills, R., & Bagnara, S. (1995). Management of fatal illness and death in children or their parents. *Pediatrics in Review, 16*(11), 419–423.

Beck, A. T. (1976). *Cognitive therapy and the emotional disorders*. New York: International Universities Press.

Benson, C., & Heller, K.. (1987). Factors in the current adjustment of young adult daughters of alcoholic and problem drinking fathers. *Journal of Abnormal Psychology, 96*, 305–312.

Brent, D. A., Moritz, G., Bridge, J., Perper, J., & Canobbio, R. (1996). The impact of adolescent suicide on siblings and parents: A longitudinal follow-up. *Suicide Life Threat Behavior, 26*(3), 253–259.

Browne, A., & Finkelhor, D. (1986). Impact of child sexual abuse: A review of the research. *Psychological Bulletin, 99*, 66–77.

Carter, R. (1998). *Mapping the mind*. Berkeley and Los Angeles: The University of California Press.

Erikson, E. (1968). *Identity, youth and crisis*. New York: International Universities Press.

Furman, E. (1984). Children's patterns in mourning the death of a loved one. In H. Wass & C. A. Corr (Eds.), *Childhood and death*. Washington, DC: Hemisphere.

Jehu, D., Gazan, M., & Klassen, C. (1984–1985). Common therapeutic targets among women who were sexually abused in childhood. *Journal of Social Work and Human Sexuality, 3*, 25–45.

Levy, D. (1945). Psychic trauma of operations in children. *American Journal of the Diseases of Childhood, 69*, 7–25.

Mulcahey, A. L., & Young, M. A. (1995). A bereavement support group for children fostering communication about grief and healing. *Cancer Practice, 3*(3), 150–156.

The National Center for Children in Poverty. (1999). New York: The Joseph L. Mailman School of Public Health, Columbia University.

Palombo, J. (1981). Parent loss & childhood bereavement: Some theoretical considerations. *Clinical Social Work, 9*, 3-33.

Piaget, J. (1965). *The moral judgement of the child*. New York: The Free Press.

Pynoos, R., & Nader, K. (1991). Posttraumatic stress disorder. In J. Weiner (Ed.), *Textbook of child and adolescent psychiatry*. Washington, DC: American Psychiatric Press.

Scipio-Bannerman, J. (1999). Nurses are the best trained detectives. *Nursing Spectrum*, 18.

Schneider-Rosen, K., & Cicchetti, D. (1984). The relationship between affect and cognition in maltreated infants: Quality of attachment and the development of visual self-recognition. *Child Development, 55*, 648–658.

Siegel, K., Karus, D., & Raveis, V. H. (1996). Adjustment of children facing the death of a parent due to cancer. *Journal of American Academy of Child Adolescent Psychiatry, 35*(4), 442–450.

Terr, L. (1990). *Too scared to cry: How trauma affects children...and ultimately us all*. New York: Basic Book.

Van Epps, J., Opie, N. D., & Goodwin, T. (1997). Van Epps themes in the bereavement experience of inner city adolescents. *Journal of Child Adolescent Psychiatric Nursing, 10*(1), 25–36.

Wallerstein, J. S., & Blakeslee, S. (1989). *Second chances*. New York: Ticknor & Fields.

Worden, J. W. (1991). *Grief counseling and grief therapy: A handbook for the mental health practitioner* (3rd ed.). New York: Springer Publishing.

Workman, C. G., & Prior, M. (1997). Depression and suicide in young children. *Issues in Comprehensive Pediatric Nursing, 20*(2), 125–132.

Depression: The Sad Child

• ENITZA D. GEORGE, MD

INTRODUCTION

A sad or dysphoric mood that generally is transient and occurs in response to negative events is common among children and adolescents. The term "depression" may refer to symptoms of depression, a depressive syndrome, or a depressive disorder. Depression as symptoms refers to the child's mood or emotional feeling. Depression as a syndrome includes vegetative, psychomotor, and cognitive changes. If a depressive syndrome lasts for 2 weeks or more and causes marked dysfunction, then it is considered a depressive disorder.

Depression can affect individuals at any time in life. Substantial differences exist, however, between children and adults in the clinical expression of depression and responses to specific treatments. Among patients who were depressed as children or adolescents, a high rate of suicide, recurrence of symptoms, and continuation of depressive illness extends into adulthood (Kent et al., 1997). Certainly, early recognition and effective management of depression are essential for all age groups but particularly in childhood when individuals acquire most of their social and cognitive skills.

Ethnic and cultural factors can influence the presentation of depression. Furthermore, these factors can make interpretation of symptoms difficult or lead to misinterpretation if the provider is not culturally aware. In addition, when assessing children, clinicians require a clear understanding of what is developmentally normal and age-appropriate to identify risk factors and diagnose pathology. The reader is referred to Chapters 8 through 12 for more information.

● Clinical Pearls:

- The clinical presentation of and assessment for depression vary across the life span.
- The most important clue in diagnosing depression in a child is a change in mood, affect, or behavior that is not easily explained.

There are no robust markers for mental illness, and given the wide range of "normal behaviors" in children, it may be difficult to make a definitive diagnosis (Jensen & Watanabe, 1999). Symptoms of sadness and low spirit are common at all ages, especially during times of rapid changes. When such symptoms are persistent and intense, however, they should alert clinicians to the possibility of depression.

ANATOMY, PHYSIOLOGY, AND PATHOLOGY

Strong evidence supports a genetic predisposition to depression. Adoption studies are compelling, documenting up to an eight-fold increase in depression among biologic relatives of adoptees with affective illness (Jellinek & Snyder, 1998). The reader is referred to Chapter 6 for more information about adoption.

Major depressive disorder in a grandparent or parent is associated with depression and other mood disorders in the child (Warner et al., 1999). The concordance rate of depression between monozygotic twins (76%) is much higher than between dizygotic twins (19%) (Jellinek & Snyder, 1998). Familial cases of major depression are characterized by earlier onset, longer duration, intermediate levels of recurrence, high levels of impairment, and recurrent thoughts of death or suicide (Kendler et al., 1999).

Several neuroendocrine abnormalities have been implicated in the pathogenesis of depression. Theorists have hypothesized that dysfunction may be found in the serotonergic, catecholaminergic, and dopaminergic systems. In particular, studies report a relative or absolute serotonergic deficiency in major depression (Lestra et al., 1998). The exact mechanism leading to a relative deficiency of serotonin is unknown. Both children and adults who are depressed are known to have cortisol hypersecretion, dexamethasone nonsuppression, hyposecretion of growth hormone in response to an insulin challenge, and sleep electroencephalographic abnormalities (Jellinek & Snyder, 1998). The clinical significance of these findings is still under evaluation.

Children with depression may have relative right posterior hemisphere dysfunction and difficulty processing receptive affective modulations in pitch, timing, and volume of speech (Emerson et al., 1999). As a result, these children have significantly decreased abilities to recognize happy, angry, sad, and neutral voice inflections within congruent and incongruent verbal statements.

Stress has long been recognized as a key element in the etiology of depression. Rejection or abuse may be a precipitating factor, especially in genetically susceptible children. Chronic diseases, emotional or financial deprivation, and loss are common antecedents to depression in children. Children with diabetes, for example, have a high incidence of depression. Early identification and treatment of the affective disorder will ease the management of the metabolic disorder (Lernmark et al., 1999). Chapters 27 and 49 may offer further insights into how exogenous issues can potentiate depression.

EPIDEMIOLOGY

The incidence and prevalence of depression in the pediatric population vary according to age group evaluated, sampling methods, diagnostic criteria, and measurement techniques. In general, the prevalence of major depression in children is about 2% and in adolescents is about 4% to 8% (Table 28-1) (AACAP, 1998).

Current statistics suggest that the prevalence of depression in children is rising. Some experts also suggest that the onset for a first major depressive episode is occurring at

Table 28–1.   PREVALENCE OF MAJOR DEPRESSION BY AGE

Age Group	Incidence
Infants	Unknown
Preschool children	<1%
School-age children	2%
Adolescents	5%
Adults (age 15–64 y)	4.9%

Adapted from Steingard, J., et al. (1995). Current perspectives on the pharmacotherapy of depressive disorders in children and adolescents. *Harvard Review Psychiatry, 2*(6), 313–326.

younger ages (Kovacs & Gatsonis, 1994). It is not clear if these observations indicate an impending epidemic of depression in the pediatric population or are a result of better diagnostic instruments.

Prepubertal rates of depression are similar for both genders. After puberty, the female to male ratio for depression is 2:1 (Jellinek & Snyder, 1998). Depression is more prevalent among children who experience emotional or financial deprivation and in children affected with chronic debilitating diseases.

HISTORY AND PHYSICAL EXAM

If parents express concerns about their child's emotional development, providers should explore both explicit and implicit concerns. History taking and physical examination should focus not only on the child's difficulties but also on the child's strengths and attributes (Thomas, 1998).

Infants, Toddlers, and Preschoolers

Differences between the child's temperament and parental expectations may contribute to stressful family relationships. The provider should gather a history of the child's past and current difficulties and how they are affecting family dynamics. The provider must ask about the parent's own childhood experiences, as well as the experiences of the child's older siblings. Finally, the clinician needs to assess the degree to which these experiences contribute to the parent's view of the child's behavior.

▲ **Clinical Warning:** In obtaining the history, providers should remember that parents often feel anxious or guilty and may fear that the provider is questioning their parenting skills. Clinicians must be cognizant that how they ask questions may influence such feelings.

In undertaking the history, the provider needs to gather data on familial medical and psychiatric disorders. To obtain a complete history, it may be necessary and appropriate to interview as many individuals as possible who have knowledge of the family and the child's current and past functioning. Besides parents, older siblings, and other caregivers, providers may include baby sitters, grandparents, aunts, and uncles.

The provider should perform a complete physical exam, ascertaining that no organic condition can explain parental concerns. Interdisciplinary assessment may unmask other areas of concern. The clinician should consider adjunctive assessment by developmental experts, as well as referrals for child psychology, neurology, genetics, nutrition, ophthalmology, audiology, speech and language therapy, occupational therapy, physical therapy, or social and educational services as indicated. Adjunctive assessment should occur in a variety of settings, including the patient's home, child care agency, school, or other settings where the child spends time. These adjunctive assessments can assist in the diagnosis and evaluation of a child and are helpful in tracking the patient's progress once treatment begins. Refer to Chapters 21 and 22 for further discussion of co-morbidity and management information.

If feasible, the provider may want to consider scheduling a session for clinical observation of the child's interaction with parents. A pediatric social worker can assist in providing for this observation, its assessment, and interpretation. Providers must inform parents of the purpose of the session, which should last at least 15 to 20 minutes. The session involves observing the family in a small carpeted room with a few age-appropriate toys. The examiner notes the quality of parent-child behavior and the child's reaction to brief parental separation and reunion. If the referral concern involves feeding problems, the professional making the assessment needs to observe the child and parent during feeding. Videotaping the session may serve as an adjunct for further discussion with the parents. When compared, serial videotapes can assist in evaluating progress after initiation of treatment (Thomas, 1998).

School-age Children

In taking the history, the provider needs to ask about family dynamics, including history of marital discord, birth of a new child, illness, or death. Questions such as "Did the family recently move?" can be illuminating. Even relatively local moves can be disturbing, especially if a child "loses" neighborhood friends and schoolmates. The clinician also needs to gather information about the child's participation in school. He or she also should ask whether the parents have noted a recent deterioration in grades. Providers also can suggest that parents question the child's teacher and as many classmates as possible for a complete picture of the child's functioning. If the child participates in sports or other extracurricular activities, the provider may want to ask coaches about recent changes in performance during these activities. The reader is referred to Chapter 27 for further understanding of situations that can trigger depression. Chapter 29 can offer further insight for providers who are dealing with children who have more serious problems.

Some depressed children try desperately to compensate for feelings of poor self-worth by attempting to please others, trying not to cause trouble, and "being good" (Jellinek & Snyder, 1998). In reality, such behavior only affords temporary relief for a sense of failure. Behind these struggles, depression persists. If a provider is considering a diagnosis of depression, he or she should investigate any inexplicable change in the child's behavior, even if seemingly "good."

Adolescents

As with younger children, obtaining the history directly from the patient is useful. Indirect information from parents, teachers, coaches, and friends also may prove helpful. Providers should keep in mind that there may be poor correlation between adolescent self-report of depression and parental report (Kent et al., 1997). When evaluating adolescents, providers must be as clear, concise, and specific as possible in history taking, within the context of the teen's developmental stage. They also must assure patients of the confidential nature of all conversations.

● **Clinical Pearl:** Providers should be available by phone or e-mail in case adolescents would like to add to any information they provided during their visit.

▲ **Clinical Warning:** It is of paramount importance for providers to ask children directly and clearly about ideas or plans for committing suicide. They also should ask about access to firearms and ammunition.

A more mature dysphoric mood is a hallmark of puberty, thus increasing the risk of acting on such feelings by committing suicide (Jellinek & Snyder, 1998). The 1997 Youth Risk Behavior Surveillance revealed that 7.7% of adolescents with depression had attempted suicide during the previous year (MMWR, 1998). Asking about ideas regarding death will not increase the risk of suicide. Instead, such questioning will give adolescents an opportunity to discuss their thoughts and feelings. Providers should remember, however, that there is no way to predict suicide among depressed children and adolescents, except in those who have made previous attempts (Jellinek & Snyder, 1998).

Besides suicide, practitioners must ask about alcohol and drug use. Not only will this information identify adolescents at risk for depression, but also will alert others to the possibility of accidental suicide while under the influence of a drug. Of similar importance is to ask about weapon availability and membership in gangs. Refer to Chapters 25, 26, and 29 on for more information.

Finally, the provider should gather information about the seasonality of symptoms, symptom clusters, atypical symptoms, psychosis, and hypomania. Such data will assist in making a differential diagnosis. They also will help identify subtypes of depression that may require special treatment strategies.

DIAGNOSTIC CRITERIA

The Diagnostic and Statistical Manual IV criteria for major depression emphasize that the "core" symptoms are the same for children and adults, but that the prevalence of certain symptoms vary with age (American Psychiatric Association, 1994). For a diagnosis of depression, five or more of the following symptoms must be present during the same two-week period and represent a change from previous functioning. At least one symptom must be either depressed mood or loss of interest or pleasure in an activity. A second (or additional) symptom must come from the following:

• Depressed or irritable mood
• Diminished interest or pleasure in activities
• Weight change or appetite disturbance
• Insomnia or hypersomnia
• Psychomotor agitation or retardation
• Fatigue or loss of energy
• Feelings of worthlessness or guilt
• Disturbed concentration or indecisiveness
• Recurrent thoughts of death, suicidal ideation, or suicide attempt

The child's symptoms must impair relationships and daily functioning. The symptoms must not be secondary to substance abuse, use of medications, other psychiatric illness, bereavement, or medical illness (AACAP, 1998).

DSM-PC (Primary Care) offers a developmental approach to the recognition and diagnosis of childhood depression (Wolraich, 1997) that is more age specific and describes a range from "normal variation" to "problem." DSM IV (1994) classifies depressive behavior during childhood and adolescence into four categories:

• Sadness variation (normal)
• Bereavement
• Thoughts of death variation/problem
• Depressive disorder

The differential diagnosis of depression in children and adolescents can be complex. Establishing this differentiation may be very difficult during adolescence because of the wide range of "normal behaviors."

An adjustment disorder is said to exist if an identifiable psychosocial stress has occurred within six months of initiation of the adolescent's symptoms and the clinical presentation does not fulfill criteria for major depression. If the psychosocial stress is the death of a loved one within the last two months, the provider should consider a diagnosis of bereavement.

Dysthymia is a persistent, long-term change in mood characterized by periods of depressive mood most of the day on most days for at least one year (AACAP, 1998). Affected individuals may report changes in appetite, sleep, self-esteem, and concentration. Dysthymia limits functioning but is not associated with the same degree of impairment as depression. A mood chart or diary may be useful in assessing dysthymia.

Depression may coexist with other psychopathologies or medical problems. Table 28-2 presents the most frequent comorbid diagnoses in children with depression. About 40% to 90% of children and adolescents presenting with depression will have a concurrent psychiatric diagnosis (Goodyer, et al., 1997).

Infants, Toddlers, and Preschoolers

Little is known about depression in infants, and true depression is difficult to define and detect. The most frequent referral concerns for infants who are suspected of being depressed include the following:

• Dysregulation of physiologic functions, such as changes in appetite, bowel function, and sleep patterns
• Irritability
• Growth retardation

Caregivers may report lag or regression in developmental milestones, which the Denver Developmental Screening Test can confirm. Infants without a stable maternal figure (eg, those raised in orphanages) may exhibit symptoms suggestive of depression (Kalinina, et al., 1997). Spitz originally

Table 28–2.   MOST FREQUENT CONCURRENT PSYCHIATRIC DIAGNOSES IN CHILDREN AND ADOLESCENTS WITH DEPRESSION

Comorbidity	Percentage
Dysthimia	30%–80%
Disruptive disorder	10%–80%
Substance use disorder	20%–30%

Adapted with permission from AACAP, 1998.

described this finding as "anaclitic depression," which is characterized by withdrawal and apathy (Jellinek & Snyder, 1998).

Differential diagnosis of depression in infants, toddlers, and preschoolers can be challenging. Display 28-1 presents information meant to assist providers in determining if a young patient is depressed. Concerns regarding developmental delays in speech, motor, or intellectual abilities also may initiate referrals. Prompt evaluation and treatment are critical. Evidence supports that even preschoolers with developmental, speech, motor, or intellectual deficits are at increased risk for depression and other psychopathologies (Dietz, et al, 1997). Thus, early identification may help prevent later school difficulties and more severe psychopathology.

● **Clinical Pearl:** Consider depression in a toddler who persistently lacks spunk, is excessively whiny and clingy, or has severe separation anxiety.

Behavioral problems in toddlers may concern parents. Problems suggestive of depression in a toddler include the following:

- More fussy, whiny, or uncooperative than seems developmentally reasonable
- Dysregulation of physiological functions (eg, reverts to early stage in toileting, eating habits, or sleep patterns)
- Developmental delays (eg, slow to take on new developmental tasks, such as being mommy's "helper")
- Other psychiatric symptoms

Changes in physiological and emotional behavior could herald normal development, an organic cause, or depression. For example, not all babies who spit up are depressed, but a depressed baby will spit up in an effort to refuse feeding. Therefore, the provider needs to collect a careful history in order to differentiate the child's problem.

School-age Children

By school age, children can become sad in response to external factors. They also begin to develop a sense of disappointment with themselves (Jellinek & Snyder, 1998). They may incorporate external events such as parental separation, poor school performance, or medical illness into a negative view of self, with accompanying loss of self-esteem. They may express feelings of worthlessness in statements such as "I'm bad; I'm stupid; No one likes me."

Frequently, providers will see these children for somatic symptoms that seem to have no cause, such as headaches, stomachaches, fatigue, or non-specific pains and aches. A detailed history of the child's illness and a complete physical exam will, in most cases, direct the need for additional diagnostic efforts. Avoidance of unnecessary, expensive, and invasive tests is necessary, since such testing will only perpetuate the syndrome and delay treatment. Display 28-2 provides information that may assist the provider in assessing for depression in the school-aged child.

▲ **Clinical Warning:** In the depression differential, sudden "improvements" in the child's grades or performance in sports can be as worrisome as any other sudden change in behavior or function.

DISPLAY 28–1 • Differential Diagnosis of Depression in Infants and Toddlers

- Variance of normal behavior for age
- Failure to thrive
  Inadequate calorie intake
  Inadequate calorie absorption
  Excessive calorie expenditure
- Medical conditions
  Gastroesophageal reflux
  Infections
  Postconcussion
  Food allergies
  Hypothyroidism
  Epilepsy (petit mal)
- Medication side effects
  Depressed mood due to sedatives (example: cold syrups, antihistaminics)
  Hyperactivity due to stimulants (example: beta agonists used to treat asthma)
  Behavioral changes (anticonvulsants)
- Sexual abuse
- Other psychiatric illnesses
  Adjustment disorder
  Separation anxiety
  Mental retardation
  Attention deficit hyperactivity disorder

DISPLAY 28–2 • Differential Diagnosis of Depression in School-Age Children and Adolescents

- Adjustment disorder with depressed mood
- Bereavement
- Anxiety disorder
- Sleep disorder
- Mental retardation or learning disability
- Attention deficit hyperactivity disorder
- Schizophrenia
- Dysthymia
- Premenstrual dysphoric disorder
- Eating disorder
- Personality disorder
- Bipolar disorder
- Post–traumatic stress disorder
- Alcohol and drug use
- General medical conditions
  Metabolic illness
  Anemia
  Hypothyroidism
  Seizure disorder
  Acquired immunodeficiency syndrome
  Addison's disease
  Post-concussion
  Tuberculosis
  Diabetes
  Brain tumor
  Chronic fatigue syndrome
- Medication side effects
  Antihypertensives
  Barbiturates
  Corticosteroids
  Oral contraceptives
  Albuterol

Clinical signs and symptoms of depression in school-age children include the following:

- Persistent sadness
- Unusual and persistent irritability (fighting in school, with other siblings, parents)
- Expressions of low self-esteem or self-worth
- Loss of interest in previously enjoyed activities
- Sudden or unusual improvement in grades and performance in sports
- Unexplained change in appetite (increase or decrease)
- Unexplained change in sleep pattern (increase or decrease)
- Unexplained somatic complaints (headaches, stomachaches, etc.)
- Poor concentration
- Recurrent thoughts of death or suicide
- Risk-taking behavior (smoking, sexual activity, alcohol, drugs)
- Nightmares
- Anxiety
- Auditory hallucinations
- Phobias

Adolescents

Compared to younger children, depression in adolescents may have a more evident clinical presentation. This stage of life is known for the normal appearance of very rapid mood shifts, which can vary from extreme sadness to grandiose self-confidence. At times, teens experience such moods nearly simultaneously. These mood shifts make it very difficult to diagnose depression in adolescents. Display 28-2 presents information that the clinician can use in forming a differential diagnosis of depression in adolescent patients.

Clinical signs and symptoms that can suggest the diagnosis of depression in adolescents include:

- Persistent boredom, anhedonia, and dyshedonia
- Anxiety and phobias
- Irritability and agitation
- Feelings of self-deprecation (worthless, useless, dumb)
- Beliefs of persecution
- Sleep disturbance
- Changes in school performance
- Early or inappropriate sexuality
- Alcohol and drug use
- School avoidance
- Eating disorders
- Somatic complaints (headaches, pelvic pain, non-specific gastrointestinal complaints)
- Poor performance or abandonment of extracurricular activities
- Suicidal ideas, plan, and attempts

DIAGNOSTIC STUDIES

Questionnaires directed at evaluating children's self-report of mood disorders tend to find high rates of depression. This finding may be more reflective of a high frequency of depressive symptoms in the pediatric population rather than the presence of the full clinical disorder (Jellinek & Snyder, 1998).

● **Clinical Pearl:** Self- or clinician-administered questionnaires have low specificity and are not useful for

diagnosing clinical depression (AACAP, 1998). They are useful to screen for symptoms, assess the severity of the disorder, and monitor clinical improvements.

Instruments based on strict research criteria and DSM-IV diagnostic criteria tend to report low rates of depression. Providers may want to supplement information obtained from these epidemiological instruments with that obtained from the child's self-administered questionnaires. Taken together, these data may add information that one instrument alone cannot capture (Kasius, et al., 1997). The Children's Global Assessment Scale and the Global Assessment of Functioning are useful instruments for tracking a child's functioning. Other assessment instruments may assist in tracking clinical improvement but tell little regarding functioning (AACP, 1998).

MANAGEMENT

For infants, toddlers, and preschoolers, primary care providers should consult with a pediatric psychiatrist, referring the child to that specialist for initiation of any necessary treatment. Co-management of the patient may be required, depending on the outcome of this consultation.

More research is needed on the treatment of depression in children and adolescents. Most of what is known stems from data on clinical experience or research in adults (AACAP, 1998). In general, treatment for depression is divided into three phases: acute, continuation, and maintenance. The clinician, patient, and parents must decide together on the best treatment modality. Treatment options available for management of depression are presented in Display 28-3.

▲ **Clinical Warning:** The clinician should consult with a pediatric psychiatrist before embarking on a course of pharmacotherapy.

Acute Treatment Phase

The choice of the initial treatment modality in the acute phase will depend on the severity of the depression, number of prior episodes, chronicity, patient's age, potential for following a treatment regimen, and family and patient's moti-

---

DISPLAY 28–3 • Treatment Options Available for Depression in Children and Adolescents

Psychotherapy
  Cognitive behavioral therapy
  Psychodynamic psychotherapy
  Interpersonal psychotherapy
  Family therapy
  Individual psychotherapy
  Group therapy
Pharmacotherapy
  Selective serotonin reuptake inhibitors
  Tricyclic antidepressants
  Heterocyclics
  Monoamine oxidase inhibitors
  Bupropion
  Venlafaxine
  Nefazodone

vation for treatment (AACAP, 1998). For children and adolescents with mild to moderate depression, the initial treatment may be psychotherapy alone. Current work suggests that positive benefits of therapy can be long-lasting.

The goals of psychotherapy are to teach the patient and family to cope with past and current stress, improve social skills and self-esteem, and help the patient develop insight. Many approaches have been recommended, of which cognitive behavioral therapy (CBT) is the most popular. CBT focuses on using cognitive restructuring to modify distorted beliefs and attitudes about self. CBT assumes that depressed patients have a distorted view of themselves, the world, and the future. CBT has been shown to be better than no intervention for children and adolescents in reducing depressive symptoms and improving self-esteem (Reinecke, et al, 1998). It is recommended for patients with mild and moderate depression but not for severe depression (Harrington, et al., 1998). A high rate of depression relapse occurs on follow-up; therefore, continuation treatment often is necessary (AACAP, 1998).

For severe depression, it is best to combine both psychotherapy and pharmacotherapy from the start. Economics and geography will play roles in treatment decisions. Generally, pharmacotherapy alone is considered insufficient treatment. Indications for using pharmacotherapy in depression treatments include:

- Depression with severe symptoms
- Unwillingness or inability to undergo psychotherapy
- Psychotic depression
- Failure to respond to psychotherapy after 8 to 12 sessions
- Non-rapid-cycling bipolar depression
- Recurrent depression

Adolescents with depressive illness have shown a more favorable response to selective serotonin reuptake inhibitors (SSRIs) than to tricyclics (Strober, et al., 1999). SSRIs are safe, have benign adverse effects, are easy to use, and present a low risk of death following overdose (Renaud, et al, 1999). If indicated, SSRIs are the treatment of choice for depression in children and adolescents. Open studies have reported 70% to 90% response rates to SSRIs in selective patients (DeVane, Sallee, 1996). The administration of SSRIs is similar in children to that in adults except for a lower initial dose (Leonard, et al., 1997).

Initial treatment should last at least four weeks before reevaluation of the dose. If the patient has not shown any clinical improvement after four weeks of treatment, the provider needs to consider increasing the dose. If after increasing the dose, no improvement has occurred by six weeks, the provider should reevaluate and change the treatment strategy (AACAP, 1998). During treatment with an SSRI, parents and teachers may notice a "behavior activation" in the child. The previously hypoactive child may now display impulsivity and agitation. Other side effects include gastrointestinal upset, diaphoresis, headaches, akathisia, bruising as well as changes in sleep, appetite, and sexual functioning (Leonard, et al., 1997).

▲ **Clinical Warning:** The provider needs to warn parents and patients against discontinuing SSRIs abruptly, especially those that have short half-lives. Abrupt withdrawal may induce symptoms of tiredness, irritability, and severe somatic complaints (Zajecka, et al., 1997).

Several randomized studies have questioned the usefulness of tricyclic antidepressants (TCAs) and other antidepressants in children. Before prescribing a TCA, providers must inform the patient and parents about side effects and the fatality of overdose (Renaud, et al., 1999). Providers must stress parental responsibility for storage, supervision, and administration of TCAs. Table 28-3 presents SSRIs currently approved for use in pediatric patients.

▲ **Clinical Warning:** Limiting the amount of medication prescribed and refills given at each appointment for all patients is important, but most especially for young children and suicidal patients.

Providers must obtain a baseline electrocardiogram, resting blood pressure, resting pulse rate, and weight before initiating treatment with a TCA. TCAs are best used in depressed children with associated attention deficit hyperactive disorder (ADHS), enuresis, and narcolepsy (AACAP, 1998). Refer to Chapter 21 for further discussion of the issues surrounding tricyclic prescription in children and adolescents.

Electroconvulsive therapy (ECT) may be effective to treat adolescents with resistant depression (Strober, et al., 1998). The pediatric psychiatrist may consider ECT as a treatment option in adolescents with primary, endogenous, psychotic depression who are resistant to antidepressant pharmacotherapy and psychotherapy.

▲ **Clinical Warning:** Referral to a pediatric psychiatrist is imperative for the seriously depressed adolescent for whom ECT is a treatment consideration. Because of the many risks associated with ECT use, including cardiac anomalies and even death, all patients must be screened beforehand for physiologic safety before ECT begins.

Continuation Treatment Phase

Continuation therapy is recommended for all patients for six to 12 months (AACAP, 1998). During this period, the patient is seen at least once monthly. Continuation of CBT may be efficacious in preventing relapses of depression in adolescents (Harrington, et al., 1998). If medications were prescribed, they should be continued at the same dose. If the patient has been asymptomatic for six to 12 months, medications can be discontinued over six weeks to prevent withdrawal effects.

Maintenance Treatment Phase

Maintenance therapy is used for selected patients to prevent relapse and recurrence. The patient must attend monthly to quarterly appointments for reevaluation and psychotherapy. Patients who respond well after a first episode of mild to moderate uncomplicated depression may not need maintenance treatment. Patients experiencing a second or third episode should receive maintenance treatment for one to

Table 28–3. SELECTIVE SEROTONIN RECEPTOR INHIBITORS (SSRIS) APPROVED FOR PEDIATRIC USE

Drug	Initial Dose	Maximum Dose
Fluvoxamine (Luvox)*	25 mg/d	200 mg/d
Sertraline (Zoloft)**	25 mg/d	200 mg/d

*Fluvoxamine is not recommended for children under 8 y.
**Sertraline is not recommended for children under 6 y.

three years. Depressed patients who experience psychosis, severe impairment, suicidal risk, or treatment resistance should receive treatment for a longer period, perhaps indefinitely (AACAP, 1998). Co-management with a psychotherapist will enhance treatment outcomes.

▲ **Clinical Warning:** Controversy exists regarding use of antidepressant medications beyond the continuation treatment phase. Long-term effects of these medications on the maturation and development of children have not been studied (AACAP, 1998).

Outcomes

The median duration of a major depressive episode in children and adolescents is 7 to 9 months (AACAP, 1998). Approximately 90% of patients experience remission one to two years after onset; 6% to 10% become protracted (Kovacs, 1996). Approximately 40% to 60% of patients will relapse after successful initial treatment (Vostanis, et al., 1998). Longitudinal studies report that the probability of recurrence is 20% to 60% at one to two years and as high as 70% after five years (Kovacs, 1996).

A protracted course with refractory or treatment-resistant depression is more common in patients who have severe symptoms, psychosis, and family history of psychiatric disorder (Botteron & Geller, 1997). Predictors of recurrence are early age at onset, multiple previous episodes, severity of index episode, psychosis, unresolved psychosocial stressors, other psychiatric comorbidities, and non-participation in the treatment regimen (Emslie, et al., 1997). Display 28-4 defines terms used to describe the clinical course of depression.

Prevention Strategies

Parents, teachers, coaches, and clinicians must be sensitive in identifying children and adolescents who are at risk for developing depression. Such children may include those who have:

- mental retardation
- attention deficit hyperactivity disorder
- parents who abuse alcohol or other drugs
- a family history of mental illness
- a past history of suicide ideation or attempts
- a family history of suicide attempts
- other mental illnesses
- conduct disorder
- a history of school problems
- a history of recent bereavement, loss, or change

Also at risk are those children who are:

- immigrants
- homeless
- ill with a chronic or debilitating illness
- physically challenged
- suffering parental loss through separation, divorce, or death
- orphans/foster children (Menker, 1998)

Schools are ideal environments for implementing preventive programs for depression. School curricula should include courses geared toward stress management and relaxation techniques, which can be taught from elementary through high schools. One study found that providing group cognitive behavioral therapy in school was useful in preventing unipolar depression in adolescents at high risk (Clarke, et al., 1995).

Parents may be able to help children through discussion of their own depression and coping styles. If needed, providers should treat or refer parents for treatment. The entire family may need to participate in family and group therapy, which can improve family dynamics and foster a more harmonious environment for the child's emotional development. Clinicians can be instrumental in providing individual and family counseling regarding stress management. Even with patients at no particular risk for depression, practitioners should inquire about coping abilities and family, job, and school stress. Providers should be available for patients and families, encouraging them to call or send e-mail, if only to "talk things out." Most importantly, practitioners need to be caring and empathetic toward patients.

DISPLAY 28–4 • Terms Commonly Used to Describe the Clinical Course of Major Depressive Disorder

Response: Significant improvement of depressive symptoms during the initial or acute phase. In general, response coincides with the onset of remission.

Remission: A period of at least 2 weeks and less than 2 months with no more than one clinically significant symptom.

Partial remission: A period of at least 2 weeks and less than 2 months with more than one clinically significant symptom but fewer symptoms than the full syndrome.

Recovery: An asymptomatic period of more than 2 months.

Relapse: An episode of depression during the period of remission.

Recurrence: The emergence of symptoms of major depression during the period of recovery (a new episode).

Adapted with permission from American Academy of Children and Adolescent Psychiatry. (1998). Practice parameters for the assessment and treatment of children and adolescents with depressive disorders. *Journal of the American Academy of Child and Adolescent Psychiatry, 37*(Suppl. 10), 63S–83S.

COMMUNITY RESOURCES

The following groups provide information for patients and their families regarding depression in children. These resources also will guide referrals to state and local chapters and support groups. All inquiries are confidential and handled by trained volunteers.

National Institute of Mental Health
6001 Executive Boulevard
Rm. 8184, MSC 9663
Bethesda, MD 20892-9663
(301) 443-4513

National Alliance for Research on Schizophrenia and Depression
60 Cutter Mill Road
Suite 404
Great Neck, NY 11021
(800) 829-8289

REFERENCES

American Academy of Children and Adolescent Psychiatry. (1998). Practice parameters for the assessment and treatment of children and adolescents with depressive disorders. *Journal of the American Academy of Child and Adolescent Psychiatry, 37*(10 Suppl), 63S-83S.

American Psychiatric Association. (1994*). DSM IV, Diagnostic and statistical manual of mental disorders* (4th ed.). Washington, DC: Author.

Botteron, K. N., & Geller, B. (1997). Refractory depression in children and adolescents. *Depression and Anxiety, 5*(4), 212-223.

Clarke, G. N., et al. (1995). Targeted prevention of unipolar depressive disorder in an at risk sample of high school adolescents: A randomized trial of a group cognitive intervention. *Journal of the American Academy of Child and Adolescent Psychiatry, 34*(3), 312-321.

DeVane, C. L., & Sallee, F. R. (1996). Serotonin selective reuptake inhibitors in child and adolescent psychopharmacology: A review of published experience. *Journal of Clinical Psychiatry, 57*, 55-66.

Dietz, K. R., et al. (1997). Relation between intelligence and psychopathology among preschoolers. *Journal of Clinical Child Psychology, 26*(1), 99-107.

Emerson, C. S., et al. (1999). Investigation of receptive affective prosodic ability in school-aged boys with and without depression. *Neuropsychiatry Neuropsychology Behavioral Neurology, 12*(2), 102–109.

Emslie, G. J., et al. Recurrence of major depressive disorder in hospitalized children and adolescents. *Journal of the American Academy of Child and Adolescent Psychiatry, 36*, 785-792.

Goodyer, I. M., et al. (1997). Short-term outcome of major depression, I: Comorbidity and severity at presentation as predictors of persistent disorder. *Journal of the American Academy of Child and Adolescent Psychiatry, 36*, 179-187.

Harrington R, et al. (1998). Meta-analysis of CBT for depression in adolescents. *Journal of the American Academy of Child and Adolescent Psychiatry, 37*(10), 1005-1006.

Kalinina, M. A., et al. (1997). [Depressive state at an early age] *Zh Nevrol Psikhiatr S S Korsakova, 97*(8), 8-12.

Kasius, M. C., et al. (1997). Associations between different diagnostic approaches for child and adolescent psychopathology. *Journal of Child Psychology and Psychiatry, 38*(6), 625-632.

Kendler, K. S., et al. (1999). Clinical characteristics of major depression that predict risk of depression in relatives. *Archives of Gen Psychiatry, 56*(4), 322–327.

Kent, L., et al. (1997). Detection of major and minor depression in children and adolescents: Evaluation of the mood and feelings questionnaire. *Journal of Child Psychology and Psychiatry, 38*(5), 565–573.

Kovacs, M. (1996). Presentation and course of major depressive disorder during childhood and later years of the life span. *Journal of the American Academy of Child and Adolescent Psychiatry, 35*, 705-715.

Kovacs, M., & Gatsonis, C. (1994). Secular trends in age at onset of major depressive disorder in a clinical sample of children. *Journal of Psychiatric Research, 28*, 319-329.

Jellinek, M. S., & Snyder, J. B. (1998). Depression and suicide in children and adolescents. *Pediatrics in Review, 19*(8), 255–266.

Jensen, P. S., & Watanabe, H. (1999). Sherlock Holmes and child psychopathology assessment approaches: The case of the false-positive. *Journal of the American Academy of Child and Adolescent Psychiatry, 38*(2), 138–146.

Leonard, H. L., et al. (1997). Pharmacology of the selective serotonin reuptake inhibitors in children and adolescents. *Journal of the American Academy of Child and Adolescent Psychiatry, 36*(6), 725-36.

Lernmark, B., et al. (1999). Symptoms of depression are important to psychological adaptation and metabolic control in children with diabetes mellitus. *Diabetic Medicine, 16*(1), 14–22.

Lestra, C., et al. (1998). Biological parameters in major depression: Effects of paroxetine, viloxazine, moclobemide, and electroconvulsive therapy. Relation to early clinical outcome. *Biol Psychiatry, 44*(4), 274–280.

Menker, E. M. (1998). The mental health of homeless school-age children. *Journal of Child and Adolescent Psychiatric Nursing, 11*(3), 87-98.

Centers for Disease Control and Prevention. (1998). 1997 Youth Risk Behavior Surveillance. *Morbidity and Mortality Weekly Review*, August 14, 1998.

Reinecke, M. A., et al. (1998). Cognitive-behavioral therapy of depression and depressive symptoms during adolescence: A review and meta-analysis. *Journal of the American Academy of Child and Adolescent Psychiatry, 37*, 26-34.

Renaud, J., et al. (1999). A risk-benefit assessment of pharmacotherapies for clinical depression in children and adolescents. *Drug Safety, 20*(1), 59-75.

Steingard, J., et al. (1995). Current perspectives on the pharmacotherapy of depressive disorders in children and adolescents. *Harvard Review Psychiatry, 2*(6), 313-326.

Strober, M., et al. (1999). The pharmacotherapy of depressive illness in adolescents: An open-label comparison of fluoxetine with imipramine-treated historical controls. *Journal of Clinical Psychiatry, 60*, 164-169.

Strober, M., et al. (1998). Effects of electroconvulsive therapy in adolescents with severe endogenous depression resistant to pharmacotherapy. *Biol Psychiatry, 43*(3), 335-338.

Thomas, J. M. (1998). Summary of the practice parameters for the psychiatric assessment of infants and toddlers (0-36 months). American Academy of Child and Adolescent Psychiatry. *Journal of the American Academy of Child and Adolescent Psychiatry, 37*(1), 127-32.

Vostanis, P., et al. (1998). Two-year outcome of children treated with depression. *European Child and Adolescent Psychiatry, 7*(1), 12-18.

Warner, V., et al. (1999). Grandparent, parent, and grandchildren at high risk for depression: A three-generation study. *Journal of the American Academy of Child and Adolescent Psychiatry, 38*(3), 289–296.

Wolraich, M. L. (1997). Diagnostic and Statistical Manual for Primary Care. (DSM-PC) Child and Adolescent Version: design, intent, and hopes for the future. *Journal of Developmental and Behavioral Pediatrics, 18*(3), 171-172.

Zajecka, J., et al. (1997). Discontinuation symptoms after treatment with serotonin reuptake inhibitors: A literature review. *Journal of Clinical Psychiatry, 58*, 291-297.

Suicide

• CYNTHIA R. PFEFFER, MD

INTRODUCTION

Suicide is among the leading causes of death in individuals 5 to 24 years old. The most important methods of preventing the tragic loss of young lives are early identification of those at risk and implementation of interventions to deter suicide attempts. Primary care providers are among the most influential professionals, serving as gatekeepers to recognize, treat, and refer at-risk youngsters. Lack of time, infrequent meetings with older children and adolescents, and, perhaps, a need for specialized clinical skills may mandate referral of at-risk patients to professionals who specialize in pediatric mental disorders. Prevention of suicide requires community-based interventions offered within a continuum of care. Practitioners often serve as links to such services for children and adolescents.

This chapter provides an overview to assist pediatric primary care providers in identifying, treating, and preventing suicide in children and adolescents. It highlights practical guidelines that address the significant risk factors for youth suicide.

ANATOMY, PHYSIOLOGY, AND PATHOLOGY

Nonfatal suicidal behavior is a complex psychiatric symptom that manifests as an episodic phenomenon. Specific co-occurring acute or chronic risk factors increase the likelihood of suicide. The basic neurobiology of suicide is currently a subject of intensive study. Promising results suggest that aspects of dysregulation of the serotonergic neurotransmitter system are prominent features of serious suicide attempts in adults, children, and adolescents (Greenhill et al., 1995; Kruesi et al., 1992; Mann & Stoff, 1997; Pfeffer et al., 1998; Pine et al., 1995).

Generally, dysregulation of the serotonergic system involves findings of low concentrations of presynaptic serotonergic neuroreceptors and dense concentrations of post-synaptic receptors (Mann, 1998). These results, with a down-regulation at the presynaptic receptors and an up-regulation at the post-synaptic receptors, suggest a functional disequilibrium. Low levels of serotonin metabolites, such as 5-hydroxy-indol-acetic acid (5-HIAA) in the cerebrospinal fluid, have been identified in adults who committed suicide and among adolescents who reported recent serious suicide attempts. Low levels of serum tryptophan, a basic precursor of serotonin, have been identified in prepubertal children with histories of recent suicide attempts (Pfeffer et al., 1998).

Postmortem neuroradiographic studies and *in vivo* biologic challenges with PET neuroimaging techniques suggest that serotonin abnormalities may involve the ventrolateral prefrontal cortex and brainstem of those who attempt and successfully complete suicide (Arango, Underwood, & Mann, 1997). The ventrolateral prefrontal cortex is involved in behavioral inhibition; impulsivity and emotional instability may be associated with dysfunctions in the ventrolateral prefrontal cortex, possibly increasing an individual's vulnerability for suicide. Research results also suggest the association of suicidal behavior with polymorphisms of the tryptophan hydroxylase gene (Mann, 1998). Validation of such results may enable the development of a blood test for suicidal behavior.

Most neurobiologic research has been with adults, and developmental differences in younger individuals may exist. Children and adolescents may not manifest these same neurobiologic dysfunctions. For example, lower levels of 5-HIAA concentrations have been found in the cerebrospinal fluid of adolescents who made serious suicide attempts, compared with levels in their adult counterparts. Conversely, low levels of cerebrospinal fluid homovanillic acid have been identified as being associated with adolescents who made serious suicide attempts (Greenhill et al., 1995; Kruesi et al., 1992).

● **Clinical Pearl:** Neurobehavioral research may someday yield tests that can predict a patient's level of risk for future suicidal behavior. Such neurobiologic testing may possibly involve an assay of cerebrospinal fluid metabolites of neurotransmitters.

Co-occurring psychopathologies significantly increase the risk for child and adolescent suicide. Only 10% of youth who commit suicide have no diagnosed psychopathology (Brent et al., 1993a; Marttunen, Hillevi, Henriksson, & Lonnqvist, 1991; Shaffer et al., 1996). This figure may overestimate the absence of clinically significant psychiatric symptoms or psychiatric disorders. The prevalent psychiatric disorders among suicidal youths include mood disorders and substance abuse (including alcoholism). Features of mood disorders include major depressive disorder, dysthymia, mania, hypomania, or mixed periods of rapid cycling. An important suicide risk for those who have a mood disorder is a mixed state of mania and depression. In males, mood disorders are frequently comorbid with conduct and substance abuse disorders. Particularly for males older than age 15 years, drug abuse, alcohol abuse, or both are significant risk factors. In general, psychiatric disorders are found to have been present for at least 2 years before the suicide.

Many suicidal youths manifest impulsivity, irritability, and outbursts of aggression. A small number of suicidal youths, however, are anxious and do not manifest signs of comorbid psychiatric disorders. They often are characterized as excellent students and well liked by peers. Their suicides are often surprises to those who know them well. Regardless, at least one third of adolescents who commit suicide have a history of suicide attempts.

According to controlled research, males and females share similar risk factors for suicide (Shaffer et al., 1996). Studies that compared completed and attempted suicides in children and adolescents failed to find significant differences in risk factors (Brent et al., 1988; Shaffer et al., 1996). A marked difference exists, however, in the relative strength of risk factors with respect to gender (Shaffer, 1988; Shaffer et al., 1996). Specifically, a previous suicide attempt increases the risk over 30-fold in males. The next significant level of risk is depression, which elevates risk 11-fold in males. Substance abuse follows, which elevates suicide risk in males approximately five-fold; and disruptive disorder, which elevates risk three-fold. In females, the presence of major depressive disorder imparts the greatest suicide risk, increasing risk 20-fold. A history of a prior suicide attempt increases risk for females approximately three-fold.

▲ **Clinical Warning:** Although schizophrenia is relatively rare in children and adolescents, its presence is a major risk factor for suicide.

Although issues regarding sexual orientation have not been identified as significant in studies of youth suicide victims, research suggests that bisexual, gay, and lesbian youths are at increased risk for suicide (Mueher, 1995; Remafedi, French, Story, Resnick, & Blum, 1998; Shaffer, Fisher, Hicks, Parides, & Gould, 1995). They are at significantly higher risk for suicidal intent, suicidal ideation, and more frequent suicide attempts than heterosexual teens. Recent instances of school violence underscore the often hidden suffering of youth who are bullied and labeled "different" by schoolmates and peers.

▲ **Clinical Warning:** Medical conditions, such as epilepsy and infection with human immunodeficiency virus (HIV), are associated with increased risk for suicide (Thiele, Gonzales-Heydrich, & Riviello, 1999). Providers must monitor closely youth with these conditions and conduct repeated evaluations of suicidal intent.

Repeated suicide attempts have been associated with hypomanic personality traits and cluster-B personality disorders (Brent et al., 1993a; 1994). Borderline personality disorder has been associated most closely with repeated suicidal behavior (Johnson et al., 1995). Controversy exists about whether borderline personality disorder is a form of bipolar disorder. Its main symptoms include repeated suicide attempts; other nonfatal self-injurious behaviors; impulsivity; unstable mood; chronic problematic interpersonal relationships; a self-concept involving grandiosity, worthlessness, or both; and irritability.

EPIDEMIOLOGY

Rates of suicide, especially among those 15 to 24 years old, have increased since the late 1960s and remain high. Suicide in adolescents and young adults in particular is considered a national public health problem (Peters, Kochanek, & Murphy, 1998).

Suicide is the third-leading cause of death in non-Caucasian youth ages 15 to 24 years among all races and both sexes, following unintentional injuries and homicide. Suicide is the second leading cause of death for Caucasians ages 15 to 24 years. In general, Caucasian males have the highest suicide rates across all ages, although rates of suicide are increasing among African American males. This increase may be related to a decrease in previously available social supports. Regional distinctions in suicide rates are evident. Higher suicide rates are found in western states and Alaska, and lower suicide rates are found in northeastern, north cen-

tral, and southern states. Urban centers have lower suicide rates than do rural regions, possibly related to the different availability of firearms used for hunting in rural communities (National Institute of Mental Health, 1999).

The most recent statistics (1997) compiled by the National Institute of Mental Health (1999) and also reported by Peters and colleagues (1998) are sobering:

- The suicide rate among children ages 10 to 14 years was 1.6/100,000, or 303 deaths among 19,040,000 children in this age group.
- The suicide rate among adolescents ages 15 to 19 years was 9.5/100,000, or 1,802 deaths among 19,068,000 adolescents in this age group, with a male to female ratio of 5:1.
- Firearms are the most common method all ages used to commit suicide (Peters et al., 1998). Multiple epidemiologic research reports indicate that females attempt suicide more frequently than males, although males are more likely to be successful.

HISTORY AND PHYSICAL EXAMINATION

Evaluation of suicidal behavior requires direct interview of the child or adolescent and interview of a parent or caregiver. Recommendations are for providers to obtain additional information from others who know the youngster, such as school professionals. Clinicians should obtain information about the suicidal behavior and risk for death or repetition of the behavior, as well as underlying problems or diagnosis. Providers also should identify the presence of any promoting factors, such as history of depression, perceived friendless state, substance use, school problems or failure, recent diagnosis of illness (eg, HIV), or recent change, such as loss of friend(s), divorce, death, or move from one area to another.

Practitioners should obtain information about the method that the patient has contemplated or used for a suicide attempt, the level of medical lethality, the degree of suicidal intent, the degree of planning, and the potential for discovery or intervention if the patient carries out the act. Clinicians can elicit suicidal intent even in children as young as 6 years (Jacobsen et al., 1994). Suicide intent involves the balance between the wish to live and the wish to die (Beck, Schuyler, & Herman, 1974; Beck, Kovacs, & Weissman, 1979a). Pervasive suicidal ideation increases the likelihood of planning suicide and usually is associated with a psychiatric disorder. An essential part of an evaluation of suicidal behavior is the determination of the availability of lethal means of carrying out suicidal impulses, such as the presence in the home of guns or firearms or knowledge of the availability of such weapons (Brent et al., 1991; 1993b).

During an evaluation, providers should strive to use a calm, reassuring, and caring tone of voice. Awareness of nonverbal cues, such as facial expression, arm placement, and sitting position in relation to the patient, can strengthen the quality of interview. Providers must ask interview questions in a manner that does not inadvertently convey a confrontational or accusing stance (Jacobsen et al., 1994). Display 29-1 provides examples of questions that clinicians may find useful when conducting this interview.

Any evaluation of suicidal risk factors must include a detailed interview about psychiatric symptoms and disorders. High-risk factors include history of mood disorders; symptoms of mania, hypomania, or mixed states of rapid cycling; anxiety disorders; substance use; conduct disorder;

DISPLAY 29–1 • Interview Questions in Assessing for Suicidality

- Did you ever feel so upset that you wished you were not alive or wanted to die?
- Did you ever do something that you knew was so dangerous that you could get hurt or killed by doing it?
- Did you ever hurt yourself or try to hurt yourself?
- Did you ever try to kill yourself?
- Did you ever think about or try to commit suicide?

Questions to identify suicidal intent may include the following:

- Did you do anything to get ready to kill yourself?
- Did you think what you did would kill you?

Other aspects of suicidal intent involve motivations, which can be addressed with the following questions:

- Did you want to get attention from someone?
- Did you hope that your relationship with (name a person) would change?
- Did you want to be with (name a person who died)?
- Did you want to get away from the problems you are having?
- Did you want to get even with (name a person)?

health professional is warranted if the practitioner determines that specialized testing with these or other instruments may help in identifying and managing the at-risk patient. The following are examples of some of the many valid and reliable instruments available:

- Beck Hopelessness Scale (Beck et al., 1974) measures level of hopeless symptoms. This self-report scale has predictive validity for suicide in adults. An adaptation has been developed for children and adolescents (Kazdin, Rogers, & Golbus, 1986; Spirito, Overholser, Ashworth, Morgan, & Benedict-Drew, 1988).
- Suicidal Ideation Questionnaire (Reynolds, 1987) is a self-report scale to measure frequency and severity of suicidal ideation in junior and senior high school students.
- Suicide Probability Scale (Tatum, Greene, & Karr, 1993) is designed for individuals 14 years and older to identify aspects of suicidal risk.
- Child-Adolescent Suicide Potential Index (Pfeffer, 2000) is a reliable and valid self-report screening questionnaire to measure level of suicidal risk in children and adolescents 6 to 18 years old.
- The Suicide Potential Scales (Pfeffer, 1986; Pfeffer et al., 1993) are used in a clinical interview format to assess suicidal and assaultive behavior and relevant associated risk factors.

DIAGNOSTIC CRITERIA

Suicidal behavior is defined as a self-destructive act with the intent to cause death. Children and adolescents use varied methods to carry out suicidal acts, including shooting, hanging, jumping from heights, stabbing, ingesting poisons, drowning, and burning. Nonfatal suicidal behavior is a self-destructive act without lethal consequences. This often is referred to as parasuicidal behavior; however, parasuicidal behavior is defined as nonfatal self-harmful behavior without the intent to kill oneself (Brooksbank, 1985).

Suicidal behavior should be differentiated from self-injurious behaviors, such as superficial cutting that often does not have intent to kill. It should be differentiated from self-destructive behaviors, such as risk taking, substance abuse, eating disorders, and autoerotic activity. Deaths in teenagers from sexual asphyxia are rare and are identified usually when sexually related materials are found at the scene of death (Shaffer et al., 1996; Johnstone & Huws, 1999).

DIAGNOSTIC STUDIES

At present, no specific biologic diagnostic studies of suicidal risk have been done. Salient to identifying suicidal risk and suicidal behavior is identification of vulnerability associated with family history of suicidal behavior, mood, anxiety, substance abuse disorders, and family violence including physical and sexual abuse. The reader is referred to Chapters 21, 22, 23, 26, and 28 for insight into these problems and their relationship to suicide risk.

MANAGEMENT

Providers should organize treatment of suicidal behavior to include a continuum of services involving outpatient, day

and prior suicide attempt (Brent et al., 1987; Pfeffer, 1986; 1997).

Providers need to evaluate for several features of cognitive distortions, including hopelessness; psychotic distortions involving hallucinations, delusions, or paranoid ideation; poor self-esteem; perceptions of isolation; and problematic coping mechanisms associated with impulsivity. Several conditions that influence suicidal risk involve environmental stresses, including family discord, family history of suicide, and history of physical or sexual abuse. Family psychopathology also is important, particularly disturbances of mood, substance use, violence, and suicidal behavior (Brent, Bridge, Johnson, & Connolly, 1996; Brent, Moritz, Bridge, Perper, & Canobbio, 1996; de Wilde, Kienhorst, Diekstra, & Wolters, 1992; Gould, Fisher, Parides, Flory, & Shaffer, 1996; Pfeffer, 1997; Pfeffer et al., 1997; Pfeffer, Normandin, & Kakuma, 1994). Children and adolescents with conditions that may enhance depression and, perhaps, induce hopelessness, include such problems as diabetes, HIV, and epilepsy. Clinicians should evaluate regularly youth who have a diagnosis of chronic disease for signs of suicidal intent or behavior. They must identify precipitating factors in vulnerable youth, such as homosexual orientation, lack of a supportive peer group, loss of a boyfriend or girlfriend, failure in school, or isolation from social activities.

Prior suicidal behavior predicts future suicidal acts (Goldston, Reboussin, Kelly, Ivers, & Brunstetter, 1996; Pfeffer et al., 1993). For example, prepubertal children who think about or attempt suicide are at significant risk for suicide attempts in adolescence (Pfeffer et al., 1993). Early onset depression, such as major depressive disorder, is associated with suicidal behavior in adolescents (Kovacs, Goldston, & Gatsonis, 1993) and adults (Harrington et al., 1994; Rao, Weissman, Martin, & Hammond, 1993). Clinicians should specifically address these issues in the evaluation and in every reassessment of a child or adolescent.

Specialized scales or interview instruments may augment evaluation. These may be used before a clinical interview to identify indicators of suicidal risk. Referral to a mental

hospital, psychiatric hospital, and residential treatment programs. Initially, gatekeepers, such as parents, peers, school professionals, pediatric providers, and others who work with children and adolescents, identify a suicidal child or adolescent.

▲ **Clinical Warning:** Once identification of suicidal behavior or risk occurs, it is considered a medical emergency. Such children and adolescents *must* be referred to a psychiatrist for evaluation, and if the evaluation confirms suicidal risk, the patient should be hospitalized for safety.

Important features of treatment involve forming an alliance with the child or adolescent and his or her parent or caregiver so that all are committed to participate in treatment. If an emergency service initially evaluates the child or adolescent, staff must interview the suicidal youth and his or her parent as a means of confirming the account of suicidal behavior and risk (Rotheram-Borus, Walker, & Ferns, 1996). In addition, the provider must discuss risk of firearms and a plan for their removal (Kruesi et al., 1999). Finally, the clinician must make a follow-up assessment, organizing treatment and ensuring its delivery. The family is most likely to follow treatment recommendations given at the time of the emergency if they match the family's expectations, are economically feasible, and the parent is medically and psychologically able to assist with follow-up attendance (Rotheram-Borus et al., 1996).

Psychotherapy

Treatment may involve a variety of psychotherapeutic interventions. Suicidal children and adolescents experience feelings of intense and distressing depression, worthlessness, anger, anxiety, hopelessness, and inability to plan solutions to their perceived and actual problems. Psychotherapeutic techniques aim to decrease such intolerable feelings, enabling patients to improve their problem-solving skills.

▲ **Clinical Warning:** Providers should refer any depressed or suicidal patient to a skilled mental health professional. Working with suicidal children and adolescents is best done by a mental health clinician who is available to the suicidal patient and family and has skill and training in administering interventions. Display 29-2 provides information on several therapeutic interventions that have been used successfully in adults, any of which mental health clinicians may use with depressed or suicidal patients.

Environmental conflicts stemming from family discord and psychopathology should be a focus of intervention. Family-oriented treatment adjunctive to individual psychotherapy can enhance family communication and support and reduce conflicts. Treatment of parental psychiatric disorders is essential as a means of stabilizing the family environment.

Pharmacotherapy

A variety of medications may be used to treat suicidal children and adolescents, although empirical studies of their safety and effectiveness in children and adolescents are lacking. The provider should forego prescribing these agents and refer any patient in need of pharmacotherapy to a psychiatrist for evaluation and medication management. The following discussion is provided as information for understanding rather than as prescriptive guidelines.

Lithium treatment has been shown to reduce recurrence of suicide attempts in studies of adults with bipolar disorder

---

DISPLAY 29–2 • Interventions With Some Empirical Evidence of Effectiveness in Suicidal Adults

- Cognitive-behavioral therapy (Beck et al., 1979b; Elkin et al., 1989) has been shown to be more effective than family or supportive therapy for depressed adolescents (Brent et al., 1997). Interventions are not specific to treatment of suicidal behavior, though by effectively reducing symptoms of depression, they may lower suicidal risk. Cognitive-behavioral therapy aims to strengthen cognitive coping skills while decreasing pessimistic, self-denigrating perceptions. Such therapy fosters behavior that enables the patient to evaluate personal situations and responses to ensure self-promoting attitudes and outcomes.
- Dialectic-behavioral therapy is the only psychotherapy that has been shown in randomized clinical trials to reduce suicidal behavior in adults (Linehan, 1993). It has not been studied regarding its efficacy for suicidal adolescents. Dialectic-behavioral therapy aims to decrease impulsivity and poor self-concepts, thus reducing the likelihood for using suicidal behavior as a coping strategy. This method uses individual and group formats to accomplish treatment goals.
- Interpersonal psychotherapy (Klerman et al., 1984) is being evaluated empirically in adolescents (Mufson & Moreau, 1998). It focuses on identifying and ameliorating distressing responses to experiences of loss. Interpersonal psychotherapy involves developing social and cognitive skills to cope with stressful losses, thereby reducing symptoms of depression.
- Psychodynamic psychotherapy is probably the most widely used therapy. This kind of intervention may help relieve poor self-esteem, enhancing understanding of underlying conflicts that led to suicidal behavior. The efficacy of such treatment has not been evaluated empirically for suicidal behavior.

(Tondo, Jamison, & Baldessarini, 1997). No such studies have been conducted with children or adolescents. Despite its promising effects, lithium has a low margin of safety if taken in overdose, so caution and close monitoring are necessary in the specialist's use of lithium as treatment in any suicidal youth (Tondo et al., 1997).

The psychiatrist should treat depressed children and adolescents who have suicidal behavior and a history of bipolar disorder with a mood stabilizer, such as valproate or carbamazepine, before an antidepressant. Doing so reduces the patient's likelihood of developing manic symptoms as a result of the effects of the antidepressant. Mood stabilizers have not been evaluated empirically for their efficacy in treating either bipolar conditions or suicidal behavior in children and adolescents.

▲ **Clinical Warning:** Primary care providers need to observe for possible induction of suicidal ideation or suicidal behavior as a result of activation or disinhibition resulting from medication. Clinical trials of selective serotonin reuptake inhibitors (SSRIs) suggest efficacy of such medications in reducing symptoms of major depressive disorder in children and adolescents (Emslie et al., 1997; Ryan & Varma, 1998). Such medications are more effective in treating depression in children and adolescents than are tricyclic medications. In fact, controlled clinical studies have not shown tricyclic medications to be effective in treating depression and suicidal behavior in children and adolescents in (Ryan & Varma, 1998). Furthermore, tricyclic antidepressants have a high lethal potential if taken in overdose and therefore are not considered usual medications for treatment of suicidal depressed children or adolescents. Because of the low lethal potential of SSRIs if taken in overdose and their efficacy in treating major depressive disorder, this class of medications is considered first-line medications to treat depressed suicidal children and adolescents. It is recommended that the clinician be particularly observant in the early stages of treatment with SSRIs, inquiring regularly about suicidal ideation before and after initiation of treatment with SSRIs. The provider needs to observe for possible suicidal ideation or acts that may be associated with akithesia resulting from medication treatment (Hamilton & Opler, 1992), discussing any signs and symptoms with the consulting psychiatrist when necessary.

Clinicians should be cautious when prescribing medications that may decrease self-control or increase impulsivity, such as benzodiazapines and phenobarbital. Some of these medications, such as phenobarbital, have high lethal potential if taken in overdose. Specifically, amphetamines should be used only when treating suicidal children or adolescents who also have attention deficit hyperactivity disorder. Clinicians must monitor their use closely, including medication amount and refills given. Tricyclics should not be prescribed for such suicidal children or adolescents unless no other intervention is indicated or effective.

Children and adolescents who are suicidal generally have a high likelihood for repeated suicidal behavior. Providers should institute a plan of follow-up as part of the intervention strategy. They may conduct such follow-up by means of completion of self-report questionnaires and subsequent interviews for patients who exhibit continued risk.

Children and adolescents who experienced the suicidal death of a friend or relative are at increased risk for major depressive, anxiety, and post-traumatic stress disorders and suicidal ideation (Brent et al., 1996a; Pfeffer et al., 1997b). In addition to acute intervention, long-term intervention is indicated for such children and adolescents because they may be likely to suffer from symptoms of depressive and anxiety disorders. Bereavement should be distinguished from depression and other psychiatric disorders. Intervention goals are to foster the bereavement processes by reducing sense of guilt, trauma, and social isolation and to decrease the likelihood of identifying with the suicidal behavior of the deceased when coping with stressful situations.

▲ **Clinical Warning:** Regardless of why they are being given, the provider needs to limit the dosage and number of pills for any potentially lethal medication prescribed for any suicidal patient.

Prevention

Providers can implement or assist with various approaches for preventing suicidal behavior among children and adolescents. Preventive measures include using crisis hotlines, controlling the availability and use of lethal methods, and counseling the media to minimize the possibility of imitation of suicidal behavior. Parents, teachers, peers, and others involved with children and adolescents should learn how to identify indicators of suicidal risk (Shaffer, Garland, Vieland, Underwood, & Busner, 1991). Practitioners can perform direct case finding among students by screening for risk fac-

tors of suicidal behavior while teaching other health professionals how to improve the recognition, intervention, and treatment of mood disorders and suicidal behavior.

Although these approaches are important in preventing suicidal behavior among children and adolescents, they have limitations. For example, crisis hotlines have not been demonstrated to reduce suicide, possibly because suicidal individuals most at risk do not use them. Restriction of firearms in the United States is limited. Thus, providers need to institute additional efforts, such as educating parents and peers about the dangers of having firearms in close proximity of those at risk for suicide and the safe use and storage of firearms. Although the Centers for Disease Control and Prevention (1994) have published guidelines for reporters and other media personnel, providing instruction about the risks of exaggerated coverage of youth suicide, use of such guidelines has not been demonstrated to reduce suicide rates in youth.

Direct case finding through screening techniques may be a valuable approach for suicide prevention because youth are willing to report suicidal states and suicidal risk factors. When followed up with more comprehensive evaluations and interventions, such screening may be useful in preventing suicide. These techniques, however, have not been subject to comprehensive empirical study. In conjunction with direct case finding, it is important to educate clinicians and other professionals in the recognition, treatment, and referral of youth who demonstrate suicidal risk. Such efforts should be subject to systematic study of their efficacy.

What to Tell Parents

One of the most important issues for parents to realize is that if they have questions about the possibility that their child may be suicidal, they should seek consultation from clinicians trained in working with such problems. Nevertheless, parents should appreciate that speaking directly with their child may clarify their concerns. A parent may want to introduce a discussion with the child by commenting as follows: "You seem to be upset about something. Can we talk about it?" "I'm here to listen to whatever you want to say." "You seem to be sad and not behaving as usual. How can I help you?" Often children and adolescents will respond to these types of questions.

Once the parent and child are conversing, the parent can ask questions about suicidal behavior, such as, "Do you feel so upset that you think you may want to die? Do you have thoughts about hurting yourself or killing yourself?" If parents elicit responses indicative of suicidal behavior, they should seek consultation from a professional to evaluate how to help the child or adolescent. Providers should make parents feel comfortable and not guilty about seeking advice. Parents must realize that consultation may be valuable in enhancing communication that may enable better resolution of a child's or adolescent's perceived problems. They must recognize that they have an important role in the treatment of their child and that family problems may require identification and resolution.

What to Tell the School

Similar issues apply to school professionals, who may be in the best position to identify suicidal children and adolescents. These professionals spend a great deal of time with youngsters, often watching them handle stressful situations, such as academic issues, peer pressures, and interpersonal relationships. These and other situations may precipitate suicidal states. Direct discussion with a child or adolescent they suspect to be at risk for suicidal behavior is the initial intervention. Referral to mental health professionals often is indicated, especially if the youngster's predictability is uncertain.

● **Clinical Pearl:** Frequently, adolescents will try to arrange for school professionals not to tell parents about suicidal tendencies. Such secrecy is not recommended. School professionals must tell a child or adolescent that it is impossible to maintain a secret if the child is in danger of self-harm. School professionals must maintain consistent involvement during the process of referral to a mental health professional.

Children and adolescents who attempt suicide and are absent from school to receive treatment require assistance to be reintegrated into school once the suicidal crisis has abated. Providers should encourage school professionals to work with the child or adolescent, parents, and the treating professional to assist with a smooth transition back to school. Often children and adolescents need help explaining their absence to peers. Providers should explore what the child or adolescent wants to tell others before he or she re-enters school. Keeping the nature of the problem private is acceptable if the child or adolescent wishes. For those whose peers know about the suicidal crisis, school professionals should assist the child or adolescent in answering questions that others may have about the current situation regarding potential for repeated suicidal behavior and minimization of possible stigma about a suicidal act. School professionals are important members of the management team who, together with the patient, parents, provider, and mental health professional, can assist the healing process.

COMMUNITY RESOURCES

Providers need to develop and maintain an up-to-date resource list for mental health and teen services in the region of practice. The following national resource may prove beneficial:

- The National Institute of Mental Health
  (800) 647-2642
  http://www.nimh.gov
  Provider, patient, and parent educational materials are available. Patient resources are also available in Spanish.

The following web-based resources can assist practitioners in obtaining continuing education programming in mental health issues, serve as a consultant finder, and provide patient educational materials:

- Mental Health Source
  http://www.mhsource.com
- The American Psychiatric Association
  http://www.psych.org

The following is a resource for patients:

- The National Adolescent Suicide Hotline
  (800) 621-4000
  This resource affords the caller in crisis with peer support.

REFERENCES

Arango, V., Underwood, M. D., & Mann, J. J. (1997). Biologic alterations in the brainstem of suicides. *Psychiatric Clinics of North America, 20,* 581–593.

Beck, A. T., Kovacs, M., & Weissman, A. (1979a). Assessment of suicide intention: The scale for suicide ideation. *Journal of Consulting and Clinical Psychology, 47,* 343–352.

Beck, A. T., Rush, A. J., Shaw, B. F., & Emery, G. (1979b). *Cognitive therapy of depression.* New York: Guilford Press.

Beck, A. T., Schuyler, D., & Herman, I. (1974). Development of suicidal intent scales. In A. T. Beck, H. L. P. Resnik, D. J. Lettieri, & M. D. Bowie (Eds.), *The prediction of suicide.* New York: Charles Press.

Brent, D. A. (1987). Correlates of the medical lethality of suicide attempts in children and adolescents. *Journal of the American Academy of Child and Adolescent Psychiatry, 26,* 87–91.

Brent, D. A., Bridge, J., Johnson, B. A., & Connolly, J. (1996). Suicidal behavior runs in families: A controlled family study of adolescent suicide victims. *Archives of General Psychiatry, 53,* 1145-1152.

Brent, D. A., Holder, D., Kolko, D., Birmaher, B., Baugher, M., Roth, C., Lyengar, S., & Johnson, B. A. (1997). A clinical psychotherapy trial for adolescent depression comparing cognitive, family, and supportive therapy. *Archives of General Psychiatry, 54,* 877–885.

Brent, D. A., Johnson, B., Bartle, S., Rather, C., Matta, J., Connolly, J., & Constantine, D. (1993a). Personality disorder, tendency to impulsive violence, and suicidal behavior in adolescents. *Journal of the American Academy of Child and Adolescent Psychiatry, 32,* 69–75.

Brent, D. A., Moritz, G., Bridge, J., Perper, J., & Canobbio, R. (1996). Long-term impact of exposure to suicide: A three-year controlled follow-up. *Journal of the American Academy of Child and Adolescent Psychiatry, 35,* 646-653.

Brent, D. A., Perper, J. A., Allman, C. J., Moritz, G. M., Wartella, M. E., & Zelenak, J. P. (1991). The presence and accessibility of firearms in the homes of adolescent suicides: A case-control study. *Journal of the American Medical Association, 266,* 2989–2995.

Brent, D. A., Perper, J. A., Goldstein, C. E., Kolko, D. J., Allan, M., Allman, C., & Zelenak, J. (1988). Risk factors for adolescent suicide: A comparison of adolescent suicide victims with suicidal inpatients. *Archives of General Psychiatry, 45,* 581–588.

Brent, D. A., Perper, J. A., Moritz, G., Baugher, M., Schweers, J., & Roth, C. (1993b). Firearms and adolescent suicide: A community case-control study. *American Journal of Diseased Children, 147,* 1066–1071.

Brent, D. A., Perper, J. A., Moritz, G., Liotus, L., Schweers, J., Balach, L., & Roth, C. (1994). Family risk factors for adolescent suicide: A case-control study. *Acta Psychiatrica Scandinavica, 89,* 52–58.

Brooksbank, D. J. (1985). Suicide and parasuicide in childhood and early adolescence. *British Journal of Psychiatry, 146,* 459–463.

Centers for Disease Control and Prevention. (1994). Prevention Guidelines Database (1994): Suicide contagion and the reporting of suicide: Recommendations from a national workshop. *Morbidity and Mortality Weekly Report, 43*(RR-6), 9–18.

de Wilde, E. J., Kienhorst, I. C., Diekstra, R. F., & Wolters, W. H. (1992). The relationship between adolescent suicidal behavior and life events in childhood and adolescence. *American Journal of Psychiatry, 149,* 45–51.

Elkin, I., She, M. T., Watkins, J. T., Imber, S. D., Sotsky, S. M., Collins, J. F., Glass, D. R., Pilkonis, P. A., Leber, W. R., Docherty, J. P., Leber, R., Fiester, S., & Parloff, M. (1989). National Institute of Mental Health Treatment of Depression Collaborative Research Program. General effectiveness of treatments. *Archives of General Psychiatry, 46,* 971–982.

Emslie, G., Rush, A., Weinberg, W., Kowatch, R., Hughes, C., Carmody, T., & Rintelmann, J. (1997). A double-blind, randomized placebo-controlled trial of fluoxetine in children and adolescents with depression. *Archives of General Psychiatry, 54,* 1031–1037.

Goldston, D. B., Reboussin, D. M., Kelly, A., Ivers, C., & Brunstetter, R. (1996). First-time suicide attempters, repeat attempters, and previous attempters on an adolescent inpatient psychiatry unit. *Journal of the American Academy of Child and Adolescent Psychiatry, 35,* 631–639.

Gould, M. S., Fisher, P., Parides, M., Flory, M., & Shaffer, D. (1996). Psychosocial risk factors of child and adolescent completed suicide. *Archives of General Psychiatry, 53,* 1155–1162.

Greenhill, L., Waslick, B., Parides, M., Fan, B., Shaffer, D., & Mann, J. (1995). Biological studies in suicidal adolescent inpatients. *Scientific Proceedings of the Annual Meeting of the American Academy of Child and Adolescent Psychiatry, 11,* 124.

Hamilton, M. S., & Opler, L. A. (1992). Akathisia, suicidality, and fluoxetine. *Journal of Clinical Psychiatry, 53,* 401–406.

Harrington, R., Bredenkamp, D., Goothues, C., Rutter, M., Fudge, H., & Pickles, A. (1994). Adult outcomes of childhood and adolescent depression, III: Links with suicidal behaviours. *Journal of Child Psychology and Psychiatry and Allied Disciplines, 35,* 1309–1319.

Jacobsen, L. K., Rabinowitz, I., Popper, M. S., Solomon, R. J., Sokol, M. S., & Pfeffer, C. R. (1994). Interviewing prepubertal children about suicidal ideation and behavior. *Journal of American Academy of Child and Adolescent Psychiatry, 33,* 439–452.

Johnson, B. A., Brent, D. A., Connolly, J., Bridge, J., Matta, J., Constantine, D., Rather C., & White, T. (1995). Familial aggregation of adolescent personality disorders. *Journal of the American Academy of Child and Adolescent Psychiatry, 34,* 798–804.

Johnstone, J., & Huws, R. (1997). Autoerotic asphyxia: A case report. *Journal of Sex Marital Therapy, 23,* 326–332.

Kazdin, A. E., Rogers, A., & Golbus, D. (1986). The Hopelessness Scale for children: Psychometric characteristics and concurrent validity. *Journal of Consulting and Clinical Psychology, 54,* 241–245.

Klerman, G. L., Weissman, M. M., Rounsaville, B. J., & Chevron, E. S. (1984). *Interpersonal psychotherapy of depression.* New York: Basic Books.

Kovacs, M., Goldston, D., & Gatsonis, C. (1993). Suicidal behaviors and childhood-onset depressive disorders: A longitudinal investigation. *Journal of the American Academy of Child and Adolescent Psychiatry, 32,* 8–20.

Kruesi, M. J., Grossman, J., Penningron, J. M., Woodward, P. J., Duda, D., & Hirsh, J. G. (1999). Suicide and violence prevention: Parent education in the emergency department. *Journal of the American Academy of Child and Adolescent Psychiatry, 38,* 250–255.

Kruesi, M. J. P., Hibbs, E. D., Zahn, T. P., Keysor, C. S., Hamburger, S. D., Bartko, J. J., & Rapoport, J. L. (1992). A two-year prospective follow-up study of children and adolescents with disruptive behavior disorders: Prediction by cerebrospinal l fluid 5-hydroxyindoleacetic acid, homovanillic acid, and autonomic measures. *Archives of General Psychiatry, 49,* 429–435.

Linehan, M. M. (1993). *Cognitive behavior therapy of borderline personality disorder.* New York: Guilford Press.

Mann, J. J. (1998). The neurobiology of suicide. *Annals of the New York Academy of Science, 4,* 25–30.

Mann, J. J., & Stoff, D. M. (1997). A synthesis of current findings regarding neurobiological correlates and treatment of suicidal behavior. *Annals of the New York Academy of Science, 836,* 352–363.

Marttunen, M. J., Hillevi, M. A., Henriksson, M. M., & Lonnqvist, J. K. (1991). Mental disorders in adolescent suicide: DSM-III-R axes I and II diagnoses in suicides among 13 to 9-year-olds in Finland. *Archives of General Psychiatry,* 834–839.

Mueher, P. (1995). Suicide and sexual orientation: A critical summary of recent research and directions for future research. *Suicide and Life Threatening Behavior, 25,* 72–81.

Mufson, L., & Moreau, D. (1998). Interpersonal psychotherapy for adolescent depression. In J. Markowitz (Ed.), *Interpersonal psychotherapy* (pp. 35–66). Washington, DC: American Psychiatric Press.

National Institute of Mental Health. (1999). *Epidemiology of suicide, 1997.* Washington, DC: Author.

Peters, K. D., Kochanek, K. D., & Murphy, S. L. (1998). *Deaths final data for 1996. National vital statistics reports, 47(9).* Hyattsville, MD: National Center for Health Statistics.

Pfeffer, C. R. (1986). *The suicidal child.* New York: Guilford Press.

Pfeffer, C. R. (1997). Childhood suicidal behavior: A developmental perspective. *The Psychiatric Clinics of North America, 20,* 551–562.

Pfeffer, C. R., Jiang, N. H., Kakuma, T. (2000). Child-adolescent suicide potential index (CASPI): A screen for risk of early onset suicidal behavior. *Psychological Assessment* (in press).

Pfeffer, C. R., Klerman, G. K., Hurt, S. W., Kakuma, T., Peskin, J. R., & Siefker, C. A. (1993). Suicidal children grow up: Rates and psychosocial risk factors for suicide attempts during follow-up. *Journal of the American Academy of Child and Adolescent Psychiatry, 32,* 106–113.

Pfeffer, C. R., Martins, P., Mann, J., Sunkenberg, M., Ice, A., Damore, J. P., Gallo, C., Karpenos I., & Jiang H. (1997). Child survivors of suicide: Psychosocial characteristics. *Journal of the American Academy of Child and Adolescent Psychiatry, 36,* 65–74.

Pfeffer, C. R., McBride, P. A., Anderson, G. M., Kakuma, T., Fensterheim, L., & Khait, V. (1998). Peripheral serotonin measures in prepubertal psychiatric inpatients and normal children: Associations with suicidal behavior and its risk factors. *Biological Psychiatry, 44,* 568–577.

Pfeffer, C. R., Normandin, L., & Kakuma, T. (1994). Suicidal children grow up: Suicidal behavior and psychiatric disorders among relatives. *Journal of the American Academy of Child and Adolescent Psychiatry, 33,* 1087–1097.

Pine, D. S., Trautman, P. D., Shaffer, D., Cohen, L., Davies, M., Stanley, M., Parsons, B., et al. (1995). Seasonal rhythm of platelet [3 H] imipramine binding in adolescents who attempted suicide. *American Journal of Psychiatry, 152,* 923–925.

Rao, U., Weissman, M. M., Martin, J. A., & Hammond, R. W. (1993). Childhood depression and risk of suicide: A preliminary report of a longitudinal study. *Journal of the American Academy of Child and Adolescent Psychiatry, 32,* 21–27.

Remafedi, G., French, S., Story, M., Resnick, M. D., & Blum, R. (1998). The relationship between suicide risk and sexual orientation: Results of a population-based study. *American Journal of Public Health, 88,* 57–60.

Reynolds, W. M. (1987). *Suicidal Ideation Questionnaire (SIQ).* Odessa, FL: Psychological Assessment Resources, Inc.

Rotheram-Borus, M. J., Walker, J. U., & Ferns, W. (1996). Suicidal behavior among middle-class adolescents who seek crisis services. *Journal of Clinical Psychiatry, 52,* 491–493.

Ryan, N. D., & Varma, D. (1998). Child and adolescent mood disorders: Experience with serotonin-based therapies. *Biological Psychiatry, 44,* 336–340.

Shaffer, D. (1988). The epidemiology of teen suicide: An examination of risk factors. *Journal of Clinical Psychiatry, 49,* 36–41.

Shaffer, D., Fisher, P., Hicks, R. H., Parides, M., & Gould, M. (1995). Sexual orientation in adolescents who commit suicide. *Suicide and Life-Threatening Behavior, 25,* 64–71.

Shaffer, D., Garland, A., Vieland, V., Underwood, M., & Busner, C. (1991). The impact of curriculum-based suicide prevention programs for teenagers. *Journal of the American Academy of Child and Adolescent Psychiatry, 30,* 588–596.

Shaffer, D., Gould, M., Fisher, P., Trautman, P., Moreau, D., Kleinamn, M., & Flory, M. (1996). Psychiatric diagnosis in child and adolescent suicide. *Archives of General Psychiatry, 53,* 339–348.

Spirito, A., Overholser, J., Ashworth, S., Morgan, J., & Benedict-Drew, C. (1988). Evaluation of a suicide awareness curriculum for high-school students. *Journal of the American Academy of Child and Adolescent Psychiatry, 27,* 705–711.

Tatum, S., Greene, A. L., & Karr, L. C. (1993). Use of the Suicide Probability Scale (SPS) with adolescents. *Suicide and Life-Threatening Behavior, 23,* 188–203.

Thiele, E. A., Gonzales-Heydrich, J., & Riviello, J. J. (1999). Epilepsy in children and adolescents. In C. R. Pfeffer, G. E. Solomon, & D. M. Kauffman (Eds.), *Neurologic disorders: Developmental and behavioral sequelae.* Philadelphia: W.B. Saunders.

Tondo, L., Jamison, K. R., & Baldessarini, R. J. (1997): Effect of lithium maintenance on suicidal behavior in major mood disorders. *Annals of the New York Academy of Science, 836,* 339–351.

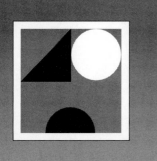

PRIMARY CARE
OF EPISODIC ILLNESS

CHAPTER 30

Viral Infections

• ELEANOR M. KEHOE, RN, MS, PNP, and THOMAS J. POWERS, MD

INTRODUCTION

Viral etiologies account for the vast majority of pediatric illnesses and are responsible for most pediatric office visits each year. Therefore, all primary care providers must learn to recognize the presenting symptoms and signs of various viral illnesses to diagnose and manage effectively these common infectious diseases. This chapter focuses on problems with classic symptomatologies: the common cold, measles, mumps, rubella, varicella, fifth disease, roseola, enteroviral illnesses, herpes simplex virus (HSV), and infectious mononucleosis.

THE COMMON COLD

Acute nasopharyngitis, also known as the common cold and upper respiratory infection (URI), is a self-limited disease of viral origin. It is the most common infectious condition of children (Behrman, Kliegman, & Arvin, 1996). Its high incidence and prevalence have long caused health care professionals and parents to seek a quick and effective treatment. The result has been the use of countless home remedies and what most experts consider the overuse of over-the-counter (OTC) and prescribed medications, both of which are addressed later in this section.

Anatomy, Physiology, and Pathology

The common cold often involves the paranasal sinuses, middle ear, and nasopharynx. Direct contact with infectious secretions by the hands, fomites, or droplets leads to viral proliferation in the mucosa and a subsequent inflammatory response. Inflammatory cytokines are thought to be of central importance in the pathogenesis of this inflammation in the respiratory tract as regulators of proliferation, chemotaxis, and activation of inflammatory cells (Nicod, 1993). Mucosal swelling and increased production of phlegm result. The swelling may then obstruct normal sinus drainage and interfere with normal aeration and drainage of the middle ear cavity.

Epidemiology

More than 200 million cases of URI occur each year in the United States, and primary care practitioners treat more than 75 million of these cases. These infections account for 26 million missed school days annually. After otitis media, URI is the most common diagnosis made by office-based clinicians.

The number of colds varies considerably among children (Katcher, 1996). Preschoolers generally have three to nine colds annually, or approximately one every 6 weeks, with increased frequency during winter months. Colds are more common among infants and young children who are enrolled in child care programs than among children who are cared for at home (Bauchner, Pellon, & Klein, 1999). Viruses that account for the vast majority of URIs in infants and children include influenza viruses, parainfluenza viruses, adenoviruses, coronaviruses, rhinovirus, and respiratory syncytial virus (Meissner, 1994). Human rhinovirus is the most common cause of cold (American Academy of Pediatrics [AAP], 1997).

History and Physical Examination

Symptoms consist primarily of rhinorrhea, nasal congestion, cough, and low-grade fever (usually less than 102.2°F [39°C]). If fever occurs, it usually is present at the onset of the illness and is associated with other constitutional symptoms, such as myalgias and headache. Fever often subsides when respiratory symptoms become prominent (Wald, 1995). In addition, occasional sneezing, chills, and scratchy throat may occur.

On physical examination, the provider observes inflammation and redness of the nasal mucosa. A clear mucous or mucopurulent discharge is present. During the course of an uncomplicated viral URI, the quality of nasal discharge changes (Gohd, 1954). It begins as a watery discharge and becomes thicker, colored, and opaque after a few days. Most often the discharge remains purulent for several days and then clears to a mucoid or watery consistency before resolving (Wald, 1995).

● **Clinical Pearl:** During the course of the common cold, the color of a child's nasal discharge has no relationship whatsoever with the presence or absence of a bacterial infection and the need for antibiotics.

Often, pharyngeal irritation and inflammation are noted as part of the clinical spectrum of the primary disease or secondary to postnasal drip. The duration of illness is usually about 1 week, but nasal discharge and cough may persist to the end of the second week.

Diagnostic Criteria

Diagnosis may be based on the following:

- Rhinorrhea
- Nasal congestion
- Cough
- Sneeze
- Low-grade fever
- Mild aches and chills

If the illness lasts beyond 10 to 14 days and shows no signs of resolving, the clinician should consider sinusitis, especially if daytime cough, fever, facial tenderness, or swelling is present. Some differential diagnoses are allergic rhinitis, sinusitis, the beginning manifestations of measles or pertussis, and less frequently poliomyelitis, hepatitis, and mumps.

Providers also should consider the possibility of drug abuse, especially inhaled solvents, cocaine, and marijuana, in older children and adolescents (Behrman et al., 1996). They also should consider rhinitis medicamentosa from the overuse of certain nasal sprays and decongestants when nasal discharge persists.

Diagnostic Studies

There are no definitive diagnostic studies for the common cold. Diagnosis is based on clinical findings.

Management

Home treatment involving OTC medications is an important part of the U.S. health care industry (Kogen, Pappas, Yu, & Kotelchuck, 1994). More than 800 OTC medications are available for treating the common cold (Lowenstein & Parrino, 1987). Consumers in the United States spend almost $2 billion per year on cough and cold remedies alone (Rosendahl, 1988). The OTC availability of numerous cold preparations promotes the perception that such medications are safe and efficacious (AAP, 1997).

● **Clinical Pearl:** Contrary to popular belief, cold preparations may not be totally benign, especially for infants younger than 6 to 9 months (Katcher, 1996).

Demonstration of the efficacy of antitussive preparations in children is lacking, and these medications may be potentially harmful (Godomski & Horton, 1992). Decongestant components of these mixtures administered to children have been associated with irritability, restlessness, lethargy, hallucination, hypertension, and dystonic reactions (Godomski & Horton, 1992). The clearance and metabolism of the components of cough mixtures may vary with age (Kearns & Reed, 1989) and disease state (Spielberg & Schulman, 1977; Larrey et al., 1989). The relative immaturity in young children of hepatic enzyme systems that metabolize drugs may enhance the risk of adverse effects of such medications, especially in those younger than 6 months (Kearns & Reed, 1989). Concurrent use of medications, such as acetaminophen, also may alter metabolism or toxicity (American Medical Association, 1995).

● **Clinical Pearl:** Most respiratory viral infections are self-limited, and infants and children require no pharmacologic treatment for URIs. Although study results are mixed, many show that young children derive no benefit from these medications; in fact, case reports show that they may harm some infants.

Perhaps even more dangerous than the indiscriminate use of OTC cold and cough preparations is the misuse of antimicrobials for URI management. From 1980 to 1996, antibiotic prescriptions by primary care practitioners increased by almost 50% from 86 to 128 million (Nyquist, 1999). The common cold or URI is the second leading condition associated with the prescription of antibiotics (McCaig & Hughes, 1995). Overuse of antibiotics has led to new patterns of resistance in virtually all the common pediatric respiratory pathogens but especially in pneumococci. Refer to Chapter 33 for a complete description of emerging drug resistance.

● **Clinical Pearl:** Millions of courses of unnecessary antibiotics are prescribed annually, which not only changes the community's bacterial ecology, but also increases an individual patient's risk of being infected with drug-resistant organisms.

According to Nyquist, Gonzalez, Steiner, and Sande (1998), who reviewed the 1992 National Ambulatory Medical Care Survey, antibiotics were prescribed unnecessarily to 44% of patients with colds and to 75% of patients with bronchitis. The reasons ranged from practitioners' desire to shorten the natural course of the illness, to prevent possible superinfection, to ease diagnostic uncertainty, and, most commonly, to deal with parents' unrealistic expectations. Parental pressure may account for more than half of the inappropriate prescriptions of antibiotics (Bauchner et al., 1999). Educational pamphlets available from the AAP attempt to fill this parental educational gap.

▲ **Clinical Warning:** In today's time-constricted environment, clinicians may find it easier to give the patient a prescription rather than taking time to explain the difference between viral and bacterial illnesses and the dangers of antibiotic overuse. Primary care practitioners must educate their patients and resist the temptation of inappropriate antibiotic treatment for the common cold ur URI.

Effective treatment modalities for infants include using a cool mist vaporizer, sleeping with the head elevated, and administering saline drops. Clinicians should encourage fluid intake and can recommend throat lozenges for older children. The common cold rarely develops into a more serious illness. The usual duration of illness is approximately 7 to 10 days, with complete or near complete resolution of all symptomatology.

Completely preventing the spread of this illness is nearly impossible, especially with present economics dictating two-income families and group day care for many children. Families should make attempts to limit unnecessary contacts for their sick children. Frequent hand washing, teaching children to cover their noses and mouths with a tissue when coughing or sneezing, and appropriately disposing contaminated materials are all measures for preventing spread of this illness.

What to Tell Parents

Most common colds resolve without any specific treatment in approximately 1 week. Although no specific restrictions from day care or school are necessary, clinicians should encourage parents to use a common sense approach about whether to send the affected child to day care or school. If the child is only mildly ill and without significant fever, parents and caregivers usually can send the child to school. If, however, the illness is more significant, keeping the child at home for a day or two may be beneficial.

Parents do not need to place any limitations on the activities of the child who has a common cold. Parents should attempt to avoid, as realistically as possible, spreading the sick child's illness to other children by limiting contacts. Parents should call the provider immediately if the child is getting sicker, any new symptoms appear, or significant fever develops. Under these circumstances, the provider should request that the child come to the office for examination. Additionally, if the sick child is not getting better within the expected time frame, the clinician should encourage a return visit.

Teaching and Self-Care

Because the common cold is so prevalent, the importance of personal hygiene cannot be overemphasized. Parents should teach their children the importance of good hand washing and the proper use and disposal of tissues at the earliest age possible. Doing so will help to instill good hygiene and to limit the spread of infection.

MEASLES

Measles is an acute, highly contagious infectious illness. Thanks to an effective vaccine, it is no longer common. Judging by the cyclical nature of measles outbreaks observed historically in the United States, however, the threat of acquiring this serious infectious disease remains very real.

Anatomy, Physiology, and Pathology

Humans are the only host to the virus, which is a *Paramyxovirus*. The organism enters the host through the respiratory tree. A susceptible person who comes into contact with infectious secretions and droplets is highly likely to contract the illness. After entering the respiratory mucosa, the organism immediately begins to replicate.

Three stages characterize the illness: an incubation period, a prodromal stage, and the rash itself. Mortality generally is low, except in the case of immunocompromised patients or patients who develop encephalitis. With measles encephalitis, mortality can be as high as 15%.

Epidemiology

More than 90% of susceptible household contacts of a patient with an acute case of measles will acquire the disease. The most infectious period is during the prodromal phase before the rash appears, although infectivity extends from 7 days after exposure to 5 days after the rash appears. The last major outbreak of measles in the United States was from 1989 to 1991. Most cases were in unvaccinated children; however, more cases were among vaccinated children than the predicted percentage of vaccine nonresponders. Such developments suggested that immunity waned and prompted the establishment of the present immunization requirement of two measles vaccines (Centers for Disease Control and Prevention [CDC], 1997a).

History and Physical Examination

The incubation period lasts for 10 to 12 days. The prodromal phase follows with the classic triad of symptoms: cough, coryza, and conjunctivitis. The cough may continue to worsen and could represent measles pneumonitis or bronchopneumonia from a bacterial superinfection. A low to moderate fever is present at this time. These symptoms last for 3 to 5 days and progressively worsen.

Children with classic measles appear ill. Koplik spots develop on the buccal mucosa at the end of the prodromal phase, lasting for 12 to 18 hours. These small, whitish-gray spots with surrounding redness most commonly are adjacent to the lower molars but may appear anywhere on the buccal mucosa. They are pathognomonic for measles. Immediately thereafter, high fevers of up to 104°F (40°C) appear along with the classic rash. At first macular then maculopapular, these red spots begin around the neck, cheeks, and face and rapidly spread to the trunk and extremities over the subsequent 3 days. In mild cases, they remain as individual spots, but in most cases, the individual lesions coalesce, covering most of the body, including the palms and soles. The rash fades thereafter in the order in which it appeared. Occasionally, petechiae or other evidence of hemorrhage are in the skin lesions. An urticarial rash sometimes occurs with measles. Splenomegaly can accompany the illness. Gastrointestinal symptoms, such as vomiting and diarrhea, are more common in infants and young children.

Diagnostic Criteria

Diagnosis rests on recognition of the classical symptoms. Clinicians often delay diagnosis until the rash appears. Prodrome includes cough, coryza, and conjunctivitis. Fever ranges between 101°F and 104°F. Diagnosis often is based on the ill appearance of the child, Koplik spots on buccal mucosa, and the erythematous macular then maculopapular rash that begins on the face and cheeks and extends downward and outward to trunk and extremities.

Diagnostic Studies

The white blood cell (WBC) count is lowered, with lymphocyte predominance. Acute and convalescent sera (immunoglobulin M [IgM] and IgG) will demonstrate a rise in antibody titers to measles. In encephalitis, cerebrospinal fluid (CSF) protein and presence of lymphocytes are increased (Behrman et al., 1996).

Management

The patient with clinically apparent measles infection should be isolated from contact with susceptible children and adults. Preventing the spread of this illness is extremely difficult due to its infectious nature. Maintaining a high level of protection through vaccination is the only way to control outbreaks. The currently licensed MMR vaccine is 90% to 95% protective. Refer to Chapter 13 for a complete discussion of measles vaccine, which normally is given at 1 year with a booster given before school entry.

In cases of endemic or epidemic outbreaks, local health departments may decide to vaccinate infants from ages 6 to 12 months, even though the efficacy of the vaccine in this age group is diminished because of the infant's competing maternal antibodies. Passive immunization using gamma globulin is effective in preventing the development of acute measles if used within 6 days of exposure. In fact, active immunization with MMR postexposure also may provide protection from development of disease if given within 72 hours of exposure (AAP, 1997).

Treatment consists of supportive therapy, including antipyretics, adequate oral fluid intake, humidified air, and prompt treatment of any complications (eg, antibiotics for bronchopneumonia). Vitamin A has been shown to ameliorate symptoms of acute infection in children in developing countries (Hussey & Klein, 1995). Most childhood cases of measles result in complete recovery.

Complication rates are highest in children younger than 1 year and in adults. Complications include pneumonia, which may be fatal in the setting of an immunocompromised patient; otitis media; and encephalitis. Encephalitis, the most feared complication, occurs at a rate of 1 to 2/1000 cases and may be demyelinating. Of those who develop encephalitis, two thirds may recover completely, one sixth may die, and one fourth may suffer permanent brain damage. Other neurologic sequelae also can occur. Disseminated intravascular coagulation may follow the acute illness but is uncommon. In adults, liver enzymes can be elevated, and jaundice may occur. Laryngitis, tracheitis, and bronchitis are frequent. Myocarditis is uncommon. Subacute sclerosing panencephalitis, a rare sequela, can appear years after the primary infection and is a devastating complication.

The differential diagnosis includes rubella, roseola, enterovirus, adenovirus, and coxsackievirus infections; infectious mononucleosis; meningococcemia; rickettsial illness; scarlet fever; Kawasaki syndrome; and drug rash. With an accompanying history of a recent infusion, serum sickness also is a consideration.

What to Tell Parents

The illness from the start of symptoms to complete resolution lasts approximately 10 to 14 days. Parents should keep the child out of day care or school until all symptoms have resolved. Rest, fever control, and hydration are important. Parents should contact the child's provider if they cannot control the fever, if a cough is getting significantly worse, or if they are unsure of how well their child is doing. Clinicians should instruct parents to return the child for an office visit at once if the child's breathing is labored or if the child seems confused or disoriented, complains of headache or neck stiffness, or is vomiting.

Teaching and Self-Care

Acetaminophen may be used to ameliorate high fever, with a dose of 10 to 15 mg/kg given every 4 hours. Additionally, ibuprofen can be used every 6 to 8 hours in a dose of 10 mg/kg. Parents should encourage oral fluid intake.

MUMPS

Mumps is a systemic disease characterized by swelling of the salivary glands. Mumps is caused by a *Paramyxovirus* and is endemic in most urban populations. It has worldwide distribution and affects both sexes equally. Clinically inapparent infection is common and has been reported to occur in more than half of infections (Falk et al., 1989). Not all cases of parotitis are due to infection with mumps virus. Other causes include parainfluenza types 1 and 3, influenza A, coxsackievirus A, echovirus, lymphocytic choriomeningitis virus, human immunodeficiency virus, and other noninfectious causes, such as drugs, tumors, immunologic diseases, and obstruction of the salivary duct. The number of reported mumps cases in the United States has decreased more than 99% since licensure of the mumps vaccine in 1967.

Anatomy, Physiology, and Pathology

The virus is spread through direct contact with airborne droplets, fomites contaminated by saliva, and possibly urine. Virus has been isolated from saliva as long as 6 days before and up to 9 days after appearance of salivary gland swelling. Transmission does not seem to occur more than 24 hours before the appearance of parotid swelling or later than 3 days after swelling has subsided. Virus has been isolated from urine from the first to 14th day after the onset of salivary gland swelling. Fever lasting for 3 or 4 days is accompanied by parotid gland swelling, which usually lasts for 7 to 10 days. Rare complications include acquired sensorineural hearing loss in children and mumps-associated encephalitis. Symptomatic meningoencephalitis may occur in 10% of cases and follows the course of benign aseptic meningitis without sequelae. According to Bang and Bang's classic study in 1944, up to 60% of cases are asymptomatic. In addition, orchitis develops in up to 38% of postpubertal male patients. Although it is often bilateral, orchitis rarely causes sterility. Rare complications include oophoritis, pancreatitis, and permanent sequelae, such as paralysis, seizures, cranial nerve palsies, aqueductal stenoses, and hydrocephalus. Deaths from mumps are rare. Although mumps infection in the first trimester of pregnancy may result in fetal loss, no evidence shows that mumps during pregnancy causes congenital malformations.

Epidemiology

Eighty-five percent of mumps infections occur in children younger than 15 years. People with mumps are considered infectious from 2 days before until 9 days after onset of parotitis. Because mumps can be asymptomatic, clinicians can easily miss the diagnosis. Epidemics appear to be primarily related to lack of immunization rather than to waning immunity. Epidemics occur during all seasons but usually are more frequent in late winter and spring. Sources of infection may be difficult to trace because 30% to 40% of infections are subclinical. Lifelong immunity usually follows clinical or subclinical infection, although second infections have been documented (Behrman et al., 1996).

History and Physical Examination

The incubation period is from 14 to 24 days, peaking between 17 and 18 days. In children, prodromal manifestations are rare but may include low-grade fever, malaise, muscular pain, and headache. Although the parotid glands alone are affected in most patients, swelling of the submandibular glands occurs frequently, usually accompanying or closely following swelling of the parotids. In 10% to 15% of patients, only the submandibular glands are swollen. Little pain is associated with submandibular infection, but swelling subsides more slowly there than in the parotids. Redness and swelling at the orifice of the Wharton duct frequently accompany gland swelling. Least commonly, the sublingual glands are infected, usually bilaterally; the swelling is evident in the submental region and in the floor of the mouth. A maculopapular erythematous rash, most prominent on the trunk, occurs infrequently; rarely it is urticarial. Some differential diagnoses include infectious mononucleosis, chronic adenitis, cat-scratch fever, leukemia, thyroglossal duct cyst, and acute cervical adenitis (Feigin & Cherry, 1998).

Diagnostic Criteria and Studies

Diagnosis may be based on the acute onset of unilateral or bilateral tender, self-limited swelling of the parotid or other salivary gland, lasting more than 2 days, without other apparent cause. These tests should be considered for the diagnosis of complicated cases:

- Serum amylase (elevated in 70% of cases)
- Saliva, throat, urine, or CSF cultures
- Enzyme immunoassay, complement fixation, or hemagglutination inhibition
- Serologic test for mumps IgM antibody (CDC, 1997b)

Management

Treatment of acute mumps infection is entirely supportive. Complications are rare. The illness is self-limited. Primary prevention through vaccination is the most effective means of controlling outbreaks of disease in communities. Mumps vaccine should be given as MMR to children age 1 year and again at age 4 years.

What to Tell Parents

The child with mumps will be well again within 2 weeks after the start of the illness. Parents should keep the child with mumps out of school for at least 9 days after noting parotid swelling. The child should be well hydrated and rest during the illness. Parents should notify their provider if the child's fever is difficult to control, the child appears significantly more ill, or at any time the child seems disoriented, confused, or complains of a stiff neck.

Teaching and Self-Care

Fever control using acetaminophen in a dosage of 10 to 15 mg/kg/dose every 4 hours as needed is recommended. For pain related to parotid swelling, ibuprofen may be used in a dosage of 10 mg/kg/dose given every 6 to 8 hours as needed. Parents should make efforts to ensure adequate oral fluid intake during the course of the illness.

RUBELLA

The incidence of rubella has declined by more than 99% since the introduction of rubella vaccine. New acute cases essentially are confined to unvaccinated populations and to individuals whose immunity has waned and who have not obtained a booster MMR vaccine. Rubella generally is a mild and often asymptomatic disease. Congenital rubella, however, can be devastating to the developing fetus. It is therefore critical to screen adults and pubertal children for protective antibodies against the virus.

Anatomy, Physiology, and Pathology

The rubella virus is shed through respiratory secretions from an infected person and comes into contact with the epithelial surface of the nasopharynx of the susceptible person. The virus propagates in the epithelium and spreads through lymphatics and possibly by transient viremia to regional lymph nodes (Green et al., 1965).

Epidemiology

Rubella virus is a togavirus and is transmitted through direct droplet contact from infected nasopharyngeal secretions. Its peak incidence is in the late winter and early spring. The proportion of cases among adults has risen steadily from 28% in 1991 to 73% in 1996. In 1996, 68% of reported rubella cases of known ethnicity were among Hispanics (CDC, 1997c). Vaccine use has effectively controlled the incidence of disease in children, but rubella outbreaks continue among adults and religious groups who refuse vaccination (CDC, 1994).

History and Physical Examination

Once viral innoculation has occurred, rubella virus incubates for 14 to 21 days, after which symptoms begin. Adults with rubella usually experience prodromal symptoms; however, children with rubella typically do not. Eye pain, sore throat, headache, swollen glands, fever, aches, chills, anorexia, and nausea are frequent prodromal symptoms in adolescents and adults (Finklea, Sandifer, & Moore, 1968). Prodromal symptoms precede the rash by 1 to 5 days; lymph node enlargement may be present from 5 to 10 days before the rash appears. An erythematous maculopapular rash of small, fine lesions follows, which then fades and coalesces, lasting for 2 to 3 days. Lymphadenopathy, especially postauricular, suboccipital, and cervical, is present. Mild fever and transient polyarthralgia and polyarthritis, especially in adolescents and females, accompany the illness. Clinical diagnosis of rubella is difficult because of the overlap of symptoms with other viral illnesses. Encephalitis and thrombocytopenia are rare complications.

Rubella acquired by the fetus during the first trimester of gestation often results in fetal death by spontaneous abortion. Congenital rubella syndrome is a multiorgan system infection. The most common manifestations include intrauterine growth retardation, cataracts, microphthalmia, structural cardiac defects and myocarditis, sensorineural hearing loss, and mental retardation (Feigin & Cherry, 1998).

Diagnostic Criteria

The clinical symptomatology is suggestive but not diagnostic of rubella. Diagnosis is based on clinical findings *plus* diagnostic studies.

Diagnostic Studies

The laboratory criteria used for diagnosis generally are not clinically useful in individual cases. Providers should use them only to investigate outbreaks for public health reasons. The following are diagnostic tests:

* Isolation of rubella virus
* A significant rise between acute and convalescent-phase titers in serum rubella IgG antibody level by any standard serologic assay
* A positive serologic test for rubella IgM antibody (CDC, 1997c)

Management

In younger children, clinical illness with rubella is generally mild and self-limited, and complications are rare. Treatment therefore is nonspecific and aims at alleviating the common symptoms. As with other illnesses, general supportive care includes fever control, adequate hydration, and bed rest as needed. Active immunization using the currently available MMR vaccine accomplishes prevention of illness. The vaccine is recommended at age 12 to 15 months, with a booster given at school entry or during middle school. All adolescents and adults of childbearing age need to have serologically protective levels of rubella antibody confirmed as part of their routine health care. If found susceptible, they should receive an additional dose of MMR vaccine. The reader is referred to Chapter 13 for further information on rubella vaccine.

What to Tell Parents

The illness will last approximately 2 weeks. Parents should keep children home from school or day care during this period. They should restrict the child's in-house activities according to the individual child's needs. Parents should call their primary care provider if a high fever persists longer than expected.

Teaching and Self-Care

Fever can be controlled as needed using acetaminophen 10 to 15 mg/kg/dose every 4 hours for a temperature above

101°F. Pain can be controlled with ibuprofen, using 10 mg/kg/dose every 6 to 8 hours as needed. Calamine lotion is helpful for the older child if the rash is itchy.

VARICELLA

Varicella-zoster virus, a human herpesvirus, manifests as primary disease (chickenpox) and reactivation of latent disease (herpes zoster or "shingles"). Most people acquire primary varicella infection in childhood. Primary infection usually invokes immunity to subsequent infection. Because the virus establishes latent infection in the dorsal root ganglia, zoster can occur at any time but is unusual in children younger than age 10 years. While most children with varicella have an uncomplicated course, moderate to severe illness is more likely in older children, adolescents, and adults. Varicella can be fatal to newborns and patients with underlying immunocompromised states. Asymptomatic primary infection is unusual, but asymptomatic reinfection can occur (AAP, 1997).

Although more than 6 million doses of varicella vaccine have been administered since its licensure in the United States during 1995, the impact of vaccination on disease incidence has yet to be documented at the national or state level. Currently, millions of cases of varicella continue to occur each year. In addition, an estimated 4000 to 9000 hospitalizations for varicella and its complications are necessary each year, with 100 to 125 deaths annually (Wharton, 1996).

Anatomy, Physiology, and Pathology

After contact with infected respiratory secretions, the organism propagates in the respiratory mucosa before entering the bloodstream through regional lymphatics, causing viremia. Distribution of the virus to viscera and skin occurs thereafter.

Epidemiology

From 8% to 9% of U.S. children younger than 10 years contract chickenpox each year, for an annual incidence of 3.5 to 4 million cases (Krause & Klinman, 1995). Varicella is most common during the late winter and early spring. Varicella virus is highly contagious. Household transmission rates are from 85% to 90%. A patient is contagious from 2 days before the onset of the rash until all skin lesions are crusted, usually 7 to 10 days.

History and Physical Examination

After exposure, the virus incubates for 10 to 21 days, with an average incubation period of about 2 weeks. The prodrome lasts for 2 days, during which the patient experiences mild to moderate fever, malaise, headache, and sometimes abdominal pain. The patient then becomes viremic, during which time successive crops of vesicles appear in a widespread distribution.

● **Clinical Pearl:** The first skin lesions usually are noted on the face, scalp, or trunk. The distribution is primarily central. The initial lesions are pruritic macules that rapidly evolve into vesicles. The vesicles typically are described as dew-drop in appearance, first filled with clear fluid and then later opaque fluid. These vesicles then rupture and crust over. During this period, a continuous crop of lesions begins to evolve. Lesions are widely distributed and commonly are found in the mouth, conjunctiva, or other mucosal sites.

● **Clinical Pearl:** A characteristic feature of varicella infection is the appearance of multiple lesions in varying stages of development (macules, papules, vesicles, and crusts) all in one anatomic region.

Fever is usually moderate but may be quite high. Pruritus can be intense. The average number of skin lesions is around 300 per illness, but as few as 10 and as many as 1500 can appear. The child with varicella is capable of transmitting the infection from 2 days before the appearance of typical lesions until all lesions are crusted over, and no new lesions are appearing.

Neonatal Disease

Neonates born to mothers who develop active varicella lesions from 5 days before to 2 days after birth are at high risk of developing neonatal varicella. Fatality rates can be as high as 30% under these circumstances. Fetuses carry a small risk of congenital varicella if the pregnant woman is exposed to live virus and develops primary infection. This risk is highest during the first half of pregnancy. Congenital varicella is associated with limb atrophy, cutaneous defects, ocular defects, microcephaly, and autonomic or CNS dysfunction.

Herpes Zoster

Varicella virus persists in a latent form and can manifest later as shingles, which results from waning immunity. Shingles presents as groups of vesicular lesions clustered along dermatomes, which may be painful. The differential diagnosis of varicella includes vesicular rashes caused by enteroviruses and *S. aureus*, contact dermatitis, insect bites, and drug reactions.

Diagnostic Criteria and Studies

Diagnosis rests on recognition of the typical rash of chickenpox. Laboratory tests usually are not performed. If laboratory testing is needed to confirm the diagnosis, immunofluorescent staining of virus gathered from scraping of lesions, using commercially available monoclonal antibodies, can be accomplished. This is more accurate than the Tzank smear, which looks for multinucleated giant cells containing intranuclear inclusions from smears of scraped lesions. Obtaining acute and convalescent sera for varicella zoster virus antibody can confirm infection. Enzyme immunoassays, latex agglutination, and indirect fluorescent antibody and fluorescent antibody-to-membrane assays have been used successfully to verify immune status of an exposed at-risk patient but are less reliable in immunocompromised patients (CDC, 1997b).

Management
General Principles

Treatment is supportive and includes control of fever and pruritus. Calamine lotion can be applied to itchy skin lesions. Systemic antihistamines, such as hydroxizine, can be given orally to control itching. Tepid baths with colloidal oatmeal also may soothe pruritus. Oral hydration should be maintained. The most common complication is bacterial superinfection of skin lesions.

▲ **Clinical Warning:** Acetaminophen given every 4 hours should be used as the antipyretic of choice, not aspirin or ibuprofen. Case reports have been made of necrotizing skin infections caused by *Streptococcus pyogenes* in patients with varicella who were treated with nonsteroidal anti-inflammatory drugs (Choo, Donahue, & Platt, 1997). Diphenhydramine-containing lotions should be avoided, because the nonintact skin of the patient with chickenpox may absorb an uncontrolled amount.

Complication

▲ **Clinical Warning:** Signs of a secondary bacterial infection complicating varicella include a sudden spike of temperature above the usual baseline, areas of erythema larger than the size of a quarter around the lesions, and a diffuse scarlatiniform rash. *Staphylococcus aureus* or group A beta hemolytic streptococci most often cause the rash and in its most severe form can result in cellulitis, scalded skin or toxic shock syndrome, or necrotizing fasciitis.

Oral antibiotics, such as cephalexin, amoxicillin clavulanate, or clindamycin, can effectively treat secondary infections if caught early. Patients who develop significant cellulitis or necrotizing fasciitis, however, should be hospitalized at once for aggressive intravenous antibiotic therapy. In adults, viral pneumonia is a frequent complication but is rare in children unless immunocompromised. Thrombocytopenia, arthritis, encephalitis or meningitis, hepatitis, and glomerulonephritis also can complicate the illness. If central nervous system (CNS) involvement is limited to its most common form, acute cerebellar ataxia, the prognosis is uniformly excellent. In the past, Reye's syndrome was a frequent and potentially fatal complication, but has virtually disappeared since discovery of its link with salicylate (Pinsky et al., 1988). Some immunocompromised children develop chronic or recurrent varicella, with eruption of lesions for weeks to months.

Antiviral Therapy

Patients with underlying immunocompromised states are at risk for severe, progressive disease. Likewise, children with malignancies or other chronic illnesses or dependent on steroids are at risk of severe disease. These patients should receive early treatment with intravenous acyclovir. Oral acyclovir may be considered in patients at risk for severe disease, such as adolescents, secondary household contacts (usually more severe cases than primary contacts), children with chronic lung or skin conditions or those receiving chronic salicylate therapy, or those on chronic inhaled steroids. Oral acyclovir given to otherwise healthy children with varicella within 24 hours of the onset of rash results in a modest decrease in the duration and magnitude of fever and in the number and duration of skin lesions.

● **Clinical Pearl:** Therapy with oral acyclovir is not routinely recommended for treatment of uncomplicated varicella in the otherwise healthy child (AAP, 1997).

Active and Passive Immunization

Varicella vaccine is a live, attenuated vaccine that has been in use in Japan for over 20 years. In the United States, it has been recommended for use in children ages 1 year and older. The vaccine has demonstrated excellent clinical and serologic protective efficacy (95%). Its safety profile is also excellent, with a low incidence of side effects. Pain, fever, and a chickenpox-like rash at the site of injection are the most common side effects. Duration of immunity is a subject of ongo-

ing study, but it appears that immunity wanes slowly. Natural ongoing exposure to wild-type varicella in the population, however, boosts the immunity of those who received the vaccine so that good serologically protective levels of antibody remain over an extended period, with a low breakthrough rate of active infection. The reader is referred to Chapter 13 for further discussion of the varicella vaccine.

Passive immunity with varicella-zoster immune globulin (VZIG) is recommended for the following patients on exposure: immunocompromised patients; unvaccinated patients with no history of chickenpox; susceptible pregnant women; newborns whose mothers demonstrate onset of active disease in the perinatal period; and exposed, hospitalized premature infants. VZIG is given IM as a single dose and should be administered within 96 hours of exposure for maximal effectiveness.

The outcome of most patients with varicella is good; however, universal vaccination is recommended based on the frequency of severe complications and death, economic impact of the disease, and efficacy and safety of the vaccine. This is increasingly true in view of the increased incidence of severe skin infections resulting from more virulent strains of *Streptococcus*.

What to Tell Parents

The child is considered contagious from 2 days before lesions appear until all lesions are dry and crusted (usually 7–10 days after their appearance) and no new lesions appear. Parents should keep the child away from day care or school until all lesions are crusted. Strict isolation of the child is not effective because of the highly contagious nature of the virus; however, parents should encourage bed rest. Parents should contact the provider if fever is difficult to control or if skin lesions appear infected.

Teaching and Self-Care

Fever control with acetaminophen only given every 4 hours is recommended. Calamine lotion (not caladryl) should be applied liberally to skin lesions. Oral systemic antihistamines, such as diphenhydramine or hydroxyzine, may be given to the child for control of pruritus if topical treatment is inadequate. Tepid baths with colloidal oatmeal preparations are soothing. Oral fluid intake should be maintained. Primary prevention of infections in susceptible children is of utmost importance through use of the varicella vaccine.

PARVOVIRUS 19 (FIFTH DISEASE)

Human parvovirus B19, a small DNA virus, is the only parvovirus known to affect humans (Portmore, 1995). Parvovirus B19 was discovered accidentally while testing healthy blood donors who were undergoing screening for hepatitis B. During electrophoresis, an abnormal band was noted in the sera from specimen 19 in panel B, which was subsequently determined to be parvovirus (Cossart et al., 1975). The virus has no lipid envelope, allowing it to survive at higher temperatures and wider pH ranges than most other viruses (Anderson, Young, & Gary, 1992). This is of some concern because parvovirus B19 can withstand superheating treatments used in some blood product preparations designed to destroy most viruses (Morfini, Azzi, & Mannucci, 1996). The virus can only grow when cultured in human marrow, fetal liver, cord blood, or erythroleukemic cells (Torok, Remington, & Klein, 1995; Anderson et al., 1992). The limited availability of these cell types makes cell culture for identification of B19 impractical. Eventually B19 was determined to be the causative agent for the childhood exanthem erythema infectiosum (EI) (also known as fifth disease), aplastic crises in patients with sickle cell disease, an arthropathy usually in adults, and some cases of vasculitis resembling Henoch-Schönlein purpura.

Anatomy, Physiology, and Pathology

B19 arrests erythropoiesis and has a cytopathic effect on erythroid precursors (Young & Mortimer, 1984). B19 viral particles also have been identified in nonerythroid tissue, such as myocardial cells (Porter, Quantrill, & Fleming, 1988). Initially, the cause for cell death was assumed to be viral-mediated cell lysis (Caul, Usher, & Burton, 1988). Evidence suggests, however, that B19 stimulates a cellular process initiating programmed cellular death, potentially accounting for the minimal inflammatory response noted in tissues infected with B19 (Morey, Ferguson, & Fleming, 1993).

Epidemiology

Outbreaks of EI can last for 2 to 6 months, and epidemics typically occur every 5 to 7 years. Epidemics usually begin in middle to late winter and can continue until school breaks for the summer.

Transmission of the B19 virus occurs through respiratory droplets, contaminated blood products, or transplacental passage from mother to fetus. The most common transmission method is presumed to be person to person through direct contact with respiratory secretions (Torok et al., 1995). Transmission may occur horizontally from a direct hematogenous route through blood transfusion or vertically from transplacental fetal inoculation. The prevalence of B19 DNA in blood donors varies from approximately 1 per 3000 if no epidemic is in the area to as high as 1 per 167 during an epidemic (Cohen, 1995).

The risk of contracting EI depends on the environment in which the exposure occurs, such as a household contact, classroom setting, or health care facility. The risk of acquiring the disease if a household member is infected is approximately 50%, whereas a seronegative individual exposed in a classroom has a 20% to 30% risk of infection (Torok et al., 1995; Chorba et al., 1986). Because of the lack of a lipid envelope in this virus, routine blood product processing for viral inactivation may be inadequate, posing an additional concern regarding the use of blood products in pregnant women (Morfini et al., 1996). Lastly, the virus can cross the placenta during maternal viremia, as has been shown by demonstrating anti-B19 specific antibody and viral DNA in amniotic fluid and fetal blood in pregnancies (Torok et al., 1995). Vertical transmission rates to the fetus have been estimated to be approximately 33% (Public Health Laboratory Service Working Party on Fifth Disease, 1990).

History and Physical Examination

A common childhood illness, EI is best recognized by its characteristic progressive rash. The illness typically begins with a URI-like prodrome that may be so mild as to go unnoticed. The typical rash evolves into three distinct phases. A bright red "slapped cheek" facial rash is followed by an erythematous diffuse macular exanthem over the trunk and proximal limbs. Lastly, a finely reticulated lacelike rash evolves by central clearing of the macules. This rash may last for up to 3 weeks but may recur in response to a number of stimuli (eg, light, heat, friction). There can be wide variation in the appearance of the exanthem, such that it may be difficult to distinguish from other viral illnesses, especially if no outbreak is occurring at the time. Young children are relatively asymptomatic except for the rash. Older children and adolescents are more likely to have associated arthralgias and pruritus. Patients with chronic hemolytic disease (eg, sickle cell disease, thalassemia, spherocytosis, and G6PD deficiency) are at risk of sustaining an aplastic crisis secondary to the profound reticulocytopenia caused by human parvovirus B19 infection.

Diagnostic Criteria

Differential diagnosis can be confused with other viral exanthemas, such as measles, rubella, and enteroviruses, or with collagen vascular diseases, drug reactions, or other allergic responses. The characteristic rash of EI, however, is classic and should enable the practitioner to distinguish it from other viral illnesses.

Diagnostic Studies

Diagnostic studies are useful only when the clinical picture is unclear, and persistent symptoms, such as arthropathy, warrant clarification. Acute or recent EI infection is best determined by the demonstration of specific IgM antibody. Obtaining acute and convalescent sera for parvovirus B19 antibody can confirm infection. Enzyme immunoassays, hemadherance, radioimmunoassay, or immunofluorescence can all be used to verify immune status. DNA hybridization, polymerase chain reaction, or electron microscopy can detect antigen (Feigin & Cherry, 1998).

Management

Treatment is symptomatic and usually not needed. Prevention of spread of the disease is through education.

● **Clinical Pearl:** Note that EI is most contagious before the onset of the rash; once the rash appears, children are not contagious. Because the diagnosis cannot be made until the rash appears, for practical purposes, control of the spread of the virus is difficult.

If contracted during pregnancy in a nonimmune woman, EI can result in spontaneous abortion or an asymptomatic intrauterine infection. Thus, a pregnant woman exposed to parvovirus B19 should be tested for IgG specific to this virus. The provider should monitor this woman carefully through ultrasound, observing for evidence in the fetus of the development of aplastic crisis and hydrops fetalis. The risk of recurrent B19 is very low; therefore, if IgG is demonstrated, no further evaluation is indicated in the pregnant woman (Markenson & Yancey, 1998).

Children with this infection usually do not require significant supportive care. The outcome in virtually all cases of EI is excellent. Colloidal oatmeal or starch baths can aid itchiness associated with the reticular rash stage.

ROSEOLA (SIXTH DISEASE)

Human herpesvirus (HHV-6) is the agent responsible for this disease, also known as exanthum subitum. Roseola infantum is a common acute illness of young infants. The classic findings of 2 to 4 days of fever followed by an evanescent rash may only be seen in a relatively small percentage of cases (Feigin & Cherry, 1998).

Anatomy, Physiology, and Pathology

The incubation period averages 10 days (Boynton, Dunn, & Stephens, 1998). Viral transmission occurs through shedding of infected secretions from a family member, caregiver, or close contact. The pathophysiologic process is unknown. It has been suggested that the rash results from neutralization of virus in the skin at the end of the period of viremia (Feigin & Cherry, 1998).

Epidemiology

Almost all young adults have serum titers positive for HHV-6. Infants and preschoolers are most susceptible; 95% of cases occur in children ages 6 months to 3 years. Cases usually do not occur in younger children, presumably due to the presence of circulating maternal antibodies against HHV-6. Ninety percent of 2-year-old children have serologic evidence of having been exposed to this organism. Transmission of the virus is through secretions of an infected individual. The illness is most common in spring and fall, although it occurs throughout the year.

History and Physical Examination

While the differential diagnosis of fever and rash is extensive, roseola can be distinguished from other causes by the timing of the appearance of the rash. The illness begins after an incubation period of 5 to 10 days with high fever, with no other symptoms to suggest the nature of the illness. The fever may persist for 3 to 6 days. During this phase, physical examination fails to reveal a source; however, otitis media is frequently and perhaps erroneously diagnosed due to tympanic membrane (TM) erythema. A rash usually begins as the fever is dropping, although it may appear before defervescence or after an afebrile period of 1 day. This rose-colored macular or maculopapular exanthem starts on the trunk and spreads to the limbs and face. It may only last hours or persist for up to 3 days. Other viruses, such as enterovirus, can cause a similar picture. The most common complication is seizure associated with high fever; occasionally, encephalopathy is seen.

● **Clinical Pearl:** The lack of symptoms and signs associated with a high fever in a child ages 6 months to 2 years and the evolution of rash as the fever subsides suggest a diagnosis of roseola.

▲ **Clinical Warning:** Providers frequently and erroneously treat children with roseola with antibiotics because of reddened TMs. When the rash appears, clinicians often mislabel these children as allergic to the prescribed medication. Providers should not diagnose acute otitis media unless otalgia and evidence of decreased TM mobility accompany TM redness.

Diagnostic Criteria and Studies

Diagnosis is based mainly on clinical findings, particularly if other cases are present in the community. The initial WBC is low and drops further by day 3 or 4 of the illness. This finding is obviously nonspecific and seen with many viral illnesses. The most reliable source of HHV-6 virus appears to be saliva. Peripheral blood mononuclear cells can carry the virus but often in a latent state (Levy, 1997). Commercial assays for antibody and antigen detection so far do not reliably differentiate between primary infection and viral persistence or reactivation (AAP, 1997).

Management

Treatment is symptomatic and in most cases, the outlook is excellent. When encephalitis occurs, the prognosis is guarded (Feigin & Cherry, 1998). One attack usually confers permanent immunity; however, the virus can persist and reactivate. Illness associated with reactivation has been described primarily in immunosuppressed hosts.

Fever control is of utmost importance, due to the increased risk of sustaining a febrile seizure. Refer to Chapter 31 for specifics. The illness is self-limited. Parents should increase the child's oral fluid intake. If the child sustains a seizure or signs of increased irritability, the parents should bring him or her to the nearest emergency room at once. They should keep the child from day care or school until the fever has subsided and the child appears well.

ENTEROVIRUSES

Enteroviruses include polioviruses, coxsackieviruses, and echoviruses. They are picornaviruses and frequent causes of human illness with protean clinical manifestations. They are worldwide in distribution. In temperate climates, enteroviral infections occur primarily in the summer and fall, but in the tropics, they are prevalent throughout the year (Feigin & Cherry, 1998). Enteroviruses cause numerous common illnesses of childhood, including the common cold, nasopharyngitis, herpangina (coxsackievirus A, B, and echoviruses), pleurodynia, aseptic meningitis, and nonspecific vomiting and diarrhea. Coxsackieviruses B1 to B5 are etiologically important in pericarditis and myocarditis in infants, children, and adults (Feigin & Cherry, 1998).

Due to the wide spectrum of clinical illness that enteroviruses cause, a clinical description of each entity is excluded from this discussion except for a few of the most common and clinically recognizable illnesses. For the most part, these illnesses are self-limited and have no specific treatments. Aseptic meningitis and myopericarditis are the most severe of the clinical spectrum of diseases that these viruses cause, and treatment is again supportive. Most of the above-mentioned infections recover completely without major sequelae. Viral shedding may occur for weeks after apparent clinical illness has subsided (AAP, 1997).

Anatomy, Physiology, and Pathology

After innoculation, viral replication occurs in the respiratory or gut mucosa. The virus then spreads to the regional lymph nodes, and viremia follows, which results in secondary infection sites (Feigin & Cherry, 1998).

Epidemiology

Infection is spread by the fecal-oral and respiratory routes; peripartum transmission from mother to infant also can occur. Enteroviruses may survive on environmental surfaces for periods long enough to allow transmission from fomites. In general, the incubation period is short (3–6 days). Infections and clinical attack rates are highest in young children (AAP, 1997).

History and Physical Examination

Because most poliovirus illness is asymptomatic, it is thought that most enteroviral illnesses also are asymptomatic. Coxsackieviruses are nonpolio enteroviruses and frequent causes of febrile illnesses in children. There are 23 group A coxsackieviruses and six group B coxsackieviruses. Among these, there are specific associations between virus and disease.

Hand, Foot, and Mouth Disease

The most common cause of hand, foot, and mouth disease is coxsackievirus A16. Other causative agents for this common illness include coxsackieviruses A5, A9, A10, B1, and B3 and enterovirus 71. Vesicular lesions anywhere in the oropharynx and on the hands and feet in association with fever characterize hand, foot, and mouth disease. Affected children are usually not terribly symptomatic. Oral lesions may ulcerate, while skin lesions remain vesicular. These vesicles are small (3–7 mm) and may involve the dorsal, palmar, and plantar aspects of the hands and feet and the buttocks. Unlike other enteroviral illnesses, vomiting is not common. Symptoms resolve within 1 week.

Herpangina

Herpangina has been commonly seen with coxsackievirus A but also may be seen with B strains and echoviruses. Clinically, the illness is associated with high fever and severe sore throat, hence the term "herpes-like pain." Vesicles progressing to ulcers are seen in the posterior oropharynx. The illness may last 5 to 8 days. Associated vomiting, high fever, and severe dysphagia make prevention of dehydration a therapeutic imperative (Rotbart, 1998).

Acute Hemorrhagic Conjunctivitis

Acute hemorrhagic conjunctivitis (AHC) occurs in epidemics. A variant of coxsackievirus A24 was isolated in 1970 and continued to cause epidemic outbreaks of AHC. Tens of millions of cases occurred in 1971. This large pandemic yielded a new virus, enterovirus 70, which continues to be the agent most associated with AHC (Ishii et al., 1989). This disease, generally localized to the eye, is characterized by subconjunctival hemorrhage and is highly contagious.

Other Manifestations

Aseptic meningitis due to enteroviruses occurs both in epidemics and as isolated cases. Epidemic disease has been most common with coxsackievirus B5 and echoviruses 4, 6, 9, and 30. A common cause of febrile illness especially in the summer and autumn, these viruses are responsible for many sepsis workups. Clinically, these viruses manifest with fever, headache, malaise, nausea, and vomiting. Skin rash is common, usually presenting as an erythematous, maculopapular rash. Frequently, particularly with echovirus 9, rash is petechial, suggesting meningococcemia (Feigin & Cherry, 1998).

Diagnostic Criteria and Studies

Due to the wide spectrum of enteroviral illness presentation and the degree of overlap of symptoms with other etiologies, the diagnosis may only be inferred based on clinical symptomatology. In most cases, diagnostic studies are not clinically useful. Viral identification should be attempted in severe complicated cases, such as myopericarditis. Viral isolation from throat, stool, or rectal swab, as well as from blood during fever, may be attempted, but the sensitivity of viral isolation varies by serotype. Viral isolation from the stool alone may or may not indicate a causal relationship to the illness. Viral RNA identified through polymerase chain reaction techniques on CSF specimens may be available in some laboratories to aid in the diagnosis of CNS infections (AAP, 1997).

Management

No specific therapy currently exists for enteroviral illness; therefore, treatment is supportive. Except for the more severe clinical diseases caused by enteroviruses, wherein symptomatology can be significant and life threatening, the vast majority of enteroviral illnesses are well tolerated by patients and short lived, with full recovery.

The patient must remain well hydrated. Fever control is through use of acetaminophen, ibuprofen, or both. Parents should call the provider if the child has poor oral intake or any signs of dehydration appear; if fever does not respond to antipyretics; if the illness does not improve within 1 week; if febrile convulsions appear; or if headache or neck stiffness becomes significant.

HERPES SIMPLEX VIRUS

Herpes simplex virus is common among humans. The two strains, HSV-1 and HSV-2, are responsible primarily for infection of the skin and mucous membranes, although disseminated infection with viremia is seen in neonates and is part of the differential diagnosis of sepsis in early infancy. HSV can infect the oral, genital, ocular, CNS, and other areas. Primary and latent, reactivated infections occur. After primary infection, people carry the infection with them, even in the absence of active disease and in the presence of circulating antibodies. Primary herpes gingivostomatitis occurs in infants, toddlers, older children, and adults. HSV-1 is the most common cause of this illness. Ocular manifestations of HSV include conjunctivitis, dendritic corneal ulcers, and keratitis. Primary genital herpes infections can be either HSV-1 or HSV-2, but recurrent genital herpes is uniformly HSV-2. Herpetic whitlow and herpes gladiatorum are two other skin manifestations of HSV infection. The first involves the digits, while the second is seen in scrapes and cuts of wrestlers and other sports players with close skin-to-skin contact. Disseminated infection with herpes can be seen in patients with altered T-cell function or generalized immunodeficiency or with nonintact skin, such as is seen with eczema herpeticum.

Anatomy, Physiology, and Pathology

The HSV tends to infect cells of ectodermal origin; in most cases, initial viral replication occurs at the portal of entry, usually in the skin or mucous membranes. As the cells manifest, injury and local inflammation supervenes, intercellular edema develops, and vesicles form in the affected area.

Epidemiology

The epidemiology of HSV is dominated by symptomatic and asymptomatic infection with resultant transmission and maintenance of a huge pool of latently infected people. The virus remains latent in the sensory ganglia. A number of triggers can activate HSV, such as emotional stress, sun exposure, drugs, menses, trauma, febrile illness, and systemic infections (Boynton et al., 1998). Their symptomatic recurrences and asymptomatic shedding ensure continued spread of HSV because it relies on humanity's need for close contact of both a sexual and asexual nature. HSV infections are global in distribution. Seroepidemiologic studies have shown that HSV infections are found in all populations, even in the most remote and isolated communities. No definite seasonal pattern to HSV infections exists. Most neonatal HSV infections are acquired from maternal genitalia strains and thus usually are caused by HSV-2. After the neonatal period, HSV-1 infections predominate, and depending on social and economic factors, 40% to 60% of young children of lower socioeconomic status are seropositive by 5 years of age. Most primary infections are asymptomatic. Approximately 30% of adults have circulating antibodies to HSV-1 and HSV-2. HSV-2 antibodies are seen in higher percentages in people from lower socioeconomic backgrounds (Feigin & Cherry, 1998).

History and Physical Examination

Generally, the incubation period for herpes infections is between 2 and 12 days, with an average of 6 days. Most primary infections are subclinical. Acute herpes gingivostomatitis presents mostly in children ages 1 to 3 years and starts with fever. Eruption of very small vesicles on the oral mucosa and gingiva follows. These lesions are painful, surrounded by erythema, and rupture to form a membrane. After sloughing of this membrane, an ulcer remains. Usually, the illness lasts between 7 to 10 days and varies in severity. In more severe cases, decreased oral intake secondary to the pain, associated with drooling and high fever, may lead to dehydration. Recurrent stomatitis can and does occur, though usually not as diffusely as the initial infection. Herpes labialis manifests with lesions to the labial mucosa. Again, these lesions are characteristically painful. Some individuals are more susceptible to recurrences than are others. HSV-1 causes 5% to 15% of initial episodes of genital herpes (Boynton et al., 1998). The differential diagnosis includes impetigo and herpangina.

Thin-walled vesicular lesions to the glans, penile shaft, and occasionally the scrotum in males and to the cervix in females characterize genital herpes. Vaginal and vulvar lesions, common in recurrent infections, often are subclinical.

▲ **Clinical Warning:** Active lesions are extremely contagious; therefore, practitioners should avoid contact with them. Neonates are especially susceptible to systemic disease. Even contact with something as apparently benign as a "cold sore" may have devastating consequences to a newborn.

Diagnostic Criteria

Practitioners should be suspicious of a diagnosis of HSV infection when the characteristic vesicular lesions, regardless of site, are grouped together on an erythematous base accompanied by tenderness. Lesions are found on mucous membranes or at the skin/mucous membrane border. A past history of herpes lesions makes the possibility of recurrence likely in the presence of new vesicular lesions. A history of recent (within past 1–2 weeks) unprotected sexual intercourse accompanied by the appearance of clustered vesicles on examination of genitalia is highly suggestive of HSV.

Diagnostic Studies

For primary gingivostomatitis and secondary oral lesions, laboratory confirmation rarely is needed. HSV can be recovered relatively easily in cell cultures, and special transport media are available. Providers should obtain cultures from all appropriate sites, including lesions, blood, urine, and CSF, to diagnose neonatal herpes infection. Direct fluorescent antibody staining of vesicle scrapings or enzyme immunoassay detection of HSV antigens can offer rapid diagnosis. They are specific but less sensitive than cell cultures (AAP, 1997).

Management

Occasionally, patients require intravenous hydration for primary herpes gingivostomatitis. In most cases, topical or systemic analgesics can maintain oral fluid balance. For secondary oral lesions, patients should avoid known triggers that cause recurrences of lesions (eg, sunburn). Some pharmacists mix Maalox and Benadryl with or without 1% to 2% viscous lidocaine. For individuals with frequent recurrences of any of these herpetic infections, oral acyclovir shortens the clinical course and is the mainstay of therapy. Acyclovir generally is not used for simple, uncomplicated HSV-1 oral disease. For genital herpes, patients can use acyclovir ointment or oral capsules, depending on the frequency and severity of recurrences. Dosing is six times a day once lesions appear. Alternatively, patients can take them orally twice a day as prophylaxis if plagued by frequent, severe recurrences. They also can use topical anesthetics, such as benzocaine aerosol or lidocaine jelly 2%, for pain. Most infections are self-limited; recurrences are common (Boynton et al., 1998).

What to Tell Parents

For primary oral HSV, fluid intake, fever control, and pain relief are of utmost importance. Providers should teach parents about the common stressors that trigger recurrent herpes infections and how to prevent the stressors that are controllable (eg, sunburn). Parents should understand that HSV is ubiquitous and, as such, unavoidable. Recurrences are common and usually occur at the same site. Autoinnoculation may spread lesions. Lesions do not leave permanent scars, but the inflammation may result in temporary loss of pigment at the lesion site. For oral lesions, transmission is through saliva or through direct contact with the lesion. For genital herpes, individuals should avoid indiscriminate, unprotected sexual contacts. Partners or prospective partners can be completely asymptomatic and still shed the virus. No cure exists for any herpes infection. Prevention of sexually acquired HSV is only through avoiding sex or having protected intercourse with a latex condom at every sexual encounter.

Teaching and Self-Care

Patients may apply idoxuridine ointment (Herplex), bacitracin, or blistex very frequently to the lesion, which may help soothe discomfort and protect skin from cracking. Acyclovir ointment can shorten the duration of HSV lesions; patients can apply it every 4 hours during the duration of the eruption. They can use topical anesthetics as described previously. Parents should watch for complications, such as bacterial superinfection of the lesions or eczema herpeticum (eruptions of clusters of lesions at sites of eczematous lesions in the atopic child accompanied by high fever). If suspicious of these problems, parents should bring the child to their provider for evaluation at once. Providers should immediately see any young infant, patient with suspicious eye lesions, or immunocompromised patient (Boynton et al., 1998).

INFECTIOUS MONONUCLEOSIS

Epstein-Barr virus (EBV), a member of the Herpesviridae, is responsible for almost all cases of infectious mononucleosis. Cytomegalovirus and toxoplasmosis may be responsible for the remainder of the "mono-like" illnesses. EBV is acquired predominantly during childhood. Infection in early childhood is usually asymptomatic, whereas infection during later childhood and adulthood demonstrates the typical triad of symptoms: fatigue, pharyngitis, and generalized lymphadenopathy. This virus has been associated with several benign and malignant tumors, including benign hairy leukoplakia, nasopharyngeal carcinoma, Burkitt lymphoma, and Hodgkin's disease.

Anatomy, Physiology, and Pathology

The principal route of transmission is through saliva. The initial infection is likely to occur in the epithelial cells of the oral pharynx and adjacent structures (Sixbey et al., 1984). Virus is then transmitted to circulating B cells passing through these lymphoepithelial tissues and organs. The EBV virion preferentially infects B lymphocytes. The viral genome circulates and is maintained in the cell nucleus as a multicopy plasmid (Lindahl et al., 1976). In response, T cells and natural killer cells proliferate, and they, not the EBV-infected B cells, represent most of the atypical lymphocytes seen on the peripheral blood smear (Katz & Miller, 1998). Purtilo (1981) referred to these two populations of cells as "combatants in an immune struggle." In cases where natural killer or T cells fail to eliminate infected B cells, lymphoproliferative diseases may result. In cases in which T cell activity is excessive, agammaglobulinemia may develop secondary to B-cell depletion. In the "normal" immune host, the clinical symptoms of mononucleosis are caused by this clash of T and B cells, and the excessive lymphoproliferation gradually subsides (Katz & Miller, 1998).

Epidemiology

Humans are the only source of EBV. Epidemiologic studies indicate that widespread infections occur in the general population, particularly in lower socioeconomic settings (Feigin & Cherry, 1998). In settings characterized by poverty, overcrowding, and poor hygiene, 80% to 90% of children demonstrate antibodies to EBV, mostly acquired through asymptomatic infections. In more privileged settings, individuals usually acquire the virus in adolescence, where "teenage" behaviors facilitate salivary spread (Peter & Ray, 1998). Virtually all older adults in the United States have acquired the virus. Worldwide, 95% of the population has serologic evidence of having had the disease. EBV is similar to other herpesviruses in that it remains latent in the person's lymphocytes and oropharyngeal epithelial cells and is excreted for prolonged periods after acute infection. It is transmitted in oral secretions (Feigin & Cherry, 1998). The period of communicability is unknown, because 10% to 20% of healthy, seropositive persons shed the virus intermittently (Boynton et al., 1998).

History and Physical Examination

The incubation period is estimated to be 30 to 50 days. The classic presentation of infectious mononucleosis is fever, accompanied by an exudative pharyngitis, lymphadenopathy, hepatomegaly (30%–50%), splenomegaly (in 50%), fatigue, and malaise. A nonspecific exanthem occurs in 10% of cases; incidence of nonspecific exanthem increases to 90% in children who are treated with ampicillin or amoxicillin (Peter & Ray, 1998). Infection in young children often is unrecognized because of a paucity of symptoms or may present simply as fever of unknown etiology. Typically, symptoms develop over 1 to 2 weeks. Physical examination reveals lymphadenopathy, especially in the neck; exudative pharyngitis resembling that of streptococcal pharyngitis; splenomegaly; and, less commonly, hepatomegaly. An erythematous maculopapular rash occurs between the fourth and sixth days of illness in 10% to 15% of cases. This rash appears on the trunk or upper arms and occasionally on the face, forearms, thighs, and legs (Hurwitz, 1993).

▲ **Clinical Warning:** A concurrent streptococcal pharyngitis may be seen in 30% of cases (Peter & Ray, 1998). Providers should screen with a rapid strep test or culture for all cases of mononucleosis.

Complications are unusual and include airway obstruction secondary to pharyngitis; neurologic manifestations, such as meningitis and ataxia; and the most feared but rare complication of splenic rupture. Rupture is usually due to trauma. Orchitis and myocarditis are also rare complications. Hematologically, thrombocytopenia, hemolytic anemia, and agranulocytosis also may occur.

Diagnostic Criteria

Diagnosis depends on history, clinical findings, and positive laboratory results. The classic triad of symptoms for infectious mononucleosis (ie, fever, pharyngitis, and cervical lymphadenopathy) should raise suspicions about EBV as the etiology of illness.

Diagnostic Studies

The "monospot" test is widely used and is 85% sensitive and 97% specific in children older than 5 years. It may not be positive in the first 10 to 14 days of illness. In children younger than 4 years, the sensitivity is only 20%. The test may remain positive for many months after the illness has resolved and should not be used as a marker of active disease (Peter & Ray, 1998).

Serum IgM or IgG against viral capsid antigen ("anti-VCA") will reveal EBV as the etiology of the illness. This expensive profile should only be used in monospot-negative patients who exhibit prolonged or complicated courses. Atypical lymphocytosis on peripheral blood smear is seen in 75% of cases (Peter & Ray, 1998). Liver enzymes are elevated in 70% to 90% of cases (Peter & Ray, 1998).

Management

Treatment is supportive. Systemic steroids can be useful in reducing tonsillar hypertrophy and inflammation and may be considered for massive splenomegaly. Providers should reserve their use for cases where massive lymphadenopathy is causing dehydration or impending upper airway obstruction. People with a recent history of infectious mononucleosis should not donate blood. The infection is self-limited.

▲ **Clinical Warning:** Even the most experienced clinicians can miss splenomegaly. Providers should order splenic precautions (eg, avoiding contact sports or situations likely to lead to trauma) in all cases of mononucleosis for at least 3 weeks from the time of diagnosis.

What to Tell Parents

The illness is self-limited and in most cases resolves within 3 weeks. Virtually all patients return to their normal state of health and activity within 4 to 6 weeks after onset of the illness. Parents should contact the primary care provider if the child has difficulty breathing or develops jaundice. The clinician should examine the child weekly until the child has recovered completely and no further splenic enlargement is noted.

Teaching and Self-Care

Providers should encourage the parents to ensure that the child receives adequate oral fluid intake. Gargles with salt water can help alleviate discomfort. Clinicians should encourage bed rest.

REFERENCES

American Academy of Pediatrics Policy Statement. (1997). Use of codeine and dextromethorphan-containing cough remedies in children (RE 9722).

American Academy of Pediatrics. (1997). *Red book: Report of the Committee on Infectious Diseases* (24th ed.). Elk Grove Village, IL: Author.

American Medical Association. (1995). *Drugs used to treat upper respiratory tract disorders. Drug evaluations annual* (pp. 493–525). Chicago: Author.

Anderson, L., Young, N., & Gary, W. (1992). Human parvovirus. In Lennette (Ed.), *Laboratory diagnosis of viral infections* (pp. 627–642). New York: Marcel Dekker.

Bang, H. O., & Bang, J.(1944). Involvement of the central nervous system in mumps. *Bulletin of Hygiene, 19*, 503.

Bauchner, H., Pellon, S. I., & Klein, J. O. (1999). Parents, physicians, and antibiotic use. *Pediatrics, 103*(7), 395.

Behrman, R. E., Kliegman, R. M., & Arvin, A. M. (1996). *Nelson textbook of pediatrics* (15th ed.). Philadelphia: W.B. Saunders.

Boynton, R. W., Dunn, E. S., & Stephens, G. R. (1998). *Manual of ambulatory pediatrics* (4th ed.). Philadelphia: Lippincott Williams & Wilkins.

Caul, E., Usher, M., & Burton, P. (1988). Intrauterine infection with human parvovirus B19: A light and electron microscopy study. *Journal of Medical Virology, 24*, 55–66.

Centers for Disease Control and Prevention. (1997a). Measles-United States, 1996 and the interruption of indigenous transmission. *Morbidity and Mortality Weekly Report, 46*, 242–246.

Centers for Disease Control and Prevention. (1997b). Case definitions for infectious conditions under public health surveillance. *Morbidity and Mortality Weekly Report, 46*(RR-10), 24–25, 29, 54.

Centers for Disease Control and Prevention. (1997c). Rubella and congenital rubella syndrome-United States, 1994-1997. *Morbidity and Mortality Weekly Report, 46*, 350–354.

Centers for Disease Control and Prevention. (1994) Rubella and congenital rubella syndrome-United States, Jan. 1, 1991-May 7, 1994. *Morbidity and Mortality Weekly Report, 43*, 391, 397–401.

Choo, P. W., Donahue, J. G., & Platt, R. (1997). Ibuprofen and skin and soft tissue superinfections in children with varicella. *Annals of Epidemiology, 7*(7), 440–445.

Chorba, T., Coccia, R., Holman, R., et al. (1986). The role of parvovirus B19 in aplastic crisis and erythema infectiosum (fifth disease). *Journal of Infectious Disease, 154*, 383–393.

Cohen, B. (1995). Parvovirus B19: An expanding spectrum of disease. *British Medical Journal, 311*, 1549–1542.

Cossart, Y., Field, A., Cant, B., et al. (1975). Parvovirus-like particles in human sera. *Lancet, 1*, 72–73.

Falk, W. A., Buchan, K., Dow, M., et al. (1989). The epidemiology of mumps in southern Alberta, 1980-1982. *American Journal of Epidemiology, 130*, 736–749.

Feigin, R. D., & Cherry, J. D. (1998). *Textbook of pediatric infectious diseases* (4th ed.). Philadelphia: W.B. Saunders.

Finklea, J. F., Sandifer, S. H., & Moore, G. T., Jr. (1968). Epidemic rubella at the Citadel. *American Journal of Epidemiology, 87*, 367–372.

Godomski, A., & Horton, L. (1992). The need for rational therapeutics in the use of cough and cold medicine in infants. *Pediatrics, 89*, 774–776.

Gohd, R. S. (1954). The common cold. *New England Journal of Medicine, 250*, 687–697.

Green, R. H., Balsamo, M. R., Giles, J. P., et al. (1965). Studies of the natural history and prevention of rubella. *American Journal of Diseases in Children, 110*, 348–365.

Hurwitz, S. (1993). *Clinical pediatric dermatology: A textbook of skin disorders of children and adolescents* (2nd ed.). Philadelphia: W.B. Saunders.

Hussey, G., & Klein, M. (1995). A randomized trial of vitamin A in children with severe measles. *New England Journal of Medicine, 323*, 160.

Ishii, K., Uchida, Y., Miyamura, K. et al. (eds.) (1989). *Acute hemorrhagic conjunctivitis.* Tokyo: University of Tokyo Press.

Katcher, M. L. (1996). Cold, cough, and allergy medications: Uses and abuses. *Pediatrics in Review, 17*, 1.

Katz, B. Z., & Miller, G. (1998). Epstein-Barr virus infections. In S. L. Katz, A. A. Gershon, & P. J. Hotez (Eds.), *Krugman's infectious diseases of children* (10th ed.). St. Louis: Mosby-Year Book.

Kearns, G. L., & Reed, M. D. (1989). Clinical pharmacokinetics in infants and children: A reappraisal. *Pharmacokinetics, 17*, 29–67.

Kogen, M. D., Pappas, G., Yu, S. M., & Kotelchuck, M. (1994). Over-the-counter medication use among U.S. preschool-age children. *Journal of the American Medical Association, 272*, 1025–1030.

Krause, P. R., & Klinman, D. M. (1995). Efficacy, immunogenicity, safety, and use of live attenuated chickenpox vaccine. *Journal of Pediatrics, 127*, 518–525.

Larrey, D., Babany, G., Tinel, M., et al. (1989). Effect of liver disease on dextromethorphan oxidation capacity and phenotype: A study in 107 patients. *British Journal of Clinical Pharmacology, 28*, 297–304.

Levy, J. A. (1997). Three new human herpes viruses (HHV 6, 7 and 8). *Lancet, 349*, 558.

Lindahl, T., Adams, A., Bjursell, G., et al. (1976). Covertly closed circular duplex DNA of Epstein Barr virus in a human lymphoid cell line. *Journal of Molecular Biology, 102*, 511–530.

Lowenstein, S. R., & Parrino, T. A. (1987). Management of the common cold. *Advances in Internal Medicine, 32*, 207–234.

Markenson, G. R., & Yancey, M. K. (1998). Parvovirus B19 infections in pregnancy. *Seminars in Perinatology, 22*(4), 309–317.

McCaig, L. F., & Hughes, J. M. (1995). Trends in antimicrobial drug prescribing among office based physicians in the United States. *Journal of the American Medical Association, 273*, 214–219.

Meissner, C. H. (1994). Economic impact of viral respiratory disease in children. *Journal of Pediatrics, 124*, S17–21.

Morbidity and Mortality Weekly Report. (1991). Measles-United States, 1990. *Journal of the American Medical Association, 265*, 3227–3228.

Morey, A., Ferguson, D., & Fleming, K. (1993). Ultrastructural features of fetal erythroid precursors infected with parvovirus B19 in vitro: Evidence of cell death by apoptosis. *Journal of Pathology, 164*, 213–220.

Morfini, M., Azzi, A., & Mannucci, P. (1996). B19 parvovirus withstands "super heating" in antihemophilic concentrate. *Thromb Haemost, 76.*

Nicod, L. P. (1993). Cytokines I overview. *Thorax, 48*, 660–667.

Nyquist, A. C., Gonzalez, R., Steiner, J., & Sande, M. (1998). Antibiotic prescribing for children with colds, upper respiratory infections and bronchitis by ambulatory physicians in the United States. *Journal of the American Medical Association, 279*, 875–877.

Nyquist, A. C. (1999). Antibiotic use and abuse in clinical practice. *Pediatric Annals, 28*, 453–459.

Peter, J., & Ray, C. G. (1998). Infectious mononucleosis. *Pediatrics in Review, 19*, 276–279.

Pinsky, P. F., et al. (1988). Reye's syndrome and aspirin: Evidence for a dose-response effect. *Journal of the American Medical Association, 260*(5), 657–661.

Porter, H., Quantrill, A., & Fleming, K. (1988). B19 parvovirus infection of myocardial cell. *Lancet, 1*, 535–536.

Portmore, A. C. (1995). Parvoviruses (erythema infectiosum aplastic crisis). In G. L. Mandell, J. E. Bennett, & R. Dolin (Eds.). *Principles and practice of infectious diseases* (4th ed.) (pp. 1439–1446). New York: Churchill Livingstone.

Public Health Laboratory Service Working Party on Fifth Disease. (1990). Prospective study of human parvovirus (B19) in pregnancy. *British Medical Journal, 300,* 1166–1170.

Purtilo, D. T. (1981). Malignant lymphoproliferative diseases induced by Epstein-Barr virus in immunodeficient patients, including X-linked, cytogenetic and familial syndromes. *Cancer, Genetics, Cytogenetics, 4,* 251–268.

Rosendahl, I. (1988). Expenses of physician care spurs OTC, self-care market. *Drug Topics, 132,* 62–63.

Rotbart, H. (1998). Enteroviruses. In S. L. Katz, A. A. Gershon, & P. J. Hotez (Eds.), *Krugman's infectious diseases of children* (10th ed.). St. Louis: Mosby-Year Book.

Sixbey, J. B., Nedrud, J. G., Raab-Traub, N., et al. (1984). Ebstein Barr virus replication in oropharyngeal epithelial cells. *New England Journal of Medicine, 310,* 1225–1230.

Spielberg, S. P., & Schulman, J. D. (1977). A possible reaction to pseudoephedrine in a patient with phenylketonuria. *Journal of Pediatrics, 90,* 1026.

Torok, T., Remington, J., & Klein, J. (1995). Human parvovirus B19. *Infectious disease of the fetus and newborn infant* (pp. 668–702). Philadelphia: W.B. Saunders.

Wald, E. R. (1995). Chronic sinusitis in children. *Journal of Pediatrics, 127,* 339–347.

Wharton, M. (1996). The epidemiology of varicella-zoster virus infections. *Infectious Disease Clinics of North America, 10,* 571–581.

Young, N., & Mortimer, P. (1984). Viruses and bone marrow failure. *Blood, 63,* 729–737.

Fever: Approach to the Febrile Child

• RICHARD BACHUR, MD

INTRODUCTION

Fever is one of the most frequently encountered pediatric problems, accounting for 25% of visits to pediatric emergency rooms (Krauss, et al., 1991; Nelson, et al., 1992). In children, most febrile illnesses are benign and self-limited. Because fever is a sign of systemic disease, however, the challenge for primary care practitioners is to determine its specific etiology. In most cases, a viral cause is evident, and careful explanation and proper instructions for supportive care and follow-up are all that parents require to care for their children appropriately. Some children with fever, however, have identifiable or suspected causes requiring specific therapy and either hospitalization or close follow-up. Only rarely, with extreme temperatures above 41.1°C (106°F), does a fever pose a danger to the child. This chapter addresses the general approach to the febrile child and the specific conditions that cause fever. Display 31-1 provides conditions associated with fever, common causes of fever, and life-threatening causes of fever.

ANATOMY, PHYSIOLOGY, AND PATHOLOGY

The hypothalamus regulates body temperature with a typical diurnal variation—high in the evening and low in the morning. The "normal" range of temperature varies among individuals. A rectal temperature of 100.4°F (38°C) generally is considered fever. Oral temperatures are 1°F (0.6°C) lower than rectal temperatures, and axillary temperatures are 2°F (1.2°C) lower than rectal measurements.

● **Clinical Pearl:** Although recent investigations have shown that tympanic temperatures may correlate well with rectal or core temperatures, providers should confirm fever by other traditional measures, such as rectal temperature. This is especially true for young infants, when the presence or degree of fever determines management.

Fever develops when exogenous pyrogens (eg, infectious agents, antibody–antigen complexes, and toxins) induce the production of endogenous pyrogen by phagocytic leukocytes. Endogenous pyrogen, traveling through the circulation, acts on the anterior hypothalamus to signal increased heat production (increased metabolism) and decreased heat loss (cutaneous vasoconstriction). Fever appears to be part of the body's adaptive response to infectious and noninfectious inflammatory challenges. It has been shown to inhibit efficient replication of many microbes and to increase phagocytic activity. Other changes, including decreased glucose production (preferred energy substrate of pathogens) and production of acute phase reactants, also contribute to this adaptive response. Antipyretics prevent production of prostaglandins, which act as signals to the anterior hypothalamus.

▲ **Clinical Warning:** The magnitude of fever reduction from antipyretics does not distinguish those with serious infections from those with simple, uncomplicated illnesses.

The organisms responsible for serious infections in infants younger than 2 months include group B *Streptococcus*, *Escherichia coli* (and less frequently other enteric gram-negative bacteria), and *Listeria monocytogenes*. In older infants and children, *Streptococcus pneumoniae*, *Haemophilus influenzae*, and *Neisseria meningitidis* account for most cases. Thankfully, invasive disease due to *H. influenzae* type b has all but disappeared due to universal vaccination. Rarely, group A *Streptococcus*, *Staphylococcus aureus*, and *Salmonella* species cause bacteremia or sepsis and usually are associated with focal infections.

HISTORY AND PHYSICAL EXAMINATION

The history and physical examination will provide the most important information in determining the urgency of the situation. Items in the history that suggest "toxicity" or an emergent situation (especially if triaging by phone) are listed in Table 31-1.

● **Clinical Pearl:** When the patient presents to the office, observation of the child from afar, in the parent's arms, or on the exam table, may suggest or dismiss concerns of toxicity. The degree of alertness and interaction, response to the parent and examiner, and respiratory status are valuable measures of illness. To the experienced practitioner, this is known as the "look test."

Because of the predictable "don't touch me" response of many toddlers and preschoolers, careful observation before attempts at examination may eliminate concerns of meningitis or encephalitis that may be less obvious once the screaming begins.

Providers should ask questions about the onset and duration of the fever, the temperature measurement and how parents obtained it, medications used, associated symptoms and signs, and infectious exposures (eg, family, daycare, school). Past medical history should focus on previous febrile illnesses, immunization status, perinatal course for young infants, and the presence of any immunodeficiency (eg, sickle cell disease, asplenia, hypogammaglobulinemia, malignancy, human immunodeficiency virus [HIV], and steroid use). The clinician should conduct a general review of systems, including feeding history, urinary output, presence of any respiratory symptoms, gastrointestinal symptoms, headache, sore throat, myalgias or arthralgias, and rashes.

During the physical examination, the provider should investigate any signs of severe, life-threatening infections. He or she should obtain a complete set of vital signs in any

DISPLAY 31-1 • Conditions Associated With Fever

- Infections
  - Upper respiratory tract
    - Common cold*
    - Pharyngitis/tonsillitis*
    - Cervical adenitis*
    - Croup*[†]
    - Epiglotittis[†]
    - Retropharyngeal abscess/cellulitis[†]
    - Peritonsillar abscess
    - Acute sinusitis*
    - Tracheitis[†]
    - Otitis media*
  - Lower respiratory tract
    - Pneumonia*[†]
    - Bronchiolitis*[†]
    - Acute bronchitis
    - Lung abscess
    - Empyema
  - Oral cavity and salivary glands
    - Dental abscess*
    - Herpangina*
    - Herpetic gingivostomatitis*
    - Parotitis*
  - Central nervous system (CNS)
    - Meningitis*[†]
    - Meningoencephalitis*[†]
    - Brain abscess[†]
    - Epidural Abscess[†]
  - Cardiac
    - Myocarditis[†]
    - Pericarditis[†]
    - Endocarditis[†]
  - Gastrointestinal
    - Viral gastroenteritis*[†]
    - Bacterial enteritis*[†]
    - Pancreatitis[†]
    - Peritonitis[†]
    - Appendicitis*
    - Cholangitis
    - Peritonitis
    - Hepatitis
    - Intra-abdominal abscess (include retroperitoneal)
  - Genitourinary
    - Urinary tract infection*
    - Renal or perinephric abscess
    - Pelvic inflammatory disease*
    - Acute salpingitis*
    - Tubo-ovarian abscess*
    - Epididymitis*
    - Orchitis
    - Prostatitis
  - Musculoskeletal
    - Septic arthritis
    - Osteomyelitis*
    - Pyomyositis
    - Discitis
    - Tetanus[†]
    - Fasciitis[†]
  - Ocular
    - Periorbital cellulitis*
    - Orbital cellulitis/abscess[†]
  - Cutaneous
    - Cellulitis*
  - Exanthems
    - Bacterial: erythroderma with toxic shock syndrome,[†] scarletina with group A streptococcal infection*
    - Viral: roseola, measles, rubella, varicella,* fifth disease,* hand-foot-mouth disease*
    - Meningococcemia*[†]
    - Rocky Mountain spotted fever[†]
    - Lyme disease*
    - Secondary syphillis
  - Systemic Infections
    - Sepsis[†]
    - "Occult" bacteremia*
    - Toxic shock syndrome[†]
    - Viruses*
    - Rickettsial (Rocky Mountain spotted fever[†]), fungal, parasitic (malaria[†]), and atypical bacteria
    - Miliary tuberculosis[†]
- CNS disorders
  - CNS lesions or malformations of hypothalamus or brainstem
  - Familial dysautonomia
  - Status epilepticus[†]
- Neoplasms
  - Leukemia*[†]
  - Lymphoma*[†]
  - Neuroblastoma*[†]
  - Sarcoma
- Vasculitic syndromes
  - Juvenile rheumatoid arthritis
  - Systemic lupus erythematosus[†]
  - Polyarteritis nodosa
  - Kawasaki disease*[†]
  - Dermatomyositis
  - Henoch-Schönlein purpura*
  - Serum sickness*
  - Stevens-Johnson syndrome[†]
  - Acute rheumatic fever*[†]
- Poisonings/drug reactions
  - Salicylate toxicity[†]
  - Atropine poisoning[†]
  - Cocaine poisoning*[†]
  - Amphetamine poisoning*[†]
  - Phenothiazines
  - Antidepressants with anticholinergic side effects
  - Malignant hyperthermia[†] associated with inhaled anesthetics and succinylcholine
- Miscellaneous conditions
  - Confined hemorrhage (eg, hematoma with long bone fracture)*
  - Heat stroke[†]
  - Intravascular hemolysis as with blood transfusion reaction[†]
  - Dehydration*
  - Inflammatory bowel disease
  - Thyrotoxicosis
  - Crush injuries
  - Other rare (familial mediterranean fever, ectodermal dysplasia, intermittent porphyria)
  - Vaccine reactions*

Common conditions (*) and potentially life-threatening conditions ([†]) are noted.

Table 31–1. INTERVIEW CLUES TO SUGGEST "TOXICITY" OR SERIOUS ILLNESS

Clue: History Item	Concern
Extreme irritability (especially parodoxical)	Meningitis, septic arthritis
Depressed sensorium	Meningitis, encephalitis, shock/sepsis
Stiff neck	Meningitis
Severe headache	Meningitis, meningoencephalitis
Breathing difficulty with stridor, especially with cyanosis, drooling	Croup, epiglottitis, tracheitis
Breathing difficulty with altered mental status, retractions/distress ("labored," "heavy" breathing), unable to speak (age dependent), cyanosis, or chest pain	Croup, epiglottitis, tracheitis, pneumonia, bronchiolitis
Unable to swallow	Retropharyngeal abscess, tonsillar abscess, epiglottitis
Nonblanchable rash (petechiae/purpura)	Sepsis, especially meningococcemia
Limp/refusal to walk	Osteomyelitis, septic arthritis, fasciitis, discitis, myositis, epidural abscess (especially with weakness)
Flank pain	Pleuritis, pyelonephritis
Seizure	Nonspecific; however meningitis/encephalitis if young infant (<1 y) or outside age range for simple febrile seizure
Rigors	Septicemia, pyelonephritis, pneumonia

ill-appearing child. Stridor, drooling, dysphonia, or leaning forward with the neck hyperextended ("sniffing" position) may be signs of impending upper airway obstruction. Tachypnea, retractions, or cyanosis may suggest severe pneumonia. Altered sensorium, meningismus, or focal neurologic deficits are seen with meningitis and encephalitis. In young infants, a bulging fontanelle may be seen with meningitis, but meningismus is rare before age 1 year. Signs of poor perfusion (eg, tachycardia, altered mental status, weak peripheral pulses, delayed capillary refill, cold or discolored extremities) can be seen with sepsis, pericarditis, myocarditis, endocarditis, as well as with dehydration. Petechial rashes often are seen with streptococccal throat infections and viruses but also may be associated with Rocky Mountain spotted fever and meningococcemia.

In most cases, the provider can focus examination on the common causes of fever in children. Common sites of infection include the eyes, ears, nose, mouth, cervical lymph nodes, chest, abdomen, skin, and skeletal system. Specific viral illnesses, such as gingivostomatitis, herpangina, varicella, bronchiolitis, and mononucleosis, may become evident by examination. Examination of the tympanic membrane, revealing erythema, loss of landmarks, opacification, and decreased mobility, suggests otitis media.

● **Clinical Pearl:** Providers should not attribute high fever to otitis media alone; most often, a viral illness or other focal bacterial infection coexists with otitis media to produce the high fever.

● **Clinical Pearl:** Streptococcal pharyngitis is a predominant cause of fever in preschoolers and school-age children; therefore, providers should suspect it in children with pharyngitis (even in the absence of exudate).

Frequently, vomiting, abdominal pain, headache, and tender cervical adenopathy are associated with streptococcal throat infections. Secondary bacterial infections frequently develop following upper respiratory infections (URIs) and include cervical adenitis (often a unilateral, swollen, and tender submandibular node), sinusitis, and otitis media. A characteristic tracheal cough (described as a honking goose or barking seal), hoarseness, and nighttime stridor are typical

findings in croup. Respiratory symptoms with lower respiratory tract signs (eg, decreased breath sounds, rales, focal rhonchi, or wheezes) may suggest pneumonia. Abdominal examination is generally innocent with gastroenteritis. Tenderness, especially if focal, can be seen with gastroenteritis, but providers also should consider mesenteric adenitis, appendicitis, and intussusception. Suprapubic pain or flank tenderness implies a urinary tract infection (UTI). Point tenderness over bone or a swollen, warm joint can be found with osteomyelitis or septic arthritis, respectively. With the exception of UTIs and pneumonias in young children, the common bacterial causes of febrile illness usually have localizing signs.

▲ **Clinical Warning:** "Occult" bacteremia has been well documented in even well appearing children with high fevers.

Approximately 3% of children ages 3 to 36 months have occult bacteremia (90% of cases due to *S. pneumoniae*); 10% of these cases lead to complications, such as sepsis, pneumonia, septic arthritis, meningitis, osteomyelitis, and cellulitis (Harper, Bachur, & Fleisher, 1995; Harper & Fleisher, 1993; Lee & Harper, 1998). Because of this issue of occult bacteremia and other occult infections, an algorithmic approach to young febrile children has been developed to identify safely those children at high risk and to provide empiric therapy pending cultures. The algorithms for different groups are presented in a later section.

Evaluation of Febrile Infants Younger Than Three Months

In general, the risk of bacteremia is inversely related to age. Roughly 7% of infants with fever in this age group have a significant bacterial infection (SBI) (eg, meningitis, bacteremia, pneumonia, UTI, bacterial enteritis, bone or soft-tissue infection), including 2.5% who have bacteremia or bacterial meningitis (Baskin, O'Rourke, & Fleisher, 1992; Baskin, O'Rourke, & Fleisher, 1994). "Toxic-appearing" infants have a 17% chance of SBI, including an 11% risk of bacteremia and a 4% chance of meningitis (Baraff, Oslund, Schriger, & Stephen, 1992).

Clinical Manifestations

Signs and symptoms of significant illness are often subtle and very nonspecific in this age group, including hypothermia or hyperthermia, poor feeding, irritability or lethargy, vomiting, or poor perfusion. Additionally, this age group is especially difficult because the diagnostic differential includes many noninfectious etiologies (Display 31-2).

▲ **Clinical Warning:** Suspicion for sepsis must be high in young infants, because of the inability of even experienced clinicians to select those with significant illness consistently from the large majority with self-limiting viral disease.

Management

The management of febrile infants is divided into those younger than 1 month and those ages 1 to 3 months. Note that definitive guidelines have not been established and that some authorities do not adhere to the intensive evaluation and cautious therapeutic approach recommended in the following paragraphs.

● **Clinical Pearl:** All patients younger than 1 month should be considered for a complete sepsis evaluation and admission for intravenous (IV) antibiotics, regardless of their appearance or identification of a seemingly minor focal infection.

The sepsis evaluation includes screening tests (complete blood count [CBC], urinalysis, cerebrospinal fluid [CSF] cell

---

DISPLAY 31–2 • Differential Diagnosis of the Septic-Appearing Infant Less Than 3 Months of Age

Infection
  Sepsis (viral or bacterial)
  Meningitis
  Urinary tract infection
Cardiac
  Congenital heart disease
  Dysrhythmias
  Myocarditis/cardiomyopathy
  Pericarditis
Hematologic
  Severe anemia from hemorrhage or hemolysis
  Methemaglobinemia
Metabolic
  Inborn errors of metabolism
  Hyponatremia, hypernatremia
  Hypoglycemia
  Hyperammonemia
  Acidosis
  Renal dysfunction
Endocrine
  Congenital adrenal hyperplasia
Gastrointestinal disorders
  Severe dehydration from gastroenteritis or pyloric stenosis
  Necrotizing enterocolitis
  Volvulus
  Intussusception
Neurologic
  Infant botulism
  Intracranial hemorrhage

---

count, CSF protein and glucose) plus cultures of blood, urine (by suprapubic aspiration or catheterization), and CSF. Antibiotic therapy includes ampicillin (50 mg/kg/dose every 6 hours) and either gentamicin (2.5 mg/kg/dose every 8 hours) or cefotaxime (50 mg/kg/dose every 6–8 hours) for 48 hours pending culture results; intramuscular (IM) or IV ceftriaxone can be used for infants older than 2 weeks without meningitis.

● **Clinical Pearl:** Clinicians also should seriously consider acyclovir in any septic-appearing infant or those with CSF pleocytosis regardless of maternal history for herpes simplex.

The management of febrile infants ages 1 to 3 months depends on whether the patient has a focal infection and his or her risk status. Patients are considered low risk based on clinical and laboratory criteria. Clinically, a low-risk infant must be previously healthy, nontoxic in appearance, with no evidence of focal bacterial infection (other than otitis media). The infant's situation must be acceptable with respect to reliable caregivers and planned follow-up. The white blood cell (WBC) count must be 5,000 to 20,000/mm³, and the band count must be less than 1500/mm³. The urinalysis should be normal. If diarrhea is present, the stool should contain fewer than 5 WBCs per high power field (hpf). A lumbar puncture should be performed with the CSF WBC count less than 10/hpf. A full sepsis evaluation is necessary for an infant to be considered low risk or to receive empiric antibiotic therapy. If the patient is low risk and the sepsis evaluation is negative, the patient may be discharged home after a dose of ceftriaxone (50 mg/kg IM/IV) is given and follow-up has been arranged. All these infants need repeat evaluation within 24 hours. Another option for infants age 1 to 3 months is to obtain a CBC, urinalysis, urine culture, and blood culture. If the CBC and urine are normal (using the low-risk criteria), the patient can be followed as an outpatient without antibiotics. Empiric administration of antibiotics should be done only after a lumbar puncture and blood culture to avoid partial treatment of bacterial meningitis or bacteremia and to avoid subsequent confusion if the patient's condition deteriorates. This latter option should be reserved for well-appearing infants who clearly meet the rest of the low-risk criteria.

● **Clinical Pearl:** Chest radiographs are not necessary in young infants without signs of respiratory illness.

Tachypnea (out of proportion to the height of fever), cough, oxygen saturation less than 95%, any lower respiratory tract signs (eg, rales, wheeze, rhonchi), or any respiratory distress (eg, grunting, nasal flaring, retracting) are indications for obtaining a radiograph. Providers should consider hospitalization and IV antibiotics pending culture results for infants who did not meet the low-risk criteria. The management of febrile infants younger than age 3 months is diagrammed in Figure 31-1.

Evaluation of the Febrile Child Ages Three Months to Three Years

Occult bacteremia has its highest incidence in this age group. By definition, these children appear well and may have fever as their only symptom, or they may have a minor infection, such as otitis media or a URI. Approximately 3% to 5% of children ages 3 to 36 months with a temperature above 102.2°F (39°C) have occult bacteremia (Baron & Fink, 1980; Dershewitz, Wigder, Wigder, &

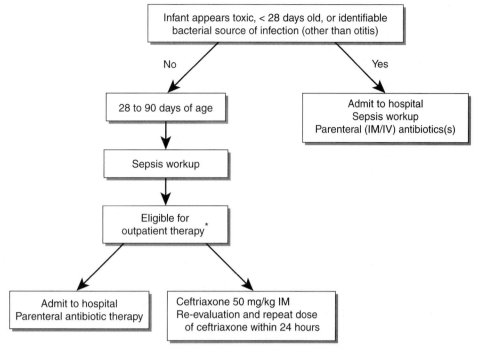

Sepsis workup includes blood culture, urine culture, and CSF culture

*Eligibility criteria for outpatient treatment:

Previously healthy
Family can be easily contacted (eg, accurate phone number)
No focal bacterial infection on examination (except otitis media)
WBC count < 20,000/mm^3
Normal urinalysis (negative dipstick or <10 WBC/hpf)
When diarrhea present < 5 WBC/hpf in stool
CSF WBC count < 10/mm^3

†See text for acceptable alternative strategies.

Figure 31–1 ■ Algorithm for the management of the previously healthy infant 0 to 90 days old with fever (T ≥ 38.0°C).[†]

Nadelman, 1983; Fleisher et al., 1994; Jaffe, Tanz, Davis, Henretig, & Fleisher, 1987; McCarthy, Jekel, & Dolan, 1977; Murray et al., 1981). Based on recent studies (Lee & Harper, 1998), the pathogens responsible for occult bacteremia are *S. pneumoniae* (90%), *Salmonella* species (5%), *N. meningitidis* (2%), *Streptococcus pyogenes* (2%), and *H. influenzae* (1%). Patients who have occult bacteremia and remain untreated are at risk for sepsis or secondary sites of infection. The complication rate depends on the patient's age and the organism's pathogenicity (6% for *S. pneumoniae*, 36% for *H. influenzae*, and 50% for *N. meningitidis*) (Alario, Nelson, & Shapiro, 1989; Bratton, Teele, & Klein, 1977; Harper et al., 1995; Korones, Marshall, & Shapiro, 1992; Shapiro, Aaron, Wald, & Chiponis, 1986). Prior to the introduction of a conjugate vaccine, *H. influenzae* accounted for approximately 13% of cases of occult bacteremia and for 40% of the complications.

Whether clinicians should try to identify and empirically treat those at risk for occult bacteremia has been debated for more than 20 years. Although consensus has not been reached, several recent "expert panel" guidelines and reviews have recommended empiric parenteral therapy in patients who are determined to be at high risk for occult bacteremia by age, height of fever, and laboratory results (Baraff & Lee, 1992; Green & Rothrock, 1999).

Clinical Manifestations

▲ **Clinical Warning:** Because occult bacteremia occurs in well-appearing, minimally symptomatic patients, clinical assessment based on the clinician's impression of toxicity or clinical scoring scales has not been shown to be either sensitive or specific for this population. The degree of temperature, however, has been helpful in assessing the risk of bacteremia. The incidence of bacteremia is directly correlated with the height of the fever. The risk of bacteremia by degree of fever is as follows: 1% for less than 38.9°C, 4% for 39.0° to 39.4°C, 8% for 39.5° to 39.9°C, 13% for 40.5° to 41.0°C, and 23% for fever above 41.1°C (Harper & Fleisher, 1993).

▲ **Clinical Warning:** Contrary to a commonly believed myth, the ease or rapidity of a febrile child's response to antipyretics has not been shown to influence the risk of bacterial disease (Baker et al., 1989).

Conclusive evidence has shown that the height of the WBC count correlates directly with the risk of bacteremia. An elevated WBC count is frequently found in patients with *S. pneumoniae* bacteremia and less reliably in those with *N. meningitidis* or *H. influenzae* bacteremia. Because *S. pneumo-*

niae accounts for the majority of bacteremias, however, the WBC count has been accepted as a useful screen. The relative risk of bacteremia is five times higher if the WBC is 15,000/mm^3 or more (13% versus 2.6%) (Jaffe & Fleisher, 1991). The percentage of bands and absolute band count has not been helpful in identifying those at risk for bacteremia except when extreme. The presence of an identifiable viral illness (eg, varicella, stomatitis, croup, bronchiolitis) lowers the risk of occult bacteremia (Greenes & Harper, 1999; Kuppermann, Fleisher, & Jaffe, 1998). The clinician must recognize, however, that "new" fever in a child who has already passed the viremic phase of an illness (such as varicella) may be a sign that a secondary infection has developed.

Management

If the history and physical examination do not identify a focal infection, the provider should consider a screening CBC if the temperature (recorded at home or at the time of visit) exceeds 39.0°C. Early in the evaluation, the clinician should decide whether to obtain a urinalysis to avoid losing the opportunity to collect a specimen. Because UTIs are often "occult" in young children, patients without respiratory signs should have placement of a urine collection bag. Chest radiographs should only be obtained in those with respiratory signs suggestive of pneumonia and in patients with leukocytosis (see below).

If the WBC count is less than 15,000/mm^3, the provider can discharge the patient with appropriate follow-up and no further testing at that point (again, clinicians should reserve this strategy for well-appearing infants only). If the WBC count is greater than 20,000/mm^3, the clinician should obtain a blood culture and consider the administration of ceftriaxone (50 mg/kg IM/IV). Patients with a WBC count between 15,000 and 20,000/mm^3 (the "gray zone") may be considered for a blood culture and empiric therapy based on age, height of fever, and other clinical factors. Although WBC counts have been shown to be useful in predicting bacteremia, the exact cutoffs represent a balance of sensitivity and specificity. Therefore, exact adherence to any strategy is never perfect. Additionally, the blood culture is not a good screening test because of the incubation period needed to identify disease, but it is currently the only reliable way to detect bacteremia. Fortunately, those at risk for bacteremia are often treated empirically in anticipation of a positive culture (and often clinically improved at the time of reevaluation). In those instances when no antibiotics were given, the positive blood culture will alert the clinicians about the necessity of immediate reevaluation. In addition to the blood culture, clinicians should obtain a urine culture (catheterization or suprapubic aspiration) in all males younger than 6 months and females younger than 2 years if empiric antibiotics are to be administered.

▲ **Clinical Warning:** A negative urinalysis is not a completely reliable screen for UTIs in young infants. Therefore, providers should obtain a culture prior to beginning empiric antibiotic therapy (Hoberman, Wald, Reynolds, Penchansky, & Charron, 1994).

Providers may avoid the urine culture in select cases: the WBC count is normal (and therefore empiric antibiotics are not to be given), the patient had onset of fever with overt respiratory symptoms, or the urinalysis from a bag specimen was completely negative in a male older than 6 months or a female older than 2 years. For patients with leukocytosis (WBC greater than 20,000/mm^3), the clinician also must reconsider the need to perform other diagnostic tests. Chest radiographs will detect "occult pneumonia" in approximately 20% of patients with fever and leukocytosis and no other major identifiable bacterial source, even in the absence of respiratory findings (Bachur, Perry, & Harper, 1999). Additionally, clinicians should consider reevaluation or further diagnostic studies for less common sites of infection (eg, meningitis; intra-abdominal abscesses; deep soft-tissue infections, including retropharyngeal or muscle abscesses; bone or joint infections) in patients with leukocytosis.

Parents should be instructed to obtain immediate follow-up if their child's condition worsens. All patients receiving outpatient therapy should be reevaluated in 24 hours. All patients who had cultures performed and were candidates for outpatient management must also be reachable, preferably by phone.

Patients in this age group with identifiable focal infections may be treated with oral or parenteral antibiotics, depending on the severity of their infections. The management of febrile patients between ages 3 and 36 months is summarized in Figure 31-2.

Evaluation of Children Older Than Three Years

Generally, older children are not considered to be at significant risk for occult bacteremia; additionally, because of improved communication with the patient, concern of occult infections is decreased. Therefore, the typical evaluation includes a thorough history and physical examination to identify any focal bacterial infections. For those in whom the clinical evaluation fails to disclose a source of the fever, providers should arrange follow-up. When the fever is persistent or the patient appears ill, a WBC count and urinalysis may be useful as a screening test. In this age group, an elevated WBC count may lead to a chest radiograph or urinalysis that were not previously "indicated," but these patients do not require empiric antibiotic therapy.

The Septic-Appearing Child

Although optimal management of a septic-appearing child is in an emergency room, offices and clinics may face the initial management and stabilization of a septic-appearing child. Preparation for such an event, as with other emergencies, is critical. When a provider cannot give initial care, prompt decisions to transport the patient to an appropriate area or facility may be life saving.

Clinicians can make a presumptive diagnosis of sepsis in any febrile child who appears ill or toxic with evidence of altered organ perfusion, such as altered mental status, tachypnea, tachycardia, hypotension, poor capillary refill, oliguria, or evidence of coagulopathy. The septic-appearing child requires aggressive evaluation and resuscitation. The immediate objective is to maximize oxygenation, support ventilation, and obtain vascular access. Cardiovascular stabilization may require generous fluid administration and vasopressors. Initial fluid boluses (20–40 mL/kg) are necessary with isotonic crystalloid to expand the intravascular space. Patients often require vasopressors, such as dopamine (5–20 µg/kg/min) or epinephrine (0.1–1.0 µg/kg/min) to increase the peripheral vascular resistance and improve myocardial function. Providers should administer antibiotics immediately and not delay them in attempts to obtain cultures; ideally, the provider should obtain blood and urine cultures prior to administering antibiotics but should defer a lumbar puncture in a patient who is clinically unstable. Infants younger than 2 months require ampicillin (200 mg/kg/d) plus either gentamicin

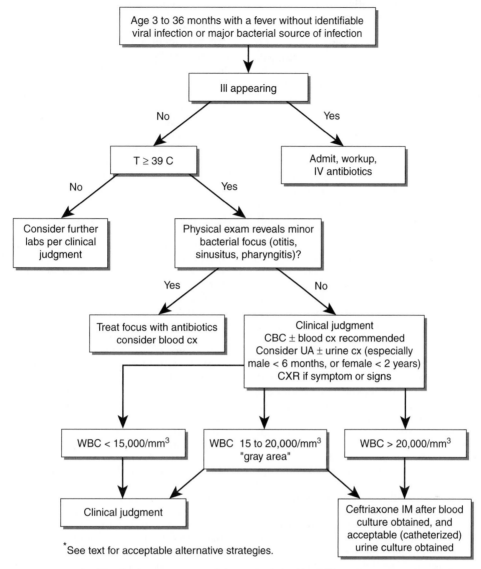

Figure 31–2 ■ Algorithm for the management of the previously healthy child aged 3 to 36 months with fever and no major bacterial source of infection.*

(7.5 mg/kg/d) or cefotaxime (150 mg/kg/d); infants older than 2 months and older children should receive ceftriaxone (100 mg/kg/d) or cefotaxime (150–200 mg/kg/d). Providers should add vancomycin (60 mg/kg/d) to standard antibiotic regimens for all life-threatening infections because of highly resistant strains of *S. pneumoniae*. The laboratory assessment of sepsis includes a CBC with a differential and platelets; electrolytes, glucose, BUN, and creatinine; an arterial blood gas; prothrombin time (PT) and partial thromboplastin time (PTT) (fibrinogen, D-dimer); urinalysis; CSF studies, including cell count, glucose, and protein Gram's stain; cultures of CSF, blood, and urine; rapid diagnostic studies of blood, CSF, and urine (eg, counterimmune electrophoresis, latex particle agglutination); and a chest radiograph. Providers should base the indications for performing these or other studies on the patient's clinical condition and age. Treatment of metabolic acidosis and hypoglycemia may be necessary for stabilization. Monitoring cardiorespiratory status, oxygen saturation, urine output, arterial blood pressure or central venous pressure, and end-tidal CO_2 in intubated patients can facilitate care.

Patients require transport to a pediatric intensive care after stabilization.

SPECIAL CONDITIONS

Fever in HIV-Positive Children

As with other children, febrile HIV-infected children require a thorough history and physical examination. Fever may merely represent simple viral infections of childhood, but many of these children will suffer recurrent and occasionally serious bacterial infections because of their immunodeficiency. Pneumonia, otitis media, sinusitis, adenitis, bacteremia, and skin and soft-tissue infections are common in these children. Additionally, providers must consider opportunistic infections. Knowledge of previous opportunistic infections and information on WBC and CD4 counts may be useful when evaluating the febrile HIV-positive individual. When this information is not readily available, use of prophylactic medications (for the prevention of *Pneumocystis carinii* pneumonia [PCP], *Mycobacterium avium-intracellulare*, and herpes) may be an indirect marker of immune function. Most of these medications are only prescribed when CD4 counts are low or the patient has had previous opportunistic infections. As described previously, the appearance of the child dictates management following a careful history and physical examination.

Evaluation of the Well-Appearing HIV-Positive Child

The evaluation of the well-appearing HIV-positive child begins with trying to identify a source of infection. When the provider can identify a focal bacterial infection, he or she can tailor treatment to that specific condition (eg, inpatient parenteral antibiotics or outpatient oral antibiotics). In the well-appearing child without a specific focus, the appropriateness of the evaluation must consider the increased risk of serious infections, such as pneumococcal bacteremia or disseminated cytomegalovirus. Fortunately, serious viral, bacterial, and opportunistic infections are uncommon among febrile HIV-infected children who appear well. Taking their increased infectious risk into account, the provider should obtain a CBC and blood culture in those with high fever. Providers should culture urine in all young infants and females up to age 2 years. Thereafter, only those with complaints of dysuria or frequency need a urinalysis or urine culture. Those with tachypnea or a relatively elevated leukocyte count should have a chest radiograph even when auscultation indicates clear lung sounds. Patients with WBC counts over 15,000/mm³ or elevated compared to baseline can begin antibiotics, such as amoxicillin, amoxicillin-clavulanic acid (Augmentin), or IM ceftriaxone (Rocephin), pending results of any cultures. As with immunocompetent children, an elevated WBC count should make the clinician reconsider the need for other cultures (eg, throat, urine) or a chest radiograph that was not indicated by history or physical examination alone. Consultation by phone with an infectious disease expert, especially if the patient has routine care from such an individual, may provide insight into the evaluation and follow-up. For these patients without a clear source of infection, daily visits are necessary until improvement is noted. The primary care clinician should be notified if the patient develops new signs or worsens.

Evaluation of the Ill-Appearing HIV-Positive Child With Fever

When ill-appearing, these patients require the same management as any other ill-appearing febrile child. Providers should order cultures of blood and urine immediately. In cases of meningismus or altered mental status, providers should perform a lumbar puncture if the patient is able to withstand the procedure. Broad-spectrum antibiotics (such as ampicillin [400 mg/kg/d every 6 hours] and cefotaxime [150 mg/kg/d every 8 hours] or ceftriaxone [100 mg/kg/d every 12 hours]) should be administered once the cultures are obtained. In those with significant respiratory findings (regardless of the chest radiograph's appearance), trimethoprim-sulfamethoxazole (20 mg/kg/d every 6 hours) should be started for the possibility of PCP. Providers should never delay treatment for PCP for fear of confusing the diagnosis of PCP. Systemic fungal infections are rare in HIV-infected patients but must be considered in those who do not improve, have indwelling central lines, or have been on prolonged courses of parenteral antibiotics.

Chronic Fevers in HIV-Positive Children

Chronic fever is frequent in HIV-infected children. As a first step, providers should conduct blood cultures, CBC, urinalysis, stool cultures, and chest and sinus radiographs to eliminate the possibility of a low-grade bacterial infection. Recurrent otitis media, sinusitis, parotitis, and adenitis can be seen. If the initial evaluation is unrevealing, then providers should consider more unusual infections, such as tuberculosis (especially in adolescents) and Mycobacterium avium-intracellulare. Chronic infections with Epstein-Barr and cytomegalovirus also can be sources of fever. Some children may require inpatient hospitalization for the coordination of their diagnostic evaluations. Of note, drug fever should be a diagnosis of exclusion.

Fever in the Neutropenic Patient

Although malignancy or its treatment can cause fever, fever is especially worrisome when patients are neutropenic because of the risk of serious bacterial infection. In children, absolute neutrophil counts below 500/mm³ define neutropenia. Certainly, patients with malignancy are immunocompromised even without neutropenia, but they require immediate evaluation when neutropenia is present. Serious infection is less likely if the dip in WBC count is expected to be transient after a course of chemotherapy (few days) and more likely in cases where the WBC count is still dropping or expected to be depressed for weeks. Along with the neutropenia, many patients have damages to their normal skin and mucosal barriers serving as portals of entry for pathogens.

Management of the fever begins with a careful history. Neutropenia and chemotherapeutic agents may mask signs of illness. The typical signs of inflammation may be absent without functional leukocytes. Providers must carefully judge any symptoms and seek possible infectious exposures. In addition to the routine physical examination, the provider must evaluate the perianal area, joints, skin, nailbeds, surgical sites, and indwelling catheter site. He or she should obtain blood cultures (including central venous catheters) along with urine and any wound cultures. Chest radiographs should be performed in any patient with respiratory symptoms, including a seemingly innocent cough. Patients do not need a lumbar puncture in the absence of meningeal symptoms because meningitis is rare in cancer patients. However, meningismus may not develop in neutropenic patients; therefore, providers should look for other signs of meningitis, such as altered mental status or headache.

▲ **Clinical Warning:** Patients with fever and neutropenia require empiric, broad-spectrum IV antibiotics and hospitalization at least until the neutropenia resolves.

For patients with previously identified bacterial or fungal infections, additional therapy aimed at those pathogens is justified. Most pathogens come from the patient's endogenous skin flora (*Staphylococcus* and *Streptococci*) and intestine (*E. coli*, *Klebsiella*, *Pseudomonas*, *Enterococcus*, and *Serratia*). Regimens for initial empiric therapy are provided in Table 31-2. Providers should recognize signs of early or compensated shock among these vulnerable patients. Along with their neutropenia, many patients may have anemia or thrombocytopenia that needs correction during the illness. Furthermore, patients who have been on adrenal-suppressive doses of steroids may need stress doses of corticosteroids during their febrile illness. The reader is referred to the table of steroid dosages in Chapter 47.

Table 31–2.   INITIAL EMPIRIC ANTIBIOTIC REGIMENS FOR NEUTROPENIC PATIENTS WITH UNEXPLAINED FEVER

Regimen	Example
Aminoglycoside + antipseudomonal beta-lactam	tobramycin* (5 mg/kg/d ÷ q8°) and ticarcillin (200–300 mg/kg/d ÷ q6°, max 24 g/d)
Third generation cephalosporin + antipseudomonal beta-lactam	cefotaxime (150–200 mg/kg/d ÷ q6–8° max 12 g/d) + piperacillin (250–400 mg/kg/d ÷ q6°, max 24 g/d)
Single drug	ceftazidime (150 mg/kg/d ÷ q8°, max 6 g/d) Or imipenem (50–100 mg/kg/d ÷ q6°, max 4 g/d)
Vancomycin + antipseudomonal beta lactam + aminoglycoside	vancomycin* (40 mg/kg/d ÷ q6°) + piperacillin + amikacin* (15–20 mg/kg/d ÷ q8°)
Vancomycin + third-generation cephalosporin	vancomycin + ceftazidime

*Check levels.

Fever of Undetermined Origin

The term fever of undetermined origin (FUO) has been used to describe the circumstance or condition of a child with fever for 8 days in whom a careful history, repeated physical examinations, and basic laboratory testing have failed to suggest a cause. Providers should refer to and evaluate fever for less than 8 days as fever without a source. The evaluation of children with a fever and no source was discussed in previous sections.

Most children with FUO do not have an exotic or rare disease. Rather, when a cause is identified before complete resolution of fever, the child is found to have one of three problems: an infectious disease, connective tissue disorder, or malignancy. Unfortunately, true FUO is often a serious condition with relatively high mortality rates. (Depending on length of follow-up, mortality rates of 9%–17% have been reported.) Pizzo, Lovejoy and Smith (1975) reviewed 100 cases of FUO (defined as recorded fever of 38.5°C at least four times over 2 weeks) and classified them as 50% infectious, 20% collagen-vascular, and 6% neoplastic, with the balance being miscellaneous conditions (10%) or no diagnosis (12%). McClung (1972) studied 99 children with FUO (defined as longer than 3 weeks outpatient or one week inpatient) and classified them as 29% infectious, 11% collagen-vascular, and 8% neoplastic, with the balance being miscellaneous conditions (11%) or no diagnosis (30%).

Providers should initiate a diagnostic evaluation as an outpatient unless the child appears ill. If the initial workup is unrevealing, further evaluation may require hospitalization. The value of hospitalization is not only for convenience of testing, but also so health care staff can document fever patterns, repeat examinations, coordinate a diagnostic evaluation, and observe the patient. The history should be exhaustive in review of any recent symptoms, exposures, and fever documentation. Elements that are vital to the history are presented in Display 31-3. The physical examination

---

DISPLAY 31–3 • History in Patients With Fever of Undetermined Origin

- Fever: pattern and documentation of temperature technique, equipment, and person's recording the temperatures
- Past medical history, including growth, previous infections, previous hospitalizations, and surgeries
- Medication use, including vitamins and holistic remedies
- Any associated symptoms or signs, even if transient (including weeks before the onset of fever)
- Travel history: include travel of family members; camping, foreign travel, imported goods
- Pets and other animal exposures: farms, house mice, neighborhood animals, zoo visits
- "Occupational" exposures related to field trips, parent's occupation
- Recent insect bites/tick exposures
- Hobbies
- Review of systems (complete)
  - Constitutional symptoms: fever, weight loss, night sweats, fatigue
  - Skin: recent or intermittent rashes, open wounds, lumps, peeling skin, changes in hair
  - Musculoskeletal: arthralgias, myalgias, swelling of joints or whole extremities, painful fingers, color change of extremities (Raynaud's), back pain, stiffness
  - Eyes: photophobia, discharge, visual changes, orbital pain, dry eyes
- Nose: recurrent epistaxis, sores in nares, discharge, sinus drip
- Mouth: ulcers, tender gums, gum bleeding, dental pain or "bad taste" from draining tooth or parotid abscess, halotosis, sore throat, painful swallowing, voice changes
- Neck: swellings, pain
- Breasts: discharge, swelling
- Respiratory: cough, sputum, hemoptysis, chest pain, previous chest radiograph, difficulty breathing, wheezing, foreign body aspiration, or choking episode
- Cardiac: palpitations, syncope, chest pain, exertional dyspnea, orthopnea, lower extremity edema
- Gastrointestinal: difficulty swallowing, anorexia, vomiting, stool pattern and consistency, abdominal pains, flatus, transient jaundice, family history of gallstones
- Genitourinary: frequency, dysuria, hematuria, polyuria, sexual activity
  - Male: testicular swelling, urethral discharge, bloody semen
  - Female: menses, dyspareunia, vaginal discharge, recent pregnancy, last PAP smear
- Neurologic: syncope, dizziness, seizures, weakness or paresthesias, tremors, memory problems
- Endocrine: heat intolerance, excessive sweating, polyuria or polydypsia
- Hematologic: bruisability, pale, epistaxis or gum bleeding, past transfusions

---

DISPLAY 31-4 • Screening Studies in Children With Fever of Undetermined Origin

---

Phase I (most patients need all)

- Complete blood count with differential
- Erythrocyte sedimentation rate
- Liver functions: ALT, AST, bilirubin, alkaline phosphatase, albumin, PT/PTT
- Blood urea nitrogen, creatinine
- Uric acid and LDH
- Blood culture
- Urinalysis (± urine culture, age dependent)
- Chest radiograph
- Tuberculin skin test
- Serologies for specific infections endemic to area
- Stool cultures (bacterial and parasitic studies)

Phase II (consider each test individually)

- Sinus radiographs or computed tomography
- Rheumatoid factor, ANA, complement panel
- Lumbar puncture (save some of specimen for special infectious studies especially if pleocytosis; consider cytology)
- Bone marrow aspiration (consult infectious disease service and oncology for testing)
- Abdominal ultrasound or computed tomography
- HIV serology
- Gallium scan
- Bone scan

ALT = alanine aminotransferase; AST = aspartate transaminase; PT/PTT = prothrombin time; PTT = partial thromboplastin time; LDH = lactate dehydrogenase; ANA = anti-nuclear antibody.

---

also should be extensive. Findings often neglected include complete examination of the skin, digits (including nailbeds), small joints, fundi, perineum, rectum, genitalia, breasts, and spine. One of the most important aspects of investigating FUOs is to pursue and completely investigate any clues revealed in the history or found on physical examination.

When the history or physical examination is suggestive of a particular problem, providers should tailor further investigation to the presumed condition. When the history and physical examination are unrevealing, however, clinicians must use screening tests (Display 31-4). Additionally, providers always must consider factitious fevers as part of the differential diagnosis. They must consider parents and other caregivers as a cause, and older patients themselves have been known to fabricate fever even under close observation. Etiologies for FUO are presented in Display 31-5.

Kawasaki Disease (Mucocutaneous Lymph Node Syndrome)

Kawasaki disease (KD) is an acute, febrile, self-limited, multisystem illness of unknown origin. It is generally a disease of young children (mean age 1–2 years, range 6 weeks–13 years) and results in serious cardiac sequelae in 20% of patients, including myocardial infarction, arrythmias, and carditis. The underlying pathology is a vasculitis mainly involving the medium-sized, extraparenchymal vessels, with a predilection for the coronary arteries. The coronary aneurysms typically develop 4 to 8 weeks after the onset of

the illness, although coronary artery changes may be seen at the time of diagnosis. Males who are younger than 1 year appear to be at highest risk for cardiac aneurysms. Fortunately, early recognition and prompt treatment of KD can dramatically diminish the risk of life-threatening cardiac sequelae.

Diagnosis and Course

Diagnosis is based on a constellation of clinical findings that may not be present simultaneously and have variable onset and duration. Providers must therefore appreciate the course of the illness and its hallmark features. Display 31-6 lists the diagnostic criteria for KD. Other suggestive but nondiagnostic findings associated with KD are listed in Display 31-7. Additionally, increasing numbers of atypical cases of KD (missing one or more criteria) are being recognized, especially in infants younger than 6 months (Rosenfeld, Corydon, & Shulman, 1995).

● **Clinical Pearl:** In all patients with prolonged fever, providers must strongly consider the possibility of KD.

Given the nonspecific signs and nondiagnostic laboratory findings, the differential diagnosis for patients is lengthy (Display 31-8). Signs that usually point away from a diagnosis of KD include exudative conjunctivitis, discrete oral lesions, diffuse adenopathy or splenomegaly, and bullous or vesicular skin lesions. Besides the physical examination, providers should include the following studies in the initial evaluation: CBC with a differential, sedimentation rate, urinalysis, electrolytes, liver profile, chest radiograph, electrocardiogram, and echocardiogram. Providers should not delay treatment when they cannot obtain an echocardiogram immediately.

The course of illness has been divided into three clinical phases: acute, subacute, and convalescent. The acute or febrile phase usually lasts 7 to 15 days and is the period when most diagnostic findings are present. After resolution of the fever, the subacute phase begins and continues for 10 to 25 days. During the subacute phase, the remaining acute symptoms resolve, but coronary aneurysms, hydrops of the gallbladder, and thrombocytosis tend to develop. Additionally, desquamation of the fingers and toes usually occurs during the subacute phase (although desquamation in the perineal area may occur during the acute phase). The convalescent phase begins following complete resolution of all clinical signs and continues until all laboratory parameters normalize (often 6–10 weeks). Complications of KD are listed in Display 31-9.

Treatment and Outcome

Although an infectious etiology has been suspected because of the epidemiology, trials of antibiotics have had no effect on the course of the illness or its sequelae. Initial attempts at using steroids have resulted in increased coronary aneurysms; therefore, they are currently contraindicated in the disease.

Immunoglobulin (IV as a single dose of 2 g/kg over 10–12 hours) has dramatically improved all clinical parameters and greatly reduced coronary aneurysms in short- and long-term follow-up (4%–5%). Its mechanisms are not exactly understood. Side effects are relatively uncommon but include allergic reactions, fever, chills, headache, transfusion reactions, and pulmonary edema requiring diuretics (due to myocardial dysfunction associated with KD). Approximately 80% of patients become afebrile within 24 to 48 hours

DISPLAY 31–5 • Etiologies of Fever of Undetermined Origin in Children

Infectious
  Common causes of occult, localized infection presenting as FUO
    Sinusitus
    Pharyngeal abscesses
    Mastoiditis
    Dental abscesses
    Urinary tract infection
    Subdiaphragmatic abscess
    Retroperitoneal abscess
    Intra-abdominal abscess
    Hepatic abscess
    Pelvic inflammatory disease
    Pelvic abscess
    Perinephric abscess
    Osteomyelitis
    Endocarditis
  Systemic infections
    Bacterial
      Tuberculosis
      Brucellosis
      Tularemia
      Leptospirosis
      Salmonellosis
      Syphillis
      Lyme disease
      Erlichiosis
    Viral
      Human immunodeficiency virus
      Epstein-Barr virus
      Cytomegalovirus
      Hepatitis viruses
      Rat-bite fever
    Rickettsial disease
      Q fever
      Rocky mountain spotted fever

Parasitic
  Malaria
  Toxoplasmosis
Chlamydial
  Lymphogranuloma venereum
  Psittacosis
Fungal
  Blastomycosis
  Histoplasmosis
Connective tissue disorders
  Juvenile rheumatoid arthritis
  Systemic lupus erythematosus
  Sarcoidosis
  Polyarteritis nodosa
  Inflammatory bowel disease
Malignancy
  Lymphoma
  Leukemia
  Neuroblastoma
  Sarcoma
Miscellaneous
  Factitious fever
  Diabetes insipidus
  Hypothalamic lesion
  Ectodermal dysplasia
  Familial dysautonomia
  Pancreatitis
  Serum sickness
  Thryrotoxicosis
  Histiocytosis
  Behçet's disease
  Familial mediterranean fever
  Immunodeficiencies without infection

of their immunoglobulin infusion. Those who remain febrile or have recrudescence of fever may need further treatments. Patients who require subsequent infusions of IV immunoglobulin (because of persistent or recurrent symptoms) have a higher chance of aneurysm formation.

DISPLAY 31–6 • The Diagnosis of Kawasaki Disease

1. Fever persisting for 5 days or more, and
2. At least four of the following findings:
   • Bilateral, nonexudative conjunctivitis
   • Polymorphous rash: morbilliform, maculopapular, or scarletiniform
   • Cervical adenopathy (>1.5 cm)—unilateral or bilateral
   • Oropharyngeal changes:
     — Erythema and cracking of lips
     — Hyperemia of oropharynx
     — Strawberry tongue
   • Erythema and swelling of the hands and feet
   • Desquamation of rash especially hands and feet
3. Findings not explained by another disease process

Anti-inflammatory doses of aspirin are recommended for the acute phase (80–100 mg/kg/d divided every 6 hours) and then changed to antithrombotic doses in the subacute phase (3–5 mg/kg/d). Aspirin is the only recommended anti-inflammatory agent and is usually discontinued when the platelet count normalizes. Management is summarized in Figure 31-3. Parents should call their provider if the child develops varicella or a flulike illness while taking aspirin because of the association with Reye's syndrome.

Fever and Petechial Rash

Providers must urgently evaluate patients with fever and petechial rash for sepsis. Although petechiae are most often seen with benign viral illness and streptococcal pharyngitis (Mandl, Stack, & Fleisher, 1997), a petechial rash also can be a marker for invasive bacterial disease, the prototype being *N. meningitidis*. Although facial petechiae are seen with coughing, forceful vomiting, or even screaming, clinicians need to consider invasive bacterial disease.

▲ **Clinical Warning:** All patients with fever and petechiae require a careful examination to exclude signs of systemic illness and meningitis. If the patient has signs of poor perfusion, unexplained tachycardia, or a rapidly progressive rash, the provider should initiate aggressive intervention immediately as described for sepsis.

DISPLAY 31–7 • Nondiagnostic Clinical Findings With Kawasaki Disease

Central nervous system
  Irritability
  Meningitis
  Sensorineural hearing loss
Ocular
  Photophobia
  Iritis
  Uveitis
Cardiac
  Coronary aneurysm
  Pericardial effusion
  Myocarditis
  ECG changes: prolonged PR or QT intervals, ST-T wave
    changes
  Gallop rhythm
  Valvular insufficiency
  Dysrhythmias
  Aortic aneurysm
Respiratory
  Cough
  Rhinorrhea
  Infiltrate
Gastrointestinal
  Diarrhea
  Vomiting
  Abdominal pain
  Gallbladder hydrops
  Elevated liver transaminases
  Mild jaundice
Genitourinary
  Dysuria
  Urethritis
  Sterile pyuria (WBCs on microurinalysis, leukocyte
    esterase negative)
  Proteinuria
Musculoskeletal
  Arthralgia
  Arthritis
Hematologic
  Anemia
  Thrombocytosis (after 7–10 days of illness)
  Elevated WBC count with left shift
  Elevated ESR
  Elevated C-reactive protein

ECG = electrocardiogram; WBC = white blood cells; ESR = erythrocyte sedimentation rate.

DISPLAY 31–8 • Differential Diagnosis of Kawasaki Disease

Viral
  Measles
  Adenovirus
  Rubella
  Epstein-Barr virus
  Enteroviruses
Bacterial
  Toxic shock syndrome (*Staphylococcus, Streptococcus*)
  Scarlet fever (*Streptococcus*)
Drug reactions
  Stevens-Johnson syndrome
Rheumatologic
  Juvenile rheumatoid arthritis

DISPLAY 31–9 • Complications of Kawasaki Disease

- Coronary aneurysms
- Dysrhythmias
- Sudden death—rupture of aneurysms or dysrhythmias
- Valvular insufficiency
- Congestive heart failure
- Myocardial infarction
- Pericardial effusion
- Large artery aneurysms
- Hydrops of gallbladder

---

than 5000 or greater than 15,000 or those with a progressive rash require admission and IV antibiotics. If the patient has any clinical deterioration or develops purpura, he or she should be admitted to a pediatric intensive care unit. Patients who appear well after several hours of observation, have only a few petechiae (which have not changed in number during observation), and normal laboratory values may be discharged home with strict instructions regarding follow-up and reasons to seek care. Many clinicians choose to give a parenteral dose of antibiotics, such as ceftriaxone, pending culture results.

▲ **Clinical Warning:** Administration of empiric antibiotic treatment to a well-appearing child with petechiae and fever is not a replacement for close and careful clinical observation over a period of hours.

Fever and Erythroderma

Providers should evaluate patients with fever and an erythroderma (diffuse macular erythema, often termed "sunburn-like") for the presence of toxin-producing *S. pyogenes* (group A *Streptococcus*) and *S. aureus*. Both organisms can produce a toxic shock syndrome. Occasionally, streptococcal pharyngitis can produce an impressive scarletinaform rash in well-appearing children, but providers must aggressively evaluate and manage patients with systemic symptoms of poor perfusion. Any child with alterations in mental status, unexplained tachycardia, acidosis, or abnormal liver or renal function requires hospitalization for IV antibiotics and monitoring. Focal infections with these bacteria may be identified.

▲ **Clinical Warning:** In the well-appearing patient with fever and petechiae, the evaluation should include a CBC with differential and platelet count, blood culture, throat culture, and PT/PTT (as a screen for early disseminated intravascular coagulation). Following this evaluation, observing the child for several hours for the progression of the rash or possible clinical deterioration is imperative.

Children younger than 1 year should be considered for a lumbar puncture because of the difficulties in assessing meningitis in infants. Patients with abnormal laboratory results, specifically thrombocytopenia or WBC counts less

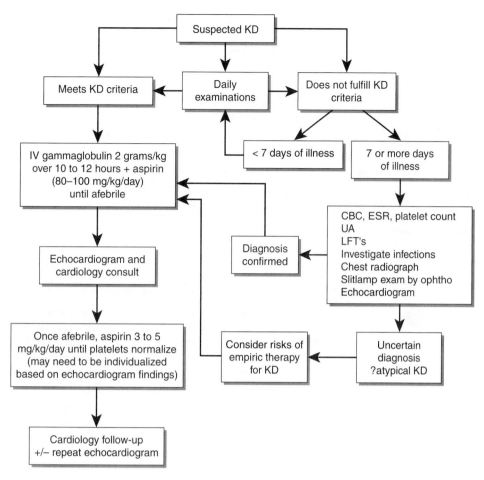

Figure 31–3 ■ The management of Kawasaki disease.

Reevaluation of the Patient With a Positive Blood Culture

All patients with proven bacteremia require reevaluation. Those who return to the provider's office ill or with serious focal infections need admission for IV antibiotics. Any patient with *H. influenzae* or *N. meningitidis* bacteremia requires a lumbar puncture and admission for parenteral antibiotics regardless of how well he or she appears. If a child with *S. pneumoniae* bacteremia returns afebrile and appears well, he or she can be discharged on a 10-day course of oral amoxicillin (plus or minus a dose of ceftriaxone) and close follow-up. If the patient with pneumococcal bacteremia initially was treated with antibiotics and returns febrile, he or she needs a careful examination to detect any new focal infections. The provider then should seriously consider lumbar puncture, a repeat blood culture, and admission for IV antibiotics. When *S. pneumoniae* bacteremia is identified in patients who were not treated with antibiotics at the initial visit, the diagnostic evaluation and treatment need to be based on the child's age, temperature at reevaluation, and whether any new foci have developed. Clinicians also must factor antibiotic resistance into decisions regarding treatment of pneumococcal bacteremia. The management of outpatients recalled for a positive blood culture is summarized in Figure 31-4.

Fever in Sickle Cell Anemia Patients

A combination of early autoinfarction of the spleen and impaired immunologic function places patients with sickle cell disease (SCD) at high risk for sepsis and other serious infections (eg, pneumonia, meningitis, septic arthritis, osteomyelitis). In these patients, the estimated risk for sepsis is several hundred times higher than in normal children (Fleisher & Ludwig, 1999). As with other patients with functional asplenia, encapsulated bacteria are the predominant pathogens. *S. pneumoniae* and *H. influenzae* are more common in young children, and *Salmonella* and *E. coli* cause more cases of bacteremia in older children. The greatest risk occurs between ages 6 months and 3 years when maternal antibody disappears, protective antibodies have not yet developed, and splenic function is minimal or absent. Immunization to *H. influenzae* and *Pneumococcus* and prophylactic penicillin can help reduce but certainly do not eliminate the risk.

When significant focal bacterial infections are identified in patients with SCD, IV antibiotics and hospitalization are necessary. In patients with fever and no clear major source of bacterial infection, the evaluation should include a CBC and blood culture.

● **Clinical Pearl:** Children with chronic hemolysis, such as SCD, may normally have elevated WBC counts, which

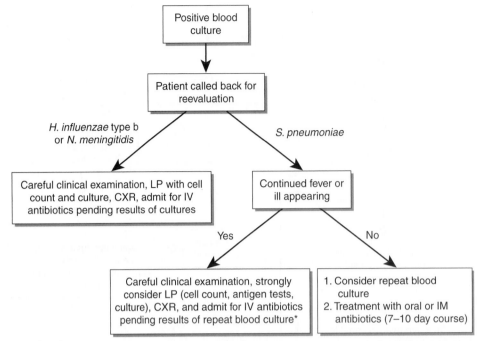

*well appearing children > 6 months old with low-grade fever may be managed as outpatients.
[LP = lumbar puncture, CXR = chest radiograph]

Figure 31–4 ■ Evaluation of a patient with a positive blood culture.

providers need to compare to baseline values for interpretation.

Additionally, increased hemolysis can occur during any illness and therefore must be addressed as part of fever evaluation. Providers should consider lumbar puncture in young or ill-appearing infants regardless of meningeal signs. They should consider chest radiographs in those with cough, tachypnea, or very high fever, even in the presence of a normal chest examination. Patients younger than 3 years and some older patients with high fever (39°C) often require hospitalization for observation and antibiotics pending cultures. An alternative approach for managing well-appearing febrile children at low risk for bacteremia (based on examination and laboratory findings, CBC, and blood culture) is to administer a long-acting cephalosporin (eg, ceftriaxone) and to discharge the patient with a clear follow-up plan for the next day or earlier based on change in condition (Wilimas et al., 1993). Patients who cannot be observed appropriately by caregivers or are unlikely to follow through with subsequent visits require hospital admission.

EDUCATING PARENTS

Clinicians should not underestimate the value of educating parents about fever regardless of the etiology. Fever phobia is entrenched in our culture because many parents have heard of or witnessed the association of fever with life-threatening illness. Some parents worry about brain damage or seizures; others will be petrified by the delirium or lethargy that fever sometimes causes. High fevers imply serious illness to parents, who therefore demand a "quick fix" unless they are properly educated. Explanation of the presumed cause and reasons to call or seek medical attention are vital to the child's subsequent care. When seeing a child

with even an innocuous viral URI, clinicians should not dismiss the family with the statement, "It's just a virus." If possible, they should name the illness and outline its anticipated course and duration. Clinicians should discuss supportive measures, such as fever management. They should advise the family when to return for reevaluation of worsening or persistent symptoms.

Any intervention that encourages communication between family and clinician will lead to better care. As a corollary, poor communication will undermine future encounters and establish barriers to care. When communication is lacking and initially unrecognized infections progress or new secondary foci develop, parents will assume maltreatment. As part of education, the primary care practitioner's efforts to review the reason for the fever, dosing and administration of antipyretics, and proper technique of sponge bathing will decrease parental anxiety and minimize unnecessary visits and phone calls.

REFERENCES

Alario, A. J., Nelson, E. W., & Shapiro, E. D. (1989). Blood cultures in the management of febrile outpatients later found to have bacteremia. *Journal of Pediatrics, 115*(2), 195–199.

Bachur, R., Perry, H., & Harper, M. (1999). Empiric chest radiographs in febrile children with leukocytosis [In Process Citation]. *Annals of Emergency Medicine, 33*(4), 480.

Baker, R. C., Tiller, T., Bausher, J. C., Bellet, P. S., Cotton, W. H., Finley, A. H., Lenane, A. M., McHenry, C., Perez, K. K., Shapiro, R. A., et al. (1989). Severity of disease correlated with fever reduction in febrile infants. *Pediatrics, 83*(6), 1016–1019.

Baraff, L. J., & Lee, S. I. (1992). Fever without source: Management of children 3 to 36 months of age. [Review]. *Pediatric Infectious Disease Journal, 11*(2), 146–151.

Baraff, L. J., Oslund, S. A., Schriger, D. L., & Stephen, M. L. (1992). Probability of bacterial infections in febrile infants less than three months of age: A meta-analysis. *Pediatric Infectious Disease Journal, 11*(4), 257–264.

Baron, M. A., & Fink, H. D. (1980). Bacteremia in private pediatric practice. *Pediatrics, 66*(2), 171–175.

Baskin, M. N., O'Rourke, E. J., & Fleisher, G. R. (1992). Outpatient treatment of febrile infants 28 to 89 days of age with intramuscular administration of ceftriaxone [see comments]. *Journal of Pediatrics, 120*(1), 22–27.

Baskin, M. N., O'Rourke, E. J., & Fleisher, G. R. (1994). Management of febrile infants 15 to 28 days of age with parenteral ceftriaxone and 24 hours of inpatient observation. *Archives of Pediatrics & Adolescent Medicine, 148*(4), 49.

Bratton, L., Teele, D. W., & Klein, J. O. (1977). Outcome of unsuspected pneumococcemia in children not initially admitted to the hospital. *Journal of Pediatrics, 90*(5), 703–706.

Dershewitz, R. A., Wigder, H. N., Wigder, C. M., & Nadelman, D. H. (1983). A comparative study of the prevalence, outcome, and prediction of bacteremia in children. *Journal of Pediatrics, 103*(3), 352–358.

Fleisher, G. R., & Ludwig, S. (1999). *Textbook of pediatric emergency medicine* (4th ed.). Philadelphia: Lippincott Williams & Wilkins.

Fleisher, G. R., Rosenberg, N., Vinci, R., Steinberg, J., Powell, K., Christy, C., Boenning, D. A., Overturf, G., Jaffe, D., & Platt, R. (1994). Intramuscular versus oral antibiotic therapy for the prevention of meningitis and other bacterial sequelae in young, febrile children at risk for occult bacteremia [see comments]. *Journal of Pediatrics, 124*(4), 504–512.

Green, S. M., & Rothrock, S. G. (1999). Evaluation styles for well-appearing febrile children: Are you a "risk-minimizer" or a "test-minimizer"? [editorial; comment]. *Annals of Emergency Medicine, 33*(2), 211–214.

Greenes, D. S., & Harper, M. B. (1999). Low risk of bacteremia in febrile children with recognizable viral syndromes. *Pediatric Infectious Disease Journal, 18*(3), 258–261.

Harper, M. B., Bachur, R., & Fleisher, G. R. (1995). Effect of antibiotic therapy on the outcome of outpatients with unsuspected bacteremia. *Pediatric Infectious Disease Journal, 14*(9), 760–767.

Harper, M. B., & Fleisher, G. R. (1993). Occult bacteremia in the 3-month-old to 3-year-old age group. [Review]. *Pediatric Annals, 22*(8), 487–493.

Hoberman, A., Wald, E. R., Reynolds, E. A., Penchansky, L., & Charron, M. (1994). Pyuria and bacteriuria in urine specimens obtained by catheter from young children with fever [see comments]. *Journal of Pediatrics, 124*(4), 513–519.

Jaffe, D. M., & Fleisher, G. R. (1991). Temperature and total white blood cell count as indicators of bacteremia. *Pediatrics, 87*(5), 670–674.

Jaffe, D. M., Tanz, R. R., Davis, A. T., Henretig, F., & Fleisher, G.
(1987). Antibioticadministration to treat possible occult bacteremia in febrile children. *New England Journal of Medicine, 317*(19), 1175–1180.

Korones, D. N., Marshall, G. S., & Shapiro, E. D. (1992). Outcome of children with occult bacteremia caused by Haemophilus influenzae type b. *Pediatric Infectious Disease Journal, 11*(7), 516–520.

Krauss, B. S., Harakal, T., & Fleisher, G. R. (1991). The spectrum and frequency of illness presenting to a pediatric emergency department. *Pediatric Emergency Care, 7*(2), 67–71.

Kuppermann, N., Fleisher, G. R., & Jaffe, D. M. (1998). Predictors of occult pneumococcal bacteremia in young febrile children. *Annals of Emergency Medicine, 31*(6), 679–687.

Lee, G. M., & Harper, M. B. (1998). Risk of bacteremia for febrile young children in the post-Haemophilus influenzae type b era. *Archives of Pediatric and Adolescent Medicine, 152*(7), 624–628.

Mandl, K. D., Stack, A. M., & Fleisher, G. R. (1997). Incidence of bacteremia in infants and children with fever and petechia. *Journal of Pediatrics, 131*(3), 398–404.

McCarthy, P. L., Jekel, J. F., & Dolan, T., Jr. (1977). Temperature greater than or equal to 40 C in children less than 24 months of age: A prospective study. *Pediatrics, 59*(5), 663–668.

McClung, H. J. (1972). Prolonged fever of unknown origin in children. *American Journal of Diseases of Children, 124*(4), 544–550.

Murray, D. L., Zonana, J., Seidel, J. S., Yoshimori, R. N., Imagawa, D. T., & St. Geme, J. (1981). Relative importance of bacteremia and viremia in the course of acute fevers of unknown origin in outpatient children. *Pediatrics, 68*(2), 157–160.

Nelson, D. S., Walsh, K., & Fleisher, G. R. (1992). Spectrum and frequency of pediatric illness presenting to a general community hospital emergency department. *Pediatrics, 90*(1 Pt 1), 5–10.

Pizzo, P. A., Lovejoy, F., Jr., & Smith, D. H. (1975). Prolonged fever in children: Review of 100 cases. *Pediatrics, 55*(4), 468–473.

Rosenfeld, E. A., Corydon, K. E., & Shulman, E. T. (1995). Kawasaki disease in infants less than one year of age. *Journal of Pediatrics, 126*(4), 524–529.

Shapiro, E. D., Aaron, N. H., Wald, E. R., & Chiponis, D. (1986). Risk factors for development of bacterial meningitis among children with occult bacteremia. *Journal of Pediatrics, 109*(1), 15–19.

Wilimas, J. A., Flynn, P. M., Harris, S., Day, S. W., Smith, R., Chesney, P. J., Rodman, J. H., Eguiguren, J. M., Fairclough, D. L., & Wang, W. C. (1993). A randomized study of outpatient treatment with ceftriaxone for selected febrile children with sickle cell disease [see comments]. *New England Journal of Medicine, 329*(7), 472–476.

CHAPTER 32

Eye Problems

- MICHELE McLEOD, MD

INTRODUCTION

Children with acute ocular problems frequently present with irritated eyes and nonspecific symptoms. The eye's anatomic considerations and the limited resources available to respond to ocular insult account for the sometimes frustratingly similar appearances of disparate entities. Therefore, the clinician must take a good history, elicit appropriate signs and symptoms, and form a reasonable differential diagnosis to separate minor eye problems from serious ocular processes that may lead to permanent visual disability. This chapter is intended to guide the reader toward the clinical signs and symptoms that, along with a careful history and physical examination, differentiate the two. When in doubt, providers immediately should refer patients to specialists. Reference to texts on pediatric ophthalmology for further detailed information is encouraged (Nelson, 1998; Taylor, 1997; Wright, 1995).

ANATOMY, PHYSIOLOGY, AND PATHOLOGY

Despite its relatively small size, the eye is one of the most complex organs of the human body. It is derived from neural crest cells, neuroectoderm, surface ectoderm, and mesoderm. The white tissue of the eye, the sclera, is a rigid connective tissue that encloses intraocular contents except at the anterior and posterior poles, where it meets the cornea and optic nerve respectively.

Conjunctiva, a diaphanous tissue that lines the inner aspect of the eyelids (tarsal conjunctiva) and reflects in the fornices to cover the sclera (bulbar conjunctiva), consists of an outer epithelial layer and underlying loose connective tissue. As a result of its rich vascularization, the conjunctiva can demonstrate dramatic injection and edema (chemosis) in response to irritation, allergies, or infection. Goblet cells within the conjunctiva secrete the mucous component of the tear film.

The cornea (more specifically, the air-tear film interface) is responsible for approximately two thirds of the eye's refractive power. Although like the sclera, the cornea is composed primarily of connective tissue (with outer epithelial and inner endothelial layers), it is transparent. This transparency is attributable to the unique characteristic arrangement of type I collagen fibrils in a regular array held in place by a proteoglycan ground substance. When damaged, corneal stroma undergoes further deposition of type I collagen; however, this secondary process occurs without fibrillar organization, and opacification (scarring) of corneal stroma occurs. When the cornea is not clear, this indicates that a pathologic event has occurred or is occurring.

Extraocular muscles attach to the globe underneath the conjunctiva and act as pulleys to effect ocular rotations. Each extraocular muscle is yoked with a muscle in the other eye, causing complementary binocular function. Strabismus (referred to in older literature as "squint" because of the tendency of individuals with strabismus to close one eye to suppress double vision) occurs when the two eyes no longer are acting in conjunction.

The eyelids and structures contained within it are derived primarily from surface ectoderm. A simplified schematic approach to eyelid anatomy would divide the eyelid into two segments (anterior/external and posterior/internal) separated by a thin fibrous structure, the orbital septum. The anatomic segments external to the septum consist of skin, loose subcutaneous connective tissue in which eyelash follicles originate, and orbicularis oculi muscle. Internal to the septum lie the levator muscle, tarsus, Müller's muscle, and tarsal conjunctiva. The lax connective tissue of the eyelid creates the potential for impressive eyelid swelling in response to infection, inflammation, trauma, allergy, and so forth. The orbital septum is noteworthy because it divides superficial processes that involve primarily skin from deeper processes that involve the orbit, with potential for damage to the globe and spread through orbital fissures to the intracranial space.

Both segments of the eyelid contain sebaceous glands that contribute to the lipid component of the trilayered tear film. Zeis' glands are associated with cilia (eyelashes), and meibomian glands located within tarsus excrete secretions through orifices in the inner eyelid margin.

The nasolacrimal system consists of inflow and outflow components. The lacrimal gland, a bilobed exocrine gland located under the temporal upper eyelid, produces aqueous secretions in response to reflex and psychogenic stimuli. Basal aqueous secretions are produced by the eccrine glands of Wolfring and Krause located adjacent to tarsus in the eyelids.

The nasolacrimal outflow tract originates at the inferior and superior puncta of the nasal aspect of the eyelids. They open into the superior and inferior canaliculi, which join to form a common canaliculus that opens into the lacrimal sac. The nasolacrimal duct exits the sac inferiorly and ends at the inferior meatus under the inferior turbinate within the nose. Tears (and topical medications) are eliminated through this canalicular and duct system. Richly vascularized nasal mucosa provides the route for systemic absorption (and possible systemic toxicity) of topical medications.

HISTORY AND PHYSICAL EXAMINATION

Primary care providers conduct pediatric eye examinations under two circumstances: during well child examinations and for episodic complaints. Primary care providers can glean information from a well child examination that point to the need for further evaluation, such as amblyopia, strabismus, and ocular pathology (ie, congenital cataracts or glaucoma).

An age-appropriate visual acuity is the essential first step in any eye examination (exception: chemical injury). Visual acuity should be checked separately for each eye. Objection to occlusion of one eye, but not the other, strongly suggests poor vision in the eye the child does not object to being covered. Children should be encouraged to read the chart despite faltering. Children with an amblyopic eye will frequently use the "occluded" contralateral eye by peeking through fingers or through extreme head positions to please the examiner. Children should be carefully monitored while reading the eye chart, because this is an excellent opportunity to pick up amblyopia.

Appropriate visual acuity varies with age. Infants up to 6 to 8 weeks of age typically avoid light. From the age of approximately 2 months, children should be able to fix and follow targets. Older children should demonstrate steady, central fixation on a target and maintain fixation with that eye when the other eye is uncovered (regardless of whether the occluded eye is straight or deviated). Some 2-year-old children may be able to read a picture chart, but by the age of 3 or 4 a child should be able to distinguish familiar pictures on the chart. Visual acuity of 20/30 is appropriate at this age. Asymmetric visual acuity or obvious disparity in ease while reading the chart is a clue to refractive error and possible amblyopia.

A penlight should be used to examine the eyelids, conjunctiva/sclera, cornea, anterior chamber, and iris. The eyes should appear symmetric; asymmetry suggests pathology. A penlight should also be used to assess the pupils both for afferent pupillary defect and similar size. The red reflex should be assessed in infants; in toddlers, the optic nerve and macula should be inspected with the direct ophthalmoscope. A white reflex is always pathologic and is associated with intraocular pathology (retinoblastoma, cataract, persistent hyperplastic primary vitreous, Coats' disease, etc.). Asymmetric retinal reflex may be caused by strabismus or by intraocular pathology.

Extraocular movements (horizontal and vertical) should be full and nonpainful.

The Bruckner (retinal light reflex) and Hirschberg's (corneal light reflex) tests may be used to screen for strabismus. Using a direct ophthalmoscope, the examiner can stand about a foot from the child and assess the red (retinal) reflex. If one red reflex is brighter than the other, either the eye with brighter reflex is deviating or intraocular pathology is present. A penlight directed at the child's eyes from a similar distance should reveal a spot of light in the pupillary space (corneal reflex) displaced slightly temporally (because the child is accommodating and converging) and appearing symmetric in placement. Asymmetric corneal reflexes suggest that one eye is deviating. These tests and observation of the child usually are adequate to evaluate for alignment. However, strabismus may be intermittent or subtle and may be uncovered during a more comprehensive ophthalmologic examination under cycloplegia and using cover testing.

● **Clinical Pearl:** Parents are excellent observers. When they report strabismus, it would be prudent to refer the child to an ophthalmologist even if a child appears orthophoric by the testing described above.

When a child presents with a specific complaint (infection, injury), a more focused examination should be carried out, but the importance of always obtaining a visual acuity, carefully assessing the anterior segment and posterior pole, checking for full extraocular movements, and ruling out an acute strabismus cannot be stressed enough. These are the minimum components of an examination when pathology is suspected, and further components of the examination depending on presentation are addressed below.

MANAGEMENT

As a general rule, management of ocular complaints related by a parent through a phone conversation may be difficult because parents often have difficulty with a precise description of the eye's appearance. If the decision is made to manage an ocular complaint over the phone, the child should be evaluated within a day, unless there is significant improvement. If a child's ocular problem does not improve after several days of initial management by a primary care practitioner, referral to an ophthalmologist should follow.

▲ **Clinical Warning:** Complaints of foreign body sensation, photophobia, or visual acuity impairment should be referred without delay to a pediatric or general ophthalmologist.

BLEPHARITIS

Pathology

Blepharitis is associated with staphylococcal colonization of the eyelids. Poor attention to eyelid hygiene contributes to the problem. Collarettes and accumulation of debris occur around the bases of eyelashes, secondary to inflammation or infection that involves the eyelid margins.

History and Physical Examination

Patients with blepharitis usually present with nonspecific complaints of irritated, itchy eyes; eyelids stuck closed in the morning; and white discharge. An examination shows crusting around eyelashes and injection of eyelid margins, and in chronic blepharitis, poliosis (whitening) or madarosis (loss) of cilia may occur. This usually is bilateral but may be asymmetric.

Blepharitis may be associated with conjunctivitis (blepharoconjunctivitis) or with a staphylococcal hypersensitivity reaction that causes tiny corneal stromal opacities. Blepharitis is often accompanied by meibomianitis, inflammation of meibomian glands, which causes meibomian dysfunction and plugging of meibomian pores along the eyelid margins. This secondarily impairs the basal lubrication of the globe and may contribute to dry eye symptoms.

Diagnostic Criteria

The diagnosis of blepharitis is made based on history of itchy eyes with morning crusting and examination of the eyelid margins. Unlike allergic conjunctivitis, blepharitis is not associated with significant eyelid edema after manipulation, patient history of atopy or asthma, and patient or family history of environmental allergies. Seasonal recurrences are useful in differentiating the two.

Management

Good lid hygiene is essential for treatment of this condition. This consists of mechanical and pharmacologic therapy. Parents should be instructed to apply frequent warm compresses to cleanse the eyelids and to gently run a moist cotton applicator along eyelid margins to dislodge crusting around eyelashes and plugs on meibomian orifices. Erythromycin or bacitracin ophthalmic ointment can be applied to the eyelid margins twice a day. Blepharitis should improve with this therapy, and children who do not respond should be referred for further management to a pediatric ophthalmologist. Blepharitis is a chronic condition, and once the acute problem has resolved, continued daily use of warm compresses to cleanse the eyelid margins helps prevent flareups.

CHALAZIA AND STYES

Pathology

The term hordeola refers to inflammatory or infectious blockage of pores of sebaceous glands in the eyelids. The term external hordeolum, often called by the lay term "stye," is a blockage of Zeis glands associated with eyelash follicles. Internal hordeola, or chalazia, occur when the meibomian orifices, which line the inner aspect of the eyelid margins, become occluded. On histopathologic examination, chalazia consist of a lipogranulomatous reaction. Children with blepharitis and meibomianitis are particularly prone to developing chalazia and styes.

History and Physical Examination

The history will depend on chronicity. Typically, parents will either describe an acute discrete eyelid swelling or a nodule that has been present for weeks or months, which may be accompanied by periodic purulent discharge and changes in size. On examination, styes are swollen at the edge of the eyelid, while chalazia are discrete firm nodules adjacent to the eyelid margin. There may be focal "pointing" on the tarsal conjunctival aspect of the lesion. Both styes and chalazia may be inflamed and tender. If chronic, they may be associated with overlying skin changes. Multiple chalazia and styes may occur and can be impressive in size.

Diagnostic Criteria

As described previously, styes and chalazia are characteristic in appearance. They occur at the eyelid margin, and the swelling and inflammation are well demarcated. If these lesions are associated with diffuse or spreading eyelid warmth and inflammation or systemic symptoms, such as fever or malaise, it may indicate progression to a cellulitis (see below).

Management

Conservative therapy, consisting of frequent warm compresses, usually is effective in eradicating chalazia and styes. Recalcitrant chalazia can be treated by an ophthalmologist with incision and drainage. Although this simple office procedure is performed under local anesthesia in adults, most children cannot tolerate the injection of local anesthetic and lid clamping that the procedure requires. Because this procedure risks perforation of the globe in unsedated children, pediatric chalazion incision and drainage necessitates a trip to the operating room under general anesthesia. Therefore, committed conservative therapy by far is the best approach. Some children are predisposed to developing chalazia, and ongoing good lid hygiene should be encouraged. Because the eye itself usually is not involved, eyedrops are not help-

ful unless the eye is injected. If there is associated blepharitis, one may augment the warm compresses with erythromycin or bacitracin ophthalmic ointment, but parents should understand that the warm compresses, not the medication, will eliminate the hordeola.

Diffuse eyelid erythema, warmth, and tenderness indicate progression to a preseptal cellulitis that will require systemic antibiotics.

CELLULITIS (PRESEPTAL AND ORBITAL)

When cellulitis involves the periocular area, it is critical to distinguish infection limited to superficial skin tissues anterior to the orbital septum (preseptal, also referred to as periorbital, cellulitis) from the far more dangerous infection that involves orbital tissues deep to the septum (orbital cellulitis). The latter not only threatens vision, but also may threaten life.

Pathology

Children with a history of sinusitis, periorbital inflammation, trauma (blunt or penetrating, including insect bites), dacryocystitis, and dental abscess are at increased risk of developing preseptal and orbital cellulitis (Rumelt & Rubin, 1996). In children, the most frequent etiology of preseptal and orbital cellulitis is ethmoid sinusitis, which is radiographically present in 96% of orbital cases and 81% of preseptal cases (Barone & Aiuto, 1997). Eyelid lesions (traumatic or related to extension of localized inflammatory processes [ie, hordeola]) are the second most common cause of preseptal and orbital cellulitis in children, followed by dacryocystitis (infection of the nasolacrimal sac).

The causative organisms involved in cellulitis may be presumptively identified based on the origin of the infection. In the absence of a history of trauma, providers should suspect organisms responsible for sinusitis, such as *Streptococcus pneumoniae*, nontypable *Haemophilus influenzae*, and *Moraxella catarrhalis* and in children with a history of chronic sinusitis, anaerobes and *Staphylococcus aureus* (Barone & Aiuto, 1997). *H. influenzae* type B, once among the most common and aggressive organisms to cause both preseptal and orbital cellulitis through bacteremic seeding, has essentially been eliminated as a source of cellulitis as a result of vaccination (Barone & Aiuto, 1997; Donahue & Schwartz, 1998). In preseptal or orbital cellulitis related to skin infections or trauma, *S. aureus* and *Streptococcus pyogenes* are the most frequent pathogens.

History and Physical Examination

Parents may give a history of recurrent sinusitis or recent respiratory infection or describe an antecedent lesion related to trauma, insect bite, chalazion, or hordeolum. Frequently, they may not recall any precipitating event.

Children with preseptal cellulitis present with eyelids that are tender, swollen, tense, warm, and red. They may exhibit some degree of malaise and be febrile. The globe itself is quiet and uninvolved with normal pupillary reflex. Extraocular movements are full, and vision (if it can be elicited) is normal.

In orbital cellulitis, the findings of swollen, inflamed, and tender eyelids appear similar to those seen in preseptal cellulitis. In contrast, however, the globe itself is proptotic, injected, and chemotic. Ocular movements typically are both painful and restricted (secondary to inflamed orbital tissues surrounding the globe); there may be papillitis (unilateral optic nerve swelling), an afferent pupillary defect, or decrease in vision secondary to swollen, infected tissues adjacent to the optic nerve. Children are febrile and appear quite ill.

● **Clinical Pearl:** Decreased and painful extraocular movements and proptosis are the most clinically apparent differentiating features between orbital and preseptal (periorbital) cellulitis.

Diagnostic Criteria

Eyelid swelling in the pediatric population typically is secondary to infection (cellulitis), trauma (with soft-tissue swelling), allergy, or infiltration. History, examination, and focal findings readily diagnose soft-tissue swelling secondary to trauma. While impressive eyelid swelling may occur secondary either to infection or allergy, infected tissues are warm and tender while allergies cause pruritus, often swell rapidly after manipulation, and are cool, nontender, and usually soft to palpation (Table 32-1).

Although infiltrative processes in children are rare, both metastatic neuroblastoma (the most common metastatic orbital tumor in children) and rhabdomyosarcoma (most common primary orbital tumor in children) cause eyelid swelling, ecchymosis, and rapidly progressive proptosis. Both may be mistaken for trauma or cellulitis.

Management

Treatment of Preseptal Cellulitis

Preseptal cellulitis can evolve rapidly into orbital cellulitis, particularly in young children. Thus, the clinician must decide whether to admit a child to the hospital for intravenous antibiotic therapy or treat as an outpatient with oral antibiotics. Among the factors guiding this management decision should be the child's age. The younger the child, the more prudent it is to admit, and children younger than 2 years should always be admitted. The severity of the infection, reliability of the child's caregivers in administering medication and noting deterioration, and the surety of close, daily follow-up examinations are important factors in deciding between inpatient versus outpatient management.

Older children with little or no fever, normal complete blood count (CBC), and who appear well may be candidates for outpatient management providing the conditions listed above are met. Patients should be closely monitored until it is clear that the infection has been controlled. In general, providers should have a low threshold for hospital admission and intravenous antibiotics.

Preseptal cellulitis should be treated with warm compresses and antibiotics tailored toward the probable source of the infection. If outpatient management is elected (see above), a broad-spectrum antibiotic, such as oral amoxicillin-clavulanate potassium, oral cefuroxime, or intramuscular ceftriaxone, would be appropriate (Donahue & Schwartz, 1998). The best choice for inpatient management would be combination of a third-generation cephalosporin (such as ceftriaxone or cefotaxime) with an antibiotic with gram-positive coverage, such as oxacillin. In patients with a history of chronic sinusitis, clindamycin should be substituted for oxacillin to provide coverage for anaerobes and gram-positive organisms (Barone & Aiuto, 1997).

Management of preseptal cellulitis should include an ophthalmologic examination if there is any doubt of the diagnosis or if the child does not rapidly improve within 24 hours on oral antibiotics. Similarly, an otolaryngology consultation should be obtained if chronic sinusitis is suspected. A computed tomography (CT) scan of the orbit and sinuses (axial and coronal views) should be ordered if there is any suspicion of orbital involvement.

Treatment of Orbital Cellulitis

Orbital cellulitis calls for immediate treatment and should be considered an emergency. Children must be admitted to a closely monitored pediatric setting. Cultures of blood (routine), purulent eye secretion if present, and abscess contents if surgical drainage is performed should be obtained. A spinal tap should be performed if central nervous system involvement is suspected (Uzcategui et al., 1998). Recent studies recommend that infants younger than 3 months undergo a full sepsis workup, including obtaining blood, cerebrospinal fluid, and catheterized or suprapubic urine cultures (Klassen & Rowe, 1992; Nozicka, 1995). After an expeditious fever workup, broad-spectrum intravenous antibiotics (ceftriaxone or cefotaxime and oxacillin or clindamycin) should be started. Axial and coronal CT scans of the orbits and sinuses should be obtained without delay both to delineate the extent of the process within the orbit and to identify the source of infection.

Both the ophthalmologic and otolaryngology services should be consulted immediately to evaluate fully children with orbital cellulitis. Further management should be guided by a multidisciplinary approach. Surgical drainage of an underlying abscess or ethmoiditis should be considered early in the course of treatment.

Orbital cellulitis can progress rapidly and may result in orbital abscess or permanent visual loss. Intracranial involvement occurs as a consequence of infection spreading through the superior orbital fissure. The devastating complications of orbital cellulitis include cavernous sinus thrombo-

---

Table 32-1. DIFFERENTIAL DIAGNOSIS OF EYELID EDEMA

Symptoms	Allergic Conjunctivitis	Preseptal Cellulitis	Orbital Cellulitis
Eyelid edema	Yes	Yes	Yes
Tender warm eyelids	No	Yes	Yes
Injected eye	Yes	No	Yes
Sinusitis	No	Often	Often
Trauma history	No	Possible	Possible
Rhinitis	Often	Possible	Possible
Pruritus	Yes	No	No
Restricted or painful extraocular movements	No	No	Yes

sis, meningitis, and brain abscess. Therefore, aggressive therapy must be instituted without delay on presentation.

NASOLACRIMAL DUCT OBSTRUCTION AND DACRYOCYSTITIS

Pathology

Congenital nasolacrimal duct obstruction occurs in approximately 6% of healthy children (Campolattaro et al., 1997). By far the most frequent cause of epiphora during the first several years of life is nasolacrimal duct obstruction. At birth, a thin membrane frequently persists at Hasner's valve, located at the junction of the nasolacrimal duct and the nasal mucosa, causing obstruction of the nasolacrimal system. When an intranasal duct cyst is present, this causes a more marked obstruction in the early perinatal period, causing congenital dacryocele (dilated lacrimal sac). Presence of a dacryocele frequently causes bouts of acute or chronic low-grade dacryocystitis.

History and Physical Examination

Epiphora secondary to nasolacrimal duct obstruction is often accompanied by an intermittent purulent discharge and crusted eyelids in the morning. Although a recent study contradicts the traditional teaching that newborns do not lacrimate at birth (Isenberg et al., 1998), symptoms usually do not manifest until 2 to 4 weeks of age. Symptoms of perinatal epiphora are usually related to a conjunctivitis (chemical or infectious). If the obstruction is above the nasolacrimal sac, only epiphora without purulent discharge may be noted. On examination, children have a prominent tear lake and may either have frank tearing or dried tear marks on their cheeks. Frequently pressure on the lacrimal sac causes expression of purulent material through the puncta.

Dacryocystitis may be either acute or chronic. In addition to epiphora and recurrent conjunctivitis as seen with simple nasolacrimal duct obstruction, dacryocystitis presents as an inflamed, tender mass over the lacrimal sac area, which may be associated with cellulitis.

Diagnostic Criteria

Epiphora is nonspecific, but the most common cause of chronic epiphora is nasolacrimal duct obstruction. This diagnosis is supported by a history of persistent tearing, recurrent conjunctivitis, and the findings on examination as described previously.

Other causes of epiphora fall under the category of overproduction of tears and occur much less frequently than obstruction. However, when evaluating for epiphora, one should inspect the eye for signs of irritation that might be the cause of excessive lacrimation, including eyelid malformations, malpositioning of eyelids or cilia, and foreign bodies.

Primary care providers should rule out congenital glaucoma in a child with epiphora. Classic symptoms of congenital glaucoma include epiphora, blepharospasm, enlarged cloudy cornea, and photophobia. Photophobia results from glare produced by corneal edema and is probably the most reliable sign of the triad. Intraocular pressure is elevated, and palpation of the globe through the eyelids reveals a firm globe and buphthalmos. Congenital glaucoma usually is bilateral. If congenital glaucoma is suspected, immediate referral to an ophthalmologist should be made. The treatment of congenital glaucoma is surgical, and

medical therapy merely temporizes until the surgery can be performed.

Management

Initial treatment of nasolacrimal duct obstruction is conservative. With lacrimal sac massage and periodic topical antibiotics (Table 32-2) as needed to control discharge, a child may be observed up to 1 year of age unless symptoms are excessive. Most studies agree that by 1 year of age, 90% of cases have spontaneously resolved. Studies also have shown that spontaneous resolution of nasolacrimal duct obstruction after 1 year of age is unlikely (Nelson, 1998).

Primary care providers should teach nasolacrimal sac massage to parents. A finger should be firmly pressed on the sac (just below the medial canthus and under the orbital rim). Gentle pressure should then be exerted inferiorly to attempt to express lacrimal sac contents through the membrane at Hasner's valve. A schedule easily remembered by parents, such as massage during each feeding period, should be recommended. Topical antibiotic drops or ointment (bacitracin ophthalmic ointment, erythromycin ophthalmic ointment, polysporin solution) should be prescribed whenever a child has purulent discharge.

Almost inevitably, a dacryocele will become infected, with a higher risk of morbidity, and children should be placed on topical antibiotics and referred expeditiously to an ophthalmologist or pediatric ophthalmologist if available. There should be no delay when the condition is observed in a neonate. Dacryocele treatment requires probing and possibly further surgical intervention.

Chronic low-grade dacryocystitis can be treated on an outpatient basis with oral and topical antibiotics (ie, amoxicillin clavulanate and polysporin drops), while more acute cases should be admitted for intravenous antibiotics (eg, a third-generation cephalosporin [cefotaxime] and penicillinase-resistant antibiotic [oxacillin]). Children who present with dacryocystitis should be monitored carefully for progression to preseptal or orbital cellulitis. Children with dacryocystitis will require surgical intervention, and all patients with dacryocystitis should be evaluated by an ophthalmologist.

When conservative therapy for simple nasolacrimal obstruction fails, children should be referred to either a pediatric or general ophthalmologist for further management. Nasolacrimal duct probing (passage of a thin probe through the nasolacrimal system, rupturing the membrane across Hasner's valve) in most cases relieves the obstruction even

Table 32-2.   ANTIBIOTIC SOLUTIONS AND OINTMENTS COMMONLY PRESCRIBED IN PEDIATRICS

Name	Age Approved for Use
Solutions	
Ciprofloxacin HCl 0.3%	>1 y
Gentamicin sulfate 0.3%	Not established
Oculofloxacin 0.3%	>1 y
Sulfacetamide sodium 10%	>2 mo
Tobramycin	No comment in PDR
Trimethoprim/polymyxin B sulfate	>2 mo
Ointments	
Erythromycin ophthalmic	Birth
Bacitracin ophthalmic	Not established
Sulfacetamide sodium	>2 mo
Polymixin B/neomycin/bacitracin	Not established

up to age 3 years (Robb, 1998; Mannor, Rose, Frimpong-Ansah, & Ezra, 1999). Further surgical intervention, including dacryocystoplasty (a recently developed technique of balloon catheter dilatation of the nasolacrimal apparatus) or placement of silicone tubes for a 6-month period to foster patency of the system, may be required (Becker, Berry, & Koller, 1996). The ultimate procedure, dacrycystorhinostomy (marsupialization of the mucosa of the nasolacrimal sac to that of the nasal mucosa), is reserved for obstruction that fails the above measures. This often is required because the nasolacrimal duct has scarred after repeated infections or secondary to anomalous anatomy.

OCULAR INFLAMMATION AND CONJUNCTIVITIS

Ocular inflammation in children is one of the most common eye problems encountered by clinicians. Because ocular injection is nonspecific, this may represent a self-limited entity or herald a vision-threatening or systemic problem. The examination and history help differentiate the two.

Conjunctivitis is a nonspecific reaction of conjunctival tissue. Common causes include infection, inflammation or irritation, allergies, foreign bodies, and toxic reactions. It may be related to lid problems, such as blepharitis or hordeola. Because conjunctivitis is nonspecific, the evaluation relies on both history and physical examination to determine the etiology and to rule out other causes of ocular irritation. As discussed below, the time course, history of exposures, presence or absence (and type) of discharge, and other symptoms provide clues to the etiology of the problem.

● **Clinical Pearl:** Whenever a child presents for evaluation of conjunctivitis, close attention should be paid to examination of the ears, because middle ear disease is associated with acute conjunctivitis in 30% to 40% of cases (Gigliotti, 1993; King, 1993).

▲ **Clinical Warning:** Under no circumstances should a primary care provider prescribe a steroid-containing topical medication to treat a red, inflamed eye. Aside from the ocular side effects from topical (and systemic) steroids (including steroid-induced glaucoma, cataracts, and ptosis), administration of a steroid-containing medication can potentiate bacterial, fungal, and herpetic infections resulting in corneal ulceration or a geographic keratitis.

Viral Conjunctivitis

The most frequent cause of infectious conjunctivitis is viral. A child with viral conjunctivitis may have an associated upper respiratory infection or gastrointestinal disturbance. Frequently a history of exposure to another child or family member with conjunctivitis can be elicited.

Common DNA and RNA viruses, including adenovirus, coxsackievirus, and enterovirus, are most often implicated in viral conjunctivitis. Herpes simplex conjunctivitis, either primarily involving the cornea and conjunctiva or secondarily caused by spillover of viral inoculum into the eye from eyelid vesicles, occurs less frequently but should always be in the differential. Sequestration of herpesvirus in the ciliary ganglion leads to recurrences.

History and Physical Examination

Patients with viral conjunctivitis present with a history of injected eyes (usually bilateral, with one eye first involved,

then the other), crusting or edema of the eyelids, and a watery discharge. Sometimes a history of ear infection or upper respiratory tract infection or exposure to other children with conjunctivitis can be elicited.

Viral infections cause a follicular conjunctival reaction (composed of aggregates of lymphocytes) in the fornices of the eye. Preauricular or submandibular nodes frequently are palpable. The eye is diffusely injected. Typically, the cornea is uninvolved (ie, does not stain with fluorescein). The notable exception is adenovirus, which causes a punctate keratopathy and subsequent subepithelial infiltrates that last for months. Some viral infections, such as those caused by enterovirus, coxsackievirus, and adenovirus, may be accompanied by extensive subconjunctival hemorrhage and chemosis. Herpetic disease causes epithelial disruptions (which often form the shape of dendrites) on conjunctiva and cornea that stain with fluorescein.

Diagnostic Criteria

Viral conjunctivitis is a diagnosis of exclusion. One should rule out the serious causes of an inflamed eye (see below). In addition to the expected findings on history and physical examination, helpful clues include the child's demeanor. Although there are exceptions, as a general rule, viral conjunctivitis usually is bothersome rather than painful. A diffusely injected eye with intact visual acuity, watery, nonpurulent discharge, preauricular or submandibular nodes, and mild discomfort most likely is secondary to viral conjunctivitis. Simple conjunctivitis does not cause significant pain, photophobia, or visual impairment.

A child with purulent discharge or with conjunctival pseudomembrane or membrane formation (fibrinoid serosanguinous accumulations) should be assumed to have bacterial rather than viral conjunctivitis.

Management

Viral conjunctivitis is highly contagious, and the process often spreads to the other eye and to other family members. It is most contagious during the first 7 to 10 days of the infection. The child and caregivers should wash their hands frequently, and towels, washcloths, pillowcases, and so forth should not be shared during this period. Cool compresses and artificial tears help relieve the symptoms.

Viral conjunctivitis, like upper respiratory system viral infections, typically does not improve on antibiotic therapy (the important exception is herpetic conjunctivitis) and runs a 1- to 2-week course before resolving. However, despite common knowledge by medical providers that viral infections do not respond to antibiotics and that overuse of antibiotics has caused significant problems with microbial resistance, most primary care providers and indeed most ophthalmologists treat viral conjunctivitis with topical antibiotics. This irony is probably attributable to the inability to be absolutely certain of the etiology of conjunctivitis and a desire to be conservative in management.

Herpes simplex vesicles involving only the eyelids with no apparent conjunctivitis should be treated with an ophthalmic ointment, such as bacitracin or erythromycin ophthalmic ointment, to prevent bacterial superinfection of skin. (Similarly, a child with varicella or other similar viral lid lesion should be placed on prophylactic antibiotic ointment.) The medical care provider should also prescribe oral acyclovir for the first herpetic episode. If the conjunctiva or cornea is involved during a herpetic infection (ie, injected eye, corneal epithelial defect), the patient should be on a topical antiviral drop (ie, vidarabine [Vira-A Ophthalmic] or trifluridine [Viroptic]) for a 2-week course under the care of an ophthalmologist.

The use of steroids is unwise in any primary medical setting. In herpetic keratoconjunctivitis, steroids lead to uncontrolled and potentially devastating spread of herpetic infection. Although herpetic keratoconjunctivitis resolves spontaneously, it recurs, and if untreated, it will cause corneal scarring. Scarring causes loss of vision through amblyopia secondary to refractive error (induced astigmatism) and corneal opacification. Repeated episodes of scarring can cause dry eye symptoms and ocular disfigurement and may necessitate corneal transplantation.

An antibiotic drop, such as ciprofloxicin, ocufloxicin, or trimethoprim and polymyxin B sulfate should be prescribed (four times per day is reasonable) if the medical provider is not sure whether the infection has a bacterial component. Topical antibiotic drops should also be used if a corneal epithelial defect is present to prevent corneal ulceration. The child should be referred to a pediatric ophthalmologist to rule out herpetic conjunctivitis.

▲ **Clinical Warning:** Although viral conjunctivitis does not subside for 1 to 2 weeks, children with progression of symptoms after 24 to 48 hours of treatment should be referred to an ophthalmologist for evaluation. Progression of symptoms may suggest possible herpetic conjunctivitis, nonviral conjunctivitis, or some other process.

Bacterial Conjunctivitis

Bacterial conjunctivitis occurs less frequently than viral conjunctivitis. The organisms most often responsible include *S. pneumoniae* and nontypeable strains of *H. influenzae.* However, bacterial infections may be secondary to a host of other species, including gram-negative organisms, such as *Neisseria gonorrhoeae* and *meningitidus* and other enteric organisms.

History and Physical Examination

The hallmark of bacterial conjunctivitis is an inflamed eye with purulent discharge. Although most primary care providers do not routinely use fluorescein to assess corneal integrity, in suspected bacterial conjunctivitis, this would be a prudent part of the examination. Fluorescein staining of the cornea indicates that the corneal epithelial integrity has been violated, and there is a risk of corneal ulcer. Some organisms (notably *Neisseria, Listeria,* and diphtheroides species) can penetrate intact corneal epithelium to cause a corneal ulcer. If there is staining of the cornea or any suggestion of opacity to the cornea, a corneal ulcer is threatened or present and requires immediate referral to an ophthalmologist.

Diagnostic Criteria

Conjunctivitis accompanied by purulent discharge typically is bacterial. Nasolacrimal duct obstruction should be considered in a child with repeated episodes of purulent conjunctivitis. Usually children do not demonstrate systemic signs unless they have an accompanying otitis media. A diffusely injected eye with intact visual acuity and purulent discharge is most likely caused by bacterial conjunctivitis.

Management

Unlike viral conjunctivitis, bacterial conjunctivitis (ie, any conjunctivitis with a purulent discharge) necessitates medical therapy with a broad-spectrum topical antibiotic. Reasonable initial antibiotic choices include ciprofloxicin, ocufloxicin, or trimethoprim and polymyxin B sulfate ophthalmic solution. Although not necessary as a routine, an extremely prurulent or atypical-appearing conjunctivitis or one not responsive to medical therapy should be cultured. Children with bacterial conjunctivitis should be followed closely. Table 32-2 lists the common topical ophthalmic antibiotics used in children.

▲ **Clinical Warning:** If there is no improvement after 1 to 2 days of topical therapy or if any corneal involvement is suspected, children should be referred without delay to an ophthalmologist to avoid the complications of corneal ulceration.

Eyes may have serosanguinous discharge during conjunctivitis secondary to the formation of membranes or pseudomembranes (inflammatory debris adherent to the surface of the conjunctiva). Generous lubrication with artificial tears and ointment should help, and this usually resolves without sequelae, although conjunctival scarring sometimes occurs.

Chronic Conjunctivitis

Chronic conjunctivitis is defined as conjunctivitis lasting more than 3 weeks. Allergic conjunctivitis falls under this category; however, this section focuses on infectious causes of chronic conjunctivitis. These include molluscum contagiosum (a DNA poxvirus), herpes simplex, *Chlamydia* (including untreated neonatal chlamydial conjunctivitis), and more unusual organisms such as *Bartonella*, tuberculosis, syphilis, tularemia, and sporotrichosis.

History and Physical Examination

Children with chronic conjunctivitis present with a history of red eye for more than 2 weeks. The onset is usually subacute. Important aspects of the history are the presence of pruritus, a history of environmental allergies or exposures, a history of waxing and waning, and the presence of any skin lesions. The examination should be detailed. Vesicles (herpetic) or lesions with central craters with central craters (molluscum) may be hidden in eyelashes and shed inoculum into the eye, causing a chronic conjunctivitis. Foreign bodies may be hidden in the fornices of the eye; the upper eyelids should be everted and inspected with penlight. Fluorescein should be used in chronic conjunctivitis to identify epithelial defects. Pruritic red eyes with swollen eyelids and white mucoid discharge suggest allergic conjunctivitis. Children may develop a toxic conjunctivitis secondary to overtreatment with topical therapy (over-the-counter or prescribed), treatment with caustic drops, or allergic reactions to the preservatives contained in a medication. Eyelid inflammatory and infectious processes (ie, blepharitis, hordeola) may cause an associated conjunctivitis. Unlike ophthalmia neonatorum, or neonatal conjunctivitis, *Chlamydia* is an unusual cause of pediatric conjunctivitis (and has been linked to sexual activity or abuse) (Hammerschlag, 1994). The appropriate diagnostic test for *Chlamydia* requires epithelial scraping.

Diagnostic Criteria

There are myriad causes of a chronic red eye, and diagnosis of the etiology of chronic conjunctivitis relies to a large extent on the history and careful examination of both eyelids and eyes. One should also consider an inflammatory allergic reaction or pharmacologica medicamentosa. Leukemia can also simulate a chronic conjunctivitis.

Management

Treatment of chronic conjunctivitis is directed toward etiology. Blepharoconjunctivitis is treated like blepharitis, with the addition of polymyxin B suflate (Polytrim) or oflaxacin drops. Molluscum lesions that cause chronic conjunctivitis should be removed by curettage or cryotherapy. If topical therapy or other medications are suspected as the causative agents, these should be discontinued and the patient observed. Chlamydial conjunctivitis not caused by neonatal exposure requires not only treatment with systemic erythromycin, but full evaluation as to risk factor for exposure to *Chlamydia* and systemic evaluation for exposure to other venereal diseases.

Chronic conjunctivitis should be referred to an ophthalmologist if there is no response to treatment within several days.

Ophthalmia Neonatorum

Neonatal conjunctivitis may be chemical or infectious and occurs within the first several weeks of birth. The infectious varieties usually result from exposure to pathogens during vaginal delivery or premature rupture of membranes. *Chlamydia* is the most frequent cause of neonatal conjunctivitis in the United States (O'Hara, 1993). Bacterial causes include *N. gonorrhoeae*, perhaps the most potentially hazardous bacterial pathogen, and *S. aureus*, the most common organism isolated from neonates in most studies (Dannevig et al., 1992). Many other gram-positive and gram-negative organisms may be involved, including *Staphylococcus epidermitis*, *Streptococcus viridans*, *S. pneumoniae*, *Enterococcus*, *Escherichia coli*, *Serratia*, and *Pseudomonas*.

History and Physical Examination

The history should include details of the timing and nature of symptoms. Chemical conjunctivitis causes a watery discharge within the first several days of life. Infectious conjunctivitis may be bacterial or viral. Purulent discharge suggests a bacterial source.

Chlamydial conjunctivitis manifests in the first 2 weeks of life with a watery discharge that becomes purulent, swollen eyelids, and chemosis. Chlamydial pneumonitis, otitis, and rhinitis also may be present (Nelson, 1998). A hyperpurulent discharge is suggestive of gonococcus. Untreated gonococcal infection may lead to corneal ulceration and perforation within 1 day. The provider should perform a complete examination of the eye, with irrigation of purulent material to assess the extent of the conjunctivitis. He or she must use fluorescein to evaluate corneal integrity.

Diagnostic Criteria

The nature of the eye discharge, the timing of its appearance, and the baby's overall health status are good diagnostic clues as to the specific etiology. Chlamydial conjunctivitis usually begins within 1 to 2 weeks of birth, but the range varies; earlier and later cases have been reported. A purulent discharge beginning within a few days of birth is more suggestive of a bacterial etiology. Infants with chlamydial ophthalmia tend not to be systemically ill, while those with gonococcal ophthalmia may range in presentation from localized ophthalmitis to full-blown septicemia. Because topical antibiotics have replaced silver nitrate for routine eye prophylaxis, chemical conjunctivitis is relatively rare.

Results of cultures obtained from the infant will establish the actual diagnosis. The provider should obtain a conjunctival scraping and send it for Gram (bacterial) and Giemsa (*Chlamydia*) stains and for bacterial cultures (blood and chocolate agar plates) and direct immunofluorescent antibody assay (*Chlamydia*). If a corneal abrasion is present, the provider should order a herpes viral culture, which usually is performed by an ophthalmologist.

Management

Once cultures are obtained, immediate treatment should begin, with therapy directed at the suspected organism and close follow-up of response to therapy and laboratory results. For infants with ophthalmia, many neonatologists recommend a blood culture prior to starting therapy. If any systemic symptoms are present, a full sepsis workup, including lumbar puncture, is necessary. Empiric therapy may begin with parenteral ampicillin and cefotaxime, as for any infant suspected of neonatal sepsis. Once culture has confirmed the etiology, gonococcal ophthalmia should be treated with parenteral ceftriaxone (50 mg/kg/d) for 7 days and hourly saline irrigation until the discharge is eliminated. Chlamydial ophthalmia should be treated with a 2-week course of oral erythromycin with a daily dose of 50 mg/kg/d divided into four doses. In all cases of neonatal conjunctivitis secondary to gonococcus or *Chlamydia*, the parents should be treated as well.

Allergic Conjunctivitis

Allergic conjunctivitis often is often associated with asthma and atopy. Seasonal allergic conjunctivitis is associated with mast cells, while vernal conjunctivitis is a more chronic condition associated with T lymphocytes (Buckley, 1998).

History and Physical Examination

The history commonly reveals other atopic disorders, such as eczema, allergic rhinitis, and asthma, either in the patient or family. Seasonal allergies frequently present with ocular symptoms, which include pruritus and conjunctival injection. Eyelid edema and chemosis can be impressive, are usually worst in the morning, and are exacerbated by rubbing. Slit lamp examination reveals a papillary tarsal conjunctival reaction. Vernal conjunctivitis presents with similar symptoms, except that they are more severe and may be year-round. Eversion of the upper eyelids in allergic and particularly in vernal conjunctivitis reveals giant papillae with a ropy white discharge. Shield ulcers (central corneal ulcers) may develop.

Diagnostic Criteria

The diagnosis is usually established on the results of the history and physical examination. As a rule, swollen, itchy, red eyes with watery or white mucoid discharge are attributable to allergic conjunctivitis. Lid edema secondary to allergies may resemble preseptal cellulitis, and this must be considered in the differential diagnosis. Table 32-1 compares the characteristics of these two entities.

Management

While allergic conjunctivitis may be treated in a primary medical setting, vernal conjunctivitis usually requires steroid therapy, and children with this disorder should be referred to an ophthalmologist.

Topical therapies available to treat allergic conjunctivitis may be grouped into mast cell inhibitors, antihistamines, vasoconstrictors, nonsteroidal anti-inflammatory drops, and steroids. The latter category of medication should be prescribed only by an ophthalmologist. Treatment of conjunctivitis should be guided by severity of ocular symptoms, response to therapy, and accompanying systemic symptoms, such as allergic rhinitis.

The use of a mast cell inhibitor or a selective H1-blocking topical ophthalmologic solutions, combined with cool compresses and avoidance of rubbing, usually can provide reasonable control of allergic symptoms. Although mast cell stabilizers treat the cause of allergic conjunctivitis, their disadvantage lies in delayed onset of action. Antihistamines treat the symptoms but not the cause. A combination of topical mast cell inhibitor and antihistamine may provide the most effective management of allergic conjunctivitis and avoids the sedative side effect of oral antihistamines. Two recently developed combination mast cell inhibitor and antihistamine ophthalmic solution, olopatadine hydrochloride 0.1% (Patanol), and nedocromil sodium 2% (Alocril) have gained acceptance as an effective first-line therapy for allergic conjunctivitis.

Vasoconstrictors decrease injection, but studies show they are less effective in controlling symptoms (Yanni, 1999). Ketorolac tromethamine ophthalmic 0.5% solution (Acular), a topical nonsteroidal anti-inflammatory drug, improves symptoms of pruritus through its antiprostaglandin effect, but it stings on application and may be less desirable in the pediatric age group for this reason.

Decisions on which medication to use are based on cost, frequency of dosing, and pediatric dosing guidelines. Severe cases of allergic conjunctivitis or children with systemic symptoms would benefit from oral antihistamines as well. The reader is referred to the section on allergic rhinitis for a full discussion on the use of oral antihistamines. Table 32-3 compares current topical medications available to treat allergic conjunctivitis.

Table 32–3.   TOPICAL ALLERGY MEDICATIONS

Name	Age Approved for Use	Dosing Schedule
Mast Cell Inhibitors		
Lodoxamide tromethamine 0.1% (Alomide)	>2 y	1–2 gtt/q.i.d
Olopatadine hydrochloride 0.1% (Patanol)	>3 y	1 gtt b.i.d.
Cromolyn sodium 4% (Opticrom)	>4 y	1–2 gtt/t.i.d.
Nedocromil sodium 2% (Alocril)	>3 y	1 gtt/b.i.d.
Antihistamines		
Emadastine difumarate .05% (Emadine)	>3 y	1 gtt/q.i.d.
Levocabastine hydrochloride 0.5% (Livostin)	>12 y	1 gtt/q.i.d.
Olopatadine hydrochloride 0.1% (Patanol)	>3 y	1 gtt b.i.d.
Nedocromil sodium 2% (Alocril)	>3 y	1 gtt/b.i.d.
Nonsteroidal Anti-inflammatories		
Ketorolac tromethamine 0.5% (Acular)	>12 y	1 gtt/q.i.d.
Vasoconstrictors		
Antazoline hydrochloride (Vasocon A)	>6 y	1–2 gtt/q.i.d.

OTHER OCULAR INFLAMMATIONS

As noted in the first paragraph of this chapter, the eye has a limited response to both minor and serious problems. Certain clues separate the two. Simple conjunctivitis does not cause significant pain, photophobia, or vision impairment.

▲ **Clinical Warning:** The symptom triad of eye pain, photophobia, or visual impairment usually suggests a serious process and should prompt immediate referral to an ophthalmologist.

In a healthy child with an intact immune system, the most common causes of a red injected eye are conjunctivitis, corneal abrasions, corneal ulcers, and foreign bodies. Congenital glaucoma is rare. Orbital infectious processes have been discussed previously. Some of the less common causes of a red eye are described in this section.

Pathology

Inflammatory processes are uncommon in children younger than 5 to 6 years (Taylor, 1997). Infectious processes frequently are linked to adnexal infections and typically are associated with antecedent processes (eg, sinusitis, trauma, chalazia, or dacryoadenitis). Infectious processes within the eye usually have a precipitating cause (eg, sinusitis, dacryocystitis, or trauma). Inflammatory processes most frequently are idiopathic but may be related to autoimmune disorders or caused by sarcoidosis, thyrotoxicosis, or similar entities.

History and Physical Examination

Orbital inflammation may be generalized and nonspecific (orbital pseudotumor) or secondary to sarcoidosis, Wegener's granulomatosis, or thyroid orbitopathy. Nonspecific inflammation also may be localized to a particular tissue of the eye, such as the extraocular muscles (myositis) or lacrimal gland (dacryoadenitis). The hallmark of inflammation is pain typically exacerbated by eye movement and may be accompanied by double vision secondary to restricted eye movements (limited by pain or swollen intraorbital tissues). This process is most commonly unilateral. On examination, significant findings include injection, painful and restricted eye movements, and proptosis. Decreased visual acuity or afferent pupillary defect is present if surrounding swollen tissues compress the optic nerve. Vision may be affected. Inflammation of the lacrimal gland causes pain, swelling, and tenderness of the lateral aspect of the eyelid.

Episcleritis occurs much less frequently than conjunctivitis. It is distinguished from conjunctivitis by sectoral (rather than diffuse) inflammation of the superficial episcleral vessels. The usual history is of sudden onset of an irritated rather than painful eye, with no vision disturbance and no pruritus or other significant symptoms.

Uveitis consists of inflammation of the uvea. It may be confined to the anterior chamber (iritis) or may be more extensive. In children, iritis is the most frequent form of uveitis. Iritis in children may be idiopathic, traumatic, or related to autoimmune disease. Symptoms include blurred vision, photophobia, and pain on pupillary constriction (elicited by accommodative targets and direct and consensual pupillary light reflex testing). Ciliary flush (injected eye particularly 360 degrees around the corneal limbus) and marked improvement of symptoms in a dark room and when under cycloplegia are essential diagnostic findings.

Reactive cells are present in the anterior chamber of the eye but not visible by penlight examination.

Diagnostic Criteria

Orbital inflammatory, infectious, and neoplastic processes share common characteristics of proptosis, injected eye, limitation of extraocular movements, and pain. One must rely on the history and physical findings to differentiate among the three. Children with inflammatory processes typically are afebrile. Infectious orbital processes frequently have an antecedent history and fever. Pediatric orbital neoplasms (eg, rhabdomyosarcoma, metastatic neuroblastoma, infiltrative leukemias, Ewing's sarcoma) present with similar findings. Imaging studies are often helpful in delineating these entities.

The sectoral vascular engorgement seen in episcleritis may be present in patients with occult foreign body or scleritis, a deep inflammation of the sclera. Scleritis, very rare (in fact reportable) in the pediatric population, is associated with pain and decreased vision and has systemic connotations (autoimmune processes).

The blurred vision and dramatic photophobia of iritis are often unmistakable. Ciliary spasm may elicit identical symptoms secondary to overaccommodation, prior injury, or uncorrected refractive error.

Management

Treatment of infectious processes is described elsewhere in this chapter. Inflammatory conditions are best managed in conjunction with a pediatric ophthalmologist. Providers should refer children with orbital inflammation to a pediatric or neuro-ophthalmologist for management and evaluation. As a general rule, inflammation requires systemic steroids and occasionally cytotoxic agents to eliminate the inflammation. Typically, a team of specialists manage neoplastic processes.

Although episcleritis is self-limited, treatment with drops of a nonsteroidal anti-inflammatory drug, such as ketorolac tromethamine ophthalmic 0.5% solution or diclofenac (Voltaren) once daily may ease symptoms and decrease the duration of the condition. Episcleritis may be related to autoimmune disease; however, it is usually idiopathic, and most practitioners order a workup only after a recurrence.

An ophthalmologist should carry out management of iritis, which consists of cycloplegia and steroid drops. Because most episodes of iritis are idiopathic and do not recur, an initial episode of iritis usually is not worked up. If a second episode of spontaneous iritis occurs, however, the child should be worked up with CBC, ANA, rheumatoid factor, FTA/VDRL, Lyme titers, and PPD.

● **Clinical Pearl:** The most common cause of repeated episodes of iritis in girls is pauciarticular juvenile rheumatoid arthritis. This autoimmune-mediated iritis occurs in eyes that are deceptively quiet. After repeated episodes, significant damage and permanent visual loss result.

STRABISMUS

Pediatric medical providers frequently are confronted with concerns of strabismus in children. This condition is extremely complex. This section is intended to help primary care providers understand why strabismus may occur, its potential significance, and management. Additional detailed information is available in pediatric ophthalmology texts.

Pathology

Binocularity develops during the first months of life and continues until about age 1 year. During the first few months of life, strabismus is common and in most cases transient (Hoyt, Mousel, & Weber, 1980). As visual maturation proceeds, most infants become orthophoric by age 3 months. Up to this age, observation of strabismus in a healthy infant is normal and does not require referral. If the child does not have a good red reflex, however, the provider should refer the child for an immediate ophthalmologic evaluation to rule out retinoblastoma, cataracts, and other intraocular conditions that require treatment to preserve vision (and possibly life).

Clinicians should be wary of new-onset strabismus. It may be secondary to a cranial nerve palsy secondary to trauma, viral infection, or intraocular or intracranial pathology. Strabismus is the second-most frequent presenting sign of retinoblastoma (the first is leukocoria).

Horizontal concomitant strabismus (strabismus that is essentially the same in all fields of gaze) in most cases is idiopathic. Strabismus is frequently seen in children with anisemetropia and high refractive errors, including hyperopia, myopia, and astigmatism. Frequently there is a positive family history of strabismus and refractive errors.

Concomitant horizontal strabismus also may occur secondary to sensory deprivation (poor vision that may be related to refractive error, unilateral cataract, optic nerve hypoplasia, or retinal macular lesion, such as retinoblastoma or toxoplasmosis scar). In very young children, this usually manifests as an esotropia, while occurrence of strabismus secondary to visual deprivation in children older than 1 to 2 years usually results in exotropia. Intraocular pathology should be ruled out in all young children with strabismus. Constant exotropia in children younger than 1 year is unusual and suggests intraocular or neurologic pathology.

Strabismus also results from cranial nerve palsies. By definition, these are incomitant (vary depending on direction of gaze), the deviation being greatest in the field of action of the affected muscle. This can result in a horizontal palsy (ie, cranial nerve six palsy causes incomitant esotropia), vertical palsy (cranial nerve IV palsy causes incomitant vertical and torsional deviation), or both (cranial nerve III palsy causes a hypodeviation and exodeviation). These may be supranuclear, nuclear, or infranuclear in origin.

Restrictive incomitant deviations also occur secondary to orbital processes (ie, orbital cellulitis, pseudotumor, myositis, and orbital fractures with entrapment and swelling of orbital contents). Incomitant strabismus denotes pathology; prompt referral to a pediatric ophthalmologist to ascertain etiology is indicated, and neuroimaging often is in order.

Epidemiology

Studies of the incidence of strabismus in children in the general population range from 3.8% to 5.3% (Graham, 1974; Simons & Reinecke, 1978; Friedman, Biedner, David, & Sachs, 1980). In children with neurologic impairment (such as cerebral palsy), the incidence of strabismus is high. Similarly, children with a history of prematurity or those with genetic (eg, trisomy 21) or craniofacial syndromes have a higher rate of strabismus than the general population.

History and Physical Examination

Aside from strabismus associated with precipitating factors, such as trauma or infection, there are two periods when esotropia frequently presents. The first (congenital or infantile) usually occurs around age 3 to 6 months and is a large-angle deviation that usually requires surgical correction. Congenital esotropia can be the most perplexing form of strabismus in the pediatric population because of the frequent confusion with pseudoesotropia.

Pseudoesotropia occurs because infants have broad flat nasal bridges accompanied by prominent epicanthal folds. Although a child with pseudoesotropia appears to have esotropia, the corneal light reflexes reveal that the eyes are straight. If by age 3 to 4 months the provider has any uncertainty about whether true strabismus is present, he or she should refer the child to an ophthalmologist for further evaluation. True strabismus does not disappear with time, and if pseudo-pseudostrabismus (true strabismus inadvertently misdiagnosed) is followed without referral to and treatment by a pediatric ophthalmologist, fusion and visual potential are lost.

The second (accommodative or refractive esotropia) usually occurs from age 6 months to 4 years, most commonly between ages 1 and 3 years. This type of strabismus usually is related to significant hyperopia or to excessive convergence. (To understand this, simply remember the triad of accommodation, convergence, and miosis. The increased accommodative demand required by high hyperopia causes excessive convergence, resulting in esotropia.) Usually hyperopic spectacles will correct the esotropia if a child is promptly treated. Again, immediate referral to an ophthalmologist will maintain visual acuity and binocularity. Some children have a combination of the two and require surgery for the nonaccommodative component of the strabismus.

As noted previously, constant exotropia in children is unusual and requires prompt investigation for etiology. Intermittent exotropia does not have the same ominous implication as a constant exotropia. Intermittent exotropia frequently is noted when children are looking at distant objects or are inattentive. The primary care provider may not notice it because the child is accommodating (and therefore converging) in a regular-sized examination room. Therefore, if a mother comments that her child's eyes appear to deviate, but the provider cannot confirm this finding, the clinician should still refer the child to an ophthalmologist for further evaluation.

Primary care providers should use the Bruckner and the Hirschberg tests to evaluate children for strabismus (described in the section on physical examination of the eye). Additionally, the provider should observe the child while speaking with the parent, because strabismus can manifest during moments of inattention on the child's part.

Diagnostic Criteria

A history of ocular misalignment, a finding of misalignment by a primary care practitioner, or both indicate true strabismus and necessitate referral to an ophthalmologist as soon as possible. Parents are usually good observers, and when they report strabismus that the clinician does not observe in the office, it is possible that the strabismus is intermittent and not uncovered during one visit. Unless a primary caregiver is very comfortable with evaluating strabismus, he or she should refer even those children they suspect to have pseudostrabismus for at least one confirmatory visit to a pediatric ophthalmologist.

Management

Surgery is only necessary if there is also a nonaccommodative component to the esotropia that does not respond to glasses. A child with a constant exotropia should have surgical correction for cosmetic reasons if this is appropriate given all other factors. Intermittent exotropia may require surgery, which should be postponed if possible until the child is 4 to 5 years old unless the deviation is very large, the child is losing binocularity, or the child is unable to control the exotropia.

● **Clinical Pearl:** As a general rule, children with congenital esotropia require strabismus surgery. Children with later onset esotropia usually have improved alignment with hyperopic spectacles.

EYE TRAUMA

▲ **Clinical Warning:** Primary care providers must handle ocular trauma with caution. Without the advantage of a slit lamp, pupillary dilation and peripheral retinal evaluation, intraocular pressure assessment, and other similar signs, clinicians should diagnose and treat only superficial injuries to the eye.

A seemingly minor external injury (eg, to eyelids) may conceal more extensive injury to the globe itself. Blunt trauma causing subconjunctival hemorrhage also may cause retinal edema (commotio), detachment or tears or rupture of the globe concealed by the hemorrhage. If a provider has any doubt as to extent of injury, he or she should refer the child immediately to an ophthalmologist for full examination.

Primary care practitioners also should be aware that long-term sequelae may result from traumatic impact to the globe. Trauma may cause angle recession and predispose to glaucoma secondary to damage to the trabecular meshwork. Angle recession glaucoma usually is asymptomatic for years until significant damage to the optic nerve has been discovered; therefore, providers should counsel parents to ensure their child has a yearly follow-up visit with an ophthalmologist following blunt trauma to the eye. Children may develop a traumatic cataract following injury and again should be followed to prevent amblyopia.

▲ **Clinical Warning:** Children with rhabdomyosarcoma frequently present with periorbital ecchymosis, proptosis, and a history of trauma yielding diagnostic confusion.

Pathology

Eye injuries are common in the pediatric population, and many injuries occur more frequently in boys than in girls (Tingley, 1999). The mechanism of injury (eg, blunt, penetrating) corresponds to the type of damage sustained. Superficial injuries often conceal more extensive damage.

History and Physical Examination

If possible, a primary caregiver should obtain a history of how the injury occurred. Pertinent information includes the mechanism and type of injury (eg, blunt versus sharp trauma).

Because examining a child with a painful eye injury is difficult, providers reasonably may instill one drop of ophthetic or tetracaine after a penlight examination reveals that the globe is intact, to numb the eye and quiet the child. The preliminary examination should establish visual acuity (which is not always easy to obtain) and the integrity of the globe. These may be prognostic of the injury's severity.

Lid Ecchymosis

Ecchymotic eyelids frequently occur after blunt trauma. Providers must visualize the eye itself (even when severe eyelid edema is present) to be sure that more extensive injuries to the eye itself have not occurred. Extraocular movements should be full. If they are not, an injury has occurred to cause either a restrictive process, which may be transient secondary to edema, or an actual injury causing restriction, such as orbital fracture. Neurologic damage also will result in limited movement. When a restrictive process is present, providers should perform orbital films to rule out a suspected orbital fracture. A floor fracture generally causes defective upward gaze, while a medial fracture impairs lateral gaze.

Lid Lacerations

Eyelid lacerations may be superficial or deep, and their location is very important. Lacerations near the medial canthus may interrupt the nasolacrimal canalicular apparatus. Lateral canthal injuries may affect lid closure. Providers should assess function of the eyelids (ability to open and close). Ptosis suggests injury to the levator muscle that lies deep to the septum. A marginal laceration is a full thickness cut through the lid margin.

Subconjunctival Hemorrhage

A subconjunctival hemorrhage occurs when subconjunctival vessels rupture (ie, secondary to trauma or Valsalva's maneuver), causing blood to accumulate under the conjunctiva. Extensive subconjunctival hemorrhage may mask more severe injuries, including a ruptured globe, and providers should perform careful examination to rule out more serious injuries.

Corneal Abrasion and Ulcers

Perhaps the most frequent minor trauma children suffer is a corneal abrasion. Corneal abrasions occur when a scrape or poke to the cornea by a fingernail or foreign object removes epithelium. By definition, abrasions are not infected and are transparent. An abrasion may be diagnosed by placing fluorescein (a drop or using a strip) in the fornix. (If the strip touches the cornea, it can cause an idiopathic corneal abrasion.) A cobalt blue light directed at the cornea will stain the cornea green if an epithelial defect is present. The examiner should distinguish diffuse nonspecific fluorescein pooling from the sharply demarcated borders and intense green stain of an epithelial defect. To differentiate the two, the provider can gently irrigate excess fluorescein from the eye with a few drops of eyewash; the eye will retain true fluorescein uptake.

Epithelial injury allows microbial access to corneal stroma and creates risk of corneal infection (corneal ulcer). Ulcers cause opacity secondary to organism invasion, corneal edema, and white cell response and may be secondary to bacterial, viral, fungal, or parasitic organisms.

Hyphema and Iritis

Cells in the anterior chamber may be red blood cells (hyphema), white blood cells (iritis), or pigmented cells from the iris. Hyphema occurs when trauma to the eye (usually blunt) causes iris vessels to bleed within the anterior chamber of the eye. A hyphema is visible often by using a penlight to illuminate a layering clot in the anterior chamber of the eye. Iritis may occur secondarily after trauma as a reactive process, usually several days after initial injury, and is marked by photophobia and painful accommodation. Blunt trauma may cause pigmented cells to be shed from the iris into the anterior chamber and usually resolve spontaneously.

Retinal Injury

Although a detailed discussion of retinal injury after trauma is beyond the scope of this chapter, primary care providers should be aware that trauma can cause vitreous hemorrhage; retinal commotio (shearing of the photoreceptors); retinal tears, holes, and detachments; and choroidal rupture. Without the aid of a dilated examination and indirect ophthalmoscope, providers often will miss these injuries.

Ruptured Globe

A ruptured globe is defined as an eye that has sustained either sharp or blunt trauma that caused perforation or rupture of the globe. The rupture may occur in the cornea, sclera, or both. A rupture site may occur at the site of impact or (particularly with blunt trauma) at the area where the sclera is thinnest (at the rectus muscle insertions) during compression of the globe. If the diagnosis is missed, the risk of endophthalmitis and sympathetic ophthalmia increases. Asymmetry of the anterior chamber, uveal protrusion through the sclera, are good indicators of subtle rupture.

Chemical Injuries

Chemical injuries are one of the few absolute ocular emergencies. Clinicians should immediately treat (see below) without any preliminary examination (including visual acuity). Acid causes burns to the lids, cornea, and conjunctiva; may cause hyphema; and, if it penetrates, can cause retinal necrosis. Alkali is worse than acid, because it saponifies and continues to penetrate into the eye. Severe long-term damage results from chemical injuries. Eyelids scar; bulbar conjunctiva adheres to tarsal conjunctiva, causing foreshortening of the fornices; goblet cells in the conjunctiva are destroyed; and severe scarring results.

Foreign Body

Either the presence of a true foreign body or disrupted epithelium may cause foreign body sensation. When there is a history of foreign body entering the eye or foreign body sensation, the provider must find and remove it or demonstrate that no foreign body is now present. When searching for a foreign body in the eye, the provider should examine eyelid fornices and flip the upper eyelid. He or she should examine the eye with fluorescein; often a foreign body may highlight with flourescein. Linear corneal fluorescence suggests the presence of a foreign body under the eyelid scraping against the cornea. The provider should try irrigating the eye with eyestream if he or she does not visualize a foreign body and inspect the cornea carefully for a possible foreign body embedded therein.

Management

Lid Ecchymoses

Eyelid ecchymoses and edema can be followed if the eye itself is not involved. Icepacks will reduce swelling.

Lid Lacerations

An ophthalmologist or emergency room physician should evaluate eyelid lacerations. Both the intricate anatomy of the eyelids and cosmetic considerations dictate referral of periocular lacerations to a surgeon familiar with such repairs. Even superficial lacerations may cause future problems (such as ectropion of eyelids) if improperly repaired. Lacerations near the medial canthus may involve the canalicular system and require repair with silicone intubation to prevent long-term problems with epiphora. Deep lacerations may involve the levator muscle and require oculoplastic attention; delay may result in permanent levator dysfunction.

Subconjunctival Hemorrhage

Subconjunctival hemorrhage usually resolves over 4 to 6 weeks without treatment or symptoms. If the hemorrhage occurs after trauma, and particularly if any significant discomfort or visual change occurs, the provider should refer the child immediately to an ophthalmologist for complete examination to rule out more extensive injury.

Corneal Abrasions and Ulcers

Treatment of corneal abrasions has changed in recent years. Current studies indicate that eye patching with antibiotics does not speed healing or decrease discomfort of corneal abrasions. Furthermore, children frequently actively resist eye patching. As a guideline, providers should patch an abrasion only when it is very large or when adults cannot restrain a child from manipulating the eyelid.

▲ Clinical Warning: Patching of an abrasion caused by a fingernail, vegetative matter, pet claw, or contact lens is contraindicated because of the possible microbial contamination by such contacts.

Treatment for corneal abrasions is antibiotic solution or ointment placed in the eye four times per day until the epithelial defect resolves. Small abrasions may heal almost overnight; larger abrasions take several days or longer. If an abrasion does not improve significantly after 1 day, the provider should refer the child to an ophthalmologist to rule out foreign body and ulceration. The practitioner may use a topical anesthetic on a one-time basis to aid in the physical examination.

▲ Clinical Warning: Although epithelial defects are very painful, a practitioner should never prescribe a topical anesthetic drop for use at home. Such drops are epithelial toxic, impede healing, and lead to corneal ulceration.

Providers should refer children with actual or suspected corneal ulcers immediately to an ophthalmologist. They may require cultures on special media and receive treatment with frequent fortified antibiotic drops. Infectious ulcers are treated with fortified antibiotic therapy and require daily ophthalmology follow-up. Corneal ulcers may result in significant scarring, and progression can result in corneal perforation. Even with treatment, the cornea may scar with permanent localized opacification. Amblyopia may result through induced astigmatism or corneal opacification.

Hyphema and Iritis

Providers should maintain children with hyphema in the upright position to allow the blood to layer inferiorly. As the blood layers, the pupillary axis clears, and vision and the ability to examine the eye may improve. Providers should place a shield over the eye to prevent further injury and rebleeding and immediately refer the child to an ophthalmologist. Treatment consists of topical medication to reduce inflammation and induce cycloplegia. The eye must be shielded at all times. Providers should place children on bed rest for 5 days, the period during which there is greatest risk of rebleed. They may consider aminocaproic acid (Amicar) 50 to 100 mg/kg every 4 hours to reduce the risk of rebleeding.

Children with hyphema are at risk of significant complications secondary to this injury both acutely and as remote sequelae. Hyphemas that rebleed are associated with increased intraocular pressure that may cause glaucomatous damage to the optic nerve. Elevated intraocular pressure also can force erythrocytes into corneal stroma, resulting in corneal blood staining that may take years to clear, causing irreversible amblyopia and permanent visual loss. In addition to a rebleed, another important risk factor associated with elevated intraocular pressure is sickle cell disease or trait caused by mechanical obstruction by sickled red blood cells of the trabecular meshwork. For this reason, a stat sickle prep should be ordered for African American or Hispanic children with hyphema. Children with positive results should be followed particularly closely.

Retinal Injury

Retinal pathology is impossible to assess in a primary care setting because it requires dilatation and use of ophthalmoscopic equipment. If visual acuity is impaired or if a significant injury has occurred, the provider should expeditiously refer the child to an ophthalmologist.

Ruptured Globe

A provider who suspects that a child has a ruptured globe from a penetrating or perforating injury should terminate the examination. He or she should tape an eye shield over the eye (providers can use a paper-drinking cup cut in half as a substitute) and request an emergency ophthalmology consultation. The provider should try to prevent emesis because of the risk of extrusion of intraocular contents.

Primary caregivers should be aware of the long-term sequelae of ocular trauma. Traumatic cataracts (partial or total) may develop months after an injury. Blunt trauma associated with significant subconjunctival hemorrhage, hyphema, or retinal pathology may induce angle recession of the trabecular meshwork and result in a silent glaucoma that causes progressive asymptomatic visual loss. Recommending yearly follow-up with an ophthalmologist is prudent for children who have incurred such injuries.

Chemical Injury

Following diagnosis of chemical injury (by history or suspicion) and before taking any other step (including a vision examination), the provider should use eyestream or normal saline to irrigate the eyes copiously, including the superior and inferior fornices, and to remove any particulate matter.

A pH test strip should reveal a neutral pH after irrigation; if not, the provider should continue irrigation. After neutralizing the pH, the provider should then immediately refer the child to an ophthalmologist for further management.

Foreign Body

If a foreign body is noted on penlight examination, copious irrigation may dislodge the object. The provider also should use copious irrigation when a child gets sand or similar material in the eye. Because penlight examination frequently is inadequate to reveal a foreign body, providers should refer children with suspected foreign bodies to an ophthalmologist for a slit lamp examination after irrigation. They also should be aware of the possibility of occult or apparent perforation of the globe by a foreign body, which would require emergency referral to an ophthalmologist.

REFERENCES

Abelson, M. B. (1998). Evaluation of olopatadine, a new ophthalmic antiallergic agent with dual activity, using the conjunctival allergen challenge model. *Annals of Allergy, Asthma, & Immunology, 81*(3), 211–218.

Barone, S. R., & Aiuto, L. T. (1997). Periorbital and orbital cellulitis in the Haemophilus influenzae vaccine era. *Journal of Pediatric Ophthalmology and Strabismus, 34*, 293–296.

Becker, B. B., Berry, F. D., & Koller, H. (1996). Balloon catheter dilation for treatment of congenital nasolacrimal duct obstruction. *American Journal of Ophthalmology, 121,* 304.

Buckley, R. J. (1998). Allergic eye disease-a clinical challenge. *Clinical and Experimental Allergy, 28*(Suppl. 6), 39–43.

Campolattaro, B. N., Lueder, G. T., & Tychsen, L. (1997). Spectrum of pediatric dacryocystitis: Medical and surgical management of 54 cases. *Journal of Pediatric Ophthalmology and Strabismus, 34*(3), 143–153.

Dannevig, L., Straume, B., Melby, K. (1992). Ophthalmia neonatorum in northern Norway. II. Microbiology emphasis on Chlamydia trachomatis. *Acta Ophthalmology (Copenhagen), 70*(1), 19–25.

Donahue, S. P., & Schwartz, G. (1998). Preseptal and orbital cellulitis in childhood: A changing microbiologic spectrum. *Ophthalmology, 105*(10), 1902–1905.

Friedman, L., Biedner, B., David, R., & Sachs, V. (1980). Screening for refractive errors, strabismus and other ocular anomalies from ages 6 months to 3 years. *Journal of Pediatric Ophthalmology and Strabismus, 17,* 315–317.

Gigliotti, F. (1993). Acute conjunctivitis of childhood. *Pediatric Annals, 22,* 353–356.

Graham, P. A. (1974). Epidemiology of strabismus. *British Journal of Ophthalmology, 58,* 224–231.

Hammerschlag, M. R. (1994). Chlamydia trachomatis in children. *Pediatric Annals, 23,* 349–353.

Hoyt, C. S., Mousel, D. K., & Weber, A. A. (1980). Transient supranuclear disturbances of gaze in healthy neonates. *American Journal of Ophthalmology, 89,* 708–712.

Isenberg, S. J., Apt, L., McCarty, J., Cooper, L. L., Lim, L., & Del Signore, M. (1998). Development of tearing in preterm and term neonates. *Archives of Ophthalmology, 116*(6), 773–776.

King, R. A. (1993). Common ocular signs and symptoms in childhood. *Pediatric Ophthalmology, 40,* 753–766.

Klassen, T. P., & Rowe, P. C. (1992). Selecting diagnostic test to identify febrile infants less than 3 months of age as being low risk for serious bacterial infection: A scientific overview. *Journal of Pediatrics, 121,* 676–681.

Mannor, G. E., Rose, G. E., Frimpong-Ansah, K., & Ezra, E. (1999). Factors affecting the success of nasolacrimal duct probing for congenital nasolacrimal duct obstruction. *American Journal of Ophthalmology, 127*(5), 616–617.

Nelson, L. B. (1998). *Harley's pediatric ophthalmology* (4th ed.). Philadelphia: W.B. Saunders.

Nozicka, C. A. (1995). Evaluation of the febrile infant younger than 3 months of age with no source of infection. *American Journal of Emergency Medicine, 13,* 215–218.

O'Hara, M. A. (1993). Ophthalmia neonatorum. *Pediatric Ophthalmology, 40,* 715–725.

Robb, R. M. (1998). Success rates of nasolacrimal duct probing at time intervals after 1 year of age. *Ophthalmology, 105*(7), 1307–1309.

Rumelt, S., & Rubin, P. A. D. (1996). Potential sources for orbital cellulitis. In F. A. Jakobiec & M. J. Lucarelli (Eds.), *Ocular and adnexal infections, International Ophthalmology Clinics* (pp. 207–221). Boston: Little, Brown.

Simons, K., & Reinecke, R. D. (1978). *Amblyopia screening and stereopsis. Symposium on Strabismus in Transactions of the New Orleans Academy of Ophthalmology* (pp. 15–50). St Louis: CV Mosby.

Taylor, D. (1997). *Paediatric ophthalmology* (2nd ed.). London: Blackwell Science.

Tingley, D. H. (1998). Eye trauma: Corneal abrasions. *Pediatrics in Review, 20*(9), 320–321.

Uzcategui, N., Warman, R., Smith, A., Howard, C. W. (1998). Clinical practice guidelines for the management of orbital cellulitis. *Journal of Pediatric Ophthalmology and Strabismus, 35*(2), 73–79.

Wright, K. W. (1995). *Pediatric ophthalmology and strabismus.* St. Louis: Mosby-Year Book.

Yanni, J. M., Weimer, L. K., Sharif, N. A., Xu, S. X., Gamache, D. A., & Spellman, J. M. (1999). Inhibition of histamine-induced human conjunctival epithelial cell responses by ocular allergy drugs. *Archives of Ophthalmology, 117*(5), 643–647.

CHAPTER 33

Ear and Sinus Problems

- MICHELLE PATRICK, RN, BSN, MSN, CPNP; KENNETH STEVEN GOTTESMAN, MD; and DARSIT K. SHAH, MD

PART 1 ▲

Ear and Sinus Problems for the Clinician

- MICHELLE PATRICK, RN, BSN, MSN, CPNP; KENNETH STEVEN GOTTESMAN, MD

INTRODUCTION

Middle ear disease is one of the most important problems that primary care practitioners encounter. It is responsible for about 25% of infant visits to practitioners, and by kindergarten age, it may account for 40% of visits (Maxon & Yamauchi, 1996). Even when a child comes for a well visit, practitioners may diagnose otitis media in up to 10% of cases, especially if an upper respiratory infection (URI) is involved.

The accurate diagnosis of middle ear disease is not simple. Ear canals can be small and inevitably occluded by cerumen. Pediatric patients are often uncooperative and screaming. Bright red tympanic membranes (TM) often match the color of the angry toddler's face but alone are not accurate predictors of the diagnosis.

The financial costs involved are immense. Even 20 years ago, the costs were approximately $2 billion for medical and surgical visits and procedures (Paradise & Rockette, 1997). Today, authorities estimate 30 million office visits and 23 million prescriptions are for otitis media in the United States alone (Klein, Marcy, & Paradise 1999).

OTITIS MEDIA

Anatomy, Physiology, and Pathology

The middle ear is a component of the upper respiratory passages. The other parts of this system are the nose, nasopharynx, eustachian tubes, paranasal sinuses, and mastoids. Respiratory mucosa lines all these structures. Researchers mostly agree that the eustachian tube is the key factor in the pathogenesis of middle ear disease. The structure and function of this conduit are almost inseparable when considering middle ear disease. The tube has three main functions:

- Ventilation to allow pressure in the middle ear to equilibrate with atmospheric pressure and provide oxygen
- Protection to keep nasopharyngeal secretions and sound pressure out of the middle ear
- Drainage of secretions produced in the middle ear

The eustachian tube connects the middle ear to the nasopharynx. Its spatial relationship in the head is one important factor. In an adult, the tube is on an angle of 45 degrees in the horizontal plane. In an infant, the tube is on an angle of 10 degrees, is half the length of an adult tube, and has less cartilagenous support. Four muscles are around the eustachian tube. One of them, the tensor veli palatini, appears to be most actively involved in tube function. In the resting state, the eustachian tube is closed. Swallowing, yawning, or sneezing cause it to open, ventilating the middle ear. The tensor veli palatini appears to cause this dilatation.

Normally a slightly negative pressure is found in the middle ear. This pressure may become more negative when obstruction impairs the tube's ventilatory function and the air in the middle ear is resorbed.

If at this point the eustachian tube opens, nasopharyngeal contents also may be aspirated into the middle ear, leading to infection. Another possible mechanism is reflux of nasopharyngeal contents, even in the absence of high negative middle ear pressure. This may occur if the tube is patulous due to abnormal muscular function. The shorter infant tube would promote both scenarios more readily, especially in the supine feeding position. A third mechanism might be insufflation of nasopharyngeal contents into the middle ear.

The tube also may be mechanically blocked. Extrinsic blockage may result from adenoidal hypertrophy or less commonly from a tumor. Intrinsic obstruction may occur due to inflammation, infection, or allergy. A classic study showed that in many cases, allergic rhinitis was contributory (Fireman, 1987). Because of immunoglobulin E (IgE) late phase reactants, frequent re-exposure to allergens may cause inflammation and secondary obstruction to persist for prolonged periods. (Intranasal challenge with house dust mites and histamine caused eustachian tube obstruction in patients with allergic rhinitis but not in normal controls). Less frequently, otitis media with effusion (OME) has been associated with immunodeficiencies, cleft palate (even postrepair), bifid uvulae (associated with a submucous cleft), and disorders affecting the normal clearance of nasopharyngeal secretions, ciliary dyskinesia, and immotile cilia syndrome.

The variety of bacterial pathogens isolated from the middle ear has remained unchanged over many years. When middle ear fluid is aspirated, bacteria are isolated in approximately two thirds of cases. Recently, the percentages of these isolates have changed, as have their resistance patterns. One must understand the concept of minimal inhibitory concentration (MIC) to understand how bacterial resistance is measured. The MIC is the minimum amount of a drug that will inhibit bacterial growth in a test tube. It is the amount that one attempts to clinically deliver to the infection site for as long as possible between doses. If the antibiotic concentration exceeds the MIC for 30% to 40% of the time, organism eradication usually occurs. The ability to deliver high concentrations of antibiotic to an anatomic area depends on multiple factors, including route of administration, dose, absorption, blood supply to the target area, and metabolic clearance. In the middle ear, the relatively limited blood supply makes it difficult to achieve adequate MICs, especially in the context of emerging bacterial resistance.

Streptococcus pneumoniae (pneumococcus) is found in 40% to 50% of isolates. Although previously exquisitely sensitive to all penicillins, incidence of resistance has been increasing in the United States in the range of 34% (Dowell et al., 1999). The method of resistance relates to penicillin-binding proteins on the bacterial cell wall and creates a new classification of pnemococcus based on its susceptibility to penicillins. The MICs for penicillin are as follows:

- Susceptible: less than or equal to 0.06 μg/mL
- Intermediate: 0.12 to 1.0 μg/mL
- Resistant: greater than 2 μg/mL

Approximately half of the resistant strains demonstrate absolute resistance and are now impervious to penicillin, however high the dose or MIC reached. The remaining half of intermediate or relatively resistant strains can be treated with higher than previously recommended doses of penicillin (Dowell et al., 1999). Factors associated with increasing pneumococcal resistance include antibiotic use within the past 3 months, age younger than 2 years, attendance in day care, recent hospitalization, and infection during the late winter or spring months (Pong & Harrison, 1998).

Haemophilus influenzae (H. flu) is found in 20% to 30% of isolates. These strains are almost all nontypeable. This organism may be more prevalent in older children and adults. Resistance is based on beta-lactam enzymes, which break down the lactam ring structure of penicillin. The percentage of lactamase producing H. flu varies by geographic locality and ranges between 30% and 90% (Dowell et al., 1999). The association of purulent conjunctivitis and otitis increases the likelihood of H. flu as an etiology (Bodor, 1982).

Moraxella catarrhalis (M. cat) is found in 10% to 15% of isolates. These are generally beta-lactamase producers and resistant to aminopenicillins in the range of 30% to 90% as well (Dowell et al., 1999).

Other bacteria may be occasionally isolated. These include group A streptococci, *Staphylococcus aureus*, and *Pseudomonas aeruginosa*. In the neonatal period, gram-negative enteric pathogens may be found; *Chlamydia trachomatis* also has been isolated in this age group. Bullous myringitis, characterized by TM blisters, is caused by the same pathogens as acute otitis media (AOM). Years ago, the etiology was thought to be *Mycoplasma pneumoniae*; however, this organism and *Chlamydia pneumoniae* may be etiologically implicated in association with disease of the lower respiratory tract.

More recently, viruses have been detected in approximately 30% to 40% of cases. The most common isolates are respiratory syncytial virus (74%), parainfluenza (52%), and influenzae virus (42%) (Heikkinen, Thint, & Chonmaitree, 1999). Some studies have found co-infection with viral and bacterial etiologies.

Epidemiology

With otitis media being one of the most common diagnoses pediatric practitioners make, one would expect many factors to be involved in its cause. This is certainly true, with genetic, familial, anatomic, allergic, and environmental components all contributing. Males have been found to have more acute and recurrent episodes in North America (Maxon & Yamauchi, 1996; Paradise & Rockette, 1997). An extremely high incidence is found in Native American and Eskimo populations. Children with Down syndrome and those with cleft palate also have a higher frequency, apparently as a result of the abnormal spatial relationship between the tensor veli palatini muscle and the eustachian tube seen in these conditions. Poor social conditions also predispose to a higher incidence of middle ear disease (Paradise & Rockette, 1997), suggesting that overcrowding, poor sanitation, and decreased access to medical care are contributing factors. Analogous to overcrowded conditions, children with older siblings and even more so, those in day care settings have a greater rate of occurrence because of their more frequent exposure to winter URIs. Infants who have their bottles propped or are fed in a supine position also have a higher incidence of MEE. Parental smoking and the use of pacifiers appear to be contributing factors as well (Niemela, Uhari, & Mottonen, 1995). Infants and children with respiratory allergies also may be at increased risk. Probably the most important determinant is a family history of middle ear disease. One important element that may help to protect against middle ear disease is if the infant is breastfed for at least 3 months (Paradise & Rockette, 1997).

History and Physical Examination

Forty percent to 50% of cases of AOM are associated with an ongoing URI, which on its own may cause irritability, fever, cough, decreased appetite, vomiting, and diarrhea.

● **Clinical Pearl:** Only half of patients with AOM have fever. Otalgia is the most specific symptom.

In the young infant, this is often represented by pulling on the ear, difficulty in swallowing, and discomfort when lying down. In the past several years, an association with purulent conjunctivitis has been noted, most often caused by nontypeable *H. influenzae*. A recent study from Finland confirmed that the most important symptom associated with AOM is otalgia (Kontiokari & Kolvunen, 1998). Sore throat and night restlessness were less strongly associated.

Being able to see the TM is not always easy. Many children do not like their ears to be examined. Cerumen is the bane of the practitioner's existence. Providers often need to irrigate wax (a Water-Pik is very good for this procedure) or curette it out of the child's ear canal (soft plastic-nylon disposable curettes are less traumatic than the older wire loop ones).

● **Clinical Pearl:** To assess the TM fully, one needs to consider its color, position, degree of translucency, and, most importantly, mobility. The diagnosis of middle ear disease cannot be made without some assessment of TM mobility.

Mobility assessment can only be accomplished with a pneumatic otoscope and insufflator or the use of tympanometry. The technique used in examining the patient depends on the child's age and degree of cooperation. In the infant, having the child lie down, with the parent holding the arms down at the patient's side, is a reasonable technique. Another option is that the parent hold the child in the arms, with the head resting on the parent's shoulder and cradled against the parent's neck. Providers should always use the largest ear speculum possible. Pulling down slightly on the pinna will allow visualization of the TM. In the older child, providers may use the same technique but pulling straight back or up slightly on the pinna.

The normal TM is grayish pink and translucent, with the characteristic cone of light progressing from the center of the drum in an anteroinferior direction. As the examiner looks at the drum, it is helpful to imagine one looking at the underside of an umbrella, with the center of the TM further away than the periphery. At the onset of AOM, the TM may be slightly retracted. As the process evolves, it becomes red, thickened, and may bulge outward. Slight redness of the upper part of the drum (pars flaccida) is usually normal, especially in the crying child. With resolution of the acute process, otitis media with effusion (OME), formerly referred to as serous otitis, commonly results and may persist for weeks. The TM is usually retracted, and fluid levels may be seen.

To evaluate mobility, one must use the insufflator by squeezing then releasing the bulb. A good example of a patient-centered technique is to gently squeeze the bulb against the child's cheek, which serves in the dual role of reassurance and distraction before insufflating the TM. When normal, the TM will move inward when positive pressure is applied and move outward (return to its original position) when the bulb is released. Any fluid in the middle ear space will cause decreased mobility. If there is high negative pressure behind the drum (seen with eustachian tube dysfunction and resolving AOM), there will be no movement with positive insufflation, only on release of the bulb. With high positive pressure of the drum (eg, a bulging TM seen with AOM or severe OME), squeezing the bulb will either yield zero or diminished movement.

Often one sees an auditory canal filled with pus. This usually represents a perforated TM associated with AOM. Once the TM has perforated, the child usually feels better because the pressure in the middle ear has been relieved. In the child with tympanostomy tubes in place, this drainage also represents AOM.

The TM of the newborn requires special consideration. It is in a different position than the older child, being more horizontal. By about 1 month of age, it has moved into the position to which practitioners are accustomed.

Diagnostic Criteria

The diagnosis of AOM is based on criteria outlined in Table 33-1. Otalgia or evidence of otalgia in the young infant is the most important consideration. For differential diagnoses,

---

Table 33–1. DIAGNOSTIC CRITERIA FOR ACUTE OTITIS MEDIA

- Otalgia
- An abnormal tympanic membrane (TM) with decreased mobility
- A draining TM with a history of otalgia
- A draining TM in a child with tympanostomy tubes
- A tympanocentesis yielding a pathogenic organism

---

providers should consider any condition that may cause otalgia. The most common conditions include the following:

- Otitis externa (see separate section).
- Pharyngitis; children often confuse throat and ear pain.
- Eustachian tube dysfunction; this diagnosis may be appropriate for the child with a URI and a normal-looking TM, possibly with decreased mobility on pneumatic otoscopy.
- Cervical adenitis.
- Temporal-mandibular joint syndrome; the mandible forms one third of the auditory canal, and this pain therefore is easily referred to the ear.
- Dental problems; teething, dental abscess, or postorthodontic adjustment may cause otalgia.

Diagnostic Studies

The following diagnostic studies may be used:

- Tympanometry. This test uses an electroacoustic impedance bridge, which presents a tone through a small probe inserted at the opening of the external auditory canal. It measures the compliance of the TM while the pressure presented to the canal varies. It produces different patterns graphically. The mean tympanometric peak pressure (TPP) is usually normal between $(-)150$ to $(+)11$. A more negative TPP or a flat tympanogram is indicative of middle ear pathology. Most commonly, tympanograms are useful in the diagnosis of middle ear pathology or as an objective test in the follow-up of AOM or OME. They also are extremely useful in assessing TM integrity, as in perforations or patency of myringotomy tubes. In these situations, the measured ear canal volume would be abnormally high. Additionally, in the case of a child with cerumenous canals whose TMs are not able to be fully visualized, a normal tympanogram would be fairly conclusive evidence against AOM or OME. The reader is referred to Figure 33-1 for common typanogram patterns and their interpretations.
- Tympanocentesis. Although usually thought of as a part of myringotomy and tubes (M&T), diagnostic tympanocentesis still has a place in the evaluation of AOM. The indications for this procedure are severe otalgia or toxic appearance, poor re-sponse to antibiotic therapy, AOM associated with suppurative complications, or the neonate or immunosuppressed patient, either of whom may harbor unusual organisms.

Management

Parents frequently have questions and concerns regarding the causes, treatment, and recurrence of otitis media. Caretakers are often unaware of preventive measures that may reduce their child's risk of AOM and OME. Education also dispels some commonly held misconceptions. Parents frequently believe cerumen buildup contributes to OM. It is also not unusual for a parent to be concerned because their child is a little cranky and ear infections are "going around" at the day care or because their preverbal child is tugging on an ear. If physical examination reveals a relatively normal-looking TM with good mobility on pneumatic otoscopy, the provider has the opportunity to discuss with parents the true causes and more reliable signs and symptoms of AOM (ie, fever, prolonged cold symptoms, complaints of pain, or hearing loss in the verbal child). Some parents, especially

Normative Tympanometric Data

Typanometric Measurement	Child's Ear (Under Age 10) 90% Range	Adult's Ear (Over Age 10) 90% Range
Peak Ya	0.2 to 0.9 mmho	0.3 to 1.4 mmho
Gradient (GR) (Tympanometric Width)	60 to 150 daPa	50 to 110 daPa
Tympanometric Peak Pressure (TPP)	-139 to +11 daPa	-83 to 0 daPa
Equivalent Ear Canal Volume (Vea)	0.4 to 1.0 cc	0.6 to 1.5 cc

NOTE: For purposes of tympanometric norms, an adult is defined as a person 10 years of age or older, and a child as under age 10. Normative data are taken from a study by Margolis and Heller (1987), and from the "Guidelines for Screening for Hearing Impairments and Middle Ear Disorders" ASHA (1990).

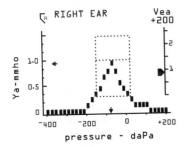

Normal Middle Ear
- Produces tympanogram within normal limits relative to height and width

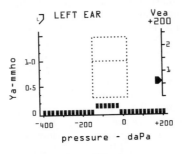

Otitis Media With Effusion
- Produces low static admittance (low peak height) tympanogram
- Tympanogram is also typical of tympanosclerosis, cholesteatoma, and middle ear tumor

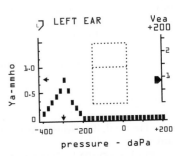

Negative Middle Ear Pressure
- Produces negative Tympanometric Peak Pressure (TTP) tympanogram
- Usually not associated with effusion when Peak Ya is normal
- Also associated with eustachian tube dysfunction, cold, or allergies

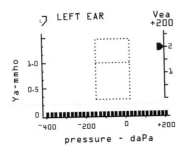

Patent Tympanostomy Tube or Perforated Tympanic Membrane
- Can produce flat tympanogram with ear canal volume higher than expected

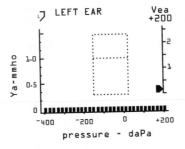

Ear Canal Occlusion
- Can produce flat tympanogram with ear canal volume lower than expected
- Requires repeating measurement

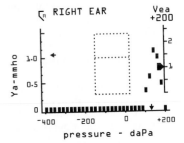

Positive Middle Ear Pressure
- Produces positive Tympanometric Peak Pressure (TTP) tympanogram
- Can be indicative of acute otitis media if peak is extremely positive

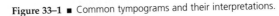

Figure 33–1 ■ Common tympograms and their interpretations.

those whose child experiences of recurrent AOM, become familiar with their child's "soft signs," such as irritability, loss of appetite, and diarrhea, when concurrent with prolonged cold symptoms.

Another area of significant parental concern is that of hearing loss due to or associated with otitis media. Serosanguinous or purulent drainage from an ear canal, as well as the diagnosis of a perforated TM, can be alarming to parents. The image of a hole in the eardrum frequently causes fear of permanent hearing loss. Parents appreciate reassurance that the eardrum should heal, and the provider has a good opportunity to reinforce the importance of follow-up visits. OME may cause a transient conductive hearing loss. The older child with OME may complain of muffled sounds or tinnitus; the younger child may seem less responsive to parents' voices. Reassurance that hearing loss is temporary and will last only as long as the effusion puts a parent's mind at ease.

● **Clinical Pearl:** Parents need to know that OME is not an acute disease. Effusions commonly last up to 3 months following AOM.

Tables 33-2 and 33-3 summarize parental instruction points regarding the nature and prevention of AOM/OME respectively.

Table 33–2. INSTRUCTION POINTS FOR ACUTE OTITIS MEDIA (AOM)/(OME)

- Pain and fever should resolve within 48–72 h of initiating antibiotic treatment; topical analgesic drops or oral analgesics can be used as needed.
- A single episode of a perforated tympanic membrane will not result in a permanent hearing loss.
- A child with AOM is likely to develop OME once the acute infection is resolved; OME may persist up to 3 mo before spontaneously resolving.
- Chronic OME (lasting more than 3–4 mo) may result in a temporary language delay, which is usually corrected with placement of tympanostomy tubes and speech therapy.
- AOM follow-up is needed 2 wk after initiation of antibiotic treatment.
- OME follow-up is needed 4–6 wk after initial diagnosis of middle ear effusion; hearing evaluation will be done if MEE persists for 3 mo.
- Criteria for antibiotic prophylaxis include > three episodes of AOM within 6 mo, or > four episodes within 12 mo.
- Criteria/candidacy for ENT referral and tympanostomy tube placement:
  - OME persisting for longer than 3–4 mo associated with a conductive hearing loss
  - Frequent recurrent AOM despite adequate prophylaxis
  - Parental choice

OME = Otitis media with effusion; MEE = Middle ear effusion; ENT = ear, nose, and throat

Pharmacologic Treatment

Before the availability of antibiotics, AOM had potentially serious suppurative sequelae. Mastoiditis, brain abscess, epidural and subdural empyema, and meningitis were complications in up to 25% of cases. The use of antibiotics in the treatment of otitis media has decreased the rate of complications to less than 3% (Fliss, Leiberman, & Dagan, 1994). Recent emergence of penicillin-resistant *S. pneumoniae* strains, however, has prompted researchers and providers to reconsider the risks and benefits of liberal antibiotic use.

A 1998 literature review (Conrad) compared five small cohort studies (n < 280) that examined antibiotic treatment versus nontreatment of AOM. These studies showed that although antibiotic use provided relief of acute symptoms, they did not decrease the frequency of either long-term effusions (OME) or acute recurrences. A meta-analysis of 33 randomized trials involving 5400 children concluded that clinical symptoms of AOM resolved spontaneously in 81% of untreated cases (Rosenfeld et al., 1994). In 1994, Klein found a spontaneous cure rate of 60%. By examining middle ear fluid obtained by tympanocentesis, researchers have found that AOM due to *M. catarrhalis* and *H. influenzae*, as well as AOM of viral etiology, are far more likely to resolve spontaneously than AOM due to *S. pneumoniae*.

AOM remains a clinical diagnosis; it is impossible for the practitioner to determine the pathogens responsible based on findings at examination. Because tympanocentesis obviously cannot be performed on every child with AOM, antimicrobials continue to be the treatment of choice for all cases meeting diagnostic criteria.

Today, many cases of otitis media occur in children at risk for infection with a resistant organism. This problem prompted the issuance of a report on the treatment of otitis media in the era of pneumococcal resistance by the Drug-resistant *Streptococcus pneumoniae* Therapeutic Work-

Table 33–3. ACUTE OTITIS MEDIA PREVENTION INSTRUCTION POINTS

- Infants breastfed for at least 3 mo are less likely to experience recurrent AOM; continued breastfeeding further decreases risk.
- Exposure to second-hand smoke greatly increases child's risk of AOM/OME (maternal smoking may increase risk as much as 70%).
- Enrollment in day care increases risk.
- Prolonged use of bottle, especially in a reclined position, increases risk.
- Prolonged use of pacifier may increase risk.

OME = Otitis media with effusion

ing Group (Dowell et al., 1999). This group emphasizes that when selecting a first-line drug for the treatment of AOM, efficacy against *S. pneumoniae* is paramount, because it is the most common bacterial cause. The other major pathogens, *H. influenzae* and *M. catarrhalis*, are more likely to produce disease with a high rate of spontaneous resolution. For these reasons, amoxicillin remains the best single choice for initial treatment of AOM (Dowell et al., 1999).

● **Clinical Pearl:** The child who is younger than 2 years, attends day care, or has been treated with antibiotics during the previous 3 months is at increased risk for infection with drug-resistant *S. Pneumoniae* (DRSP). For these children with AOM, amoxicillin 80 to 90 mg/kg/d (twice the usual recommended dose) should be the initial treatment.

The older child who does not have any other risk factors may be treated with what was previously considered the standard amoxicillin dose of 40 to 45 mg/kg/d (Dowell et al., 1999).

● **Clinical Pearl:** Treatment failure can be defined as a lack of clinical improvement in signs and symptoms, such as ear pain, fever, and TM findings (eg, redness, bulging, or otorrhea) after 3 days of treatment (Dowell et al., 1999).

▲ **Clinical Warning:** Children with signs or symptoms that are not specific to an acute otitis, such as a persistent MEE, cold symptoms, or other accompaniments to a viral URI, should not be considered treatment failures. A persistent MEE is an expected finding in 70% of patients evaluated after 2 to 3 weeks and should not be considered a treatment failure (Dowell et al., 1999).

The child who remains symptomatic after 72 hours of amoxicillin therapy or the child with a bulging, immobile TM and recurrence of acute symptoms after a full course of amoxicillin requires retreatment with a second-line agent. Table 33-4 lists common antibiotics and their in vitro efficacy.

Retreatment of a child at risk for resistant infection should be limited to agents known to be efficacious against both resistant pneumococci and beta-lactamase producing pathogens, based on comparative clinical trials. It should be noted, however, that many antibiotics listed in Table 33-4 may well have equal but not yet proven efficacy to those that are described below. However, until each has been studied in comparative clinical trials, the clinician should be circumspect regarding their use. At the time of publication, only the following antibiotic regimens have met the above criteria of

Table 33–4.   RELATIVE IN VITRO ACTIVITY OF VARIOUS ANTIBIOTICS AGAINST COMMON ACUTE OTITIS MEDIA PATHOGENS

Antibiotic	*Streptococcus pneumoniae*			*Haemophilus influenzae*		*Moraxella catarrhalis*	
	S	I	R	BL −	BL+	BL −	BL+
Amoxicillin (Amoxil)	+++	++	+	+++	−	+++	−
Amoxicillin-clavulanate (Augmentin)	+++	++	+	+++	+++	+++	+++
Azithromycin (Zithromax)	+++	+	−	++	++	+++	+++
Cefixime (Suprax)	+++	−	−	+++	+++	+++	+++
Cefpodoxime (Vantin)	+++	+	−	+++	+++	NE	NE
Cefprozil (Cefzil)	+++	+	+/−	++	++	++	++
Ceftibuten (Cedax)	+++	−	−	+++	+++	+++	+++
Ceftriaxone (Rocephin)	+++	+++	++	+++	+++	+++	+++
Cefuroxime (Ceftin)	+++	+	−	+++	++	+++	+++
Clarithromycin (Biaxin)	+++	+	−	+	+	+++	+++
Loracarbef (Lorabid)	++	−	−	++	+/−	++	+
TMP-SMX (Septra/Bactrim)	++	−	−	+	+	+	+

BL− = β-lactamase negative; BL+ = β-lactamase positive; I = intermediate; NE = not evaluated; R = resistant; S = susceptible; TMP-SMX = trimethoprim-sulfamethoxazole; +++ = excellent; ++ = good; + = fair; − = poor or none.
  Data updated from susceptibility studies by Jones et al.,[15] Barry et al.,[16] Doern et al.,[17] Washington,[18] and Wise et al.[19]
  Courtesy of (1998). *Otitis media: Management strategies for the 21st century.* 1998 Meniscus Educational Institute.

clinically proven efficacy in comparative trials against both DRSP and beta-lactamase producing pathogens:

- Amoxicillin-clavulanate (in its newer formulation containing 80–90 mg/kg/d of amoxicillin and 6.4 mg/kg/d of clavulinic acid)
- Cefuroxime axetil
- Intramuscular ceftriaxone (1–3 daily intramuscular doses)

Combining amoxicillin (40–45 mg/kg/d), with amoxicillin-clavulanate (45 mg/kg/d) achieves the same effect as the newer single preparation.

According to the Therapeutic Working Group (Dowell et al., 1999), other agents, cefprozil and cefpodoxime, have been proven effective against beta-lactamase producers but have only demonstrated in vitro activity against some DRSP. Studies may yet show their efficacy in comparative clinical trials but have not done so to date. Pneumococcal resistance to trimethoprim/sulfamethoxazole may be more common than that to penicillin, making this class of previously effective drugs less so today. Pneumococcal resistance to erythromycin is more absolute than to penicillin, calling into question this macrolide's part in its combination with sulfasoxizole. The role of the newer macrolides, clarithromycin and azithromycin, in the treatment of otitis in this age of DRSP remains to be studied. In the future, newer agents in the fluoroquinolone class of antimicrobials may prove safe and efficacious for children. The reader is referred to an algorithm for treatment of AOM in the era of emergent drug resistance (Fig. 33-2).

Analgesia is an important part of the overall management; the provider must keep in mind that ineffective pain control can lead to the misdiagnosis of treatment failure. Otalgia is usually well managed with acetaminophen, nonsteroidal anti-inflammatory drugs, or topical analgesic otic drops.

AOM not responding to appropriate antimicrobials may be due to factors other than resistant organisms. It was recently found by tympanocentesis that in 50% of persistent AOM cases, no pathogen could be isolated from middle ear fluid

(MEF); in 52% to 80%, the cultured organism was susceptible to the prescribed antibiotic (Pichichero & Pichichero, 1995). A persistently red, immobile TM may be due to a postinfectious inflammatory response and can be distinguished from persistent AOM by the lack of acute signs and symptoms.

● **Clinical Pearl:** In the absence of symptoms, an abnormally red TM or one manifesting decreased or absent mobility does not warrant antibiotic treatment.

● **Clinical Pearl:** A child with fever, achiness, rhinitis, and questionable ear pain, whose examination fails to demonstrate an abnormal TM, does not warrant antibiotic treatment.

AOM complicated by TM perforation requires the same treatment as AOM without perforation. Some providers also prescribe topical antibiotic suspensions for use in children with AOM and TM perforation. Theoretically, those containing neosporin should be used with caution because of the extremely rare possibility of ototoxicity. Although far more expensive, the newer quinolone otic drops avoid this potential problem.

The incidence of antibiotic resistance has increased at an alarming rate over the past few years. Future changes in the patterns of resistance will dictate changes in recommended treatments. It is imperative that practitioners keep up to date in their knowledge of epidemiology and current recommendations.

● **Clinical Pearl:** Overtreatment of otitis media has resulted in a significant increase in resistant strains; decreasing the frequency of antibiotic use will, over time, reverse patterns of antibiotic resistance (Seppala et al., 1997).

Prevention

The most common risk factors for recurrent or persistent otitis media include attendance in day care, exposure to second-hand smoke, prolonged bottle drinking, and pacifier use. Of these, in pragmatic terms, day care attendance is the only risk

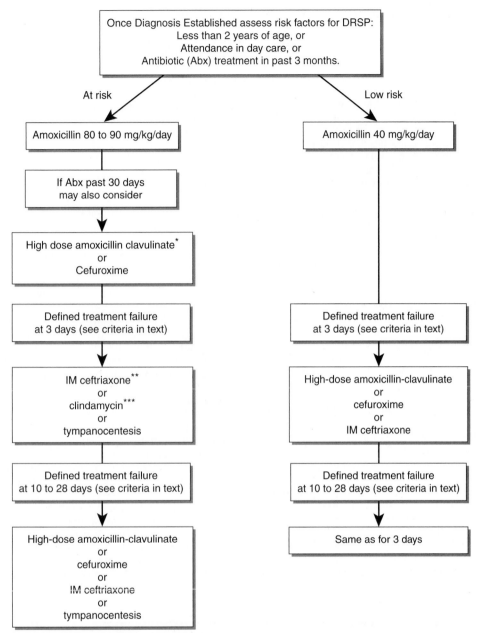

This algorithm incorporates drugs for which there is strong evidence for efficacy. Future studies may well demonstrate efficacy for other antibiotics. Please see text for details.

*Contains 80 to 90 mg/kg/day of the amoxicillin component and 6.4 mg/kg/day of clavulinic acid (requires newer formulation or combination with amoxicillin).

**Documented efficacy in treatment failures if 3 daily IM doses given.

***Clindamycin not effective against *H.influenza* or *M. catarrhalis*; should only be used after completion of three days of effective treatment for these pathogens with lactamase resistant antibiotics.

Figure 33–2 ■ Management of acute otitis media in the era of antibiotic resistance. Adapted from Dowell, S. F., Butler, J. C., Giebink, G. S., et al. (1999). Acute otitis media: Management and surveillance in an era of pneumococcal resistance—a report from the Drug-resistant *Streptococcus pneumoniae* Therapeutic Working Group. *Pediatric Infectious Disease Journal, 18,* 1–9.

factor that usually cannot be eliminated. As for the others, providers can fairly easily impress on parents that weaning to a cup, "losing" the pacifier, and smoking outdoors (if at all) are much more sensible strategies than long-term antibiotics or surgical interventions, with their attendant anesthetic risks.

● **Clinical Pearl:** Counseling the family on risk factors is often very effective in decreasing the frequency of recurrent AOM. Providers should perform such counseling before considering either medical or surgical interventions (see Table 33-3).

Medical Prophylaxis of Acute Otitis Media

Several prophylactic measures are available for children with recurrent AOM, defined as more than three distinct episodes within 6 months or more than four episodes within 12 months. Prophylactic antibiotic use recently has become more controversial because of the rising incidence of resistant bacteria. A child with recurrent AOM usually has several other risk factors for colonization or infection with resistant *S. pneumoniae*; therefore, providers must carefully consider the appropriateness of daily antibiotics. For children deemed candidates for this method of prophylaxis, sulfisoxazole (60 mg/kg/dose) given once daily during the winter months has been shown to decrease significantly the number of recurrences. Prophylaxis usually is discontinued from May through September, when URIs are less frequent. In an attempt to decrease further the spread of resistant organisms, however, many authorities are recommending the initiation of prophylaxis only at the first signs of URI and then discontinuance when cold symptoms have resolved. Some parents may not be comfortable with the idea of long-term antibiotic use or may find it difficult to administer antibiotics regularly for an extended period. They may want to explore myringotomy with tympanostomy tubes as a therapeutic option.

The new pneumococcal polysaccharide conjugate vaccine, should prove beneficial to the high-risk population younger than 2 years and has been projected to reduce the overall incidence of AOM by 10% and recurrent episodes by 20% (Klein et al., 1999). Recommendations call for a schedule of immunization at ages 2, 4, and 6 months and between ages 12 and 15 months. Influenza vaccine also has been shown to decrease the incidence of AOM and may be considered for children with a history of frequent recurrences.

When discussing preventive options with the parents of a child with recurrent AOM, providers should consider the time of year. Recurrent AOM is most likely to plague children during the seasons when respiratory syncitial virus, rhinovirus, adenovirus, and influenza are common; only a small percentage of children develop AOM during the summer. Winter is most appropriate for placement of tympanostomy tubes or a trial of antibiotic prophylaxis. As previously discussed, clinicians always should address environmental risk factors when discussing preventive measures with parents.

OTITIS MEDIA WITH EFFUSION

Two thirds of children with AOM will subsequently develop OME. Spontaneous resolution occurs within 90 days in 80% to 90% of cases. Chronic OME (effusions lasting more than 3 months) not only is associated with hearing loss, but also presents the possibility of language delay and behavioral problems in younger children and poor academic performance in older children. In an attempt to minimize variations in treatment, the Agency for Health Care Policy and Research (AHCPR) issued guidelines in 1994 for the management of OME (Stool, Bert, & Berman, 1994). In conjunction with the American Academy of Family Physicians and the American Academy of Otolaryngology Head and Neck Surgery, the American Academy of Pediatrics developed guidelines and an algorithm. The guidelines and algorithm are for the child from ages 1 to 3 years, without craniofacial or sensory deficits, and who is healthy except for OME (Fig. 33-3). Follow-up is recommended at 6, 9, and 12 weeks. Evaluations should include the use of pneumatic otoscopy or tympanometry. Management for OME per-

sisting at the 6-week follow-up is either continued observation or a trial of antibiotics. Although the AHCPR guidelines do not recommend specific antibiotics, the same criteria used to select the appropriate agent for treatment of AOM may apply to OME. Environmental risk factor counseling (especially the effects of second-hand smoke) and hearing evaluation are optional at the 6-week follow-up. Management for OME persisting at the 9-week follow-up, diagnosed by either pneumatic otoscopy or tympanometry, may again be observation or a trial of antibiotics.

● **Clinical Pearl:** Surgical intervention is not indicated until OME has persisted for at least 4 months, with bilateral conductive hearing loss of at least 20 dB.

Some studies have shown that adenoidectomy, especially in conjunction with tympanostomy tube placement, may be efficacious in treating OME. Only bilateral myringotomy with tube placement is specifically recommended. The guidelines specifically discourage the use of oral steroids, decongestants, and antihistamines in the management of OME. Studies have shown that antibiotics combined with prednisone 1 to 2 mg/kg/d for 5 to 7 days may be effective in clearing OME in some children. Though not recommended in the AHCPR guidelines, this treatment may be appropriate for the child whose parents view surgery as the last resort. Steroid therapy always is contraindicated for the child exposed to varicella due to the possibility of life-threatening disseminated disease.

Most treatment and management of OME lies within the scope of the primary care provider's expertise. Referral to an otolaryngologist should occur when a child becomes a candidate for tympanostomy tube placement. Myringotomy with tube placement is the most common surgical procedure performed on children in the United States. The 1994 AHCPR recommendations on tympanostomy tube placement are based on analysis of efficacy and cost-effectiveness.

Recurrent AOM (three or more episodes in 6 months or four or more episodes in 12 months) resulting in significant morbidity also may benefit from tube placement, especially if antibiotic prophylaxis has failed. Providers must consider each child individually when assessing the appropriateness of tube placement. They must consider parental preference, time of year, and bilateral versus unilateral disease.

OTITIS EXTERNA

Otitis externa (OE), also known as swimmer's ear, is an infection and inflammation of the auditory canal. This form of ear infection is often more painful than otitis media. For many pediatric practitioners, it may be a year-round occurrence to include in the differential diagnosis of otalgia; for others, otitis externa is a seasonal event.

Anatomy, Physiology, and Pathology

The auditory canal usually is well protected by cerumen produced there. If, however, the canal is exposed to a large inoculum of offending organisms, it is a good locus for bacterial reproduction and infection, because it is a warm and relatively enclosed space. The most common precipitant is swimming, more commonly in lakes and ponds, and often during heat waves, which induce more luxuriant growth of the normally occurring flora. The most common infectious organisms are *S. aureus, Pseudomonas aeroginosa,*

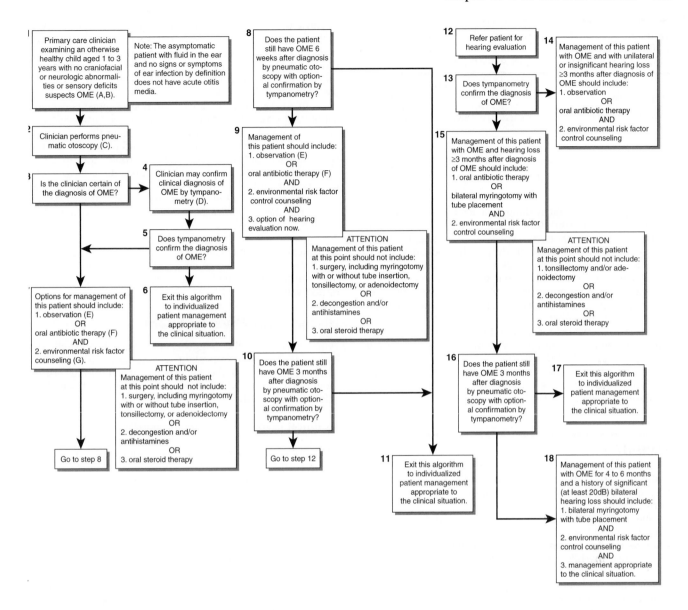

Figure 33–3 ■ Algorithm for managing otitis media with effusion in an otherwise healthy child aged 1 to 3 years. From Steel, S. E., Bert, A. O., & Berman, S. Otitis Media with Effusion in Young Children. Clinical Practice Guideline #12 AHCPR publication #94-062.

and any of the common fungi inhabiting the external auditory canal.

History and Physical Examination

Otalgia is the universal complaint. A history of swimming is readily obtained. Children are very aware that touching the affected ear elicits exquisite pain. Therefore, the provider must examine the affected ear(s) very cautiously and gently. Even before using the otoscope, the practitioner will have a firm idea of the diagnosis, as gently pulling on the pinna or tragus will evoke significant pain. The ear canal will appear red, often rough, and significantly swollen and may exude a mucopurulent discharge. The degree of any of the above findings may make it impossible to visualize the TM. If seen, the TM may appear red, rough, or thickened. This usually represents extension of the inflammation from the auditory canal onto the membrane and not a true middle ear infection. If the provider suspects the presence of a concomitant

middle ear infection, he or she should perform gentle typanometry in an attempt to exclude that diagnosis. In the era of antibiotic resistance, providers should prescribe systemic antibiotics only when the presence of a true middle ear infection is certain.

Management

Treatment for otitis externa consists of topical antibiotic drops. An informal survey of topical otic preparations in Dutchess County, NY, revealed a wide variation in retail cost (Table 33-5). Clinicians would be wise to ascertain cost variations in their own locales. The advantage of the newer quinolone preparations appears limited to children whose TMs are not intact, because of perforation or tube placement. In these cases, the quinolones may prevent potential neomycin ototoxicity, thus justifying their higher cost.

While being treated, the child should avoid situations that might allow water into the ear canal. Occasionally, OE can

Table 33–5. AN INFORMAL SURVEY OF COMMON TOPICAL OTIC ANTIBIOTIC PREPARATION RETAIL COST IN DUTCHESS COUNTY, NY, IN AUGUST 1999

Preparation	Pharmacy A	Pharmacy B
Vosol HC 10 mL	$20.00	$14.97
Corticosporin otic 10 mL	$23.00	$28.99
Cipro HC 10 mL	$76.69	$73.99
Floxin 5 mL	$49.98	$42.00

cause significant edema, making visualization of the canal or administration of drops difficult. An ear wick (a spongefoam that expands when moistened) placed in the canal facilitates the administration of antibiotic drops. The wick may stay in place for a few days and also allows the otic preparation to remain in contact with the canal for a prolonged period. Some patients may not respond to topical treatment. They may require an oral antibiotic with good *S. aureus* coverage.

Preventive measures include nightly administration of otic solution, especially if the child swam that day. Using a hair dryer on a cool setting may reduce excess moisture in the canal. Opinions differ on the use of earplugs as a preventive measure. Some feel earplugs are effective; others argue that earplugs trap small amounts of water in the canal, increasing the potential for OE.

SINUSITIS

Until the early 1980s, when Wald's articles about sinusitis first appeared, a chronic runny nose in a child usually was attributed to frequent URIs or was ignored. Now sinusitis has become one of the most common pediatric diagnoses. Unfortunately, because of overdiagnosis or misdiagnosis, sinusitis also has become one of the prime reasons for antibiotic misuse in children. It probably is the most common cause of a persistent cough in children, but its true incidence is uncertain. Researchers disagree about which group of symptoms is characteristic of sinusitis. Many practitioners may order more sinus films than chest x-rays. Sinusitis is classified as follows:

* Acute sinusitis: symptoms lasting more than 10 days but less than 30 days
* Subacute sinusitis: symptoms lasting up to 4 months
* Chronic sinusitis: extremely protracted symptoms

Anatomy, Physiology, and Pathology

Sinuses are outpouches of the nasal mucosa and therefore have mucosal lining identical to that of the nose. The four pairs of paranasal sinuses are the maxillary, ethmoidal, sphenoidal, and frontal. The sinuses develop embryologically and are visible radiologically at different ages (Goldenhersh & Rachelefsky, 1989). The ethmoid and maxillary are anatomically present from 3 to 5 months of intrauterine life; radiologically, they are present at birth. The frontal sinuses anatomically develop by age 1 year and radiologically by ages 3 to 7 years. The sphenoids develop anatomically by ages 4 to 5 years and radiologically by age 9 years. The maxillary, anterior ethmoidal, and frontal sinuses drain into the nose's middle meatus. The posterior ethmoidal and sphenoidal sinuses drain into the superior meatus. The most fre-

quently involved sinus is the maxillary. More importantly, it is the only sinus whose ostia is located high on the sinus wall, and the cilia must work against gravity to cleanse it (Wald, 1995). The normal physiology of the sinuses depends on ciliary function, quality of secretions, and patency of the ostia (Yogev & Tan, 1998).

As in AOM, the three most common organisms causing acute (and probably chronic) sinusitis are *S. pneumoniae*, *H. influenzae*, and *M. catarrhalis*. Other organisms that have been isolated include *Streptococcus pyogenes* and peptostreptococci species. Bacteroides species and anaerobic gram-positive cocci were reported in one study of subacute or longer lasting cases of sinusitis; however, other studies, including that of Otten and Autrelink (1994), found *S. pneumoniae*, *H. influenzae*, and *M. catarrhalis* to predominate as isolates (Tinkelman & Silk, 1989).

● **Clinical Pearl:** In children, cultures of the nasopharynx show absolutely no correlation with those obtained directly from the sinuses and middle ear in acute sinusitis and AOM respectively.

History and Physical Exam

When considering the diagnosis of sinusitis, it is usually the history that is most important. The common URI presents identically, but it is the persistence of symptoms lasting longer than 10 to 14 days without improvement that is characteristic of sinusitis.

● **Clinical Pearl:** Contrary to popular belief, the color and character of a child's nasal discharge during a cold has little relationship to the presence or absence of a secondary bacterial infection. During an uncomplicated URI, the nature of the nasal discharge changes sequentially from clear and watery, to foul, cloudy, thick, and greenish, and then gradually reverts to watery and clear near the end of the cold.

The character of the nasal discharge in sinusitis can vary from clear to purulent. The cough should be present during the day but is usually worse at night. Parents often state that there is periorbital edema, but this finding usually resolves as the day progresses. Other historic findings include foul breath, otalgia, sore throat, sinus tenderness, and periorbital headache. When the symptoms are chronic, there may be minimal rhinorrhea, postnasal drip (cough and throat clearing), or nasal congestion.

The adolescent may present with a more acute and toxic presentation. Following a 3- to 4-day history of a URI, there is the acute onset of fever, headache, and tenderness over the involved sinuses.

In sinusitis, the physical examination is often very unrewarding and nonspecific. The provider may find nasal mucosal injection and purulent discharge. He or she may note facial or periorbital swelling and possible sinus tenderness. The clinician may see any degree of TM abnormality.

Diagnostic Criteria

The diagnosis is based purely on clinical grounds. The following are common differential diagnoses for sinusitis:

* Streptococcal nasopharyngitis (streptococcosis) caused by group A beta-hemolytic strep usually is seen in children younger than 3 years. This presents as a purulent rhinitis that may last for weeks and is diagnosed by nasal or throat culture.

- Nasal foreign body usually presents with a unilateral rhinitis and a foul odor in young children who enjoy plugging various body orifices. It may require nasopharyngoscopy for diagnosis and removal.
- In allergic rhinitis, there often is a family history of respiratory allergy or a personal history of eczema, food allergy, colic, or asthma. There is usually a clear, watery, itchy rhinitis, often associated with conjunctivitis. The classic allergic salute and shiners may be present. The nasal mucosa tends to be pale or bluish in color, and a nasal smear will show many eosinophils.
- For recurrent URIs, obtaining an accurate history to determine a respite in symptoms, even if only for a few days, is very important to distinguish persistent symptoms as seen in sinusitis versus those seen with recurring colds.
- Vasomotor rhinitis is rare in children and characterized by the abrupt onset and cessation of profuse rhinorrhea, perhaps on an autonomic basis.

● **Clinical Pearl:** In a young child, the diagnosis of sinusitis is established when cold symptoms last longer than 10 to 14 days without improvement and are associated with a day- and night-time cough and occasionally bad breath.

The above characterizes the vast majority of presentations of pediatric sinusitis. Occasionally in older children, sinusitis may present as a cold that suddenly worsens with respect to fever, headache, and congestion. In adolescents, sinusitis may have a more adult-like presentation with headache, photophobia, and significant facial tenderness.

● **Clinical Pearl:** Radiographic studies usually are not reliable in assisting with the diagnosis of sinusitis or determining the effectiveness of treatment.

Available radiographic methods cannot distinguish bacterial sinusitis from viral infection. The American College of Radiology Appropriateness Criteria recommends no imaging for acute sinusitis (Kronener & McAlister, 1997). Many studies have shown that a significant percentage of children without clinical symptoms of sinusitis have "abnormal" sinus x-rays (Abbasi & Cunningham, 1996). One study found that 10% of "normal" children between ages 1 and 16 years without a history of URI had abnormal sinus x-rays. Of those with a history of URIs, only 52% had abnormal x-rays (Kovatch et al., 1984). Computed tomography (CT) scans are no more reliable than x-rays, and there may be as much as a 75% discrepancy between plain films and coronal CT. Although CT is considered the gold standard, Diament et al. (1987) found that 5% to 55% of children without suspected sinus disease had abnormal CT scans showing moderate or severe opacification in the maxillary or ethmoid sinuses. Ultrasound lacks sensitivity and specificity; the high cost and need for sedation involved with magnetic resonance imaging limits its usefulness in the pediatric population.

Management

The treatment for a child diagnosed with sinusitis is oral antibiotics. In most cases, the pathogens responsible for sinusitis are the same as those responsible for AOM; thus, considerations in choosing an agent are the same for both illnesses. Amoxicillin remains the first-line treatment of choice. The reader is referred to the section on pharmacologic treatment of AOM and Table 33-4.

The only controlled trial of antibiotic treatment in children with cold symptoms for at least 10 days (clinical sinusitis) compared amoxicillin with amoxicillin/clavulanate (Wald, Chiponis, & Ledesma-Medina, 1986). Both agents were equally effective in providing modest short-term benefits and resolution of symptoms (cure rate: 79% antibiotics, 60% placebo). Some authorities also recommend extending treatment to 14 to 21 days if symptoms persist at the completion of the 10-day course. Once again, antibiotic overuse and the prevalence of resistant pathogens must be considered when diagnosing and treating the young child with prolonged cold symptoms.

REFERENCES

Abbasi, S., & Cunningham, A. S. (1996). Are we overtreating sinusitis? *Contemporary Pediatrics, 13*(10), 49–62.

Adderson, E. E. (1998). Preventing otitis media: Medical approaches. *Pediatric Annals, 27*(2), 101–107.

Bluestone, C. D., & Klein, J. O. (1998). *Otitis media in infants and children.* Philadelphia, W.B. Saunders.

Bodor, F. F. (1982). Conjunctivitis-otitis syndrome. *Pediatrics, 69*, 695–698.

Byington, C. L. (1998). The diagnosis and management of otitis media with effusion. *Pediatric Annals, 27*(2), 96–100.

Clements, D. A., Langdon, L., Bland, C. B., & Walter, E. (1995). *Archives of Pediatric and Adolescent Medicine, 149*, 1113–1117.

Chartrand, S. A., & Pong, A. (1998). Acute otitis media in the 1990s: The impact of antibiotic resistance. *Pediatric Annals, 27*(2), 86–95.

Conrad, D. A. (1998). Should acute otitis media ever be treated with antibiotics? *Pediatric Annals, 27*(2), 66–74.

Diament, M. J., Senac, M. O., Gilsanz, V., et al. (1987). Prevalence of incidental paranasal sinuses opacification in pediatric patients: A CT study. *Journal of Computed Assisted Tomography, 11*, 426.

Dowell, S. F., Butler, J. C., Giebink, G. S., et al. (1999). Acute otitis media: Management and surveillance in an era of pneumococcal resistance—a report from the drug-resistant *Streptococcus pneumoniae* Therapeutic Working Group. *Pediatric Infectious Disease Journal, (18)*, 1–9.

Fireman, P. (1987). Newer concepts in otitis media. *Hospital Practice,* 85–91.

Fliss, D. M., Leiberman, A., & Dagan, R. (1994). Medical sequelae and complications of acute otitis media. *Pediatric Infectious Disease Journal, (Suppl. 13)*, S34–40.

Goldenhersh, M. J., & Rachelefsky, G. S. (1989). Sinusitis: Early recognition, aggressive treatment. *Contemporary Pediatrics, 6*, 22–42.

Howie, V. M. (1993). Otitis media. *Pediatrics in Review, 14*(8), 320–323.

Klein, J., Marcy, S. M., & Paradise, J. L. (1999). Controversies in otitis media. Pediatric Academic Societies' Annual Meeting. *Infectious Diseases in Children, 12*, 11–22.

Kontiokari, T., & Koivunen, P. (1998). Symptoms of acute otitis media. *Pediatric Infectious Disease Journal, 17*(8), 676–679.

Kovatch, A. L., Wald, E. R., Ledesma-Medina, J., et al. (1984). Maxillary sinus radiographs in children with nonrespiratory complaints. *Pediatrics, 73*, 306.

Kronener, K. A., & McAlister, W. W. (1997). *Pediatric Radiology, II*, 837–846.

Maxon, S., & Yamauchi, T. (1996). Acute otitis media. *Pediatrics in Review, 17*(6), 191–195.

Niemela, M., Uhari, M., & Mottonen, M. (1995). Pacifier increases the risk of recurrent acute otitis media in children in day care centers. *Pediatrics, 96*(5), 884-888.

Otten, H. W., & Autrelink, J. B. (1994). Is antibiotic treatment of chronic sinusitis effective in children. *Clinical Otolaryngology, 19* 215–217.

Paradise, J. L., & Rockette, H. E. (1997). Otitis media in 2253 Pittsburgh area infants: Prevalence & risk factors during the first two years of life. *Pediatrics, 99*(3), 48–54.

Pichichero, M. E., & Pichichero, C. L. (1995). Persistent acute otitis media I: Causative pathogens. *Pediatric Infectious Disease Journal, 214*, 178–188.

Pitkaranta, A., Jero, J., Arruda, E., et. al. (1998). Polymerase Chain Reaction-based detection of rhinovirus, RSV, and coronavirus in otitis media with effusion. *Journal of Pediatrics, 133*(3), 390–394.

Pong, A., & Harrison, C. J. (1998). A practical approach to drug-resistant *Streptococcus pneumoniae. Contemporary Pediatrics, 15*(9), 154–165.

Seppala, H., Klaukka, T., Vuopio-Varkila, J. et al. (1997). The effect of changes in the consumption of macrolide antibiotics on erythromycin resistance in group A streptococci in Finland. *New England Journal of Medicine 337,* 441–492.

Stool, S. E., Bert, A. O., & Berman, S. (1994). Otitis media with effusion in young children. *Clinical Practice Guidelines, 12,* AHCPR publication 94-0622.

Teele, D. W., & Klein, J. O. (1989). Epidemiology of otitis media during the first 7 years of life in children in Greater Boston: A prospective study. *Journal of Infectious Disease, 160*(1), 83–94.

Tinkelman, D. G., & Silk, H. J. (1989). Clinical and bacteriologic features of chronic sinusitis in children. *American Journal of Diseases of Children, 143,* 938–941.

Rosenfeld, R. M., Vertrees, J. E., Carr, J., et al. (1994). Clinical efficacy of antimicrobial drugs for acute otitis media: Meta analysis of 5400 children from thirty-three randomized trials. *Journal of Pediatrics, 124,* 355–367.

Wald, E. R. (1995). Chronic sinusitis in children. *Journal of Pediatrics, 127*(3), 339–347.

Wald, E. R., Chiponis, D., & Ledesma-Medina, J. (1986). Comparative effectiveness of amoxicillin and amoxicillin-clavulanate potassium in acute paranasal sinus infections in children: A double-blind, placebo-controlled trial. *Pediatrics, 77*(795).

Yogev, R., & Tan, T.Q. (1998). Rhinosinusitis in children: Avoiding diagnostic pitfalls. *Journal of Respiratory Diseases, 19*(10), 858–876.

P A R T   2   ▲

Surgical Options in Chronic Otitis Media With Effusion

• DARSIT K. SHAH, MD

INTRODUCTION

Acute otitis media and otitis media with effusion are responsible for many health care dollars spent for the care of children younger than 5 years. More than 90% of children have at least one episode of otitis media, and 75% of children have three or more episodes (Klein et al., 1988). Primary care practitioners spend one third of their time treating children younger than 5 years who have infections of the middle ear (Howle & Schwartz, 1983). In fact, estimates are that 30 million prescriptions are written each year for the treatment of otitis media in children (Nelson & Kennedy, 1988). Significant controversy has surrounded the use of myringotomy with ventilation tube placement in these settings. Nonetheless, this procedure is the most frequently performed operation requiring general anesthesia in all children, with an estimated 1 million tubes placed annually (Derkay, 1993).

PATHOLOGY

The development of acute and chronic otitis media with effusion (COME) results from multiple intrinsic and extrinsic disorders. The main contributing factor is abnormal eustachian tube function. The eustachian tube in children typically undergoes both functional and mechanical obstruction, resulting in otitis media with effusion. Other important factors that contribute to the development of chronic otitis media include male gender, day care attendance, exposure to second-hand smoke, prolonged bottle-feeding, cleft palate, nasal allergy, and pacifier use.

Chronic and acute otitis media carry the potential for serious sequelae and complications. In the times before antibiotics, the most lethal of these included meningitis, intracranial abscess, sigmoid sinus thrombosis, and extracranial abscess development. These now occur relatively infrequently. Hearing loss of some degree, however, accompanies almost all episodes of otitis media. The sequela of prolonged or long-term hearing loss in children is the most worrisome consequence of otitis media in the modern era. The vast majority of children exhibit a conductive, reversible hearing loss due to otitis. Otitis media, however, can result in conductive hearing loss due to TM perforation or cholesteatoma. Rarely, sensorineural hearing loss can occur as a result of diffusion of inflammatory products through the oval or round window (Johansson & Hellstrom, 1993; Daly, Hunter, & Giebnik, 1999).

Children undergo rapid language and speech development between ages 1 month and 3 years. They acquire speech discrimination as early as 1 month and begin babbling by 5 or 6 months. In addition, other intellectual and cognitive skills have accelerated development during this critical period. Normal speech perception is crucial in allowing the acquisition of these developmental milestones.

Numerous studies have examined the impact of COME on hearing and cognitive development. Many support the notion that children with COME have impaired speech development, lower cognitive abilities, and poorer performance in school compared with children without middle ear pathology. Teele studied 207 children from birth to age 3 years who had COME for variable lengths of time. This study analyzed cognitive ability measured by IQ scores at age 7 years. In children with COME for more than 130 days, IQ scores were significantly lower than for those with effusion less than 130 days (Teele & Klein, 1990). The issue is very controversial, however, because other studies have failed to demonstrate a link between COME and behavior or language development. In fact, two very recent studies fail to support a causative relationship between cumulative duration of middle ear effusion and parent–child stress and behavior problems (Paradise et al., 1999) and parent-reported language skills (Feldman et al., 1999) in children ages 1 to 3 years.

SURGICAL INDICATIONS

Because of these cognitive concerns, COME should be managed more aggressively in high-risk groups. Initial management includes an intensive medical regimen, which is covered in Part 1. Ideally, a formal audiogram should be obtained at the termination of a prolonged medical treatment of at least 3 months.

● **Clinical Pearl:** Myringotomy and pressure equalization tube (PET) insertion are indicated when conservative measures fail to reverse and correct bilateral OME after 4 months, and the obtained audiogram demonstrates conductive hearing loss, or a soundfield test in the ear with better hearing shows a hearing loss of greater than 20 dB.

Recently, guidelines were established and published regarding PET placement by a consensus of otolaryngologists and pediatricians. The Otitis Medial Guideline Panel (1994) stated that myringotomy with PET becomes an additional option when OME persists beyond 3 months and becomes recommended after a total of 4 to 6 months of COME.

The management of children with either bilateral COME without conductive hearing loss or unilateral COME with normal contralateral hearing is unclear. Although tympanostomy tubes are not formally indicated in these settings, the long-term effects of unilateral COME on cognition, language development, and behavior are unknown. Only a few studies have addressed these issues, and future study is necessary. The role of adenoidectomy in the management of COME has been an area of significant debate (Gates, 1987).

● **Clinical Pearl:** Adenoidectomy may only be currently recommended in conjunction with a second tube placement when children have recurrent COME despite primary myringotomy and tube surgery.

In 1990, Paradise evaluated 213 children requiring a second set of tympanostomy tubes. Those children having concomitant adenoidectomy and PET placement had fewer episodes of otitis media compared with those undergoing only PET placement. The size of the adenoid bed, whether small or large, played no role in determining whether an adenoidectomy was of benefit in this setting. It should be noted, however, that the only surgery recommended by the Otitis Media Guideline Panel (1994) is PET placement.

MANAGEMENT

Surgical Technique and Complications

Tympanostomy tube placement in children requires a general anesthetic. Rarely, however, it can be performed under local anesthetic in the office. With binocular microscopic magnification, a small radial incision is made in the anterior, inferior quadrant of the TM. Fluid from the middle ear space is atraumatically suctioned. A PET is then placed through the myringotomy site. Various types and sizes of PET have been used. Grommet-type tympanostomy tubes are most commonly placed. T-shaped tubes are used less frequently but tend to extrude less quickly (Shah, 1971; Mandel, 1992).

When indicated, the benefits of tympanostomy tube placement far outweigh any potential risks. Complications can and do result from this procedure, the most common of which is postoperative otorrhea. The incidence varies from 5% to 40% and is usually the result of water contamination or otitis media development. This complication is usually easily managed with ototopical antimicrobial drops. Rarely intravenous antibiotics or tube removal is necessary to halt otorrhea. Persistent TM perforation is the most problematic consequence of PET surgery. The incidence is 1% to 5%. Rare complications of tympanostomy tube placement also include the development of cholesteatoma, tinnitus, sensorineural hearing loss, vertigo, or jugular bulb injury.

▲ **Clinical Warning:** Children who receive "long-term" tubes, such as T and larger grommet tubes, tend to have a higher incidence of perforation. Repair is necessary and should be delayed until eustachian tube function improves.

Management of the Child With Tubes

Most children who have pressure equalization tubes require no significant additional postoperative care. The primary care provider, however, often faces the management of two relatively common scenarios in the child with myringotomy tubes: water contamination and otorrhea.

Water Contamination

Water contamination of the middle ear space is an ongoing concern. As can be expected, little true scientific evidence guides management. Recommendations are often contradictory.

Many specialists suggest earplugs to prevent unsterile water from traversing the tube, entering the middle ear space, and causing a purulent otitis media with otorrhea. Advocates of plugs claim a reduction in the incidence of post-tube otorrhea with their use. Validation is difficult because acute otitis media unrelated to middle ear contamination also may cause post-tube otorrhea. Others suggest no protection for children with PET. They claim that the ear canal is an s-shaped structure that does not allow water to easily reach the TM. Recent studies support that at least 30 cm of water pressure are required to force water to the TM. For this reason, some authorities suggest earplugs only when children are exposed to either high-pressure water or underwater head submersion.

Earplugs, at times, are difficult to maintain in the ears of children. Despite this, they carry little risk and are inexpensive. For these reasons, despite their questionable value, the general consensus is to suggest them for children with PET when exposed to water of any kind.

Otorrhea

The management of the child with PET and post-tube otorrhea is also not standardized. The incidence of post-tube otorrhea is fairly common and ranges from 30% to 50% (Johansson & Hellstrom, 1993). In the face of a tympanostomy tube, middle ear infections have an easy path of egress resulting in otorrhea. Left untreated, however, they may result in an external otitis or a loculated middle ear or mastoid process. As such, treatment is recommended for post-tube otorrhea.

Unless a child has mastoid tenderness or periauricular erythema, treatment should consist solely of ototopical drops. The only ear drop that is formally indicated in this circumstance (when the TM is not intact) is ofloxacin (Floxin) otic suspension, which eliminates the rare potential for ototoxicity that may be seen with other ototopicals. Other ototopical drops containing gentamycin, tobramycin, or neomycin should be reserved for children with persistent otorrhea despite ofloxacin.

▲ **Clinical Warning:** Oral antibiotics have no role in the routine management of post-tube otorrhea and should not be prescribed for initial management of uncomplicated cases.

Children who have persistent infection despite multiple treatment courses of ototopical drops or who have developed a complication of otitis media should receive oral antibiotics. Rarely, children have persistent otorrhea and may require removal of the tube, intravenous antibiotics, or tympanomastoidectomy to halt the discharge.

REFERENCES

Daly, K., Hunter, C., & Giebink, S. (1999). Chronic otitis media with effusion. *Pediatrics in Review, 20,* 85–93.

Derkay, C. S. (1993). Pediatric otolaryngology procedures in US: 1978-1987. *International Journal of Pediatric Otorhinolaryngology, 25,* 1–12.

Feldman, H. M., Dollagan, C. A., et al. (1999). Parent-reported language and communication skills at one and two years of age in relation to otitis media in the first two years of life. *Pediatrics, 104,* e52.

Gates, G. (1987). Effectiveness of adenoidectomy and tympanostomy tubes in the treatment of COME. *New England Journal of Medicine, 317,* 1444.

Howle, V. M., & Schwartz, R. W. (1983). Acute OM: One year in general pediatric practice. *American Journal of Diseases in Children, 137,* 155–158.

Johansson, U., & Hellstrom, S. (1993). Round window membrane in serous and purulent otitis media. Study in the rat. *Annals of Otololgy, Rhinology, and Laryngology, 102,* 227–235.

Klein, J. O., Teele, D. W., et al. (1988). Epidemiology of acute OM. In D. J. Lim & C. D. Bluestone (Eds.), *Recent advances in OM.* Philadelphia: BC Decker.

Mandel, E. M. (1992). Efficacy of myringotomy with and without tympanostomy tubes for COME. *Pediatric Infectious Disease Journal, 11,* 270–277.

Nelson, W. L., & Kennedy, D. L. (1988). Outpatient systemic antibiotic use by children in the United States, 1977 to 1986. *Pediatric Infectious Disease Journal, 7,* 505–509.

The Otitis Media Guideline Panel. (1994). Managing otitis media with effusion in young children. *Pediatrics, 94,* 766.

Paradise, J. (1990). Efficacy of adenoidectomy for recurrent otitis media in children previously treated with tympanostomy tube placement. *Journal of the American Medical Association, 263,* 2066.

Paradise, J. L., Feldman, H. M., et al. (1999). Parental stress and parent-rated child behavior in relation to otitis media in the first three years of life. *Pediatrics, 104,* 1264–1273.

Shah, N. (1971). Use of grommets in glue ears. *Journal of Laryngology and Otology, 85,* 283–287.

Teele, D. W., & Klein, J. (1990). Greater Boston OM Study Group. OM in infancy and intellectual ability, school achievement, speech and language at 7 years. *Journal of Infectious Diseases, 162,* 685–694.

Mouth and Throat Infections

• DANIEL Z. ARONZON, MD

INTRODUCTION

Sore throats represent a leading cause of visits to the primary care office for children and adolescents. After otitis media, upper respiratory infections (URIs), and bronchitis, it is the fourth leading diagnosis prompting a prescription for antibiotics (Nyquist et al., 1998). Fortunately, with the proliferation of rapid streptococcal antigen testing and the ease and availability of throat cultures, little or no reason exists for diagnostic uncertainty and unnecessary prescription of antibiotics.

In general, tonsillitis, pharyngotonsillitis, and pharyngitis all mean the same thing, because throat infections are never so ideally localized. For the purposes of this discussion, the term acute pharyngitis is used to denote all three.

Etiologically and practically, acute pharyngitis can be divided into two broad categories: viral and bacterial. Viruses as a group account for 15% to 40% of cases of acute pharyngitis in children and 30% to 60% of cases in adolescents. Rhinovirus, adenovirus, influenza, parainfluenza, coronovirus, enteroviruses (EVs), herpes simplex, Epstein-Barr, and cytomegalovirus are commonly implicated (Pichichero, 1998). Only acute pharyngitis caused by the EV group, herpes simplex, Epstein-Barr, and cytomegalovirus is clinically distinctive enough to warrant specific discussion. Other causes may be responsible for a wide variety of clinical diseases but are indistinguishable with respect to pharyngeal findings and therefore are not discussed further.

Group A beta-hemolytic *Streptococcus* (GABHS) is the most important of the bacterial etiologies, accounting for 8% to 40% of cases of acute pharyngitis in children and 5% to 9% of cases in teenagers (Pichichero, 1998). Other less prevalent primary bacterial etiologies include group C and G streptococcal species, *Neisseria gonorrhoeae*, *Corynebacterium diphtheriae*, *Arcanobacterium haemolyticus*, and *Mycoplasma* and *Chlamydia pneumoniae*. In practical terms, all fall into the differential diagnosis of GABHS and are discussed in that section. An algorithm illustrating in general terms the clinical decision making for a child or adolescent with acute pharyngitis is presented in Figure 34-1.

ENTEROVIRAL PHARYNGITIS

The EV family consist of polio, echo, and Coxsackie viruses. Polio has been eradicated from much of the developed world through active immunization efforts beginning in the 1950s. The nonpolio EVs are frequent pathogens in children (Pichichero, 1998). They produce three very common clinical scenarios associated with acute pharyngitis: a nonspecific febrile illness characterized by myalgia and malaise, stomatitis classically known as herpangina, and the aptly termed hand, foot, and mouth (HFM) disease (Zaoutis & Klein, 1998). Herpangina means herpes-like pain and etiologically should not be confused with herpes simplex.

Other clinical manifestations of EV include aseptic meningitis, pleurodynia, myocarditis, pericarditis, meningoencephalitis, hemorrhagic conjunctivitis, and orchitis. EVs are responsible for a large proportion of infants admitted for sepsis workups during the summer (Rotbart, 1998). This section focuses on the clinical manifestations of EV associated with acute pharyngitis.

Pathology

The EVs are single-stranded RNA viruses belonging to the *Picornaviridae* family. The incubation period varies between 3 and 10 days. Upon entering the host though the gastrointestinal tract, initial viral replication occurs in the intestinal Peyer's patches, leading to a minor viremia, with seeding of central nervous system (CNS), heart, liver, pancreas, skin, and mucous membranes. Parents often report that the child has some mild intestinal symptoms associated with the initial intestinal replication. Viral replication at these secondary sites accounts for a second or major viremia with further opportunity for CNS seeding. The two viremias described in this model help to explain the often biphasic symtomatology: fever for a day or two, followed by an afebrile period of 2 to 3 days, and finally an additional 2 to 5 days of fever. Neutralizing antibodies appear after about 6 to 12 days of symptoms, peak after 3 to 4 weeks, and result in resolution of symptoms (Zaoutis & Klein, 1998). For most EVs, the variety of clinical presentations results in symptoms lasting 7 to 10 days (Pichichero, 1998).

Epidemiology

In temperate climates, EV infections predominantly are seen in the warmer months. In tropical climates, they occur year-round. Transmission is primarily by the fecal-oral route and less commonly by respiratory droplet. Crowded living conditions, poor sanitation, and low socioeconomic class are all risk factors for infection. Risk factors for young children are day care attendance, poor hygiene, and lack of natural immunity (Zaoutis & Klein, 1998). A recent study emphasized that spread to family members of affected children is very common, occurring in 50% of siblings and 25% of parents (Pichichero, 1998).

History and Physical Examination

Clinicians should remember that up to 50% of EV infections may be asymptomatic. The remainder of the discussion focuses on clinical presentations associated with acute pharyngitis, namely the nonspecific febrile illness, herpangina, and HFM.

Enterovirus-Associated Nonspecific Febrile Illness

All EVs are associated with a nonspecific febrile illness. Typical manifestations include a rather sudden onset of fever (which may be biphasic as described above), accompanied by muscle aches, headache, and mild intestinal symptoms, including nausea, vomiting, mild diarrhea, and abdominal pain. Physical findings are not terribly specific but may include pharyngitis, cervical adenopathy, conjunctivitis, and a rash in 23% of patients (Rotbart, 1998; Zaoutis & Klein, 1998).

Herpangina

Findings include abrupt onset of fever associated with sore throat pain and difficulty swallowing. The fever may be extremely high, especially in younger patients. The classic enanthema begins a day later and consists of vesicles that ulcerate and are located posteriorly on the soft palate, tonsillar pillars, and posterior pharyngeal wall. In younger children, fluid intake may be severely compromised, which, along with increased insensible losses due to fever, contributes to the possibility of dehydration. Symptoms last for approximately 7 days.

A variant of herpangina consists of firm white nodules in the same distribution as the vesicles, termed lymphonodular pharyngitis. Herpangina is commonly associated with coxsackie A viruses but coxsackie B and echoviruses also have been implicated (Zaoutis & Klein, 1998).

Hand, Foot, and Mouth Disease

Systemic symptoms of fever and dysphagia tend to be milder. The child may have a mild sore throat with or without fever, but the most frequent reason for presentation is the classic rash. The enanthema consists of scattered vesicles that ulcerate on the pharynx, buccal mucosa, and tongue. The ulcerations are much less painful than those seen in either herpangina or herpetic gingivostomatitis. The classic exanthem consists of vesicles on the palms, soles, and especially the periungual and interdigital surfaces. Nonvesicular lesions also may be seen on the buttocks and perineum (Rotbart, 1998; Zaoutis & Klein, 1998). Because of the milder constitutional symptoms, dehydration is almost never a concern. HFM is usually associated with coxsackie A 16, but other EVs also have been implicated.

Diagnostic Criteria and Studies

The diagnosis is established based on the clinical presentation and in the context of patterns of similar illness in other children, especially during warm weather. Although viral cultures are diagnostic, they are not practical or suitable for the primary care setting. PCR technology may soon become available; its cost and ease of use will determine how helpful it will become to primary care providers. For the foreseeable future, the diagnosis hinges on eliminating treatable forms of pharyngitis, namely GABHS pharyngitis, which can be simply and economically achieved with a throat culture or rapid streptococcal antigen test.

▲ **Clinical Warning:** Providers should exclude the presence of GABHS pharyngitis by throat culture in patients with all but the most classic enteroviral presentation, such as HFM.

● **Clinical Pearl:** Establishing the presence of mild intestinal symptoms (initial site of viral replication) at the onset of symptoms is an important diagnostic clue for all EV infections but especially for EV-associated nonspecific febrile illness, in which classic enanthemas or exanthems are not apparent.

● **Clinical Pearl:** Herpangina produces high fevers, painful posterior intraoral vesicles, and the potential for dehydration. It can be distinguished clinically from HFM, which is a much milder illness, and from herpes simplex gingivostomatitis, in which the ulcers are classically anterior and predominantly gingival.

Management

Management of EV infections is supportive, consisting of hydration and antipyretics as needed to maintain the child's level of comfort. Providers should pay particular attention to the young child with severe herpangina, because dehydration is not uncommon. They should instruct parents to offer frequent fluids. Parents should avoid giving carbonated or acidic juices and should favor blander beverages. The toddler with severe dysphagia may more readily accept cold drinks, pops, or ice cream. Education as to signs of dehydration and when to seek reevaluation is also important. Most EV infections will run a 7-day course, and providers should alert parents to this fact, thereby avoiding needless reevaluations, emergency room visits, and the potential for unnecessary antibiotics.

HERPES SIMPLEX GINGIVOSTOMATITIS

Herpes simplex virus (HSV) produces a wide variety of clinical diseases, including sexually transmitted genital infections; disease in the neonate and immunocompromised host, leading to encephalitis and systemic dissemination; gingivostomatitis; and the ubiquitous cold sore. This section focuses on the oral and pharyngeal manifestations of herpes simplex.

Pathology

The HSV is a double-stranded DNA virus belonging to the herpesvirus group that also contains Epstein-Barr virus (EBV), cytomegalovirus, and varicella-zoster virus. All members of the family share the distinct characteristic of becoming latent after primary infection and then reactivating periodically in response to various apparent (eg, infection, fatigue, stress, sunlight) or unknown triggers. Primary and recurrent infections can either be symptomatic or asymptomatic, and any combination of one can exist with another (Annunziato, 1998).

Pathologically, HSV produces skin vesicles and mucous membrane ulcers. Infected cells become multinucleated giant cells, and intranuclear inclusions become visible. During primary infection, the virus reaches nerve ganglia through sensory nerve endings in the infected skin. The virus can then remain latent within the nerve cells, only to reactivate later. The interplay between the host immune system and reactivation of HSV and the mechanism for reactivation remain unclear.

Symptomatic primary infections display vesicular eruptions and may show some systemic signs, such as fever. Symptomatic recurrent infections usually are characterized by cutaneous or mucous membrane eruptions but lack systemic findings. The incubation period varies between 2 days and 2 weeks.

● **Clinical Pearl:** The virus is so ubiquitous that after either a symptomatic or inapparent primary infection, 50% of the population is thought to harbor latent HSV (Annunziato, 1998).

Epidemiology

Herpetic infections have a worldwide distribution. The infection is transmitted from either primary or recurrent infections, either from symptomatic or asymptomatic individuals by direct contact with infected oral secretions or lesions (American Academy of Pediatrics [AAP], 1997). Oral herpes also may be acquired through genital contact during oral sex. In lower socioeconomic groups, oral infection tends to occur at younger ages; in higher socioeconomic groups, it is mostly acquired in adolescence.

There are two antigenically distinct types: human HSV type I (HSV-1), primarily responsible for oral, eye, and CNS infections, and human HSV type II (HSV-II), primarily implicated in genital and neonatal infections. There are no strict distinctions, however, and both types can commonly cause infections at all sites.

History and Physical Examination

Herpetic gingivostomatitis is the clinical manifestation of a primary infection with HSV. The vast majority of children who are primarily infected have no distinguishable symptoms at all. The patients with symptomatic gingivostomatitis represent only about 5% of all those primarily infected (Annunziato, 1998).

As with herpangina due to enteroviral infection, the onset tends to be abrupt with high fever and poor oral intake. Physical examination reveals multiple small ulcers with a surrounding erythemetous base on the lips, gums, tongue, and inner cheeks, which may progress posteriorly to the soft palate and tonsils. Vesicles occasionally are seen on the perioral skin or the fingers of children who suck their thumbs.

The spectrum of severity varies, but children with severe disease may become dehydrated and require intravenous rehydration. In mild cases, the illness may last a week, but with severe disease, symptoms may persist for as long as 14 days (Annunziato, 1998). Recurrent herpes stomatitis presents as herpes labialis, more commonly referred to as a cold sore.

Diagnostic Criteria and Studies

Diagnosis is based on clinical grounds and the classic appearance of the intraoral lesions. Because early isolated posterior pharyngeal HSV lesions may be confused with those of GABHS, the provider should obtain a throat culture. Ultimately, the development of anterior ulcers will clarify the diagnosis.

● **Clinical Pearl:** HSV gingivostomatitis causes ulcers of the gums, lips, and tongue and less commonly lesions of the posterior pharynx. The presence of anteriorly located ulcers distinguishes HSV gingivostomatitis from enteroviral herpangina, which almost never causes anterior lesions.

Specimens for viral cultures may be obtained, with results usually available in a few days. They usually are not practical in the primary care setting. Providers may obtain faster results by newer enzyme immunoassay antigen techniques, but their applicability to the office setting remains to be demonstrated (AAP, 1997).

Management

Studies are lacking as to the use and efficacy of oral acyclovir in children with primary gingivostomatitis. Information inferred from the adult literature demonstrates that acyclovir, valacyclovir, and famciclovir all shorten the duration of symptoms and decrease viral shedding in cases of genital herpes. Valacyclovir and famciclovir offer no improved efficacy compared to acyclovir but do offer the advantage of less frequent dosing. No pediatric formulations, however, are available (AAP, 1997).

Given the above, its safety profile, and how well it is tolerated, providers should prescribe acyclovir at a dose of 80 mg/kg/d divided in five to six daily doses for all moderate and severe cases of HSV gingivostomatitis. To be effective, therapy should begin early (first 72 hours) in the course of illness. Topical acyclovir is not recommended.

Moderate to severe cases may benefit from the use of topical viscous xylocaine, swabbed on to the ulcers preprandially. This will allow a short window of time for the child to be able to eat but more importantly drink. Clinicians must caution parents not to overuse this topical anesthetic due to the dangers of systemic absorption.

Milder cases will require nothing more than supportive care consisting of hydration and antipyretics as needed to maintain the child's level of comfort. As in the case of herpangina, providers should instruct parents to offer frequent fluids. Parents should avoid giving carbonated or acidic juices and favor blander beverages. The toddler with severe mouth pain may more readily accept cold drinks, pops, or ice cream. Education as to signs of dehydration and when to seek reevaluation is also important. As with any acute illness, providers should counsel parents as to the anticipated duration of the illness.

Because viral shedding in primary herpetic gingivistomatitis is considerable, parents should keep children away from day care or school until symptoms resolve. Children with common cold sores pose little risk and should go to daycare or school. Because HSV infection may be potentially life threatening to a neonate or other immunocompromised host, clinicians must caution caregivers not to expose their child with gingivostomatitis to others in these two vulnerable categories.

The treatment of the recurrent lesions of herpes labialis has not been adequately established in children. Topical acyclovir appears to have little efficacy, perhaps because by the time the lesions become apparent, it is too late to influence viral replication.

INFECTIOUS MONONUCLEOSIS

In children and particularly adolescents, infectious mononucleosis (IM) is an important consideration when the clinician is confronted with a patient with acute pharyngitis. Epstein-Barr virus (EBV) is the cause of IM, yet clinically indistinguishable syndromes of fatigue, pharyngitis, and generalized lymphadenopathy may be seen with either acute cytomegalovirus infection or toxoplasmosis. All three may be termed "mono-like" illnesses.

The reader is referred to the excellent discussion of the epidemiology and pathophysiology of IM in chapter 30. This section focuses on the clinical presentation, diagnosis, differential considerations, and management of the patient with IM.

History and Physical Examination

Infectious mononucleosis may begin either abruptly with fever and a severe sore throat or less dramatically with fatigue and malaise. For most primary care practitioners, it will present in the context of an acute pharyngitis.

● **Clinical Pearl:** In general terms, younger children tend to have milder symptoms and signs. The older the patient, the more severe and dramatic is the symptomatology.

Clinical presentation of IM is the result of an immune system battle between EBV activated B lymphocytes seeking to proliferate and the host's natural killer and T-cell response. Presumably, the older the patient, the more mature is his or her immune system, and hence the more "violent" the battle.

Sore throat is a cardinal symptom of IM, and tonsillar exudates are observed in 50% of cases. Palatal petechiae reminiscent of those with GABHS pharyngitis are common (Katz & Miller, 1998). Fevers and headaches of variable degree are commonly seen and may last up to 3 weeks. Lymphadenopathy is another characteristic symptom commonly seen in the cervical, axillary, epitrochlear, and inguinal regions.

Splenomegaly is seen in 50% of cases. Some controversy exists about whether the incidence is higher but clinically inapparent. Rupture of an enlarged spleen is a dreaded and life-threatening complication that usually follows trauma, although spontaneous ruptures have been reported (Rutkow, 1978).

Hepatomegaly may be seen in 10% to 40% of cases (Peter & Ray, 1998; Katz & Miller, 1998). Jaundice is rare. Abdominal pain is fairly common and may be due to a coexistent GABHS infection, stretching of the splenic capsule, hepatic tenderness, or mesenteric lymphadenopathy, which may be severe enough to mimic a surgical abdomen.

A polymorphic dermatitis appearing during the first few days of symptoms may be seen in anywhere from 5% to 19% of cases (Peter & Ray, 1998; Katz & Miller, 1998). It may be macular, papular, petechial, morbiliform, scarlatiniform, or even vesicular.

● **Clinical Pearl:** An itchy maculopapular eruption is seen in almost all patients with IM who are given ampicillin, amoxicillin, or related penicillins. The association is strong enough to be considered diagnostic and occurs 7 to 10 days after administration of these drugs (Peter & Ray, 1998; Katz & Miller, 1998). This rash is not an allergic reaction, and children can safely take these medications in the future.

Periorbital edema may be an early physical finding of IM; however, if mild, patient, parents, and clinician may overlook it. Less frequently, a clinical and x-ray picture are indistinguishable from atypical pneumonia can complicate IM. Rarely, infection is associated with signs of a bleeding diathesis due to thrombocytopenic purpura. Various neurologic manifestations, such as aseptic meningitis, encephalitis, Guillain-Barré syndrome, transverse myelitis, acute cerebellar ataxia, and peripheral neuropathy, are also rare complicaitons (Katz & Miller, 1998).

Diagnostic Criteria and Studies

Given a teenager with a 2-week history of fatigue, sore throat, and swollen glands recently back from college or camp, the diagnosis becomes fairly obvious. In most cases, however, the provider will need to consider IM in the context of acute pharyngitis. Providers should obtain a throat culture or rapid strep antigen test for all patients, because 30% of patients with IM will also have "strep throat" (Peter & Ray, 1998).

● **Clinical Pearl:** Providers should consider IM in patients with pharyngitis who have negative throat culture or rapid strep antigen tests and whose symptoms do not resolve in 7 to 10 days, the expected course of most viral pharyngitides.

● **Clinical Pearl:** Because 30% of patients with IM are also positive for GABHS, providers also should suspect it in patients being treated for strep who do not show a rapid clinical response to therapy.

Providers should obtain a complete blood count (CBC) to both rule in the possibility of IM and help exclude the possibility of leukemia in a child with fever, generalized lymphadenopathy, and possibly hepatosplenomegaly. The CBC in IM will usually reveal an absolute lymphocytosis defined as a white blood cell (WBC) count greater than 5000 with more than 50% lymphocytes. The differential count will show atypical lymphocytes commonly greater than 10% (Peter & Ray, 1998). A normal hemoglobin, hematocrit, and platelet count will help to distinguish IM from leukemia and other myeloinvasive diseases.

● **Clinical Pearl:** IM is one of the most common causes of anicteric or subclinical hepatitis in children and adolescents. Elevated liver enzymes are present in 70% to 90% of cases (Peter & Ray, 1998).

Clinically apparent jaundice is rare, occurring in less than 5% of cases; hyperbilirubinemia may be seen in 25% of cases (Katz & Miller, 1998).

Given a strong clinical suspicion for IM, the clinician should then consider obtaining confirmatory testing, which usually consists of a monospot slide test or an EBV antibody panel.

▲ **Clinical Warning:** The utility, interpretation, and limitations of both tests is predicated on the child's age, the duration of symptoms, and in the case of EBV titers, the high cost of the test itself.

The monospot slide test correlates well with the classic heterophile test, is available as a diagnostic kit with results ready in minutes, and is easily and inexpensively performed. Its sensitivity and specificity are respectively 85% and 97%, but only in older children and only by the second or third week of illness. The monospot may remain positive for up to 1 year following clinical resolution and as such, is not a good marker of active disease.

▲ **Clinical Warning:** Children younger than 4 years commonly do not develop a heterophile antibody to EBV infection, and in this age group, the monospot's sensitivity is less than 20% (Peter & Ray, 1998). Early in the illness, the test is also not useful, becoming positive in 80% of patients only by the third week of illness (Katz & Miller, 1998).

EBV titers are difficult to interpret and very expensive. A 2000 survey of commercial laboratories serving primary care practitioners in Dutchess County, NY, revealed a price range between $136.00 and $191.00. Anti-VCA immunoglobulin M (IgM) antibodies appear early in the course of illness and last for months. Anti-VCA IgG also appears early but lasts for life. Anti-EBNA appears after the acute phase of the illness and also lasts for life. EBV early antigens that appear during the acute stage of illness may disappear and reappear for unknown reasons. An acute infection is marked by a positive anti-VCA IgM and IgG and a negative anti-EBNA. In the context of a negative monospot in an older child, it is very rare to obtain positive EBV titers.

● **Clinical Pearl:** The monospot, performed 2 to 3 weeks into the illness, should be the primary confirmatory test. EBV titers should only be used in young children or older patients with negative monospots who exhibit severe or unusual symptoms.

Obtaining liver function studies in young patients or older patients with negative monospots may also be useful diagnostically, given their purported 70% to 90% sensitivity and the previously mentioned limitations of the monospot and EBV titers.

Management

For the vast majority of children with IM, treatment is supportive, consisting of rest, fluids, and fever control. Many will need to be home from school for a period of time. The patient's energy level will determine a gradual resumption of normal activities. Too much activity too soon may lead to clinical relapses. Constitutional symptoms of fatigue and malaise may persist for up to 3 months in severe cases.

During the acute phase of illness, the provider should reevaluate the patient frequently, primarily to assess hydration. Once symptoms have reached a plateau, follow-up is as needed. Clinicians should assess splenomegaly every 10 to 14 days. Care of the enlarged spleen entails avoidance of any activity in which the likelihood of inadvertent trauma may lead to rupture and serious hemorrhage. In most cases, this includes gym and sports. School attendance depending on the patient's energy level is usually safe. Affected individuals may resume normal activities gradually once splenomegaly has resolved.

▲ **Clinical Warning:** Because even the most experienced clinicians may miss splenomegaly, all patients with IM should observe splenic precautions for a minimum of 3 weeks.

Systemic steroids have been shown to shrink tonsillar hypertrophy dramatically and reduce the sore throat pain in acute IM. A theoretical concern, however, exists that steroids may interfere with the "battle" between activated B cells and T cells in EBV infections (see Chap. 30), potentially increasing the risk of lymphoproliferative processes or other complications. Steroid use should be limited to patients in whom dysphagia and inanition are severe enough to yield dehydration or to those in whom tonsillar and adenoidal hypertrophy are severe enough to cause upper airway obstruction. Prednisone at a dose of 2 mg/kg/d for 5 to 7 days (maximum dose 60–80mg/d) yields dramatic and rapid improvement.

Because IM is transmitted through the saliva, transmission from patient to sibling or other family member is extremely unlikely, given even the most basic hygienic measures. Little else is required to prevent spread. Transmission among teenagers is very common, however, because of typical adolescent behaviors, which include sharing drinks, food, and lips.

"STREP" THROAT AND GROUP A BETA-HEMOLYTIC STREPTOCOCCAL INFECTIONS

The leading bacterial cause of sore throats in children, GABHS pharyngitis is by far the most important because of its suppurative and nonsuppurative sequelae. Although differential considerations include some other bacterial etiologies, for all practical purposes and with rare exceptions, only acute pharyngitis due to GABHS requires specific antibiotic treatment.

● **Clinical Pearl:** In simple terms, for a child with sore throat, the pediatric primary care practitioner must identify and treat those who are GABHS positive and resist the temptation and parental pressures to prescribe antibiotics for those who are not.

Over the past 20 years, GABHS has become more virulent, accounting for increasing incidences of suppurative complications, including various head and neck abscesses, toxic shock, and necrotizing fasciitis (Altemeier, 1998). A thorough and detailed understanding of the pathology, epidemiology, clinical scenarios, sequelae, treatment and treatment failures, recurrences, carrier state, and referral considerations will equip the clinician to deal with this increasingly complex topic.

Pathology

The term beta-hemolytic streptococci refers to the ability of these organisms to produce clear hemolysis of red blood cells. These are further subdivided into serologic groups based on group-specific polysaccharide antigens, termed Lancefield groups. Group A is the subject of this chapter. Group B strains are major pathogens in neonates. Groups C and G, the *Enterococcus* species, the nongroupable viridans, and anaerobic species, are also human pathogens. Either serologic techniques or growth inhibition on red blood cell agar by a bacitracin disk can identify group A strains.

The GABHS is uniquely suited to cause disease. The cell wall of group A strains contains surface proteins, of which type M is the most virulent because of its antiphagocytic effect (Kaplan, 1998). M proteins determine the type specificity, more than 80 of which have been identified to date. GABHS secretes enzymes that aid in bacterial spread, tissue necrosis, and resisting phagocytosis, such as streptokinase, proteinases, nucleases, and hyaluronidase. Exotoxins also are produced, such as hemolysins, responsible for red cell hemolysis on throat culture plates; erythrogenic toxins, which cause the scarlet fever rash; and streptococcal pyrogenic exotoxins, hypothesized as factors in the pathogenesis of invasive infections and streptococcal toxic shock (Ahmed & Ayoub, 1998).

Certain strains (1, 3, 5, 6, 18, and 24) have been designated "rheumatogenic" in that they are commonly isolated in patients with acute rheumatic fever (ARF). Others have been termed nephritogenic (types 4 and 12), because of their relationship with poststreptococcal acute glomerulonephritis (PSAGN).

Three percent of untreated cases of GABHS pharyngitis may result in ARF (Kaplan, 1998). The exact mechanism by which GABHS leads to ARF remains unknown. An abnormal immune response to some component of the bacterium is the most popular hypothesis. The absence of ARF in children younger than 3 years who are "immunologically immature" and the duration between GABHS infection and development of ARF are important clues. The cross-reactivity between M proteins and heart valve glycoproteins, cross-reactivity between streptococcal proteins and the brain's caudate nucleus, and the known difference in human susceptibility to ARF because of unclear host factors also favor the immunologic model (Todd, 1999).

● **Clinical Pearl:** Both ARF and PSAGN may follow GABHS pharyngitis. Only PSAGN follows streptococcal skin infections, not ARF.

● **Clinical Pearl:** ARF is preventable with adequate antibiotic therapy initiated within 9 days of disease onset (Pichichero, 1998). PSAGN may not be preventable despite adequate treatment.

Antibodies to M-specific protein and erythrogenic toxins provide immunity (Kaplan, 1998). The problem is that immunity is type specific to each of more than 80 M protein serotypes. Only with repeated infections throughout life does a child acquire immunity to a greater number of subtypes, explaining the decreased incidence of GABHS pharyngitis in adolescents and adults.

The mechanisms by which GABHS may persist in the nasopharynx or oropharynx despite seemingly adequate treatment have not been clarified. Some theoretical hypotheses relating to persistence and development of the carrier state include the absence of alpha hemolytic streptococci as part of the normal nasopharyngeal flora. These produce bacteriocins that protect against infection with GABHS. Other postulates include deep-seated tonsillar foci of infection, which commonly used antimicrobials may not reach, and the elaboration of lactamases by normal pharyngeal flora, which may inactivate penicillins. Uncommonly tight adherence of GABHS to the pharyngeal mucosa also has been hypothesized as a reason for carriage (Tanz & Shulman, 1998; Pichichero, 1998).

Epidemiology

In children and adolescents, GABHS accounts for approximately 15% of cases of acute pharyngitis. In patients with fever, sore throat, and pharyngeal inflammation, GABHS is the cause in 8% to 40% of children and in 5% to 9% of adolescents (Pichichero, 1998). Teens have a lower incidence, presumably because of increased contact with GABHS and the development of some protective immunity.

Infections are rare in infants, due to transplacental maternal immunity, and in toddlers younger than 2 years, perhaps because of the bacteria's inability to attach to nasopharyngeal or oropharyngeal epithelial cells (Pichichero, 1998). GABHS pharyngitis is predominantly a disease of school-age children, with incidence peaking between 5 and 15 years. Recently, however, perhaps because of increased reliance on day care, reports of infection in younger children have been published (Nussinovitch, Finkelstein, Amir, & Varsano, 1999). Given that ARF and PSAGN probably do not occur in children younger than 3 years (Kaplan, 1998; Berstein, 1999), the relevance of identifying and treating GABHS in this age group should be viewed skeptically (see section on diagnosis and management).

The infection is spread through contact with nasopharyngeal and oropharyngeal secretions. In temperate climates, "strep season" for pharyngitis is late winter and early spring. A secondary peak is commonly seen in the early fall, as children return to school. In tropical climates, GABHS acute pharyngitis is seen all year. Skin infections due to GABHS are most common in preschoolers and favor warmer climates or seasons (Kaplan, 1998).

Depending on the study, 8% to 11% and in some reports up to 15% of the population are asymptomatic carriers of GABHS (Tanz & Shulman, 1998). Carriers are not felt to be at risk for either suppurative complications or the development of either ARF or PSAGN. Early during the carrier state, transmissibility of GABHS to others is a concern, but bacterial numbers decline after the first few weeks, markedly reducing this risk (Pichichero, 1998). In the past, family dogs were implicated as a source of recurrent infections in humans; newer evidence disproves the idea that animal carriage is a reservoir for human infection (Wilson, Maroney, & Gander, 1995).

History and Physical Examination

The clinical presentation of GABHS pharyngitis varies with age. The classic presentation of sudden onset of high fever, sore throat, and cervical adenopathy tends to be limited to the school-age group. In younger children, a more indolent presentation predominates, termed streptococcosis.

Streptococcosis in Children Six Months to Three Years

The presentation is gradual with mild or absent constitutional symptoms, low-grade or no fever, some degree of anterior cervical adenopathy, and mild nasopharyngitis. The nasal discharge may either be clear or cloudy, and symptoms may persist for up to 2 months. In some cases, the symptom constellation is indistinguishable from the common cold. In others, fever and pharyngeal symptoms are more pronounced, resembling the presentation in older children (Nussinovitch et al., 1999). The clinical and diagnostic significance of streptococcosis is controversial.

● **Clinical Pearl:** For all practical purposes, nonsuppurative complications (ARF and PSAGN) do not occur in children younger than 3 years. The development of possible but rare suppurative complications, such as cervical adenitis or parapharyngeal or retropharyngeal abscesses, would prompt treatment in their own right. The question then arises: Does the clinician need to diagnose and treat GABHS infections in this age group? If a sibling has recurrent infections or a household contact has a history of rheumatic fever, treatment will be useful for transmissibility reasons. Otherwise, some would argue that diagnosis and treatment serve no purpose and in fact might preclude the development of protective immunity.

GABHS Pharyngitis in School-Age Children

Classic clinical features of GABHS pharyngitis include a sudden onset of symptoms, consisting of sore throat, difficulty swallowing, fever, and headache. Physical findings include a red and inflamed pharynx and tonsils with or without exudate, soft palate petechiae or red enanthems, and tender, swollen anterior cervical nodes. If an erythrogenic toxin-producing strain causes the infection, the classic scarlatiniform rash will also be present, as described below.

● **Clinical Pearl:** Abdominal pain, nausea, and vomiting are common features especially in children and may be severe enough to mimic a surgical abdomen.

● **Clinical Pearl:** When discussing the clinical features of GABHS pharyngitis, remember that all the above positive findings (with the exception of scarlet fever) lack diagnostic specificity (Gerber, 1998). The diagnosis cannot be excluded by the absence of fever, tonsillar exudate, soft palate findings, or adenopathy.

▲ **Clinical Warning:** GABHS pharyngitis can and does occur with milder signs and symptoms and cannot be discounted on the basis that the child is not that ill or the throat is not that red.

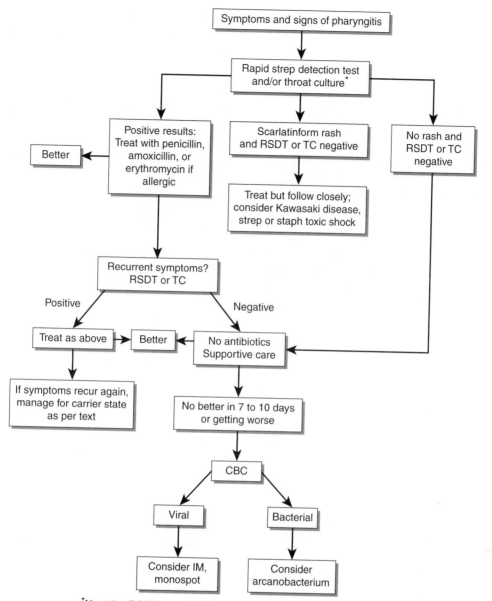

Figure 34–1 ■ Management of pharyngitis.

In contrast to the lack of specificity regarding the above, the presence of other findings, such as conjunctivitis, cough, hoarseness, diarrhea, anterior stomatitis, and discrete mouth ulcers, tends to suggest but not prove a viral etiology.

● **Clinical Pearl:** Even without treatment, GABHS pharyngitis is a self-limited illness with symptoms abating after 1 week.

Scarlet Fever

The elaboration of an erythrogenic toxin by certain strains produces the classic scarlatiniform rash. The texture is characteristic, alternatively described as either peach fuzzy or like fine sandpaper, over confluent erythema. Patients complain of mild pruritus. The rash tends to spare the face, giving the appearance of perioral pallor that stands out in contrast to flushed-appearing cheeks. In mild or early cases, the rash may not be terribly noticeable on the trunk but is much more visible on the lower abdomen and groin when lifting the waistband of the patient's underpants or panties. In more pronounced cases, a coalescence of petechiae in the antecubital fossa forms the classic Pastia's lines. In African American patients, the rash may be difficult to appreciate and the diagnosis only established retrospectively with desquamation.

Other classic findings include a "strawberry" tongue, pharyngeal erythema with or without exudate, soft palate findings, and abdominal pain. Desquamation begins centrally, spreads peripherally, and varies in intensity. Peeling of the hands and feet may not occur for weeks following the acute illness.

Streptococcal Vaginitis and Anitis

Perianal and vaginal streptococcal infections produce an intensely red and at times moist, pruritic, halo-like rash. Vaginitis produces dysuria that can be confused with signs of a urinary tract infection. Some rapid streptococcal detection tests may not be positive for these scenarios, which are often seen in conjunction with streptococcal pharyngitis but at times are isolated phenomena.

Suppurative Complications

The incidence of suppurative complications has increased over the past 15 years, presumably due to increased GABHS virulence (Altemeier, 1998; Ahmed & Ayoub, 1998). These can be divided into local extensions and systemic complications.

Localized extensions, including peritonsillar, parapharyngeal, and retropharyngeal abscesses, are discussed in the ensuing section on suppurative complications. Cervical adenitis is discussed in Chapter 35.

Systemic complications consist of streptococcal toxic shock and necrotizing fasciitis (discussed in Chap. 45). Briefly, hypotension, shock, and multiple organ system failure characterize streptococcal toxic shock. In children, it differs from adults because of its high association with varicella and the high frequency with which GABHS pharyngitis is identified as the only antecedent event. A complete discussion of streptococcal toxic shock is beyond the scope of this chapter, and the reader is referred to an excellent review article by Ahmed and Ayoub (1998).

Nonsuppurative Complications

Nonsuppurative complications include ARF, PSAGN, pediatric autoimmune neuropsychiatric disorder associated with strep (PANDAS), and poststreptococcal reactive arthritis (PSRA). Of these, ARF is the most serious, necessitating years of prophylaxis and potentially leading to the permanent valvular damage of rheumatic heart disease. Children with ARF will require years of prophylactic penicillin; intramuscular benzathine penicillin given every 3 to 4 weeks is the regimen of choice.

Although a serious acute illness, PSAGN fortunately carries an excellent long-term prognosis. ARF and PSAGN are discussed in detail in Chapters 37 and 39, respectively.

Associated with streptococcal infections, PANDAS is discussed briefly in relation to tic disorders and obsessive-compulsive disorder (OCD) in Chapter 46, and PSRA, alluded to in Chapter 47, is discussed further.

Pediatric Autoimmune Neuropsychiatric Disorder Associated With Strep

In 1998, Swedo, Leonard, and Garvey published a paper describing the clinical features of 50 children with childhood onset OCD and tic disorders in whom GABHS infections (and occasionally other illnesses) periodically exacerbated their neuropsychiatric symptoms. This subset of patients shared the following characteristics:

- Tics or OCD
- Early age at onset (usually between 6 and 7 years)
- Sudden and dramatic symptom exacerbation with GABHS infections
- Neurologic abnormalities, such as abnormal movements similar to chorea

Additionally, frequent associations were found with hyperactivity, impulsivity, and distractibility, meeting criteria for the diagnosis of attention deficit hyperactivity disorder and other symptoms characterized by emotional lability, separation anxiety, and inappropriate behavior for age. The patho-

physiology was presumed to be autoimmune and hypothesized to resemble Sydenham's chorea (SC), one of the major diagnostic features of ARF. Both OCD and SC show neuroimaging evidence of basal ganglia dysfunction and similar antineuronal antibodies. Host factors also were felt to play a large role in pathogenesis, with males predominating and, similar to ARF, certain populations being more susceptible. They also suggested that in a small group of patients, intensification of symptoms was associated with a two-fold or higher rise in antistreptolysin-O titers. Further study on larger groups will be needed to establish this principle firmly and to clarify whether symptom amelioration coincides with falling titers.

▲ **Clinical Warning:** The authors were careful to note that obtaining a single positive ASO titer at the time of exacerbation of either OCD or tics is insufficient to establish the diagnosis of PANDAS. A clear association between GABHS infection and exacerbation must exist on at least two occasions.

A later paper by the same authors (Garvey, Perlmutter, & Allen, 1999) attempted to determine whether oral penicillin prophylaxis might prevent symptom exacerbation in PANDAS. Unfortunately, because the incidence of GABHS infections was equal in both the study and control groups, no conclusions could be drawn.

This disorder presents an entirely new set of challenges and questions for practitioners. Does PANDAS represent a form frust of ARF or SC, in that the autoimmune insult was insufficient to cause frank chorea? Do children with PANDAS deserve a cardiac workup to look for carditis? What should the clinician do with respect to penicillin prophylaxis if he or she identifies a child with PANDAS? Is monthly intramuscular prophylaxis necessary? Do all children with prepubertal onset of OCD or tics require baseline and serial ASOs? The answers await further study.

Poststreptococcal Reactive Arthritis

In a 1995 review, Moon, Greene, and Katona described PSRA as an arthritis or arthralgia following GABHS infection, unassociated with the carditis or chorea seen in ARF. Qualitatively, the arthritis in PSRA is different than that in ARF. It tends to be more prolonged, lasting up to 3 to 5 months, compared with the self-limited variety seen in classic ARF that lasts only 2 to 3 weeks. As opposed to the arthritis in ARF that responds dramatically to aspirin or nonsteroidal anti-inflammatory drugs, PSRA tends to be more resistant to treatment. From this point of view, PSRA seems to resemble the reactive arthritis that follows certain enteric infections. A small percentage of children with PSRA may develop carditis when reinfected with GABHS (Moon et al., 1995). As with PANDAS, unanswered questions regarding PSRA include whether the child requires long-term intramuscular penicillin prophylaxis.

● **Clinical Pearl:** All patients with PSRA should undergo a basic cardiac workup, consisting of an electrocardiogram and perhaps a 2D echocardiogram.

Diagnostic Criteria and Studies

Numerous authors have attempted to develop clinical scoring systems to establish the diagnosis without obtaining confirmatory testing (DiMatteo, 1999). Classic scores by Breese in 1977 and Stillerman and Bernstein in 1961 at best only predicted positive results 77.6% and 70% of the time respectively, which is clearly inadequate. Others developed guidelines that suggest empiric treatment based on positive physical findings, even though the probability of a positive throat culture was only 50% (Perkins, 1997). In the era of rapidly emerging antimicrobial resistance, these clearly have no place in the management of acute pharyngitis in childhood, especially given the ease and availability of throat cultures and other rapid detection tests. Throat cultures and rapid streptococcal detection tests (RSDTs) form the basis for confirmatory testing and are mandatory for anyone whose practice deals with illness in children and adolescents.

▲ **Clinical Warning:** The use of any clinical scoring system to either include or exclude the diagnosis of GABHS pharyngitis without confirmatory testing is dangerous and cannot be recommended. Even experts cannot diagnose or exclude GABHS pharyngitis on clinical grounds alone and must rely on bacteriologic confirmation (Gerber, 1998).

Throat Cultures

Throat cultures remain the gold standard for isolation of GABHS from the nasopharynx (Gerber, 1998). If providers use good technique, throat cultures will identify GABHS with 90% to 95% sensitivity, a degree of accuracy many other commonly used laboratory tests rarely achieve. Culture plates are inexpensive, as are small incubators specifically made for office use. How the culture is obtained, plated, and incubated will influence the accuracy of a throat culture.

Almost all children and adolescents dislike throat cultures because of the discomfort and gagging they precipitate. Regardless, clinicians must insist on impeccable technique in obtaining the swab, which includes carefully immobilizing uncooperative patients before obtaining swabs. With the child supine on the examining table, the clinician should ask the parent to hold the child's arms above the head, pressing the elbows against the ears. Doing so effectively prevents sudden side-to-side or backward head movements. The clinician or assistant can then slide a tongue blade to the posterior portion of the tongue, producing a gag and widening of the mouth opening. The clinician or assistant then rapidly but systematically obtains a swab from both tonsillar surfaces and the posterior pharyngeal wall. He or she should take care to avoid touching the swab to any other portion of the oropharynx either upon entering or leaving.

▲ **Clinical Warning:** It is totally unacceptable to swab a throat blindly in a moving and frightened child. Providers must perform all cultures under direct visualization to ensure that they obtain a proper specimen, preventing false-negative results and the small but real possibility of untreated GABHS progressing to ARF. All but the most cooperative patients will require some assistance in immobilizing the head and neck.

The next step is plating on sheep red blood agar according to the manufacturer's recommendations. Although anaerobic incubation and the use of selective media have been reported to increase sensitivity, they are not generally recommended as necessary for practitioners processing their own cultures (Gerber, 1998).

Hemolysins elaborated by beta-hemolytic strains will produce crystal clear hemolysis of red blood cells. Alpha-hemolytic strains by distinction produce a green hemolysis that is not crystal clear. Placing a bacitracin disk on the plate is an inexpensive and highly effective means of distinguishing between group A beta-hemolytic strains and non-group A strains, which are not implicated in development of ARF.

Group A strains are sensitive to bacitracin and will effectively demonstrate a zone of inhibition around the disk, which will appear as a red circle in the middle of crystal clear hemolysis.

Providers should incubate the plates for 18 to 24 hours at 35° to 37°C and then for an additional 24 hours at room temperature. Initial reading may occur between 18 and 24 hours. They should reexamine negative plates at 48 hours, during which time a considerable number of additional positives will appear (Gerber, 1998). In all cases, the manufacturer's recommendations should be followed.

Presumably cultures obtained from patients with true infection are more strongly positive than those obtained from carriers, but the distinction is not clinically practical (Gerber, 1998). When providers use only throat cultures, it is perfectly acceptable not to initiate antibiotic treatment until culture results are known. Exceptions to the above might include cases in which providers cannot ensure follow-up, either by phone or in person. Increased use of RSDTs in emergency rooms and large walk-in clinics will effectively minimize even this last scenario.

▲ **Clinical Warning:** In the vast majority of cases, providers should not initiate empiric treatment pending culture results, because continuation of this common practice will no doubt contribute to the selection and propagation of antimicrobial resistance.

Rapid Streptococcal Detection Tests

Commercially available RSDTs use techniques varying from latex agglutination, enzyme immunoassay, and most recently optical immunoassay. They are more expensive than throat culture plates, at $1.93 versus $0.37 per test. As a group, they offer the distinct advantage of available results in minutes rather than days, translating to decreased absences from school and work for patients and parents. These tests are particularly suited for walk-in facilities and emergency departments, where they have been shown to reduce inappropriate antibiotic treatment (Gerber, 1998). As a group, their specificity is very high, averaging 90% to 96%, but their sensitivity is low, ranging from 76% to 87%. This disparity prompts the recommendation that if using RSDTs, providers should use a two-swab technique to obtain the culture, saving the second for plating a culture if the RSDT is negative.

● **Clinical Pearl:** Due to its high specificity, if the RSDT is positive, the provider can treat the patient without further testing. Due to its low sensitivity, however, if the RSDT is negative, the provider should plate a regular throat culture.

The newer optical immunoassays are being promoted as having sensitivities high enough to preclude the need for throat cultures following negative results. The literature is still contradictory on this matter (Schlager, Hayden, Woods, Dudley, & Hendley, 1997; Gerber et al., 1997). Until further definitive evidence becomes available, the clinician would be prudent to follow negative RSDTs with standard throat cultures.

Diagnostic Considerations if the Throat Culture is Negative

Because viral infections as a group account for most sore throats in all age groups, it is reasonable to assume a viral etiology when throat cultures or RSDTs are negative. Providers need to consider gonococcal pharyngitis as a possibility in sexually active adolescents or in pediatric victims of sexual abuse. Diphtheria thankfully has been eliminated from most of the developed world, but occasional outbreaks occur, and providers should consider it in this context.

Mycoplasma and *Chlamydia* also cause acute pharyngitis but not with pharyngitis as an isolated finding. Other manifestations of these pathogens, such as pneumonia, conjunctivitis, and occasionally otitis, will invariably be present as well, leading the clinician to the proper diagnosis and treatment.

Groups C and G streptococci have been listed as etiologies for acute pharyngitis and URIs (Pichichero, 1998; AAP, 1997). It is not completely clear whether they are colonizers or cause true infection (Kaplan, 1998) and if so, whether the infection is self-limited as with GABHS. In any event, they are insignificant in the clinical decision-making process.

▲ **Clinical Warning:** Providers should treat a scarlatiniform rash regardless of throat culture or RSDT results. In the face of a negative throat culture, the provider should follow the patient closely, however, because Kawasaki syndrome and streptococcal (nonpharyngeal) and staphylococcal toxic shock may present this way.

● **Clinical Pearl:** When the signs and symptoms of throat culture negative pharyngitis do not abate in 7 to 10 days, clinicians should consider the possibility of IM, even in the absence of classic findings of exudative pharyngitis, generalized adenopathy, and splenomegaly.

Arcanobacter haemolyticus (formerly known as *Corynebacterium haemolyticum*) is a gram-positive bacillus that produces a clinical picture virtually indistinguishable from GABHS. Exudative pharyngitis, fever, and cervical adenopathy characterize this rare cause of acute pharyngitis seen primarily in adolescents. A maculopapular pruritic exanthem beginning on the extensor surfaces of the extremities and spreading to the trunk but sparing the palms, soles, and face is present in 50% of cases (AAP, 1997). *Arcanobacterium* is sensitive to erythromycin and under very specific circumstances, providers should consider treatment. Figure 34-1 presents an algorithm illustrating the clinical approach in a patient with primary symptoms of pharyngitis.

● **Clinical Pearl:** Providers should consider *Arcanobacterium* in the symptomatic adolescent whose throat culture is negative. When pursuing the diagnosis of mononucleosis, the provider will discover a negative monospot and an elevated WBC count and nonviral differential.

▲ **Clinical Warning:** The clinician must remember that poor technique in obtaining a throat swab and surreptitious use of leftover antibiotics initiated by a parent, are significant causes of false-negative throat cultures.

Management

In the past, practitioners learned that treatment of GABHS did not alter the natural course of the illness, which was self-limiting after 7 to 8 days. It is clear today that treatment shortens the course and decreases the severity of symptoms. However, this is not the major reason for treatment.

● **Clinical Pearl:** The primary purpose of treatment is to decrease the incidence of suppurative and nonsuppurative sequelae and to decrease transmissibility.

Management of the Patient With a Positive Throat Culture or RSDT

Fortunately, GABHS is still sensitive to many antibiotics, including simple penicillin. A 10-day course has been the gold standard for treatment and ARF prevention. The dosage frequency of any medication obviously influences cooperation with a treatment plan, with once- or twice-a-day dosing most likely to achieve compliance. To this end, many studies have examined treatment efficacy using a variety of antibiotics in an attempt to achieve efficacy with less frequent dosing regimens and shorter lengths of treatment. Cefuroxime, cefpodoxime, and azithromycin are currently Food and Drug Administration (FDA) approved for 5-day courses of treatment. Additionally, cefadroxil, cefixime, ceftibuten, and azithromycin have been granted FDA approval for once-a-day treatment of GABHS (Feder et al., 1999). As a group, cephalosporins have been shown to have lower treatment failure rates than penicillin (Pichichero, 1998). These results must be tempered with the knowledge that cephalosporins are significantly more expensive than penicillin. Another major consideration is the effect on emerging bacterial resistance to antibiotics, by using more broad-spectrum antimicrobials when more narrow-spectrum drugs will do almost as well.

A recent meta-analysis concluded that 10 days of penicillin twice daily was equally as effective as more frequent regimens, but that once-a-day dosing had a 12% lower cure rate. A lower cure rate was not seen with once-a-day dosing of amoxicillin, however (Lan, Colford, & Colford, 2000). Another study showed that 750 mg of amoxicillin given once a day was equally as effective as penicillin given three times a day (Feder et al., 1999).

The 1997 AAP *Red Book*, which serves as the "bible" of pediatric infectious disease, recommends that GABHS be treated with penicillin V 250 mg two or three times a day for 10 days in children and 500 mg two or three times a day for 10 days in adolescents. Alternatively, long-acting intramuscular benzathine penicillin (LA preparation) or combined with procaine penicillin (CR preparation) may be given at a dose of 600,000 U for children who weigh less than 60 lb and 1.2 million U for those above this weight. This injection, though quite painful, eliminates the concern about cooperation with the treatment plan. For children allergic to penicillins, erythromycin at a dose of 20 to 40 mg/kg/d in two to four divided doses or azithromycin 10 mg/kg/d as a single dose for 5 days are reasonable choices.

The major problem with the current AAP recommendations concerns the taste of the liquid preparations of penicillin V. Uniformly, they taste terrible, which precludes adequate completion of a treatment regimen for many children. With more studies reporting successful therapy with once-daily amoxicillin (Feder et al., 1999; Lan, 2000), this author recommends using amoxicillin 40 mg/kg/d two or three times a day for children unable to swallow pills, and penicillin at the same intervals for those who can. As more studies of once daily dosing of amoxicillin are published, it is possible that a regimen of once-a-day amoxicillin will supplant penicillin as the gold standard in the treatment of GABHS.

There is universal agreement that follow-up cultures are not recommended after completion of treatment in patients who are asymptomatic. Obtaining follow-up cultures will undoubtedly pick up a number of carriers of GABHS, raising the likelihood of streptophobia but accomplishing little else, because for the most part, carriers are not at risk to develop sequelae and are unlikely to transmit the organism to others.

As with any other disease, there are treatment failures, which have been attributed to renewed exposure, especially common in crowded conditions, such as within a family, child care setting, or school. Other reasons include lack of cooperation with the antibiotic regimen, the theoretical presence of beta lactamase producing co-colonizers, and the loss of protective oropharyngeal flora, such as alpha-hemolytic streptococci. These last two are discussed in more detail in the previous section on pathology.

Of the 5% to 35% of patients who exhibit a bacteriologic treatment failure (Pichichero, 1998), a much smaller percentage may exhibit persistent symptoms compatible with the clinical picture of GABHS. Whether these clinical treatment failures represent reinfection, failure of eradication due to deep-seated foci of infection, lactamase protection by co-colonizers, or increased bacteriologic adherence can only be theorized. The most likely explanation is that most treatment failures were not real GABHS infections. They really represented a carrier with an intercurrent viral infection who was misdiagnosed because of a positive throat culture. Management of recurrences and the carrier state is discussed in the following section. Regardless of the reason, providers should counsel parents to return if symptoms recur, even if the range of signs and symptoms is milder than the original infection (Pichichero, 1998).

▲ **Clinical Warning:** Providers should reculture only symptomatic patients; routine reculturing of asymptomatic children will accomplish little except to increase anxiety in both patient and parent.

Management of Patients With Recurrences and the Carrier State

Traditionally, the carrier state was defined as the asymptomatic presence of GABHS in the nasopharynx without evidence of an immune response. Theorists believe it is acquired in one of two ways. It may develop following a symptomatic or asymptomatic infection. In this model, ASO titers are elevated initially and gradually decrease proportionately to the length of time the carrier state has existed. It also may develop as the result of colonization without infection. In this model, no ASO response occurs.

● **Clinical Pearl:** Regardless of how the carrier state developed, carriers will culture positive for GABHS, whether they are truly infected or just have an intercurrent viral illness.

Because GABHS is still very sensitive to antibiotics, the most likely reason for its persistence in adequately treated patients is the treatment of a presumed infection that was actually a carrier state. The theorized mechanisms for bacteriologic treatment failure and the carrier state are similar (see section on pathology). Practically, the distinction between carriers and treatment failures blurs, as the persistence of GABHS in the throat despite adequate therapy is the route by which patients come to a provider's attention. Therefore, clinicians should approach bacteriologic treatment failures and the carrier state in the same manner (Tanz & Shulman, 1998).

● **Clinical Pearl:** When a child or adolescent has had multiple "strep" episodes, providers should suspect the carrier state, especially if symptoms are mild, atypical, or absent.

▲ **Clinical Warning:** A positive ASO does not exclude the possibility of the carrier state, because some chronic carriers will demonstrate elevated results. In the face of multiple recurrences, only a negative ASO is diagnostic for the carrier state.

Streptococcal carriers are not at risk for developing ARF or suppurative complications (Kaplan, 1980). Transmissibility to others seems to wane after 1 or 2 months (Pichichero, 1998). Therefore, major problems related to the carrier state include parental and patient anxiety (streptophobia), unnecessary repeated courses of antibiotics leading to the development of resistant bacteria, and unnecessary referrals to surgical specialists for tonsillectomies.

Management of the chronic carrier state is a challenge for even the most experienced practitioners. In most cases, it entails patient education and selective use of diagnostic tests and treatment modalities.

● **Clinical Pearl:** Successful treatment is predicated on the clinician's ability to communicate effectively the nature of the condition and the fact that it poses little or no risk either to the patient or others.

In carriers, providers should perform throat cultures and RSDTs only if the clinical scenario is suggestive of GABHS. Practitioners should avoid these tests in circumstances that would suggest a viral infection (Tanz & Shulman, 1998). In case of positive results, providers should prescribe only narrow-spectrum antibiotics (ie, penicillin or amoxicillin).

The *Red Book* recommends a number of treatment regimens in cases of extreme family anxiety and streptophobia, patients with a history of or family member with ARF, or families experiencing "ping-pong" spread among members. Clindamycin 20 mg/kg/d divided twice daily (maximum daily dose 1.8 g) for 10 days provides 92% eradication rates (Tanz & Shulman, 1998). Another regimen combines intramuscular benzathine penicillin with rifampin 20 mg/kg/d divided twice daily (maximum daily dose 600 mg) for 4 days beginning on the day of the injection. Providers should warn families that the child taking rifampin will have bright orange urine, tears, and saliva. Providers should certainly not consider tonsillectomy in even the most streptophobic of situations, without first attempting the pharmacologic interventions outlined above (Tanz & Shulman, 1998).

▲ **Clinical Warning:** Many families and ear, nose, and throat specialists mistakenly believe that tonsillectomy is a cure for chronic streptococcal carriage. Acute streptococcal pharyngitis and the carrier state occur with or without tonsils. Management of pharyngitis is illustrated in Figure 34-1.

Referral Criteria

Tonsillectomy continues to be used as a treatment modality for repeated infections with GABHS. Fortunately, its use continues to decline, and in this era is used more frequently for obstructive sleep apnea. Prospective studies have shown benefits of tonsillectomy in repeated cases of culture-documented GABHS infections, and tonsillectomy may be considered for those with six infections in a year. This author's bias is to use either clindamycin or benzathine penicillin in combination with rifampin (as outlined above) in these recurrent cases before considering tonsillectomy. This approach is directed toward eradication of the theoretically deep-seated GABHS infection.

REFERENCES

Ahmed, S., & Ayoub, E. M. (1998). Severe invasive group A streptococcal disease and toxic shock. *Pediatric Annals, 27*(5).

Altemeier, W. A. (1998). A brief history of group A beta hemolytic strep—A pediatrician's view. *Pediatric Annals, 27*(5), 264–267.

American Academy of Pediatrics. (1997). *Red book: Report of the Committee on Infectious Diseases* (24th ed.). Elk Grove Village, IL: Author.

Annunziato, P. W. (1998). Herpes simplex virus. In S. L. Katz, A. A. Gershon, & P. J. Hotez (Eds.), *Krugman's infectious diseases of children* (10th ed.). (pp. 189–203). St. Louis: Mosby-Yearbook.

Bergstein, J. M. (1999). Glomerular disease. In R. E. Behrman, R. M. Kliegman, & H. B. Jenson (Eds.), *Nelson textbook of pediatrics* (16th ed.). (pp. 1581–1582). Philadelphia: W.B. Saunders.

Breese, B. B. (1977). A simple scorecard for the tentative diagnosis of Streptococcal pharyngitis. *American Journal of Diseases of Children, 131*, 514–517.

DiMatteo, L. (1999). Managing streptococcal pharyngitis: A review of clinical decision-managing strategies, diagnostic evaluation, and treatment. *Journal of the American Academy of Nurse Practitioners, 11*(2), 57–62.

Feder, H. M., Jr., Gerber, M. A., Randolf, M. F., et al. (1999). Once daily therapy for Streptococcal pharyngitis with amoxicillin. *Pediatrics, 103*, 47–51.

Garvey, M. A., Perlmutter, S. J., & Allen, A. J. (1999). A pilot study of penicillin prophylaxis for neuropsychiatric exacerbations triggered by Streptococcal infections. *Biologic Psychiatry, 45*, 1564–1571.

Gerber, M. A. (1998). Diagnosis of group A streptococcal pharyngitis. *Pediatric Annals, 27*(5), 269–273.

Gerber, M. A., Tanz, R. R., Kabat, W., Dennis, E., Bell, G. L., Kaplan, E. L., & Shulman, S. T. (1997). Optical immunoassay for Group A Beta Hemolytic Streptococcal pharyngitis. *Journal of the American Medical Association, 277*(11), 899–903.

Kaplan, E. L. (1980). The group A streptococcal upper respiratory tract carrier state: An enigma. *Journal of Pediatrics, 97*, 337–345.

Kaplan, E. L. (1998). Streptococcal infections. In S. L. Katz, A. A. Gershon, & P. J. Hotez (Eds.), *Krugman's infectious diseases of children* (10th ed.). (pp. 487–500). St. Louis: Mosby-Yearbook.

Katz, B. Z., & Miller, G. (1998). Epstein-Barr infections. In S. L. Katz, A. A. Gershon, & P. J. Hotez (Eds.), *Krugman's infectious diseases of children* (10th ed.). (pp. 37–56, 98–113). St. Louis: Mosby-Yearbook.

Lan, A. J., Colford, J. M., & Colford, J. M. Jr. (2000). The impact of dosing frequency on the efficacy of 10-day penicillin or amoxicillin therapy for streptococcal tonsillopharyngitis: A meta-analysis. *Pediatrics, 105*(2), E19.

Moon, R. Y., Greene, M. G., & Katona, I. M. (1995). Poststreptococcal reactive arthritis in children: A potential predecessor of rheumatic heart disease. *Journal of Rheumatology, 22*, 529–532.

Nussinovitch, M., Finkelstein, Y., Amir, J., & Varsano, I. (1999). Group A beta-hemolytic Streptococcal pharyngitis in preschool children aged 3 months to 5 years. *Clinical Pediatrics (Phila), 38*(6), 357–360.

Nyquist, A., Gonzalez, R., Steiner, F. J., et al. (1998). Antibiotic prescribing for children with colds, upper respiratory tract infections, and bronchitis. *Journal of the American Medical Association, 279*, 875–877.

Perkins, A. (1997). An approach to diagnosing the acute sore throat. *American Family Physician, 131–138.*

Peter, J., & Ray, G. C. (1998). Infectious mononucleosis. *Pediatrics in Review, 19*(8), 276–279.

Pichichero, M. E. (1998). Group A beta hemolytic streptococcal infections. *Pediatric Review, 19*(9), 291–302.

Pichichero, M. E., McLinn, S., Rotbart, H. A., et al. (1998). Clinical and economic impact of enterovirus illness in private pediatric practice. *Pediatrics, 102*(5), 1126-1134.

Rotbart, H. (1998). Krugman's enteroviruses. In S. L. Katz, A. A. Gershon, & P. J. Hotez (Eds.), *Infectious diseases of children* (10th ed.). (pp. 81–97). St. Louis: Mosby-Yearbook.

Rutkow, I. M. (1978). Rupture of the spleen in infectious mononucleosis. *Archives of Surgery, 113*, 718.

Schlager, T. A., Hayden, G. A., Woods, W. A., Dudley, S. M., & Hendley, J. O. (1996). Optical immunoassay for rapid detection of group A beta hemolytic streptococci. *Archives of Pediatric Adolescent Medicine, 150*, 245–248.

Stillerman, M., & Bernstein, S. H. (1961). Streptococcal pharyngitis. *American Journal of Diseases of Children, 101*, 476–489.

Swedo, S. E., Leonard, H. L., & Garvey, M. (1998). Pediatric autoimmune neuropsychiatric disorders associated with Streptococcal infections: Clinical description of the first 50 cases. *American Journal of Psychiatry, 155*(2), 264–271.

Tanz, R. R., & Shulman, S. T. (1998). Streptococcal pharyngitis: The carrier state, definition and management. *Pediatric Annals, 27*(5), 281–285.

Todd, J. K. (1999). Rheumatic fever. In R. E. Behrman, R. M. Kliegman, & H. B. Jenson (Eds.), *Nelson textbook of pediatrics* (16th ed.). (pp. 806–810). Philadelphia: W.B. Saunders.

Wilson, K. S., Maroney, S. A., & Gander, R. M. (1995). The family pet as an unlikely source of Group A Beta Hemolytic Streptococcal Infection in humans. *Pediatric Infectious Disease Journal, 14*, 372–375.

Zaoutis, T., & Klein, J. D. (1998). Enterovirus infections. *Pediatrics in Review, 19*(6), 183–191.

Suppurative Complications of Pharyngitis and Neck Masses

• DARSIT K. SHAH, MD

P A R T 1 ▲

Suppurative Complications of Pharyngitis

INTRODUCTION

Suppurative complications, although uncommon, are the most frequently seen complications resulting from tonsillitis and pharyngitis. These suppurative sequelae include peritonsillar abscess (PTA), parapharyngeal abscess (PPA), and retropharyngeal space abscess (RPA). Other rare sequelae can occur but are beyond the scope of this chapter.

ANATOMY, PHYSIOLOGY, AND PATHOLOGY

The palatine tonsil is situated between the tongue base inferiorly, the superior constrictor laterally, and the palate superiorly. A tight fibrous capsule surrounds the tonsil in its entirety except at its palatal interface. Here, approximately 20 to 30 mucous glands, named Weber's glands, lubricate the tonsil and create a potential communication between the tonsil and palate. This potential area is called the peritonsillar space (Fig. 35-1).

The parapharyngeal space (PPS) extends from the skull base to the hyoid bone and is surrounded by the pharynx and vertebral bodies. It is mainly hidden in the retromandibular area. It does communicate posteriorly with the retropharyngeal space (RPS). The RPS is the most dangerous space in the neck because it can extend from the skull base to the sacrum. It is essentially devoid of any important anatomic structures outside of an abundance of lymph nodes in children.

Peritonsillar abscess develops through two potential mechanisms. The first entails direct spread of infection from the tonsil through the capsular dehiscence at its superior pole into the palate, with subsequent suppuration. The second mechanism entails suppuration of Weber's mucous glands present in the palate adjacent to the tonsil, resulting essentially in a salivary abscess. PPA or RPA, however, rarely result from direct spread of infection. The more likely scenario in the face of tonsillitis is the development of nodal adenitis with suppuration within the node, leading to abscess formation.

EPIDEMIOLOGY

The most common cervical space infection is PTA. Its incidence is approximately 30/100,000 or about 45,000 cases per year (Kitirat et al., 1995). The occurrence of PPA or RPA is less common, with ill-defined incidence.

HISTORY AND PHYSICAL EXAMINATION

Typically, children with PTA present with severe odynophagia or painful swallowing. They usually can only tolerate liquids and many times not even their own saliva. In addition, otalgia and trismus are also frequent. Examination demonstrates a toxic patient with a high fever.

● **Clinical Pearl:** The combination of hot potato voice due to soft palate edema, drooling, trismus, and uvular deviation is extremely suggestive of a diagnosis of PTA (Table 35-1).

Both PPA and RPA are associated with suppurative neck masses. Children with PPA appear toxic with a high fever and have dysphagia, trismus, and a muffled voice with varying degrees of airway symptoms. Physical examination demonstrates a palatal bulge and most importantly a high cervical neck mass obscuring visualization and palpation of the mandibular angle. In addition, when airway impingement is present, children may assume a sniffing posture to maximize air exchange. Because RPA is usually an extension from a lower suppurative adenitis, the classic clinical findings include a neck mass, fever, and some degree of upper airway obstruction, leading to the sniffing position and some shortness of breath.

If incompletely or inadequately treated, PTA, RPA, and PPA have potential serious and life-threatening sequelae. These include airway obstruction, jugular vein thrombosis, carotid artery rupture, sepsis, and mediastinitis.

DIAGNOSTIC CRITERIA

The diagnosis of PTA usually is established on the basis of the classic findings on physical examination as mentioned previously. The diagnosis of PPA or RPA may be suspected on clinical grounds by the presence of a tender neck mass in association with systemic toxicity and some signs of upper airway embarrassment, such as shortness of breath and the "sniffing position." Imaging studies are needed to confirm the diagnosis of PPA or RPA.

Various benign and malignant disorders can simulate abscess occurrence within the RPS or PPS. The differential

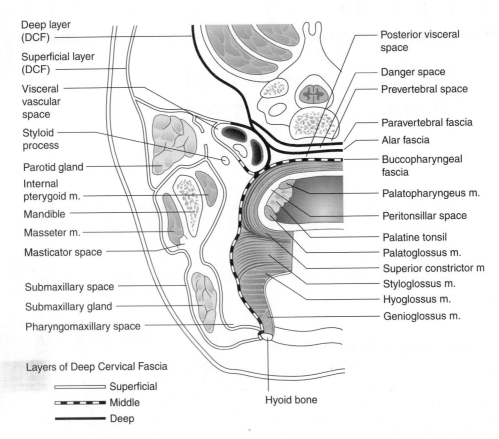

Figure 35–1 ■ Axial section through the neck demonstrating the various deep neck spaces. (Adapted from Bailey B: Principles of Otolaryngology—Head and Neck Surgery, p. 827.)

diagnosis should include infected congenital cyst, lymphoma, rhabdomyosarcoma, or granulomatous disease (Nicklaus & Kelley, 1996). When the clinical scenario is atypical, these other disorders should be considered in the management of the child with RPA or PPA.

DIAGNOSTIC STUDIES

Before the advent of computed tomography (CT) scanning, only plain AP and lateral neck x-rays were used to assist in diagnosing neck abscesses. Lateral neck films, in cases of

RPA, demonstrated RPS of greater than 7 mm at C2 and 14 mm at C6. Other nonsuppurative processes, such as adenitis, could give the same findings. For this reason, when RPA or PPA is suspected, children should undergo a CT scan with contrast. Typical findings when a neck abscess is present include low attenuation areas with ring enhancement. Providers should pay particular attention to the vascular structures and mediastinum to exclude venous thrombosis and mediastinitis.

No purulence is found in 5% to 10% of neck explorations, even with the classic findings on CT scan. This implies that necrotic lymph nodes can occasionally give the same image findings as an abscess. Despite this occasional false-positive, CT scanning has revolutionized the management of the child with a suspected neck abscess (Lazor, 1994).

MANAGEMENT

Multidisciplinary consultation from the primary care practitioner, otolaryngologist, and radiologist is essential in the management of a potential PTA, RPA, or PPA. Initial assessment of a child should exclude imminent or potentially imminent airway obstruction. Further workup and intervention can proceed when the airway has been stabilized.

When a diagnosis of PTA, RPA, or PPA has been confirmed on clinical and radiographic grounds, the provider should obtain a CBC and blood and throat cultures and start the child on broad-spectrum antibiotics with anaerobic coverage.

The bacteriology of neck abscess is usually polymicrobial, with GABHS and *Staphylococcus aureus* being the most com-

Table 35–1. COMPARISON OF THE PRESENTATION OF VARIOUS NECK ABSCESSES

Neck Abscess	Symptoms/Signs
Peritonsillar	Fever, dysphagia, drooling, hot potato voice, trismus, palatal bulge, uvular deviation
	No significant neck mass
Parapharyngeal	Fever, dysphagia, shortness of breath, trismus, palatal/tonsillar bulge
	Neck mass (usually fluctuant)
Retropharyngeal	Fever, neck stiffness, dysphagia, sniffing position, shortness of breath
	Neck mass

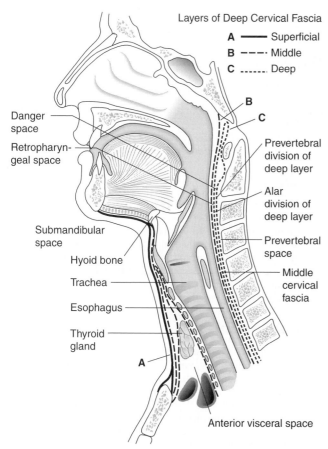

Layers of Deep Cervical Fascia

A ——— Superficial
B - - - - Middle
C .... Deep

Danger space

Retropharyngeal space

Submandibular space

Hyoid bone

Trachea

Esophagus

Thyroid gland

A

B

C

Prevertebral division of deep layer

Alar division of deep layer

Prevertebral space

Middle cervical fascia

Anterior visceral space

Figure 35–2 ■ Sagittal section of the neck demonstrating the various spaces between the pharynx and vertebrae. (Adapted from Bailey B: Principles of Otolaryngology—Head and Neck Surgery, p. 827.)

mon organisms. Unfortunately, there is a high incidence of beta-lactamase production. *Bacteriodes* species, an anaerobic organism, is frequently present concomitantly (Kitirat et al., 1995). Because of these factors, broad-spectrum coverage is necessary in the treatment of neck abscesses in children. Providers should select drugs that combine excellent gram-positive coverage for staphylococci and streptococci with anaerobic coverage. Examples include ampicillin (Unasyn) or a combination of clindamycin or vancomycin and a third-generation cephalosporin.

Traditional teaching has recommended external incision and drainage for all cases of RPA or PPA and internal incision and drainage for all cases of PTA. In select cases, however, other options are available, including treatment with intravenous antibiotics alone, needle aspiration, or transoral drainage.

▲ **Clinical Warning:** An external surgical incision and drainage should be performed in all cases in which airway obstruction is present, the child has failed to improve on 24 hours of intravenous antibiotics, or other neck complications accompany the abscess (Gidley & Ghorayeb, 1997).

Surgical Treatment of Peritonsillar Abscess

In the past, PTA was treated with drainage and "quinsy" or immediate tonsillectomy. More contemporary management includes drainage and elective (interval) tonsillectomy. Recent data, however, suggest that the incidence of subsequent abscesses is actually low, and a planned tonsillectomy may not be indicated.

Drainage for PTA usually can be performed under local anesthesia through a transoral route in most children. Recent studies have supported the efficacy of needle aspiration alone in multiple locations to drain PTA (Wolf et al., 1994). The other option would be cold-knife drainage under local anesthesia. Both options carry a 5% to 10% incidence of persistent or recurrent abscess. When children are uncooperative, providers should use general anesthesia to perform a transoral drainage procedure without a "quinsy" tonsillectomy. Most children experience an immediate and rapid improvement in symptoms when the PTA is drained. Some, however, require admission for intravenous fluids and antibiotics.

Surgical Treatment of Parapharyngeal Abscess and Retropharyngeal Space Abscess

Generally, PPA should be drained using an external approach to allow visualization of and prevent injury to the great vessels and neural structures. Transoral drainage should only be performed when the abscess is medially placed and the great vessels are at minimal risk. Resolution of PPA with intravenous antibiotics alone can occur in 5% to 10% of cases (Nicklaus & Kelley, 1996). This approach is reasonable for the initial 24 hours of treatment. If the patient's clinical course fails to improve or worsens, then immediate incision and drainage are required. A drain is left to prevent persistent or recurrent abscess. Continued antibiotics are necessary to allow complete resolution of the infection.

Either a transoral or external drainage procedure can be used to manage RPA safely. Recent opinion favors transoral drainage in nearly all cases, unless airway obstruction is present (Nagy et al., 1997). Studies have demonstrated similar efficacy using either approach with less cosmetic deformity associated with an intraoral approach. The transoral option is not without potential risk, however, including uncontrolled rupture of the abscess with aspiration of pus and subsequent pneumonitis.

REFERENCES

Gidley, P., & Ghorayeb, B. (1997). Contemporary management of deep neck space infections. *Otolaryngology and Head and Neck Surgery, 116,* 16–22.

Kitirat, U., Yellon, R., et al. (1995). Head and neck space infections in infants and children. *Otolaryngology and Head and Neck Surgery, 112,* 375–382.

Lazor, J. (1994). Comparison of computed tomography and surgical findings in deep neck infections. *Otolaryngology and Head and Neck Surgery, 111,* 746–750.

Nagy, M., Pizzuto, M., et al. (1997). Deep neck infections in children: A new approach to diagnosis and treatment. *Laryngoscope, 107,* 1627.

Nicklaus, P., & Kelley, P. (1996). Management of deep neck infections. *Pediatric Clinics of North America, 43,* 1277–1294.

Wolf, M., Chen, I., et al. (1994). Peritonsillar abscess: Repeated needle aspiration versus incision and drainage. *Annals of Otolaryngology, Rhinology, and Laryngology, 103,* 554–557.

P A R T   2   ▲

Neck Masses

INTRODUCTION

This chapter focuses on the evaluation and management of various disorders that affect the neck in children and adolescents. It discusses midline neck masses, torticollis, adenopathy, and cervical adenitis, with special emphasis on clinical differentiation.

MIDLINE NECK MASSES

The differential diagnosis of midline neck masses in children includes thyroglossal duct cyst (TGDC), dermoids, thyroid nodules, fourth brachial cleft cyst, and plunging ranula. By far, TGDC is the most common (Table 35-2).

Thyroglossal Duct Cyst

Pathology

After reactive lymphadenopathy, TGDCs are the second most frequently encountered neck mass (Josephson & Spencer, 1998). They develop from a remnant of the thyroglossal duct. In utero, the thyroid gland descends from the tongue base to its position in the lower neck. When a portion of the duct remains, a cyst eventually may form.

History and Physical Examination

Most TGDCs present in children between ages 5 and 20 years, usually after an upper respiratory infection (URI). They usually are asymptomatic; however, TGDCs can become infected, resulting in a midline neck abscess. If incision and drainage are required, ultimate surgical excision becomes more difficult. Physical examination reveals a midline neck cyst that is

Table 35–2.   DIFFERENTIAL DIAGNOSIS OF MIDLINE NECK MASSES

Position of Midline Neck Mass	Differential Diagnosis
Suprahyoid	Dermoid cyst
	Ranula
	Cystic hygroma
	Adenopathy
Infrahyoid	Thyroglossal duct cyst
	Fourth brachial cleft cyst
	Thyroid nodule
	Adenopathy

usually found in an infrahyoid position. The cyst moves with glutiton and ascends in the neck with tongue protrusion.

Diagnostic Criteria and Studies

The clinical presentation is unique; therefore, imaging usually is not necessary to confirm a diagnosis of TGDC. Some authors, however, recommend the routine use of preoperative thyroid scanning or sonogram to exclude the possibility that TGDC contains the patient's only functioning thyroid tissue (Josephson & Spencer, 1998).

Management

The ultimate management of TGDC is surgical. The definitive procedure is termed the Sistrunk operation. It entails complete resection of not only the cyst, but also the thyroglossal duct remnant leading from the cyst wall through the hyoid, with resection of the central hyoid bone up to the base of the tongue. In cases of more limited removal, children almost uniformly develop recurrent cyst formation in the remnant thyroglossal duct.

Thyroid Nodules

Thyroid nodules also may present as midline neck masses in children. Although the vast majority of these nodules are benign, the incidence of malignancy in children is 20%, significantly higher than the incidence in adults (Brown & Azizham, 1998). Factors that increase the risk of malignancy for children with thyroid nodules include prior irradiation, family history of thyroid malignancy, presence of vocal cord paralysis, and nodal enlargement. Routine evaluation should include thyroid function tests, serology to exclude thyroiditis, and fine needle aspiration biopsy. If cytology is inconclusive and no evidence of thyroiditis is found, the clinician should seriously consider thyroidectomy to exclude definitively thyroid carcinoma. Further management depends ultimately on histopathology found at the time of thyroidectomy.

Dermoids

● **Clinical Pearl:** Suprahyoid midline masses almost always represent dermoids and dermoid cysts.

The submental region is, in fact, the most common location for dermoids in the head and neck (Howard, 1998). Dermoids can be confused easily with TGDCs, but their suprahyoid location makes them easily distinguishable. Dermoids arise from trapped ectodermal elements during gestation. Management is surgical with preservation of normal anatomic structures when possible.

TORTICOLLIS

Neonatal torticollis most likely begins in utero and is the cause, many times, of a difficult delivery. The etiology of this disorder remains uncertain but may result from intrauterine abnormalities. Affected children usually present between ages 4 and 8 weeks with a mass in the upper sternocleidomastoid muscle. A characteristic head position is found, with the child's chin tilted away from the affected side and the occiput toward it.

Pathology reveals extensive fibrosis of the sternocleido-mastoid muscle. The provider should exclude other causes of secondary torticollis, including infectious and inflammatory processes and upper motor neuron disease. Prolonged untreated torticollis can result in hemifacial underdevelopment. In children in whom physical therapy fails and progressive craniofacial abnormalities develop, surgical sectioning of the sternocleidomastoid muscle should be undertaken.

▲ **Clinical Warning:** Treatment should be initiated quickly, and aggressive physiotherapy is the management of choice (Brown & Azizham, 1998).

CERVICAL ADENOPATHY

Benign Adenopathy

Cervical lymph node enlargement in children is common. Almost all children at some time have cervical adenopathy. Fortunately, more than 90% of cases are either benign lymph gland enlargement secondary to URIs, scalp inflammation, or part of the entity of physiologic lymphoid hyperplasia. Physiologic lymphoid hyperplasia is enlargement of all lymphoid tissue, including lymph nodes, tonsils, adenoids, and spleen. It commonly is seen between ages 2 and 8 years as part of immune system maturation.

● **Clinical Pearl:** Adenopathy that is mobile, nonmatted, and soft ("shotty"); present for less than 3 months; smaller than 2 cm; and not associated with systemic symptoms, such as night sweats, weight loss, pruritus, or fever, is not likely to represent a neoplastic process.

● **Clinical Pearl:** Small cervical glands that get slightly bigger and tender with colds or illness, then become smaller, only to enlarge again with the next URI are also extremely common and completely benign, giving credence to the adage that "bad things don't get smaller."

Adenopathy that does not fit the above criteria can result in a provider overlooking a malignancy or other systemic disorder. A high index of suspicion is necessary to diagnose less common entities. When those circumstances are present, the provider should consider open nodal biopsy (Park, 1995).

▲ **Clinical Warning:** Providers should never consider supraclavicular adenopathy benign. It always warrants further investigation and biopsy.

Chronic Adenopathy Secondary to Infection

The differential diagnosis of the child with a chronically enlarged lymph node is vast and includes chronic infections, such as toxoplasmosis, Epstein-Barr virus (EBV), cytomegalovirus (CMV), histoplasmosis, human immuno-deficiency virus-related disease, and cat scratch disease (CSD). Granulomatous disorders, in particular mycobacterial disease, are not uncommon. Clinicians also must exclude neoplastic disorders, such as lymphoma and sarcoma.

Chronic viral-induced lymphadenopathy from EBV, CMV, or parasite-induced toxoplasmosis results in diffuse cervical and, many times, axillary and inguinal adenopathy. Systemic symptoms, such as malaise, arthralgias, and lethargy, also may accompany these disorders at onset. When serologic studies for mononucleosis are negative, nodal biopsy may be necessary to exclude more serious entities.

Cat Scratch Adenopathy

Cat scratch disease can present with solitary, tender, cervical lymphadenopathy. An antecedent history of feline exposure (especially kittens) is common. A raised inoculation site usually is found but may be absent in 20% to 30% of children afflicted with CSD. The causative organism is a gram-negative bacillus known as *Afipia felis*.

Diagnosis of CSD is usually based on clinical grounds, but a positive Hanger Rose skin test can support it. Serologic confirmation is now available and has greatly facilitated the diagnosis of CSD. When a nodal biopsy is performed, characteristic appearance is achieved with a Warthin Starry stain of the specimen. The natural history of CSD is self-resolution over 1 to 2 months. More rapid improvement may be possible with a course of ciprofloxin for adults and rifampin for children (Park, 1995).

Mycobacterial Adenopathy

The incidence of cervical mycobacterial disease once again has increased dramatically. Unlike adults who predominately manifest with typical *Mycobacterium tuberculosis* disease, children tend to be infected with atypical mycobacteria. Groups of nodes that appear matted on examination are found particularly in the submandibular and posterior triangles. Draining fistulas are much less common in children but still found occasionally. Establishing a diagnosis of atypical mycobacterial disease in children can be difficult. A positive purified protein derivative (PPD) or chest x-ray is present in only 30% to 50% of patients afflicted with atypical mycobacterial disease.

● **Clinical Pearl:** Most children with mycobacterial cervical lymph node disease present with nodal enlargement, no systemic symptoms, and a negative PPD and chest x-ray.

Although a fine needle aspirate biopsy occasionally yields a diagnosis of mycobacterial disease, more commonly open biopsy is necessary. Because atypical mycobacterial infection is commonly resistant to standard antituberculosis treatment, most surgeons recommend excisional biopsy of all diseased nodes with preservation of normal anatomy at the time of a diagnostic biopsy. Surgery rarely leads to a postoperative cutaneous fistula, unlike surgery on tuberculosis (MacKellar, 1976). Children with systemic disease will require postoperative multidrug treatment based on the results of culture and sensitivity.

Adenopathy Secondary to Neoplasia

Fortunately, malignancy presenting as cervical adenopathy is uncommon in children. Only 10% of abnormal cervical lymph node enlargement represents carcinoma (Park, 1995). The most common of these carcinomas are lymphomas and sarcomas. If a provider discovers such entities, he or she must refer the child for oncologic evaluation immediately.

CERVICAL ADENITIS

Acute nonsuppurative cervical adenitis is the most common cause of cervical adenopathy. Children typically present with acutely enlarged and painful lymph nodes after having tonsillitis or pharyngitis. They generally are systemically ill and can have high fever. Examination usually demonstrates enlarged and tender lymph nodes with no evidence of fluctuance. The cause is usually bacterial, with *Staphylococcus aureus* being most common, followed by group A beta-hemolytic *Streptococcus*. Oral antibiotics are the usual treatment. First-line therapy should include coverage for the above two pathogens and consist of either a semisynthetic penicillin (eg, cloxacillin or dicloxacillin) or a first-generation cephalosporin (eg, cephalexin). For children who are unable to swallow pills, experienced clinicians usually will prescribe a first-generation cephalosporin, because liquid formulations of either cloxacillin or dicloxacillin are unpalatable to the point of compromising cooperation with the therapeutic regimen. Amoxicillin-clavulinate is a reasonable but more expensive alternative. When treating a child on an outpatient basis, the provider must ensure close clinical follow-up. When nodal disease persists, the provider should consider a trial of clindamycin. If the child is systemically ill or a nodal abscess is possible, hospital admission for intravenous antibiotics and further evaluation may be necessary. With treatment, the nodes generally will recede in size over a short period. If nodal enlargement persists, the provider must consider and exclude other previously discussed entities.

REFERENCES

Brown, R., & Azizham, R. (1998). Pediatric head and neck lesions. *Pediatric Clinics of North America, 45*, 889–905.

Howard, R. (1998). Congenital midline lesions: Pits and protuberances. *Pediatric Annals, 27*, 150.

Josephson, G., & Spencer, W. (1998). Thyroglossal duct cyst: The NY eye and ear infirmary experience. *ENT Journal, 77*, 642.

MacKellar, A. (1976). Diagnosis and management of atypical mycobacterial lymphadenitis in children. *Journal of Pediatric Surgery, 11*, 85–89.

Park, Y. (1995). Evaluation of neck masses in children. *American Family Physician, 51*, 1904.

Approach to the Child With a Cough

• DIANA LOWENTHAL, MD, FAACP

INTRODUCTION

Cough is a frequent pediatric complaint. Most episodes of coughing in children are benign and self-limited, yet families frequently are concerned that their coughing child may have pneumonia or another serious illness. In addition, coughing can interrupt a family's sleep, disrupt the classroom, and provoke stares or comments from strangers. Health care providers who work with coughing children must be adept at discerning the cough associated with mild viral illness from that associated with a more serious malady. In addition, they must be able to reassure families that coughing is a normal part of the host defense to acute respiratory illness. This chapter will review the pertinent history, physical examination, and diagnostic evaluation of a child with a cough. In addition, it will discuss in detail the treatment of pneumonia, croup, and bronchiolitis.

ANATOMY, PHYSIOLOGY, AND PATHOLOGY

Coughing occurs in response to excess mucus secretion or the presence of foreign matter in the nasopharynx, larynx, trachea, or bronchi. The act of coughing moves mucus to the pharynx, where it can be expectorated, sneezed out, or swallowed. An effective cough requires a deep inhalation, a narrowing of the proximal airways, and then a marked, coordinated contraction of all muscles of exhalation. The process demands a profound effort, and can be affected by muscular weakness or chest or abdominal pain.

HISTORY

Ascertaining the nature, severity, and triggers of a cough is important. A detailed guide to important aspects of the history can be found in Table 36-1. Some general points follow.

Acute or Chronic

Chronic coughing has been defined as a cough lasting for 3 weeks or more. The basic tenet is that acute coughing is likely to be a viral or self-limited process, while chronic coughing merits an evaluation for an underlying illness. This distinction, however, is not always simple. Pediatric providers must recognize the child who presents with a cough that is acute yet recurrent—not an uncommon scenario. For example, the child who develops 10 days of "acute" coughing every month still warrants an evaluation for chronic cough.

● **Clinical Pearl:** Children with chronic respiratory problems can present with acute respiratory illness, which may or may not be related to the underlying condition.

In a child who has chronic respiratory problems, it is extremely helpful to ask the parent: "Is this the same type of cough your child usually gets with asthma (or allergies, sinusitis, etc.), or is the cough different this time?" It is helpful to see if a pattern to the cough exists and how it fits into the child's overall health history. Regardless of the duration of the cough, providers must use good clinical judgment to evaluate the severity of the illness.

Timing

Ascertaining the time of day that the cough is most severe is one of the most important and helpful tasks. Coughing from postnasal drip can occur at any time but tends to be most prominent when the child first wakes up in the morning. It also may be troublesome when the child first lies down. Bronchospasm is likely to cause a cough that is most annoying in the middle of the night; however, postnasal drip, pertussis, and gastroesophageal reflux also strike at night. On the contrary, the cough that occurs all day—especially during times of stress—yet disappears completely the instant the child falls asleep, may be a habit cough, also called a cough tic or psychogenic cough.

Seasonal Pattern

In temperate climates, coughing is a far more common complaint during the winter, especially in those with viral respiratory illnesses, asthma, or sinusitis. Bronchiolitis from respiratory syncytial virus (RSV) usually occurs between October and March but can happen at other times as well. A pattern of coughing in the fall, spring, or both should raise suspicions about allergic rhinitis and allergy-triggered asthma.

Sound

Families and providers often point out the nature of the cough, using terms such as dry, moist, loose, tight, barking, honking, or hacking. This element of the history can be helpful but usually is not specific enough to help pin down the diagnosis. Some practitioners have come to label all children with a dry, barking cough as having "croup". This practice should be avoided unless one is explicitly referring to a specific acute viral illness characterized by inspiratory stridor. Patients diagnosed as having "recurrent croup" are likely to have asthma, postnasal drip, or sinusitis.

Coughing fits, or paroxysms, often followed by posttussive vomiting are common in patients with pertussis. Similar coughing fits can occur in patients with asthma, bronchi-

Table 36–1. PERTINENT HISTORY

Aspect of the Patient's History	Possible Significance
Coughing during sleep	Asthma, postnasal drip, GER
Coughing when waking up	Postnasal drip (allergies, sinusitis, viral illness)
Coughing loudly, only when awake; cough is distractible	Habit cough ("cough tic")
Coughing during feeds	Dysphagia, GER, aspiration, vascular ring, TE fistula, food allergy (if other signs of atopy)
Coughing after feeds	GER, aspiration, vascular ring, food allergy
Coughing after exercise, laughing, or exposure to cold air	Asthma
Paroxysmal cough	Pertussis, asthma, sinusitis, CF
Post-tussive vomiting	Asthma, pertussis, sinusitis, CF
Spitting up, colic, heartburn	GER
Dry, barky cough	Croup, asthma, laryngospasm (associated with postnasal drip), foreign body in airway, airway anomaly
Prolonged cough with viral illness	Reactive airways, asthma, sinusitis, CF
Mild cough with runny nose resolves within 10 days	Viral respiratory illness
Snoring, mouth breathing or noisy breathing	Postnasal drip (allergies, sinusitis, adenoidal hypertrophy)
Exposure to others who are coughing	Viral illness, TB, pertussis
Production of clear or white secretions	Asthma
Production of purulent secretions	Bronchiectasis, CF, sinusitis
Hemoptysis	Bronchiectasis, CF, nosebleed, hematemesis, pulmonary hemorrhage, coagulopathy, TB

GER: gastroesophageal reflux; TE fistula: Tracheoesophageal fistula; CF: cystic fibrosis; TB: tuberculosis

olitis and other viral infections, sinusitis, and cystic fibrosis (CF).

A loud, brassy cough is seen in patients with cough tic (a habit cough) or tracheomalacia. Many patients with residual tracheomalacia associated with tracheoesophageal fistula will have a troublesome brassy cough. Patients with asthma will often report a change in cough from dry to wet (or tight to loose) as they improve.

Relationship to Feeding

Coughing that is triggered primarily by food intake always warrants evaluation. These patients may develop aspiration, laryngospasm, choking, or apnea. Newborns with suck-and-swallow incoordination may cough and sputter upon initiation of feeds, perhaps accompanied by oxyhemoglobin desaturation, cyanosis, or apnea. Patients with neuromuscular disease may have varying degrees of dysphagia, most commonly presenting with respiratory difficulty when drinking thin liquids. Infants or young children with coughing or choking during feeding and a history of stridor or wheezing may have a vascular ring. Babies with an H-type tracheoesophageal fistula may present with aspiration episodes and abdominal distension from swallowing air. Gastroesophageal reflux (GER) may occur at any age but is most likely to elicit respiratory symptoms in infants. The child may cough, choke, or have apnea toward the end of a feed or even an hour or longer afterward. Choking, nasal congestion, arching of the back, drooling, hoarseness, and irritability may characterize the event. The child may appear to be in pain or seem to have a bad taste in the mouth. If there is associated laryngospasm, bronchospasm, or aspiration, the child may have respiratory distress. The diagnosis

of GER is more likely when these symptoms occur in association with vomiting.

▲ **Clinical Warning:** Some infants with prominent respiratory symptoms from GER have reflux up to the larynx or pharynx only and may never actually display significant vomiting. They are essentially "spitting up internally."

Finally, children with coughing during feeds accompanied by signs of allergy (eg, rhinitis, conjunctivitis, puffy eyelids, eczema, hives, or wheezing) may have an underlying food allergy. Food allergy is seen most commonly in infants and young children.

Past Health History

Clues to the etiology and significance of the cough may be found in the patient's personal or family health history or in the environment. Has the child presented with coughing before? If so, what was the cause and what worked to make it better? Equally important, which medications were tried in the past for coughing and did not work? Does the child generally wheeze or go into respiratory distress after the onset of coughing? Does the child have a history of asthma, allergies, or sinusitis?

The child's past medical patterns are important. It is alarming when a child who was never prone to respiratory problems in the past begins to have such symptoms. While this scenario may only indicate the late onset of asthma or allergies, it also can be the presentation for a collagen vascular disease or an airway tumor. While most providers will consider CF in the child with a cough, failure to thrive, and malabsorption, it is important to remember that CF is quite variable. Ten percent of

Table 36–2. PERTINENT PAST MEDICAL HISTORY

Aspect of Past Medical History	Possible Significance
Coughing with viral illnesses	Asthma, RAD, sinusitis, postnasal drip
Asthma, allergies, sinusitis	Cough-variant asthma, allergic rhinitis, sinusitis
Eczema or hives	Allergic rhinitis, asthma
Otitis media	Adenoid hypertrophy, immunodeficiency, ciliary dyskinesia
Sinusitis	Adenoid hypertrophy, immunodeficiency, CF, ciliary dyskinesia
Pneumonia	Asthma, RAD, CF, immunodeficiency, foreign body in airways, congenital anomaly of lungs, aspiration, ciliary dyskinesia
Bronchopulmonary dysplasia	RAD, airway stenosis, or granulation tissue
Vomiting, colic, heartburn	GER
Failure to thrive	CF
Obesity, overfeeding	GER
Malabsorption, rectal prolapse, intestinal obstruction	CF
Prolonged neonatal jaundice	CF
Situs inversus	Primary ciliary dyskinesia
Neuromuscular impairment	Aspiration, GER
Absence of pertussis vaccine	Pertussis
Absence of *Hemophilus influenza* B vaccine	Pneumonia

RAD: reactive airway disease; CF: cystic fibrosis; GER: gastroesophageal reflux.

patients with CF do not have malabsorption, and some patients with CF are overweight. Table 36-2 lists some important aspects of past medical history and their implications.

Family History

Most children with asthma have a positive family history. Uncovering a family history of asthma can be trickier than it seems, however, as many patients are undiagnosed or have been mislabeled as having various forms of chronic or recurrent "bronchitis." Siblings may have been diagnosed with "recurring croup." Display 36-1 lists important aspects of the family history to explore.

● **Clinical Pearl:** Providers should ask the following questions:

Does anyone in the family have a history of severe or prolonged coughing when they have a cold, wheezing, or "having things go to their chest" easily?
Does anyone in the family use an inhaler, puffer, or nebulizer machine?

Environmental History

The environmental history should include the home, neighborhood, school, daycare center or babysitter's home, as

appropriate. It also should include the work site of employed adolescents. If the parents are divorced, there may be two home environments to consider. It is gratifying to cure a chronic cough by making appropriate modifications to the home environment. Display 36-2 lists important aspects of the environmental history.

PHYSICAL EXAMINATION

The office examination can help pinpoint whether the cough is from the upper or lower airway, or both. It is an ideal opportunity for noting the severity and character of the cough. Although time consuming, reproducing the cough in the office, perhaps by having the child perform some exercise or watching the infant feed, can be extremely revealing.

Initially, providers should observe the patient from afar for signs of respiratory distress, tachypnea, pallor, cyanosis, retractions, or nasal flaring. They should try to perform physical examination of the chest with the child quiet and relaxed. For infants and toddlers, the parents should hold the child comfortably in their arms. Providers should auscultate the chest carefully for the presence, quality, and symmetry of breath sounds. They should listen for adventitious

---

DISPLAY 36–1 • Pertinent Family History

Asthma, bronchitis, chronic cough, use of inhalers
Allergies (environmental or food), eczema, hives
Sinusitis
Cystic fibrosis
Ciliary dyskinesia
Heartburn, gastroesophageal reflux
Tuberculosis
Histoplasmosis or other fungal illness (in endemic areas)

DISPLAY 36–2 • Clues in the Environment

Pets or farm animals
Cigarette smoke
Mildew, dampness (especially bathroom, basement, roof, haystacks, stable)
Dust (cluttered rooms, stuffed animals, construction, renovation)
Fumes
Wood-burning stove
Cockroaches
Occupational exposures (for employed adolescents)

Table 36–3. PERTINENT ASPECTS OF THE PHYSICAL EXAM

Aspect of the Physical Exam	Possible Significance
Nasal secretions, clear or white	Viral illness, allergic rhinitis, adenoidal hypertrophy
Nasal secretions, purulent	Viral illness, sinusitis
Nasal polyps	CF, allergic rhinitis
Mouth breathing, noisy breathing, adenoid facies	Adenoidal hypertrophy, allergic rhinitis, viral illness
Shiners, eye puffiness, conjunctivitis, eczema	Allergies
Fluid in middle ear	Adenoidal hypertrophy, allergic rhinitis
Cobblestoned appearance of oropharynx	Postnasal drip, GER
Cervical lymphadenopathy	Viral respiratory illness
Wheezing	Asthma, RAD, tracheomalacia, vascular ring, foreign body in airway, CF, bronchiolitis, mycoplasma pneumonia, airway tumor
Prolonged expiratory phase	Asthma, RAD, tracheomalacia, bronchomalacia
Rales or crackles	Pneumonia, CF, interstitial lung disease, pulmonary edema
Stridor	Croup, foreign body in the airway or esophagus, vascular ring, laryngomalacia, tracheomalacia
Barrel-chested (↑ AP diameter of chest)	Asthma, RAD, CF
Decreased breath sounds	Pneumonia, pleural effusion, atelectasis, foreign body
Clear chest	Does NOT rule out asthma or pneumonia
Murmur, diaphoresis, hepatomegaly	Congenital heart disease, heart failure
Clubbing of digits	CF

RAD: reactive airway disease; CF: cystic fibrosis; GER: gastroesophageal reflux.

sounds: rales, ronchi, and wheezes. A particularly important portion of the respiratory cycle is the end of inspiration, during which fine rales are common. Table 36-3 lists some notable aspects of the physical examination.

● **Clinical Pearl:** Clinicians also should focus on the inspiratory to expiratory (I:E) ratio. The expiratory phase is commonly prolonged in children with reactive airway disease or asthma and may be the only positive finding on exam.

DIAGNOSTIC CRITERIA

In the vast majority of cases, providers will establish the correct diagnosis based on the findings of the history and physical exam. Additionally, the patient's age will affect the various diagnostic considerations, as certain diagnoses tend to be more age-specific than others.

In young infants, coughing can be a sign of congenital anomaly, such as tracheomalacia, a vascular ring, pulmonary sequestration, or tracheoesophageal (TE) fistula. In addition, GER commonly presents in young infants. Providers also should consider *chlamydia pneumonitis* in young infants with a cough, eye discharge, or otitis media.

While toddlers are prone to laryngotracheobronchitis (croup) from parainfluenza virus, adenovirus, or RSV, providers should consider aspiration of a foreign body as well, especially when the onset of symptoms is particularly abrupt. Children in daycare and school-age children share numerous respiratory ailments, such as viral illnesses, mycoplasma pneumonia, and even tuberculosis (TB).

Adolescents with waning pertussis titers, children who did not receive pertussis vaccine, and infants awaiting vaccination are all at risk for weeks of severe coughing spasms if they contract whooping cough. Additionally, providers should ask preteens or teens with chronic cough if they smoke.

DIAGNOSTIC STUDIES

Most children with a cough require no diagnostic testing. Providers should initiate an evaluation if the cough is persistent, frequently recurring, or severe. Evaluation should proceed in a stepwise fashion, depending on the probable yield and risk of the test. The most basic tests should include a chest x-ray and a complete blood count with differential.

Imaging Studies

When ordering a chest radiograph, it is important to order films in both the posterior–anterior (PA) and lateral positions. It is not uncommon to miss findings if only the PA film is ordered. It is always worthwhile to provide the radiologist with clinical information. The chest x-ray may reveal pneumonia, an unsuspected aspirated foreign body, bronchiectasis in a patient with CF, or lymphadenopathy suggestive of TB. Commonly, the chest x-ray may reveal signs of hyperinflation or atelectasis as a result of mucus plugging, findings suggestive of bronchiolitis or asthma. Peribronchial cuffing or central perihilar densities also suggest asthma. The x-ray also may detect pleural disease, interstitial disease, pulmonary edema, congenital pulmonary anomalies, or a mass. If a mass is detected, a chest CT may be useful in further delineating the lesion. Serial radiographs can be helpful in determining whether or not an abnormality is persistent.

Localized hyperinflation suggests an endobronchial foreign body. In such cases, decubitus films, or, in cooperative older children, inspiratory and expiratory films may be ordered to enhance findings of unilateral hyperinflation secondary to a retained foreign body. A mucus plug in the airway due to asthma or bronchiolitis may yield the same radiographic appearance as a foreign body. If the clinical history is suggestive, and there is no history of foreign body aspiration, the provider may elect to treat for asthma and repeat the chest x-ray to see if the localized hyperinflation has disappeared. A normal chest radiograph can give reassurance, narrow the diagnostic possibilities, and reduce the use of unnecessary antibiotics.

A soft tissue x-ray of the neck can reveal adenoidal hypertrophy or various forms of upper airway obstruction. Sinus films may detect air-fluid levels or opacification, but a sinus CT scan has greater sensitivity for sinus disease and anatomy.

The upper gastrointestinal (GI) series, or barium swallow, is helpful in the child with cough related to feedings. It is less sensitive in detecting GER as the pH probe but can detect associated anatomical problems, such as hiatal hernia, and is very sensitive for cases of vascular ring. Finally, an upper GI series can sometimes detect an H-type tracheo-esophageal fistula, although these are notoriously difficult to find. For obvious reasons, a technician and radiologist accustomed to performing this study on infants and young children should perform the GI series.

A modified barium swallow, or cinefluoroscopy, is helpful in the evaluation of the child who may be aspirating oral feedings. In this study, the patient eats and drinks barium-coated drinks and foods in various textures. Fluoroscopy is performed while the child swallows, so that abnormalities in the swallowing mechanism and any tracheal aspiration can be documented.

Laboratory Evaluation

The complete blood count (CBC) may reveal an elevated number of eosinophils in patients with asthma, allergies, or chlamydia. Neutrophils will be elevated in bacterial pneumonia, sinusitis, or CF, and lymphocytes will be high in viral illness or pertussis. Quantitative immunoglobulins (IgG, IgA, and IgM) may be useful to measure in the patient with recurring cough and frequent infections. The quantitative subclasses of IgG also can be determined, but there is significant variability in the reliability of results from different laboratories. Serum IgE can be measured to detect allergies. Blood cultures can occasionally establish the etiology of bacterial pneumonia.

Testing for Cystic Fibrosis

Currently, three states perform CF screening in all newborns, and several other states are considering initiating these programs. Elsewhere, testing is ordered when providers suspect the condition. The most sensitive test is the sweat test, which should be ordered whenever a child has a history of repeated lower respiratory infections with or without malabsorption or failure to thrive. Whenever possible, providers should choose a laboratory with extensive experience and credentials for performing the sweat test, such as a Cystic Fibrosis Foundation–accredited laboratory. Genetic testing (mutation analysis) has lower sensitivity, depending on the particular laboratory and the patient's ethnic background. The reader should refer to Chapter 55 for more information about CF.

Allergy Testing

Children with a cough from asthma, rhinitis, or sinusitis often have underlying allergies. In the past, referral for allergy testing and desensitization was almost a knee-jerk reaction to a diagnosis of asthma. Today, it is clear that allergy testing and desensitization demonstrate very limited utility for children with asthma. They may be moderately useful for youngsters with allergic rhinitis unresponsive to

medical therapy with nonsedating antihistamines and intranasal steroids.

Testing may be warranted in certain situations, such as when the family needs evidence that a family pet is causing the problem or if food allergies are suspected. Skin tests have the greatest sensitivity in detecting allergies. Specific IgE radioallergosorbent technique (RAST) tests are less sensitive and more expensive, particularly if a large panel of tests is requested. Skin or RAST tests should check for the most likely allergens related to the patient's environmental exposures and seasonal pattern of illness. In young infants, foods are the most likely allergens; the likelihood of environmental allergies increases with age.

Mantoux (Tuberculin) Testing

A reliable method of tuberculin testing, such as the Mantoux (PPD) test, is a basic part of the evaluation of coughing children. This testing becomes more important if there is a history of exposure, suggestive findings by radiograph, or any documented pneumonia.

MANAGEMENT: GENERAL PRINCIPLES

Treatment of the cough will clearly depend upon the etiology, which is not always apparent upon initial presentation. The most common cause of cough is postnasal drip associated with a viral illness. No medical treatment is mandated if the child is breathing, feeding, and sleeping comfortably. Providers should educate families that not all coughing requires medicine.

If the cough is severe or persistent, initial treatment approaches should reflect the most common etiologies: bronchospasm, rhinitis, or sinusitis, or associated with a viral illness or allergies. While pursuing a diagnostic evaluation, as described above, it is reasonable to give a trial of bronchodilators if asthma is the suspected etiology. If sinusitis is suspected and the symptoms have persisted for at least 7 to 10 days, a course of antibiotics may be useful.

Providers should minimize the use of cough suppressants. They should explain to families that cough is a normal part of the body's defense against viral illness. If a cough is severe enough to warrant treatment, it is preferable to treat the cause of the cough, such as nasal congestion, bronchospasm, or sinusitis. A rare dose of a cough suppressant, such as dextromethorphan or a mild codeine preparation, may allow an exhausted family to get some sleep. If a child requires more than a rare dose of cough suppressant, however, an evaluation to find out the root of the cough is needed. Cough suppressants should be avoided in patients with impaired mucociliary clearance, asthma, pertussis, or CF. Narcotics, such as codeine, should be avoided in patients with significant snoring, upper airway obstruction, or chronic lung disease, as they can worsen ventilation. Expectorants, found in numerous over-the-counter cold and cough medications, are not effective in relieving cough.

In a child with cough secondary to allergic rhinitis, a trial of antihistamines is often very helpful, both in treating the symptoms and "confirming" that an allergy is likely. Control or containment of common environmental allergens may also be useful. Perennial symptoms may reflect dust mite, cockroach, or pet allergy. Simple maneuvers such as keeping furry pets out of the child's bedroom, minimizing stuffed animals and other dust collectors, and encasing the bedding may also be beneficial.

SPECIFIC CAUSES OF COUGH

No discussion of cough in children would be complete without a brief discussion of upper respiratory infections (URIs), asthma (also termed reactive airway disease), and bronchitis. Croup, bronchiolitis, and pneumonia are discussed in greater detail in the sections that follow.

Upper Respiratory Infection

By far, the most common etiology for a cough in an otherwise healthy child is an acute respiratory viral illness. The cough in this case is the result of postnasal drip and mucus hypersecretion. The afflicted child may develop a runny or stuffy nose, perhaps some fever, and cough. Generally, the cough is not severe, and the child has minimal interruption in sleep or other daily activities. The child may appear well or only mildly ill. The chest examination will be normal. Often, other family members will be affected as well. The cough generally resolves itself within 10 days and requires no specific treatment. If the fever persists for several days or if the child appears ill or has a marked loss of appetite or persistent vomiting, the provider must consider the possibility of pneumonia, even if the examination is normal.

Asthma/Reactive Airway Disease (RAD)

If the cough is disturbing the child's sleep or associated with post-tussive vomiting, providers should consider the possibility of asthma or reactive airway disease (RAD). This is true even if the child is not wheezing.

▲ **Clinical Warning:** A common error is to dismiss the possibility of RAD or asthma in a child whose chest exam is clear. Many times, children with these conditions may not wheeze.

Infants cannot cooperate in taking a deep breath for chest examination, so providers may miss mild wheezing on auscultation. They also can miss wheezing on examination of a screaming, fussy baby. Children may wheeze mainly at nighttime and sound completely clear during the day. Many children with RAD present with a cough and perhaps coarse breath sounds and a prolonged expiratory phase, but no overt wheezing. Finally, patients with severe bronchospasm may not be moving enough air to generate a wheeze.

Young children often show evidence of airway reactivity with nearly every viral respiratory illness. If the cough is disturbing to the patient and family or does not clear up after 10 days, a trial of asthma medications (eg, a bronchodilator, perhaps with a short course of an oral corticosteroid) may be warranted. Another option, if nasal congestion is prominent, is to try a decongestant or antihistamine. Coughing that restricts a child's sleep, activity, or school attendance and prevents parents from attending work is worth treating. A more detailed discussion of asthma and cough-variant asthma is presented in Chapter 55.

Bronchitis

Bronchitis, defined as inflammation of the bronchial epithelium, occurs as part of the clinical spectrum of many different diseases. As such, its existence as an isolated illness is unusual during childhood. Most children who are experiencing bronchial inflammation have antecedent or current viral illness. Inflammation and spasm of the bronchi also occur as part of the spectrum of asthmatic illness. *Bordatella pertussis*, measles, influenza and diphtheria, can all involve the tracheobronchial airway and as such produce the harsh cough that is observed with inflammation of this part of the respiratory tree. With croup, a relatively common illness in early childhood, there is inflammation of the trachea, bronchi, and larynx. (Please refer to the ensuing discussion of croup.) Environmental allergens, irritants, pollutants, and toxins can also affect the bronchi and cause acute or chronic symptoms.

History and Physical Exam

The usual course of viral bronchitis begins with nasal congestion and rhinitis, followed by a cough. Low-grade fever may be present. Initially, the cough is dry and hacking, causing significant retrosternal discomfort as it progresses. After several days of a dry cough, a wet and productive cough with purulent sputum follows. This thick sputum begins to thin at about the 10th day of illness, with steady resolution of the cough. Most children and adults can expect resolution of all symptoms within 2 weeks from the start of symptoms.

Auscultation of the chest may reveal coarse breath sounds, ronchi, and rales. The cough may persist briefly after all mucus is cleared. For most children, the cough and discomfort that it causes become the prominent symptoms and complaints.

Diagnostic Criteria

Findings gleaned from the history and physical exam usually establish the diagnosis. Viral illnesses and the spectrum of RAD/asthma account for the vast majority of cases. More rarely, anatomical or functional problems of the airways cause a persistence of or recurring pattern of symptoms of bronchitis. Providers should consider ciliary dyskinesias, bronchiectasis, TB, and CF in patients whose symptoms do not resolve or are recurrent. They also should rule out a foreign body or local or systemic immune deficiency. In older children and adolescents, providers must consider cigarette smoking, marijuana use, and inhalation of noxious gases (eg, from spray cans) as possible causes of ongoing or frequently recurring symptoms.

Management

Although *Streptococcus pneumonia*, *Moraxella catarrhalis* and non-typeable *Haemophilus influenza* may cause superinfection of the bronchi, antibiotics generally have not been found to be useful in producing a speedier resolution of symptoms. Antihistamines and decongestants have also not been proven helpful in relieving symptoms. Coexisting illness such as sinusitis or pneumonia may contribute to or be complications of bronchitis. Lack of resolution of symptoms after 10 to 14 days should prompt consideration of these conditions.

● **Clinical Pearl:** In a normal child, bronchitis as an entity for which to prescribe antibiotics does not exist. There is little justification for the practice of treating otherwise healthy children with antibiotics for bronchitis.

Immunocompetent children with normal mucociliary function do not develop bacterial bronchitis. On the other hand, antibiotics certainly have a role for children with pneumonia, sinusitis, or CF.

Viral Croup (Laryngotracheobronchitis)

Croup is technically a syndrome, the hallmark of which is upper airway obstruction and stridor. Congenital airway anomalies, smoke inhalation, postintubation stridor, measles, and diphtheria can all cause a croup syndrome. In common parlance, however, the term croup refers to the most frequently occurring variety, laryngotracheobronchitis (LTB), or viral croup. While most children with LTB have mild illnesses that can be treated at home, the potential exists for severe airway obstruction or even respiratory failure.

Pathology

Viral infection of the airways produces inflammation and edema of the larynx, trachea, and bronchi, which clinically manifests as hoarseness, stridor, and coughing respectively. The pathology is primarily subglottic, as opposed to the now rare condition of epiglottitis in which the pathology is supra-glottic. Clinically there is primarily upper airway obstruction, with variable degrees of lower airway obstruction.

Epidemiology

Croup is seen most commonly in children ages 6 months to 3 years, with peak incidence between ages 1 and 2 years. It is more common in males. When the clinical features of croup are seen in an infant younger than age 6 months, providers should consider the possibility of a congenital airway anomaly.

Parainfluenza virus is the most common cause of croup, but RSV, adenovirus, and influenza virus are also possibilities. Cases appear throughout the year, but peak in the fall and spring. Reinfection can occur but is generally milder. Croup is diagnosed in 1.5% to 4.7% of 1-year-olds, based on reports from two American pediatric practices (Foy, et al., 1973; Denny, et al., 1983).

History and Physical Exam

The illness begins with a brief prodrome of a runny nose, perhaps accompanied by a low-grade fever. Next, symptoms develop related to airway edema: a loud, barking, hoarse-sounding cough; and inspiratory stridor. These problems often start quite suddenly, most commonly at night. In more severe cases, marked retractions, particularly sternal, may occur. Stridor may be noted when the child is crying or excited, but in more severe cases it may be present even at rest. There also may be expiratory wheezing. In mild cases the child feeds well, appears comfortable, and plays normally. In moderate cases, the stridor is more pronounced, and the child may appear somewhat uncomfortable, as if the throat is irritated from speaking or coughing. In severe cases, the child may have tachycardia and tachypnea and appear anxious and uncomfortable associated with decreased activity and poor feeding. Pulse oximetry may reveal hypoxemia on the basis of hypoventilation and mucus plugging, which is always a worrisome sign. The child with stridor and retractions at rest has significant airway obstruction. Younger children, having a narrower airway, are most severely affected.

Diagnostic Criteria

The diagnosis of croup is made clinically; its features, however, often overlap with those of other conditions causing stridor and dry cough (eg, foreign body aspiration, congeni-tal airway anomaly, laryngospasm associated with allergies, or postnasal drip). Providers should suspect older patients with a barky cough or any patient with "recurrent croup" of having asthma, allergies, or postnasal drip. The term "recur-rent croup" is a description, not a diagnosis. Epiglottitis is in the differential diagnosis but has become rare in the era of *Haemophilus influenza B* vaccination. While epiglottitis can cause the sudden onset of stridor and respiratory distress, it generally does not produce significant hoarseness or cough.

The child with croup often has a history of noisy breathing occurring after a brief respiratory illness. The noisy breath-ing is generally worse at night and often sudden in onset. If the noise is not apparent on physical examination, it is important to determine if the noise was stridor, wheezing, snoring, or a stuffy nose. To most parents, any breathing noise is a wheeze. Asking the family if the noise was there on inhalation or exhalation may help, although they are often unsure. It can be extremely useful to imitate the sounds of stridor or wheeze, and to ask the family to identify the cor-rect sound.

Viral croup can be more confidently diagnosed if and when the patient fulfills the following criteria:

Is age 6 months to 3 years
Has had a prodrome of runny nose and low-grade fever for up to 5 days
Presents with a loud, barking cough, especially with agi-tation and some degree of hoarseness; often worse at night
Presents with symptoms of stridor with agitation or exertion
Demonstrates variable expiratory wheezing
Has been sick for up to 10 days
Has no history suggestive of foreign body aspiration or allergic reaction
Stridor or retractions at rest suggest a more severe disease

Diagnostic Studies

Children who fulfill the typical diagnostic features of croup do not necessarily require any diagnostic testing. Most patients have a mild self-limited illness. Since agitation worsens airway obstruction, the fewer frightening or painful tests conducted the better. If deemed necessary, providers can obtain a soft tissue neck film in the AP and lateral posi-tions. Medical personnel, however, should observe patients with severe airway obstruction during the radiography. Neck radiographs may reveal evidence of subglottic tracheal narrowing ("steeple sign") and a dilated hypopharynx. The degree of radiographic abnormality, however, does not nec-essarily correlate with the degree of clinical airway obstruc-tion. Neck radiographs are most helpful in cases of sus-pected aspirated foreign body. This suspicion may arise if the child's symptoms begin while eating, or if no antecedent respiratory illness occurred. Neck radiographs can also reas-sure the clinician that the epiglottis is not inflamed. A med-ical emergency exists when a patient with severe airflow obstruction is suspected of having epiglottitis. Rather than delaying treatment by performing radiographs, the patient requires urgent visualization of the larynx in a controlled environment, with preparation for emergency endotracheal intubation.

● **Clinical Pearl:** Croup is often worse at night, and commonly the child who manifested symptoms of mild or moderate severity at night, is relatively asymptomatic the next morning at the time of the evaluation. If the parental account appears reliable, the prudent practitioner will assess the severity of the illness and select treatment based on both the previous night's history and the actual physical assessment.

Management

Mild Croup

Patients with mild cough and minimal stridor need no specific therapy beyond observation. Providers can prescribe antipyretics as necessary, as the work of breathing increases with fever. Analgesics can relieve an irritated throat. Traditional maneuvers, such as having the patient breathe while in a steamy bathroom or outdoors in cool air, seem to help some patients feel better, although clinical studies have not supported these treatments. These traditional treatments may soothe the patient, and if they give the family a sense of helping the child, may help the whole family to stay calm.

If the child manifests minimal findings, but a reliable history is consistent with a significant degree of stridor the previous night, many clinicians will choose to prescribe a short course of oral steroids. This is particularly valid if the encounter occurs early in the course of the illness, as croup tends to increase in severity for the first few days. Most important is to teach the family the signs of worsening disease (ie, worsening stridor, tachypnea, and agitation) and to arrange for appropriate follow-up.

Providers should advise parents about the following:
- Croup can worsen over the first few days, then generally improves over 10 days.
- The child should be kept calm and comfortable. Remain calm yourself!
- The provider should be contacted immediately if any of the following occur: worsening stridor; increasing respiratory rate (especially over 50 breaths per minute); indrawing of neck, chest, or abdomen with breathing; agitation or lethargy; poor fluid intake.
- If the condition worsens, the child may require special medications. Sometimes children need to be hospitalized to receive oxygen and to closely monitor their breathing.

Moderate Croup

These patients have inspiratory stridor and retractions. They may be somewhat agitated. Pulse oximetry may reveal hypoxemia. Appetite may drop, and assessment of hydration status is necessary. Medical treatment includes corticosteroids. In some cases, epinephrine by inhalation, oxygen, and a trial of bronchodilators are warranted.

Corticosteroids

Corticosteroids reduce airway inflammation. While their use has been controversial over the years, most well-designed studies have supported it. Corticosteroids can both reduce hospitalization rates and decrease the length of hospitalization for inpatients. They should be administered to all inpatients with croup and all outpatients with disruptive stridor or cough. Recent placebo controlled, double blind studies have demonstrated the efficacy of corticosteroids for croup (Klassen, Craig, et al., 1998; Johnson, Jacobson, et al., 1998; Godden, Campbell, et al., 1997; Klassen, 1997). Dexamethasone has a long half-life and has been most widely studied.

By injection: A single intramuscular injection of 0.6 mg/kg of dexamethasone

Orally: A single dose of dexamethasone is effective and avoids a painful injection. Dose range: 0.15–0.6mg/kg.

Another option is prednisone or prednisolone at a dose of 2 mg/kg/day divided twice daily for a total of four doses.

Inhaled: Nebulized budesonide (2 mg or 4 mg) appears to be effective in several recent studies, but this preparation has only recently become available in the United States. A small randomized study comparing inhaled fluticasone administered by metered dose inhaler and spacer to placebo revealed no difference in outcome (Roorda & Walhof, 1998).

Inhaled Epinephrine

Inhaled epinephrine or vaponephrine (racemic epinephrine) is a vasoconstrictor that presumably reduces airway vascular permeability; it is also a bronchodilator. It can provide rapid and marked relief of upper airway obstruction; yet, its effects are short-term. Thus, patients given epinephrine require observation for several hours to determine if obstruction recurs. Inhaled epinephrine should be given to patients with stridor at rest and respiratory distress. The dose is 0.5 mL of the 2.25% solution of racemic epinephrine diluted in 2 mL of saline. Repeat doses can be given as often as every 2 hours as needed. L-epinephrine appears to be equally effective. The dose of L-epinephrine is 2.5 mL of the 1:1000 solution diluted in 2 mL of saline.

Bronchodilators

Providers should consider a trial of bronchodilators, especially if the patient has a personal or family history of asthma or if expiratory wheezing is present. Providers should assess response to bronchodilators critically. While many patients respond favorably, others do not improve or even worsen.

Oxygen

Hypoxemia can be assessed noninvasively with pulse oximetry. Hypoxemia can reflect lower airway involvement (bronchiolitis) or upper airway obstruction (hypoventilation). Treatment of hypoxemia with oxygen can reduce the work of breathing. Mist tents are popular ways to provide oxygen to young children (see below). Other options include oxygen by hood, nasal cannula, or face mask.

Humidification/Mist Tents

Mist tents are frequently prescribed as therapy for children with croup, although no actual benefits have been documented. They have the liability of limiting the patient's visibility to medical personnel and contact with family. The patient's own nose is an excellent humidifier of air, and it is unlikely that mist tents further enhance laryngeal or tracheal moisture.

Severe Croup

These patients have stridor at rest, hypoxemia, and retractions. Increased oxygen requirement, decreased breath sounds, agitation, and lethargy are signs of impending respiratory failure. Fortunately, it is uncommon for a child to require airway intubation for croup. Treatment includes the following.

Admission to a pediatric intensive care unit
Administration of corticosteroids
Administration of frequent doses of inhaled epinephrine
Administration of fluids as needed to prevent both dehydration and fluid overload
For patients with respiratory failure or impending failure, intubation by personnel skilled at working with an obstructed pediatric airway and placement on mechanical ventilation

While airway protection is always the most important concern, it must be balanced against the risk of intubation complications, such as subglottic stenosis. Pulmonary edema has been reported following intubation for severe croup, presumably related to post-obstructive edema.

▲ **Clinical Warning:** An elevated arterial pCO_2 is always alarming; a pCO_2 even in the "normal range" is abnormal in the face of tachypnea and may signal ventilatory failure.

The following are admission criteria:

The child presents with persistent stridor at rest, defined as resting in the parent's arms, not being poked or prodded.
The child requires multiple doses of racemic epinephrine.
The child is very young.
The child has a history of previous intubation or other airway compromise.
Stridor has been present for less than 2 days, as distress will frequently worsen before it improves.
The family lives far from medical facilities or cannot be relied upon to call or return appropriately for follow-up.
The child shows signs or symptoms of respiratory distress

Consider referral to a pediatric pulmonologist for cases of severe or recurring croup, particularly if an underlying cause cannot be determined, or if the patient is not responding rapidly to treatment. Recurring stridor or barking cough can be quite stressful for families, who may have sleepless nights, emergency room visits, or fears that their child's airway may "close up". These patients often will be found to have asthma, allergies, or postnasal drip and respond well to treatment. Others may have congenital airway anomalies or an occult aspirated foreign body that bronchoscopy can diagnose.

Bronchiolitis

Bronchiolitis is a common illness presenting to pediatric providers. Although most cases are treated on an ambulatory basis, it is responsible for a large number of pediatric hospital admissions. Today, bronchiolitis is not only treatable but also frequently preventable.

Pathology

Infection with RSV is the most common cause of bronchiolitis, but other viral illnesses also cause a similar clinical picture. The bronchiolar walls are inflamed, with cellular infiltration. Epithelial cells secrete copious mucus. There is resultant mucus plugging, air trapping, and ventilation-perfusion mismatching.

Epidemiology

In temperate regions of the United States, outbreaks occur annually between November and April, although sporadic cases occur throughout the year. Although nearly all children have had a viral illness caused by RSV by age three years, most children experience only runny nose and cough. Infection does not provide complete protective immunity. Reinfection is common at any age and can even occur in the same season, but is generally milder with each episode. Full-blown bronchiolitis with wheeze peaks at ages 6 to 12 months. Glezen and colleagues (1981) reported the risk of hospitalization for RSV bronchiolitis among infants to be 5 in 1,000. Boys are affected slightly more than are girls. Kim and colleagues (1973), in a study of children hospitalized in Washington, DC, detected RSV infection in 43% of inpatients with bronchiolitis, 25% of inpatients with pneumonia, and 23% of all inpatients with acute respiratory tract disease. The greatest morbidity occurs in children younger than age 2 years, particularly those born prematurely, and those with bronchopulmonary dysplasia, congenital cardiac disease, or immunodeficiency. Children with other forms of chronic respiratory disease, such as asthma, CF, tracheoesophageal fistula, airway malacia, or a history of immunodeficiency are also at increased risk. Severe bronchiolitis may be an early manifestation of CF.

The vast majority of cases are mild or moderate. With advances today in supportive care and modern pediatric intensive care units, mortality from RSV bronchiolitis is quite low.

History and Physical Exam

A prodrome for 1 to 3 days consists of runny nose and cough, sometimes accompanied by a low-grade fever. The next stage is heralded by the onset of lower airway obstruction: wheezing and increased work in breathing. Otitis media often occurs concomitantly. Most children younger than age 2 years with wheezing associated with a respiratory illness have bronchiolitis. The differential diagnosis includes other causes of wheezing such as foreign body aspiration, asthma, vascular ring, and *Mycoplasmal pneumonia* infection. The signs of bronchiolitis overlap with those of asthma exacerbation and may occur together.

Diagnostic Criteria

The following are diagnostic criteria for bronchiolitis:

Prodrome of runny nose, with or without low-grade fever, for 1 to 4 days
Onset of coughing and expiratory wheezing, generally worse at night, worsening over 5 days, then improving
Respiratory distress in more severe cases, including tachypnea, retractions, and nasal flaring
Hypoxemia in more severe cases
Infants younger than age 6 months can present with central apnea

Diagnostic Studies

Most young children with typical features of bronchiolitis require no diagnostic testing. Diagnostic evaluation becomes increasingly important, however, if the diagnosis is uncertain or the case is severe.

Imaging Studies

On chest radiograph (PA and lateral views), bilateral hyperinflation is the most common finding. There may be atelectasis, central densities (mucus plugging), or peribronchial cuffing. In a wheezing child, the finding of a lobar infiltrate, perhaps with pleural effusion, should raise the possibility of *M. pneumonia* infection. Radiographic findings may raise the possibility of foreign body aspiration, congenital lung anomalies, TB, or CF.

RSV Antigen Testing

RSV antigen testing of nasal washings or nasopharyngeal secretions can confirm RSV infection quickly. Cultures take several days and are not universally available. Testing can be useful if the diagnosis is unclear or severe and should be performed on young infants with apnea associated with a viral illness. It is mandatory for inpatients for cohorting purposes, to ensure that patients with RSV are isolated from other high-risk patients in the hospital. Confirmation of the diagnosis is also important when contemplating treatment with ribavirin (see below).

Management

Most children with mild bronchiolitis and no respiratory distress can be managed at home with no pharmacological interventions. Appropriate follow-up, educating the family about the signs of worsening respiratory distress, and ensuring adequate fluid intake are essential interventions.

Bronchodilators

Many studies have found no or modest benefits from the use of bronchodilators. One study found a lower hospitalization rate following two doses of nebulized epinephrine, compared to two doses of nebulized salbutamol (Menon, Sutcliffe, et al., 1995). It is reasonable to try bronchodilators if the child has a history of asthma or bronchopulmonary dysplasia, or a family history of asthma.

Corticosteroids

Studies have not found benefits of corticosteroid administration to children with bronchiolitis (Klassen, et al., 1997; Berger, 1998; Richter & Seddon, 1998). A subset of patients may respond, perhaps those with asthma or bronchopulmonary dysplasia, but this has not been determined.

Oxygen

Oxygen should be provided to hypoxemic patients to reduce the work of breathing. Children with oxygen saturations below 93% will require supplemental oxygen.

Fluids

Babies in significant respiratory distress will often feed poorly. Intravenous fluids may be given as required to maintain adequate hydration, but fluid overload should be avoided.

Monitoring

Pulse oximetry can easily determine blood oxygenation status. An arterial blood gas should be obtained if there is severe distress, impending respiratory failure, exhaustion, or inadequate oxygenation despite oxygen therapy. Infants presenting with apnea require close observation in the hospital and placement on an apnea monitor.

Ribavirin

Ribavirin has antiviral activity. Some studies have associated ribavirin with mild improvement in oxygenation status; many, however, used inappropriate placebo control or had other flaws. Other studies have shown no benefits of ribavirin administration. Long-term benefits, if any, are still being investigated (Long, et al., 1997; Edell, et al., 1998). There are concerns about the cost of ribavirin, potential for teratogenicity, and difficulty of administration. For all these reasons, the use of ribavirin is highly variable and controversial.

The new AAP guidelines in the 1997 *Red Book* have softened substituting the phrase that ribavirin "should be considered for" rather than "is recommended for" certain patient groups (AAP, 1997). Ribavirin may be considered for patients with severe illness or potential for severe illness. This includes patients with bronchopulmonary dysplasia (BPD) or other underlying congenital respiratory disease, congenital heart disease, or immunodeficiency.

Administration of ribavirin is through a small particle aerosol generator (SPAG) via an oxygen tent, oxygen hood, or ventilator tubing. Meticulous care is required when ribavirin is administered through ventilator tubing, because of the risk of crystallization. Aerosol delivers ribavirin over 12 to 18 hours per day. The solution is made with 6 grams of ribavirin diluted in 300 mL of preservative-free sterile water. Alternatively, 2 grams may be administered over 2 hours, 3 times per day.

What to Tell Parents

Bronchiolitis causes cough, wheezing, and chest congestion. Children generally grow sicker over the first 5 days, then improve rapidly. Coughing and congestion may persist for 10 to 14 days.

Control fever, if it occurs, as breathing becomes more labored in the presence of fever.

Call the provider immediately if any of the following occur: drawing in of chest, neck, or abdominal muscles with breathing; rapid breathing (over 50 breaths per minute); blueness of lips or nail beds; lethargy or agitation; trouble drinking fluids.

Determine the child's breathing rate by counting how many breaths he or she takes in thirty seconds (feel the belly or watch it move in and out) and doubling it. This is easiest to do when the child is still or sleeping. Call the provider if the respiratory rate is 50 or higher. Keep fever down, since fever also increases respiratory rate.

If the infant with bronchiolitis is able to drink fluids well from breast or bottle, breathing is not dangerously compromised. Call the provider if the baby has a difficult time drinking.

A virus causes bronchiolitis. Antibiotics are not helpful in treating it, unless an ear or sinus infection also is present.

While many babies have bronchiolitis and then never wheeze again, some babies go on to have asthma, especially if asthma is in the family. During a first episode of wheezing, it is not possible to tell if the child will show an asthmatic tendency in the future.

Admission Criteria

The following are admission criteria:

Respiratory distress or oxyhemoglobin saturation is less than 94%.
Respiratory rate is over 60 breaths per minute.
The child is not taking fluids well.
The family is overwhelmed, lives far from medical facility, or is unreliable for follow-up.

Referral Criteria

Bronchiolitis is an extremely common pediatric diagnosis. Consider referral to a pediatric pulmonologist if the case is unusually severe or recurrent.

Prevention

Recently, two products have become available for RSV prophylaxis for high-risk patients younger than age two years: RSV-IVIG (Respigam) (The PREVENT Study Group, 1997) and RSV monoclonal antibody (Synagis) (The

IMPACT Study Group, 1998). RSV-IVIG is administered by monthly intravenous infusion, while RSV monoclonal antibody is administered by monthly intramuscular injection (15mg/kg).

Treatment is generally given during the peak RSV season. In a study of over 1,500 babies with BPD younger than age 2 years and premature babies younger than age 6 months, RSV monoclonal antibody prophylaxis reduced the rate of hospitalization for RSV by 55% compared to placebo (The IMPACT Study Group, 1998). RSV monoclonal antibody is the preferred product for most children at risk of severe RSV bronchiolitis, because of the ease of the intramuscular injections. RSV-IVIG, however, offers additional protection against other common pathogens and may warrant the inconvenience of monthly intravenous administration in immunocompromised or other fragile patients. RSV-IVIG is contraindicated in children with cyanotic congenital heart disease. Use of RSV monoclonal antibody for cyanotic congenital heart disease is under investigation. Both products are expensive. For example, a single injection of RSV monoclonal antibody costs between $900 and $1000, depending on the child's size and dosage. The American Academy of Pediatrics (1998) and a consensus report (Meissner, et al., 1999) have published detailed recommendations regarding the use of RSV monoclonal antibody (Synagis).

Another important aspect of prevention of RSV bronchiolitis is basic infection control measures, both at home and in the hospital. The importance of avoiding sick contacts and remembering to wash hands cannot be overstated.

Pneumonia

Pneumonia is a common worldwide condition that ranges from a mild illness to one associated with severe morbidity, complications, or mortality. Children who are immunocompromised, critically ill, weak, malnourished or who have underlying cardiac or respiratory disease are at greatest risk of severe disease. While viral lower respiratory infections are far more common, the likelihood of severe illness and complications is highest with bacterial infections. Antibiotic choices, both new and old, abound. One challenge today is to minimize unnecessary use of antibiotics. Another challenge is to choose antibiotics wisely when they are required, considering the severity of illness, underlying medical conditions, and increasing presence of antibiotic resistance. Detailed reviews of pneumonia in infants and in children were published in 1996 (Churgay, 1996; DeMuri, 1996; Latham-Sadler & Morell, 1996).

Pathology

Pneumonia can occur when a person inhales or aspirates pathologic organisms. This may occur through airborne droplets or direct person-to-person contact. Organisms also may be aspirated from oropharyngeal secretions, particularly in children with neuromuscular impairment, dysphagia, laryngeal or vocal cord abnormalities, cleft palate, tracheostomy, or impaired cough reflexes. Less commonly, organisms enter the lungs hematogenously from other sites of infection. Healthy individuals have a variety of defense systems to clear the lungs of invading organisms, including mucociliary clearance, alveolar and tissue macrophages, and cellular and humoral immunity. Pneumonia will occur if the invading organisms overwhelm the host defense systems.

Inflammation and consolidation of alveoli and cellular infiltration of the pulmonary interstitium characterize pneumonia. Viruses are the most common cause of lower respiratory infection. In healthy children, *Streptococcus pneumonia* is the most common bacterial cause. *Haemophilus influenza* pneumonia is now uncommon, thanks to routine vaccination of infants against *Haemophilus influenza B*. Mycoplasma pneumonia is common in school-age children and adolescents. The etiology of pneumonia in children varies with age and underlying medical conditions.

Epidemiology

In temperate areas of North America, pneumonia occurs most commonly during the colder months. Boys are affected slightly more often than are girls. Most pneumonia occuring in children is viral. Foy et al. (1973) found evidence of viral illness in 37% of children sick enough to be hospitalized with pneumonia. Evidence suggests that 3% to 4% of children ages 1 to 5 years are diagnosed with pneumonia. The incidence of bacterial pneumonia in children is not known precisely, as young children cannot expectorate sputum for culture, blood cultures are not always positive, and serologic studies and radiographic findings may be inconclusive. The incidence of pneumonia increases in the presence of crowded living conditions and contact with large numbers of children.

History and Physical Exam

While typical signs of pneumonia include fever, tachypnea, and cough, these findings vary, and atypical presentations are not uncommon. The illness may begin gradually, precipitously, or following a viral illness. The higher the fever and white blood count and the more ill the child appears, the greater is the likelihood of a bacterial etiology. In the case of viral pneumonia, a runny nose or other evidence of URI may be present.

The child with pneumonia may look well or, particularly if the pneumonia is bacterial, may look ill and be feeding poorly or dehydrated. There may be retractions, nasal flaring, or pleuritic chest pain. Cough may be productive or dry, severe, or minimal. While older children and adolescents may cough up sputum, younger children swallow it and occasionally vomit it. Rarely do they cough it out.

● **Clinical Pearl:** In pneumonia, abdominal pain, nausea, vomiting, and anorexia are quite common, and may be prominent enough to generate an erroneous diagnosis of acute abdomen.

Pneumonia may be discovered in a child with an unexplained fever. Signs of respiratory distress, such as tachypnea, retractions, nasal flaring, and grunting may be absent, mild, or severe. Chest examination may reveal tachypnea, fine rales, or diminished breath sounds. There may be signs of consolidation, such as egophony (in which a vocalized letter "e" sounds like the letter "a") and dullness to percussion. These findings are usually localized, so it is critical to listen to all lung fields and compare one side to the other. There may be pain on inhalation (pleuritic pain) or abdominal pain. Neonates and infants may not have localizing findings but may have nonspecific signs of sepsis, such as fever, hypothermia, irritability, inconsolability, or poor feeding.

It may take considerable time and patience to perform an adequate chest examination if the child is initially squirming, fussing, or crying. Providers may need to try various maneuvers to gain the child's trust and cooperation. These include allowing the child to stay in the parent's arms, using various distraction techniques, or briefly playing with the child. Numerous ways to encourage young children to take deep breaths during the chest examination including asking them to blow on a piece of paper or a pinwheel toy or to breathe hard like a dog. Another technique is to ask the child to blow hard enough to "blow the parent away," or blow the parent's hair. (This technique often elicits smiles from both child and parent.)

Group B *streptococcus* is the leading cause of pneumonia among neonates. Infection occurs through the birth canal during delivery. Early onset infection may produce symptoms as soon as several hours after birth. The newborn may develop respiratory distress, apnea, hypoxemia, temperature instability, or fever. Respiratory failure rapidly ensues.

Chlamydia trachomatis is a common cause of pneumonia among young infants, classically ages 2 to 3 months. Infection occurs through the birth canal. The infant develops a prodrome of rhinorrhea followed by a staccato cough and tachypnea. Conjunctivitis is common but not invariable. The chest may be clear or show crackles and rales. The illness is usually mild and resolves gradually over a few weeks.

Pneumococcal Pneumonia

Pneumococcus is the most common cause of bacterial pneumonia in children. Children are commonly colonized with pneumococcus in the upper respiratory tract, especially during the winter. Antecedent viral illness may predispose the patient to pneumococcal disease. The patient may have a concomitant ear or sinus infection or conjunctivitis. The illness tends to present quite abruptly, with the sudden appearance of fever, chills, respiratory distress, tachycardia, restlessness, or lethargy. Abdominal symptoms, such as vomiting, diarrhea, distention, and pain may be prominent. Cough is generally mild initially but may increase over the first few days. There may be signs of respiratory distress, such as grunting, flaring, retractions, and tachypnea. Chest examination may reveal tachypnea, fine crackles and rales, or diminished breath sounds. Chest pain on inspiration is common, particularly if pleural fluid is present. Patients who are susceptible to severe pneumococcal disease, such as those with sickle cell disease or asplenia, may rapidly develop respiratory failure or cardiorespiratory collapse.

Atypical Pneumonia

Mycoplasma pneumonia and *chlamydia pneumonia* cause clinically similar illnesses common among school-age children and adolescents. As these illnesses are frequently mild, they have earned the title "walking pneumonias". Outbreaks in families, schools, and communities are common. The incubation period is 2 to 3 weeks. Illness from mycoplasma frequently starts with sore throat or earache, low-grade fever, and cough. The cough may be dry or productive. Chest auscultation may reveal crackles, rales, or wheezes. Pleural effusions are not uncommon but usually small to moderate in size. Mycoplasma also may be associated with a rash, neurologic abnormalities, or myocarditis. Children with sickle cell disease are prone to mycoplasma pneumonia, as well as infection from encapsulated organisms.

Complications

Regardless of cause, complications of pneumonia include pleural effusion, empyema, lung abscess, and bronchiectasis. The incidence of purulent pleural effusion (empyema) appears to be increasing. Decreasing pneumococcal sensitivity to commonly used oral antibiotics may be fueling this increase.

Diagnostic Criteria

The following are diagnostic criteria for pneumonia:

- Pneumonia is generally diagnosed in the setting of fever, cough, and localized signs of consolidation or infection, such as crackles, rales, and diminished breath sounds. There may also be respiratory distress and abdominal complaints.
- High fever and white count and toxicity suggest bacterial etiology. Radiographic findings range from patchy, segmental consolidations, to rounded infiltrates (so-called round pneumonia) to lobar consolidations, often with air bronchograms. Bulging fissures and pleural effusions suggest bacterial infection as well.
- Runny nose, cervical lymphadenopathy, and lymphocytosis suggest a viral etiology. Radiographs may reveal hyperinflation, peribronchial cuffing, atelectasis, or small central densities.
- If expiratory wheezing is detected, the diagnosis is likely to be RAD/asthma associated with viral illness or mycoplasma.
- The differential diagnosis of a child with chest crackles and rales includes pneumonia, asthma, CF, congestive heart failure, interstitial lung disease, and pulmonary hemorrhage. If asthma seems likely, an in-office treatment with inhaled bronchodilators may result in prompt resolution of the rales and clinical improvement.

Diagnostic Studies

Providers must assess the need for diagnostic studies in each individual patient. The otherwise healthy child with typical signs of pneumonia and mild severity of illness requires no diagnostic studies.

Blood Work

In more puzzling or severe cases, a white blood cell count with differential and blood culture can be helpful. The higher the white blood cell count and number of polymorphonuclear cells and bands, the greater is the likelihood of bacterial infection. Blood cultures may yield the offending organism in 10% or more of cases of bacterial pneumonia. Knowing the specific infecting organism and antibiotic sensitivities is enormously helpful, particularly in this era of antibiotic resistance.

Sputum Cultures

● **Clinical Pearl:** Sputum cultures are not frequently helpful, as young children will only rarely expectorate purulent sputum from the chest.

If a young child produces purulent secretions, they most commonly are nasopharyngeal secretions, but providers should still consider CF. If *Staphylococcus aureus* or *Pseudomonas* is cultured, providers should consider CF or immotile cilia syndrome. They should send sputum, if possible, along with gastric aspirates, for acid-fast bacilli if a Mantoux test is positive and radiographic abnormalities are compatible. They may send cultures from endotracheal or tracheostomy tube aspirates. Because these sites usually are colonized with organisms, it is difficult to differentiate colonization from infection.

Chest Radiographs

Previously healthy children who have a mild illness suggestive of pneumonia but no prior history do not necessarily require a chest radiograph upon initial presentation. Radiographic evidence of pneumonia may lag behind the clinical picture, particularly if the child is dehydrated. Clinicians should consider obtaining a chest radiograph when the results could alter management. Since antibiotics have been overused for viral illnesses, a serious problem with antibiotic resistance has developed. Use of the chest radiograph may help prevent unnecessary use of antibiotics. Regardless of whether antibiotics are prescribed, all patients require close follow-up, and providers should order a radiograph if improvement has not been prompt. Currently, since the incidence of resistant pneumococcal infections and associated empyema is increasing, clinicians must follow the clinical course and radiographic progression of patients very closely. The expense and inconvenience of radiographs are certainly justified if providers can start appropriate antibiotics early and avoid empyema or necrotizing pneumonia.

A chest radiograph, taken in two positions, is very important when the child is severely ill or has underlying medical problems. Providers should order radiographs early in the evaluation of immunocompromised children, such as those with AIDS, on chemotherapy, or on chronic corticosteroids. They should order radiographs early when they suspect pneumonia in children with underlying cardiac or respiratory disease, such as asthma, bronchopulmonary dysplasia, or CF.

X-ray findings may influence therapy. A lobar infiltrate, perhaps with pleural effusion, pneumatocele, or abscess may be present, prompting the use of intravenous antibiotics. If the pleural effusion is significant, providers may consider draining it, for either diagnostic studies or therapeutic relief. The radiograph also may alert clinicians to the possibility of CF, TB, aspirated foreign body, congenital lung abnormality, or cardiomegaly with congestive heart failure.

Lobar consolidation is highly suggestive of bacterial pneumonia, as is the presence of a pleural effusion. Pneumococcal pneumonia may be associated with a patchy infiltrate, lobar consolidation, or round infiltrate. Pneumatoceles, thin-walled air pockets, are suggestive of *Staphylococcus aureus* pneumonia but can be seen with other infections as well. Hilar adenopathy may be seen with bacterial pneumonia but is also suggestive of TB or histoplasmosis. In chlamydia pneumonia, the radiograph may show patchy infiltrates and hyperinflation; the radiograph typically "looks worse" than the patient. In Group B *streptococcal pneumonia* in neonates, there may be localized infiltrates or a diffuse reticulonodular pattern virtually indistinguishable from the findings in respiratory distress syndrome. Viral infections are associated with hyperinflation, central infiltrates, peribronchial, cuffing or atelectasis. Diffuse interstitial infiltrates are seen in cases of *Pneumocystic carinii* pneumonia. Lung abscess suggests anaerobic infection. Bronchiectasis, seen most commonly in CF, can also be seen following other infections, such as adenovirus, TB, or pertussis.

Unfortunately, chest radiographs are frequently inconclusive. There may be vague areas of haziness or "possible" infiltrate. These small or vague abnormalities do not help distinguish reactive airways from pneumonia, or viral from bacterial pneumonia. Providers must then use their best clinical judgment. They may attempt a repeat chest radiograph if the child's clinical status worsens. Radiographic abnormalities resolve slowly after bacterial pneumonia, generally taking 6 to 8 weeks. Viral and mycoplasma pneumonia resolve much faster, often within 10 days. The need for follow-up chest radiograph in routine cases of pediatric pneumonia is controversial. If the pneumonia is recurrent, complicated, or severe, ensuring complete radiographic resolution is worthwhile.

Viral Studies

Viral studies are not worth the expense in most cases of pneumonia in healthy children. They may be warranted for hospitalized patients. For example, rapid detection of RSV might prompt consideration of treatment with ribavirin. Rapid RSV detection testing will allow for proper isolation or cohorting of patients. A positive viral study does not eliminate the possibility of bacterial superinfection. Bacterial antigen testing and cold agglutinins have suboptimal sensitivity and specificity. Mycoplasma titers may be worth obtaining, particularly in patients with sickle cell anemia, but they are frequently inconclusive and results may take days.

Testing in Children With Chronic Diseases

Children with severe pneumonia, those who are immunocompromised, and those with underlying respiratory or neuromuscular disease warrant more aggressive testing to determine the precise etiology of the pneumonia. Pneumonia remains a common cause of severe morbidity and mortality among immunocompromised patients, including organ transplant recipients, those with AIDS or sickle cell disease, and patients on chronic corticosteroid therapy. These patients are also more likely to have unusual organisms, such as *Pneumocystis carinii*, mycobacteria, cyto-megalovirus, and fungal infections.

Referral to a subspecialist for flexible bronchoscopy with bronchoalveolar lavage can be helpful. This procedure can be performed even on children receiving mechanical ventilation. It can also be performed as an ambulatory procedure under conscious sedation or anesthesia. During this procedure, the bronchoscope is wedged in various bronchi. Saline is then administered through the bronchoscope and suctioned back, essentially washing and sampling millions of alveoli. The samples are then sent for cultures or rapid organism detection studies. This procedure can be a powerful tool to determine the precise etiology of pneumonia. It is extremely sensitive in cases of *Pneumocystis carinii* infection. Since the scope enters the mouth or nose, however, upper airway flora may contaminate the specimens. Patients generally tolerate the procedure well, even those on mechanical ventilation. Potential risks include increased respiratory distress and adverse reactions to any sedatives or anesthetics employed.

Management

The first priority is to decide if the child is ill enough to be hospitalized. Then, clinicians must decide if the patient is likely to have a bacterial or viral infection. If the child is only mildly ill and seems to have a viral illness, providers should avoid the use of antibiotics. If coughing or wheezing is significant, a trial of a bronchodilator may help. If a provider suspects a bacterial infection but the child is not very ill, he or she may try narrower spectrum, less expensive antibiotics first, and move to more broad spectrum antibiotics if the child does not respond. In severely ill children or those with underlying disease, providers should start with more broad-spectrum antibiotics. The key in every case is to arrange appropriate follow-up.

Mild to Moderate Disease in a Healthy Child

If the child is older than age three months and not in respiratory distress, providers may treat empirically with appropriate oral antibiotics. Typical selections might include amoxicillin, amoxicillin-clavulanic acid, erythromycin, azithromycin, clarithromycin, or cefuroxime. Clinicians should consider coverage for atypical mycoplasma in school age patients (ie, erythromycin, azithromycin, clarithromycin, or, if the child is older than age eight years, tetracycline).

● **Clinical Pearl:** Assuring appropriate follow-up is just as critical as choosing the antibiotic for initial treatment of a child with pneumonia.

For a child with evidence of a bacterial etiology, clinicians should appoint a return visit in 1 to 2 days. In children with signs of an atypical pneumonia, practitioners should arrange follow-up in 2 to 7 days. As a part of any follow-up, providers must educate the family about the signs of respiratory distress and worsening illness.

If the child does not improve rapidly, clinicians should obtain a chest radiograph and consider a blood count and culture. In addition, they should broaden antibiotic coverage to include partially resistant pneumococcus, such as through high-dose amoxicillin (80 mg/kg/day), amoxicillin plus amoxicillin-clavulanic acid (40 mg/kg/day of each), or, especially if the child is vomiting, intramuscular ceftriaxone (50-100 mg/kg/day).

The incidence of resistant pneumococcus varies in different locations. Treatment approaches are evolving. Providers may wish to contact local infectious disease specialists for current recommendations. Table 36-4 lists some appropriate antibiotic choices and Figure 36-1 portrays a suggested algorithm for the outpatient care of pneumonia in an otherwise healthy child.

Providers should perform a Mantoux test in children with pneumonia, especially if they are at high risk or have hilar adenopathy by chest radiograph. Clinicians must avoid the common practice of prescribing antibiotics to asthmatics with a wheezy or congested chest, for presumed "bronchitis" or "pneumonia." Bacterial bronchitis does not occur in otherwise healthy children, including asthmatics. With the exception of mycoplasmal pneumonia, wheezing is very uncommon in cases of bacterial pneumonia. When asthmatics do have recurrent pneumonia, it is often a sign that their asthma is under suboptimal control. Another possibility is that they have CF, immotile cilia syndrome, or immunodeficiency, such as hypogammaglobulinemia.

Neonates

In neonates with fever and pneumonia, providers should perform a sepsis evaluation, including lumbar puncture. Infants should be hospitalized and treated with intravenous antibiotics, such as ampicillin and cefotaxime, pending culture results. Clinicians should order a culture of nasopharyngeal secretions or eye drainage for chlamydia, and consider adding erythromycin for treatment of presumed chlamydia pneumonia.

Severe Pneumonia or Pneumonia in an Immunocompromised Host

Clinicians should hospitalize the patient and administer intravenous antibiotics as quickly as possible. They must consider treatment for pneumococcus that is resistant or only partially sensitive to penicillin. Currently, partial resistance is far more common than complete penicillin resistance. Thus, beginning treatment with high-dose cefotaxime or ceftriaxone is reasonable, in an effort to minimize the use of vancomycin. In the most immunocompromised or critically ill patients, providers can add vancomycin initially to treat resistant pneumococcus. Providers should change antibiotics to more narrow-spectrum choices as culture results dictate. Oxygen should be administered if oxyhemoglobin saturation is less than 94%. Providers should order arterial blood gas analysis if the patient is in respiratory distress or has an altered mental status and is requiring more than low-dose supplemental oxygen. They should obtain a blood culture and, if possible, sputum culture. If clinically appropriate, clinicians should check for RSV virus, and isolate afflicted patients from other susceptible patients in the hospital. They should check electrolyte concentrations, as inappropriate antidiuretic hormone secretion can occur. Providers should consider consulting a subspecialist for flexible bronchoscopy with bronchoalveolar lavage, especially if the patient is critically ill or not responding to therapy. They should consider consultation with pediatric pulmonology or pediatric infectious disease specialists.

Table 36–4. ANTIBIOTIC THERAPY FOR BACTERIAL PNEUMONIA

Patient Population	Antibiotic Options
Infant, 0–3 months	IV ampicillin and cefotaxime (or ampicillin and gentamicin)
Infant with *Chlamydia trachomatis*	IV or PO erythromycin or PO clarithromycin
Child, 4 months–18 years	IV cefuroxime or PO erythromycin, clarithromycin, azithromycin or amoxicillin–clavulanic acid (can start with IM ceftriaxone if vomiting)
Pneumococcus partially resistant to penicillin	PO amoxicillin (80–90 mg/kg/day) or PO amoxicillin–clavulanic acid (40 mg/kg/day) PLUS amoxicillin (40 mg/kg/day)
	PO cefuroxime (30 mg/kg/day), or PO or IV clindamycin
	IV high-dose cefotaxime or IV ceftriaxone or IV high-dose penicillin
Pneumococcus resistant to penicillin and other antibiotics	IV vancomycin
Atypical pneumonias: Mycoplasma and Chlamydia	IV or PO erythromycin or PO clarithromycin or azithromycin (or PO or IV tetracycline if over age 8 years)
Aspiration pneumonia	IV cefoxitin or IV ticarcillin–clavulanic acid or IV high dose penicillin or PO or IV clindamycin

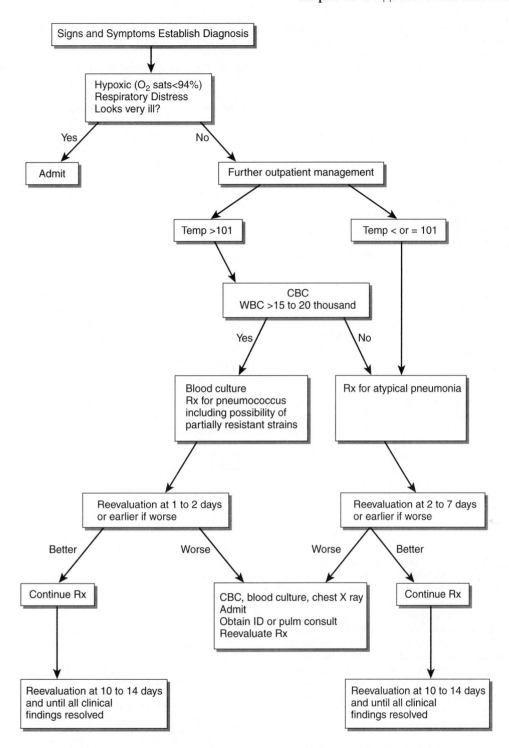

Figure 36–1 ■ Suggested outpatient management of pneumonia in a normal host.

Complications, Pleural Effusions, and Empyema

Large pleural effusions may require drainage for diagnostic or therapeutic purposes. Lateral decubitus films can determine if the fluid is "free-flowing." Freely flowing fluid implies that the fluid is thinner and less organized into loculations. If the radiograph reveals a nearly opacified hemithorax, providers should obtain an ultrasound or chest CT scan to differentiate the amount of consolidation and infiltrate

from the amount of pleural effusion. If the pleural fluid has loculated, thoracentesis and chest tube drainage may not be adequate to control the infection, and the patient may require surgical decortication, either by thoracoscopy or an open procedure.

Management of large pleural effusions is complicated. Options range from intravenous antibiotics alone, which sometimes requires a long course, to chest tube drainage and thoracoscopic or open decortication. Providers should manage these patients in consultation with pediatric specialists experienced in the care of empyema. Such specialists include pediatric pulmonologists, pediatric surgeons, and pediatric infectious disease specialists. Fortunately, complete resolution over time is the outcome in the vast majority of cases of pediatric empyema.

Admission Criteria

Admission decisions depend largely on the patient's age, severity of illness, presence of underlying disease, and family circumstances. The following circumstances should prompt hospitalization:

Age younger than 4 months
Room air oxyhemoglobin saturation less than 94%
Respiratory distress, especially nasal flaring, grunting, respiratory rate over 50 (40 in older child)
Pleural effusion that is more than minimal
Poor response to oral antibiotics
Family that is unreliable, lives far from medical facility, or lacks transportation or telephone
Immunocompromised host
Patient with impaired cough reflex, neuromuscular disease, sickle cell anemia, or underlying cardiac or respiratory illness

Referral Criteria

Providers should consult a pediatric pulmonologist and pediatric infectious disease specialist for patients with severe pneumonia, particularly if they are immunocompromised. They should consult a pulmonologist and immunologist if the patient is having recurring bacterial pneumonia without an explanation. If the patient is immunocompromised or severely ill, clinicians should prepare for the possibility of respiratory failure and need for ICU admission, intubation, and mechanical ventilation.

Recurrences

Patients with recurring bacterial pneumonia warrant evaluation. They may have underlying asthma, immunodeficiency, CF, immotile cilia, foreign body aspiration, airway tumor, or a congenital anomaly such as pulmonary sequestration or H-type tracheoesophageal fistula. The most basic evaluation should include pulmonary function tests before and after bronchodilators, serum immunoglobulins, sweat test, and PPD Mantoux test. Providers should repeat the chest radiograph to ensure that it clears after each episode. They should consider consultation with a pediatric pulmonologist and immunologist.

What to Tell the Family

Providers should discuss the following with the family:

The child has a lung infection, which is caused by a virus or bacterium. Antibiotics will not help viral infections. If antibiotics are prescribed, the child must take the entire course of antibiotics, even if he or she seems better before it is complete.
Call the provider if the child is having a hard time breathing. Call if the infant is breathing more than 50 breaths per minute, toddler is breathing more than 40 breaths per minute, or older child is breathing more than 35 breaths per minute. Call if the child is pulling in the ribs or abdomen while breathing, or if the lips or fingernails are blue.

Call if the child is not drinking well, not urinating normally, if the inside of the mouth is dry, or if crying does not produce tears.
Call if fever, cough, chest discomfort, and activity level do not improve within 2 days, or if the child seems worse at any time.
If the child has a history of asthma, the child should start using their prescribed bronchodilator (such as albuterol) during treatment for pneumonia.
Contact the provider if the child is coughing up colored phlegm (not just clear or white).

Prevention

The following are preventive measures against pneumonia:

Encourage *Haemophilus influenza B* vaccination for all infants.
Pneumococcal vaccination is extremely important for children at increased risk of pneumococcal pneumonia, such as patients with sickle cell disease, asplenia, renal failure, immunosuppressed patients, and HIV infection. Administer at age 2 years and repeat every 5 years in children younger than age 10 years. Young children with sickle cell anemia should receive daily prophylactic penicillin. The currently available pneumococcal vaccine is ineffective in children younger than age 2 years. The new conjugated pneumococcal vaccine, however, is immunogenic even for children younger than age 2 years. Universal immunization will be recommended in the United States for all infants at a 2, 4, and 6 month schedule with a booster at 12 to 18 months. Recommendations for the use of the conjugated vaccine in older children at risk for invasive pneumococcal disease are being developed.
Consider pneumococcal vaccine for children with underlying respiratory disorders, such as CF.
Encourage annual influenza vaccination for children with underlying cardiac or respiratory disease, including asthma, diabetes, sickle cell disease, and immunosuppressed patients. Health care workers should also receive annual influenza vaccination.

REFERENCES

American Academy of Pediatrics. (1997). Respiratory syncytial virus. Report of the Committee on Infectious Diseases. *1997 Red Book*. Elk Grove Village, IL: Author.

American Academy of Pediatrics Committee on Infectious Diseases. (1998). Prevention of respiratory syncytial virus infections: Indications for the use of palivizumab and update on the use of RSV-IVIG. *Pediatrics 102*, 1211–1216.

Berger, I., Argaman, Z., Schwartz, S. B., et al. (1998). Efficacy of corticosteroids in acute bronchiolitis: short-term and long term follow-up. *Pediatric Pulmonology, 26*, 162–166.

Churgay, C. A. (1996). The diagnosis and management of bacterial pneumonias in infants and children. *Primary Care, 23*, 821–835.

DeMuri, G. P. (1996). Afebrile pneumonia in infants. *Primary Care, 23*, 849–860.

Denny, F. W., Murphy T. F., Clyde, W. A., et al. (1983). Croup: An 11-year study in a pediatric practice. *Pediatrics, 71*, 871–876.

Dershewitz, R. A., & Dorkin, H. L. (1999) Persistent cough. In R. A. Dershewitz (Ed.), *Ambulatory pediatric care* (3rd ed.). Philadelphia: Lippincott-Raven Publishers.

Edell, D., Bruce, E., Hale, K., et al. (1998). Reduced long-term respiratory morbidity after treatment of respiratory syncytial virus bronchiolitis with ribavirin in previously healthy infants. *Pediatric Pulmonology, 25*, 154–158.

Foy, H. M., Cooney, M. K., Maletzky, A. J., et al. (1973). Incidence and etiology of pneumonia, croup and bronchiolitis in preschool children belonging to a prepaid medical care group over a four year period. *American Journal of Epidemiology, 97*, 80–92.

Glezen, W. P., Paredes A., Allison, J. E, Hussey, M., et al. (1981). Risk of respiratory syncytial virus infection for infants from low-income families in relationship to age, sex, ethnic group, and maternal antibody level. *Journal of Pediatrics, 98*, 708–715.

Godden, C. W., Campbell, M. J., Hussey, M., et al. (1997). Double blind placebo controlled trial of nebulized budesonide for croup. *Archives of Disease in Children, 76*, 155–158.

The IMPACT Study Group. (1998). Reduction of respiratory syncytial virus hospitalization among premature infants and infants with bronchopulmonary dysplasia, using respiratory syncytial virus monoclonal antibody prophylaxis. *Pediatrics 102*, 531–537.

Johnson, D. W., Jacobson, S., Edney, P. C., et al. (1998). A comparison of nebulized budesonide, intramuscular dexamethasone, and placebo for moderately severe croup. *New England Journal of Medicine, 339*, 498–503.

Kim, H. W., Arrobio, J. O., Brandt, C. D., et al. (1973). Epidemiology of respiratory syncytial virus infection in Washington, D.C. *American Journal of Epidemiology, 98*, 216–225.

Klassen, T. P., Craig, W. R., Moher, D., et al. (1998). Nebulized budesonide and oral dexamethasone for treatment of croup. *Journal of the American Medical Association, 279*, 1629–1632.

Klassen, T. P. (1997). Recent advances in the treatment of bronchiolitis and laryngitis. *Pediatric Clinics of North America, 44*, 249–259.

Klassen, T. P., Sutcliffe, T., Watters, L. K., et al (1997). Dexamethasone in salbutamol-treated inpatients with acute bronchiolitis: A randomized, controlled trial. *Journal of Pediatrics, 130*, 191–196.

Latham-Sadler, B. A., & Morell, V. W. (1996) Viral and atypical pneu-

monias. *Primary Care, 23*, 837–848.

Long, C. E., Voter, K. Z., Barker, W. H., et al. (1997). Long term follow-up of children hospitalized with respiratory syncytial virus lower respiratory tract infection and randomly treated with ribavirin or placebo. *Pediatric Infectious Disease Journal, 16*, 1023–1027.

Meissner H. C., Welliver R. C., Chartrand, S. A., et al. (1999). Immunoprophylaxis with palivizumab, a humanized respiratory syncytial virus monoclonal antibody, for prevention of respiratory syncytial virus infection in high risk infants: a consensus opinion. *Pediatric Infectious Disease Journal, 18*, 223–231.

Menon, K., Sutcliffe, T., Klassen, T. P. (1995). A randomized trial comparing the efficacy of epinephrine with salbutamol in the treatment of acute bronchiolitis. *Journal of Pediatrics, 126*, 1004–1007.

The PREVENT Study Group. (1997). Reduction of respiratory syncytial virus hospitalization among premature infants and infants with bronchopulmonary dysplasia using respiratory syncytial virus immune globulin prophylaxis. *Pediatrics, 99*, 93–99.

Richter, H., & Seddon, P. (1998). Early nebulized budesonide in the treatment of bronchiolitis and the prevention of postbronchiolitic wheezing. *Journal of Pediatrics, 132*, 849-853.

Roorda, R. J., & Walhof, C. M. (1998). Effects of inhaled fluticasone propionate administered with metered dose inhaler and spacer in mild to moderate croup: a negative preliminary report. *Pediatric Pulmonology, 25*, 114-117.

Wilmott, R. W. (1990). Cough. In M. W. Schwartz (Ed.), *Pediatric primary care: A problem-oriented approach* (2nd ed.). Chicago: Year Book Med. Publishers, Inc.

Heart Problems

• FREDRICK Z. BIERMAN, MD

INTRODUCTION

Successful management of heart problems in the pediatric population depends on timely diagnosis and initiation of appropriate medical or surgical intervention. While most practitioners are familiar with congenital and acquired pediatric cardiovascular anomalies, the confounding variability in their clinical presentation is an ongoing challenge. The intent of this chapter is to provide a guideline for pediatric primary care practitioners confronting the varied presentations of infants with congenital heart disease, well children with murmurs, children and adolescents with chest pain or syncope, and patients with acute rheumatic fever (ARF).

CONGENITAL HEART DISEASE IN INFANTS

Cardiovascular examination of the newborn begins with assessment of respiratory status, oxygenation, and exercise tolerance. Tachypnea, cyanosis, and feeding performance are nonspecific parameters of cardiopulmonary physiology in the newborn. During the first month of life, clinicians, either in the nursery or the office, use auscultation to identify systolic and diastolic murmurs and to assess ventilation; palpation to evaluate peripheral perfusion and hepatic size; pulse oximetry to quantitate systemic saturation and saturation gradients; and chest x-ray to assess cardiac size, abdominal viscera laterality, and pulmonary parenchyma. Clinicians must recognize that murmurs are not a universal finding with either simple or complex cardiovascular anomalies. Normal variations or coexisting pulmonary disease can distort the chest x-ray, particularly in neonates.

Pathology

Murmurs reflect pressure gradients across anatomic partitions (interventricular septum), cardiac valves and vascular channels (ductus arteriosus, coarctation), or simply turbulent blood flow. While the absence of a murmur suggests that the interatrial or interventricular septum is intact and the cardiac valves and great vessels are normal, their absence in the neonate does not exclude clinically important cardiovascular anomalies. The limitations of the physical examination and alternative diagnostic resources available to practitioners are illustrated in the following clinical scenarios:

- Interventricular septal defect (VSD)
- Tetralogy of Fallot (TOF)
- Left heart obstructive anomalies
- Meconium aspiration with persistence of fetal circulation

Interventricular Septal Defect

The murmur of VSD depends on a pressure gradient between the right and left ventricles. Pulmonary artery pressure at systemic levels in utero declines over the first few weeks of life, with thinning of the muscular wall of the smaller pulmonary arterioles. When right ventricular pressures drop below left-sided pressures, left-to-right shunting occurs across the septal defect, creating the characteristic holosystolic murmur. The appearance of a VSD murmur depends on the rapidity of this vascular maturation process.

● **Clinical Pearl:** The classic pansystolic murmur of a VSD may not become apparent until after a newborn has been discharged home.

During the perinatal period, the size of the communication, coexisting right ventricular outflow obstruction, or persistence of fetal-type cardiopulmonary circulation may mute audibility of the VSD. The clinical course of most VSDs, particularly those located in the muscular segment of the interventricular septum, is often benign. As the duration and intensity of the systolic murmur decrease on serial follow-up, uncomplicated spontaneous closure of the VSD usually follows.

Complications

Infrequently, spontaneous closure of a VSD may lead to undesirable changes in intracardiac anatomy or pulmonary physiology. Closure of VSDs, particularly those in the subaortic membranous septum, normally is accomplished with fibrous thickening of the defect's border or adjacent septal tricuspid valve leaflet and formation of a windsock-like aneurysm on the right septal surface. Undesirable herniation of an aortic cusp into the septal defect, however, may initiate closure. In this sequence, the aortic cusp seals the communication, but secondary distortion of the valve results in aortic regurgitation.

● **Clinical Pearl:** As the VSD systolic murmur decreases in intensity and duration, a pandiastolic, high-frequency murmur of aortic insufficiency becomes audible with herniation of the aortic cusp.

Another variation in the natural history of the relatively small membranous VSD is the spontaneous development of anomalous muscle bundles in the right ventricle. As the VSD spontaneously decreases in size, muscle bundles within the body of the right ventricle hypertrophy, partitioning the chamber into higher and lower pressure segments. The softer systolic murmur of the closing VSD becomes obscured by a harsh ejection murmur. This murmur results from the intraventricular pressure gradient that the anomalous muscle bundles generate. While the left-to-right shunt is not a hemodynamic burden, surgical intervention in the toddler or younger child may be necessary to resect the obstructing anomalous muscle bundles.

Undesirable changes in pulmonary vascular physiology may simulate spontaneous closure of a VSD. While timely surgical intervention during infancy has reduced the frequency of this clinical problem, certain patients experience accelerated maladaptive changes in the pulmonary arterioles in response to increased pulmonary blood flow due to moderate or large VSDs. The media of the arterioles thicken, increasing pulmonary artery pressure and pulmonary vascular resistance. In addition, this thickening reduces left-to-right shunting across the VSD. The pansystolic VSD murmur recedes as right and left ventricular pressures equilibrate, and the left-to-right intracardiac shunt is minimized. Subsequent physical examination reveals no systolic or diastolic murmur. The second heart sound (S_2) increases in intensity, and a palpable right ventricular impulse is apparent.

Interventricular Septal Defect as Part of Atrioventricular Canal Defect

In neonates with trisomy 21, a complete common atrioventricular (AV) canal defect (unrestrictive atrial septal defect [ASD], VSD, mitral and tricuspid valve anomalies) may be clinically silent during their physical examination. The pansystolic murmur, which results from left-to-right shunting, is blunted until pulmonary vascular maturation reduces pulmonary vascular resistance and right ventricular pressure. Therefore, newborns with Down syndrome require more than just a careful physical examination. Screening for an AV canal, also known as an endocardial cushion defect, begins with the standard 12-lead electrocardiogram (ECG). In most cases, the neonatal ECG is too nonspecific to identify cardiovascular anomalies; however, the superior QRS axis and counterclockwise depolarization loop associated with an AV canal is characteristic for this anomaly. As with other cardiovascular anomalies whose clinical expression depends on maturation of pulmonary circulation, exclusion of an AV canal anomaly or more complex interventricular septal communications warrants cardiac ultrasound examination.

Tetralogy of Fallot

Although listening for a murmur is a common focus of the practitioner's assessment when screening for newborn cardiovascular anomalies, TOF illustrates how variable such findings may be. The anomalies in TOF consist of a large malalignment-type VSD; an aortic valve overriding the interventricular septum; obstruction of the pulmonary circulation below, at, or above the pulmonary valve; and right ventricular hypertrophy. Although a large VSD is part of the complex, it does not typically contribute to the auscultatory findings in an affected neonate. The systolic ejection murmur at the left upper sternal border associated with TOF is secondary to the obstruction and attendant pressure gradient across the right ventricular outflow tract.

Variations in the auscultatory findings in TOF reflect the dynamic and static nature of the right ventricular outflow tract obstruction. Patients vary in the degree of fixed obstruction across the hypertrophied, right ventricular outflow, stenotic pulmonary valve, and bifurcation of the branch pulmonary arteries. Obstruction at or below the valve is manifested by a systolic ejection murmur at the left upper sternal border. Distal branch pulmonary artery stenosis radiates this ejection murmur to the axillae and posterior lung fields. An individual patient's physical examination

may vary over time as progressive hypertrophy of the right ventricular outflow increases subvalvar obstruction. Auscultatory findings also may suddenly change with superimposition of reactive dynamic obstruction and virtual occlusion of the right ventricular outflow.

The VSD associated with TOF is a lesion that is seen rather than heard. The typically large defect equalizes both right and left ventricular systolic pressure, and accordingly, no shunt murmur is audible. The defect decompresses the obstructed right ventricle by shunting desaturated blood into the left ventricle and the systemic circulation.

There is considerable anatomic variation with TOF. While many affected patients present with a systolic ejection murmur and cyanosis, some are clinically acyanotic. In such cases, a fortuitous physiologic balance exists between the large VSD and the degree of right ventricular outflow obstruction. The potential for excessive pulmonary blood flow with left-to-right shunting across a large VSD is moderated by right ventricular outflow tract obstruction. These infants may have an uneventful course until elective surgical intervention is performed to close the VSD and relieve the outflow obstruction. Until surgical correction is performed, however, these children remain at risk for hypercyanotic episodes due to acute increase in dynamic obstruction of the right ventricular outflow.

One of the most clinically challenging variations of TOF is the neonate who also has atresia of the pulmonary valve. This infant may be minimally cyanotic at birth as a result of persistent shunting across the patent ductus arteriosus (PDA) or the presence of systemic-to-pulmonary artery collaterals that preserve pulmonary blood flow.

When pulmonary blood flow is totally ductal dependent, the infant may become rapidly and profoundly cyanotic with spontaneous closure of the ductus arteriosus. These infants require emergency intervention with initiation of prostaglandin E-1 therapy and surgical placement of a systemic-to-pulmonary artery shunt.

Those infants with TOF and pulmonary atresia whose pulmonary blood flow depends on multiple systemic-to-pulmonary artery collaterals may not present clinically for several weeks following discharge home. These infants often have complex pulmonary artery anatomy, with marked hypoplasia or even absent branch segments.

Left Heart Obstructive Anomalies That are Ductal Dependent

In utero, the ductus arteriosus effectively bypasses anomalies of the great vessels (Fig. 37-1), AV and semilunar valves, and hypoplasia of the ventricles. Congenital cardiovascular anomalies of the left heart that are well palliated in the fetus and newborn by the PDA and placental circulation may present acutely and precipitously in the newborn period following spontaneous closure of the ductus arteriosus. Following birth, patency of the ductus arteriosus can transiently preserve systemic or pulmonary circulation. In neonates with critical aortic stenosis or coarctation of the aorta, closure of the ductus in the first 48 to 96 hours of life is followed by progressive metabolic acidosis and myocardial dysfunction. The challenge is to identify affected infants before clinical deterioration alters the opportunity for successful surgical management.

Meeting the challenge of early diagnosis of ductal-dependent cardiovascular anomalies requires more than a clinician's high index of suspicion. The neonate with clinically occult coarctation of the juxtaductal aorta is an example of how a large PDA can obscure clinical acumen (Fig. 37-2). Right-to-left shunting across a neonate's unrestrictive PDA provides effective sys-

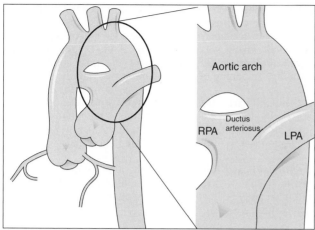

Figure 37–1 ▪ Normal ascending aorta, transverse aortic arch, and descending aorta with large ductus arteriosus bridging the main pulmonary artery. The diameter of the normal ductus arteriosus in the fetus and newborn, prior to closure, approximates that of the transverse aortic arch.

temic blood flow distal to the severest of aortic arch anomalies. Femoral pulses are preserved, and the discrepancy in saturation between the upper and lower extremities may not be clinically apparent. Subtle respiratory changes due to progressive left ventricular failure may not be appreciated until spontaneous closure of the PDA compromises peripheral perfusion. Metabolic acidosis then results. A similar clinical pattern occurs with hypoplasia of the left heart where right-to-left shunting across the ductus arteriosus is necessary to palliate aortic or mitral atresia (see Fig. 37-2).

Identification of congenital cardiovascular anomalies when patency of the PDA preserves systemic or pulmonary (Fig. 37-3) blood flow is a challenge for the pediatric clinician. It is critical to identify ductal-dependent lesions so that prostaglandin E-1 therapy can be initiated to keep the ductus arteriosus patent and preserve pulmonary or systemic blood flow.

▲ **Clinical Warning:** Ductal-dependent anomalies may not be apparent during initial physical examination in the newborn nursery.

The infant's subsequent presentation following spontaneous closure of the PDA is heralded by either significant cyanosis or, in the case of left-sided obstruction, profound metabolic acidosis and shock. Fetal echocardiography allows antenatal diagnosis of most ductal-dependent anomalies. However, cost and availability limit its application as a universal screening procedure.

Diagnostic Studies

It is obvious that a small but significant number of newborns with either cyanotic congenital heart anomalies or those with defects that depend on the ductus arteriosus to maintain critical systemic or pulmonary blood flow will be missed by even the most careful of physical examinations. Pulse oximetry, however, can identify ductal-dependent lesions and systemic oxygen desaturation in neonates with right-to-left intrapulmonary or intracardiac shunts.

Most clinicians are familiar with the partial pressure of oxygen (pO_2) reported on arterial blood gas samples. This is a measure of the oxygen concentration dissolved in plasma regardless of hemoglobin binding. Arterial oxygen satura-

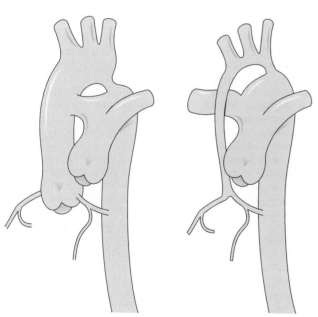

Figure 37–2 ▪ *(Left)* Simple coarctation of the juxtaductal aorta with unrestrictive ductus arteriosus confluent with proximal descending thoracic aorta. *(Right)* Aortic valve atresia with hypoplastic proximal ascending aorta originating at confluence of right and left main coronary arteries and continuing as hypoplastic transverse aortic arch. The confluence of an unrestrictive ductus arteriosus preserves antegrade blood flow to the descending aorta and retrograde flow to the transverse aortic arch, ascending thoracic aorta and coronary arteries.

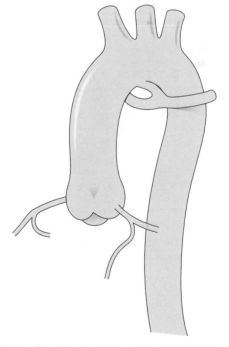

Figure 37–3 ▪ Dilated proximal ascending aorta continuous with transverse aortic arch from which a "reverse" ductus arteriosus communicates with hypoplastic, confluent branch pulmonary arteries in a neonate with atresia of the main pulmonary artery and pulmonary valve. The reverse ductus, so called because of its more anterior origin from the inferior aspect of the transverse aortic arch, preserves antegrade branch pulmonary artery blood flow.

tion, however, is a measure of the percent of oxygen bound to hemoglobin. Oxygen capacity is the maximum predicted volume of oxygen that can be bound to hemoglobin (1.34 mL oxygen per gram of hemoglobin) in a sample of blood. The oxygen content is the measured amount of oxygen actually bound to hemoglobin in blood from a specific vessel (eg, the aorta). The oxygen saturation, expressed as a percent is the simple fraction relating oxygen content and capacity:

$$\% \text{ oxygen saturation} = \frac{\text{oxygen content}}{\text{oxygen capacity}} \times 100$$

Pulse oximetry offers a repetitive, noninvasive measure of systemic oxygen saturation using the distinctive light absorption properties of oxygenated and deoxygenated hemoglobin in pulsating tissue (Poets & Martin, 1996). Sampling can be performed from the upper and lower extremities as well as the nares or ear lobes.

In the normal neonate, virtually all arterial hemoglobin is bound to oxygen, and the systemic arterial (aortic) saturation is greater than 95%. Right-to-left shunting, either due to pulmonary parenchymal disease or intracardiac/extracardiac shunting reduces the aortic oxygen saturation. If the right-to-left shunt occurs in the lungs or within the heart, then the systemic oxygen saturation is decreased no matter where the pulse oximetry probe is applied to the infant. If, however, right-to-left shunting occurs across the PDA, then the pulse oximetry oxygen saturations in the upper extremities will be higher than those recorded in the lower extremities (Fig. 37-4). Along with other surveillance protocols,

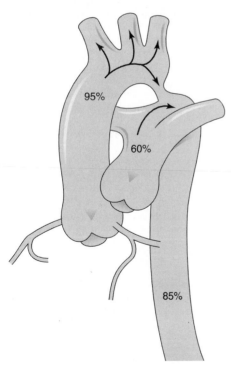

Figure 37–4 ■ Illustration of oxygen saturations in the ascending aorta, main pulmonary artery, and descending aorta associated with right-to-left shunting across an unrestrictive ductus arteriosus with critical juxtaductal coarctation of the aorta. Simultaneous pulse oximetry of the right upper and right or left lower digits would reveal an oxygen saturation gradient between the upper extremities (95%) (perfused by subclavian arteries arising proximal to the right-to-left ductus arteriosus shunt) and the more distal lower extremities (85%) perfused by the descending aorta.

pulse oximetry screening is an efficient technology applicable to large well child nurseries. The procedure can be performed during customary nursing assessment with results recorded during routine charting of vital signs. The algorithm in Figure 37-5 summarizes the protocol for pulse oximetry screening of the neonate.

● **Clinical Pearl:** Pulse oximetry is performed at 36 hours of age on the lower extremity to identify all intrapulmonary, intracardiac, and ductal-dependent shunts. A lower extremity saturation less than 95% is considered abnormal.

● **Clinical Pearl:** A lower extremity pulse oximetry saturation less than 95% with higher upper extremity saturations is the pulse oximetry hallmark of a ductal-dependent aortic coarctation.

The neonate with critical coarctation of the aorta will have a saturation gradient between the upper and lower extremities due to right-to-left ductal shunting. However, the upper extremity saturation may not be normal if the infant has pulmonary venous congestion that interferes with normal gas exchange and lowers the saturation of pulmonary venous blood.

● **Clinical Pearl:** In neonates with hypoplastic left heart complex and aortic atresia, global systemic desaturation is present with no saturation gradient between the upper and lower extremities.

The absence of a pulse oximetry gradient between the upper and lower extremities and the globally reduced systemic saturation reflect common mixing of pulmonary venous and systemic venous blood in the atria in the presence of mitral and aortic atresia or single ventricle.

The utility of pulse oximetry extends beyond screening in the management of congenital heart disease. It also provides effective surveillance following interventions to stabilize neonates with ductal-dependent circulation. Prior to medical intervention, the acidotic neonate with critical coarctation and spontaneous closure of the PDA will have no saturation gradient between the upper and lower extremities. In the absence of pulsatile flow due to the proximal coarctation, no saturation in the lower extremity can be documented. Following initiation of prostaglandin E-1 therapy, pulse oximetry of the lower extremity provides evidence of pulsatile flow as ductal patency is restored and a systemic oxygen saturation gradient is established.

Right-to-left shunting across the PDA and its surveillance with pulse oximetry is not restricted to neonates with complex congenital heart disease. A common application of this clinical tool is in newborns with persistence of fetal-type circulation (Walsh-Sukys et al., 2000). Neonates with persistent elevation of pulmonary artery resistance and pressure following meconium aspiration or birth asphyxia often demonstrate right-to-left shunting across both the interatrial septum and PDA. Medical therapies for management of this problem (Davidson et al., 1998) are directed to increase effective pulmonary blood flow while the infant recovers from related pulmonary parenchymal injury. Reduction in pulmonary artery pressure and resistance, as oxygenation and gas exchange improve, can be monitored with surveillance of the oxygen saturation gradient between the upper and lower extremities. As pulmonary artery pressure and resistance decrease, the oxygen saturation gradient between the upper and lower extremities will fall until right-to-left shunting across the PDA ceases.

Pulsed Oximetry Newborn Screening

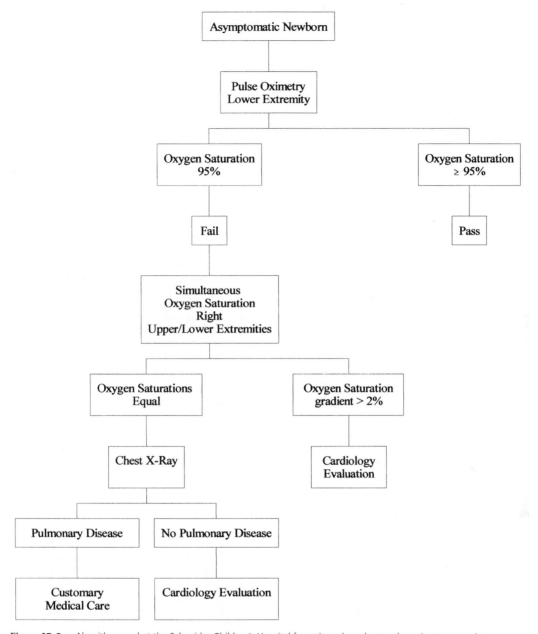

Figure 37–5 ■ Algorithm used at the Schneider Children's Hospital for universal newborn pulse oximetry screening to identify cyanotic and ductal-dependent congenital heart disease.

THE INNOCENT MURMUR

Evaluation of the preschool child with a nonradiating, vibratory systolic ejection murmur at the left mid and upper sternal borders remains a common problem for the primary care practitioner (Sapin, 1997) and a debatable cause for pediatric cardiology referral. This auscultatory finding in an otherwise normal child at a well child examination, or the child with normal past medical history presenting with an intercurrent febrile illness, often escalates beyond its clinical relevance due to parental concern.

The term innocent murmur refers to an auscultatory finding heard in the majority of children at some time in their lives. Many clinicians prefer to label these murmurs "innocent" rather than "functional," because the former is a much more reassuring term to parents and patients. The critical issue for the primary care provider is to be able to distinguish these murmurs from those caused by true organic heart problems.

History and Physical Examination

● **Clinical Pearl:** The innocent murmur's quality and timing, the changing intensity from supine to sitting, and the presence of normal splitting of the second heart sound are critical differentiating characteristics.

Quality and Timing

The physical examination of the normal infant, toddler, and young child is often punctuated by the discovery of "functional" murmurs. They are ejection type and have a vibratory or musical quality.

These murmurs are always systolic; diastolic murmurs are never innocent. In the majority of toddlers and young children, the left upper/midsternal border "innocent" or vibratory systolic ejection murmur is evidence of accelerated blood flow across the right ventricular outflow tract or central systemic veins. The truncated shape of the right ventricle due to continuity of its capacious tricuspid valve annulus and body with a conical shaped tapering outflow accelerates blood flow. The change in velocity of blood flow through the normal right ventricle is similar to that of water in a stream whose channel narrows. The sound of water accelerating as the stream's banks converge parallels the functional murmur, audible at the left upper sternal border of the heart, as blood accelerates across the normal right ventricular outflow tract.

If the volume of blood returning to the right heart is increased, either by febrile illness, anemia, or posture, the intensity of the murmur increases much as the sound of the stream does with runoff following a rainfall. This explains the frequent discovery of a "new" or "never heard before" murmur during the evaluation of a routine febrile illness.

Change from Supine to Sitting

● **Clinical Pearl:** Distinguishing the normal, typically grade 1 to 2/6, vibratory, systolic ejection flow murmur from that of a cardiovascular anomaly begins with altering the patient's posture. Arising from a supine to an upright posture decreases systemic venous return to the right heart, reducing the intensity and possibly silencing the systolic ejection murmur.

While murmurs secondary to structural cardiovascular anomalies can be influenced by changes in systemic venous return to the heart, simple postural changes usually have a minimal effect on the intensity of organic murmurs.

● **Clinical Pearl:** Murmurs related to structural cardiovascular anomalies, particularly the systolic ejection murmur of dynamic left ventricular outflow tract obstruction or the insufficiency murmur of mitral valve prolapse, will often increase in intensity with decreased venous return to the heart (supine to upright).

Postural changes in intensity help identify most murmurs of "functional origin." Interpretation of the response to such maneuvers, however, may be confusing. While upright posture decreases venous return from the inferior vena cava, it accelerates superior vena cava as well as innominate, subclavian, and internal jugular venous blood flow. This acceleration in blood flow often results in a continuous, infraclavicular venous hum that may simulate a PDA in the toddler or young child. Discriminating the continuous murmur of the venous hum from that of a PDA is straightforward. The venous hum continuous murmur is exquisitely sensitive to maneuvers reducing superior venous blood flow velocity. The transition from upright to supine posture, contralateral rotation of the head, or gentle supraclavicular compression eliminates the venous hum murmur but does not influence the continuous murmur of the PDA.

Physiologic Splitting of the Second Heart Sound

● **Clinical Pearl:** The single first and the softer, variably split second heart sound (S2) are the auscultatory hallmarks of the normal heart.

Being able to identify variability or physiologic splitting of S2 is often a challenge, especially in younger children. Concentrating on that particular phase of the cardiac cycle requires patience. In older cooperative children, asking for deep breathing in and out and holding the breath may make variable splitting more apparent.

Hearing variability in the splitting of S2 commonly differentiates between the ejection-type flow murmur of an innocent murmur, an ASD, and those murmurs caused by right sided outflow tract obstruction. All of these murmurs sound the same in that they are typical ejection type murmurs; S2 splitting differentiates between the three. Innocent murmurs have variable splitting.

The murmur of an ASD is caused by relative pulmonic stenosis. This is due to increased blood volume across a normal pulmonic valve due to inter-atrial left-to-right shunting, and it sounds like a typical pulmonic ejection-type murmur (the sound of the murmur is not caused by flow across the ASD). Because of the increased flow, closure of the pulmonic valve lags behind aortic valve closure, resulting in a fixed and widely (nonvariable) split S2. With the murmur of pulmonic stenosis, it is typically difficult to identify any normal splitting of S2.

Diagnostic Criteria

The experienced provider will be able to differentiate innocent (functional) murmurs from their organic counterparts by the three auscultatory characteristics described previously. If all three criteria are not met or if there is clinical uncertainty, then further evaluation is recommended. Depending on local circumstances, this may involve two-dimensional echocardiography, referral to a pediatric cardiologist, or both.

Functional murmurs are encountered in the newborn and younger infant. It is imperative, however, to remain vigilant for subtle clinical evidence of congenital heart disease. A short systolic ejection murmur with no diastolic component and localized at the left upper sternal border may accompany normal closure of the ductus arteriosus in the first few days of life. A restrictive, pinhole sized apical or midmuscular VSD may produce a short, regurgitant murmur at the left lower sternal border shortly after birth. Peripheral pulmonic stenosis, the normal perinatal discrepancy between the main and branch pulmonary arteries' diameters during the first few weeks of life, accelerates blood flow, resulting in a systolic ejection murmur audible at the left upper sternal border and radiating to the axillae and interscapular areas.

Management

Once the provider establishes the diagnosis of an innocent murmur, he or she must be clear and precise in explaining to both parent and patient that the murmur is truly a normal variant. A good explanation is that the sound is caused by blood rushing through a healthy, young, elastic, and normal heart. The provider must emphasize that there is no need for any further testing, referral to a cardiologist, limitation of activity, or endocarditis prophylaxis.

The diagnosis should be clearly documented in the health record, however. Any future intercurrent illness, particularly with fever, will no doubt reveal a louder but also completely innocent murmur. If this evaluation is performed by someone other than the usual provider, having the parent or patient fully informed of the previous finding, as well as having it documented clearly in the record, will alleviate undue anxiety and eliminate the need for further unnecessary testing.

CHEST PAIN

Chest pain is a common chief complaint encountered in the primary care practice office. Nontraumatic chest pain is rarely associated with structural cardiovascular disease in this population. Most chest discomfort in older children and adolescents is secondary to transient musculoskeletal or esophageal dysfunction.

However, certain organic problems can occur in children and adolescents that do require prompt assessment and intervention. They include pericardial inflammation, myocardial ischemia secondary to accelerated atrial or ventricular arrhythmias, pulmonary parenchymal or pleural disease, and spontaneous vascular injury. The usually aggressive diagnostic and therapeutic interventions applied to the symptomatic adult patient with chest pain must be modified in the evaluation and management of the more benign etiologies of chest discomfort in children.

Unlike the adult describing crushing anginal symptoms of myocardial ischemia, the child or adolescent frequently has difficulty characterizing the symptomatology that prompted medical evaluation. The practitioner is often confronted with a report of nonspecific, transient, anterior chest discomfort that is vague in quality, poorly localized, and variably associated with activity or posture. While such ill-defined chest pain in the pediatric population is often functional, there is a subset of neonates, children, and adolescents with organic chest discomfort that may be obscured by the patient's communicative skills.

The precordial discomfort of sustained supraventricular tachycardia with ventricular pre-excitation of Wolf-Parkinson-White in a young child, the aching sensation of pericardial inflammation in an adolescent awakening in the middle of the night, or colic-like symptoms secondary to myocardial ischemia of coronary artery anomalies in an infant require timely diagnosis and intervention. Discrimination between the chest pain of self-limiting, benign musculoskeletal or gastroenteric dysfunction in an otherwise well pediatric patient and that due to far less common, but potentially life-threatening, organic disease is a clinical challenge.

History and Physical Examination

Management of chest pain is guided by pertinent findings in the patient's medical and family history and description of symptoms in terms of their duration, location, quality, and the circumstances provoking discomfort. Figure 37-6 illustrates clinical cues for assessment of chest pain in this population.

History

Antecedent viral illness is commonplace during the winter and spring months. Temporal relationship to symptoms help pinpoint the prodrome, which precedes pericardial or pleu-

ral disease. Marfan syndrome in first- or second-degree relatives of a phenotypically suggestive, tall adolescent presenting with a spontaneous pneumothorax should direct the clinician's attention to connective tissue disease, especially when scoliosis, pectus excavatum, or abdominal wall hernias have been treated or noted in the past. Such patients may present with acute chest pain radiating to the neck or back secondary to spontaneous injury of an aortic aneurysm (Groenink et al., 1999). Past medical history of Kawasaki syndrome or an atypical febrile illness associated with a perineal rash, edema of the hands and feet, or mucoconjunctivitis warrants investigation of coronary artery anatomy. A history of intractable colic and poor weight gain in the young infant may be the only manifestation of abnormal coronary artery (anomalous origin of the left coronary artery from the pulmonary circulation). The child or adolescent reporting a tapping sensation in the chest or vague chest discomfort with irregular heartbeats may be experiencing tachyarrhythmias related to atrial or ventricular ectopy.

Discrimination between benign functional and organic chest pain can often be accomplished with review of the symptoms' duration, location and quality of the discomfort, and circumstances provoking the complaint.

Duration of Symptoms

Patients with benign, fleeting chest discomfort of musculoskeletal or transient gastrointestinal etiology find it difficult to be precise about the onset of symptoms that are fleeting in quality and rarely interrupt their activity. In contrast, those with organic chest pain can often pinpoint the onset of symptoms and are emphatic about its chronicity.

● **Clinical Pearl:** The more precise and specific the description of the chest pain is, the more likely the etiology is truly organic. For example, patients with inflammatory pain, such as pericarditis, report how the persistent discomfort interferes with sleep throughout the night.

The timelines of chest pain in the pediatric population vary according to etiology. Pain due to self-limiting musculoskeletal or gastrointestinal etiologies is fleeting, lasting only seconds. A spontaneous pneumothorax results in acute penetrating pain that wanes. Myocardial ischemia results in minutes of provocable anginal discomfort. Pleuropericardial inflammation and costochondritis result in an incessant ache.

Location

The ability to localize chest pain in the pediatric patient is limited by age and communicative skills. Localization of recurrent, but transient musculoskeletal pain is often vague and described by the patient with a sweeping hand gesture across the entire anterior chest. The absence of laterality and localization to the precordium or shoulders is indicative of the benign nature of the discomfort.

● **Clinical Pearl:** The pain of costochondritis secondary to nonspecific focal inflammation, or Tietze's complex, is best localized during the physical examination. Typically the adolescent patient will generalize the location of discomfort to the anterior chest wall until right or left parasternal palpation elicits point tenderness at a costochondral junction.

Localization of pleural or pericardial chest pain depends on the site and source of discomfort. Pleural pain corre-

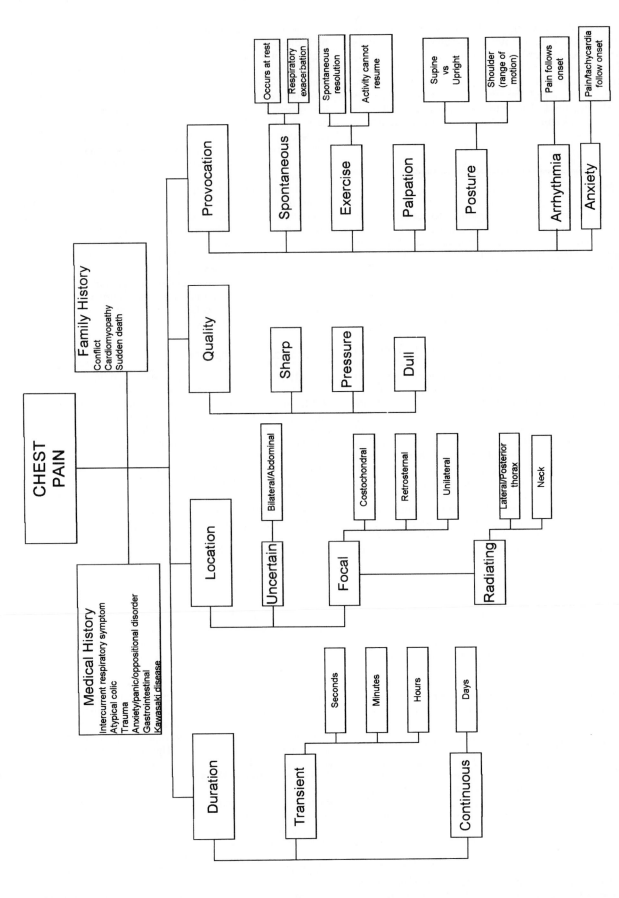

Figure 37-6 ■ Algorithm for assessment of chest pain in the pediatric population. There is considerable overlap in clinical expression of functional and organic causes of chest pain. Their discrimination, however, is facilitated by a systematic approach that begins with the patient's medical and family history, followed by determination of symptom duration, localization, quality, and inciting or provocative factors. The majority of benign chest pain referred for pediatric cardiology assessment includes a noncontributory medical history with no organic family history. The duration of pain is reported as seconds, the location is vague and referred primarily to anterior chest wall bilaterally, and the quality is sharp or knife-like and exacerbated by deep respiration. It resolves spontaneously in minutes with voluntary resumption of full activity.

sponds to the site and extent of inflammatory reaction or in the case of spontaneous pneumothorax, the site of the pleural injury. Localizing pain due to pericardial inflammation is dependent on the extent of pericardial inflammation and innervation of adjacent noncardiac structures. The visceral and parietal pericardium have few pain receptors; however, secondary inflammation of well innervated, contiguous parietal pleura radiates pericardial discomfort along the anterior and posterior intercostal muscle segments and upper abdomen. Shoulder pain with pericarditis is secondary to inflammation of the inferior parietal pericardium and contiguous central tendon of the diaphragm.

Anginal pain of myocardial ischemia is rare in the pediatric population. Esophageal dysfunction or inflammation may simulate angina-like discomfort. In older communicative patients, angina is reported as being retrosternal or parasternal, radiating across the precordium and extending to the arm, neck, or jaw. Coronary artery anomalies that may present with angina-like symptoms can be anticipated with knowledge of the patient's medical or surgical history. Coronary artery stenosis related to coronary artery aneurysms following Kawasaki syndrome (Kato et al., 1996); less commonly, narrowing of coronary arteries after reimplantation during surgical correction of congenital cardiac anomalies (anatomic correction of D-transposition of the great arteries, Ross procedure for complex aortic stenosis); and congenital anomalies of the coronary arteries provide the small subset of pediatric patients at risk for coronary artery ischemic symptoms.

Quality of Pain

The quality of chest pain (ie, sharp, aching, or pressure-like) is also influenced by the patient's communicative skills.

● **Clinical Pearl:** Benign musculoskeletal chest pain is sharp or stabbing in quality but lasts only seconds. The quality of the pain is often amplified with inspiration, resulting in the patient's observation that the pain is associated with shortness of breath. The transitional waning quality following the sharp pain of pleural injury from spontaneous pneumothorax is lacking with benign chest discomfort.

The quality of chest pain associated with pleural or pericardial inflammation is nonspecific. It typically lacks the sharpness of transient musculoskeletal discomfort or crescendo/decrescendo quality of acute pleural injury. Pleural and pericardial pain are usually reported as a persistent aching discomfort amplified by respiratory movement and supine posture.

In contrast to adults, the pressure-like tightness of angina is uncommon, reflecting the rarity of coronary artery ischemia in children and adolescents.

● **Clinical Pearl:** A complaint of chest tightness, in the absence of relevant medical or family history, is often related to reactive airway disease. The frequent association of reactive airway disease with exercise creates a distracting scenario of exercise-induced chest tightness in a pediatric patient.

While the adult with similar symptoms will likely require evaluation for coronary artery disease, exercise-induced reactive airway disease requiring appropriate bronchodilator therapy is more likely in the younger population.

Rarely, angina-like chest pain is reported in older adolescents with classic mitral valve prolapse. The discomfort is precordial and may radiate to the left arm. The cause of this symptom complex is uncertain; however, it is usually observed only in patients with clear evidence of mitral valve prolapse on physical examination.

▲ **Clinical Warning:** Crying and diaphoresis, particularly with feeding; atypical colic; and poor weight gain are indicative of the precordial pain experienced by the young infant with anomalous origin of the left coronary artery and its attendant myocardial ischemia.

These infants experience recurrent myocardial ischemia secondary to diversion of coronary blood from the myocardium through an anomalous communication to the lower pressure pulmonary circulation. Recognition of this uncommon anomaly is challenging and requires a high index of suspicion when an infant has atypical colic.

Provocation

The provocation of chest pain by palpation, activity, particular posture, or anxiety related to stressful situations assists the provider in identifying its cause.

● **Clinical Pearl:** Pain evoked with palpation of the chest along the anterior costochondral junctions is relatively specific for benign costochondritis or Tietze's syndrome (Mukamel et al., 1997).

● **Clinical Pearl:** Chest pain in the older child and adolescent provoked by sustained exercise is most commonly of benign musculoskeletal origin. Unlike the angina complex experienced by the adult with coronary artery disease, the chest pain in pediatric patients provoked by exercise is typically sharp in quality, localized to the right or left anterior inferior chest, and transiently amplified with inspiration.

Resolution of discomfort and respiratory symptoms follows discontinuation of activity. These patients often resume the activity that precipitated the symptoms with no return of discomfort.

Respiratory effort or posture classically provokes chest pain secondary to pleural or pericardial inflammation or injury.

● **Clinical Pearl:** Patients with viral pericarditis will typically prefer sitting, leaning slightly forward to avoid the accentuation of discomfort provoked by recumbent posture (Reese & Betts, 1996).

The sudden acute pleural pain associated with spontaneous pneumothorax may follow intense coughing or Valsalva's maneuver. The pain following the acute pleural injury is exacerbated with inspiratory chest motion.

Chest discomfort may be preceded by palpitations or sustained acceleration of the heart rate. It is necessary for the clinician to identify clearly the pain-rhythm sequence. Acute anxiety attacks or anxiety about benign chest pain is often associated with a rapid pulse rate that gradually returns to normal. Chest pain associated with accelerated atrial or ventricular tachyarrhythmias follows the onset of the abnormal rhythm, is crescendo-like if the rate remains high, and resolves following an acute change in the pulse rate.

Physical Examination

Physical examination of a patient following an episode of chest pain is often inconclusive. Frequently no abnormalities, except perhaps for tenderness over a costochondral junction, are identified in subjects with benign musculoskeletal pain. Physical examination of a patient reporting chest pain with an accelerated rhythm will be unrevealing unless the rapid rhythm persists or the pulse is irregular. Phenotypic features of Marfan syndrome, including abnormal visual acuity with arachnodactyly, pectus excavatum, thoracolumbar scoliosis, and abdominal wall hernias, should be noted in patients presenting with spontaneous pneumothorax. Asymmetry of peripheral pulses may reveal past vasculitis secondary to earlier Kawasaki syndrome. Resting or sleeping tachycardia with auscultatory evidence of a pericardial friction rub supports a diagnosis of myopericarditis, particularly with the patient reluctant to remain recumbent during the examination. Physical examination of the patient with pericarditis must include precordial auscultation with the subject in supine, left lateral decubitus, and upright positions.

▲ **Clinical Warning:** The absence of a pericardial rub does not necessarily exclude the diagnosis of pericarditis. A pericardial friction rub is audible when there is apposition of visceral and parietal pericardium or pericardial adhesions. No rub may be audible if a large, circumferential pericardial effusion is present.

Findings on physical examination of the infant with anomalies of coronary circulation vary according to the degree of myocardial dysfunction. The abnormal communication between the coronary artery and pulmonary circulation will not likely be audible. However, as myocardial dysfunction evolves due to increasing myocardial ischemia or infarction over the first few months of life, the infant will be pale, diaphoretic, tachycardic, and tachypneic with an apical systolic murmur of mitral insufficiency and congestive heart failure.

Diagnostic Criteria

A complete medical and family history and a thorough review of the symptomatology are usually sufficient to establish a diagnosis and minimize the need for additional studies or consultations. When the patient history, description of discomfort, and physical examination suggest benign musculoskeletal discomfort, including costochondritis, no further testing is necessary. Diagnostic investigations are advised for the evaluation of chest pain in patients with medical or family histories that increase the probability of an organic etiology.

Diagnostic investigation of chest pain related to pericarditis includes an ECG to identify ST-T wave abnormalities and a chest x-ray to assess cardiac size and exclude pulmonary parenchymal disease. A two-dimensional echocardiogram to examine the size of the pericardial effusion, presence of pericardial thickening, and status of left ventricular function is indicated. Symptoms due to pericardial irritation may not be proportionate to the volume of pericardial effusion demonstrated on two-dimensional echocardiogram. It is not uncommon for the initial cardiac ultrasound to demonstrate a nominal pericardial collection despite notable symptoms. Initial laboratory data should also include a complete blood count and an erythrocyte sedimentation rate to be used for monitoring the clinical response to anti-inflammatory therapy.

With pericarditis, acquisition of additional diagnostic studies, including liver function profile, serum amylase, monospot, and viral titers, is guided by the patient's subsequent clinical course. While commonly acquired during the acute and convalescent phase of the illness, viral titers primarily provide epidemiologic surveillance. Their results have limited impact on the management of uncomplicated acute pericarditis.

Laboratory studies for atypical chest pain related to tachycardia or associated with irregular rhythm begins with an ECG to identify cardiac rhythm and AV conduction. Absence of pre-excitation on the routine ECG does not exclude an AV node bypass tract. Twenty four-hour Holter monitoring of the cardiac rhythm or, depending on clinical suspicion and frequency of symptoms, patient-activated event recorder surveillance for extended periods of observation will help identify rhythm and conduction anomalies not apparent on routine ECG. Dynamic exercise testing is reserved for patients with exercise-provoked chest pain and evidence of rhythm or conduction anomalies.

Management

Patients with chest pain due to benign musculoskeletal etiologies require only reassurance. The clinician should emphasize that the cause of the pain is muscular and is not of cardiac origin. Costochondritis may be treated with nonsteroidal anti-inflammatory drugs.

▲ **Clinical Warning:** Patients presenting with chest pain, palpitations, and sustained tachycardia or syncope; evidence of large pericardial effusion on cardiac ultrasound; or anginal symptoms should be referred for immediate pediatric cardiology consultation.

Referral to a pediatric cardiologist should be considered in cases of diagnostic uncertainty or when parental or patient anxiety appears excessive.

SYNCOPE

Syncope, a transient loss of consciousness and postural tone, is a common clinical problem (Driscoll et al., 1997; Tanel & Walsh, 1997). The causes span the clinical spectrum of benign breath-holding spells in toddlers to the ominous syncope varsity athletes experience during athletic competition. Practitioners must triage symptomatic patients with an understanding of etiologies ranging from benign to potentially life threatening. This discussion focuses on syncope of cardiac origin that yields decreased effective systemic blood flow, resulting in cerebral hypoperfusion or hypoxemia.

Pathology

Cardiac syncope may be a consequence of abnormal neurocardiogenic reflexes, abnormal cardiac anatomy, or abnormal cardiac rhythm. Whatever the cause, it alters systemic venous tone, systemic arterial blood pressure, or heart rate.

Neurocardiogenic Reflexes

Neurocardiogenic syncope is a term that includes vasovagal syncope or simple fainting. It is characterized by a transient loss of consciousness related to a noxious situational stimulus, such as blood drawing, high ambient temperature, or acute or prolonged upright posture. Prodromal features include lightheadedness, visual changes, nausea, and pallor. Neurocardiogenic syncope is classified according to the primary hemodynamic perturbation: cardioinhibitory syncope if sinus bradycardia is dominant, vasodepressor if systemic hypotension is dominant, or mixed response when both sinus bradycardia and systemic hypotension are present. Neurocardiogenic syncope mediated by a cardioinhibitory response begins with profound sinus bradycardia, sometimes continuing to a brief period of asystole (Fig. 37-7). Systemic hypotension, regardless of the dominant hemodynamic problem, results in cerebral ischemia and loss of consciousness. Tonic-clonic activity of the extremities may occur with neurocardiogenic syncope if cerebral hypoperfusion and hypoxia are sustained. In contrast to the postictal confusion following a generalized seizure, recovery from reflex-mediated cardiac syncope is rapid when the individual returns to a recumbent position with no motor deficits following the episode.

● **Clinical Pearl:** Syncope in patients ages 8 to 21 years is usually secondary to a neurocardiac-mediated reflex response to upright posture (exaggerated Bezold-Jarisch reflex) (Lewis & Dhala, 1999) or noxious stimulus.

Anomalies of Cardiac Anatomy

Syncope due to abnormal cardiovascular anatomy is a consequence of inadequate pulmonary blood flow and hypoxia, left ventricular outflow obstruction, or arrhythmias secondary to myocardial ischemia. Prior to surgical intervention, TOF is the most common cause of cardiac syncope in infants and toddlers. Syncope due to fixed left ventricular outflow obstruction (eg, valvar or subvalvar aortic stenosis) is uncommon in children and adolescents. Usually, the systolic ejection murmur of fixed left ventricular outflow tract stenosis prompts early referral to a pediatric cardiologist before outflow tract obstruction is severe enough to compromise cardiac output.

▲ **Clinical Warning:** In patients with idiopathic hypertrophic cardiomyopathy, dynamic left ventricular outflow obstruction may be more subtle and not clinically apparent until syncope or death occurs.

Syncope due to primary pulmonary hypertension is an uncommon but life-threatening manifestation of occlusive changes in the intraparenchymal pulmonary arterioles.

Abnormal proliferation of the media and endothelium of the pulmonary arterioles reduces pulmonary blood flow and left ventricular diastolic filling, resulting in reduction of cardiac output. Syncope may occur with an acute increase in pulmonary vascular resistance and reduction in pulmonary blood flow or peripheral systemic vasodilatation.

● **Clinical Pearl:** Congenital anomalies of coronary artery anatomy are uncommon, but when present, they may be arrhythmogenic and cause syncope.

While anomalous origin of the left coronary artery from the pulmonary circulation is typically a clinical problem in infancy, it may first manifest itself with ventricular ectopy and possible syncope in later childhood or adolescence. Arrhythmogenic congenital coronary artery anomalies also include those where a coronary artery arises from the aorta but courses abnormally between the great vessels. Vigorous physical activity, particularly in adolescence, compresses the coronary artery between the aorta and main pulmonary artery, producing myocardial ischemia and possible high-grade ventricular ectopy.

Anomalies of Cardiac Rhythm

Arrhythmias, particularly sustained tachyarrhythmias or bradyarrhythmias, may be responsible for syncope at any age in the pediatric population. These rhythm-related syncopal episodes may initially but falsely be considered neurocardiogenic in origin.

● **Clinical Pearl:** Abnormality in cardiac rhythm should be considered in patients with seizures having an atypical or absent prodrome, unusual tonic-clonic activity, or an absent postictal recovery phase. While breath holding and seizures are more common, atypical presentations of either should prompt cardiology consultation.

The practitioner should consider complicating arrhythmias when seizures are reported in a patient following surgical correction or palliation of congenital cardiovascular anomalies. This is particularly relevant in TOF and left ventricular outflow reconstruction.

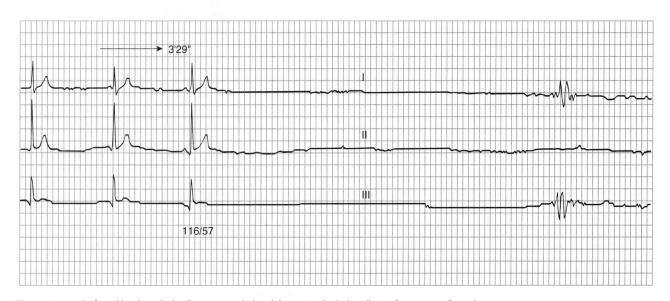

Figure 37–7 ■ Profound bradycardia leading to asystole in adolescent male during tilt test for neurocardiogenic syncope.

● **Clinical Pearl:** In general, the practitioner should consider rhythm-related cardiac syncope when a patient experiences unprovoked, precipitous loss of consciousness.

Wolf-Parkinson-White syndrome, prolonged QT syndrome, arrhythmogenic right ventricular dysplasia, sinus node dysfunction, and AV block all may present with syncope. Syncope due to ventricular arrhythmias is an ominous event (Leenhardt et al., 1995). The idiopathic varieties are most common; however, a subgroup of such patients has been identified with fibro-fatty infiltration and thinning of the right ventricular myocardium on MRI examination. The practitioner also must recognize that syncope with complex ventricular arrhythmias, including polymorphic ventricular tachycardia with torsades de pointes, may be a consequence of drug therapies combining histamine blockers and macrolide antibiotics or intentional antidepressant overdosing (Fig. 37-8).

Syncope related to complete heart block is uncommon in the absence of previous cardiac surgery. Trauma to the AV node or adjacent His bundle during surgical closure of a subaortic or AV canal type of VSD may result in transient or permanent AV block. This typically occurs in the immediate postoperative period. Spontaneous heart block may occur in otherwise asymptomatic patients with L transposition of the great vessels ("corrected transposition") and ventricular inversion. Complete heart block in the neonatal population with normal cardiac architecture is most often associated with immune-mediated maternal connective tissue disease. Infants of mothers with variants of systemic lupus erythematosis are exposed in utero to teratogenic transplacentally acquired anti-Ro and anti-La antibodies. These antibodies preferentially injure the fetal AV node, resulting in complete heart block in the fetus and neonate.

● **Clinical Pearl:** Autoimmune studies should be performed on an asymptomatic mother who gives birth to an infant with complete heart block to identify occult systemic lupus erythematosis (Waltuck & Buyon, 1994; Saleeb et al., 1999).

Acquired complete heart block may complicate bacterial, rickettsial, or viral infections. Diphtheria is now virtually absent from western clinical pediatrics, but Lyme disease, Rocky Mountain spotted fever, and viral myocarditis are seen in many regions. These diseases have been associated with acquired AV conduction anomalies.

History and Physical Examination

Clinical evaluation of the pediatric or adolescent patient following a syncopal episode begins with documentation of the circumstances related to the event. The clinician must consider the patient's past medical and family history, time of day and activity immediately preceding the episode, prodromal symptoms, duration of syncope, and pattern of recovery.

History

Benign neurocardiogenic syncope is most common in adolescence with a peak incidence of 15 and 19 years of age (Driscoll et al., 1997). It is typically associated with a noncontributory past medical history. A temporally related noxious stimulus, intercurrent viral illness, prolonged upright posture (sitting or standing), warm ambient temperature, pallor, sweating, and nausea are often identified. Such syncopal episodes are self-limiting with spontaneous recovery once the patient is supine. Immediate recurrences may occur when the patient does not remain recumbent long enough during recovery. Tonic-clonic activity may be observed when the duration of hypotension and cerebral hypoperfusion is prolonged. Following recovery, the patient should be able to resume customary activities without the fatigue or somnolence that follows generalized seizures of epileptiform etiology.

While the prodrome preceding syncope due to hypoglycemia may parallel that of neurocardiogenic syncope, discriminating between the two should be possible by reviewing the patient's dietary schedule. Benign neurocardiogenic

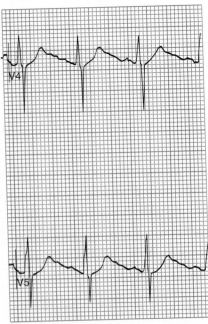 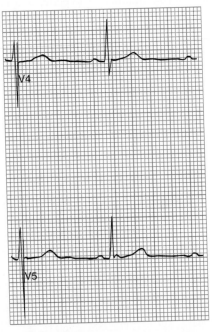

Figure 37–8 ■ *(Left)* Precordial leads recorded on adolescent female following imipramine (Tofranil) overdose demonstrating distortion of T wave and prolongation of QT interval. *(Right)* Same patient following treatment with magnesium and normalization of T wave morphology and QT interval.

syncope may occur at earlier ages. However, added consideration should be given to rhythm abnormalities and arrhythmogenic congenital cardiac anomalies when syncope is reported in patients younger than 8 years.

▲ **Clinical Warning:** Sudden loss of consciousness or change in sensorium, particularly with exercise, should expedite evaluation of a cardiac etiology for the syncopal event.

It is not uncommon for the family history of an adolescent with benign syncope to include a history of syncope in a parent during adolescence or young adulthood. A positive history in first- or second-degree relatives of early death in childhood or adolescence or of syncope with deafness should direct attention to arrhythmogenic prolonged QT syndrome, hypertrophic cardiomyopathy, and Wolf-Parkinson-White syndrome.

Syncope with exercise or activity should prompt evaluation for a dynamic cause of left ventricular outflow obstruction, such as idiopathic hypertrophic cardiomyopathy.

Physical Examination

The physical examination following transient syncope is often unremarkable unless an underlying anatomic anomaly is present.

Tetralogy of Fallot

During a hypercyanotic episode in an infant with TOF, variation in the auscultatory findings is common. As the hypercyanotic episode evolves, the initial coarse systolic ejection murmur at the left upper sternal border softens and may disappear. It is generally accepted that this transition in the physical examination is due to reversible, dynamic subpulmonic obstruction superimposed on the fixed right ventricular outflow obstruction.

Left Ventricular Outflow Obstruction

The systolic crescendo/decrescendo ejection murmur at the left midsternal and right upper sternal borders due to fixed valvar or subvalvar aortic stenosis is relatively constant in intensity. A palpable thrill at the suprasternal notch and active apical impulse may accompany auscultatory findings.

Findings on physical examination of patients with near syncope due dynamic subaortic stenosis are similar to those with fixed left ventricular outflow obstruction but vary more with reduction in left ventricular diastolic filling associated with Valsalva's maneuver and changing posture. These include variation in intensity of the left midsternal and right upper sternal systolic ejection murmur generated by left ventricular outflow obstruction. Upright posture and Valsalva's maneuvers decrease systemic venous return to the heart, decrease left ventricular volumes, and exaggerate obstruction of the left ventricular outflow tract, increasing the intensity of the ejection type murmur.

Coronary Artery Anomalies

The physical examination of patients with congenital coronary artery anomalies is usually unrevealing, unless an apical systolic mitral insufficiency murmur secondary to papillary muscle dysfunction is present. When the left coronary artery arises from the right sinus of Valsalva of the aorta and courses between the great vessels, myocardial ischemia and related arrhythmias due to mechanical compression with vigorous exercise are not apparent at rest.

▲ **Clinical Warning:** It is imperative for the clinician to appreciate that the patient with hypertrophic cardiomyopathy or a congenital coronary artery anomaly may present with a deceptively innocent physical examination. Absence of a systolic ejection murmur does not exclude hypertrophic cardiomyopathy. Coronary artery anomalies responsible for myocardial ischemia with dynamic exercise are typically silent on routine physical examination or resting ECG. Identifying such potentially life-threatening abnormalities requires pursuing the reason for the syncopal episode despite the normal findings on physical examination.

Pulmonary Hypertension

The physical examination of patients with idiopathic pulmonary artery hypertension (pulmonary hypertension not due to a preexisting intracardiac anomaly and shunt) reflects right ventricular hypertrophy and dilation, elevation in pulmonary artery pressure, and tricuspid or pulmonary valve insufficiency. These findings are a consequence of the thickening of pulmonary arterioles, increasing pulmonary vascular resistance, and decreasing pulmonary blood flow. A prominent cardiac impulse due to right ventricular enlargement is often palpable along the left sternal border with a loud, single second heart sound, tricuspid insufficiency systolic regurgitant murmur at the left lower sternal border, or high-frequency pulmonary insufficiency diastolic murmur at the left upper sternal border murmur. If the foramen ovale is patent, the patient may be cyanotic due to right-to-left interatrial shunting.

Patency of the foramen ovale in a patient with primary pulmonary artery hypertension is somewhat protective in preventing syncope and symptoms of low systemic cardiac output. Severe pulmonary vascular disease reduces pulmonary venous return to the left atrium. This decreased pulmonary venous return reduces the filling pressure of the left atrium, allowing shunting of desaturated blood from the right to left atrium. This shunting preserves diastolic filling of the left ventricle systemic cardiac output at the expense of cyanosis. A curious but infrequent finding in patients with primary pulmonary artery hypertension is the presence hoarseness. This uncommon finding is secondary to mechanical distortion of the recurrent laryngeal nerve as it courses around the ductal ligament adjacent to the markedly dilated branch pulmonary arteries.

Abnormal Cardiac Rhythms

The physical examination is typically normal with syncope related to anomalies in sinus and AV node function or atrial and ventricular tachyarrhythmias. An irregular pulse may be the only indication of an underlying rhythm anomaly. Bradycardia is associated with sinus or AV node dysfunction. However, it is a nonspecific finding common among adolescent athletes. As a normal variant, sinus bradycardia is readily accelerated with low-level exercise during the physical examination. Sustained sinus bradycardia with prominent U wave and prolongation of the QT interval is a feature of prolonged QT syndrome in the neonate. The neonate is at the same risk as older patients with prolonged QT syndrome for torsades de pointes with polymorphic ventricular tachycardia. Sinus bradycardia is not a feature of prolonged QT syndrome in the older child or adolescent. The physical examination in these patients is typically unremarkable unless there is associated deafness, which suggests that the Jervell-Lange-Nielsen variant of the syndrome is also present.

Diagnostic Studies

Laboratory investigation of the adolescent patient reporting an isolated episode of syncope related to a sudden change in posture, noxious stimuli, or prolonged upright posture in a warm environment with a noncontributory medical or family history and a normal physical examination should be limited. The indications for tilt testing of older children and adolescents are not standardized, and such investigation is usually reserved for individuals with recurrent episodes of neurocardiogenic syncope requiring medical, or rarely surgical (pacemaker implantation), intervention (Benditt et al., 1996).

Electrocardiogram Findings

Obtaining cardiovascular consultation of a syncopal event is warranted when the syncopal prodrome is atypical, the event is precipitous, or there is an obvious rhythm anomaly. Initial evaluation by the primary clinician should include a standard 12-lead ECG. Prominent right ventricular forces, right axis deviation, and evidence of right ventricular strain suggest pulmonary hypertension. Prominent left ventricular hypertrophy and septal Q waves with intraventricular conduction anomalies are consistent with hypertrophic cardiomyopathy (Fig. 37-9). Ventricular pre-excitation with Wolf-Parkinson-White syndrome includes a shortened PR interval, "slurring" of the QRS upstroke by a delta wave, and nonspecific ST-T wave anomalies. The ECG in Figure 37-10 was recorded on an adolescent male with no history of cardiovascular abnormalities who experienced cardiac arrest after running the bases during a baseball game. Typical slurring of the R wave due to an accessory pathway bypassing the AV node is present. Following successful cardiopulmonary resuscitation, the patient underwent electrophysiologic cardiac catheterization and radio-frequency ablation of the abnormal bypass tract (see Fig. 37-10). Prolongation of the rate-corrected and age-adjusted QT interval, often with a prominent U wave, is evident in patients with prolonged QT syndrome and certain drug ingestions. Figure 37-11 was recorded in a newborn noted to have persistent fetal sinus bradycardia. The slow sinus rate with abnormal T-U wave morphology and prolonged QTc interval reflect the repolarization anomaly. A pacemaker was placed in this patient to

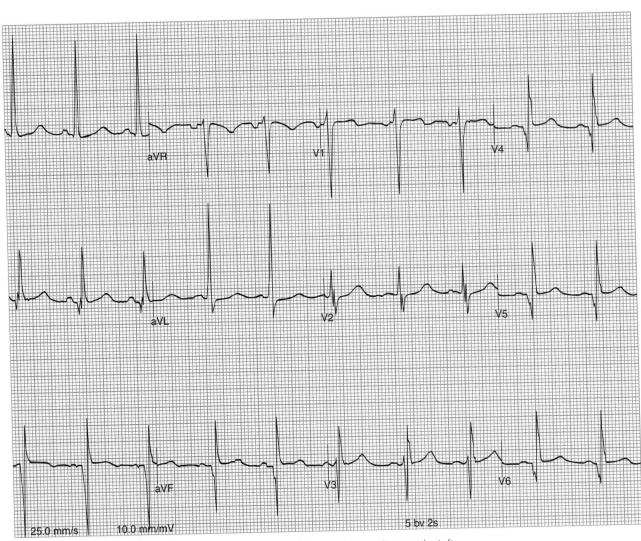

Figure 37–9 ■ Twelve-lead electrocardiogram in adolescent female with hypertrophic cardiomyopathy. Left ventricular hypertrophy with prominent Q waves in limb and precordial leads suggest significant thickening of the interventricular septum and global left ventricular hypertrophy.

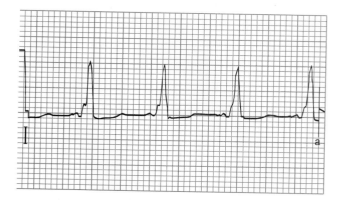

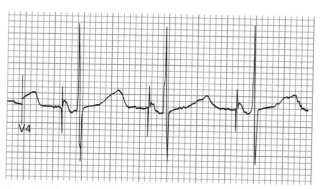

Figure 37–11 ■ Lead V4 from electrocardiogram of neonate with long QT syndrome requiring transvenous atrial pacemaker implantation to control associated bradycardia.

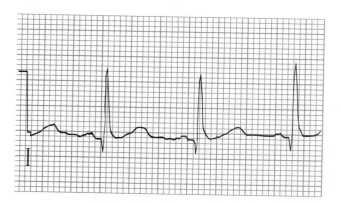

Figure 37–10 ■ *(Upper panel)* Lead I from electrocardiogram in adolescent male with previously unrecognized Wolff-Parkinson-White syndrome. The PR interval is shortened with slurring of the R wave secondary to a bypass tract between the atrium and ventricle. *(Lower panel)* Lead I from electrocardiogram of above patient following successful ablation of the bypass tract with catheter delivered radio-frequency "burn" to anomalous conduction pathway.

control a progressively decreasing heart rate following initiation of beta blockade therapy to prevent polymorphic ventricular tachycardia (ie, torsades de pointes). Aggressive intervention was guided by a family history of unexplained death in childhood in two second-degree relatives.

Abnormalities in sinus node function or AV conduction may not be manifest on the standard ECG. Additional ECG surveillance includes ambulatory 24-hour Holter monitoring to identify asymptomatic rhythm anomalies. Longer term, patient-activated, ambulatory surveillance using a transtele-

phonic event recorder (Fig. 37-12) is a consideration for patients with a negative Holter recording and a compelling clinical suspicion of rhythm-related syncope.

Other Diagnostic Tests

Exercise-related syncope may be due to prolonged QT syndrome, idiopathic hypertrophic cardiomyopathy, an uncommon variant of neurocardiogenic syncope (Tanel & Walsh, 1997), or arrhythmogenic congenital coronary artery anomalies. Dynamic exercise testing may contribute to the evaluation of patients with bypass tracts that do not manifest on ECG. Exercise testing of patients in which idiopathic hypertrophic cardiomyopathy is a consideration should only be performed after cardiac ultrasound. Exercise testing of patients with equivocal prolongation of the QT interval should be approached with caution given the arrhythmogenic quality of such provocation when abnormal repolarization is present.

Imaging

The contribution of noninvasive cardiac imaging to management of patients with an isolated episode of syncope associated with a noncontributory past medical or family history, normal physical examination, and normal 12-lead ECG is limited. The standard chest x-ray typically does not contribute to the evaluation of benign syncope in patients with a normal physical examination and a 12-lead ECG. Primary pulmonary hypertension is often associated with dilatation of the right atrium, right ventricle, and main pulmonary artery segment on the routine chest x-ray; findings with idiopathic hyper-

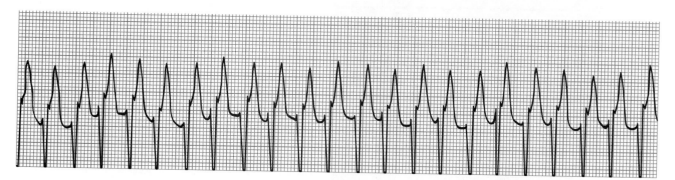

Figure 37–12 ■ Transtelephonic electrogram obtained with event recorder by adolescent male who reported sudden acceleration of his heart rate and near syncope while standing in outfield during baseball game. Tracing documents a relatively narrow complex tachycardia at a rate of 180 beats per minute.

trophic cardiomegaly are usually limited, consisting of mild cardiomegaly with left ventricular prominence.

● **Clinical Pearl:** Two-dimensional echocardiography is the noninvasive screening imaging modality of choice for patients with syncope.

It should, however, be reserved for patients with a relevant family history, organic systolic ejection or regurgitant murmurs, or ECG findings of ventricular hypertrophy or strain. Two-dimensional echocardiography readily displays the magnitude of left ventricular hypertrophy and outflow tract stenosis associated with either fixed or dynamic obstruction (Fig. 37-13). In patients with primary pulmonary artery hypertension, two-dimensional echocardiography displays the dilated, hypertrophied right ventricle; dilated central pulmonary artery vessels; and abnormal posterior systolic bowing of the interventricular septum. Simultaneous Doppler quantitation of tricuspid and pulmonary valve pressure gradients provides an estimate of pulmonary artery pressure.

Arrhythmogenic congenital anomalies of the coronary arteries are identified by combining two-dimensional and color flow Doppler imaging. Anomalous origin of a coronary artery from the pulmonary circulation with retrograde blood flow in the vessel and the anomalous course of a coronary artery between the great vessels are visible with cardiac ultrasound imaging techniques used in most pediatric echocardiography laboratories (Johnsrude et al., 1995).

Management

Management of all but simple neurocardiogenic syncope should be initiated in consultation with a pediatric cardiologist. In patients with isolated neurocardiogenic syncope, initial management should address control of inciting events with appropriate oral fluid and salt supplementation (Salim & DiSessa, 1996). Therapies beyond such basic interventions should be guided by findings on tilt testing that discriminate between vasodepressor, cardioinhibitory, and mixed types of mechanisms for neurocardiogenic syncope (Balaji et al., 1994; Salim et al., 1998).

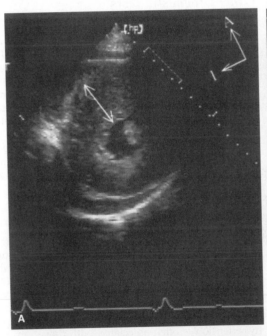

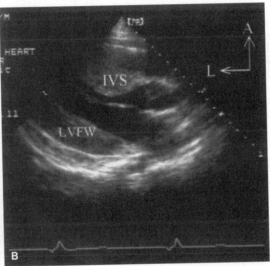

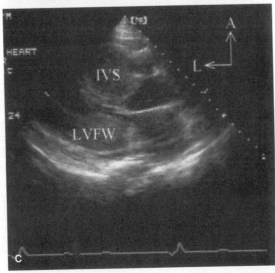

Figure 37–13 ■ *(A)* Parasternal short axis echocardiogram in adolescent female with severe hypertrophic cardiomyopathy. The interventricular septum (IVS) is greater than 3.5 cm in thickness. A, Anterior; I, inferior. *(B)* Same patient with left heart displayed in parasternal long axis projection demonstrating anterior, opened position of the anterial mitral leaflet between the interventricular septum (IVS) and left ventricular free wall (LVFW). A, Anterior; L, Left. *(C)* During systole the mitral leaflets buckle and obstruct the subaortic left ventricular outflow tract.

Diagnosis and management of syncope due to anomalies of sinus or AV node conduction (complete heart block, ventricular pre-excitation), ventricular repolarization (prolonged QT syndrome), arrhythmogenic hypertrophic cardiomyopathy, congenital coronary artery anomalies, and pulmonary artery hypertension require close collaboration between the primary clinician and pediatric cardiologist.

Treatment of tachyarrhythmias must include identification of provocative medications, including bronchodilators and decongestant sympathomimetics, and excessive consumption of caffeine-containing beverages. Pediatric cardiology referral is customary once provocative iatrogenic or dietary causes have been excluded in the patient presenting with a history of recurrent episodes of accelerated heart rate.

Therapy for supraventricular and ventricular tachyarrhythmias must balance the rate, frequency, and severity of symptoms with the potential complications of therapy. A diverse clinical spectrum of pediatric tachyarrhythmias exists. The clinician must be prepared to evaluate the clinically compromised infant with a narrow complex tachycardia of >180 beats per minute requiring intravenous adenosine therapy; the adolescent with anecdotally brief, self-limiting episodes of narrow complex supraventricular tachycardia; or the adolescent with sustained supraventricular tachycardia with pre-excitation on resting ECG requiring interventional electrophysiologic bypass tract ablation. Syncope associated with such anomalies requires expedited assessment and timely medical or surgical intervention. Patients with atypical syncope, particularly that related to exercise, should modify their participation in competitive athletics until the risk from such provocative activity is assessed.

● **Clinical Pearl:** The familial component of idiopathic hypertrophic cardiomyopathy and prolonged QT syndrome warrants screening of asymptomatic first-degree relatives by two-dimensional echocardiography and ECG respectively.

Investigation is ongoing to identify genetic markers associated with both these abnormalities, and the practitioner should monitor and apply advances in such research to index cases and family members (Towbin et al., 1994).

RHEUMATIC FEVER

Acute rheumatic fever is a diagnostic and therapeutic challenge for clinicians; its incidence in North America and Europe has decreased over the past 50 years. In 1944, Dr. T. Duckett Jones recognized the diagnostic dilemma posed by ARF and proposed guidelines for its diagnosis that have endured to date with only modest revisions. Successful management of a primary attack and appropriate surveillance following recovery require accurate initial diagnosis and appropriate intervention. Failure to identify ARF may result in profound cardiac sequelae; however, its inaccurate, premature diagnosis will result in years of unnecessary antibiotic prophylaxis and medical stigma.

Pathology

Rheumatic fever is a multisystem disease of toddlers, children, adolescents, and adults occurring 2 to 6 weeks after a pharyngeal, not cutaneous, infection with group A beta-hemolytic *Streptococcus* (GABHS). It is extremely uncommon in people younger than 3 years. It is immunomodu-

lated, involving antibodies to the M protein coat of group A *Streptococcus* that cross-react with myocytes, cartilage, chondrocytes, synovium, connective tissue, and thalamic and subthalamic nuclei of the central nervous system (Janavs & Aminoff, 1998). This histologically broad band cross-reactivity contributes to the diagnostic dilemma of distinguishing ARF from post-streptococcal reactive arthritis, toxic synovitis of the hip, fibromyalgia, hysterical conversion reactions, and even neoplastic infiltration of bone (Schaller, 1996).

Epidemiology

Acute rheumatic fever is not a disease of the ages (Markowitz, 1998). Surveillance reports by Siegel and colleagues in 1961 identified a 3% occurrence rate of ARF following GABHS pharyngitis. While the incidence of ARF has decreased in developed countries, it remains a common cause of hospitalization for cardiac disease in patients ages 5 to 24 years worldwide (Ledford, 1997). The decline in incidence of ARF in the United States is purportedly due to an antigenic drift of GABHS and improved social conditions and access to medical care. The occurrence of ARF in North America is multifactorial and not completely moderated by family finance or social standing. Veasy et al. reported in 1994 that 84% of 274 confirmed cases of ARF referred to the Primary Children's Hospital of Salt Lake City over 7 years were from middle-class families, with only 17% having sought medical care for an antecedent sore throat. Endemic areas prevail in the United States at rates comparable to those in the 1960s, and immigration of populations from undeveloped countries provides a durable source of new cases.

History and Physical Examination

Arthritis

Arthritis is the most commonly encountered major manifestation of ARF. Its occurrence varies with age: adults, 95% to 100%; adolescents, 82%,; and children, 66% (Ledford, 1997). Joint involvement is a true arthritis, not arthralgia, and includes swelling, redness, tenderness, and limited mobility. It is a self-limiting process, which untreated lasts for 4 to 6 weeks with few sequelae.

Carditis

The likelihood of developing carditis with an initial episode of ARF varies inversely with age. It is present in more than 90% of children, one third of adolescents, and less than 20% of adults with ARF. The cardiac examination during an acute or recurrent episode of rheumatic fever depends on the degree of cardiac involvement. The course of acute rheumatic carditis appears more fulminant in younger patients; the need for ionotropic support and afterload reduction therapy is a frequent consideration. Pancarditis with involvement of the pericardium, myocardium, and valvular endocardium is the hallmark of rheumatic carditis.

● **Clinical Pearl:** When ARF is a consideration, the clinician's examination should begin with simple observation of the patient's supine resting (or sleeping) pulse rate. An accelerated pulse rate that is out of proportion to fever or cardiac function is a nonspecific but useful marker of myocarditis.

Evaluation of the pericardium requires auscultation of the precordium with the patient supine, in lateral decubitis position, and in upright postures to identify the rub between the visceral and parietal pericardium and examine jugular venous distension. The presence of myopericarditis, even with ECG findings of decreased ventricular forces or ST-T wave changes, does not confirm a diagnosis of rheumatic carditis. Myopericarditis can be viral and may be associated with arthralgia and serologic findings that parallel those of ARF.

● **Clinical Pearl:** Valvulitis is the index finding of rheumatic carditis.

The more common blowing, apical systolic regurgitant murmur and mid-diastolic rumble of mitral insufficiency or the less frequent decrescendo diastolic murmur of aortic insufficiency at the right upper and left midsternal borders provide compelling diagnostic support for rheumatic carditis when large-joint, migratory polyarthritis is present. The practitioner should consider the potentially confounding auscultatory findings of functional, hemic flow murmurs and preexisting anomalies of the aortic (bicuspid valve) or mitral (classical prolapse with multiple apical systolic clicks) valves.

Chorea, Erythema Marginatum, and Subcutaneous Nodules

Sydenham's chorea, erythema marginatum, and subcutaneous nodules complete the clinical panorama of ARF. Central nervous system injury secondary to cross-reactivity of M protein antibodies with the thalamic and subthalamic nuclei results in purposeless, involuntary rapid choreiform movements of the trunk and extremities. Unilateral or bilateral choreiform activity may not be apparent for weeks to months following initial group A streptococcal pharyngitis. This delayed onset of chorea may obscure the temporal link between an antecedent streptococcal pharyngitis and neurologic symptoms. The prolonged latency between infection and development of symptoms may confuse the diagnosis between Sydenham's chorea and behavioral tics, athetosis, metabolic anomalies, psychiatric pathology, and PANDAS (pediatric autoimmune neuropsychiatric disorder associated with *Streptococcus*). The reader is referred to Chapter 34 for further discussion.

Erythema marginatum and cutaneous nodules are major manifestations of ARF that add little to the morbidity of an attack. The primary diagnostic consideration regarding the rare evanescent, pink rash that spares the face while involving the trunk and proximal extremities is its confusion with the cutaneous manifestations of rheumatoid arthritis. The nontender, firm subcutaneous nodules on the extensor surfaces of the extremities of patients with ARF are rare but reportedly associated with a greater incidence of carditis (Dajani, 1993).

Diagnostic Criteria

The diagnosis of ARF must conform to criteria established by Jones in 1944 and the modest contemporary revisions that others have added (Shiffman, 1995; Dajani, 1995). A high probability of ARF exists when two major criteria or one major criterion and two minor manifestations are present. Both diagnostic formulas require evidence of a preceding streptococcal infection. Major criteria include carditis, arthritis, chorea, erythema marginatum, or subcutaneous nodules. Minor diagnostic criteria include fever, arthralgia, a prolonged PR interval, and elevated acute phase reactants. According to these guidelines, carditis identified by physical examination should include auscultatory findings of mitral or aortic insufficiency.

Documentation of antecedent group A *Streptococcus* infection may be difficult when (1) medical attention is delayed, (2) a streptococcal carrier state exists (reportedly 15% in children up to age 4 years), or (3) chorea, occurring weeks or months after streptococcal infection, is the only clinically apparent major criterion. A positive throat culture or rapid strep antigen test may diagnose either current infection or the presence of a carrier state. Streptococcal antibody tests, including those for streptolysin O, deoxyribonuclease B, nicotinamide adenine dinucleotidase, hyaluronidase, and streptokinase antigens, also provide supportive evidence of antecedent streptococcal infection. Eighty percent of patients with group A *Streptococcus* infection will have a positive antistreptolysin-O (ASLO) assay with peak values at 2 to 6 weeks after exposure (Kaplan et al., 1998). Interpretation of ASLO and anti-DNAase B must consider subject age and regional prevalence of group A streptococcal infection. Kaplan and colleagues in 1998 examined ASLO and anti-DNase B titers in sera acquired within 1.8 days of onset of signs and symptoms of acute-onset documented GABHS pharyngitis among 1131 children. Geometric mean normal ASLO titers in this population from 23 states ranged from 100 todd units for 2- to 4-year-olds to 140 todd units for 12-year-olds with upper normal limit values of 120 and 320 todd units respectively. A similar age-related lower mean titer pattern was noted for anti-DNase B levels.

Exceptions to the established guidelines for diagnosis of ARF apply to patients with Sydenham's chorea, indolent carditis, or recurrence of rheumatic carditis. Chorea is a late-onset major manifestation of ARF and in some situations, may be the only criterion identified. The diagnostic problem is compounded by ambiguity in laboratory documentation of antecedent streptococcal exposure due to the time interval between exposure and onset of chorea. In patients with indolent rheumatic carditis, the initial attack was not recognized, and cardiac involvement has continued beyond the period during which major or minor manifestations can be identified. Definitive diagnosis of a recurrence of rheumatic fever is particularly difficult when findings from previous cardiac involvement persist. In those cases of recurrence where new onset aortic insufficiency is identified, this issue is less problematic. A certain diagnosis may not be possible in these three clinical circumstances and therefore a presumptive diagnosis of ARF is made, supported only by evidence of a single major or several minor manifestations.

Other common forms of arthritis in children need to be considered in the differential diagnosis. They include septic and rheumatoid arthritis, Lyme disease, reactive arthritis secondary to enteric bacterial infections or *Streptococcus*, or postinfectious arthritis secondary to a myriad of viral infections. In children, septic arthritis tends to be monoarticular, the exception being gonococcal arthritis. Lyme arthritis looks worse to the examiner than it feels to the patient, whereas the arthritis of ARF is exquisitely painful and feels worse than it looks. In juvenile rheumatoid arthritis, the joint stiffness tends to get better as the day wears on.

● **Clinical Pearl:** In ARF, the migratory polyarthropathy of the elbows, wrists, knees, or ankles is exquisitely sensitive to salicylate therapy, so much so that the diagnosis of ARF arthritis should be questioned in cases unresponsive to adequate salicylate therapy.

Reactive arthritis following a documented group A streptococcal pharyngitis may be difficult to distinguish from ARF in the absence of clinically apparent carditis. Short-term observation of such a patient is a reasonable alternative to premature exclusion or diagnosis of rheumatic fever. Earlier studies (Catanzanro et al., 1954) have demonstrated no substantive effect on outcome when rheumatic fever therapy was postponed for up to 9 days following onset of pharyngitis. Judicious use of anti-inflammatories may discriminate between the responsive arthritis of rheumatic fever and the more refractory arthropathy of post-streptococcal reactive arthritis. This problem with differential diagnosis is mitigated somewhat by the customary practice of penicillin prophylaxis for 1 year following an episode of post-streptococcal reactive arthritis (Dajani, 1995). From a practical clinical standpoint, the latter does not resolve the diagnostic dilemma so much as postpone a diagnostic commitment by the clinician and allow an extended period of observation.

As stated previously, myopericarditis is not specific to ARF and may be commonly seen in a variety of viral infections. The presence of endocarditis manifested by acute valvular disease excludes most viral infections but does not eliminate from consideration cases of bacterial endocarditis.

Diagnostic Studies

An ECG will demonstrate a prolonged PR interval reflecting myocardial inflammation. The role of noninvasive cardiac technology is limited. Cardiac ultrasound provides an indispensable window into cardiac anatomy and function for the general practitioner and pediatric cardiologist; however, its contribution to the diagnosis of ARF is restricted to confirmation but not diagnosis of carditis. Physiologic mitral and aortic insufficiency with no associated auscultatory findings are well recognized normal variants of valve function in the general pediatric and adult population. The only independent contribution of echocardiography to diagnosis and management of ARF is its documentation of pericardial inflammation and assessment of left ventricular dysfunction.

● **Clinical Pearl:** Doppler echocardiographic evidence of mitral or aortic insufficiency should only be considered confirmatory evidence of valvulitis when appropriate auscultatory findings are present on physical examination.

Management

Treatment of ARF is relatively straightforward. It focuses on the eradication of pharyngeal streptococcal infection, control of multiorgan inflammation, and prevention of recurrence secondary to GABHS reinfection. Prevention of an initial episode of ARF can be accomplished with a single weight-adjusted dose of intramuscular benzathine penicillin G or 10 days of oral penicillin administered within 9 days of the onset of symptoms of GABHS pharyngitis (Stollerman & Rusoff, 1952; Catanzanro et al., 1954). Therapy can be effected in penicillin-allergic patients with erythromycin estolate or azithromycin. The reader is referred to Chapter 34 for a more complete discussion of GABHS management.

Cardiac and joint inflammation is controlled with age- and weight-adjusted oral salicylate therapy. The use of corticosteroids, particularly methylprednisolone, is reserved for patients with carditis complicated by congestive heart failure due to either progressive mitral insufficiency or myocarditis. Supportive parenteral ionotropic therapy for myocardial dysfunction with afterload reduction to palliate mitral insufficiency is individualized according to the patient's clinical course. Bed rest is a mainstay of supportive therapy during recovery from clinically evident carditis. Anti-inflammatory therapy is continued until clinical evidence of arthritis and carditis has resolved and peak acute

phase reactant values have receded. The clinician should be wary of a recrudescence of inflammatory changes while weaning the recovering patient from anti-inflammatory therapy.

Acute rheumatic fever is a preventable disease if providers can counsel parents to seek prompt evaluation of sore throats in their children. Every practitioner is responsible to be vigilant in the diagnosis of GABHS.

▲ **Clinical Warning:** All clinicians should have a very low threshold for obtaining rapid strep antigen tests or throat cultures in their patients who either complain of sore throat or have pharyngitis on examination, even in the absence of fever.

Prevention of recurrences of ARF due to re-exposure to GABHS is founded in tradition and somewhat uncertain. Stollerman and Rusoff in 1952 reported their early experience with a repository penicillin therapy for the prophylaxis of rheumatic fever patients against group A streptococcal infection. Since then, monthly penicillin G benzathine (Bicillin Long-Acting) therapy has remained the standard of rheumatic fever prophylaxis. Alternative therapies include twice-daily oral erythromycin estolate when penicillin allergy is present and less desirable oral penicillin therapy for those reluctant to receive monthly intramuscular injections. Clinical studies in regions where rheumatic fever is prevalent have reviewed the conventional rheumatic fever prophylaxis schedule. In 1996, Lue et al. studied rheumatic fever recurrence rates in Asian patients comparing 3- and 4-week prophylaxis programs. These investigators identified a fivefold greater risk of prophylaxis failure in their population when administered at 4-week intervals.

● **Clinical Pearl:** Providers should consider the protection afforded by the 3-week interval for patients in endemic regions and those in nonendemic areas experiencing recurrent attacks on the customary 4-week protocol.

The duration of prophylaxis therapy to prevent recurrences of rheumatic fever is controversial. Currently the duration of prophylaxis is extended for young children and those in professions at risk for GABHS infection, such as school teachers and medical personnel. Current guidelines suggest a minimum of 10 years of prophylaxis extending to 40 years of age for those having had carditis (Dajani, 1995).

REFERENCES

Balaji, S., et al. (1994). Neurocardiogenic syncope in children with a normal heart. *Journal of the American College of Cardiology, 23,* 779–785.

Benditt, D. G., et al. (1996). Tilt table testing for assessing syncope. *Journal of the American College of Cardiology, 28,* 263-75.

Dajani, A. S., et al. (1993). Special Report: Guidelines for the diagnosis of rheumatic fever: Jones criteria, updated 1992: Special writing group of the Committee on Rheumatic Fever, Endocarditis, and Kawasaki disease of the Council on Cardiovascular Disease in the Young, American Heart Association. *Circulation, 87,* 302–307.

Dajani, A. S., et al. (1995). Treatment of acute streptococcal pharyngitis and prevention of rheumatic fever: A statement for health professionals. *Pediatrics, 96,* 758–764.

Davidson, D., et al. (1998). Inhaled nitric oxide for the early treatment of persistent pulmonary hypertension of the term newborn: A randomized, double-masked, placebo-controlled, dose-response, multicenter study. *Pediatrics, 101,* 325–334.

Driscoll, D. J., et al. (1997). Syncope in children and adolescents. *Journal of the American College of Cardiology, 29,* 1039–1045.

Groenink, M., et al. (1999). Survival and complication free survival in Marfan's syndrome: Implications of current guidelines. *Heart, 82,* 499–504.

Janavs, J. L., & Aminoff, J. J. (1998). Dystonia and chorea in acquired systemic disorders. *Journal of Neurology, Neurosurgery, and Psychiatry, 65,* 436–445.

Johnsrude, C. L., et al. (1995). Differentiating anomalous left main coronary artery originating from the pulmonary artery in infants from myocarditis and dilated cardiomyopathy by electrocardiogram. *The American Journal of Cardiology, 75,* 71–74.

Jones, T. D. (1944). Diagnosis of rheumatic fever. *Journal of the American Medical Association, 126,* 481–484.

Kaplan, E. L., et al. (1998). Antistreptolysin O and anti-deoxyribonuclease B titers: Normal values for children ages 2 to 12 in the United States. *Pediatrics, 101,* 86–88.

Kato, H., et al. (1996). Long-term consequences of Kawasaki disease: A 10- to 21-year follow-up study of 594 patients. *Circulation, 94,* 1379–1385.

Ledford, D. K. (1997). Immunologic aspects of vasculitis and cardiovascular disease. *Journal of the American Medical Association, 278,* 1962–1971.

Leenhardt, A. et al. (1995), Catecholaminergic polymorphic ventricular tachycardia in children. A 7-year follow-up of 21 patients. *Circulation, 91,* 1512–1519.

Lewis, D. A., & Dhala, A. (1999). Syncope in the pediatric patient: the cardiologist's perspective. *Pediatric Clinics of North America, 46,* 205–216.

Lue, H-C, et al. (1996), Three- versus four- week administration of benzathine penicillin G: Effects on incidence of streptococcal infections and recurrences of rheumatic fever. *Pediatrics, 97,* 984–988.

Markowtiz, M. (1998). Rheumatic fever—a half-century perspective. *Pediatrics, 102,* 272–274.

Mukamel, M., et al. (1997). Tietze's syndrome in children and infants. *The Journal of Pediatrics, 131,* 774–775.

Poets, C. F., & Martin, R .J. (1996). Noninvasive determination of blood gases. In J. Stock (Ed.), *Infant respiratory function testing* (pp. 411–443). New York: Wiley-Liss.

Reese, R. E., & Betts, R. F. (1996). Pericarditis and myocarditis. In R. E. Reese & R. F. Betts (Eds.), *Practical approach to infectious disease* (4th ed.) (pp. 371–373). Philadelphia: Lippincott Williams & Wilkins.

Saleeb, S., et al. (1999). Comparison of treatment with fluorinated glucocorticoids to the natural history of autoantibody-associated congenital heart block: Retrospective review of the research registry for neonatal lupus. *Arthritis & Rheumatism, 42,* 2335–2345.

Salim, M. A., et al. (1998). Syncope recurrences in children: relation to tilt-test results. *Pediatrics, 102,* 924–926.

Salim, M. A., & DiSessa, T. G. (1996). Serum electrolytes in children with neurocardiogenic syncope treated with fludrocortisone and salt. *The American Journal of Cardiology, 78,* 228–229.

Sapin, S. O. (1997). Recognizing normal heart murmurs: A logic-based mnemonic. *Pediatrics, 99,* 616–619.

Schaller, J. G. (1996). Nonrheumatic conditions mimicking rheumatic disease of childhood. In Behrman (Ed.), *Nelson textbook of pediatrics* (15th ed.) (pp. 689–690). Philadelphia: W.B. Saunders.

Shiffman, R. N. (1995). Guideline maintenance and revision: 50 years of the Jones criteria for diagnosis of rheumatic fever. *Archives: Pediatrics and Adolescent Medicine, 149,* 727–732.

Siegel, A. C., et al. (1961). Controlled studies of streptococcal pharyngitis in a pediatric population. Factors related to the attack rate of rheumatic fever. *New England Journal of Medicine, 265,* 559–565.

Stollerman, G. H., & Rusoff, J. R. (1952). Prophylaxis against group A streptococcal infections in rheumatic fever patients. Use of a new repository penicillin preparation. *Journal of the American Medical Association, 150,* 1571.

Tanel, R. E., & Walsh, E. P. (1997). Syncope in the pediatric patient. *Cardiology Clinics, 15,* 227–294.

Towbin, J. A., et al. (1994). Evidence of genetic heterogeneity in Romano-Ward long QT syndrome. Analysis of 23 families. *Circulation, 90,* 2635–2644.

Veasy, L. G., et al. (1994). Persistence of acute rheumatic fever in the intermountain area of the United States. *Journal of Pediatrics, 124,* 673–674.

Walsh-Sukys, M. C., et al. (2000). Persistent pulmonary hypertension of the newborn in the era before nitric oxide: Practice variation and outcomes. *Pediatrics, 105,* 14–20.

Waltuck, J., & Buyon, J. P. (1994). Autoantibody-associated congenital heart block: Outcome in mothers and children. *Annals of Internal Medicine, 120,* 544–551.

Abdominal Pain, Vomiting, and Diarrhea

• SAMUEL SANDOWSKI, MD, and ROSEMARY M. JACKSON, MD

INTRODUCTION

"Mommy, my tummy hurts!" is a complaint heard frequently from children. Abdominal pain plagues almost all children at some point in their lives. For some, the pain is an acute, limited experience of viral gastroenteritis; others experience recurrent or chronic pain, such as in Familial Mediterranean Fever or Henoch-Schönlein purpura. Most cases require nothing more than observation and reassurance, although some require extensive evaluations or surgical interventions. Regardless of etiology, the provider will face the challenge of determining the best course of action for each patient with abdominal pain.

PATHOLOGY

All people perceive pain differently. The perception of pain varies among individuals and cultures. The perception of pain may even vary for the same individual from one day to the next. Though perceptions and responses to pain vary, however, the pain stimulus is the same. Abdominal pain is caused by stimulation of afferent fibers within cells in the dorsal root ganglia. Some fibers cross the midline and ascend to the medulla, midbrain, and thalamus. The pain is perceived in the post-central gyrus of the cerebral cortex.

Organs in the abdomen do not detect painful stimuli caused by cutting or burning; yet they are sensitive to distention, compression, and torsion. It is the peritoneal covering and the skin and muscles overlying the abdomen that detect painful stimuli as a sharp sensation. Inflammation and infarction also cause pain when they affect the peritoneum.

The peritoneum, of mesodermal origin, covers the organs within (visceral layer) and the inner surface (parietal layer) of the abdominal cavity. Autonomic nerves innervate the visceral layer, and the pain detected tends to be midline. Somatic nerves of spinal origin innervate the parietal layer, and the pain is perceived at its location (Martin & Rossi, 1997). Additionally, different types of nerve fibers, originating at T7-L2, innervate the two peritoneal layers. The visceral peritoneum contains C fibers, which are slow and give the sensation of dull, aching pain. A-λ fibers innervate the parietal peritoneum; these fibers are much quicker and cause the sensation of sharp, severe pain. Thus, in early appendicitis, abdominal pain first is dull and central due to visceral peritoneal inflammation. As the process progresses, the parietal peritoneum becomes inflamed. The pain localizes to the right lower quadrant and becomes sharper and more severe.

The etiologies of abdominal pains can be divided into acute, chronic, and acute on chronic. They also can be divided into surgical, medical, and idiopathic. They may further be subdivided into age groupings, such as infant, toddler, and adolescent (Table 38-1).

EPIDEMIOLOGY

Gastroenterological complaints are found in 5.4% to 13% of all children ages 17 years and younger [Centers for Disease Control and Prevention, 1994]. Abdominal pain may be acute, chronic, or recurrent. Recurrent abdominal pain is defined as three or more episodes of abdominal pain over a 3-month period (Seller, 1996). Patients with recurrent abdominal pain, however, may present with a new episode as "acute abdominal pain".

Acute abdominal pain usually is defined as abdominal pain lasting less than 3 days. It accounts for approximately 5% of all unscheduled visits to primary care providers, urgent care centers, and emergency rooms (Scholer, Pituch, Orr, & Dittus, 1996). Fever, vomiting, anorexia, cough, and sore throat often accompany it. Most often, a "self-limiting" or medical condition such as "abdominal pain of uncertain etiology," gastroenteritis, or constipation causes acute abdominal pain (Mason, 1996).

● **Clinical Pearl:** Often, extra-abdominal sources cause abdominal pain, including pharyngitis (especially cases caused by group A β-hemolytic streptococci), otitis media, pneumonia, lead poisoning, and diabetes (see Table 38-1).

In most cases, medical treatment, supportive therapy, appropriate antibiotics, and observation are sufficient. In 1% to 2% of cases, however, surgical intervention is necessary (Scholer, Pituch, Orr, & Dittus, 1996).

Appendicitis is the most common reason that older children with abdominal pain require surgical intervention (74%). In 50% to 60% of cases of children admitted for possible appendicitis, however, observation and further evaluation preclude the need for surgical intervention. When surgery is performed, 10% of cases reveal no pathology (Holland & Gollow, 1996). In children younger than age 4 years, diagnosing appendicitis is often more difficult. In children younger than age 5 years, incarcerated hernias and intussusception are the most common reasons for abdominal pain requiring surgical intervention.

HISTORY AND PHYSICAL EXAM

As with all diseases, the history and the physical exam are the guides to establishing a clinical diagnosis. Common questions to answer are the "PQRSTs" of pain:

Table 38–1.   ETIOLOGIES OF ABDOMINAL PAIN IN CHILDREN

Diagnosis	Nature/location of Pain	Additional Symptoms and Findings
Non-surgical		
Gastroenteritis	Non specific, diffuse, crampy	Associated with vomiting, diarrhea, and/or fever
Irritable bowel	Crampy, periumbilical, or diffuse	Relief with bowel movements/flatulence
Peptic Ulcer Disease	Burning, epigastric	May have blood in stool
Inflammatory bowel disease	Diffuse, left-lower quadrant	Diarrhea and/or hematochezia
Mesenteric adenitis	Diffuse, may mimic surgical abdomen	
Pancreatitis	Boring pain radiating to back, epigastric and/or left-lower quadrant	Vomiting, elevated amylase, often infectious, familial, or drug-induced
Lead poisoning	Diffuse	Neuropathy, learning disabilities, constipation
Henoch-Schönlein purpura	Crampy, diffuse	Blood in stool, rash, proteinuria, arthralgia
C1 esterase deficiency	Crampy, diffuse	Swelling of face and lips
Lactose intolerance	Crampy, diffuse	Flatulence/diarrhea from milk products
Mittleschmerz	Cyclical, lower abdomen	Associated with ovulation
Diabetes		
Constipation	Diffuse	Appropriate history
Pelvic inflammatory disease (PID)	Severe, constant, lower right or left quadrants	Appropriate history, vaginal discharge (not always present)
Urinary tract infections (UTI)	Constant, dull, suprapubic or back pain	Dysuria and/or frequency, or fever
URI/pharyngitis and otitis media	Intermittent, diffuse	Rhinorrhea, cough, dysphagia, sore throat, otalgia
Lower-lobe pneumonia	Constant, upper quadrants	Cough, sputum, fever
Sickle cell anemia	Constant, diffuse or periumbilical	Precipitated by fever/crises, more common in persons of African descent
Nephrolithiasis	Severe, crampy, flank	Hematuria
Familial Mediterranean Fever	Severe, intermittent, diffuse	Fever, arthralgia
Gastroesophageal reflux disease (GERD)	Burning, epigastric	Worse at night, sour taste in mouth, cough
Porphyria	Intermittent, severe	
Surgical		
Incarcerated hernia	Periumbilical/lower abdomen	Vomiting
Appendicitis	Right-lower quadrant, originally started periumbilically	Anorexia
Intussusception	Periumbilical, lower abdomen cramping	Currant jelly stools, vomiting, quiet infant 6 mo–2 y (idiopathic; no leading point) > 2 years (lipoma, lymphoma, polyp, leiomyoma; may act as leading points)
Torsion of testes/ovaries	Lower abdomen, groin	
Obstruction	Dependent on level of obstruction	Abdominal distention, vomiting usually bilious

P—place of pain. Where is it? Can the child point to it with one finger? Surgical etiologies tend to be more localized.

Q—quality of pain. Is it sharp? dull? aching? burning? colicky? crampy?

R—radiation of the pain. Does the pain stay in one place or go to the back? to the chest? Has the pain itself migrated?

S—symptoms associated with the pain. Is there vomiting? fever? anorexia? diarrhea? sore throat? The provider must explore a sexual history in all patients (including abuse as well as consensual activities).

T—timing of the pain. When did it start? How long does it last? How often does it occur? Has it happened before? —things that make the pain better or worse. Does position, bowel movement, or medication affect the pain?

The provider must do the physical exam carefully and kindly, remembering that the patient is in pain. Since the abdomen is hurting, it is often best to examine it last. A thorough exam, starting with vital signs and including respiratory rate, pulse, blood pressure, and temperature, is essential. Tachypnea is seen with pneumonia. Tachycardia and hypotension occur with sepsis, peritonitis, or profound anemia and hemorrhage. Observing the skin, looking for any rash or pallor, may help identify hemolytic or sickle cell anemia, as well as purpura. A cardiac evaluation may reveal a murmur secondary to anemia (from GI bleeding, sickle cell disease, or other etiologies). Auscultation of the lungs may uncover lower lobe pneumonia.

The abdominal exam should begin with observation. The provider should approach the child gently. This is best done after first talking with the child and parent and establishing trust. The clinician should note the child's facial expression, so he or she can compare it to a "grimace" while palpating the abdomen. A grimace is often a more sensitive tool than any verbal acknowledgment of pain (Wagner, McKinney, & Carpenter, 1996). The clinician should observe the patient's position, noting if he or she is bent over or writhing with pain. The provider should note the skin over the abdomen. Discoloration of the flank (Gray-Turner sign) or periumbilical discoloration (Cullen sign) occurs with hemorrhagic pancreatitis.

Auscultation should precede palpation; palpation that elicits pain may cause a paralytic ileus, and the provider may not be able to hear bowel sounds. The absence of bowel sounds indicates ileus and thus requires hospital admission. High pitched/hyperperistaltic sounds suggest mechanical obstruction. Prior to auscultation, allowing the child to touch the stethoscope and even place it on his or her abdomen eases anxiety.

The provider should perform palpation gingerly, starting with an area that is not painful and moving clockwise toward the painful area. The patient should lie supine, with knees slightly flexed. Engaging the child in conversation helps to distract him or her from the pain and the exam. Superficial palpation should precede deep palpation.

● **Clinical Pearl:** Instead of palpating with the hands, palpating with the stethoscope head may reduce fear and anxiety in a young child, since the stethoscope is not expected to produce as much pain as does manual palpation. This technique also may aid in identifying an exaggerated pain response. Patients expect pain when someone presses the abdomen with the hand and thus may exaggerate their response. They may not do so, however, when the abdomen is pressed with the head of the stethoscope, because they think that the provider is auscultating and not palpating.

The clinician should note signs of guarding, rebound, and any masses. The cough test (in which voluntary coughing elicits abdominal pain) has a sensitivity of 78% and a specificity of 79% for diagnosing peritonitis (Bennett, Tambeur, & Campbell, 1994) and is more sensitive than the manual test for rebound. The "heel drop jarring test," in which the patient drops onto his or her heels after standing on the toes for 15 seconds, or to have the patient hop on one leg several times also may be used to diagnose peritonitis.

A rectal exam is part of the routine exam when the provider suspects a diagnosis of an acute abdomen. It may not aid in diagnosis, however, and is not always necessary (Mason, 1996). Though generally the rectal exam is uncomfortable, reproducing the pain on rectal exam when pressing on the appendix increases the suspicion of appendicitis. Stool guaiac testing reveals occult blood. Sexually active females should have a gynecological (speculum and bimanual) exam.

DIAGNOSTIC STUDIES

After performing the history and physical exam, the provider should begin a diagnosis-specific approach. He or she may treat obvious etiologies for abdominal pain, such as simple gastroenteritis, irritable bowel syndrome (IBS), upper respiratory illness, and otitis media without further testing. When testing is appropriate, the clinician should perform tests to confirm or exclude specific diagnoses.

Laboratory Testing

In children with pharyngitis, the provider should obtain a rapid strep test or throat culture. He or she should do blood testing methodically, not with a "shotgun" approach. In children with recurrent vomiting and diarrhea, the provider should draw an "SMA 6" or "Astra 7". Electrolyte abnormalities may occur, and a measurement of blood urea nitrogen (BUN) and serum creatinine may help assess levels of dehydration. Elevated glucose levels suggest diabetes mellitus, and low serum bicarbonate (CO_2) suggests sepsis or dehydration with secondary metabolic acidosis.

When the provider suspects hepatic involvement, he or she should evaluate liver function tests. Elevation of serum transaminases indicates hepatitis, which may be Hepatitis A, B, C, or numerous other viruses, such as Epstein-Barr. When the provider suspects pancreatitis, amylase levels usually are elevated.

Providers should routinely check lead levels on all young children, especially those who live in housing where leaded paint and dust continue to pose environmental hazards. Providers should query children with elevated levels about abdominal pains as a manifestation of lead poisoning. Additionally, older children with known exposures to lead require testing as well. Clinicians must report cases of elevated lead levels to the local Health Department.

The complete blood count (CBC) is not specific for identifying the etiology of abdominal pain but aids in evaluation. A low hematocrit suggests anemia (sickle cell or from GI bleeding). An elevated white blood cell (WBC) count suggests an inflammatory or infectious process, such as pelvic inflammatory disease (PID), gastroenteritis, mesenteric adenitis, or surgical emergencies, such as appendicitis and peritonitis.

The urine analysis (UA) may reveal blood (urolithiasis) or WBCs (urinary tract infections/pyelonephritis). Proteinuria found on UA may suggest target organ damage secondary to diabetes mellitus or connective tissue disorders (eg, Henoch-Schonlein purpura). The UA is normal in appendicitis but checked routinely to exclude genitourinary causes of abdominal pain.

Imaging

Plain Films

Plain x-rays are often the first imaging studies performed in patients with abdominal pain (Lee, 1976). While often unrevealing, a collection of plain films of the abdomen, such as the kidney-ureters-bladder (KUB), an upright abdomen, and an upright chest film, can identify emergent, potentially fatal conditions. The provider should note air distribution. Free intraperitoneal air (often seen as a crescent of lucency under the diaphragm) or air in the retroperitoneum suggests perforation of a viscus. If a child is unable to maintain the position required for an upright film or even a decubitus film, a supine film may suggest free intraperitoneal air in 59% of cases (Levine, Scheiner, & Rubesin, 1991). Common signs on these supine films include Riglers sign (air on both sides of the intestinal wall) and the right upper quadrant sign (air outlining the peritoneal cavity) (Gupta & Dupuy, 1997).

Air fluid levels, especially in a "ladder fashion," suggest obstruction. The lack of air may represent late stages of obstruction. Excessive amounts of air in the colon (toxic megacolon) could be found in ulcerative colitis.

Foreign bodies and stones can be seen on plain films. Stones may be gallstones in the gallbladder or bile ducts, kidney stones in the kidney or ureter, or appendicoliths, which may correlate with appendicitis (Martin & Rossi, 1997).

Ultrasonography

Ultrasonography (US) has become a common imaging modality for patients with acute abdominal pain. It is the modality of choice for gynecological and obstetric imaging (Gupta & Dupuy, 1997). However, it is only useful in adding to the diagnosis in 50% of cases of acute abdominal pain (Walsh, Crawford, & Crossing, 1990). For appendicitis, US is highly specific (about 90%) and sensitive (about 95%). The provider's clinical suspicion, however, always should guide treatment and decision making. US is best used as an adjunct when the provider's clinical findings and suspicion are equivocal (Wilcox & Traverso, 1997). Therefore, in younger children in whom the diagnosis of appendicitis may be more difficult to make, US may play a larger role in establishing a diagnosis. Other diseases in which ultrasonographic findings may help establish or confirm a diagnosis in patients with abdominal pain are noted in Table 38-2.

When requesting US, providers must convey clinical questions and concerns to the sonographer, because not all US is the same. Regular/abdominal sonography looks at solid viscera, including the liver, spleen, pancreas, and kidneys, but usually not the appendix. Graded-compression sonography evaluates the GI tract only and measures "compressibility" of the bowel. Doppler flow sonography measures blood flow.

Computed Tomography

The use of Computed Tomography (CT) is useful in the diagnosis of appendicitis, diverticulitis, intestinal ischemia, pancreatitis, intestinal obstruction, and perforated viscus (Gupta & Dupuy, 1997). It is associated with greater cost and radiation exposure than US. The introduction of the helical CT, which images the patient during a single spiral scan and then reconstructs the images by computer, has eliminated the need for repeat images and additional radiation.

CT is a useful adjunct to US, and providers should consider it when the diagnosis remains equivocal. They also should use it as a guide to medical management of complications of appendicitis (such as evaluation and treatment of abscesses and phlegmon), especially when perforation occurs (Sivit, 1997).

MANAGEMENT

Treatment of acute abdominal pain depends on its etiology. First and foremost is the necessity to identify the causes and development of the pain. Even if a diagnosis is not possible, the provider must determine a disposition. Is the patient stable enough to be sent home, or does he or she require hospitalization? If a child is found to have signs of an acute abdomen, then hospitalization, observation, and consultation with a surgeon is needed. If symptoms seem benign and recurrent (as suggestive of irritable bowel), then counseling and reassurance are appropriate. In all cases, the clinician must address severity of the pain, employ appropriate analgesics (when warranted), and correct and maintain hydration status. Specific treatments are described below for each disease.

APPENDICITIS

Appendicitis is the most common diagnosis considered when children younger than age 14 years present with abdominal pain to the emergency room or provider's office (Simpson & Smith, 1996). Only a small percentage of patients, however, actually have appendicitis. Because of the high morbidity and mortality that can result from a perforated appendix, it is a diagnosis that must not be missed. The incidence of pediatric patients with perforated appendices at the time of diagnosis ranges from 30% to 65%. The diagnosis becomes even more difficult when the child is younger (Mason, 1996).

Table 38–2.   COMMON ULTRASONOGRAPHIC FINDINGS IN ACUTE ABDOMINAL PAIN IN CHILDREN

Disease	Ultrasonographic Findings
Appendicitis	Noncompressible, inflamed appendix
Bacterial ileocecitis	Mural thickening of the terminal ileum, cecum and ascending colon. Large mesenteric lymph nodes and nonvisualization of the appendix, as found in appendicitis.
Mesenteric adenitis	Large mesenteric nodes (> 4 mm). Its presence does not exclude appendicitis.
Crohn's disease	If appendix is involved, may be thickened and mimic appendicitis.
Colitis	Thumb-printing along the thickened colonic wall.
Cholelithiasis	Gall stones in the gall bladder.
Hemorrhagic ovarian cyst	"Fishnet weave" appearance caused by septations in a cystic ovary. Fluid/debris levels may be noted.
Pelvic inflammatory disease	Used to assess complications, not establish diagnosis. Distended fallopian tubes; tubo-ovarian abscess; may be bilateral.
Adnexal torsion	May have ovarian mass. Poor or no blood flow with doppler sonography.
Nephrolithiasis	Stone, possibly with proximal hydroureter and/or hydronephrosis.
Pancreatitis	Abnormal, nonspecific swelling of the pancreas.

History and Physical Exam

The typical history is abdominal pain that starts periumbilically, migrates to the right lower quadrant, and gradually intensifies. The pain is constant, though sometimes the patient feels slight relief when flexed at the waist. The patient's gait may be stooped. He or she may have anorexia and vomiting. Classically, the patient will present with fever and an acute abdomen, including rebound tenderness (called Rovsing's sign), guarding, a positive cough test, and tenderness over the right lower quadrant on rectal exam.

Diagnostic Criteria

The diagnosis of appendicitis is challenging because not all patients present with typical and classical features. Often the history is vague and the physical exam findings are equivocal. Scoring systems have been created to help guide providers to the probability of making a diagnosis (eg, the MANTRELS Score - Table 38-3). The diagnosis of appendicitis is based on pathological examination of the removed appendix, but the decision to operate is based on clinical findings.

● **Clinical Pearl:** Persistent right lower quadrant tenderness in a child is the most specific, important, and diagnostic clinical finding.

Diagnostic Studies

Laboratory tests are used to support or aid in the direction of a diagnosis when clinical findings are equivocal. The WBC count usually is elevated, with an increased percentage of neutrophils and immature bands, "a shift to the left." Though appendicoliths, also known as fecoliths, may suggest appendicitis, plain x-ray films usually yield little diagnostic value, unless a perforation has occurred, revealing free air.

Advanced imaging procedures have been used more commonly over the past decade. For all ages, US was found to have a sensitivity and specificity of 85% and 92% respectively (Orr, Porter, & Hartman, 1995). In children, however, sensitivity is about 90% and specificity is 97% (Ramachandran, Sivit, Newman, et al., 1996). The classic finding on US is that of a non-compressible, inflamed (> 6 mm) appendix. Computerized tomography (CT), especially spiral or helical CT, has proven to be a useful and accurate method of diagnosing appendicitis, with even higher sensitivities and specificity than US.

Management

Treatment of appendicitis is surgical. A false positive (white appendix) rate of less than 15% is often considered acceptable.

● **Clinical Pearl:** A surgeon should promptly evaluate all suspected cases. If unsure, the patient is probably best served by being admitted and observed, especially very young children, in whom the diagnosis is very difficult to make.

IRRITABLE BOWEL SYNDROME

Up to 22% of the U.S. adult population has irritable bowel syndrome (IBS). Most of these individuals are diagnosed in young adulthood and adolescence (Lynn & Friedman, 1995). These patients comprise up to 25% of referrals to gastroenterologists. The condition is twice as common in females than in males (except in India and Sri Lanka, where it is more common in males). Ten to 15% of school-aged children have recurrent abdominal pain, 52% of whom were diagnosed with IBS (Hyams, 1995).

Pathology

Patients with IBS have increased bowel motility and altered bowel contractions in response to stress. Some patients (often those who complain of pain) tend to have increased activity in the distal colon and rectum, while others (often those of who complain of diarrhea) have increased transit time of the colon with less water resorption. No one finding, however, has proved to be a consistent marker for the disease.

Patients with IBS may have different thresholds for pain. In these patients, balloon distention of the rectum, sigmoid colon, and small intestine causes pain at lower volumes as compared to controls. This observation led to the theory that patients with IBS have a lower threshold for visceral pain but not necessarily somatic pain (Accarino, Azpiroz, & Malagelada, 1995). It is still unclear, however, if this is normal perception to abnormal physiology, or abnormal perception to normal physiology. This question is further confused by not knowing if certain medications, such as serotonin inhibitors that are sometimes used in treatment, are acting centrally, altering the perception of pain, or locally on the gut at yet unidentified sites.

History and Physical Exam

In neonates, colic may be the first symptom. Young children may display frequent bouts of loose and watery stools, lasting for weeks, labeled as chronic diarrhea of childhood or "toddler's diarrhea." Others may have functional constipation. Chronic recurrent abdominal pain is also a frequent finding. Older patients usually complain of altered bowel habits, diarrhea alternating with constipation, and abdominal pain. In this age group, stress often aggravates and bowel movements or flatulence often relieve symptoms. The reader is referred to Chapter 57 for a complete discussion of IBS.

▲ **Clinical Warning:** Signs and symptoms of weight loss, fever, rectal bleeding, and abdominal pain while sleeping suggest a diagnosis other than IBS.

Table 38–3. MANTRELS SCORE* FOR EVALUATION OF PATIENTS WITH SUSPECTED APPENDICITIS

Clinical Findings		Value
M	Migration of Pain	1
A	Anorexia (acetone in urine)	1
N	Nausea, vomiting	1
T	Tenderness in right-lower quadrant	2
R	Rebound tenderness or Rovsing sign	1
E	Elevation of temperature	1
L	Leukocytosis	2
S	Shift to the left (increased bands or segmented neutrophils)	1

*A score of 5–6 is compatible with acute appendicitis; 7–8 probable appendicitis; 9–10 very likely to have appendicitis. (Taken from Alvarado, A. (1986). A practical score: the early diagnosis of acute appendicitis. *Annals of Emergency Medicine, 15,* 557–564.)

PEPTIC ULCER DISEASE

Peptic ulcer disease most frequently occurs in adults. It may afflict adolescents and children but is rare in toddlers. The bacteria *Helicobacter pylori* usually is found. Research shows it to be more common in patients from lower socioeconomic status, but some studies have challenged this finding (Macarthur, Saunders, & Feldman, 1995). Symptoms range from chronic abdominal pain to GI bleeding. Treatment consists of eradication of *H. pylori* with proton pump inhibitors and antibiotics. Short-term continuation of acid reduction (with proton pump inhibitors, H_2 blockers or antacids) is usually necessary. If the diagnosis is questionable, treatment seems suboptimal, or complications are suspected, a gastroesophagoduodenoscopy (EGD) or an upper GI series is warranted.

PANCREATITIS

Pancreatitis may occur throughout childhood and most commonly results from a mumps infection. When secondary to other etiologies, pancreatitis in childhood is rare and often associated with trauma, medications (eg, thiazides, steroids, estrogens), diseases (eg, diabetes mellitus, cystic fibrosis, hemolytic uremic syndrome, or liver diseases), or familial causes.

The pain is usually epigastric, and boring, drilling straight to the back. Nausea and vomiting are often present. Laboratory evaluation must include a CBC, amylase, lipase, serum glucose, BUN, electrolytes (SMA 6), liver function tests, and calcium. Additionally, an arterial blood gas is warranted. Treatment includes appropriate analgesia and sufficient hydration. Hospitalization, with intravenous hydration and bowel rest with nasogastric suction, is usually necessary. Complications include pseudocysts, abscesses, thrombosis, and necrosis of intraabdominal vessels and organs.

HENOCH SCHÖNLEIN PURPURA

Henoch Schönlein Purpura—also known as anaphylactoid purpura or nonthrombocytopenic purpura—is a vasculitis of unknown etiology. Children present with abdominal and joint pain and a characteristic rash. The rash classically begins as large patches of urticaria predominantly on the lower extremities but also on the arms and ears. The trunk is relatively spared. The rash then progresses to purpuric lesions, which become edematous, hence the term, palpable purpura. Gross hematuria and bloody stools also may be seen. Intussusception, as a result of edematous nubbins of intestinal mucosa acting as leading points, is a dangerous complication. Evaluation of the urine may reveal signs of a glomerulonephritis (proteinurea and hematuria); fortunately, this resolves without permanent renal damage in the vast majority of cases. Treatment with systemic steroids is useful for the child with severe GI symptoms but does not appear to help either the arthritis or nephritis. Nor does treatment appear to alter the natural course of the illness, which may last for 3 to 4 weeks. Fortunately, the prognosis in almost all children is uniformly excellent.

CONSTIPATION

Constipation is one of the most common reasons for acute abdominal pain in the child. Though patients may have their own definition of constipation, it is generally considered less than one bowel movement every third day, consisting of hard stool. The causes of constipation are many and may present at any age, from newborn to adult (Display 38-1). The provider must exclude dangerous etiologies, such as bowel obstruction, anatomical and neurological conditions, and systemic disorders.

The diagnosis of constipation is made by history. Usually, the common complaints are inability to move one's bowels, painful bowel movements, or both. Additionally, severe, soft, liquid stool may slide around the impacted stool, and the patient may complain of diarrhea or encopresis. A history of vomiting should raise the suspicion of intestinal obstruction.

The physical examination for "simple" constipation may be unremarkable or reveal a distended abdomen or a mass (of stool-filled bowel). Rectal exam may be normal or reveal a rectal vault full of stool with impaction. The provider should carefully examine the rectum (noting fissures) prior to palpating the rectal vault. Laboratory testing, including

---

DISPLAY 38–1 • Common Causes of Constipation in Children

Functional
Variation of the norm
Fear of painful bowel movements
Desire to use "own" and not "foreign" bathroom
Anorexia nervosa

Anatomic
Anal fissure
Anal-rectal stenosis
Anterior displacement of the rectum
Chagas' disease
Colonic strictures (eg, secondary to Crohn's disease)
Hirschsprung's disease
Pseudo-obstruction
Obstruction
Volvulus

Systemic
Cystic fibrosis
Dehydration
Diabetes mellitus
Hypercalcemia
Hypothyroidism
Hypokalemia
Lead poisoning

Medications
Narcotics
Antidepressants (type)
Thorazine (class)

Neurologic
Amyotonia congenita
Spinal cord tumor
Spina bifida occulta
Neuronal intestinal dysplasia

blood work, is unremarkable, but an abdominal x-ray may demonstrate stool in the bowel.

FAMILIAL MEDITERRANEAN FEVER

Patients with familial Mediterranean Fever (FMF) often present with abdominal pain, fever, and arthralgia. Work-up for the abdominal pain or connective tissue disorders are often extensive but unrevealing. The condition is believed to result from an autosomal recessive genetic trait. There is usually a history of family members with similar symptoms. FMF is commonly found in people of Mediterranean descent, such as Northern Africa, Italy, and Armenia. Treatment consists of patient education and colchicine.

GASTROESOPHAGEAL REFLUX DISEASE (GERD)

Gastroesophageal reflux disease (GERD) is found most commonly in infants, but often resolves by age 12 to 18 months (Squires, 1996). It may reappear in children older than age 3 years. Symptoms range from abdominal pain (classically a burning sensation in the epigastrium) and regurgitation, to nocturnal cough, to apnea and bradycardia. Complications of GERD include poor weight gain, wheezing, aspiration pneumonia, apnea, bradycardia, anemia, Sandifer's syndrome, esophageal stricture, and Barrett's esophagus (Squires, 1996). Any infant or child with signs or symptoms of these complications, as well as those with excessive spitting or excessive post-feeding discomfort, deserves further investigation and intervention, and would benefit from consultation with a pediatric gastroenterologist.

The diagnosis is made clinically. Providers should suspect it in any infant with poor weight gain, apparent discomfort during or after feeds, frequent lower respiratory infections, apnea, or excessive spitting up. Empiric therapy is usually sufficient. In mild cases, therapy usually consists of patient education, including upright and thickened feedings for infants. Parents can accomplish such feedings by adding one tablespoon of rice cereal to every two ounces of formula. Parents should keep the child upright after meals. Providers should use antacids, cimetidine, or ranitidine when simple measures do not provide relief. In refractory cases or cases with complications, fundoplication surgery may be appropriate. Persistence or recurrence of symptoms or complications requires further evaluation. Some modalities used to diagnose GERD include endoscopy, barium swallow and upper GI series, US of the lower esophagus, and esophageal pH probes.

MESENTERIC LYMPHADENITIS

Mesenteric lymphadenitis is a diagnosis describing enlarged mesenteric lymph nodes. The etiology is usually viral but may be bacterial. Affected children often present with acute abdominal pain, often localized to the right lower quadrant, mimicking appendicitis. In fact, mesenteric adenitis may be the most common reason for surgery when the suspected diagnosis was appendicitis, but no inflamed appendix was found at surgery (Sivit, 1997). US reveals enlarged (> 4 mm)

nodes; these large nodes, however, may also be found in appendicitis. The presence of mesenteric lymphadenitis on US should not exclude the diagnosis of appendicitis.

INTUSSUSCEPTION

Intussusception is the process by which part of the bowel (intussusceptum) telescopes into another part (intussuscipiens). Most cases are idiopathic (often in children between age 5 months and 2 years), but some are secondary to a "lead point" (children older than age 2 years). A lead point is any growth or anomaly found in the bowel that provides a potential site where the bowel invaginates, and with normal peristalsis, may fold into other parts of the bowel. Some common lead points are lipomas, Meckel's diverticuli, lymphomas, edematous mucosa (as in Henoch-Schönlein purpura), polyps, leiomyomas, neoplasms, and foreign bodies.

● **Clinical Pearl:** A lead point should be sought in all cases of intussusception above 2 years of age.

Intussusception most commonly occurs between ages 5 and 9 months (Winslow, Westfall, & Nicholas, 1996) and is more common in males than in females. Most cases occur near the ileocecal junction (ileocolic). Other types of intussusceptions are ileoileocolic, colocolic, jejunojejunal, and cecocolic.

Typically, the patient with intussusception will present with a triad of abdominal pain, vomiting, and bloody stools. The pain is colicky or cyclical, with periods of relief between the bouts of excruciating pain. Patients may appear ill, lethargic, and severely dehydrated; though these manifestations may not appear until later stages. Classically, the patient will have bloody stools (the color of currant jelly), but these may be absent in more than half of all cases (Losek, 1993). On physical exam, the provider should note vital signs, including fever, which may be markedly elevated. The patient may show all the signs of an acute abdomen, including guarding and rebound. A sausage-shaped abdominal mass may be present and noted on the rectal exam.

Laboratory data may be normal. The WBC count, however, can be elevated, and the SMA 6 may suggest dehydration. Radiographically, plain films of the abdomen may reveal an absence of air, usually in the right lower quadrant, and perhaps a mass. Sonographically, the doughnut or pseudokidney signs are present. The barium enema, however, is considered the gold standard for diagnosing intussusception (Winslow, Westfall, & Nicholas, 1996). A filling defect is noted, along with a "coiled spring" appearance, caused by trapping of barium between the intestinal walls of the intussusceptum and the intussuscipiens.

Barium enemas are therapeutic in 75% of cases (Losek, 1993). The force of the barium reduces the intussusceptum and barium can be seen refluxing freely into the small intestines. Hydrostatic reduction of intussusceptions also have been successful (especially with ileocolic intussusception) with Hartmann's solution (Peh, Khong, Lam, et al., 1997). If "conservative measures" of hydrostatic or barium reduction are unsuccessful, surgery is warranted. Laparoscopic surgery has been attempted but was successful in only about half of all cases (Schier, 1997). Open reduction is still the surgical procedure of choice. Monitoring of fluid status is always necessary.

VOMITING

Vomiting is a highly integrated, forceful expulsion of gastric contents through the mouth. It is not to be confused with the more common problem of regurgitation (GERD). GERD is a passive movement of gastric contents into the esophagus, associated with inappropriate opening of the lower esophageal sphincter (LES).

Nausea and retching respectively usually precede vomiting. Although vomiting is an unpleasant symptom, the body uses it as a defense to expel unwanted toxins. Nausea is a sensation or urge to vomit. Retching is spasmodic yet rhythmic respiratory movements against a closed epiglottis, with simultaneous abdominal muscle contraction. As with retching, abdominal contractions and spasmodic respiratory movements facilitate the vomiting process. There is also relaxation of the diaphragm, with subsequent expulsion of gastric content.

Pathology

Two areas of the central nervous system mediate vomiting: the floor of the fourth ventricle (area *postrema*) and the reticular formation of the medulla. The chemoreceptor trigger zone (CTZ) is located in the area *postrema* and responds only to chemical stimuli. All drugs or toxins must pass through this zone to emit a vomiting response. The CTZ is located outside the blood brain barrier and therefore is permeable to polar molecules in both the blood and CSF.

The CTZ cannot function independently of the Vomiting Center (VC), which is the final integrating pathway that mediates all vomiting. The vomiting center also receives stimuli from other areas, such as the afferent vagal fibers in the gut (ie, abdominal distension) and pharynx (ie, gag reflex), vestibular labyrinth, and cerebral cortex. The VC lies in the lateral reticular formation of the medulla, which is anatomically near the medullary center (salivation, vasomotor, and respiratory centers) and the cranial nerves (somatic and visceral efferent). The VC receives and integrates stimuli and in turn stimulates the medullary center and cranial nerves. The vagal efferent fibers synchronously cause relaxation of the proximal stomach, retrograde contraction of the mid-small intestine (abdominal contraction), and relaxation of the diaphragm. The diaphragm descends on the stomach in the presence of increased intra-abdominal and intragastric pressure and expels gastric content.

The differential diagnosis for the causes of vomiting is vast (Table 38-4). The provider can limit the diagnostic possibilities by considering the patient's age, the nature of the vomitus, and how the vomitus is expelled.

Neonate to Two Months

Innocent vomiting occurs in nearly half of all infants (Gartner & Zitelli, 1997). It is usually secondary to aerophagia, improper formula preparation (too little water), or postcibil handling. Again it is important to differentiate this type of vomiting from the very common and almost universal phenomenon of "spitting up". Frequent, effortless regurgitation in the baby who is growing and developing normally, does not have apnea or frequent respiratory infections, and seems to be comfortable during and after feeds is a normal, albeit somewhat messy occurrence. Any persistent true vomiting during the neonatal period, however, should raise concern of a life-threatening disease, such as obstruction or infection.

Obstructive disorders, depending on their anatomical location, may present with bilious or nonbilious vomiting.

Bilious vomiting is a sign of an obstructive disorder regardless of age. Causes include malrotation, volvulus, incarcerated hernia, meconium ileus, and duodenal atresia. All these occur anatomically below the ligament of Treitz.

▲ **Clinical Warning:** In the infant, bilious vomiting signals an ominous event, either intestinal obstruction or sepsis, and requires urgent evaluation and treatment. In any age group, it is the *sine qua non* of intestinal obstruction.

Esophageal obstructive disorders may present with nonbilious vomiting but more commonly present with the classic triad of coughing, choking, and cyanosis. Pyloric stenosis and antral webs also are obstructive disorders that present with non-bilious vomiting because of their more proximal location.

Hypertrophic pyloric stenosis usually presents initially as intermittent, then persistent projectile vomiting in a first-born male infant by ages 4 to 8 weeks. In 90% of these infants, the provider can palpate an enlarged pyloric muscle (the size of an olive) in the upper abdomen, after the stomach has been emptied. If the condition persists undiagnosed, infants classically present with hypokalemic and hypochloremic dehydration and metabolic alkalosis because of the continued loss of both hydrogen and chloride ions in the vomitus. These infants usually require fluid resuscitation to restore metabolic homeostasis before surgery.

Not all obstructive processes that present with bilious vomiting require surgical intervention. Meconium plugs and left microcolon are nonsurgical obstructive processes. Meconium plug is inspissated meconium in the distal colon, which can be evacuated by a barium enema (both diagnostic and therapeutic). Left microcolon syndrome presents as a functional obstruction secondary to an area of narrowed colon located between otherwise normal colonic tissue. Mild forms of this disorder respond to electrolyte-balanced and warmed enemas.

The preterm infant is at risk for necrotizing enterocolitis (NEC), GI perforation, and vomiting associated with prolonged total parenteral nutrition. Young infants who have hemolytic disorders or who have had an ileal resection are at risk of developing cholelithiasis and cholecystitis, both of which also cause vomiting.

Infants with central nervous system disorders also may present with vomiting. Those with increased intracranial pressure (ICP) secondary to hydrocephalus, subdural hematomas, or kernicterus may present with vomiting. If infants present with lethargy, hypotonia, or convulsions, the clinician must consider inborn errors of metabolism.

Although infection is not the leading cause of vomiting in this age group, it may be present in neonates who develop meningitis, pyelonephritis, or enteral infections. By far, the most common causes of persistent vomiting in children younger than age 2 months are anatomical GI abnormalities, inflammatory conditions (NEC), and disorders of the CNS.

Infancy: Two Months to Twelve Months

During this time, innocent vomiting as well as late manifestations of congenital GI abnormalities persist. Patients continue to present with torsion of a Meckel diverticuli, malrotation, incarcerated hernias, and intussusception.

As infants develop, begin to crawl, and experience the world via the mouth, providers will see a higher incidence of infectious causes of vomiting. Although gastroenteritis is by far the most common cause of vomiting during this time, other nongastrointestinal infections also may present with

Table 38–4   ETIOLOGIES OF VOMITING

	Neonate	Infancy	Older Children
Obstruction	Tracheoesophageal fistula	Pyloric stenosis	Foreign bodies
	Esophageal stenosis or web	Malrotation of bowels	Malrotation (volvulus)
	Esophageal duplication	Foreign bodies	Intussusception
	Volvulus	Intussusception	Meckel's diverticulum
	Meconium ileus	Meckel's diverticulum	Incarcerated hernia
	Meconium plug	Incarcerated hernia	
	Malrotation		
	Hirschsprung's disease		
	Incarcerated hernia		
	Intestinal stenosis		
	Pyloric stenosis		
	Left microcolon		
Infectious Disorders (extra-gastrointestinal disorders)	Sepsis	Sepsis	Meningitis
	Meningitis	Meningitis	Otitis media
		Otitis media	Hepatitis
		Pneumonia	Urinary tract infections
		Pertussis	Pharyngitis
		Urinary tract infections	Pneumonia
			Thyrotoxicosis
Inflammatory/Infectious (gastrointestinal disorders)	Necrotizing enterocolitis	Gastroenteritis	Appendicitis
	Peritonitis	Appendicitis	Gastroenteritis
	Paralytic ileus	Peritonitis	Peptic ulcer disease
		Celiac disease	
Neurological	Hydrocephalus	Hydrocephalus	Hypertension
	Kernicterus	Intracranial hemorrhage	Intracranial hemorrhage
	Subdural hematoma	Subdural hematoma	Mass lesion
		Mass lesion	Migraines
			Motion sickness
Other	Inborn errors of metabolism	Adrenal insufficiency	Diabetic ketoacidosis
	Milk allergy	Food poisoning	Eating disorders
	Urea cycle defects	Ingestion accidents	Ingestion accidents
			Ingestion of illicit drugs
			Pregnancy

vomiting. Otitis media with stimulation of the vestibular nerve may present with vomiting. Pertussis and pneumonia that present with paroxysms of cough may stimulate the gag reflex or irritate the diaphragm to precipitate vomiting. As with neonates, sepsis, meningitis, and urinary tract infection also may cause vomiting in infants.

Childhood to Adolescence

Throughout childhood and adolescence, causes of vomiting are obstructive, such as intussusception, Meckel's diverticuli, and incarcerated hernias. The incidence of obstruction secondary to foreign body increases during this time, particularly in toddlers.

During the toddler years, providers also will see an increased incidence of vomiting secondary to accidental ingestion of medication and lead poisoning. Toddlers who attend day care and are not toilet trained have an increased incidence of infections that may precipitate vomiting. Providers should not overlook extra-abdominal causes of

vomiting and abdominal pain, such as strep pharyngitis and lower lobe pneumonia.

Older children have a higher incidence of peptic ulcer disease, migraine headaches, motion sickness, appendicitis, and hypertension as causes of vomiting. During adolescence, there is a higher incidence of vomiting secondary to illicit drug ingestion, pregnancy, and eating disorders.

Epidemiology

Vomiting is not a diagnosis but a symptom that presents diagnostic challenges for providers. The cause may be a benign, self-limited process, or vomiting may be a symptom of a serious underlying disorder. Vomiting occurs in all age groups but is more common in infancy and childhood. It is usually acute, short-lived, and associated with GI infections. It can be persistent, chronic, or cyclic.

Acute vomiting episodes are the most common presentation the provider will see. A viral illness, such as Rotavirus and Norwalk virus, usually precipitates such episodes.

Infants infected with Rotavirus who were admitted to the hospital presented with vomiting 2 to 3 days before diarrhea in 96% of cases (Nelson, 1986). Other conditions that precipitate acute emesis include meningitis, pneumonia, bacterial enteritis, and a host of other infectious processes, including otitis media and streptococcal pharyngitis.

Persistent vomiting is less common than acute vomiting and may be secondary to a protracted infection or an obstructive process. An even smaller percentage of children have a chronic low-grade pattern of emesis daily. In 76% of individuals with chronic vomiting, the etiology was GI in origin (40% peptic disorders, 26% infectious, 10% IBS) (Li, 1996).

Cyclic vomiting syndrome in children is least common. Although the incidence of cyclic vomiting has increased in the past decade, this is only secondary to improved recognition of the syndrome. The causes of cyclic vomiting are predominantly nongastrointestinal in origin (eg, abdominal migraine, chronic sinusitis, metabolic, or endocrine). Only in 12% of patients with cyclic vomiting is the etiology GI in origin (eg, peptic disorders, infection, IBS). Twenty three percent of the cases are idiopathic.

History and Physical Exam

In the presence of signs suggestive of significant dehydration (Table 38-5), providers must quickly assess the need for any emergent fluid resuscitation. Only then should clinicians proceed with a more methodical, detailed history of the patient, followed by a physical exam. The primary goal is to determine whether the child has a significant or life-threatening disease.

As part of the history, a description of the vomitus—whether bilious, coffee-ground, bright red blood (hematemesis), mucus, or just food—is important in determining the level of the problem. The mode of vomiting (ie, whether it is projectile) gives a clue as to the obstructive nature of the disease. The frequency and volume of vomitus, as well as any precipitating factors, helps in assessing the severity of the problem. The provider must note other associated GI symptoms, such as constipation, diarrhea, jaundice, pain, or distension. The clinician should inquire about other non-GI symptoms, such as headaches, fever, hives, dietary habits, and last normal menstrual period. He or she should obtain a list of all surgeries, as adhesions may lead to obstruction. A family history of acute and chronic GI symptoms or diseases

is necessary, too. In the history, the clinician must document whether the patient cries tears, voids, and tries to drink.

The patient's general appearance and mental status help to determine the severity of his or her condition. In addition, body language and level of discomfort may suggest the diagnosis. For example, a patient in a flexed, bending position, writhing with pain may be a sign of peritoneal irritation.

The vital signs reflect the level of dehydration (Table 38-5). The first objective sign of dehydration is an increase in pulse rate by 10% to 15%. Blood pressure usually is preserved (compensated) until the patient is severely dehydrated (10% to 15%). The provider must remember that the younger the child, the greater the percentage of the body weight is fluid. Therefore, the smaller the child, the easier it is for him or her to become dehydrated.

The provider must assess the child systematically, checking for a depressed fontanel (if present), sunken eyes, decreased tears, and dry mucus membranes. If the child is quiet, the provider can proceed by listening to the heart, lungs, and then to the abdominal exam.

The clinician should first inspect the abdomen, auscultate for bowel sounds, and finally palpate the abdomen, distracting the child during the process. He or she should notice any masses, enlarged organs, and areas of tenderness. An olive-like mass in a neonate with projectile vomiting is indicative of pyloric stenosis. A sausage-like mass, in a child with intermittent abdominal pain and currant-jelly stool, is suggestive of intussusception.

Examination of the skin may help assess hydration status. Capillary refill is determined by squeezing the blood out of the nail bed, then observing how quickly it returns. Normal capillary refill time is less than 2 seconds. Skin turgor is similarly determined by tenting the skin and observing its return to normal position. In a normally hydrated person, it returns back into position immediately (note this is very subjective). When an infant approaches 10% body fluid weight loss, elasticity of the skin decreases, and the skin does not snap back to its normally taut position after being pinched.

The rectal exam is not always necessary, especially if the provider suspects an acute, self-limiting process, such as gastroenteritis. If the provider suspects an obstructive process, GI bleeding, or appendicitis, a rectal exam is warranted. In addition to assessing sphincter tone, the clinician must note any masses and stool in the ampulla (hard, soft, empty), and blood, both fresh and occult.

Table 38–5. CLINICAL SIGNS AND SYMPTOMS OF DEHYDRATION

Dehydration		< 5% (mild)	5–10% (moderate)	> 10% (10–15%) (severe)
Amount of dehydration	Body fluid lost	50 cc/kg	50–100 cc/kg	100–150 cc/kg
	Mental status	alert	+/− altered	+ altered
Cardiovascular	Heart rate	slight increase^	^^	^^^
	Blood pressure	normal	normal	decreased
	Orthostatic hypotension	− (absent)	+/−	+ (present)
	Capillary refill	< 2 seconds	2–5 seconds	> 5 seconds
Skin	Turgor	normal	sluggish	slow
	Elasticity	normal	slight decrease	decreased (tenting)
	Mucus membranes	normal/slightly dry	dry	very dry
	Eye appearance	normal	sunken	sunken
Secretions	Tears	normal/decreased	decreased/absent	absent
	Urine output	concentrated/decreased	oliguria	oliguria/anuria

Diagnostic Studies

Laboratory Testing

The choice of laboratory testing depends greatly on the hydration status of the patient and the suspected age-related diagnosis. If the provider suspects that the patient has a simple, non-invasive gastroenteritis and is less than 5% dehydrated, no chemical work-up is necessary. If vomiting persists and dehydration progresses beyond 5%, though, the provider should obtain serum electrolytes (Na+, K+, Cl-, bicarbonate, BUN) to determine metabolic status and to classify the dehydration based on the serum sodium (ie, isotonic, hypotonic, hypertonic). In addition to serum electrolytes, serum bicarbonate, or more accurately, an arterial blood gas may indicate the presence of metabolic acidosis.

Certain disease processes present with classic electrolyte changes. Pyloric stenosis presents with hypochloremic hypokalemic metabolic alkalosis. Diabetic ketoacidosis may present with acidosis and hyperkalemia. If the provider suspects liver disease or Reye's syndrome, then he or she should obtain liver function tests, serum ammonia, and glucose levels.

The UA may be helpful in detecting the degree of dehydration, metabolic diseases, and urinary tract infections.

▲ **Clinical Warning:** Urine-specific gravity is an indication of hydration status. Its use is limited, however, in infants younger than age 6 months, in whom maximum concentrating ability may only be 1.010 or 1.015 despite the presence of severe dehydration.

Glucosurea will be present with diabetic ketoacidosis. Urinary tract infections may show nitrites, protein, blood, and leukocytes on dipstick, and WBCs and bacteria on microscopic exam.

Regardless of the disease process, a base line CBC is recommended in patients with moderate to severe dehydration or who have obstructive disease. An elevated leukocyte count suggests inflammation, infection, sepsis, or systemic "stress." Anemia may be secondary to GI blood loss (eg, bleeding peptic ulcers) or malabsorption (eg, Crohn's disease). Even if normal, the CBC will serve as a baseline as the disease process continues. A sedimentation rate, although nonspecific, is usually elevated in inflammatory bowel disease.

Radiographic Studies

The type of imaging ordered depends on the patient's age and whether the provider suspects an obstructive process. Patients thought to have bilious vomiting or obstruction should first have an abdominal plain film series, which includes radiographs in supine, upright, and left lateral decubitus positions. Free air in the abdomen denotes a perforated viscus. Air fluid levels are suggestive of obstruction. This study should be followed by an upper GI series (UGI), US, or both in patients suspected of anatomic abnormalities or gastric outlet obstruction.

A barium enema can be both diagnostic and therapeutic in cases of intussusception, left small colon syndrome, and meconium plugs. Abdominal US is recommend for the initial evaluation of infants suspected of having hypertrophic pyloric stenosis. It remains controversial, however, whether this should be the initial imaging prior to contrast study for all infants with persistent vomiting. Two thirds of vomiting infants will have a negative sonogram and subsequently require an UGI series to determine the diagnosis (Ramos & Tuchman, 1994).

Other imaging techniques may be helpful in specific cases. Computerized tomography (CT) scanning or magnetic resonance imaging (MRI) aids in establishing the diagnosis of abdominal tumors or abscess. Endoscopy can be considered when radiographic studies are negative and the provider suspects intestinal obstruction. It is also useful in assessing peptic ulcer disease, esophagitis, and inflammatory bowel disease.

Management

The initial therapeutic goal is to restore circulatory and metabolic homeostasis. The amount of fluid lost (in mL) is calculated by multiplying the child's body weight (gm) by the percentage of dehydration. (For example, a child weighing 10 kg with 10% dehydration has lost 1 liter—10,000 grams x 10% = 1000 mL.)

In mild dehydration (< 5%) not due to an obstructive process, patients can be orally rehydrated using a balanced electrolyte solution (see Table 38-6). Providers should give special attention to the amount of sodium and potassium available in the rehydrating solutions. The fluid replaced should reflect the amount of fluid, sodium, and potassium lost. Children lose 40 to 70 mEq/L of sodium and 10-20 mEq/L of potassium in diarrheal stools. They may lose more potassium and hydrogen ion in the vomitus.

Solutions are available in several flavors as well as ices and are available over the counter (OTC). Most OTC fluids have a lower sodium and chloride concentration than prescription rehydration fluids and are adequate for acute, mild dehydration. Rehydralyte is ideal for the initial rehydration phase, but the amount of sodium supplied should be decreased (by adding free water to the diet) as the viral illness runs it course. Therefore, continuous monitoring of fluid and electrolyte status is important. The World Health Organization's (WHO) formula is particularly useful in

Table 38–6.   ORAL-REHYDRATION SOLUTIONS

	Pedialyte	Resol	Infalyte	Lytren	Rehydralyte	WHO
Na+ (mEq/L)	45	50	50	50	75	90
K+ (mEq/L)	20	20	25	25	20	20
Cl− (mEq/L)	35	50	45	45	65	80
Glucose (gm/dL)	2.5	2.0	0*	2	2.5	2
COST	$	$	$	**	$$$	***
AVAIL	OTC	OTC	OTC	**	OTC	Rx

* Contains rice syrup 30
** Lytren not available in the U.S.; available in Canada
*** WHO is available in the U.S. only through UNICEF

undeveloped nations, where diseases such as cholera (with high sodium losses) predominate. WHO's formula is not easily obtained in the United States.

Parents should use caution when giving children more palatable "home foods and liquids" as fluid replacement. They should not use chicken broth, loaded with sodium, alone. Ginger ale, commonly administered during vomiting, is a good source of fluids but lacks electrolytes. Parents should not, therefore, use it to excess alone but in combination with oral rehydration fluids. Jell-O and apple juice often serve as a source of liquids, but providers should caution parents when children have concomitant diarrhea about the osmotic effects due to their high carbohydrate content, which may actually exacerbate diarrheal losses. Additionally, soft drinks, Jell-O, and chicken broth have insufficient potassium concentrations (usually < 1mEq/L).

In the infant, parents should interrupt formula feeding temporarily, but should continue breast-feeding, alternating with an oral rehydration solution. Initially parents should administer fluids slowly and in small doses (eg, spoon-feeding one teaspoon every few minutes). They should increase administration gradually to prevent abdominal distention and stimulation of the vomiting center. Giving fluids immediately after an episode of vomiting will commonly result in further vomiting. Allowing the stomach to "rest" for about 20 to 30 minutes after vomiting will usually allow for a more successful oral rehydration regimen. When vomiting has resolved, the parent may advance the diet to full liquids, then to a soft diet, and finally to the usual age-appropriate diet.

● **Clinical Pearl:** Parents appreciate a strict recipe for achieving or maintaining hydration. The more specific the provider's instructions, the better. Instructing caregivers just to give clear fluids is less than optimal care. Providers must specify the type, amount, and frequency of fluids.

In cases of moderate to severe dehydration, initial parenteral resuscitation with isotonic fluid is necessary to rapidly restore metabolic and circulatory homeostasis. This is accomplished by administration of a 20 cc/kg bolus of either normal saline or lactated Ringer's solution, followed by a regimen calculated to replace the estimated fluid and electrolyte deficit. These children usually are admitted and hydrated intravenously until they are able to tolerate oral fluids.

If the patient presents with projectile or bilious vomiting or the provider suspects an obstructive process, the child should receive nothing by mouth. He or she should be admitted to the hospital, with placement of a nasogastric tube connected to intermittent suction. The provider should then obtain a surgical consultation.

Most children usually do not require antiemetic drugs because acute vomiting is often associated with a self-limiting infectious process. Such drugs, however, may be indicated in patients receiving chemotherapy or radiation or for postoperative emesis and motion sickness.

Several classes of drugs are used to treat nausea and vomiting. The antihistamines (eg, diphenhydramine, dimenhydrinate) or anticholinergic drugs (eg, scopolamine) are helpful in treating motion sickness. Phenothiazenes are effective in treating vomiting due to radiation, drugs, or cyclic vomiting. Selective 5-Hydroxytriptamine (5-HT3) receptor antagonists (eg, odansetron) have been used to reduce the occurrence of vomiting secondary to chemotherapy and radiation.

The most common causes of vomiting in children are infections, which are usually acute and short-lived. Occasionally,

---

> **DISPLAY 38–2 • Parental Guideline: When to Seek Medical Attention for a Vomiting Child**
>
> - If the vomiting persists despite attempts at spoon-feeding small amounts frequently and offering clear liquids
> - If the child consistently vomits all fluids ingested
> - If the vomiting becomes bilious
> - If urine output becomes drastically reduced
> - If the child is younger than age 4 months
> - If there are any signs or symptoms that the child is more than 5% dehydrated (see Table 37-5)

a patient may have severe or protracted symptoms, which should alert the provider to the possibility of a more serious etiology. Providers should educate parents to inform them in the event of protracted, severe, or bilious vomiting or in cases in which signs of dehydration appear (Display 38-2).

DIARRHEA

Almost everyone experiences diarrhea, characterized by many loose and frequent bowel movements. It is often defined as greater than 10 grams/kg in a day in infants or greater than 200 grams per day in children. A few loose bowel movements do not constitute diagnosable diarrhea. Like vomiting, diarrhea is a symptom of an underlying disease process. It is usually self-limiting and benign, but severe cases may lead to dehydration and death (1%–4% of cases worldwide) (Behrman, 1996). Approximately 5% of all children require an emergency room (ER) visit for diarrhea by age 5 years. Diarrhea was associated with 6.3% of hospitalizations and 4% of ER visits for children ages 1 month to 4 years. In winter months, 92.9 % of hospitalizations for diarrhea were due to viral or non-infectious etiologies (Parashar, Holman, Bresee, et al., 1998).

PATHOLOGY

Diarrhea occurs by one of the following four mechanisms:

> Increased osmotic load in the bowel, causing increased fluid in the intestine
> Excess secretion of electrolytes and water into the bowel lumen
> Exudation of protein and fluid from the intestinal mucosa
> Increased transit time of bowel contents, caused by increased motility

While these four mechanisms causing diarrhea are independent, several may occur simultaneously.

Osmotic Diarrhea

Osmotic diarrhea often results from increasing the osmotic load by ingesting certain foods or medications or because of malabsorption. An increased osmotic load is noted when a person takes laxatives. Malabsorption can be secondary to common entities, such as lactose intolerance, or rarer diseases, such as those causing pancreatic insufficiency.

Secretory Diarrhea

Secretory diarrhea is commonly seen in infectious processes that cause diarrhea. The intestinal mucosa secretes increased amounts of water and electrolytes. This is classically associated with cholera, but other agents also may cause it, such as enterotoxigenic *Escherichia coli*. Non-infectious agents, such as bile acids and long chain fatty acids, also may cause secretory diarrhea.

Exudative Diarrhea

An inflammatory process usually results in exudative diarrhea. Often blood is present. The cause may be an invasive, infectious agent or inflammation, as in Crohn's disease.

Motility Disorders

Diarrhea from motility disorders stems from an increased transit time of food and water in the intestine. It is seen in diseases such as IBS, thyrotoxicosis, and dumping syndrome. Chronic nonspecific diarrhea (toddler's diarrhea) may be a motility disorder modulated by dietary factors, such as excess fruit juice (Kneepkens & Hoekstra, 1996).

Epidemiology

A variety of entities may cause diarrhea. The most common reason for acute diarrhea in all age groups is gastroenteritis. A study of severe and protracted diarrhea requiring hospitalization in infancy revealed that 50% of cases were caused by infectious agents— Rotavirus, Salmonella, and Staphylococcus (Guarino, Spagnuolo, Russo, et al., 1995). Another study showed that a cause could be found in 56% of children hospitalized for gastroenteritis, no infectious agent could be identified in 46% of cases (the number rose to 60% of cases in children younger than age 6 months). When identified, 40% of children had Rotavirus, especially in the winter months, 6% had adenovirus, and 10% had bacterial infections (Salmonella and Campylobacter) (Barnes, Uren, Stevens, et al., 1998). Other causes of gastroenteritis include Norwalk virus (watery diarrhea), Shigella (bloody diarrhea), *Entamoeba histolytica* (bloody diarrhea), Cryptosporidium (bloody diarrhea), *Vibrio cholera* (bloody diarrhea), Cyclospora (intermittent chronic diarrhea), and *Giardia lamblia* (chronic diarrhea). *Escherichia coli* (*E. coli*), the most common cause of traveler's diarrhea, may cause watery diarrhea from the enterotoxins it produces. Other serotypes of *E. coli* may be enteroinvasive, causing inflammation, ulceration, and bleeding from the bowel. *E. coli* serotype O157:H7 has been associated with hemolytic uremic syndrome. *Clostridium difficile* is associated with antibiotic-induced pseudomembranous colitis.

History and Physical Exam

The provider must first establish if the diarrhea is chronic and recurrent or acute and isolated. He or she also must assess the type (eg, watery, mucous, blood, fatty) of diarrhea and the amount. Gastroenteritis is the most common reason for patients to present with acute diarrhea. Once a determination of dehydration status is made, further questioning may ensue.

The history of acute gastroenteritis is usually straightforward. The usual bowel pattern changes to one of frequent, watery stools. Nausea and vomiting may be concurrent and often precede the first episodes of diarrhea, especially when the cause is Rotavirus. Bouts of abdominal pain, relieved by often explosive bowel movements are common. The provider should ask about recent travel of the child or family members or friends who have similar symptoms. Agents that cause invasiveness may cause fever, blood or mucus in the diarrhea, and a toxic appearance. Providers must question about recent antibiotic use as well as the use of other medications.

The physical examination is often unrevealing. The provider should assess vital signs, including temperature, pulse, and blood pressure, to evaluate the possibility of sepsis. There may be a diffusely tender abdomen and active bowel sounds. At times, gastroenteritis mimics an acute abdomen. A rectal exam need not always be done, unless the provider is concerned about fecal impaction or a history of bloody diarrhea. Most importantly, the provider should assess hydration status (see Table 38-5).

Diagnostic Studies

For acute diarrhea, a stool collection for weight and fat analysis and special staining is not needed. This may be useful in cases of protracted or chronic diarrhea. If acute diarrhea has occurred and the child is less than 5% dehydrated, laboratory testing is generally not indicated. However, when the child has bloody diarrhea or fever or appears septic, laboratory assessments are prudent.

The CBC may show an elevated WBC count, with a predominance of immature neutrophils. This is more common when enteroinvasive agents are causing bloody diarrhea. The amount of blood loss is usually not significant, but a CBC will provide a baseline hematocrit.

Providers should measure serum electrolytes, BUN, creatinine levels, and serum bicarbonate in patients who are more than 5% dehydrated (Eliason & Lewan, 1998). If the provider suspects *E. coli* O157:H7, he or she should order serotyping. Measurements of clotting studies and LDH also are needed. The provider should seek *Clostridia difficile* toxin B in suspected cases of pseudomembranous colitis. Radiological studies are rarely necessary in the assessment of acute diarrhea. Stool is assessed for leukocytes seen on the stool smear (5 WBCs/high power field is significant).

● **Clinical Pearl:** Stool cultures and rectal swabs are of value when providers suspect invasive agents, as in the case of bloody or mucus diarrhea, or if the child appears toxic.

● **Clinical Pearl:** The provider should specifically request identification of *E. coli* 0:157, Yersinia, Camphylobacter, Shigella, and Salmonella when ordering stool cultures, since many commercial labs do not routinely test specimens for all of these pathogens.

If bacteria grow, providers should identify and test them for sensitivities to antibiotics. When they request stool chemistry analysis, however, providers must properly instruct patients on how to obtain the sample, because up to one third of samples that patients provide are inadequate for analysis (Phillips, Donaldson, Geisler, et al., 1995).

Management

Mild Illness

▲ **Clinical Warning:** In children, antidiarrheal agents are generally not indicated and may increase enterotoxin absorption in those cases due to bacterial enteritis. In fact, the American Academy of Pediatrics' practice guideline specifically discourages the use of antidiarrheals (Nazarian, 1997).

Mild cases of diarrhea (< 5% dehydration) should be treated in the outpatient setting. The mainstay of treatment is oral rehydration therapy (see Table 38-6). Candidates for oral rehydration therapy should fulfill the following criteria:

* Have mild to moderate dehydration
* Are older than age 4 months
* Have no persistent vomiting
* Are unlikely to have a cause other than viral gastroenteritis
* Are isonatremic
* Are not acidotic (serum bicarbonate is 18 mEq/L) (Eliason & Lewan, 1998).

Rehydration, in general, should follow the same guidelines as discussed in the section on vomiting. The concept of complete bowel rest is usually not necessary, but parents should not force the child to eat. They should encourage, however, drinking fluids. In the nursing infant, breast-feeding should continue. In formula-fed babies with mild diarrhea, regular formula feedings may continue; in more severe cases, parents should use oral rehydration solutions.

▲ **Clinical Warning:** In diarrheal states when vomiting is not present, the prolonged withholding of food is inappropriate. In fact, once hydration is assured, parents should limit the exclusive feeding of oral rehydration solutions or other clear liquids to 12 to 24 hours. Prolonged use of clear liquids, to the exclusion of other foods, will actually prolong diarrhea and promote the development of small, frequent, green, mucousy stools commonly known as "starvation stools."

Once hydration is assured, the diet should return to normal as quickly as possible. The traditional practice of withholding milk products or switching to non-lactose containing formulas for as long as the diarrhea persists in an attempt to treat secondary lactase deficiency is no longer recommended.

● **Clinical Pearl:** Recent evidence has shown that lactase deficiency is not clinically significant in 80% or more of pediatric patients. Early introduction of the child's regular form of milk or formula is recommended and will usually prove beneficial (Nazarian, 1997).

Moderate to Severe Illness

Children with moderate to severe dehydration (5%) should be referred immediately to an acute care setting, where intravenous access can be established. These patients should be admitted and monitored. Aggressive fluid replacement, as discussed in the section on vomiting, is appropriate for these patients.

Antibiotic treatment is not necessary in cases of gastroenteritis caused by viruses or enterotoxin-producing bacteria and may even be harmful. It may prolong the carrier state of patients with Salmonella and has been associated with an increased risk of hemolytic uremic syndrome in patients with E. coli 0:157 gastroenteritis.

▲ **Clinical Warning:** In a child with bloody diarrhea, providers should not initiate empiric antibiotic therapy until a definitive microbiological diagnosis can be established.

Some invasive bacteria, however, may be treated with antibiotics. Trimethoprim-sulfamethoxazole has been used with success in certain enteroinvasive diarrheas, such as Shigella. In one study, however, Shigella was found to be significantly (90%–95% of the time) resistant to trimethoprim-sulfamethoxazole and ampicillin. They were all (100%) sensitive to nalidixic acid (Townes, Quick, Gonzales, et al., 1997). In practical terms, however, by the time the results of stool cultures and sensitivities are reported, most children with Shigellosis have become asymptomatic and will not require treatment. The infant or immunodeficient child with salmonella or signs of true enteric fever should receive antibiotics. Children with Yersinia or Campylobacter who are still symptomatic by the time cultures are reported also should be treated. As stated above, children with E. coli O:157 should not be treated with antimicrobials, because of the increased risk of hemolytic uremic syndrome, presumably due to the release of bacterial endotoxins.

The use of zinc (Fuchs, 1998) and lactobacillus reuteri (Shornikova, Casas, Isolauri, et al., 1997) has been suggested in the treatment of acute diarrhea in children. Further studies are necessary before these agents can be universally recommended (Nazarian, 1997).

Travelers' Diarrhea

Avoiding water, ice, and washed fresh vegetables is an important method of prophylaxis for gastroenteritis when traveling. Use of probiotics, such as lactobacilli, also has been advocated. Taking along bismuth subsalicylate may be of benefit, although the use of this agent in children due to the salicylate moiety poses at least theoretical risk for Reye's syndrome. When necessary (eg, in patients with impaired health), prophylactic antibiotics such as trimethoprim-sulfamethoxazole may be given, but the risk of photosensitivity, especially in tropical and subtropical climates, must be considered (Scarpignato & Rampal, 1995). More recently, in adults, floroquinolones have been used, but the current formulations cannot be recommended in children, because of their effect on growing cartilage. Most effective is the combination of antimicrobial agents and an antidiarrheal agent (such as Loperamide) (Ericsson, 1998). Nonabsorbed antimicrobial agents, such as rifaximin, are currently being studied, as are vaccines for enterotoxigenic E. coli and Shigella.

REFERENCES

Accarino, A. M., Azpiroz, F., & Malagelada, J. R. (1995). Selective dysfunction of mechanosensitive intestinal afferents in irritable bowel syndrome. *Gastroenterology, 108,* 636–43.

Alvarado, A. (1986). A practical score for the early diagnosis of acute appendicitis. *Annals of Emergency Medicine, 15,* 557–564.

Andrew, P. L. R. (1992). Physiology of nausea and vomiting. *British Journal of Anesthesiology, 69* (suppl:1), 2S-19S.

Barnes, G. L., Uren, E., Stevens, K. B., et al. (1998). Etiology of acute gastroenteritis in hospitalized children in Melbourne, Australia, from April 1980 to March 1993. *Journal of Clinical Microbiology, 36*(1), 133–8.

Behrman, R. E., Kliegman, R. M., & Arvin, A. M. (1996). *Nelson textbook of pediatrics* (15th ed.). Philadelphia: W. B. Saunders.

Bennett, D. H., Tambeur, L. M., & Campbell, W. B. (1994). Use of coughing test to diagnose peritonitis. *British Medical Journal, 308,* 1336.

Centers for Disease Control and Prevention. (1994). *Health of our nation's children.* Vital and Health Statistics, Series 10, No. 191.

Drossman, D. A. (1995). Diagnosing and treating patients with refractory functional gastrointestinal disorders. *Annals of Internal Medicine, 123,* 668–697.

Eliason, B. C., & Lewan, R. B. (1998). Gastroenteritis in children: Principles of diagnosis and treatment. *American Family Physician, 58*(8), 1769–76.

Ericsson, C. D. (1998). Travelers' diarrhea. Epidemiology, prevention and self-treatment. *Infectious Disease Clinics of North America, 12*(2), 285–303.

Fuchs, G. J. (1998). Possibilities for zinc in the treatment of acute diarrhea. *American Journal of Clinical Nutrition, 68*(2Suppl), 480S–483S.

Gartner, J. C., Jr., & Zitelli, B. J. (1997). *Common and chronic systems in pediatrics.* St. Louis: Mosby.

Guarino, A., Spagnuolo, M. I., Russo, S., et al. (1995). Etiology and risk factors of severe and protracted diarrhea. *Journal of Pediatric Gastroenterologic Nutrition, 20*(2), 173–178.

Gupta, H., & Dupuy. (1997). Advances in imaging of the acute abdomen. *Surgical Clinics of North America, 77*(6), 1245–1263.

Harris, M. S. (1997). Irritable Bowel Syndrome: A cost effective approach for primary care physicians. *Postgraduate Medicine, 101*(3), 215–226.

Holland, A., & Gollow, I. J. (1996). Acute abdominal pain in children: An analysis of admissions over a three year period. *J Cal Clinical Practice, 16*(3), 151–5.

Hyams, J. S. (1995). Recurrent abdominal pain in children: Commentary. *Current Opinion in Pediatrics, 7*, 529–532.

Kneepkens, C. M., & Hoekstra, J. H. (1996). Chronic nonspecific diarrhea of childhood: Pathophysiology and management. *Pediatric Clinics of North America, 43*(2), 375–90.

Lee, P. W. R. (1976). The plain x-ray in the acute abdomen: A surgeons evaluation. *British Journal of Surgery, 63*, 763–766.

Levine, M. S., Scheiner, J. D., Rubesin, S. E., et al. (1991). Diagnosis of pneumoperitoneum on supine abdominal radiographs. *American Journal of Roentgenology, 156*, 731–5.

Li, B. U. K. (1996). Cyclic vomiting: New understanding of an old disorder. *Contemporary Pediatrics, 13*, 48–62.

Losek, J. D. (1993). Intussusception: Don't miss the diagnosis. *Pediatric Emergency Care, 9*, 46–51.

Lynn, R. B., & Friedman, L. S. (1995). Irritable Bowel Syndrome: managing the patient with abdominal pain and altered bowel habits. *Medical Clinics of North America, 79*(2), 373–391.

Macarthur, C., Saunders, N., & Feldman, W. (1995). Helicobacter pylori, gastroduodenal disease and recurrent abdominal pain in children. *Journal of the American Medical Association, 273*, 729–734.

Martin, R., & Rossi, R. (1997). The acute abdomen: An overview and algorithms. *Surgical Clinics of North America, 77*(6), 1227–1243.

Mason, J. D. (1996). The evaluation of acute abdominal pain in children. *Emergency Medicine Clinics of North America, 14*(3), 629–643.

Nazarian, L. F. (1997). A synopsis of the American Academy of Pediatrics' practice parameter on the management of acute gastroenteritis in young children. *Pediatrics in Review, 18*, 221–223.

Nelson, J. D. (1986). *Current therapy in pediatric infectious disease.* Toronto: Decker.

Orr, R. K., Porter, D., & Hartman, D. (1995). Ultrasonography to evaluate adults for appendicitis: Decision making based on meta-analysis and probabilistic reasoning. *Academy of Emergency Medicine, 2*, 644–5.

Parashar, U. D., Holman, R. C., Bresee, J. S., et al. (1998). Epidemiology of diarrheal disease among children enrolled in four west coast health maintenance organizations. Vaccine Safety Datalink Team. *Pediatric Infectious Disease Journal, 17*(7), 605–11.

Peh, W. C., Khong, P. L., Lam, C., et al. (1997). Ileoiliocolic intussusception in children: Diagnosis and significance. *British Journal of Radiology, 70*(837), 891–6.

Phillips, S., Donaldson, L., Geisler, K., et al. (1995). Stool composition in factitial diarrhea; a six-year experience with stool analysis. *Annals of Internal Medicine, 123*(2), 97–100.

Ramachandran, P., Sivit, C. J., Newman, K. D., et al. (1996). Ultrasonography as an adjunct in the diagnosis of acute appendicitis: a 4-year experience. *Journal of Pediatric Surgery, 31*, 164.

Ramos, A. G., & Tuchman, D. N. (1994). Persistent vomiting. *Pediatrics in Review, 15*, 24–31.

Scarpignato, C., & Rampal, P. (1995). Prevention and treatment of travelers' diarrhea: A clinical pharmacological approach. *Chemotherapy, 41* (Suppl. 10), 48–81.

Schier, F. (1997). Experience with laparoscopy in the treatment of intussusception. *Journal of Pediatric Surgery, 32*(12), 1713–4.

Scholer, S. J., Pituch, K., Orr, D. P., & Dittus, R. S. (1996). Clinical outcomes of children with acute abdominal pain. *Pediatrics, 98*(4 Pt 1), 680–5.

Seigel, L. J., & Longo, D. L. (1981). The control of chemotherapy-induced emesis. *Annals of Internal Medicine, 95*, 352–359.

Seller, R. H. (1996). *Differential diagnoses* (3rd ed.). Philadelphia: W. B. Saunders.

Shornikova, A. V., Casas, I. A., Isolauri, E., et al. (1997). Lactobacillus reuteri as a therapeutic agent in acute diarrhea in young children. *Journal of Pediatric Gastroenterological Nutrition, 24*(4), 399–404.

Simpson, E. T., & Smith, A. (1996). The management of acute abdominal pain in children. *Journal of Pediatric Child Health, 32*, 110–112.

Sivit, C. (1997). Imaging children with acute right lower quadrant pain. *Pediatric Clinics of North America, 44*(3), 575–589.

Squires, R. H., Jr. (1996). Common problems in pediatric gastroenterology. *Comprehensive Therapy, 22*(12), 767–775.

Townes, J. M., Quick, R., Gonzales, O. Y., et al. (1997). Etiology of bloody diarrhea in Bolivian children: Implications for empiric therapy. Bolivian Dysentery Study Group. *Journal of Infectious Disease, 175*(6), 1527–30.

Wagner, J. M., McKinney, W. P., & Carpenter, J. L. (1996). Does this patient have appendicitis? *Journal of the American Medical Association, 276*, 1589–1594.

Walsh, P. F., Crawford, D., Crossing, F. T., et al. (1990). The value of immediate ultrasound in acute abdominal conditions: A critical appraisal. *Clinical Radiology, 42*, 47–49.

Wilcox, R. T., & Traverso, L. W. (1997). Have the evaluation and treatment of acute appendicitis changed? *Surgical Clinics of North America, 77*(6), 1355–1369.

Winslow, B. T., Westfall, J. M., & Nicholas, R. A. (1996). Intussusception. *American Family Physician, 54*(1), 213–217.

Acute Nephrology

• ROBERT A. WEISS, MD

INTRODUCTION

Disorders of the urinary tract are common in pediatric practice. This chapter reviews the most common conditions that are likely to be encountered by the practitioner. Their mode of presentation, diagnosis, differential diagnosis, pathophysiology, and treatment are discussed, emphasizing office approach. Indications for referral to a specialist are also covered.

Urinary Tract Infection

Second only to respiratory tract infection in frequency, urinary tract infection (UTI) occurs in approximately 0.5% to 1% of all boys and 3% to 5% of all girls during the pediatric years (Winberg, Andersen, Bergorrom, et al., 1974). In the newborn period extending into infancy, the male-female ratio is 1:1 (Ginsburg & McCracken, 1982). The uncircumcised state is a risk factor for UTI in male infants (Wiswell & Hachey, 1993); UTI in boys after infancy, however, is rare. The peak age for UTI in girls is around the time of toilet training (Winberg, et al.). It is distinctly uncommon in girls older than 8-years-old (Winberg, et al.). These epidemiological features may, in part, be explained by the differences in pathogenesis of UTI between boys and girls.

ANATOMY, PHYSIOLOGY AND PATHOPHYSIOLOGY

UTI occurs when bacteria, usually of bowel origin (approximately 80% *Escherichia coli*) (Jodal, 1987), colonize the periurethral area. Bacteria that are characterized by hair-like structures on the cell wall (p-fimbriae or pili), allowing them to adhere to the urinary tract epithelium, are most likely to be pathogenic. Another reservoir of bacteria is the prepuce beneath the uncircumcised foreskin in infant boys. After the urethra is colonized, bacteria replicate in bladder urine. If the infection is confined to the bladder, the symptoms are usually those of bladder irritation: frequency, urgency, dysuria, and wetting in children who are already toilet-trained.

Bacterial infection may ascend to the kidneys in one of two ways. Normally, each ureter enters the bladder in a way that prevents regurgitation of bladder urine into the ureter and, by extension, the kidney itself.

● **Clinical Pearl:** In approximately one third of all children with UTI (Smellie, Normand, Katz, et al., 1981), this ureterovesical junction valve is incompetent, creating a condition called vesicoureteral reflux (VUR).

The second potential mechanism that can allow infected bladder urine to ascend to the kidney is the elaboration of a toxin by the infecting bacteria that prevents the normal peristaltic action of the ureter, thus allowing bladder bacteria to ascend the ureter to the kidney. In addition, any mechanical obstruction to the drainage of urine, such as hydronephrosis, will allow bacterial access and replication, producing UTI.

HISTORY AND PHYSICAL EXAM

● **Clinical Pearl:** The clinical features of UTI are nonspecific during infancy and in preschool-aged children. Fever and irritability, without obvious origin in the respiratory tract, is the most common mode of presentation.

Often, gastrointestinal symptoms such as vomiting, diarrhea, and abdominal pain are present. The urine is often foul-smelling or cloudy. The child who had been successfully toilet trained may have wetting accidents. In the school-aged child, the signs and symptoms are more directed to the urinary tract. There may be symptoms of bladder irritation (frequency, dysuria) with cystitis. If the kidney(s) is involved, there is usually significant fever, and the diagnosis of acute pyelonephritis is used. Currently, the $_{99m}$Tc-DMSA scintiscan is the best tool available to accurately diagnose acute pyelonephritis. In one study, 75% of children had unilateral pyelonephritis; 25%, bilateral lesions (Bjorgvinsson, Majd, Eggli, et al., 1991).

DIAGNOSTIC CRITERIA AND STUDIES

Because the diagnosis of UTI, particularly in infants, commits the clinician to a diagnostic evaluation to determine potentially correctable risk factors, the importance of an accurate diagnosis cannot be underestimated.

The diagnosis of UTI is based on significant bacterial growth in a properly collected urine specimen. The traditional significant colony count is greater than 100,000 colonies/mL.

▲ **Clinical Warning:** The presence or absence of white blood cells (pyuria) in the urinalysis (UA) is too unreliable for making or discarding the diagnosis of UTI.

Children who are able to void on command can provide a midstream clean catch urine sample. When compared with the gold standard of a catheterized or bladder puncture specimen, the midstream clean catch is only 80% reliable (Ogra & Faden, 1985). That is, 20% of the time, contamination is the reason for a positive midstream clean catch culture result.

459

▲ **Clinical Warning:** In infants, the results of a urine culture from a specimen obtained by a plastic bag applied to the perineum is helpful only when negative. If the diagnosis of UTI is entertained in an infant, the urine specimen should be obtained by catheterizing the bladder per urethra or by directly aspirating urine from the distended bladder (suprapubic puncture).

● **Clinical Pearl:** Virtually any bacterial growth is significant when a urine specimen is obtained by suprapubic tap. Intermediate growth (<100,000 colonies/mL) from a catheterized specimen may be significant.

Occasionally, specific clinical scenarios may cloud the diagnosis. The child with symptoms of urgency and frequency is an example. In this scenario, a negative culture in the face of a very dilute urine may actually be a false-negative result. This should prompt a repeated culture obtained from a first morning specimen, which is more likely to be concentrated and thus yield a higher colony count. Additionally, dysuria in the face of a true negative culture may be caused by bubble baths or other bath additives, representing a chemical urethritis.

MANAGEMENT

Acute Antibiotic Treatment

After the results of urine culture are known, or while pending, acute treatment for the less toxic, older child is usually amoxicillin, 40 mg/kg per day, divided into three doses daily, for 10 days. An alternative is a trimethoprim-sulfamethoxazole preparation: 8 mg/kg per day of the trimethoprim moiety, divided into two daily doses. Hospitalization for intravenous treatment is indicated for the infant and/or toxic-appearing patient. Ceftriaxone, 75 mg/kg parenterally every 24 hours at least until the child is afebrile, is a first-line drug, with other cephalosporins available as acceptable alternatives, depending on antibiotic sensitivities. The urine will usually become sterile within 48 to 72 hours, accompanied by a clinical response, including resumption of a healthy demeanor. The remainder of the 10-day antibiotic course may be completed with amoxicillin or an oral cephalosporin, such as cefixime, 8mg/kg per day, divided into two daily doses.

Evaluation for Risk Factors

After acute treatment of the infection, the diagnostic evaluation for risk factors must begin. The purpose of imaging studies is to identify those patients at risk for recurrence of UTI, with its attendant acute morbidity and risk of pyelonephritic scarring (American Academy of Pediatrics [AAP], 1999). While the yield of ultrasonography of the kidneys and bladder is approximately 40% (AAP, 1999), it presents no risk to the patient. Kidney size, number, and position can be determined, as well as dilatation of the pelvis and calyces (hydronephrosis) or ureter (hydroureteronephrosis). The bladder can be evaluated for wall-thickness and for postvoid residual. Ultrasonography is an excellent screen for abnormal urinary tract anatomy, but it provides no functional information.

● **Clinical Pearl:** The frequency of VUR is such that any infant or child with a febrile UTI merits investigation for this condition with a voiding cystourethrogram (VCUG).

VCUG should be performed as soon as the urine is sterile. The bladder is catheterized with an 8F feeding tube, and radiographic contrast fills the bladder by gravity. Under fluoroscopic control, the radiologist determines if the contrast enters one or both ureters and goes up into the kidney. Figure 39-1 illustrates the clinical grading of VUR as seen on VCUG. Because the likelihood of detecting VUR declines precipitously after age 5 years; those girls older than 5 with a first episode of cystitis who respond promptly to antibiotic treatment need not undergo VCUG. The yield from ultrasonography is so low as to make this examination also unnecessary. However, below the age of 5, many authorities recommend both sonography and a VCUG with the first UTI in respect of the presence or the absence of fever.

Management of Vesicoureteral Reflux

VUR can be unilateral or bilateral, mild, moderate, or severe. When severe, it is frequently associated with kidney scarring from one or more episodes of acute pyelonephritis. Scarring is best seen by the use of a radionuclide renal scan using

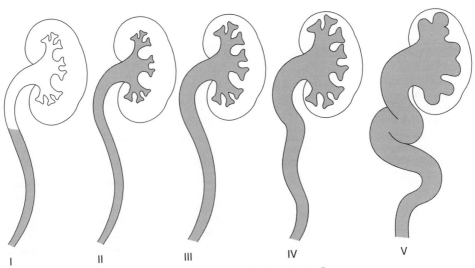

I   II   III   IV   V

Figure 39–1 ■ Grades of vesicoureteral reflux.

$_{99m}$Tc-DMSA. VUR, when mild or moderate, will often disappear over several years. The patient can be successfully protected against UTI with antibiotic prophylaxis during this period. The preferred agent is trimethoprim-sulfisoxazole, 4 mg/kg per day, administered at bedtime. When VUR is severe, referral to a pediatric urologist is indicated for possible surgical reimplantation of the refluxing ureter(s).

Ancillary Management

In addition to imaging studies, a more detailed history of the child's bladder habits may reveal a pattern of dysfunctional voiding. This condition is often observed in preschool- and school-aged children who void infrequently, often have to rush to the toilet when the urge to void overcomes them, and may wet during the day. Often these symptoms are accompanied by chronic constipation. Such children will frequently benefit from a bladder re-education program of timed voiding and anticonstipation therapy. Occasionally, anticholinergic medication, such as oxybutynin (Ditropan), 5 mg two or three times daily, is helpful.

What to Tell Parents

▲ **Clinical Warning:** Regardless of the outcome of the imaging studies, unless antibiotic prophylaxis is prescribed, UTI recurrence rate is at least 50% (Hellerstein, 1982).

Parents should be counseled that after the diagnosis and treatment of a first UTI, monthly surveillance urine cultures are recommended for 3 months, followed by quarterly urine cultures for at least 2 years.

▲ **Clinical Warning:** Any febrile illness is an indication to repeat the urine culture (UC) in a child with a past history of even one UTI. Parents must be reminded to report the history of UTI, if they are seeking care for a febrile illness away from the provider's usual office.

Hematuria

Hematuria must be described as either gross (ie, so many red blood cells [RBCs] that the threshold for visual detection is exceeded) or microscopic (ie, requiring either chemical testing for hemoglobin [dipstick] or microscopy to identify RBCs).

PATHOPHYSIOLOGY

RBCs can originate either from kidney parenchymal disease, such as glomerulonephritis, or from outside the nephron (eg, from the urinary drainage system). The former requires a nephrologic perspective and the latter a urologic perspective. Table 39-1 depicts the clinical and laboratory features that might assist the provider in distinguishing between these two categories.

DIAGNOSTIC CRITERIA AND STUDIES

A visual or microscopic examination of the urine establishes the diagnosis. Not all dark urine is gross hematuria. Two conditions that are not hematuria can be associated with dark urine, reacting with the occult blood pad on the dipstick.

- Active hemolysis may release sufficient hemoglobin into the plasma, and thus glomerular filtrate, that the urine is dark, but RBCs are not seen on microscopy. Frequently, bilirubin is found in the urine under such conditions as well.

Table 39–1   DIFFERENTIATION BETWEEN NEPHROLOGIC AND UROLOGIC HEMATURIA

	Nephrologic	Urologic
History		
Pain (flank or dysuria)?	No	Possibly
Urine color?	Brown, rust, "Coke"	Red or pink
Clot(s) in urine?	No	Possibly
Urine stream?	Normal	Initial/terminal hematuria
Family history of hematuria?	Possibly	Possibly
	Familial nephritis	Hypercalciuria
	Hypercalciuria	Urolithiasis
Physical Exam		
Hypertension?	Possibly	Rarely
Edema?	Possibly	Rarely
Mass?	No	Possibly
Laboratory		
Proteinuria?	Frequently > 2+	Rarely > 2+
Dysmorphic RBCs?	Frequently	Rarely
RBC casts?	Frequently	No
GFR?	Possibly decreased	Rarely decreased
Serum albumin?	Frequently decreased	Normal

GFR = glomerular filtration rate; RBC = red blood cell

- Massive muscle trauma or disorders of muscle metabolism may release enough myoglobin to darken the urine; again, no RBCs are seen by microscopy.

▲ **Clinical Warning:** Neither visual description nor the dipstick alone is sufficient to diagnose gross hematuria; urine microscopy is required.

MANAGEMENT

Gross Hematuria

▲ **Clinical Warnings:**

- The child with gross hematuria who is suspected of having a nephrologic process, typically glomerulonephritis, needs evaluation for hypertension, edema, and oliguric renal failure (see section on glomerulonephritis).
- The child whom the provider suspects has bleeding from outside the nephron needs an immediate imaging study, typically ultrasonography of the kidneys and bladder, because bleeding may stem from anywhere in the urinary tract.

Microscopic Hematuria

● **Clinical Pearl:** Screening microhematuria is rarely associated with significant urinary tract pathology (Feld, et al., 1998).

A positive dipstick reaction for "blood" requires confirmation by urine microscopy, because frequently the dipstick reaction is out of proportion to the quantitation of RBCs per high powered field. Should urine microscopy be negative for RBCs, the patient and family can be reassured that no pathology is present, and thus there is no need for follow up surveillance urinalyses.

In the past, children with confirmed microscopic hematuria were subjected to extensive imaging and serologic evaluations, including renal biopsy (Trachtman, et al., 1984). The yield from these diagnostic investigations is so low that they are no longer recommended, except for patients with a history of gross hematuria, significant proteinuria, or a family history of hematuria (gross or microscopic).

What to Tell Parents

For microscopic hematuria, no more than reassurance is usually indicated. Such patients, however, should be instructed to notify their provider if and when gross hematuria occurs, because this event is much more likely to be associated with significant uropathology. For patients with documented microscopic hematuria, regular (at least annual) surveillance UAs should be continued for the purpose of detecting proteinuria, a much more serious marker of glomerular disease. Figure 39-2 depicts an algorithm for the evaluation and management of hematuria.

Proteinuria

Proteinuria is the hallmark of glomerular disease. The urinary dipstick is highly efficient as a screening tool, because it is sensitive primarily to albumin, the most important type of urinary protein; the pediatric population is spared from the paraproteinemias seen in adults that can result in urinary excretion of pathologic proteins not detectable by the dipstick.

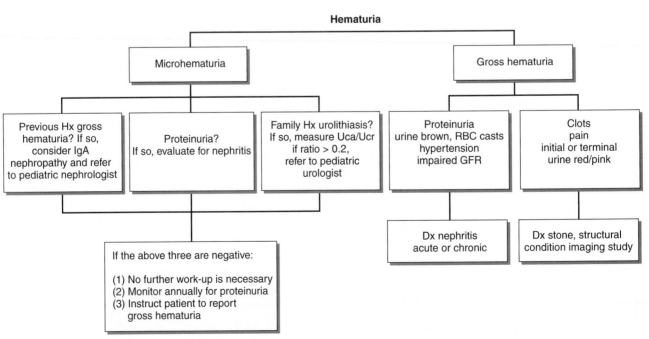

Figure 39–2 ■ Algorithm for the evaluation and management of hematuria.

DIAGNOSTIC CRITERIA AND STUDIES

The dipstick records urinary proteinuria concentration, which will vary with the degree to which the urine is concentrated or diluted.

● **Clinical Pearl:** A negative or trace reading for protein on the dipstick needs no further investigation.

A value of 1 or greater is an indication for quantitation of urine proteinuria concentration by measuring the ratio of urine protein concentration to urine creatinine (Upr/Ucr). A ratio of less than 0.2 is physiologic, while 0.2 or greater is pathologic, requiring investigation as to the etiology.

Orthostatic Proteinuria

Orthostatic (or postural) proteinuria is the most common cause of screening proteinuria, particularly in adolescents. This benign physiologic condition is characterized by increased urine protein excretion in the upright posture that reverts to normal when the subject is recumbent. Thus, measuring 24-hour urine protein excretion, as is commonly done in adults, will not diagnose this condition.

● **Clinical Pearl:** Should a child or adolescent have a screening urine with 1+ proteinuria or greater on the dipstick, a timed overnight urine collection is indicated.

For a timed overnight urine collection, the patient is instructed to empty his or her bladder into the toilet immediately before going to bed and record the time. If the patient awakens during the night to void, this urine should be voided into the collection container. This can be any clean, nonsterile household receptacle. Immediately upon arising, the patient voids into the collection container and the time is recorded. This provides a timed urine collection, reflecting urine formed by the kidneys in the recumbent posture, for analysis. A "first morning" urine sample may include urine formed by the kidneys from the time of the last evening void, until bedtime, which may be proteinuric. This will contribute to the first morning specimen and may confuse the provider.

● **Clinical Pearl:** A properly collected, timed, overnight urine sample that is negative or trace on the dipstick establishes the diagnosis of orthostatic or postural proteinuria.

Parents can be reassured that this is a benign physiologic condition of late childhood and adolescence, without any clinical significance. Should this urine sample test 1+ or greater on the dipstick, however, it should be sent to the laboratory for Upr/Ucr. By extrapolation, a 24-hour urine protein excretion can be derived.

Nonorthostatic Proteinuria

Significant proteinuria detected on screening examination, or at any other time, requires diagnostic investigation. Careful attention should be paid to other markers of glomerulonephritis such as edema and/or hypertension. Additional laboratory testing should include measurement of serum albumin concentration and glomerular filtration rate (GFR, as estimated by BUN and serum creatinine concentrations) and serum complement (C3) concentration. Hypoalbuminemia, even of a modest degree, will clearly point to glomerular disease, whereas depressed GFR can be seen with any

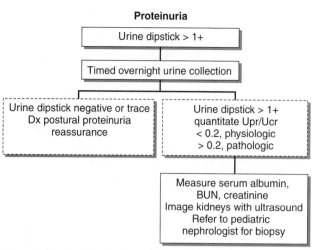

Figure 39–3 ■ Algorithm for the evaluation and management of proteinuria.

condition that involves enough nephrons. Timely referral to a pediatric nephrologist will usually result in the recommendation for renal biopsy. Because this procedure is typically done with ultrasound guidance, the small proportion of patients with proteinuria due to structural urinary tract conditions will be diagnosed as well.

The differential diagnosis of glomerular disease is extensive, but the most common conditions that present with screening proteinuria are focal segmental glomerulosclerosis (FSGS) and membranous glomerulopathy. A third cause of screening proteinuria is membranoproliferative glomerulonephritis (MPGN), although this condition is usually accompanied by significant hematuria. Figure 39-3 depicts the approach to the child with screening proteinuria.

Hypertension

Systemic arterial blood pressure (BP) increases almost linearly with age, height, and weight. Since all three generally occur at the same rate during normal growth, the primary determinant of increasing BP cannot be distinguished. As depicted in Figures 39-4 and 39-5, epidemiological studies of the blood pressure of normal (and primarily Caucasian) infants, children, and adolescents have been divided into centiles. Blood pressure measurements less than the 90th percentile for age and sex are considered normal, while those at the 90th percentile or higher are divided into borderline hypertensive (90th-95th percentile) and hypertensive (≥ 95th percentile). Although those children who are tall for age are allowed a slightly higher BP (Rosner, et al., 1993), more frequently patients in the former category are characterized by excessive weight for age or for height, with or without a family history of hypertension. Unfortunately, the only way to determine with certainty that a high reading is weight-related is to have the patient lose sufficient weight to restore body mass index (BMI; a measure of weight for height) to normal, and see if the BP normalizes. As any pediatric practitioner knows, this is often very difficult.

Regardless of height, weight, or age, a significant proportion of normal children will have hypertensive readings in the provider's office but will be normotensive in less stressful situations. This condition is well described in adults as "white coat" hypertension. Any child or adolescent with screening hypertension, as determined in the provider's office or any health care facility, should have their BPs measured elsewhere, such as the school nurse's office or at home. The latter is preferable, because most school-aged children and adolescents can use a standard, off-the-shelf, digital BP machine. The patient (or parent) should be instructed to measure blood pressure at least twice daily for several weeks and record the readings. Only those patients who are consistently at the 95th percentile or higher by this method merit investigation.

Hypertension in the pediatric population can be divided into two broad categories: primary, characterized by no identifiable etiology, and secondary, due to a diagnosable condition. The proportion of pediatric-aged patients with secondary hypertension is directly correlated to the severity of hypertension and inversely correlated to age, with most adolescents having primary hypertension, similar to adults. The initial diagnostic evaluation for the child or adolescent with significant hypertension (≥ 95th percentile, with normal BMI) should start with a careful personal and family history, particularly noting previous BP measurements, because primary hypertension is usually a process that evolves over many years.

▲ **Clinical Warning:** The patient whose blood pressure jumps one or more quartiles from one yearly measurement to the next requires careful evaluation.

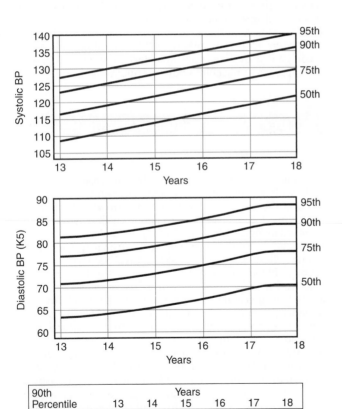

90th	Years					
Percentile	13	14	15	16	17	18
Systolic BP	124	126	129	131	134	136
Diastolic BP	77	78	79	81	83	84
Height cm	165	172	178	182	184	184
Weight kg	62	68	74	80	84	86

Figure 39–4 ■ Age-specific percentiles of blood pressure measurements in boys ages 13 to 18 years. Adapted with permission from Task Force on Blood Pressure Control in Children. (1987). Report of the Second Task Force. *Pediatrics 79*, 1–25.

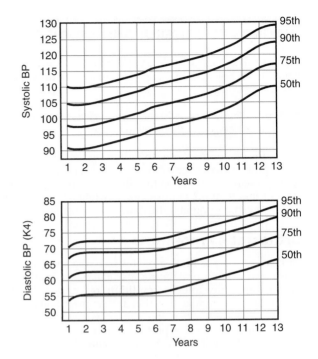

90th	Years												
Percentile	1	2	3	4	5	6	7	8	9	10	11	12	13
Systolic BP	105	105	106	107	109	111	112	114	115	117	119	122	124
Diastolic BP	67	69	69	69	69	70	71	72	74	75	77	78	80
Height cm	77	89	98	107	115	122	129	135	142	148	154	160	165
Weight kg	11	13	15	18	22	25	30	35	40	45	51	58	63

Figure 39–5 ■ Age-specific percentiles of blood pressure measurements in girls ages 1 to 13 years. Adapted with permission from Task Force on Blood Pressure Control in Children. (1987). Report of the Second Task Force. *Pediatrics 79*, 1–25.

HISTORY AND PHYSICAL EXAM

Rarely do children and adolescents have any complaints that are directly due to hypertension. Children of families with a history of early cardiovascular morbidity and mortality also require extra attention. Because most adults do not have regular BP surveillance, it may be difficult to determine the result of their last BP measurement; alternatively, measure the parent(s) blood pressure directly.

The upper extremity BP measurement should be confirmed with a proper size cuff. Obese and/or very muscular adolescents may require a large adult cuff for accurate BP measurement.

▲ **Clinical Warning:** A cuff width that is too small may result in a BP reading that is falsely high; conversely, a cuff width that is too large will not result in a BP reading that is falsely low.

● **Clinical Pearl:** The recommendation is to use the largest cuff width that will allow access to the antecubital fossa.

The clinician should palpate the femoral pulses and measure BP in the thigh to exclude coarctation of the aorta. The skin should be examined for the neurocutaneous lesions of neurofibromatosis or tuberous sclerosis. Pallor suggests the anemia of chronic renal failure. Edema may be present with nephrotic syndrome. Rarely, a Wilm's tumor, palpable as a flank mass, may present with hypertension.

Laboratory testing should include the following:

- UA to screen for renal disease. The kidney is the organ most commonly involved in the etiology of secondary pediatric hypertension. The detection of proteinuria alone or proteinuria and hematuria should prompt measurement of GFR and serum albumin concentration (see Proteinuria section).
- Imaging the urinary tract by ultrasound of the kidneys and bladder. Careful attention should be paid to kidney size (a report of normal size is insufficient; there are norms for kidney size versus age and versus height) and whether or not the collecting system is dilated (hydronephrosis). One of the most common causes of pediatric hypertension is reflux nephropathy (see UTI section), characterized by small, deformed kidney(s) with hydronephrosis. On occasion, autosomal-recessive polycystic kidney disease (ARPKD), diagnosable by ultrasound, will present during childhood or even adolescence with hypertension. Although somewhat insensitive and nonspecific, measurement of renal artery blood flow velocity by Doppler technology, to begin the evaluation for renovascular hypertension, can be done at the same ultrasound examination.
- If both UA and ultrasound are normal, renal scan (DTPA radionuclide) and arteriography can be done to test further for renovascular hypertension. The role of spiral CT and magnetic resonance angiography (MRA) are still unclear. The advantage of arteriography (usually intra-arterial digital subtraction) is that not only can a diagnosis be made, but also if the renovascular lesion is amenable to balloon dilatation, it can be done at the same time.

DIAGNOSTIC CRITERIA AND STUDIES

Extrarenal conditions that should be considered include catecholamine-secreting tumor, such as pheochromocytoma. The diagnosis requires measurement of urine catecholamines, such as VMA, HVA, epinephrine, norepinephrine, metanephrine, normetanephrine, dopamine, and creatinine (the latter to assess the completeness of the urine collection).

Typical phenotype or other signs and symptoms characterize other endocrine conditions, such as hyperthyroidism, congenital adrenal hyperplasia, and Cushing's syndrome. Hyperaldosteronism (primary or secondary), the syndrome of apparent mineralocorticoid excess (AME), and glucocorticoid remediable hypertension (GRH) are almost always accompanied by hypokalemic hypochloremic metabolic alkalosis. Thus, serum electrolytes should be measured at some point in the diagnostic evaluation.

Figure 39–6 depicts an algorithm for the diagnostic evaluation of hypertension in the pediatric patient.

MANAGEMENT

The treatment of hypertension in adults has benefited immeasurably from data generated by large clinical trials that have tested antihypertensive drugs. Because there are measurable outcome variables, such as cardiovascular morbidity and mortality, efficacy and safety of treatment regimens have been established. In contrast, the treatment of hypertension in the pediatric patient is empiric, both as to indications for drug treatment and safety/efficacy data.

●**Clinical Pearl:** Nonpharmacological treatment of pediatric hypertensive patients has received scant attention. Lifestyle

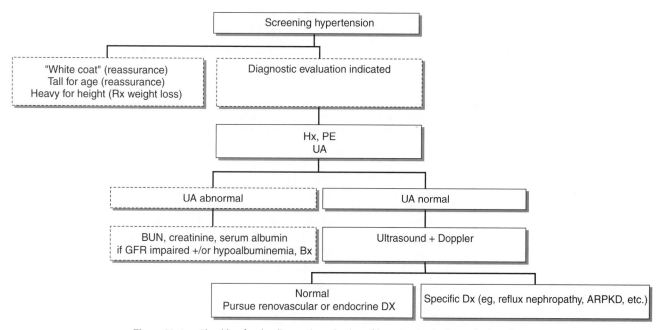

Figure 39–6 ■ Algorithm for the diagnostic evaluation of hypertension in the pediatric patient.

changes, including calorie and salt reduction sufficient to restore and maintain body weight to that appropriate for height, with regular exercise, should be strongly encouraged.

Adolescents should be counseled about the additive adverse health effects of cigarette smoking and hypertension. In addition to patients who fail nonpharmacologic treatment, those with a strong family history of cardiovascular morbidity and mortality, as well as those with left ventricular hypertrophy by echocardiography, are more likely to be candidates for drug therapy.

Pharmacotherapy

At present, both calcium channel blockers (CCBs) and angiotensin-converting enzyme (ACE) inhibitors are widely used, safe, and efficacious. They have overtaken thiazide diuretics and adrenergic inhibitors (β-blockers) as first-line drug therapy in the pediatric hypertensive population. Unfortunately, there are no data in either adults or children as to the consequences of potentially decades of such drug therapy. In contrast, there are overwhelmingly positive data that effective treatment of hypertension in adults dramatically decreases the rate of cardiovascular morbidity and mortality. Possibly, a significant proportion of those pediatric hypertensive patients relegated to drug therapy could be maintained normotensive with only lifestyle modifications, and compliance with the latter may be encouraged by the prospect of discontinuing drug therapy. Commonly used antihypertensives and their doses are listed in Table 39-2.

Acute Nephritis

■ Acute Poststreptococcal Glumerulonephritis

PATHOPHYSIOLOGY

Acute nephritis typically presents after an infection, most frequently streptococcal (strep) throat or skin infection. The interval between strep exposure and onset of acute nephritis can be up to 3 weeks, but some children present with acute nephritis without any previous signs or symptoms to suggest strep infection. Approximately 3% of those with a diagnosed strep infection will get acute poststreptococcal glomerulonephritis (APSGN) (Sagel, et al., 1973), but only the more serious cases come to medical attention with the aforementioned presentation. As opposed to acute rheumatic fever, effective antibiotic treatment has no effect on the risk of acquiring APSGN, or on its course or severity, once established.

HISTORY AND PHYSICAL EXAM

Clinical features may include gross hematuria, edema, low urine output, and hypertension; constitution symptoms such as fever, abdominal pain, and headache may also be present.

DIAGNOSTIC CRITERIA AND STUDIES

The diagnosis of APSGN is confirmed by the following laboratory studies:

- Proteinuria
- Red blood count (RBC) casts seen on urine microscopy
- Low serum C_3
- Evidence of preceding streptococcal infection:
  Bacteriologic, such as positive throat or skin lesion culture
  Serologic, such as increased ASO titer or Streptozyme test
- Serum albumin concentration and GFR may be depressed. The latter may be sufficient for the diagnosis of acute renal failure (ARF) (see p. 471).

Other conditions that often present with an acute nephritic syndrome and low serum C_3 concentration include the following:

- Postinfectious glomerulonephritis due to pneumococcus
- Systemic lupus erythematosus (SLE)
- Idiopathic chronic membranoproliferative glomerulonephritis
- Chronic infections such as infected ventriculoatrial shunts, visceral abcess, or endocarditis
- Idiopathic vasculitis

Table 39–2 ANTIHYPERTENSIVE DRUG THERAPY FOR CHILDREN AND ADOLESCENTS

Class	Drug	Starting Dose	Maximum Dose
ACE inhibitor	Captopril (Capoten)	1.5 mg/kg/day, div TID	6 mg/kg/day, div TID
	Enalapril (Vasotec)	0.15 mg/kg/day	0.5 mg/kg/day, QD or div BID
Calcium channel blocker	Nifedipine (Procardia) XL or Adalat CC	0.25 mg/kg/day	3 mg/kg/day, QD or div BID
	Amlodipine (Norvasc)	0.1 mg/kg/day	0.1–0.5 mg/kg/day
β-Blocker	Atenolol (Tenormin)	1 mg/kg/day	8 mg/kg/day
α-Blocker	Prazosin (Minipress)	0.05–0.1 mg/kg/day	0.5 mg/kg/day
Peripheral vasodilator	Minoxidil (Loniten)	0.1–0.2 mg/kg/day	1 mg/kg/day, div BID
Diuretic	Hydrochlorothiazide (Hydrodiuril)	1 mg/kg/day	2 mg/kg/day, QD or div BID
	Furosemide (Lasix)	1 mg/kg/day	10 mg/kg/day

ACE = angiotensin-converting enzyme; BID = twice daily; div = divided; QD = once daily; TID = three times daily.
Adapted with permission from Sinaiko, A.R. (1996). Hypertension in children. *New England Journal of Medicine 335*, 1968–1973.

MANAGEMENT

The management of the child with APSGN is guided by the expected clinical course. Hypertension and ARF are the most important complications. The former is unpredictable in its severity and is a frequent reason for hospitalization of the child with ASPGN. A short-acting CCB, such as nifedipine (see Table 39-2), is effective; those children with edema due to oliguria may have an antihypertensive effect from the use of loop diuretic therapy as well.

▲ **Clinical Warning:** The absence of both hypertension and ARF at the time of diagnosis is no guarantee of a benign course. Daily outpatient follow-up is mandatory for the measurement of BP and weight, as markers of fluid balance.

● **Clinical Pearl:** GFR measurement should be repeated 24 to 48 hours after diagnosis; if this second measurement is normal as well, ARF is unlikely to evolve.

Dietary salt restriction to 1 g per day is essential for prevention of edema accumulation because any acute nephritis is characterized by low urinary sodium excretion. Treatment of edema, both by diet and diuretic therapy, will also reduce the risk of hypertension. In the child with uncomplicated APSGN, gross hematuria, impaired GFR, and hypertension should resolve by the second week, followed by resolution of proteinuria. Serum C_3 concentration should return to normal by 6 to 8 weeks and microhematuria should disappear within 6 months. The long-term outcome of APSGN is generally good, with fewer than 1% of patients having any significant permanent renal disease.

■ Other Acute Nephritides

Acute nephritis may also complicate Henoch-Schönlein purpura. The presentation and clinical course are usually the same as those of APSGN, but without the hypocomplementemia or evidence of strep infection. It too has a high spontaneous resolution rate with a low risk of permanent renal injury. The principles of management are the same as APSGN.

Chronic glomerulonephritis can present either acutely (eg, with gross hematuria, edema, hypertension, and impaired GFR) or with only screening proteinuria and/or hematuria. The most common type of chronic glomerulonephritis is immunoglobulin A (IgA) nephropathy. It is characterized by recurrent gross hematuria, and each episode occurring with a febrile respiratory illness.

▲ **Clinical Warning:** The first attack of chronic glomerulonephritis may mimic acute nephritis, but the UA does not return to normal. Therefore, every patient with what may seem to be uncomplicated acute nephritis must be followed until the UA has returned to normal.

Typically, hematuria is persistent; proteinuria is minimal and may be present only during an episode of gross hematuria.

DIAGNOSTIC CRITERIA AND STUDIES

● **Clinical Pearl:** A diagnostic kidney biopsy is indicated for any child with a persistently abnormal UA following a first episode of gross hematuria or if a second episode of gross hematuria recurs.

IgA is the predominant protein detected in the glomerular mesangium when the tissue is examined by immunofluorescence.

MANAGEMENT

Currently, there no standard treatment of chronic glomerulonephritis exists, and a significant proportion of patients are anticipated to progress to renal failure over several decades.

Other primary forms of chronic glomerulonephritis include, as mentioned in the proteinuria section (and below in the nephrotic syndrome section), FSGS, MPGN, and membranous glomerulopathy. All require kidney biopsy for definitive diagnosis, none has a uniformly safe and effective therapy, and all have significant risk of progressive renal failure. There are several types of chronic glomerulonephritis that are part of systemic or multiorgan conditions. The most common of these is SLE. Please see Chapter 62, Chronic Urinary Problems, for further discussion of chronic glomerulonephritis.

Nephrotic Syndrome

PATHOPHYSIOLOGY

Nephrotic syndrome (NS) is a condition characterized by increase in permeability of the glomerular capillary wall to plasma proteins and a marked reduction in the ability of the kidney tubules to excrete sodium (and water). The latter causes the accumulation of edema fluid. The etiology remains unknown. More than 80% of children will have normal kidney biopsy (International Study of Kidney Disease in Children, 1981), thus the term minimal change disease. A similar proportion of patients will respond (lose their proteinuria) to the administration of corticosteroid within 1 to 2 weeks.

HISTORY AND PHYSICAL EXAM

Every few years, a typical pediatric practice might see a child, usually of preschool age, who presents with generalized edema of several days' or sometimes weeks' duration. The parents may report periorbital edema in the morning and resolution during the day, followed by swelling of the feet or legs by the end of the day due to the effect of gravity. Distention of the abdomen due to ascitic fluid accumulation may be persistent. Urine output is usually less than normal, and the child may have been observed to have a gain of weight due to fluid accumulation. Gross hematuria is not present, nor is hypertension. Less commonly, NS may present with serious bacterial infection, because proteinuria makes the nephrotic child deficient in important immunoglobulins owing to urinary losses. Children with ascites due to active NS are particularly susceptible to bacterial peritonitis, usually characterized by fever, abdominal pain, and vomiting.

DIAGNOSTIC CRITERIA STUDIES

The pathognomonic diagnostic findings of NS are significant proteinuria (2-4+ on the dipstick and Upr/Ucr > 3), low serum albumin concentration (typically < 2.0 g/dL), and hyper-cholesterolemia. GFR is usually normal.

MANAGEMENT

Hospitalization is recommended for children with severe edema and/or children whose parents seem overwhelmed and need the reassurance of a hospital setting until they can come to grips with their child's condition. Because NS is likely to be a relapsing condition that will last throughout childhood, the clinician must be attentive to the need for support to the family of such patients. Speaking to another family with a nephrotic child can be very helpful. A recommended approach to the newly diagnosed child with NS is outlined in Figure 39-7.

Prednisone (or prednisolone) in tablet or liquid formulation should be started immediately, at a dose of 2 mg/kg per day, given once every morning with food. The parents should be instructed to test the child's urine daily for protein, using a urine dipstick and to record the results in a permanent format (eg, a notebook). When the child responds, there will be a diuresis and all the water weight will be lost. Around this time, however, the effect of steroid treatment on appetite will become apparent, and slow but steady weight gain should be expected. Fat accumulation occurs primarily in the face and trunk. A small proportion of children will have an increase in blood pressure, so this should be measured weekly, for at least the first 2 months of therapy. Parents should also be advised that steroid therapy is likely to cause a change in their child's behavior and personality; the most common pattern is lowered frustration tolerance and crying easily.

●**Clinical Pearl:** Referral to a pediatric nephrologist for kidney biopsy is indicated only for patients who fail to respond to therapy.

The immunosuppressive nature of steroid treatment will place the child at higher risk for adverse outcomes from certain viral infections, especially varicella. Should an unimmunized patient be exposed, he or she should receive varicella-zoster immune globulin (VZIG) immediately, followed by high-dose acyclovir. According to the *Red Book*, the varicella vaccine should be administered to nonimmune patients during remissions, after the child has been off high-dose steroid therapy for at least 30 days. Children receiving systemic steroids at a lower dose (less than 2 mg/kg per day of prednisone) may receive the vaccine, although some experts recommend discontinuing steroid use for 2 weeks after immunization, if possible.

After 4 to 6 weeks (depending upon tolerance) of daily prednisone treatment, the same dose is to be given every other morning for an additional 4 to 6 weeks, then discontinued. No tapering schedule is necessary, although many pediatric nephrologists do taper the medication.

Parents should be advised that more than 50% of children with NS will suffer from frequent relapses—every few weeks or months. Each is characterized by recurrence of proteinuria, often coincident with the onset of URI. The caretakers should be trained to test their child's urine daily so that a relapse will be detected and treatment can be initiated to prevent edema accumulation. Relapses can be treated with prednisone, 2 mg/kg per day until proteinuria has disappeared for 3 consecutive days, at which point therapy can be abruptly discontinued. Usually less than 2 weeks of daily treatment is needed. Alternatively, additional treatment with a tapering, alternate-day prednisone schedule over several weeks can be administered. Although this method delays the interval between relapses, the price is more unwanted steroid effects.

Unfortunately, those NS patients who relapse frequently are likely to accumulate unwanted effects, such as obesity and growth retardation, from recurrent courses of steroid therapy. Such patients should be referred to a pediatric nephrologist for evaluation. The treatment of steroid toxicity is steroid withdrawal. A course of alkylating agents—cyclophosphamide (Cytoxan), 2.5 mg/kg per day for 3 months or more potent immunosuppressive therapy with drugs like cyclosporine (Neoral), 5 mg/kg per day for 6 to 12 months, is frequently successful in this regard.

●**Clinical Pearl:** The parent(s) should be advised that regardless of the number of relapses, as long as each responds to steroid treatment, there is no permanent kidney injury and no risk of progressive renal failure.

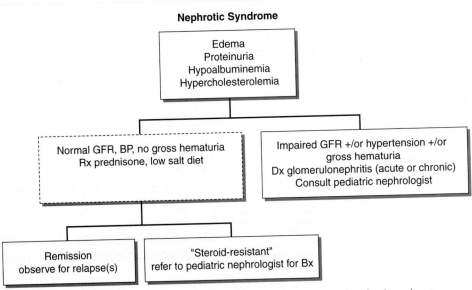

Nephrotic Syndrome

Edema
Proteinuria
Hypoalbuminemia
Hypercholesterolemia

Normal GFR, BP, no gross hematuria
Rx prednisone, low salt diet

Impaired GFR +/or hypertension +/or gross hematuria
Dx glomerulonephritis (acute or chronic)
Consult pediatric nephrologist

Remission
observe for relapse(s)

"Steroid-resistant"
refer to pediatric nephrologist for Bx

Figure 39–7 ■ Management approach for the child with newly diagnosed nephrotic syndrome.

The great majority of children who relapse will enter spontaneous permanent remission by adolescence.

Acute Renal Failure

Acute renal failure (ARF) is quite uncommon in pediatric practice. It can be defined simply as low urine output and impaired GFR characterized by accumulation of BUN, creatinine, potassium, phosphorous, uric acid, etc. Gross hematuria, edema, hypertension, and proteinuria easily diagnose inflammatory conditions responsible for ARF, such as acute glomerulonephritis. ARF can also result from hemodynamic insults, such as severe diarrheal dehydration, shock, sepsis, or trauma.

MANAGEMENT

Depending on the severity and/or duration of the reduction in kidney blood flow, ARF can be reversible if the abnormal hemodynamic situation is effectively treated. Tubular function, the ability to conserve sodium and water, is most easily measured in the office setting by the urine specific gravity (Usg). For example, if the patient with diarrheal dehydration and preserved tubular function, as measured by a high Usg of 1.025, is rehydrated, one would expect the urine output to increase, Usg to decrease, and an increased BUN and creatinine to return to normal. Such a patient would then be diagnosed as "pre"-renal failure. However, if impairment of both glomerular function and tubular function (eg, Usg < 1.015) is already apparent at presentation, or the patient is already edematous, nothing is to be gained by giving fluids in an attempt to increase urine output. Such patients, as well as those with acute glomerulonephritis, require meticulous management of fluids and electrolytes until, as is usually the case, renal function recovers.

In such cases, water is administered only in amounts to replace insensible losses (450-500 mL/m² per day) and whatever urine the patient makes. As edema indicates accumulation of total body sodium, none should be administered, nor should potassium, which typically accumulates with ARF.

High-dose loop diuretic (eg, furosemide) therapy can also be tried. It is more likely to be effective in patients with acute glomerulonephritis than in those with ARF due to hemodynamic injury. Indications for dialytic support until renal function recovers include hyperkalemia and/or severe edema, unresponsive to diuretic treatment.

Figure 39-8 outlines the evaluation and management of the child with acute renal failure.

Hemolytic Uremic Syndrome

One cause of ARF that does not fit into either the inflammatory or hemodynamic category is hemolytic uremic syndrome (HUS). The toxin elaborated by E. coli 0157:H7 causes this condition. Occasionally, ingestion of potentially contaminated food, most frequently undercooked hamburger, can be identified. HUS develops in approximately 10% of people infected with this organism. The usual presentation is bloody diarrhea in a toddler or young school-aged child.

▲ Clinical Warnings:

- In a child with bloody or mucusy diarrhea, the clinician should not prescribe empiric antibiotic therapy until the results of stool cultures are known, because antibiotic treatment for E. coli 0157:H7 has been identified as a risk factor for the development of HUS.
- Many labs do not routinely culture for E. coli 0157:H7. The clinician should request specific identification for this pathogen when ordering stool cultures on a child with bloody diarrhea.

Such children should be carefully monitored for anemia and thrombocytopenia, as well as oliguria, proteinuria, hematuria, and rising levels of BUN/creatinine. The clinical presentation includes pallor due to microangiopathic hemolytic anemia, petechiae due to thrombocytopenia, and edema because patients may receive advice to encourage oral fluids or have received intravenous fluids to prevent or treat dehydration from diarrhea. Treatment is identical to that for ARF of other causes, but these patients frequently need blood products and are at risk for hypertension, neurologic symptoms, pancreatitis, and bowel perforation from HUS as well. Approximately 50% will require dialysis for ARF, compared with fewer than 20% in ARF from other causes.

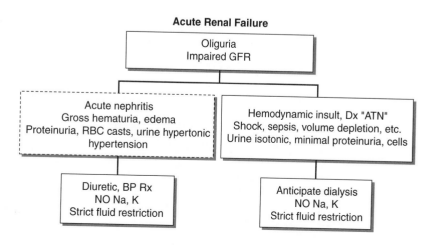

Figure 39–8 ■ Algorithm for the evaluation and management of acute renal failure.

REFERENCES

American Academy of Pediatrics (1999). Committee on Quality Improvement. Subcommittee on UTI. Practice parameter: The diagnosis, treatment, and evaluation of the initial UTI in febrile infants and young children. *Pediatrics, 103,* 843–852.

Bjorgvinsson, E., Majd, M., Eggli, D.K., et al. (1991). Diagnosis of acute pyelonephritis in children: Comparison of sonography to 99mTc-DMSA scintigraphy. *American Journal of Roentgenography, 157,* 539–543.

Feld, L., Mexers, K.E.C., Kaplan, B.S., et al. (1998). Limited evaluation of microscopic hematuria in pediatrics. *Pediatrics, 102,* e42.

Ginsburg, C.M., & McCracken, G.H., Jr. (1982). UTIs in young infants. *Pediatrics, 69,* 409–412.

Hellerstein, S. (1982). Recurrent UTIs in children. *Pediatric Infectious Diseases, 1,* 271–281.

Jodal, U. (1987). The natural history of bacteriuria in childhood. *Infectious Disease Clinics of North America, 1,* 713–729.

Ogra, P., & Faden, H. (1985). UTIs in childhood: An update. *Journal of Pediatrics, 106,* 1023–1028.

Rosner, B., Prineas, R.J., Loggie, J.M.H., et al. (1993). Blood pressure nomograms for children and adolescents, by height, sex, and age, in the United States. *Journal of Pediatrics, 123,* 871–876.

Sagel, I., Treser, G., Yoshizawa, N., et al. (1973). Occurrence and nature of glomerular lesions after group A *streptococci* infections in children. *Annals of Internal Medicine, 79,* 492–498.

Smellie, J.M., Normand, I.C.S., Katz, G., et al. (1981). Children with UTI: a comparison of those with and without vesicoureteric reflux. *Kidney Int, 20,* 717–722.

Task Force on Blood Pressure Control in Children. (1987). Report of the Second Task Force. *Pediatrics, 79,* 1–25.

The primary nephrotic syndrome in children. Identification of patients with minimal change nephrotic syndrome from initial response to prednisone. A report of the International Study of Kidney Disease in Children. (1981). *Journal of Pediatrics, 98,* 561–64.

Trachtman, H., Weiss, R., Benett, B., et al. (1984). Hematuria in children-indications for renal biopsy. *Kidney Int, 25,* 94–99.

Winberg, J., Andersen, H., Bergorrom, H.T., et al. (1974). Epidemiology of symptomatic UTI in childhood. *Acta Paediatr Scand Supplement 252,* 1–20.

Wiswell, T.E., & Hachey, W.E. (1993). UTIs and the uncircumcised state: an update. *Clinical Pediatrics, 32,* 130–134.

Acute Urology

• STANLEY J. KOGAN, MD, and PENNY COLBERT-KOGAN, RN, BSN

INTRODUCTION

Genitourinary (GU) problems are frequently encountered in general pediatric practice. With the prenatal diagnosis of GU problems made in 0.1% to 1% of pregnancies (Johnson et al., 1992) and the presence of cryptorchidism found in about 3% of term boys (Gill & Kogan, 1997), primary care providers are commonly expected to have basic knowledge of these and related conditions. Urinary tract infections (UTIs), occurring in 1% to 2% of school girls; vesicoureteral reflux; acute scrotal inflammation; and penile disorders all constitute additional frequently encountered problems demanding basic expertise. This chapter provides information for understanding, recognizing, referring, and treating patients with these problems.

CONGENITAL HYDRONEPHROSIS, MULTICYSTIC KIDNEY, AND VESICOURETERAL REFLUX

Anatomy, Physiology, and Pathology

Abnormal ureteral bud development is the clue to understanding congenital hydronephrosis, multicystic kidney, and vesicoureteral reflux. At about the 4 mm embryonic stage, the ureteral bud grows out of the cloaca (which ultimately forms the bladder and rectum) cephalad into the developing metanephric cell mass (which ultimately forms the kidney). According to one theory (Mackie & Stephens, 1975), if the bud enters the metanephric cell mass in too cranial of a position, an obstructed or cystic kidney will result. If it enters in too caudal (inferior) a position, kidney dysplasia is the consequence. At the same time, if the lower end where the ureteral bud originates grows out of the cloaca from a lateralized position, the resulting tunnel through the subsequent bladder wall is too short. Vesicoureteral reflux is the outcome.

The cysts in multicystic kidneys vary in size and usually do not communicate with one another. Often the ureter is atretic or absent, and there may be no renal pelvis. Obstruction leads to progressively abnormal branching of the developing calyces and thinning of the renal parenchyma, changes that ultimately affect renal function.

Fortunately, many neonatally confirmed ureteropelvic junction obstructions have a huge distended renal pelvis with relatively well preserved parenchyma. The distensible pelvis "protects" the parenchyma from markedly increased pressures, at least for a while, and renal function is initially preserved in many (Fig. 40-1).

Epidemiology

Whereas only a few decades ago, the usual presentation of hydronephrosis was as a silent abdominal mass, now virtu-

ally all are discovered prenatally. Most cases are cystic or hydronephrotic kidneys, with obstruction or underlying vesicoureteral reflux as the cause. Physiologic dilatation, which spontaneously subsides in the postnatal period, constitutes another significant group of patients.

Some cystic diseases of the kidneys and vesicoureteral reflux are associated with genetic tendencies. Reflux risk is increased in some families, especially those with blond females and of Scandinavian descent.

▲ **Clinical Warning:** The overall risk of a sibling having reflux when it has been identified in an index patient increases to about one in four in some series, even if there is no history of urinary infection. This fact should prompt the clinician to investigate the possibility of reflux in at-risk siblings of an affected child.

Similarly, there is a significant increased genetic risk involved with autosominal dominant, "adult polycystic" (AD-PKD) and autosomal recessive, "infantile polycystic" kidney disease (AR-PKD). If a parent has AD-PKD, each child has a 50% chance of inheriting the disease. If neither parent has the disease, none of the children will inherit the disease, even if history of the disease is in the family. With AR-PKD, if both parents have the recessive gene, one in four children can inherit the disease despite no findings of the disease in the parents. Multicystic kidney disease, which is the most common variety of cystic disease seen in children, occurs sporadically and is not associated with an increased genetic risk.

History and Physical Examination

Most cases are now diagnosed prenatally. Occasionally, an abdominal mass may be evident at birth or become evident subsequently. Providers should observe the urinary stream and seek evidence for bladder distension in males. Urinary infection may occur sometime during the first year of life or after and usually is a sign of underlying vesicoureteral reflux. Children with multicystic kidneys have an increased risk (between 10% and 20%) of associated vesicoureteral reflux.

Diagnostic Criteria

Because there are usually no symptoms or physical findings, the diagnosis is usually based on prenatal sonography. Postnatal radiologic studies are indicated for any child with a history of prenatal urinary tract dilatation, because the frequency of underlying pathology is significant.

● **Clinical Pearl:** For unilateral hydronephrosis, it is best to defer postnatal sonographic imaging until 2 to 3 weeks after birth. Sonography during the first few days after birth notoriously underestimates the extent of hydronephrosis because newborns lose a significant amount of water weight. Later imaging more accurately indicates the true extent of the problem.

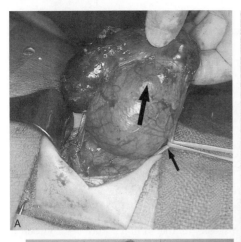

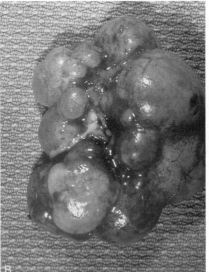

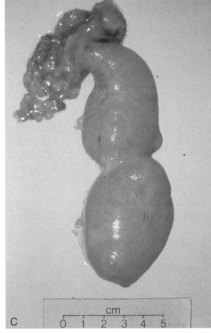

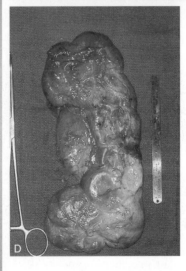

Figure 40–1 ■ Examples of congenital hydronephrotic kidneys. *(A)* Congenital ureteropelvic obstruction. Large arrow indicates dilated renal pelvis. Small arrow indicates normal size ureter with loop around it. *(B).* Congenital multicystic dysplastic kidney associated with absent ureter. *(C)* Multicystic dysplastic kidney and dysplastic ureter. *(D)* Example of non-functional giant hydronephrotic kidney destroyed because of silent ureteropelvic junction obstruction. Kidney contained over 1000 mL of urine prior to decompression for removal.

▲ **Clinical Warning:** If bilateral hydronephrosis is present and severe at birth, a voiding cystourethrogram (VCUG) and sonogram should be performed within 24 hours of birth to determine whether outlet obstruction is present (posterior urethral valves in boys and ureterocele or urethral/urogenital sinus obstruction in girls).

A VCUG is indicated in all instances of prenatally diagnosed hydronephrosis to determine the presence of vesicoureteral reflux and to image the urethra in males. If kidney obstruction is suspected, a renal scan is indicated at times to confirm obstruction in a dilated kidney and to quantitate kidney function and excretion. This study is not usually done before age 3 to 4 weeks, because neonatal glomerular filtration rate is markedly decreased initially and does not normalize completely until about age 6 months. Multicystic kidneys typically are found to be devoid of all function, as are some dysplastic kidneys. Diminished function in a nonrefluxing hydronephrotic kidney usually indicates significant obstruction. Figure 40-2 refers to an algorithm for the evaluation of prenatal hydronephrosis.

Management

Reflux

When reflux is documented, antibiotic prophylaxis is indicated as initial treatment for all grades except the most severe (grade V). Antibiotics do not cure reflux; rather, they prevent urinary infections from occurring. Treatment is based on the premise that reflux will often disappear spontaneously by ages 4 to 6 years in most instances, providing that no breakthrough urinary infections occur. Reflux without urinary infection usually does not damage the kidney. As determined on the VCUG, the lower the reflux grade, the more likely the reflux will ultimately self-cure (American Urological Association, 1997).

The sonogram and VCUG are repeated 12 to 15 months later. Reflux persisting beyond ages 4 to 6 years usually requires surgical correction, because reflux persisting thereafter has a markedly reduced chance of spontaneous resolution. When surgical correction is required, the ureter is reimplanted into the bladder in a manner to lengthen its course through the bladder wall, enabling it to act in a one-way-

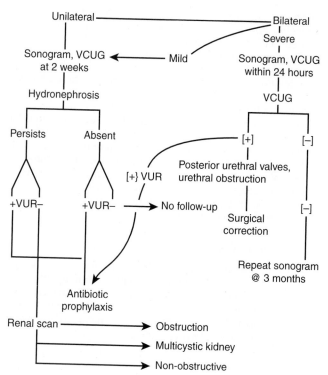

Code: VCUG = Voiding cystourethrogram
VUR = Vesico ureteral reflux

Figure 40–2 ■ Algorithm for evaluation of prenatally diagnosed hydronephrosis.

low-up sonography in 3 and in 6 months with an additional renal scan if necessary. Antibiotic prophylaxis is indicated for the more severe cases, although not all practitioners uniformly recommend this approach. If follow-up imaging indicates deterioration, surgical correction is indicated, because obstruction is usually progressive and compromises renal function. Pyeloplasty is eminently successful in childhood and preserves renal function from further deterioration.

What to Tell Parents

Parents must be counseled that continued low-dose antibiotic prophylaxis is important because omission increases the risk of febrile UTIs and kidney damage. Repeated radiologic imaging is essential and cannot be omitted. Chronic (albeit infrequent) follow-up is essential because late deterioration does occur.

SCROTAL AND TESTICULAR ABNORMALITIES

Developmental disorders predispose testes to later problems. Boys with abnormally descended testes are subject to rapid germ cell loss and ultimate sterility if the problem is not corrected early in life. Scrotally located testes with abnormal fixation are subject to increased risk of testicular torsion, atrophy, and subfertility. A persisting processus vaginalis and hydrocele may expand with time into a hernia, necessitating surgical correction. Knowledge of childhood scrotal and testicular problems is essential in preventing later health mishaps and medicolegal problems.

For all problems involving the scrotum and testes, the primary care practitioner will need to consider various diagnoses and interventions. Scrotal swelling may be caused by a hydrocele, hernia, testicular torsion, torsion of the appendix testis, epididymitis, varicocele, hematocele, and rarely tumors. Loss of a testicle may be a tragic consequence if diagnosis of testicular torsion is missed. The following is a list of general considerations that may be useful in establishing the correct diagnosis and consequent course of action.

Determine the following about the swelling:

- Acute or chronic
- Painful or painless
- Fluctuating in size or stable
- Associated with GU symptoms, systemic symptoms, or trauma

On physical examination, note the following:

- Look for signs of inflammation (eg, erythema, heat, swelling, tenderness).
- Determine if the swelling is moveable, reducible, present only in upright position.
- Transilluminate to determine if swelling is lucent (fluid-filled) or solid.

Cryptorchidism

Pathology

Testicular descent is a function of fetal development and correlates with gestational age and fetal weight. Cryptorchidism occurs in about one in three premature boys. By term, most testes will descend, with about 3% remaining

valve fashion. Surgical methods vary, but all now are associated with a reduced hospital stay, usually varying between 1 and 4 days. Results of surgery are highly successful; once the reflux is corrected, it is very unlikely to recur.

Multicystic Kidneys

Multicystic kidneys are functionless on renal scan. Most will involute with time, literally "shriveling" into a minute or indiscernible mass on follow-up sonography. Observant follow-up with periodic sonography is the appropriate initial treatment. Rarely, multicystic kidneys will grow, sometimes to very significant size, requiring surgical excision. Hypertension, infection, and neoplastic change are additional rare causes for nephrectomy. Conventional large incisions are no longer needed for nephrectomy in infants with multicystic kidneys. Mini-incision nephrectomy and laparoscopic nephrectomy now allow for markedly reduced morbidity and even same-day surgery in many instances.

Obstruction

Considerable judgment is required with kidneys demonstrating an obstructive pattern on renal scan. For those that are clear-cut, pyeloplasty for relief of ureteropelvic obstruction should be done as soon as the infant is thriving and fit, usually between ages 1 and 2 months. Early repair is feasible in skilled pediatric urologic hands when skilled pediatric anesthesia can be provided as well. This approach maximizes preservation of renal function.

Infants demonstrating an "equivocal" or indeterminate pattern on renal scan should be followed carefully by fol-

cryptorchid. Probably resulting from the physiologic burst in testosterone noted in boys at age 6 to 8 months, most testes that are cryptorchid at birth descend subsequently, with only 1% remaining cryptorchid at age 1 year (Table 40-1).

If not treated within the first year, germ cells rapidly deteriorate. At 2 years, about one third of untreated cryptorchid testes are completely devoid of germ cells, one third have significant germ cell loss, and one third have testes with normal germ cell numbers (Houissa, dePape, Diebold, et al., 1979). Testes remaining cryptorchid at puberty are uniformly oligospermic or azoospermic. Leydig cell function usually remains adequate, though persistent cryptorchid adults may suffer premature androgen failure.

▲ **Clinical Warning:** Because spontaneous descent occurs minimally beyond age 1 year and the onset of deterioration is noted at the same time, medical or surgical treatment is indicated by the first birthday (American Academy of Pediatrics, 1997).

History and Physical Examination

When evaluating cryptorchid testes, clinicians should determine whether a parent has ever visualized the testis in the scrotum. Surprisingly, parents or older boys often know that the testicle has been felt within the scrotum even though the testis is not evident during the pediatric office examination. Testicular retraction causes confusion in diagnosis. Some boys have a hyperactive cremasteric muscle reaction, causing a truly descended testis to retract rapidly into the inguinal region at the slightest provocation (retractile testis).

● **Clinical Pearl:** Retraction may be avoided if the clinician places two fingers over both inguinal rings before examining the scrotal contents, thereby blocking testicular escape into the canal.

Another technique involves positioning the boy cross-legged and leaning forward, which relaxes the cremasteric muscles and often allows the testicle to fall into the scrotum and become palpable. If these means do not place the testicle in the scrotum, true cryptorchidism exists. Making this distinction is important because retractile testes usually develop normally, and conversely, treatment must be provided to truly cryptorchid testes to prevent deterioration.

Besides this distinction, secondary or delayed ascent of a previously descended testis occurs in about 5% of cryptorchid boys, further confounding diagnosis. These testes are exposed to the same risk of deterioration as those that are congenitally cryptorchid, though occurring at a slower rate. Retraction of the testis may occur due to reabsorption of an occult patent processus vaginalis (PPV) (Rabinowitz & Hulbert, 1997). Examination and documentation of the position of both testes through the end of pubertal development is absolutely essential to prevent medicolegal problems in these instances. In the case of retractile testes, the clinician should document and demonstrate to the parent their scrotal position at each preventive visit.

Diagnostic Criteria

About 20% of all cryptorchid testes are impalpable despite all posturing and positioning maneuvers. Impalpable testes are either present within the abdomen or inguinal canal, or they are atrophic or absent. Bilateral impalpable testes in a phenotypic male should raise the suspicion of an occult female adrenogenital syndrome.

Diagnostic Studies

When testes are impalpable, inguinal, pelvic, and scrotal ultrasound can be used to aid in diagnosis. Technical limitations sometimes occur, limiting the reliability, and "negative" sonograms have been seen indicating an absent testis when the testis was easily palpable in the groin or scrotum. A sonogram indicating that an impalpable testis is actually present is usually accurate. If the sonogram does not identify a testis, an impalpable testis may still be present (false-negative examination). In these instances, laparoscopy preceding surgical exploration is the most reliable test to determine whether the testis is present. Computed tomography and magnetic resonance imaging examinations are not routinely used in these instances because they are costly and not completely reliable and diagnostic. In highly selected cases (ie, in which a previous surgical exploration failed to reveal an impalpable testis) these examinations may have some utility (Kogan, 1992).

When the examination reveals bilateral impalpable testes, endocrinologic diagnostic evaluation is indicated. Measurement of plasma follicle-stimulating hormone, luteinizing hormone, and the testosterone response to human chorionic gonadotropin stimulation is indicated to determine whether bilateral testicular absence (bilateral anorchia) is present (Jarow, Berkowitz, Migeon, et al., 1986). In these circumstances, when all endocrinologic criteria are fulfilled, surgical exploration for confirmation of testicular absence is not required. These evaluations should be made in conjunction with a pediatric endocrinologist, pediatric urologist, or both.

Management

Palpable undescended testes are amenable to ambulatory orchidopexy in virtually all instances. Potential complications include testicular retraction, arterial or vas deferens injury, and subsequent atrophy, all of which are exceedingly rare. Treatment of impalpable testes is more complex, and complications occur more commonly in this group (Kogan, 1992). A variety of surgical techniques now exist that can bring even the highest abdominal testis into a scrotal location. Surgical options vary according to the individual sur-

Table 40-1.   PREVALENCE OF CRYPTORCHIDISM AT VARIOUS AGES

Age	Weight (g)	Incidence (%)
Premature	451–910	100.0
	911–1810	62.0
	1811–2040	25.0
	2041–2490	17.0
		Total 30.3
Full term	2491–2720	12.0
	2721–3630	3.3
	3631–5210	0.7
		Total 3.4
1 y		0.7–0.8
School age		0.76–0.95
Adulthood		0.7–1.0

Data from Scorer, G. C., & Farrington, G. H. (1971). *Congenital deformities of the testis and epididymis*. London: Butterworths. Printed with permission, Kogan S. J. Cryptorchidism. In P. P. Kelalis, L. R. King, A. B. Belman (Eds), *Clinical pediatric urology*, (3rd ed.). (p. 1059). Philadelphia: W.B. Saunders.

geon's preferences: high transabdominal dissection, laparoscopic orchidopexy, and microvascular autotransplantation are all capable of achieving successful results.

Hernias and Hydroceles

When a testis descends, the processus vaginalis precedes it as it descends to the scrotum, usually obliterating subsequently. A persisting or PPV often terminates in a cystic dilatation above the testicle (hydocele), which may fill and empty through the PPV (Fig. 40-3). If the processus widens, a hernia occurs.

Inguinal hernias and PPVs occur more commonly in premature infants. At birth, the incidence of unilateral or bilateral PPVs is high. When a unilateral inguinal hernia is present, a PPV is present on the opposite side in more than 50% of cases. One study indicated that 59% of boys up to age 16 years were found to have an occult contralateral PPV when bilateral explorations were performed. Another study indicated that older children with a repaired left hernia had a 40% chance of a subsequent hernia on the right. Conversely, when a hernia was repaired on the right, there was only a 14% chance of a subsequent hernia on the left. These frequencies diminish with age, but clinical experience indicates that routine surgical exploration of the opposite groin or some method of evaluation (eg, pneumoperitoneum, laparoscopic examination) should be done in boys whose examination reveals a unilateral hernia or hydrocele. Hernias also occur more commonly when an undescended testis is present (Skoog et al., 1995).

History and Physical Examination

Most scrotal disorders other than torsion are painless, though childhood inguinal hernias may be uncomfortable, and incarcerated inguinal hernias are usually exceedingly painful. The presence of a painful inguinal mass in an inconsolable infant is pathognomonic of an incarcerated inguinal hernia. If the testis is not palpable in the scrotum, torsion of an undescended testis is another similar rare cause.

● **Clinical Pearl:** Bilateral inguinal hernias in a male infant with hypospadias or in a phenotypic female should raise suspicion of an underlying genetic or intersex disorder, such as male pseudohermaphroditism, true hermaphroditism, or testicular feminization.

Diagnostic Criteria

Hernias and hydroceles are diagnosed by physical examination, without the need for any adjunctive testing. Transillumination of the scrotum with a focused penlight in a darkened room is helpful to distinguish fluid-filled (hydrocele) from solid inguinal and scrotal swellings. Hydroceles usually fluctuate in size and are readily transilluminable.

Management

Hydroceles are common at birth and resolve spontaneously in most instances. If they persist beyond or enlarge significantly before age 15 to 18 months, ambulatory surgical repair is indicated because a PPV remains present. The contralateral side is evaluated by a diagnostic pneumoperitoneum or intraoperative peritoneoscopy or is explored at the same time because subsequent risk of a hydrocele or hernia increases.

Hernias, by contrast, pose a clear risk to the patient and must be repaired when diagnosed, regardless of the patient's age, due to the risk of incarceration. The risk of testicular infarction from an incarcerated hernia in premature infants and neonates is significant. Bowel incarceration represents an additional risk if the condition is not treated emergently. If a hernia cannot be reduced, a temporizing option is to sedate the patient and place him in Trendelenburg's position and attempt reduction again in half an hour. If this is not successful, hospital admission and surgical evaluation are indicated. A hernia that is not incarcerated requires no immediate treatment, though a surgical referral should be made to schedule an elective repair. Bilateral evaluation or repair is indicated at surgery in young boys, as with hydroceles (Skoog, 1997).

Testicular Torsion

Testicular torsion causes progressive venous congestion, diminished arterial inflow, and ultimately, edema, swelling of the testis, hypoxia, and hemorrhagic infarction. Torsion usually results from poor fixation of the testicle within the surrounding tunica vaginalis sac, resulting in the "bell-clapper" deformity.

Testicular survival relates to the duration of torsion. Many testes will recover when detorsion occurs within 6 hours, but survival markedly decreases after 12 hours of complete tor-

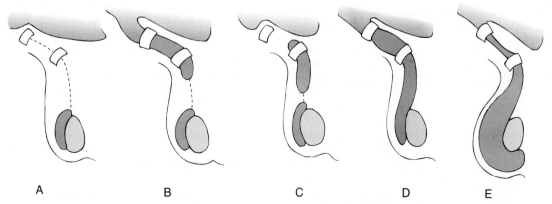

Figure 40–3 ■ Diagrammatic representation of persisting patent processus vaginalis and hernia. (A), normal obliteration of patent processus. (B), patent processus proximally with inguinal bulge; processus obliterated distally. (C), closure proximal and distal with loculated hydrocele of cord. (D), complete patency with hernia sac extending into scrotum. (E), partial proximal closure, resulting in scrotal hydrocele and proximal patent processus.

sion and is nonexistent at 24 hours (Donohoe & Utley, 1978). At times, torsion may be noted at birth, and it is not possible to know the duration. Most of these testes will be lost, with at best a 10% survival (Stone, Kass, Cacciarelli, et al., 1995).

Testicular or epididymal appendiceal torsion may mimic torsion of the testis, though pain and swelling may be more localized to the superior pole of the testis ("blue-dot sign"). These appendages can twist spontaneously, becoming congested, edematous, and ultimately undergoing infarction without damaging the testes as a whole.

History and Physical Examination

Boys with testicular torsion may relate a history of previous episodic intermittent acute scrotal pain without swelling (intermittent torsion). Examination in the upright standing position during painless interludes may reveal that the testis has an anterior lie (ie, it has "flopped forward"), offering a clue that the classical "bell-clapper deformity," predisposing to torsion, is present. During acute episodes of torsion, sudden pain progresses to erythema and swelling of the testis and scrotum. Within hours, a hard "egg-shell" mass emerges. Often there is associated nausea and vomiting but usually no fever or urinary complaints. About 5% of episodes of testicular torsion are painless.

Diagnostic Criteria

▲ **Clinical Warning:** In boys with acute hemiscrotal pain, swelling, or both, testicular torsion is the underlying diagnosis until proven otherwise.

Torsion of a testicular or epididymal appendage must be distinguished from torsion of the testis. In some instances, a small blue nodule may be visualized and felt at the superior testis pole ("blue dot sign"); at other times, the entire hemiscrotum may be tender and swollen, indistinguishable from the appearance noted in torsion of the testis.

Epididymo-orchitis causes diffuse swelling and pain and may be associated with fever, systemic signs, and sometimes signs of urinary infection and pyuria. Prehn's sign (relief of pain with elevation of the testis) and elevated white blood cell count may be present. Table 40-2 describes the differential diagnosis of an acutely inflamed scrotum.

Varicoceles are another cause of intermittent scrotal swelling. Present in about 15% of adolescent boys, varicoceles are dilated testicular veins that result in a "bag of worms" appearance within the scrotum. Varicoceles are prominent only in the upright position, so standing the patient for examination is a necessary part of diagnosing this condition. Ninety percent occur on the left side as a result of drainage of the testicular vein directly into the renal vein. Most are painless; rarely patients will describe a "nagging, dragging" sensation. Varicoceles are important to recognize because they may cause ipsilateral testicular atrophy and bilateral testicular dysfunction (subfertility) if left untreated into late adolescence and adulthood (Skoog, Roberts, Goldstein, et al., 1997).

Testicular tumors seldom present with inflammatory signs, though rarely pain or a surrounding hydrocele may be present. Hematoceles (blood within the tunic vaginalis surrounding the testicle) may follow a direct traumatic incident.

Diagnostic Studies

Torsion must be distinguished from epididymitis, tumors, and incarcerated inguinal hernias. When a clinical diagnosis of testicular torsion is obvious, emergent surgical detorsion is indicated because testis survival relates directly to duration of torsion. When the diagnosis is equivocal, Doppler ultrasound and radionuclide scrotal scanning are helpful adjunctive tests, but only if they are available on an emergent basis. Both are subject to interpretive errors, however. False-negative Doppler studies occur, and radionuclide imaging is not uniformly technically satisfactory, so these tests should be used only to supplement the clinical impression. Figure 40-4 illustrates an algorithm for evaluating the acutely painful inflamed scrotum.

● **Clinical Pearl:** Epididymitis is rare in prepubertal boys.

Management

When acute scrotal inflammation is present, diagnosis and treatment must be performed expeditiously. Practitioners dealing with this condition should consult a pediatric urologist and determine if immediate referral and adjunctive diagnostic tests are indicated. Time is of the essence. When the diagnosis is confirmed, surgical exploration and detorsion are performed immediately. At surgery, when the testicle is found to be viable, it is sutured in place; the opposite testis is also sutured to prevent sequential torsion, which definitely occurs with increased frequency. If the testicle is necrotic, it is removed. After the scrotum heals, placement of a testicular prosthesis may be considered.

Torsion of a testicular appendage is usually self-limited, requiring treatment with anti-inflammatory medications, such as ibuprofen. In very rare instances, the inflammation does not resolve, and delayed surgical removal of the appendix is necessary.

Epididymo-orchitis requires medical treatment once the diagnosis of testicular torsion is firmly excluded. After a urine culture is obtained, treatment with trimethoprim/sulfa or amoxicillin; anti-inflammatory medications, such as ibuprofen; and bed rest with scrotal elevation is indicated. A pediatric urologic surgeon should evaluate varicoceles, testicular tumors, and other miscellaneous scrotal conditions.

Table 40–2. DIFFERENTIAL DIAGNOSIS OF THE ACUTELY INFLAMED SCROTUM

	Testicular Torsion	Epididymorchitis
Age	Through puberty	More common after puberty
Recurrent pain	May be present	Absent
Fever	Generally absent	Usually present
Scrotal examination	Abnormal testis position	More discrete mass
	Generalized scrotal swelling	
Urine and WBC	Normal	May be abnormal
Ultrasound	Absent blood flow	Normal or increased flow

PENILE ABNORMALITIES

As with other pediatric urologic conditions, knowledge of penile development and anatomy helps providers to understand disorders that occur. Penile structural formation occurs during the first trimester of pregnancy. During this

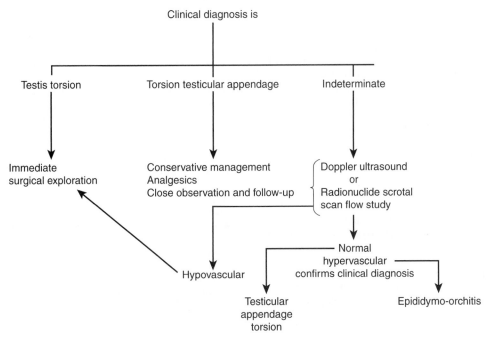

Figure 40–4 ■ Algorithm for managing acute scrotal swelling.

time, the urethra extends itself completely to the tip of the glans. The sizes of the penis and the clitoris in the female are similar at this point, but during the subsequent two trimesters, the penis grows dramatically under the influence of testosterone, while clitoral size remains stable.

These observations are significant, because endocrinologic or developmental events during the first trimester result in abnormal penile formation (eg, hypospadias), whereas disorders of penile size (eg, micropenis) result from conditions later in pregnancy, causing disrupted growth. In both situations, providers must look for other associated causes. These include genetic or intersex conditions, such as male pseudohermaphroditism, which affects androgen production or action; central nervous system disorders; or endocrinologic abnormalities, such as growth hormone deficiency. Sometimes the cause is unusual, such as maternal ingestion of progestational agents early in pregnancy, which disrupts normal penile morphogenesis. In some instances, familial genetic conditions are present (eg, inherited androgen insensitivity syndromes, familial rudimentary testis development). Questions regarding other family members having abnormal genital development and obtaining a pregnancy history are important.

Anatomy, Physiology, and Pathology

At birth, the penis is normally straight, with the urethral meatus at the tip and a full foreskin completely enveloping the glans. The foreskin is normally nonretractable; adhesions between the glans and inner foreskin are present. Phimosis, therefore, is a normal physiologic occurrence at birth. These adhesions usually lyse spontaneously by age 4 to 5 years in most boys. In cases that do not spontaneously resolve or in which the foreskin is long and tight, smegma may form, presenting as a pearly white cheesy collection seen or felt under the skin. Smegma is a mixture of sheared cells from the glans

and inner foreskin, mixed with secretions from glands on the glans. Though unsightly at times, this naturally occurring substance does not represent infected material, cyst, tumor formation, or a "growth."

Balanitis

Uncircumcised boys are at increased risk for development of inflammation of the foreskin (posthitis) and inflammation of the glans (balanitis). These conditions usually occur when the foreskin is long, tight, and unretractible. Urine trapping occurs in some, resulting in overgrowth of the normal bacteria under the foreskin. Inflammation follows, with edema, swelling, localized pain, and dysuria. With treatment and healing, adhesions result, setting the stage for recurrence of similar episodes.

Meatitis

One "purpose" of the foreskin is to envelop and protect the glans and urethral meatus from the surrounding environment (eg, urine, diapers). Ammoniacal dermatitis from urine and chemicals within the diaper causes meatitis, visible at times as a "cherry-red spot" at the meatus. The inflammation eventually heals but with scarring, which is not visible until later years when the urethra and penis grow. The scarred meatus remains stationary in size. A narrowed, upward-deflected urinary stream results, sometimes with associated dysuria.

● **Clinical Pearl:** While boys who are uncircumcised are at increased risk of smegma formation, balanitis, and posthitis, circumcised boys are at significantly increased risk for developing stenosis of the urinary meatus. Meatal stenosis occurs virtually exclusively in circumcised boys; congenital narrowing is extremely rare.

Hypospadias

When the urethra does not reach the tip of the penis and falls short on the underside, hypospadias exists. The urethra may be positioned anywhere on the undersurface (Fig. 40-5), though most cases of hypospadias are more distally located. Chordee, a downward bend of the penile shaft, often accompanies hypospadias; the more severe the hypospadias, in general, the worse the chordee. At times hypospadias may be present without chordee, and the opposite may occur as well. In these situations, the foreskin is virtually always incompletely formed on the undersurface of the glans and is part of the whole maldevelopment of this area.

Epispadias

Epispadias is a very rare condition that in many ways can be considered a mirror image of hypospadias. In these cases, the urethra falls short of the tip of the glans on the upper (dorsal) surface of the shaft. Dorsal chordee (ie, an upward bend) is present. The developmental defect in epispadias may be more extensive, however, because it may extend into the bladder neck region, causing maldevelopment of the neck and sphincter with urinary incontinence.

Management

Hypospadias

When hypospadias is present, providers should inquire whether a family history exists and whether the mother ingested any medications during the first trimester. They should inspect the testes to determine whether they are present, descended, and palpably normal. Cryptorchidism or absence (even unilaterally) should raise the suspicion of an underlying intersex condition. Clinicians should ensure that urination is normal. Boys with minor degrees of hypospadias, descended testes, and normal urination do not need immediate pediatric urologic consultation, though sometimes parents are appreciative and relieved when in-hospital consultation is provided. Boys with more severe hypospadias, cryptorchidism, or other associated congenital malformations should be evaluated urologically at birth with renal and pelvic sonography and urologic consultation. In some instances, a VCUG and blood karyotyping may be required.

Management of the Uncircumcised Penis

In older boys, foreskin-related problems occur commonly. In uncircumcised boys, providers should ask about inflamma-

tory symptoms (eg, dysuria, swelling, discharge from beneath the foreskin). They should inquire about "ballooning" of the foreskin with voiding or significant dripping after urination, which occurs as a result of a tight phimosis with urine trapping within. These boys are at increased risk of developing inflammatory conditions, such as balanitis, which is usually treated with sitz baths and careful attention to hygiene. Systemic antibiotics are not needed.

If the foreskin is easily retractable, cleaning during baths or showers may easily be accomplished. In those with true phimosis without symptoms and signs of inflammation and urinary infections, the foreskin should not be retracted. In these instances, bathing the outside skin alone is sufficient. Forcible retraction creates bleeding, scarring, and more importantly, pain and avoidance between parent and son. Outcomes from this "treatment" are worse than the risks associated with not retracting the foreskin.

Sometimes the foreskin can become trapped behind the glans (paraphimosis) and cannot be replaced, leading to progressive edema and potential glans gangrene. Emergency treatment consists of reducing the foreskin back to its natural position to prevent serious sequelae.

Management of the Circumcised Penis

Circumcised boys are subject to a different set of problems. Adhesions between the penile shaft skin and glans occur, especially in infants, in whom the penis retracts naturally into the often generous peripubic fat. Penile adhesions after circumcision are often obvious, especially when extra skin remains. At other times, they may be subtle and can be identified only by following the normal dark coronal rim around the glans circumferentially. If the rim margin cannot be seen, adhesions are covering it and obscuring it from view. Adhesions may lead to smegma collection. In most cases, clinicians may easily lyse them by gentle traction. In some instances, the adhesions between the penile skin and glans can become literally "grafted" to the glans and are inseparable. Surgical excision and repair are necessary. Incomplete circumcision leaving extra or redundant eccentric skin sometimes occurs, leaving a very unfavorable cosmetic appearance. Removal of too much skin is much more serious, leading often to scarring or a "trapped" or "buried" penis as the skin heals around it. Figure 40-6 illustrates some of potential complications of circumcision.

THE CIRCUMCISION CONTROVERSY

The decision whether to circumcise at birth is often difficult, tumultuous, and conflicting. Medical recommendations have wavered over the years to each extreme. Presently, data indicate that the risk of urinary infection is increased in uncircumcised boys, perhaps by a 10-fold factor; however, the absolute risk of urinary infection remains small (Wiswell, Smith, & Bass, 1985). Additional increased risks of epididymitis, balanoposthitis, sexually transmitted diseases, and penile cancer in older uncircumcised males have been suggested. The validity of some of these statements, however, has been questioned. Body rights advocates argue that patients should be allowed to make their own decisions about removal of this body part, claiming that body image is unfairly altered and important sexual nerves are removed. Problems outlined above (eg, incompletely removed foreskin, increased meatal stenosis risk, adhesions) occur, confirming that circumcision is clearly not problem free. Parents often look to clinicians for guidance and recommendations

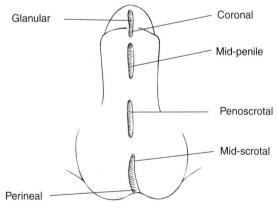

Figure 40–5 ■ Classification of hypospadias.

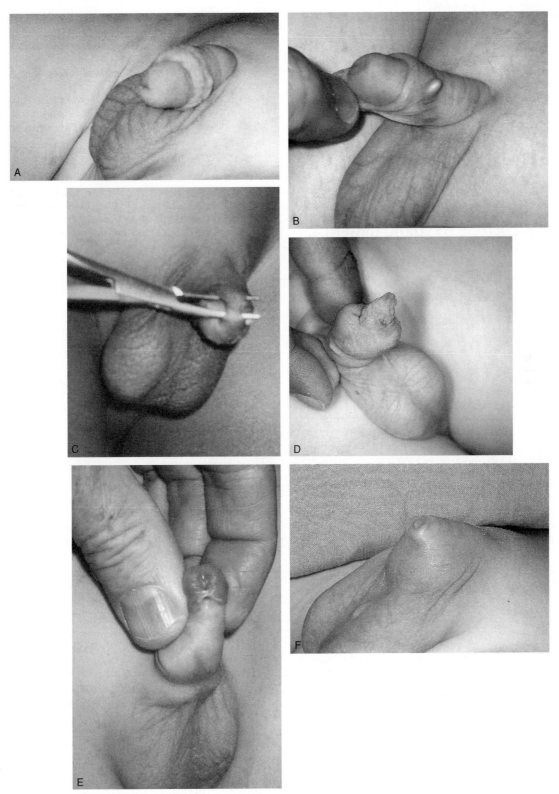

Figure 40–6 ■ Complications of circumcision. *(A)* meatal stenosis (note ventral meatal lip); *(B)* epithelial inclusion cyst; *(C)* severe adhesion between penile skin and glans; *(D)* incomplete disfiguring foreskin removal; *(E)* ventral urethral fistula; *(F)* buried (trapped) penis.

within this morass of conflict and confusion, and it is often difficult to make recommendations that are totally unbiased and helpful.

In these circumstances, it is best to explain the pros and cons of circumcision and involve the parents in the decision-making process. It is helpful to indicate that circumcision is not totally risk free but has benefits as well as risks. One of the most important benefits of circumcision is a practical one: penile hygiene is much easier to perform. Parents must come to appreciate that all considerations are "relative" in the overall decision-making process. The 1999 Task Force on Circumcision by the American Academy of Pediatrics gives a full and cogent description of these pros and cons.

NEGATIVE-CULTURE DYSURIA, URGENCY, AND URINARY FREQUENCY

Pathology

Anything that causes bladder and urethral inflammation, even in the absence of infection, may cause dysuria and frequent urination. These conditions differ from those that have been previously described in that they are descriptions of symptoms rather than of specific conditions.

Conceptually, it is helpful to consider that there are endogenous and exogenous causes for these complaints. Endogenous etiologies include culture-negative acute or chronic cystitis, urethritis, and bladder calculi. Structural and anatomic causes include meatal stenosis, urethral stricture, female urethral prolapse, or overflow urinary incontinence in which frequent overflow may be confused with frequent voiding. Exogenous causes include environmental upset and transference of psychosomatic unrest, bubble baths or other environmental irritants, and occasionally, hypercalciuria with resultant urethral inflammation. Finally, besides exogenous and endogenous causes, a great number of children have idiopathic urinary frequency with no identifiable cause.

Idiopathic or Daytime Urinary Frequency Syndrome (DUFS)

A vast number of boys in particular suffer from sudden onset of diurnal urinary frequency and urgency in the absence of identifiable urinary infection. Postvoiding urgency and frequency may last several weeks, but then usually resolves spontaneously. The symptoms may be extremely upsetting and disruptive to the child and family. When symptoms persist or are extreme and diagnostic testing (eg, ultrasound or VCUG) is undertaken, specific reasons for the frequency are not identified. When otherwise healthy boys with these symptoms are seen, therefore, a conservative approach to diagnosis and treatment is indicated.

● **Clinical Pearl:** Absence of nocturnal frequency (ie, the child sleeps through the night without the need to void) indicates that the problem is not organic.

Cystitis Follicularis

This type of chronic cystitis occurs in about 10% to 15% of girls with urinary infections. It also occurs rarely in boys, usually who have structural abnormalities or a neurogenic bladder with poor bladder emptying.

Urinary infection need not be present, but the pathogenesis is believed to be urinary infection inducing an unusual inflammatory response in the bladder mucosa, which then sets the stage for recurring infections. Recurring infections then worsen the inflammation, setting up a vicious repetitive cycle. Bladder inflammation may persist, causing symptoms during infection-free periods. At times, besides dysuria and frequency, wetting and even strangury are present. The diagnosis is made by cystoscopy, which reveals multiple raised salmon-colored lesions mostly on the bladder trigone, which at pathologic examination reveals dense collections of lymphocytes.

Bulbar Urethritis

Occurring exclusively in boys, terminal hematuria or postvoid urethral bleeding is the hallmark characteristic of this condition. Frequent urination may occur. Urine cultures are always sterile. Cystoscopic examination reveals inflammatory changes in the bulbar urethra, sometimes leading to urethral stricture formation. The cause of this condition is unknown. Though resolution may occur within a few weeks of onset, reactivation may occur several weeks or months later.

Bubble Bath or Chemical Urethritis

Use of any bath additives or soaps can lead to urethral pain and dysuria. At times, visible inflammatory signs are lacking. Diagnosis is based on obtaining a positive history of bath additive use and ensuring that a negative urine culture is obtained. Elimination of the offending additive causes symptoms to disappear. Urines should be repeated subsequently if the symptoms persist.

Hypercalciuria

Some children excrete excessive amounts of calcium in the urine. This condition manifests itself with symptoms of urinary frequency, urgency, and dysuria. At times, microhematuria or crystalluria may be present, even in the absence of urinary calculi. The cause is irritation to the urinary mucosa by the high urinary calcium.

Psychosomatic or Environmentally Induced Urinary Frequency

The bladder and urethra should be considered "target organs" for psychosomatic illnesses. Just as headaches, diarrhea, nausea and vomiting, itchy skin, and visual disturbances may have a psychosomatic basis, the urinary system may be affected as well, with resultant frequency and urgency. The diagnosis is made by excluding all other possible organic causes and identifying specific family or other environmental stressors.

History and Physical Examination

Any child having symptoms of dysuria, frequency, or urgency should have an initial thorough physical examination. Clinicians should especially look for signs of introital or urethral inflammation in girls and meatal stenosis or inflammation of the foreskin or glans in boys. They should examine the abdomen as well for abdominal masses (eg, ovarian cyst), compressing the bladder, or for signs of a continually full bladder with incomplete emptying. Constipation at times also can cause frequency by significantly compressing the bladder or urethra. Systemic diseases are usually obvious (ie, febrile illnesses will sometimes cause nonspecific urethral discomfort and urgency that resolve as the illness improves). Observation of the urinary stream may demonstrate narrowing, diminished force, or intermittency.

Diagnostic Criteria

Clinicians should initially evaluate these symptoms with a urinalysis and culture. At times, pyuria may be present in the absence of culture-proven bacteriuria, representing findings of inflammation rather than infection. In these instances, any of the above conditions may be present.

Microhematuria suggests that hypercalciuria may be the underlying cause. Clinicians should evaluate those with infection further as indicated in Chapter 39. A concentrated urine specimen is essential to determine properly whether true bacteriuria (>100,000 colonies/mL on a voided specimen) is present. Further evaluation depends somewhat on the specific presenting symptoms, their chronicity, and whether abnormal physical findings are present.

▲ **Clinical Warning:** A false-negative culture may be obtained if the urine is very dilute (eg, low specific gravity), as commonly seen in many of the above conditions. A first-morning specimen (usually more concentrated) should be obtained for culture when the suspicion for infection is high.

Management

For boys with frequency and urgency who have no additional identifiable abnormal physical findings or laboratory tests, reassuring the parents that the symptoms are temporary usually suffices. If the symptoms are lasting or debilitating, symptomatic treatment with pyridium (100 mg three times a day for the prepubertal child) may be tried. If ineffective, oxybutinin (0.1–0.2 mg/kg body weight) may be helpful in some cases. If the symptoms continue for more than 8 to 10 weeks, screening for hypercalciuria should be undertaken. A renal and bladder sonogram may be obtained at this point if the urine calcium is normal (less than 4 mg/kg body weight over 24 hours).

Children reaching this point in their management require pediatric urologic evaluation to assess their continuing symptoms. Voiding cystourethrography and cystoscopy are reserved for those with chronic severe symptoms, those with associated urinary stream abnormalities, and those who have no identifiable cause.

When pyuria is present but repeated cultures are sterile, sonography should be performed to look for a structural cause for the symptoms. In patients with negative evaluations, cystoscopy may be indicated (eg, the symptomatic girl with normal sonography who may be found to have cystitis follicularis as the cause of her symptoms).

REFERENCES

American Academy of Pediatrics. (1997). Action Committee Report of the Urology Section, Timing of elective surgery on the genitalia of male children with particular reference to the risks, benefits and psychological effects of surgery and anesthesia. *Pediatrics, 97,* 590.

American Academy of Pediatrics. (1999). Task Force on Circumcision. Report of the Urology Section. *Pediatrics, 103,* 686.

American Urological Association, Inc. (1997). *Caring for children with primary vesicoureteral reflux: A guide for parents.* Author.

Donohoe, R. E., & Utley, W. L. (1978). Torsion of the spermatic cord. *Urology, 11,* 33.

Gill, B. G., & Kogan, S. J. (1997). Cryptorchidism. Current concepts. *Pediatric Clinics of North America, 44*(5), 1211.

Houissa, S., de Pape, J., Diebold, N., et al. (1979). Cryptorchidism: Histologic study of 220 biopsies with clinico-anatomical correlations. In J. C. Job (Ed.), *Cryptorchidism: Diagnosis and treatment. Pediatric and Adolescent Endocrinology* (Vol. 6). Basel, S Karger.

Jarow, J. P., Berkowitz, G. D., Migeon, C. J., et al. (1986). Elevation of serum gonadotropins establishes the diagnosis of anorchia in cryptorchid boys. *Journal of Urology, 136,* 277.

Johnson, C. E., Elder, J. S., Judge, J. E., et al. (1992). The accuracy of antenatal ultrasonography in identifying renal abnormalities. *American Journal of Diseases in Children, 146,* 1181.

Kogan, S. J. (1992). Cryptorchidism. In P. P. Kelalis, L. R. King, & A. B. Belman (Eds.), *Clinical pediatric urology* (3rd ed.). Philadelphia: W.B. Saunders.

Mackie, G. G., & Stephens, F. D. (1975). Duplex kidneys: A correlation of renal dysplasia with position of the ureteral orifice. *Journal of Urology, 114,* 274.

Rabinowitz, R., & Hulbert, W., Jr. (1997). Late presentation of cryptorchidism: The etiology of testicular re-ascent. *Journal of Urology, 157,* 1892.

Skoog, S. J. (1997). Benign and malignant pediatric scrotal masses. *Pediatric Clinics of North America, 44*(5), 1234.

Skoog, S. J., Roberts, K. P., Goldstein, M., et al. (1995). Pediatric hernias and hydroceles. *Urology Clinics of North America, 22,* 119.

Skoog, S. J., Roberts, K. P., Goldstein, M., et al. (1997). The adolescent varicocele: What's new with an old problem in young patients. *Pediatrics, 100,* 112.

Stone, K. T., Kass, E. J., Cacciarelli, A. A., et al. (1995). Management of suspected antenatal torsion: What is the best strategy? *Journal of Urology, 153,* 782.

Wiswell, T. E., Smith, F. R., & Bass, J. W. (1985). Decreased incidence of urinary tract infections in circumcised male infants. *Pediatrics, 75,* 901.

CHAPTER 41

Sexually Transmitted Infections

• EVAN R. GOLDFISCHER, MD; DANIEL M. KATZ, MD; and
ANN BOLLMANN , RN-C, MSN, FNP, RPA-C

INTRODUCTION

The term sexually transmitted infections (STIs) denotes more than 25 infectious organisms transmitted by sexual activity and the myriad clinical manifestations that they can cause. The health consequences range from mild acute illnesses (eg, urethritis or vaginitis) to severe long-term complications (eg, urethral stricture, permanent compromise of reproductive ability) to life-threatening conditions (eg, cancer). Adolescents are particularly vulnerable to STIs because they frequently have unprotected intercourse, are biologically more susceptible to infection, and are likely to have social pressures that substantially increase their risk (Eng & Butler, 1997).

The hidden nature of the processes and the sociocultural taboos related to sexual activity make STIs difficult health problems. These concerns clearly present obstacles to treatment and prevention. Lack of awareness, fragmentation of STI-related services, inadequate training of health care providers, lack of health insurance, and inadequate investment in STI prevention also hinder prevention efforts (Centers for Disease Control and Prevention [CDC], 1995b). Because of their knowledge of patients' social, cultural, and familial relationships, primary care practitioners who treat adolescents are perfectly poised to have a major impact on the management and prevention of STIs (Lappa, Coleman, & Moscicki, 1998).

ANATOMY, PHYSIOLOGY, AND PATHOLOGY

The male phallus and its associated ejaculate are ideally suited for transmission of STIs. The skin covering the shaft is a prime location for the festering wounds that accompany many STIs, including herpetic ulcers, syphilitic chancres, and genital warts (human papillomavirus [HPV]). The skin-to-skin or mucous membrane contact that occurs during sexual activity allows for easy transmission of viral, bacterial, or parasitic elements necessary for the propagation of many diseases. Also, the seminal emission during sexual activity can be deposited orally, vaginally, or anally, allowing for passage of various disease-causing agents. Equally damaging is the fact that while the penis can be free of any obvious abnormalities and the affected male asymptomatic, he can still transfer infective organisms to his sexual partner.

These infections often affect the male urethra, testes, and epididymis. These structures are contiguous, so simple urethritis can easily evolve into a serious case of epididymoorchitis. Furthermore, long-term consequences of infection of these structures can lead to significant health problems, such as urethral stricture, scrotal/testicular abscess, and male-factor infertility. In the female, vaginal and cervical infections may lead to pelvic inflammatory disease (PID) and the potential for tubo-ovarian abscess, ectopic pregnancy, and infertility.

EPIDEMIOLOGY

Because STIs are the most commonly reported infectious diseases in the world, they constitute a persistent major public health problem (World Health Organization, 1992). More than 68 million Americans (25% of the population) now have an incurable STI, including herpes, HPV, hepatitis B, and human immunodeficiency virus (HIV). By age 24 years, one in three sexually active people in the United States has had an STI. One in five Americans older than 12 years has genital herpes (Hopkins, 1998). The impact on individuals, their contacts, and society is staggering. Each year, an estimated 15 million new STIs occur, and approximately 3 million American adolescents will contract an STI (Joffe, 1997). Without even considering the tremendous impact of HIV, the average yearly cost of STIs in the United States is about $10 billion. Annually, the cost of HIV alone is nearly $7 billion (Gunn, Rolfs, Greenspan, et al.,). In terms of human suffering, the cost is immeasurable.

Adolescents (ages 15–19) are second only to young adults in terms of numbers of STIs reported annually. More young people are developing STIs during their teen years than ever before. In many countries, more than half of the adolescent population has unprotected intercourse before age 16 years (The World's Youth, 1994). Furthermore, more than 60% of HIV infections in many developing countries occur among individuals ages 15 to 24 years (Sernderowitz, 1995).

As huge numbers of teenagers engage in sexual activity and with adolescents often having nonchalant attitudes for risk-taking behaviors, it is no wonder that 3 million cases of adolescent STIs occur every year. A recent publication regarding adolescent perceptions noted that 59% did not believe that oral sex constituted having "had sex." An astounding 19% responded similarly regarding penile–anal intercourse (Sanders & Reinisch, 1999).

HISTORY AND PHYSICAL EXAMINATION

The clinical and sexual histories are the primary components that help providers effectively and efficiently estimate a patient's risk for STIs. Seventy percent of adolescents state that they would like to discuss sexual health with their practitioners, but less than 50% say that they have done so (Moscicki, Millstein, Broering, et al., 1993). The purpose of the history in an asymptomatic adolescent is to elicit behavioral risks that guide clinicians in ordering appropriate screening tests and to provide the opportunity for preventive counseling. In symptomatic patients, the history should elicit symptoms and behavioral risks. While simple on the surface, these discussions can be quite challenging (Lappa et al., 1998).

The practitioner must establish a trusting alliance with the patient to facilitate an open discussion on very sensitive and private matters. For some adolescents, a primary care practitioner who has a long-term relationship with the family already may have established that trust. For others, however, this family relationship may engender the fear of disclosure to the patient's parents. The caregiver must be aware of these concerns and assure the adolescent of confidentiality. It is often necessary and appropriate to excuse the parent during the sexual history evaluation. Studies demonstrate that adolescents guaranteed confidentiality are far more likely to volunteer sensitive information vital to the success of taking the sexual history (Ford, Millstein, Halpern-Felsher, et al., 1996).

● **Clinical Pearl:** To facilitate open communication regarding sexual behavior, it is most helpful if discussions begin during early adolescence, prior to the onset of sexual behavior. This allows the clinician to develop a trusting relationship with the patient before the time when crises might occur. In addition, it allows for promoting preventive measures as a basis for the development of sexual health.

Once the practitioner–patient relationship is solid, sexual history taking should first focus on a general discussion of normal physical development, a primary concern to most adolescents. Providers should discuss variations in development and discourage comparisons to peers.

Once suspicions for STIs arise or patients volunteer such information, then providers should undertake specific questioning to elicit behavioral risks. Behavior risks that are key to STI history are early age of sexual activity, multiple partners, history of sexual abuse or rape, lack of condom use, homosexuality or bisexuality, anal sex, history of past STIs, substance abuse, and use of sex in exchange for money or food (Lappa et al., 1998).

Male Physical Examination

The physical examination of the male adolescent should include a complete genital examination and an external perianal evaluation. The provider must carefully inspect the pubic area, groin lymph nodes, penile shaft, foreskin (if present), glans, and urethral meatus. Next, he or she should direct attention to the scrotal skin and underlying testes, epididymes, and vas deferens. Finally, he or she addresses the perineal, perianal, and rectal areas. Actual digital rectal examination is not necessary on a routine basis unless the caregiver suspects or is told of an abnormality. Clearly the provider should evaluate any teen who admits to receptive anal intercourse with a digital examination to evaluate for lesions or trauma.

The provider should make specific notice of the Tanner stage, and sexual history taking can continue based on cues from the developmental stage. Early stage development may prompt questions regarding early adolescent development and family life, while Tanner stage V (adult characteristics) may stimulate discussion of sexual identity and actual sexual activity (Lappa et al., 1998).

● **Clinical Pearl:** Advanced physical maturity does not necessarily imply developmental maturity. The caregiver must be cognizant of this dichotomy to help the patient work through the possible confusion (Bishop-Townsend, 1996).

Female Physical Examination

In the immature female, lack of estrogen greatly increases the susceptibility of the external genitalia to infection and the effects of trauma. In the adolescent menarchal patient, however, the concerns are different. Usually, estrogen and progesterone imbalances are partly responsible for some visits these teens will make to a provider. Pelvic examinations can be done at this age, with anesthesia rarely necessary. Confidence, gentleness, and reasonable care are major assets.

The essentials of the examination include inspection with ample separation of the labia. Endoscopy is included when conditions require visualization of the upper vagina and the cervix. In the younger female, the posterior vaginal fornix is considerably short. Accordingly, a palpating finger in the vagina cannot advance high enough to outline pelvic structures even under anesthesia. The provider may explore the uterus more definitively on rectal examination in a bimanual examination with one hand above the symphysis pressing in a downward motion and one finger in the rectum pushing upward and moving laterally in both directions to identify the pelvic organs fully.

For visualization of the vagina and cervix, a vaginal scope, the Kelly cystoscope, or a tiny speculum is necessary. Makeshift instruments, such as otoscopes or nasal speculums, are totally inadequate. When positioning a child for the inspection and for the internal visual examination, the provider can rely on a frog position lying supine. Sometimes, if the child feels more comfortable, a knee-chest position provides the examiner with adequate visualization. As the patient grows older into adolescence, the usual stirrup position on the table with a more adult form of female examination is the appropriate methodology for examination.

MANAGEMENT: GENERAL PRINCIPLES

Specific conditions and their management are discussed in the following section. With any condition, providers should always approach the patient with sensitivity and understanding.

Prevention of STIs among sexually active adolescents is of the utmost importance, given the significant health and financial issues involved. In addition, viral STIs, such as herpes, condyloma, hepatitis, and HIV, must be prevented, because no true cures exist. Effective prevention programs must be multidisciplinary, involving the clinical, basic, and social sciences.

While abstinence will clearly prevent the transmission of STIs, this goal seems unrealistic. According to the CDC, two thirds of 12th graders and nearly 40% of eighth graders report having had sexual intercourse. Seventy percent of male teenagers ages 14 to 19 years who attended teen health clinics reported having more than one sexual partner during the previous year (Kegeles, Adler, & Irwin, 1988). Furthermore, nearly 25% of high school males report having more than four sexual partners during their adolescence (Kann, Warren, Harris, et al., 1995).

Three levels of prevention exist. Primary prevention involves reducing the actual incidence of new cases of STIs. This level of prevention should take place in arenas easily accessible to adolescents, such as schools and the media. Secondary prevention is aimed at reducing the number of current cases of STI through early detection and effective treatment. Finally, tertiary prevention is aimed at diminishing the biologic and psychological complications of STIs and preventing the long-term sequelae of these diseases (Ehrhardt, Fishbein, Washington, et al., 1990).

Specific prevention messages must be tailored to each patient and his or her specific risks. Caregivers should be direct and clear when giving advice on measures one can take to prevent the acquisition and transmission of STIs (Bishop-Townsend, 1996). While it is easy to tell an adolescent that abstinence is the best way to avoid STIs, programs espousing this approach have never been shown to delay intercourse or reduce its frequency (Christopher & Roosa, 1990).

Some programs, often led by adolescents themselves, have attempted to deter early intercourse by emphasizing the risks and consequences of STIs and unwanted pregnancies. Studies have shown that these programs did consistently raise the knowledge level but also failed to reduce unprotected intercourse or pregnancy (Dawson, 1986). Other programs promote safer sex as a means of decreasing the transmission of STIs. The promotion of condom use is easy, yet data from the national Youth Risk Behavior Surveys revealed that only 50% of adolescents between 1991 and 1995 used condoms "at last intercourse" (Warren et al., 1998). A more extensive discussion of these prevention programs is beyond the scope of this chapter. It should be noted that recently, the first randomized controlled trial of an abstinence intervention compared with a safer-sex intervention revealed that the latter program was clearly superior in reducing unprotected sexual intercourse among adolescents (Jemmott, Jemmott, & Fong, 1998). No other programs have yet proved successful in reducing the level of unprotected sexual intercourse among adolescents.

While the problem remains rampant, signs are encouraging. Between 1993 and 1996, gonorrhea rates dropped 35% among males ages 15 to 19 years. In addition, between 1991 and 1997, the percentage of adolescents who reported ever having had intercourse decreased, and the prevalence of condom use among sexually active teenagers increased (CDC, 1998). The combined efforts of families, schools, community organizations, religious organizations, and health professionals have made these improvements possible.

While some gains have been made in terms of reducing unprotected sexual intercourse, many of today's adolescents remain at risk. Only through the continued efforts of the above groups can we begin to eradicate the serious health problems related to STIs and their sequelae. Primary caregivers should continue to emphasize sexual health during visits with their adolescent patients. Only through a trusting relationship and thorough history and physical examination skills can clinicians obtain the information necessary to have an impact on the sexual health of the adolescents under their care.

SPECIFIC CONDITIONS

Male Urethritis

Urethritis is divided into two broad categories based on the causative organism. At one time, the most commonly reported STI was *Gonococcal urethritis* (GU) caused by *Neisseria gonorrhoeae*, a gram-negative *Diplococcus*. Adolescents younger than 19 years account for 32% of reported cases of GU (CDC, 1995). The other broad category is nongonococcal urethritis (NGU), which can be attributed to several organisms, including *Chlamydia trachomatis*, the most common bacterial STI in the United States, and *Ureoplasm urealyticum* (CDC, 1995; Taylor-Robinson & McCormack, 1980).

● **Clinical Pearl:** Because GU and NGU coexist in a large percentage of patients, identification and treatment of one requires empiric treatment of the other.

Gonococcal Urethritis

Gonococcal urethritis can be transmitted through vaginal intercourse or during oral sex if the partner's pharynx is infected (Edwards & Carne, 1998). Thus, GU can easily be prevented through the use of a condom. Only 54% of sexually active adolescents, however, actually use condoms (Warren et al., 1998). The incubation period ranges from 12 hours to as long as 3 months. Typically, gonorrhea produces a copious and purulent urethral discharge, burning on urination, frequency of urination, and erythema of the urethral meatus. Up to 60% of men may be asymptomatic.

● **Clinical Pearl:** Treatment for GU should be based on the history and not on symptoms alone.

Diagnosis

Diagnosis is typically made by examination under a microscope. A specimen is taken with a noncotton urethral swab of a Gram stain showing intracellular gram-negative diplococci or by culture on Thayer-Martin or New York City media. These chocolate agar culture media contain antibiotics that inhibit nonpathogenic *Neisseria* and normal flora found on mucosal surfaces. They are used when culturing nonsterile sites (eg, urethra, vagina, rectum, pharynx).

▲ **Clinical Warning:** Culture specimens need to be plated immediately, because the organism will not survive if not immediately inoculated onto specific culture medium incubated with carbon dioxide or specific transport media for *Gonococcus* (American Academy of Pediatrics [AAP], 1997a).

The use of DNA probes and polymerase chain reaction (PCR) techniques in the diagnosis of male GU is still controversial. These tests may well prove to be comparable to culture in sensitivity and specificity, but in general for males, Gram stain and cultures are diagnostic gold standards.

Management

The current treatment regimen considers the emergence and spread of penicillin-resistant species. Ceftriaxone 125 mg IM is the first-line drug; however, other effective agents include oral ciprofloxacin 500 mg, norfloxacin 800 mg, and Ofloxacin 400 mg. Because up to 30% of men are coinfected with *C. trachomatis*, the main cause of NGU, patients are empirically treated with doxycycline or azithromycin as well (Youngkin, 1995).

Nongonococcal Urethritis

The incubation period for NGU can be up to 4 weeks. Many teens will be either asymptomatic or have only mild symptoms instead of a urethral discharge.

Diagnosis

Diagnosis is made by Gram stain of a urethral swab with microscopic observation of more than four polymorphonuclear leukocytes in a high-power field. For *Chlamydia*, the definitive diagnosis is established by isolating the organism in tissue culture. Because this is not practical, other techniques for detection include direct fluorescent antibody staining, enzyme immunoassay, DNA probe, and PCR (Biro & Rosenthal, 1995).

The clinician should be familiar with the identification technique used and its limitations. The above techniques are useful for urethral specimens from symptomatic males, cervical specimens from both symptomatic and asymptomatic females, and infant conjunctival specimens. They have not been validated for nasopharyngeal specimens and should not be used for rectal, vaginal, or urethral specimens in children due to cross-reaction with fecal flora. All positive non–cell-culture results need verification if a false-positive test is likely to impact the patient adversely medically, socially, or psychologically (AAP, 1997).

Management

Treatment is usually with oral doxycycline 100 mg twice daily for 7 days or azithromycin 1 g orally as a single dose. As with GU, treatment is initiated based on the history, not just clinical symptoms and examination (Youngkin, 1995).

Epididymitis

Acute epididymitis usually presents with acute onset testicular pain coupled with testicular swelling and inflammation. In older men, it is usually caused by common urinary pathogens; however, in sexually active males younger than 35 years, it should be considered an STI that can lead to testicular infarction, abscess, and infertility if left untreated (Berger et al., 1979). The diagnosis is often mistaken for testicular torsion, which is common in the same age group. If the diagnosis is unsure, radionuclide scanning of the scrotum or Doppler ultrasonography should be performed (Lappa & Moscicki, 1997).

The most common causes are the same organisms that cause urethritis or an enteric organism if the individual is engaged in anal intercourse. A small minority of men, however, may have epididymitis due to tuberculosis, *Cryptococcus*, or *Brucella*. Treatment is directed at the causative organism (CDC, 1992).

Vaginitis

Vaginal infections are among the most common problems in clinical medicine. Commonly, they are categorized into three different types: candidal vaginitis (CV), trichomonal vaginitis (TV), and bacterial vaginosis (BV). BV is not the result of a single pathogen, but rather represents bacterial colonization and in some cases overgrowth with *Gardnerella vaginalis*, among others. CV and BV are not necessarily STIs, but because they can be, they are included in this discussion.

History and Physical Examination

Effective management of vaginitis depends on obtaining a detailed history, including characteristics of any vaginal discharge (eg, odor, amount, color) and examination of the external genitalia, vagina, and cervix. Patients with vaginitis frequently complain of increased abnormal vaginal discharge, odor, itching, and dysuria. Oral contraceptive use, pregnancy, menstruation, antibiotic use, corticosteroid use, diabetes mellitus, and immunosuppression (including an HIV history) are all factors predisposing to candidiasis. They should certainly be recorded in the patient's history.

Physical inspection and examination of the discharge usually establish the diagnosis. The provider should obtain a sample of the discharge from the vaginal wall, noting its color in comparison with the white background of the swab and determining the pH by rolling the swab onto a pH indicator paper. These techniques combined with microscopy using both a KOH slide and a normal saline slide (wet prep) will often yield the correct diagnosis. In some cases, however, classic presentations may be absent or clouded by the coexistence of multiple etiologies, requiring laboratory confirmation.

Diagnosis

The pH of the discharge with CV is usually less than 4.5, while a pH of greater than 4.5 is seen with TV or BV. Candidal vaginitis classically presents with a white, cottage cheese-like thick discharge and a KOH prep showing budding pseudohyphae. The discharge with *Trichomonas* tends to be frothy yellow green and the cervix "strawberry like." A wet prep reveals rapidly moving flagellated trichomonads. With BV, the discharge is grayish white and profuse and classically gives off a strong fishy odor. The wet prep may reveal "clue cells," large epithelial cells coated with bacteria.

▲ **Clinical Warning:** All adolescents with vaginitis should also have an endocervical sample tested for *Chlamydia* and gonorrhea.

Management

In the case of vulval or vaginal candidiasis, treatment consists of topical anticandidal agents, such as nystatin, ketoconazole, miconazole, and clotrimazole. In younger patients, ointments are better tolerated than the creams, which tend to have a burning sensation. Older adolescents, however, can tolerate creams and oral agents. Oral fluconazole, in a single dose of 150 mg, may be used for older adolescents. Males who are exposed to females with vulvovaginal candidiasis may also develop candidiasis of the penis, penile-scrotal fold, and inner thighs. The treatment is the same as for females.

Metronidazole is used to treat TV and BV. For TV, a single dose of 40 mg/kg with a maximum dose of 2 g is curative in 95%. For BV, the recommended dose is 500 mg twice daily for 7 days. BV also may be treated by metronidazole gel intravaginally twice a day for 5 days or clindamycin cream 2% given by vaginal applicator at bedtime for 7 nights. In most males, trichomoniasis is generally asymptomatic, although it sometimes presents as urethritis. If female partners are found to be positive for *Trichomonas*, however, their male partners also should be treated. In cases of recurrent BV, male partners may be treated as well. Oral treatment for partners is the same—metronidazole. Patients taking metronidazole should be cautioned about its antabuse effect and its metallic taste.

Patients with *Candida* and BV should understand that their condition is not necessarily the result of sexual behavior. Indeed it has just as much, if not more, to do with their vaginal pH and personal ecology. Education relating to personal hygiene is important adjunctive treatment.

Cervicitis

Symptoms of cervicitis may include a vaginal discharge, postcoital bleeding, dyspareunia, and dysuria, or there may be no symptoms. The diagnosis is established clinically on pelvic examination by finding a mucopurulent discharge at the cervical os. The organisms primarily responsible are the same as in male urethritis, namely *C. trachomatis* and *N. gonorrhoeae*.

As opposed to males, in whom the Gram stain is specific diagnostically for *Gonococcus*, the genital tract in females (and the pharynx in children) may be normally colonized by other closely related bacterial species, making this technique unreliable. After wiping the outside of the cervix, cultures should be obtained using a noncotton swab twirled inside the cervical os. Specimens should be handled as described in the section on male urethritis for both *Gonococcus* and *Chlamydia* testing.

Because of high rates of coinfection, and as for male urethritis, treatment for cervicitis should include coverage for both chlamydial and gonococcal disease. Treatment specifics are described in the section on male urethritis.

Pelvic Inflammatory Disease

Pelvic inflammatory disease results from the ascending spread of pathogens from the vagina and the cervix to the uterus, fallopian tubes, and ovaries. It is a syndrome of polymicrobial etiology, which includes *C. trachomatis* and *N. gonorrhoeae* predominantly but also *G. vaginalis*, coliforms, group B *Streptococcus*, various mycoplasma, and anaerobes. Results obtained from cervical cultures are not representative of organisms isolated by direct cultures obtained surgically.

Infertility, the most significant consequence of PID, has been estimated at 11%, 34%, and 54% after one, two, and three episodes, respectively. Other consequences include tubo-ovarian abscess, ectopic pregnancy, chronic pain, and repeated episodes (Brodnax, 1999).

The most important decision the practitioner needs to make is the choice between inpatient or outpatient treatment. In general, patients with systemic symptoms of high fever, who appear toxic, and who are too ill to comply with oral treatment should be hospitalized. Patients with peritoneal findings, a suspicion of an adnexal abscess, or another surgical condition should also receive inpatient care and gynecologic and surgical consultation. Associated conditions of pregnancy or HIV should also prompt admission (Brodnax, 1999). The reader is referred to Displays 41-1 and 41-2 for treatment guidelines and practice guidelines.

Genital Ulcers

Genital ulcers can be caused by several organisms, including syphilis, herpes simplex virus (HSV), chancroid, lymphogranuloma venereum, and donovanosis (Berger, 1998). Only the two most common, syphilis and HSV, are discussed in this chapter.

Syphilis

Primary syphilis is caused by the spirochete *Treponema pallidum*. The primary or chancre stage appears 2 to 4 weeks after exposure. The secondary stage appears 1 to 2 months after the chancre has healed. This is manifested by fever; a rash that is variable in appearance, usually maculopapular and classically involving the palms and the soles; condylomata lata; and systemic symptoms of fever, sore throat, athralgia, lymphadenopathy, and spenomegaly. These findings spontaneously resolve within 2 to 6 weeks, although they may recur periodically during the latent stage. Latency is the time in which infected people have no symptoms. Tertiary syphilis occurs several years to decades after exposure if the syphilis is left untreated. Congenital disease is a manifestation of secondary syphilis.

History and Physical Examination

The male will present with a painless sore, known as a chancre, on his genitalia. The chancre will break down to form an ulcerated lesion. In females, typically the external genitalia and cervix are involved. A chancre can also form on other

---

DISPLAY 41–1 • Summary of 1998 CDC Guidelines for the Treatment of Pelvic Inflammatory Disease

Parenteral Regimen A
Cefotetan (2 g IV every 12 hours)
  or
Cefoxitin (2 g IV every 6 hours)
  plus
Doxycycline (100 mg orally or IV every 12 hours)

Parenteral Regimen B
Clindamycin (900 mg IV every 8 hours)
  plus
Gentamicin (2.0 mg/kg as IV or IM loading dose followed by 1.5 mg/kg IV or IM every 8 hours in patients with normal renal function)

Alternative Parenteral Regimens
Olfloxacin 400 mg IV every 12 hours
  plus
Metronidazole 500 mg IV every 8 hours
  or
Ampicillin/Sulbactam 3 g IV every 6 hours
  plus
Doxycycline 100 mg IV or orally every 12 hours
  or
Ciprofloxacin 200 mg IV every 12 hours
  plus
Doxycycline 100 mg IV or orally every 12 hours
  plus
Metronidazole 500 mg IV every 8 hours

Oral Regimen A
Ofloxacin 400 mg orally twice a day for 14 days
  plus
Metronidazole 500 mg orally twice a day for 14 days

Oral Regimen B
Ceftriaxone 250 mg IM once
  or
Cefoxitin 2 g IM plus Probenecid 1 g orally in a single dose concurrently once
  or
Other third-generation cephalosporin (e.g., ceftizoxime or cefotaxime)
  plus
Doxycycline 100 mg orally twice a day for 14 days (include this regimen with one of the above regimens)

---

areas of sexual contact, such as the lips, tongue, or anal area. By 2 to 6 weeks, the chancre spontaneously disappears. There is usually impressively painless lymphadenopathy, which may persist for longer than the chancre. Differential considerations must include the multiple and very painful vesicles and adenopathy of genital herpes and the tender and suppurative adenopathy associated with chancroid, the result of infection with *Haemophilus ducreyi*.

Diagnosis

In primary syphilis, the diagnosis can be made by examining scrapings taken from the base of the chancre or by serologic tests. The fluorescent treponemal antibody absorption test (FTA-ABS) is a treponemal test, and the Venereal Disease Research Laboratory (VDRL) or rapid plasma reagin (RPR) tests are nontreponemal.

**DISPLAY 41–2 • Pelvic Inflammatory Disease
Practice Guideline**

**Patient MUST meet *all* of the following criteria,
in the absence of another established cause:**
☐ lower abdominal pain
☐ cervical motion tenderness
☐ adnexal tenderness

**Patient MUST meet *at least one* of the
following criteria:**
☐ oral temp > 38.3 C
☐ WBC ≥ 13,000 K/mm³
☐ abnormal cervical or vaginal discharge
☐ ESR > 20 mm/hr
☐ laboratory documentation of cervical infection with
   N gonorrheae or *C. trachomatis*

**All patients should have the following as part
of the initial evaluation:**
☐ pelvic exam
☐ endocervical culture for *gonorrheae*
☐ endocervical EIA or culture for chlamydia
☐ CBC with differential
☐ ESR or C reactive protein
☐ RPR
☐ urine *BhCG*
☐ urine dipstick
☐ urine culture

The following should be considered
☐ serum *BhCG* if urine *BhCG* is negative and suspect
   ectopic
☐ U/S if mass or difficult exam
☐ GYN consult immediately if pregnant or if needs U/S
☐ surgical consult if suspect appendicitis or other surgical
   problem

Differential Diagnosis (partial list):
GI–appendicitis, constipation, diverticulitis, gastroenteritis,
   IBD, irritable bowel syndrome
GYN–rupture or torsion of ovarian cyst, endometriosis,
   dysmenorrhea, ectopic pregnancy, mittelschmerz,
   ruptured follicle, septic or threatened abortion, tubo-
   ovarian abscess
Urinary tract–cystitis, pyelonephritis, urethritis,
   nephrolithiasis

☐ Check box if patient was placed on the PID clinical
   practice guideline

From: Emans, Laufer, & Goldstein (1998): *Pediatric and adolescent
gynecology* (4th ed). Philadelphia: Lippincott-Raven.

Nontreponemal tests (VDRL and RPR) are readily available, inexpensive screens. They provide quantitative results that are useful measures of disease activity, response to therapy, and detection of reinfection and relapse. They may be falsely negative in early primary disease and in longstanding latent and congenital syphilis. False-positive results may be seen with common viral infections, such as mononucleosis, hepatitis, and varicella, and with a variety of other common diseases. With successful treatment, quantitative nontreponemal tests will become negative within 1 to 2 years for primary and secondary syphilis respectively (AAP, 1997).

Treponemal tests (FTA-ABS) are used to establish the diagnosis in the face of an abnormal screening nontreponemal test. They may remain positive for life and as such, are not good markers of disease activity or adequacy of therapy. False-positives may occur with other spirochetal diseases, such as Lyme disease and leptospirosis. As a distinguishing test, a VDRL is nonreactive in Lyme disease (AAP, 1997).

Because the VDRL and RPR tests are nontreponemal, they can be nonreactive in up to 28% of men with primary syphilis. In secondary and tertiary syphilis, it is often necessary to sample the cerebrospinal fluid to provide greater sensitivity for the nontreponemal tests. Thus, the FTA-ABS, which has a 90% sensitivity, is often necessary (Johnson & Farnie, 1994).

Management

First-line treatment for both primary and secondary syphilis is 2.4 million U of benzathine penicillin G, given intramuscularly in one dose. Alternative therapies with doxycycline 100 mg orally twice daily for 14 days or tetracycline 500 mg orally four times daily can be used in patients with penicillin allergies but are contraindicated in pregnant women. It is unlikely that an adolescent would be diagnosed with tertiary syphilis given the long latent phase, and discussion of this entity is beyond the scope of this chapter. All recent sexual partners of a person diagnosed with primary syphilis should be screened (Lappa & Moscicki, 1997).

Herpes Simplex Virus

Herpes simplex virus, a double-stranded DNA virus, is more prevalent in college students than gonorrhea or syphilis. It is transmitted by genital-genital or oral-genital contact. Most patients with genital lesions have HSV type II virus, but up to 25% can have type I virus (Smith & Elton, 1993). The first outbreak is the most severe, especially in patients with a history of oral herpes. Urethritis can develop, as can painful genital ulcers. Neurologic complications include urinary retention, constipation, and weakness. Examining the classic lesions by Tzanck smear or viral culture establishes the diagnosis. Topical, intravenous, and oral acyclovir, which acts as a guanine analogue, can be used for the first episode. Oral acyclovir (400 mg twice daily) or famcyclovir (250 mg twice daily) given orally can decrease the recurrence rate (Hatcher et al., 1994).

Genital Warts

Genital warts are caused by one of many strains of HPV, a DNA virus. Types 6 and 11 are usually responsible for visible warts. Types 16, 18, 31, 33, and 35 have been associated with cervical dysplasia in women, which can lead to cervical carcinoma. Hence, what was once thought to be an unsightly affliction could possibly lead to a deadly disease (McNab, Walkinshaw, Cordiner, & Clements, 1996). Almost 46% of college women undergoing routine pelvic examination were shown to be infected with HPV. It is impossible to "cure" the patient with this virus; hence, the goal is to remove the exophytic warts. This can be performed with cryosurgery, electrocauterization, laser vaporization, or application of podophyllin weekly for 4 weeks (Cowsert, 1994). Application of 5% acetic acid to the male genitalia has been shown to expose subclinical flat condylomas as whitish areas. Due to the high false-positive rate of this test, however, treatment of these lesions is not recommended (Hatcher et al., 1994).

Hepatitis

Hepatitis A is more prevalent in homosexual men than in heterosexual men. It can be spread through sexual contact, particularly through anal intercourse and analingus. Hepatitis B is attributed to homosexual transmission in 33% of cases and heterosexual transmission in 25% of cases. It also is associated with rape and intravenous drug use. Hepatitis B is often asymptomatic in adolescents. Universal vaccination is now recommended (Corey & Holmes, 1980).

● **Clinical Pearl:** Any adolescent presenting for the diagnosis and management of an STI should be counseled and tested for HIV and for hepatitis B if not immunized.

REFERENCES

American Academy of Pediatrics. (1997a). *Gonococcal infections. Report of the Committee on Infectious Diseases* (24th ed.) (pp. 212–219). : Author.

American Academy of Pediatrics. (1997b). *Chlamydial Infections. Report of the Committee on Infectious Diseases* (24th ed.) (pp. 170–174). : Author.

American Academy of Pediatrics. (1997c). *Syphilis. Report of the Committee on Infectious Diseases* (24th ed.) (pp. 504–514). : Author.

Berger, R., Alexander, E., & Harnish, J., et. al. (1979). Etiology, manifestations and therapy of acute epididymitis: Prospective study of 50 cases. *Journal of Urology, 121,* 750–754.

Berger, R. (1998). Sexually transmitted diseases: The classic diseases. In Walsh et al. (Eds.), *Campell's urology* (pp. 673–677).

Biro, F., & Rosenthal, S. (1995). Adolescents and sexually transmitted diseases: Diagnosis, developmental issues, and prevention. *Journal of Pediatric Health Care, 9,* 256–262.

Bishop-Townsend, V. (1996). STDs: Screening, therapy, and long-term implications for the adolescent patient. *International Journal of Fertility, 41*(2), 109–114.

Brodnax, J. (1979). Pelvic inflammatory disease. In Dershowitz, R. A. (Ed.). *Ambulatory pediatric care* (4th ed.). Philadelphia: Lippincott-Raven.

Centers for Disease Control and Prevention. (1998). Trends in sexual risk behaviors among high school students—United States, 1991–1997. *Morbidity and Mortality Weekly Report, 47,* 36.

Centers for Disease Control and Prevention. (1996). Youth risk behavior surveillance, United States, 1995. *Morbidity and Mortality Weekly Report, 45,* 64.

Centers for Disease Control and Prevention. (1995a). Summary of notifiable diseases, United States 1994. *Morbidity and Mortality Weekly Report, 43.*

Centers for Disease Control and Prevention. (1995b). Sexually Transmitted Disease Surveillance.

Centers for Disease Control and Prevention. (1992). Sexually transmitted diseases treatment guidelines. *Morbidity and Mortality Weekly Report, 42,* RR-14.

Christopher, S., & Roosa, H. (1990). An evaluation of an adolescent pregnancy prevention program: Is "just say no" enough? *Family Planning Perspectives, 39,* 68–72.

Corey, L., & Holmes, K. (1980). Sexual transmission of hepatitis A in homosexual men: Incidence and mechanism. *New England Journal of Medicine, 302,* 445.

Cowsert, L. (1994). Treatment of papillomavirus infections: recent practice and future approaches. *Invervirilogy, 37,* 226–230.

Dawson, D. (1986). The effect of sex education on adolescent behavior. *Family Planning Perspectives, 18*(4), 162–170.

Edwards, S., & Carne, C. (1998). Oral sex and the transmission of non-viral STIs. *Sexually Transmitted Infections, 74,* 95–100.

Ehrhardt, A. A., Fishbein, M., Washington, E., et al. (1990). Issues in designing behavioral interventions. *Sexually Transmitted Diseases, 17,* 204–207.

Eng, T. R., Butler, W. T. (Eds.). (1997). *The hidden epidemic: Confronting sexually transmitted diseases.* National Academy Press: Washington, DC.

Ford, C., Millstein, S., Halpern-Felsher, B., et al. (1996). *Confidentiality and adolescent disclosure of sensitive information.* 28th Annual Meeting Society of Adolescent Medicine, Arlington, VA, March 1996.

Gunn, R. A., Rolfs, R. T., Greenspan, J. R., et al. *Journal of the American Medical Association, 279,* 680–684.

Hatcher, R., Trussell, J., Stewart, F., Stewart, G., Kowal, D., Guest, F. Cates, W., & Policar, M. (1994). *Contraceptive technology* (16th ed.). New York: .

Hopkins, J. H. (1998). Report based on article from BMJ. *British Medical Journal, 317,* 1616.

Jemmott, J. B., Jemmott, L. S., & Fong, G. T. (1998). Abstinence and safer sex HIV risk-reduction for African American adolescents: A randomized controlled trial. *Journal of the American Medical Association, 279,* 1529–1536.

Joffe, A. (1997). Worth a careful look. *Archives of Pediatrics and Adolescent Medicine, 151,* 637.

Johnson, P., & Farnie, M. (1994). Testing for syphilis. *Dermatology Clinics of North America, 12,* 9–17.

Kann, L., Warren, C., Harris, W., et al. (1995). Youth risk behavior surveillance: United States, 1993. *Morbidity and Mortality Weekly Report, 44*(ss-1).

Kegeles, S., Adler, N., & Irwin, C. (1988). Sexually active adolescents and condoms: Changes over one year in knowledge, attitudes, and use. *American Journal of Public Health, 78,* 460–461.

Lappa, S., Coleman, M. T., & Moscicki, A.-B. (1998). Managing sexually transmitted diseases in Adolescents. *Adolescent Medicine, 25*(1), 71–110.

Lappa, S., & Moscicki, A. (1997). The pediatrician and the sexually active adolescent. *Pediatric Clinics of North America, 44,* 1405–1445.

McNab, J., Walkinshaw, S., Cordiner, J., & Clements, J. (1996). Human papillomavirus in clinically and histologically normal tissue of patients with genital cancer. *New England Journal of Medicine, 315,* 1052–1058.

Moscicki, A. B., Millstein, S., Broering, J., et al. (1993). Risks of human immunodeficiency virus infection among adolescents attending three diverse clinics. *Journal of Pediatrics, 122,* 813.

Sanders, S. A., & Reinisch, J. M. (1999). Would you say you "had sex" if...? *Journal of the American Medical Association, 281,* 275–277.

Sernderowitz, J. (1995). Adolescent health: Reassessing the passage to adulthood. *World Bank Discussion Paper, 272.*

Smith, R., & Elton, R. (1993). The epidemiology of herpes simplex types 1 and 2 infection of the genital tract in Edinburgh 1978-1991. *Genitourinary Medicine, 69,* 381.

Taylor-Robinson, D., & McCormack, W. (1980). The genital mycoplasmas. *New England Journal of Medicine, 302,* 1003.

Warren, C., et al. (1998). Sexual behavior among U.S. high school students, 1990–1995. *Family Planning Perspectives, 30,* 170–172, 200.

World Health Organization. (1992). *Women's health: Across age and frontier.* Geneva: Author.

The World's Youth. (1994). *A special focus on reproductive health.* Washington, DC: Population Reference Bureau and the Center for Population Options.

Youngkin, E. (1995). Sexually transmitted diseases: Current and emerging concerns. *Journal of Obsteric and Gynecology Nursing, 24,* 743–758.

CHAPTER 42

Hematology Disorders

• SOMASUNDARAM JAYABOSE, MD

INTRODUCTION

Anemia is defined as a reduction in the hemoglobin or hematocrit values below the lower limit of normal for age (see Table 42-1). Possible causes include blood loss, increased destruction of red cells (hemolysis), and decreased production of hemoglobin or red cells. In most cases, it is possible to determine the cause of anemia with a methodical approach to diagnosis. Iron deficiency anemia, thalassemia minor, and anemia of infection or inflammation are among the most common anemias in children. In the vast majority of cases, primary care providers can diagnose and manage these conditions. A consultation with a pediatric hematologist is necessary when anemia is severe (hemoglobin less than 8 gms/dL) or when there is associated thrombocytopenia, neutropenia, or both. Children with inherited anemia require regular visits with both the primary care provider and the pediatric hematologist.

A careful history and physical exam can offer several clues to the anemia's cause (see Tables 42-2 and 42-3). By evaluating a few initial laboratory data (ie, mean corpuscular volume (MCV), red cell distribution width (RDW), reticulocyte count, blood smear findings, serum lactic dehydrogenase (LDH), and indirect bilirubin level), providers can classify most anemias into one of the following five groups:

Microcytic anemias
Normocytic anemias
Macrocytic anemias
Hemolytic anemias
Anemias caused by bone marrow failure

The differential diagnosis for each group and the necessary confirmatory tests are given in Tables 42-4, 42-5, 42-6, and 42-7. The differential diagnosis of neonatal anemia is provided in Table 42-8.

● **Clinical Pearl:** An easy way to remember the lower limit of normal MCV is to add the child's age in years to the number 70.

Anemia is considered microcytic when the MCV is less than the lower limit of normal for age (see Table 42-1). Microcytic anemia, when mild (hemoglobin not less than 8 gms/dL) and not associated with any systemic illness, is most often secondary to iron deficiency anemia (IDA) or thalassemia minor (trait).

● **Clinical Pearl:** In an anemic child, a low MCV with a high RDW usually is associated with iron deficiency.

Even more specifically, an RDW index (MCV/RBC × RDW) greater than or equal to 220 supports the diagnosis of IDA with more than 90% sensitivity and specificity (Jayabose, 1999). Such a patient can be empirically started on iron

therapy. A response to iron therapy (an increase in the hemoglobin level of at least 1 gm/dL in 2 weeks and to normal values within 4 to 6 weeks) confirms the diagnosis. An algorithm for the diagnosis of mild microcytic anemia is given in Figure 42-1.

● **Clinical Pearl:** Patients with microcytosis and a normal or low RDW, or those who fail empiric iron therapy, may have thalassemia minor and should be evaluated by a hemoglobin electrophoresis. An RDW index (MCV/RBC X RDW) less than 220 is strongly suggestive as well.

● **Clinical Pearl:** A hemoglobin A_2 level greater than 4.0% is diagnostic of β-thalassemia trait.

Hemoglobin electrophoresis is also diagnostic in cases of Hemoglobin E disease, which is most common in persons of Southeast Asian descent. Presence of microcytic anemia in one or both parents supports this diagnosis. Parents and siblings of a child diagnosed with thalassemia trait (α or β) should be evaluated by a complete blood count (CBC), and those who have microcytic anemia should be evaluated by hemoglobin electrophoresis. If both parents have thalassemia trait, they should receive formal genetic counseling because of the risk of thalassemia major in future progeny.

● **Clinical Pearl:** A normal hemoglobin electrophoresis (with normal Hb A_2 and Hb F) in a patient with microcytic anemia not responding to iron therapy is very suggestive of alpha thalassemia trait.

This chapter discusses in detail the various types of anemia. It also provides information about the various neutropenias. Finally, it examines different bleeding disorders.

MICROCYTIC ANEMIAS

Iron Deficiency Anemia (IDA)

Iron deficiency anemia (IDA) occurs because of inadequate intake of iron or blood loss. IDA from inadequate intake occurs most commonly between ages 9 months to 24 months. To maintain positive iron balance during childhood, the body must absorb 0.8 mg of elemental iron each day from the diet. Because the body absorbs less than 10% of dietary iron, the daily diet should contain at least 10 mg of iron (Schwartz, 1996).

Pathology

In the full-term newborn, iron stores present at birth are sufficient to prevent iron deficiency during the first 6 months of life. In premature infants, however, iron deficiency can develop in the first few months of life because of low iron

Table 42–1.   AGE RELATED NORMAL VALUES—HEMOGLOBIN (HB), HEMATOCRIT (HCT), AND MEAN CORPUSCULAR VOLUME (MCV)

	Hb	g/dL	Hct (%)		MCV (u³)	
Age	Mean	Lower Limit	Mean	Lower Limit	Mean	Lower Limit
newborn	18.5	14.5	56	45	108	95
1 month	14	10.0	43	31	104	85
2 months	11.5	9.0	35	28	96	77
0.5–1.9 year	12.5	11.0	37	33	77	70
2–4 years	12.5	11.0	38	34	79	73
5–7 years	13.0	11.5	39	35	81	75
8–11 years	13.5	12.0	40	36	83	76
12–14 years						
female	13.5	12.0	42	36	85	78
male	14.0	12.5	43	37	84	77
15–17 years						
female	14.0	12.0	41	36	87	79
male	15.0	13.0	46	38	86	78
18–49 years						
female	14.0	12.0	42	37	90	80
male	16.0	14.0	47	40	90	80

From Brugnara, C. (1998). Reference values in infancy and childhood. In D.G. Nathan & S.H. Orkin (eds), *Nathan and Oski's hematology of infancy and childhood* (Appendix p. viii). Philadelphia: WB Saunders.

Table 42–2.   DIAGNOSIS OF ANEMIA—CLUES FROM HISTORY

History	Diagnostic Possibilities
Neonatal jaundice	Hemolytic disease: Rh or ABO incompatibility, hereditary spherocytosis, G6PD or pyruvate kinase deficiency
Race & ethnicity	Sickle cell and hemoglobin C disease (common in people of African descent); alpha thalassemia (in people of African descent and Asians); β-thalassemia in whites
Family history	Autosomal dominant-spherocytosis; X-linked recessive-G6PD deficiency
Diet-excessive intake of whole cow's milk	Iron-deficiency anemia
Blood loss; gastrointestinal symptoms	Inflammatory bowel disease; malabsorption with B_{12} or folate deficiency
Drugs: anticonvulsants	Megaloblastic anemia
Dark colored urine (suggestive of hemoglobinuria)	Intravascular hemolysis-autoimmune hemolytic anemia G6PD, hemolytic uremic syndrome
Extremity pains	Leukemia; lymphoma; neuroblastoma; and other malignancies

Adapted from Oski, F.A., Brugnara, C., & Nathan, D.G. (1998). A diagnostic approach to the anemic patient. In D.G. Nathan & S.H. Orkin (eds), *Nathan and Oski's hematology of infancy and childhood* (p. 377). Philadelphia: WB Saunders.

Table 42–3.   DIAGNOSIS OF ANEMIA—CLUES FROM PHYSICAL EXAMINATION

Findings	Causes of Anemia
Growth retardation	Renal disease, malabsorption
Hypertension	Hemolytic uremic syndrome, renal disease
Jaundice and splenomegaly	Hemolytic anemia
Purpura, lymphadenopathy, hepatosplenomegaly	Leukemia, lymphoma, other malignancies
Edema with severe pallor	Protein-losing enteropathy

Table 42–4. DIFFERENTIAL DIAGNOSIS OF MICROCYTIC ANEMIA

	Diagnostic Considerations	Initial Laboratory Data	Confirmatory Tests
Common			
	Iron deficiency anemia	RDW markedly increased (> 16); mild anemia (Hb > 9 gm/dL)	$\downarrow$ serum iron, $\uparrow$ TIBC, $\downarrow$ transferrin saturation $< 16\%$; or response to empiric iron therapy.
	β-thalassemia trait	RDW normal or slightly decreased (< 16); MCV/RBC ratio < 11; RDW index (MCV/RBC $\times$ RDW) < 220	$\uparrow$ Hb A_2 and/or $\uparrow$ Hb F. Family studies; no response to empiric iron therapy.
	α-thalassemia trait	Same as above	Normal Hb A_2 and Hb F; Family studies
	Anemia of chronic inflammation	RDW and severity of anemia variable	Evidence of systemic disease. $\uparrow$ ESR, CRP, Fibrinogen
Rare			
	Lead poisoning	RDW normal or increased	Lead level
	Hemoglobin H disease (a form of α-thalassemia)	Evidence of hemolysis— $\uparrow$ retic count, $\uparrow$ indirect bilirubin, $\uparrow$ LDH	Hb. H(β_4) 5%–30%
	Hereditary elliptocytosis	Presence of hemolysis	Blood smear; family studies
	Sideroblastic anemia	Hypochromic red cells	$\uparrow$ serum iron, ringed sideroblasts in the bone marrow
	β-thalassemia major	Severe hemolytic anemia, jaundice, hepatosplenomegaly, delayed growth	Markedly $\uparrow$ Hb F ($> 75\%$); markedly $\downarrow$ or absent Hb A

Table 42–5. DIFFERENTIAL DIAGNOSIS OF NORMOCYTIC ANEMIAS

Diagnostic Considerations	Initial Laboratory Data	Confirmatory Tests
Anemia of acute infections, chronic inflammation or systemic disease such as renal disease	Normal RDW, $\downarrow$ serum iron, $\downarrow$ TIBC, $\uparrow$ serum ferritin	Urinalysis, BUN, creatinine; evidence of other systemic diseases; $\uparrow$ ESR, CRP and fibrinogen; $\downarrow$ serum erythropoietin level
Transient erythroblastopenia of childhood (TEC)	Normal RDW, markedly decreased reticulocyte count ($< 0.5\%$) except during recovery phase, $\uparrow$ iron serum	Observation
Physiologic anemia of infancy	Normal RDW	Observation
Anemia of recent blood loss	Normal RDW	Look for gastrointestinal lesions and bleeding disorder
Hypersplenism or splenic pooling	Splenomegaly	Investigations for the cause of splenomegaly
Hemolytic disease	$\uparrow$ retic, indirect bilirubin, and LDH	See Table 41-7

Table 42–6. DIFFERENTIAL DIAGNOSIS OF MACROCYTIC ANEMIAS

Diagnostic Considerations	Initial Laboratory Data	Confirmatory Tests
Megaloblastic anemias		
Folate or B_{12} deficiency	$\uparrow$ RDW, markedly $\uparrow$ LDH, $\pm$ neutropenia, and/or thrombocytopenia	$\downarrow$ Serum folate (< 3 ng/mL), $\downarrow$ serum B_{12} (< 100 pg/mL), $\uparrow$ serum methyl malonic acid and homocysteine in B_{12} deficiency, megaloblastic bone marrow
Macrocytic anemia without megaloblastic bone marrow		
Aplastic anemia, Diamond Blackfan syndrome, stomatocytosis, hypothyroidism, liver disease, alcoholism, congenital dyserythropoietic anemias		Bone marrow aspirate study; thyroid and liver function studies
Bone marrow failure syndromes (may be normocytic)		
Aplastic anemia, leukemia, neuroblastoma	$\downarrow$ platelets, $\downarrow$ neutrophils, $\downarrow$ reticulocyte counts	Bone marrow aspirate study
Diamond Blackfan syndrome	No thrombocytopenia or neutropenia	Bone marrow aspirate study

Table 42–7.   DIFFERENTIAL DIAGNOSIS OF HEMOLYTIC ADEMIAS

Diagnostic Considerations	Initial Laboratory Data	Confirmatory Tests
Extravascular hemolysis (Hemoglobinopathies, Thalassemias, membrane disorders)	↑ Reticulocyte count, ↑ LDH ↑ indirect bilirubin	
Sickle cell disease	Sickle cells, target cells on smear	Hb electrophoresis—see Table 41–19
β-thalassemia major	Microcytosis, anisocytosis, poikilocytosis	Hb electrophoresis—markedly elevated Hb F (> 75%) and markedly decreased Hb A
Hemoglobin H disease	Microcytosis, hypochromia, and fragmented red cells	5%–30% Hb H (β_4) on Hb electrophoresis
Hereditary spherocytosis	> 15% spherocytes on smear	Increased osmotic fragility, family studies
Hereditary elliptocytosis	> 15% elliptocytes on smear	↑ osmotic fragility in severe cases, family studies
Intravascular hemolysis (Enzyme deficiencies, extracellular defects)	Hemoglobinuria, ↑ LDH, ↓ haptoglobin, fragmented cells on smear	
G6PD deficiency	Blister cells, spiculated	Quantitative assay of G6PD and Pyruvate kinase
Pyruvate kinase deficiency	Pyknocytes	
Autoimmune hemolytic anemia	Spherocytes	Positive Direct Coombs' test
Hemolytic uremic syndrome	Fragmented cells, thrombocytopenia	Clinical syndrome of hemolytic anemia, thrombocytopenia & uremia
Cardiac hemolytic anemia	Fragmented cells, congenital heart disease	Presence of cardiac prosthesis
Paroxysmal Nocturnal Hemoglobinuria (PNH)	Thrombocytopenia, neutropenia	Acid serum test; sugar water test

stores at birth. In some infants, intolerance to whole cow's milk protein can cause a protein losing enteropathy, with occult blood loss leading to severe IDA and hypoproteinemia.

● **Clinical Pearl:** Infants who consume large amounts of cow's milk are particularly susceptible to develop IDA because of poor intake of iron-rich solids and a microscopic loss of heme in the gut.

In adolescents, increased requirements during pubertal growth spurt and menstrual blood loss in females are contributing factors to IDA. Less common causes of IDA related to occult blood loss in children include inflammatory bowel disease, peptic ulcer disease, Meckel's diverticulum, polyps, and hemangiomas. Hookworm infestation and trichuriasis are common causes of IDA in developing countries.

Epidemiology

Iron deficiency remains the most common cause of anemia in children around the world. In the United States, the incidence of IDA in children has decreased considerably due to iron fortification of most infant formulas and the American Academy of Pediatrics' (AAP) recommendation that bottle-fed infants remain on formula till age 1 year. The incidence of IDA in 12-month-old American infants fed iron-fortified formulas is 0%, compared to 4% in those who received whole cow's milk and iron-fortified cereals (Fuchs, 1993). In the United Kingdom, the incidence of anemia in 12-month-old infants fed whole cow's milk from age 6 months was noted to be 31%, compared to only 3% in those who were fed fortified formulas from age 6 months (Daly, MacDonald, Aukett, 1996).

Table 42–8.   DIFFERENTIAL DIAGNOSIS OF ANEMIA IN THE NEWBORN

Initial Data	Diagnostic Considerations	Confirmatory Tests
Evidence of hemolysis (Jaundice + ↑ retic count)		
Positive Coombs	Rh or ABO incompatibility	Rh or ABO set up
Negative Coombs	Hereditary spherocytosis	Positive family history, ↑ osmotic fragility
	Deficiency of G6PD, pyruvate kinase, or other red cell enzymes.	Assay of G6PD and pyruvate kinase, and if necessary other enzymes
No evidence of hemolysis		
Signs of hypovolemia	Recent perinatal blood loss	Obstetric history
No signs of hypovolemia, microcytosis	Chronic fetomaternal hemorrhage	Positive Kleihauer-Betke test

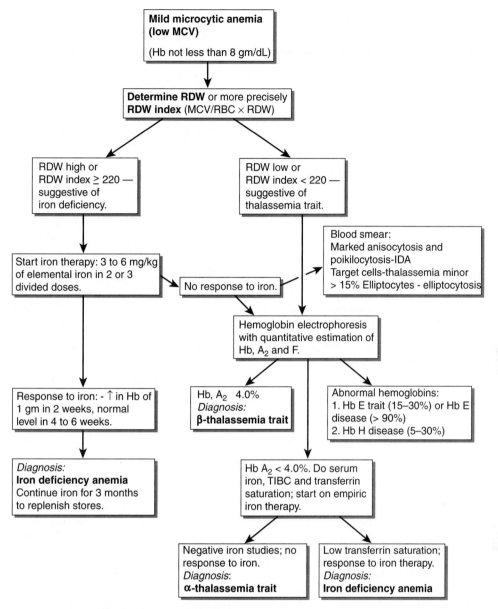

Figure 42–1 ■ Algorithm for the diagnosis of mild microcytic anemias.

History and Physical Exam

Symptoms of IDA include irritability, pallor, and anorexia. These symptoms usually do not appear until the hemoglobin level is less than 7 gms/dL. Irritability may improve within a few days of starting iron, even before any hematological improvement. In mild cases the physical examination is unrevealing. In more severe cases, the clinician may note pallor, tachycardia, and a systolic flow murmur.

▲ **Clinical Warning:** IDA may impair attention span, alertness, and learning in infants and adolescents. These symptoms may not be completely reversible with treatment—hence the importance of prevention.

Diagnostic Studies

The diagnosis of IDA should be strongly considered according to red cell indices and blood smear findings. Studies of plasma iron and storage iron or response to iron therapy can

confirm diagnosis. Diagnostic criteria for IDA are listed in Display 42-1.

Management

Oral iron in the form of ferrous sulfate or gluconate (3–6 mg/kg of elemental iron per day, in two to three divided doses) is effective in most patients. Providers should become familiar with the contents of a few preparations, all of which are listed in Table 42-9. A reticulocyte response is usually seen within 4 days of beginning therapy. The hemoglobin level begins to rise within a week, reaching normal levels in 4 to 6 weeks.

● **Clinical Pearl:** After initiating empiric treatment, clinicians must arrange for follow-up. In IDA, a CBC obtained a month after therapy begins will demonstrate a significant rise in hemoglobin or hematocrit, thereby confirming the diagnosis. Iron therapy should continue for an additional 2 months after the patient achieves normal hemoglobin in order to replenish depleted iron stores.

DISPLAY 42–1 • Iron Deficiency Anemia—Diagnostic Criteria

Suggestive

1. *MCV*—decreased proportionate to the degree of anemia. Increased RDW indicates anisocytosis.
2. *Blood smear*—microcytosis, hypochromia, anisocytosis, poikilocytosis

Diagnostic

3. *Transferrin saturation*—< 16% in children; < 10% in infants. (Serum iron is usually < 40 ug/dL and TIBC > 400 ug/dL.)
4. *Serum ferritin*—decreased (< 10 ng/mL)
5. *Response to iron therapy*—increase in hemoglobin of at least 1 gm/dL in 2 weeks, and to normal values in 4 to 6 weeks

---

DISPLAY 42–2 • Patient Instructions for Iron Therapy

- Administer iron between meals.
- Liquid preparations may stain teeth; rinse with water.
- GI symptoms (eg, constipation) are rare.
- Antacids and H_2 blockers interfere with iron absorption.
- In deficiency states, take iron for three months to replenish stores.

Oral iron therapy is effective in almost all patients. Failure to respond to iron therapy usually indicates ongoing blood loss or poor compliance. Poor tolerance to oral iron or defective gastrointestinal absorption of iron, requiring parenteral iron therapy, is extremely rare in children. Patients should follow the instructions given in Display 42-2.

Prevention of IDA in infants is of utmost importance. Primary care providers should educate parents regarding the various preventive measures listed in Display 42-3.

● **Clinical Pearl:** Breast milk alone is an insufficient source of iron after age 6 months. Infants exclusively breast-fed should receive iron supplements of 1 mg/kg per day.

Anemia of Lead Poisoning

Lead interferes with heme synthesis, which is essential for erythropoiesis and for basic cellular respiration through the mitochondrial cytochrome system. Thus, lead poisoning can cause microcytic hypochromic anemia in addition to its detrimental effects on the central nervous system. The hematologic effects of lead poisoning, however, do not appear until the lead level is greater than 50 mcg/dL. The microcytic anemia seen in patients with mild lead poisoning is frequently due to associated IDA.

Thalassemias

In thalassemia, partial or complete failure to synthesize globin chains (β or α) results in decreased hemoglobin produc-

tion. The resulting anemia, therefore, is microcytic and hypochromic. Most individuals with the heterozygous defect have mild microcytic anemia; some have microcytosis with no anemia. In homozygous thalassemia, the synthesis of globin chains is severely impaired, causing imbalance in polypeptide chain production. The polypeptide chains produced in excess precipitate in the cell membrane, causing hemolysis. A high frequency of thalassemia genes is seen in Mediterranean countries, Africa, the Middle East, the Indian subcontinent, and Southeast Asia. From 3% to 8% of Americans of Italian or Greek ancestry and 0.5% of African Americans carry a gene for β-thalassemia (Honig, 1996).

Heterozygous-β thalassemia (β-thalassemia trait)

In this condition, there is marked microcytosis, hypochromia, and poikilocytosis; ovalocytosis and basophilic stippling also may be seen. RDW is normal to slightly elevated. Hb A_2 is elevated (>4.0 %) in most patients, and Hb F is slightly increased (2%–6%) in about 50% of cases. In the most common form, $β^+$-thalassemia trait, the anemia is mild, with hemoglobin levels in the range of 9 to 12 gms/dL. Affected children are asymptomatic. In the less common form, $β^0$-thalassemia trait, the anemia may be moderate in severity. Not all patients with the thalassemia trait have microcytosis. Patients with the rare δβ-thalassemia trait have normal MCV, normal or slightly decreased Hb A_2 levels, and increased Hb F levels (5%–15%).

Homozygous $β^0$-thalassemia (Cooley's anemia, Thalassemia major)

Thalassemia major, a severe, progressive, hemolytic anemia, usually presents between ages 6 and 12 months. Clinical features include jaundice secondary to hemolysis and hepatosplenomegaly due to extramedullary hematopoiesis.

Table 42–9. COMMONLY USED PREPARATIONS OF IRON (FERROUS SULFATE)

Preparation (strength)	Amount of Elemental Iron
Drops (75 mg/0.6 mL)	15 mg/0.6 mL*
Syrup (90 mg/5 mL)	18 mg/5 mL
Sulfate elixir (220 mg/5 mL)	44 mg/5 mL*
Tablets (325 mg)	65 mg*
Tablets (160 mg) (slow release)	50 mg
Capsules (200 mg)	65 mg
Capsules (250 mg) (time release)	50 mg

*Indicates most frequently used preparations in pediatrics

DISPLAY 42–3 • Prevention of Iron Deficiency in Infants

1. Breast-fed infants should receive iron supplements of 1 mg/kg/day from age 6 months.
2. Non-breast fed infants should receive iron-fortified formula (12 mg of elemental iron per liter) until age 1 year.
3. Iron-fortified cereals should be started at age 6 months in all infants.
4. Avoid whole cow's milk in the first year of life.
5. Start iron supplements at age 4 weeks in premature babies (2 mg/kg/day).

The hemoglobin level continues to drop to less than 5 gms/dL. Growth is impaired because of severe anemia, and bone marrow hyperplasia causes head bossing and prominent malar eminences. Unless regular transfusions are given, the life expectancy is no more than a few years. The anemia is microcytic and hypochromic. The blood smear shows many poikilocytes, target cells, and nucleated red cells. Indirect bilirubin and LDH are elevated. Hemoglobin electrophoresis reveals very high levels of fetal hemoglobin, elevated hemoglobin A_2, and markedly decreased or no hemoglobin A.

Monthly transfusions to maintain a hemoglobin level higher than 10gms/dl allow normal growth and development. Within a few years of transfusion therapy, however, chelation (with daily subcutaneous infusion of deferoxamine) is needed to prevent transfusion-induced hemosiderosis. After several years, splenectomy becomes necessary for most patients to decrease the increasing transfusion requirement caused by hypersplenism. Bone marrow transplantation from an HLA-identical sibling can cure most patients. This procedure, however, is not routinely performed because of the risk of morbidity and mortality from bone marrow transplantation.

α-Thalassemia

Four genes—two gene loci on each of chromosome 16—control the synthesis of α chains. Thus, α-thalassemia presents in four degrees of severity according to the number of gene deletions: silent carrier, α-thalassemia trait, Hemoglobin-H disease, and hydrops fetalis (Table 42-10).

α-thalassemia trait usually presents as a mild microcytic anemia that does not respond to iron therapy. Newborns with α-thalassemia trait have elevated levels of hemoglobin Barts (γ_4). Southeast Asians commonly carry α^0 thalassemia gene mutations, and α^+ thalassemia mutations are generally seen in people of African ancestry. Thus, the severe forms of the disease (Hemoglobin-H disease and hydrops fetalis) usually are not seen in African Americans. Nearly 30% of African Americans are silent carriers, and 2% have α-thalassemia trait (Dozy, 1979).

NORMOCYTIC ANEMIAS

Anemia of Inflammation

Acute or chronic inflammation is one of the most common causes of anemia in children. During acute infections, hemo-globin may drop by as much as 2.4 gms/dL, depending upon the severity of the illness.

● **Clinical Pearl:** Anemia of inflammation may be normocytic or microcytic. Serum iron is low in both anemia of inflammation and iron deficiency.

With chronic inflammation, the release of stored iron from the reticuloendothelial system to the serum decreases; iron stores are normal as evidenced by a normal or high serum ferritin and a low total iron binding capacity (TIBC). Conversely, in IDA, the TIBC is increased, while serum iron and serum ferritin are decreased. The resolution of anemia coincides with that of the inflammation, and may take longer than a month.

● **Clinical Pearl:** In children, delaying investigation of a mild normocytic anemia by at least 4 weeks is wise when the child has a history of a recent infection. Anemia of inflammation may take this duration to resolve.

Physiologic Anemia of Infancy

In the normal full-term infant, the hemoglobin level drops from a mean of 18.5 gms/dL (−2SD = 14.5 gms/dL) on the first day of life to 11.5 gms/dL (−2SD = 9.0 gms/dL) between ages 8 to 12 weeks. Three factors contribute to this physiologic drop in the hemoglobin, often referred to as physiologic anemia of infancy:

Decreased production of red cells during the first 8 to 12 weeks of life
Decreased life span of fetal red cells
Hemodilution caused by increasing plasma volume associated with rapid growth

Thus it is not uncommon to see normal infants with a hemoglobin of 9 to 10 gm/dl at age 2 to 3 months, especially in association with minor infections. The MCV and RDW are normal. The reticulocyte count may be normal or slightly increased during the recovery phase.

In premature infants, the physiologic anemia occurs earlier, and the degree of anemia is more severe. In infants with birth weight less than 1500 gms, the hemoglobin level drops to 7 to 8 gms at age 3 to 6 weeks. Nutritional deficiencies may exacerbate the physiologic anemia.

▲ **Clinical Warning:** Premature infants should receive folic acid (1 mg/day) and iron supplements (2 mg/kg of elemental iron/day) beginning at age 4 weeks.

Table 42–10 α-THALASSEMIA GENOTYPES AND CLINICAL SYNDROMES

Genotype Abbreviation	Genotype	Clinical Type	Clinical Features
αα/αα	Normal	Normal	None
α/αα	Heterozygous α^+ thalassemia	Silent carrier	None
--/αα	Heterozygous α^0 thalassemia	α-thalassemia trait —Asian type	Mild microcytic anemia
-α/-α	Homozygous α^+ thalassemia	α-thalassemia trait—African type	Mild microcytic anemia
--/-α	Compound heterozygous α^+/α^0 thalassemia	Hemoglobin H disease (β^4)	Moderately severe hemolytic anemia
--/--	Homozygous α^0 thalassemia	Hydrops fetalis-Hemoglobin Barts (γ_4)	Death in utero

Adapted from Embury, S.H. & Steinberg, M. (1994). Genetic modulators of disease. In Embury, S.H., Hebbel, R.P., Mohandas, N., & Steinberg M., (Eds.), *Sickle cell disease: Basic principles and clinical practice* (p. 281). New York: Raven Press.

Transient Erythroblastopenia of Childhood (TEC)

A transient but marked suppression of erythropoiesis, usually following viral infections, causes TEC. The mechanism may be immune-mediated suppression of the erythroid progenitor cells. Parvovirus has been shown to be the etiology in some patients.

The peak incidence is between ages 1 to 3 years. Children with TEC have few symptoms other than pallor at the time of presentation, and physical examination does not reveal any abnormal findings except for pallor and tachycardia. The anemia is usually severe, with hemoglobin levels less than 8 gm/dl. The red cell count is decreased; MCV, MCH, and RDW are normal. The reticulocyte count is less than 1% in most patients. In some patients, the absolute neutrophil count (ANC) may be less than $1000/mm^3$ at diagnosis (Cherrick, 1994). The platelet count is increased in most patients, especially during the recovery phase. Most children recover within one to two months from diagnosis. About 5% to 10% of patients are in the recovery phase when they first see the provider. These patients have normal or increased reticulocyte counts and elevated MCV.

Diagnosis of TEC is based on excluding other causes of anemia; spontaneous recovery confirms the clinical impression. Diamond-Blackfan syndrome (congenital pure red cell aplasia) should be suspected in the presence of the following features: age younger than 6 months, macrocytosis, increased HbF, and lack of recovery within 2 months. No specific therapy is available for TEC. Transfusion of red cells is indicated only if there is evidence of cardiac decompensation secondary to the severe anemia. Recurrence of TEC is rare.

MACROCYTIC ANEMIAS

Megaloblastic Anemias

Both vitamins B_{12} and folate are essential for DNA synthesis, and a deficiency of either or both will cause failure of DNA synthesis and disordered cell proliferation. The increased interval between cell divisions allows more cell growth but fewer divisions, leading to macrocytosis. In the bone marrow, the macrocytosis is most apparent in the erythroid precursors. The megaloblastic picture is characterized by a nucleus that looks less mature than the cytoplasm; the nuclear chromatin appears stippled and lacy, while the cytoplasm appears normally mature and hemoglobinized.

Folic Acid Deficiency

Folate is abundant in many foods including whole wheat, green vegetables, carrots, fruits, egg yolk, and animal organs (eg, kidney, liver). The normal adult requirement of folate is about 100 mcg /day. The causes of folate deficiency in children are given in Display 42-4.

▲ **Clinical Warning:** Human milk and cow's milk provide adequate amounts of folic acid; goat's milk and powdered milk are poor sources of folate. Babies receiving only goat's milk require supplementation, which usually can be achieved with a multivitamin containing the B group.

● **Clinical Pearl:** Serum folate levels drop within 2 weeks after cessation of folate intake. Red cell folate, which better

---

> **DISPLAY 42–4 • Causes of Folate Deficiency**
>
> - Low birth weight
> - Deficient intake: goat's milk, powdered milk
> - Defective absorption:
>   Malabsorption syndromes: Celiac disease, kwashiorkor, marasmus, chronic infectious enteritis, enteroenteric fistulas
>   Congenital folate malabsorption
> - Increased requirements: pregnancy, hemolytic anemia
> - Drugs:
>   Anticonvulsant drugs: phenytoin, primidone, phenobarbital
>   Methotrexate, trimethoprim, oral contraceptives pyrimethamine
> - Congenital dihydrofolate reductase deficiency

represents body folate stores, may remain within normal limits for up to 3 months of deficient folate intake.

History and Physical Exam

The peak incidence for megaloblastic anemia of infancy is ages 4 to 7 months. Irritability, poor weight gain, and chronic diarrhea are common symptoms. Infants with congenital folate malabsorption present with mouth ulcers, progressive neurologic deterioration, and immune deficiency in addition to the above symptoms. In infants with poor nutrition, IDA may coexist.

Diagnostic Criteria and Studies

MCV is markedly increased (>100). The blood smear shows hypersegmented neutrophils and marked anisocytosis and poikilocytosis of red cells. The reticulocyte count is decreased. Neutropenia and thrombocytopenia may be present in some cases. Serum LDH is markedly elevated. Bone marrow shows erythroid hyperplasia with megaloblastic changes and giant metamyelocytes.

The diagnosis is confirmed by a serum folate less than 3 ng/mL (normal range 4–20 ng/mL) and a red cell folate less than 150 ng/mL (normal range 200–800 ng/mL). The provider should exclude concomitant presence of B_{12} deficiency before starting treatment.

Management

Folic acid in a dose of 100 mcg/kg per day, given orally or parenterally for 3 to 4 weeks, is sufficient for most patients. Larger doses of folic acid can exacerbate neurologic damage in patients with cobalamin (B_{12}) deficiency. Patients with congenital folate malabsorption will require intramuscular folinic acid (5-formyl tetrahydrofolate) therapy, which should be instituted early to prevent neurologic deterioration.

Vitamin B₁₂ Deficiency

Vitamin B_{12} is a cobalt containing porphyrin, named cobalamin. It is found in foods of animal origin (eg, liver), fish, and dairy products, but not in fruits, cereals, or vegetables. A normal diet contains a large excess of B_{12} in comparison to daily needs. B_{12} combines with intrinsic factor (a glycoprotein synthesized by the gastric mucosa) and is absorbed to the receptors in the distal ileum. B_{12} alone is then absorbed into the portal blood, where it attaches to transcobalamin II and is transported to the bone marrow and other tissues. The total body content of vitamin B_{12} is 3 to 5 mg, and the rate of daily loss of vitamin B_{12} is less than 0.1% of the total body stores.

● **Clinical Pearl:** As opposed to nutritional folate deficiency, which becomes clinically apparent within months, it takes more than 2 years of poor absorption of vitamin B_{12} before clinically significant B_{12} deficiency develops (Hughe-Jones & Wickramasinghe, 1991).

Deficiency of vitamin B_{12} occurs in various clinical conditions (see Display 42-5). Juvenile pernicious anemia is a megaloblastic anemia caused by absence of effective intrinsic factor (IF). In some patients, IF is present but functionally defective. Gastric acid secretion is normal.

History and Physical Exam

The presenting symptoms may be those of *severe anemia* (ie, weakness, listlessness, anorexia, and irritability) or of *neurologic involvement* (ie, failure to reach milestones, slow mental development, parasthesias, hyporeflexia, ataxia, extensor plantar reflexes, and clonus). Most children with juvenile pernicious anemia present between 1 to 5 years of age.

Diagnostic Criteria and Studies

Peripheral blood picture and bone marrow findings are identical to that seen in folate deficiency (see above). Serum B_{12} levels are usually decreased (< 100 pg/mL) but by themselves are not diagnostic. A Schilling test differentiates juvenile pernicious anemia (IF deficiency) from other causes of vitamin B_{12} deficiency.

▲ **Clinical Warning:** Plasma levels of methylmalonic acid and total homocysteine are markedly increased. Providers should routinely obtain these levels when they suspect B_{12} deficiency, since serum B_{12} levels can be normal in the presence of significant B_{12} deficiency.

Management

Initial treatment consists of an intramuscular injection of 1 mg of vitamin B_{12}. Children with neurologic involvement should receive 1 mg of B_{12} daily for 2 weeks. They will need maintenance doses of 1 mg given monthly for life.

DISPLAY 42–5 • Causes of Vitamin B_{12} Deficiency

- Intrinsic factor (IF) deficiency (juvenile pernicious anemia)
- Transcobalamin II deficiency
- Intestinal malabsorption of B_{12}
  Familial absence of receptor for IF-B_{12} (Imerslund-Grasbeck syndrome)
  Surgical resection of terminal ileum
  Crohn's disease
  Diverticulitis
  Diphyllobothrium latum (fish tape worm) infestation

Aplastic Anemia (Pancytopenia)

Acquired Aplastic Anemia

Pancytopenia resulting from bone marrow failure is referred to as aplastic anemia. Acquired aplastic anemia may result from direct damage to the stem cell or bone marrow microenvironment or from immune-mediated insult to the progenitor cells. Known causes include drugs, toxins, and viruses (Display 42-6). Patients present with symptoms of severe anemia, bleeding due to thrombocytopenia, or frequent infections secondary to neutropenia. The aplastic anemia is considered severe when two of the following three criteria are present: absolute neutrophil count (ANC) < 500/mm³, platelet count < 20,000/mm³, or reticulocyte count < 1% after correction for hematocrit.

Differential diagnosis of aplastic anemia includes leukemia, collagen vascular disorders, and paroxysmal nocturnal hemoglobinuria (PNH). PNH often presents with pancytopenia without other manifestations of the disorder. Fanconi's anemia can be mistaken for acquired aplastic anemia if the patient lacks the characteristic congenital abnormalities. Thus, all patients should have a chromosomal fragility test done to rule out Fanconi's anemia. A bone marrow biopsy that shows markedly decreased cellularity of all marrow elements confirms the diagnosis of aplastic anemia.

Bone marrow transplantation (BMT) from an HLA-identical sibling has a 92% chance of cure (Storb, 1994). For those who lack an HLA-identical sibling, immunosuppressive therapy (IST) with antithymocyte globulin (ATG) and cyclosporine is recommended. IST offers complete remission to about 72% of patients and is thus preferable to a BMT from a matched unrelated donor; however, 10% to 20% of those who receive IST may develop late complications: PNH, myelodysplastic syndrome, or acute myeloblastic leukemia.

Constitutional Aplastic Anemia Syndromes

This rare group of disorders includes Fanconi's anemia, dyskeratosis congenita, Shwachman syndrome, and amegakaryocytic thrombocytopenia. Fanconi's anemia, the most common, is characterized by short stature, absent or hypoplastic thumb, hyperpigmentation, and café-au-lait spots. Patients with Fanconi's anemia may not manifest pancytopenia until later in childhood. The diagnosis is confirmed by demonstrating increased chromosomal breakage in the peripheral blood lymphocytes. Bone marrow transplantation is the only curative treatment.

HEMOLYTIC ANEMIAS

The term *hemoglobinopathy* refers to the presence of an abnormal hemoglobin. The cause is an altered amino acid structure of the polypeptide chains that form the globin fraction of the hemoglobin.

DISPLAY 42–6 • Causes of Acquired Aplastic Anemia

- Radiation
- Drugs: cytotoxic drugs, chloramphenicol, antiinflammatory drugs, anticonvulsants, gold
- chemicals: benzene
- Viruses: Hepatitis B and C virus, Parvovirus, HIV

Sickle Cell Disease

Sickle cell disease is a group of hemoglobinopathies characterized by production of hemoglobin S (Hb S), chronic hemolytic anemia, acute painful crises, and chronic organ damage. The three most common types of sickle cell disease and their incidence are given in Table 42-11. The homozygous state of Hb S is known as Hb SS disease or *sickle cell anemia*. Hb SC disease and S-β thalassemia are double heterozygous states of Hb S with Hb C or thalassemia trait respectively. S-β thalassemia has two subtypes: S-β$^+$ and the more severe S-β^0 thalassemia.

Approximately 8% of African Americans carry the sickle cell trait (Schneider 1976). Individuals with sickle cell trait are generally asymptomatic and do not have any anemia, vaso-occlusive crises, or chronic organ damage. The following complications may occur occasionally: gross hematuria, hyposthenuria, splenic infarcts in high altitude, bacteriuria, and pyelonephritis in pregnancy (Sears, 1994). Extremely rare cases of sudden unexplained death following exertion also have been reported (Kark, Poshey, Schumacher, 1987). Diagnosis of sickle cell trait is confirmed by hemoglobin electrophoresis: Hb S concentration (range 35%–45%) is lower than that of Hb A (range 50%–60%). In contrast, in sickle-β$^+$ thalassemia, the concentration of Hb S is higher than that of Hb A. Since the mid-1970s, diagnosis of sickle cell trait has routinely been made at newborn screening.

● **Clinical Pearl:** Most adolescents with sickle cell trait are unaware of their condition. Parents and physicians should counsel adolescents and young adults with sickle cell trait regarding its genetic implications. No restrictions on physical activities or sports are warranted in individuals with sickle cell trait (Pearson, 1989).

Pathology

When deoxygenated, the molecules of sickle hemoglobin polymerize to form pseudo-crystalline structures known as "tactoids," which distort the red cell membrane and produce the characteristic sickle-shaped red cells. Initially, this process of sickling is reversible with reoxygenation; with repeated deoxygenation-oxygenation cycles, however, the red cells become irreversibly sickled. Cells that are sickled increase blood viscosity, traverse capillaries poorly, and slow blood flow. The sluggish circulation and resulting hypoxia lead to sickling of more red cells, eventually leading to complete obstruction of blood flow and tissue infarction.

The clinical picture of acute episodes of ischemia and infarction, called vaso-occlusive or painful crisis, consists of severe pain, swelling, and tenderness. Ongoing low-grade ischemia may cause irreversible damage to vital organs such as kidneys and lungs, which usually becomes apparent when the patient reaches the fourth or fifth decade of life. In addition, the markedly reduced life span of sickled red cells results in a chronic, moderately severe, but well-compensated hemolytic anemia.

The hallmark of sickle cell disease is recurrent episodes of acute vaso-occlusive or painful crisis. Other acute manifestations are acute chest syndrome, infections, aplastic crisis, splenic sequestration crisis and stroke.

VASO-OCCLUSIVE CRISES

These crises are characterized by episodes of severe pain commonly involving the extremities, joints, back, chest, or abdomen and may be precipitated by fever, dehydration, acidosis, exposure to cold, or hypoxia. In infants, they classically cause swelling of hands and feet (hand-foot syndrome). Mesenteric infarction may present as acute abdomen. When an extremity or joint crisis is associated with marked swelling and tenderness, it may mimic osteomyelitis. Mild crises of the extremities may be managed at home with oral fluids and analgesics. Lack of improvement with such therapy, inadequate fluid intake, or presence of fever warrants hospitalization. With intravenous (IV) fluids and analgesics, most patients recover within seven days.

ACUTE CHEST SYNDROME (ACS)

Children with acute chest syndrome (ACS) present with chest pain, fever, and respiratory distress. In many patients, pain in the extremities or joints precedes signs of ACS by a few days. Chest radiographs show infiltrates or consolidation of the lungs. Pulmonary infarction, infection, or both cause ACS. All patients should be hospitalized. Aggressive therapy with IV fluids, antibiotics, oxygen, and red cell transfusions may prevent progression of mild ACS. Children with severe ACS should receive immediate exchange transfusion and be managed in the intensive care unit (ICU).

INFECTIONS

Because of poor or absent splenic function, children with sickle cell disease are prone to develop severe bacterial sepsis, especially with encapsulated organisms like *S. pneumoniae* and *H. influenzae*. In the past, this concern of overwhelming sepsis prompted hospitalization and treatment with IV antibiotics for all febrile children with SS disease. This approach has been modified. Febrile children should be hospitalized when at a high risk for sepsis: if the temperature is greater than or equal to 103^0 F or if the child looks ill. In addition, children with infiltrates on chest radiograph or WBC counts greater than or equal to 30,000/mm^3 also should be hospitalized for IV antibiotic therapy and close observation for signs of septic shock. Children with a temperature less than 103°F, a normal chest x-ray, a WBC count less than 30,000/mm^3, and reliable parents may be treated with parenteral ceftriaxone after obtaining blood cultures and may be discharged home on oral antibiotics. Close, daily outpatient follow-up is mandatory when providers contemplate this type of management.

▲ **Clinical Warning:** Providers must consider children with SS disease as immunocompromised. They must regard any febrile illness in this population as potentially life-threatening. Prompt evaluation and treatment of the febrile child with SS disease is critical.

STROKES

About 10% of all children with sickle cell anemia develop strokes before reaching adulthood. Affected children present

Table 42–11.   INCIDENCE OF MAJOR TYPES OF SICKLE CELL DISEASE

Genetic Types	Frequency Among African American Live Births
Hb SS disease	1 in 375
Hb SC disease	1 in 835
Sickle-β thalassemia	1 in 1667

Management and Therapy of Sickle Cell Disease (September 1989) U.S. Department of Health and Human Services. Public Health Service. National Institutes of Health. NIH publication No. 89-2117 p1.

with sudden onset of hemiplegia, usually secondary to occlusion of large blood vessels. Hemorrhagic stroke is more common in adults. Such patients require immediate exchange transfusion, followed by monthly transfusion therapy to prevent further episodes.

ANEMIA

The severity of anemia in sickle cell disease varies widely, with the hemoglobin level ranging from 5 to 9 gms/dL. Most children have a hemoglobin level of 7 to 8 gm/dL. Although most children appear normally active, their exercise tolerance is decreased proportionately to the degree of anemia. Clinicians should instruct them to avoid competitive sports and strenuous exercise. Because of chronic hemolysis, they are prone to develop gallstones, especially after age 10 years.

SPLENIC SEQUESTRATION CRISES (SSC)

Sudden enlargement of the spleen with pooling of large amounts of blood forms the basis of SSC. It is most common between ages 8 months and 5 years and may affect up to 30% of children with sickle cell disease. These children present with splenomegaly, severe anemia, and in severe cases, hypovolemic shock. Immediate transfusion of red cells is essential to prevent death.

APLASTIC CRISES

The red cell life span in sickle cell disease is about 15 days, which is markedly less than the normal red cell life span of 120 days. In this context, even transient viral-induced suppression of marrow erythropoiesis results in a rapid drop in the hemoglobin level— 1 gm/dL per day. The most common viral infection that can trigger an aplastic crisis is parvovirus. Children with aplastic crisis present with severe anemia (Hb 3–4 gms/dL). Diagnosis is made by a markedly decreased (usually < 1%) or absent reticulocyte count. Transfusion is often necessary, although erythropoiesis returns to normal in 7 to 10 days.

Diagnostic Criteria and Studies

Commercially available hemoglobin solubility tests are effective for screening for Hb S. These tests, however, do not differentiate between the disease and the trait, and they are not reliable in the first few months of life. The common laboratory abnormalities in sickle cell anemia are listed in Display 42-7. Hemoglobin electrophoresis is necessary not only

> **DISPLAY 42–7** • Laboratory Findings in Sickle Cell Anemia
>
> WBC: increased: 12,000–20,000/mm^3
> Hemoglobin: 5–9 gms/dL
> Reticulocyte count: 5%–15%
> Platelets: increased
> Sedimentation rate: decreased
> Blood smear: target cells, poikilocytes, sickle cells
> Serum LDH: increased
> Serum bilirubin: increased (usually > 2 mg/dL)

to confirm the diagnosis of sickle cell disease but also to differentiate the various sickling disorders. The various hemoglobin electrophoresis patterns of sickle cell disease in newborns, older infants (older than age 6 months), and children are given in Table 42-12. In most states, newborn screening programs identify infants with any sickle hemoglobinopathy, including sickle cell trait, and notify the infant's primary care provider.

Management

Apart from the care of patients with various forms of crisis, children with sickle cell disease requires the same routine well–child-care visits and immunizations recommended for all children. Additionally, they should receive the preventive measures outlined in Display 42-8.

In addition to regular visits to the primary care provider, sickle cell patients should attend a multi-disciplinary comprehensive sickle cell clinic at least semiannually. In such a clinic, a nurse coordinator provides education for patients and parents regarding sickle cell disease. He or she holds support groups for parents and adolescent patients and reinforces the need for all the preventive measures outlined in Display 42-9. Genetic counseling for the parents and sexually active adolescents is also vital.

Children who suffer from frequent (more than three each year) painful crises are more likely to die as young adults due to chronic organ damage. Such patients are likely to benefit from one of the following three treatment options:

1. Monthly transfusions of red cells decrease the concentration of sickle cells in blood and thus decrease the frequency of crisis. Potential risk of transfusion-associated viral infections, development of alloantibodies, and need

Table 42–12. DIFFERENTIAL DIAGNOSIS OF SICKLE CELL SYNDROMES BY HEMOGLOBIN ELECTROPHORESIS AND HEMATOLOGIC FEATURES

Sickle Cell Disorder	Hb Electrophoresis Pattern in Newborn	Hemoglobin Electrophoresis in Older Infants and Children						Hb gms/dL	Severity of painful crises
		Hb S %	Hb C %	Hb F %	Hb A %	Hb A$_2$ %	MCV		
Hb SS disease	FS	80–95	0	2–20	0	Normal	Normal	6–10	2+–4+
Sickle β^0 thalassemia	FS	75–90	0	5–25	0	> 3.5%	Low	6–10	2+–4+
Sickle β$^+$ thalassemia	FSA	65–85	0	—	10–30	> 3.5%	Low	9–11	1+–3+
Hb SC disease	FSC	45–48	45–48	2–5	0	Normal	Normal	10–12	1+–3+
S/HPFH	FS	65–80	0	15–30	0	Normal	Normal	12–14	0–1+
Sickle cell trait (Hb AS)	FAS	32–45	0	—	52–65	Normal	Normal	12–14	0–1+

for iron chelation therapy in chronically transfused patients make transfusion therapy less than ideal for most patients.

2. Hydroxyurea, a cancer chemotherapeutic drug, increases the intracellular fetal hemoglobin concentration, which reduces sickling. The decreased number of irreversibly sickled cells in the circulation reduces the frequency and severity of vaso-occlusive crises (Jayabose, 1996). In addition, hydroxyurea increases the hemoglobin level in most patients, thus improving their tolerance for exercise. The long-term safety of hydroxyurea, however, has yet to be established for children.

3. Bone marrow transplantation from an HLA-identical sibling donor has been curative in most patients who have undergone this therapy. The risk of bone marrow transplantation, however, may not be acceptable to many patients. In addition, an HLA-identical sibling match may not be available.

Hemoglobin SC Disease

In Hb SC disease, the anemia is mild or absent. Vaso-occlusive crises occur less frequently and tend to be milder. Severe bacterial infections are less common than with Hb SS disease. Cerebrovascular accidents and leg ulcers are rare. Aseptic necrosis of the femoral head, retinal vein thrombosis, and painless hematuria are common complications. Therapeutic and preventive measures are similar to those described for Hb SS disease. Transcranial doppler (TCD) screening, however, is not mandatory because of the rarity of cerebrovascular accidents.

Sickle-Beta Thalassemia

In patients with S-β thalassemia, the anemia is mild and microcytic. The severity of the disease in S-β^0 thalassemia is similar to that of sickle cell anemia. However, patients with

S-β^+ thalassemia have a much milder course because of the presence of variable amounts of hemoglobin A. Management is similar to that of sickle cell anemia. TCD screening is not indicated for patients with S-β^+ thalassemia.

Hemoglobin C Syndromes

Approximately 2% of African Americans have the heterozygous form or Hb C trait (AC) (Honig, 1996). They are asymptomatic and have no anemia, but the blood smear shows an increased number of target cells. Patients with the homozygous form (Hb CC disease) have mild, chronic hemolytic anemia (Hb 10 to 12 gms/dL), splenomegaly, and abundant target cells on the blood smear. Unlike sickle cell disease, no vaso-occlusive process is associated with Hb CC disease.

Hemoglobin E Syndromes

Because of the growing number of people of Southeast Asian origin in the United States, Hb E has become a common abnormal hemoglobin detected by screening programs. Individuals with Hb E trait (Hb AE) are asymptomatic and have no anemia. The red cells may be microcytic (MCV 74±10.6), however, and target cells are on the blood smear. Hemoglobin electrophoresis reveals 19% to 34% Hb E. Patients with the homozygous form (Hb EE disease) have mild hemolytic anemia, marked microcytosis, target cells on the blood smear, and an Hb E concentration greater than 90% on electrophoresis.

Red Cell Membrane Disorders

Hereditary Spherocytosis (HS)

Hereditary spherocytosis is the most common congenital hemolytic anemia, affecting approximately one in 5000 individuals in the United States (Segal, 1996; Beck & Tepper, 1991). It is usually transmitted as an autosomal dominant but sometimes as an autosomal recessive disorder. In about 25% of patients, the disease may be the manifestation of a new mutation, and thus the family history is negative.

Pathology

The primary defect is membrane instability due to deficiency or dysfunction of spectrin, a red cell membrane protein. Membrane weakness leads to formation of spherocytes, which are more rigid and more permeable to sodium than normal red cells. In the spleen, because of sluggish circulation, glucose levels in the spherocytes fall, and ATP generation declines. Intracellular sodium accumulates, causing osmotic swelling and increased membrane rigidity. In addition, lipids are readily lost from the membrane when red cells are deprived of energy. Repeated passages through the splenic circulation eventually lead to destruction of these rigid cells by phagocytosis as well as osmotic lysis.

History and Physical Exam

The neonate with HS often presents with significant jaundice and anemia. The severity of HS in infants and children varies. About 25% of patients have no anemia; the only evidence of hemolysis is an elevated reticulocyte count and a mild hyperbilirubinemia. Most patients have mild to moderate anemia (Hb 8–12 gms/dL), along with mild jaundice and splenomegaly. Less than 10% of patients have moderately severe (Hb 6–8 gms/dL) or severe anemia (Hb < 6 gms/dL). Patients with severe anemia are transfusion-dependent.

Exacerbations of anemia due to increased hemolysis or decreased production of red cells may punctuate the clinical course. Because of the shortened life span of the spherocytes, even a brief duration of decreased or absent erythroid activity causes the hemoglobin to drop to very low levels, requiring red cell transfusions. Such transient but complete suppression of erythropoiesis, referred to as *aplastic crisis*, is usually caused by parvovirus, although other viruses may cause milder suppression of erythropoiesis (hypoplastic crisis). Pigmentary (bilirubin) gallstones are only seen in 5% of children younger than age 10 years but are much more common in older children and adults.

Diagnostic Criteria and Studies

Reticulocyte counts and indirect bilirubin levels are increased as in any hemolytic anemia. (The differential diagnosis of hemolytic anemia is listed in Table 42-7.) During episodes of aplastic crisis, however, the reticulocyte count is markedly decreased or absent. Mean corpuscular hemoglobin (MCH) is normal; mean corpuscular hemoglobin concentration (MCHC) is increased (36–38). The blood smear usually shows at least 15% spherocytes. In patients with the mildest form of disease, the typical spherocytes are sparse; in these patients, the *unincubated* osmotic fragility test may be normal. The *incubated* osmotic fragility test, however, is almost always abnormal and is most reliable.

Management

Splenectomy increases the red cell life span, eliminating anemia and hyperbilirubinemia in almost all patients with HS. Thus, it is indicated in children with chronic severe anemia or repeated episodes of severe anemia, poor exercise tolerance, or impaired growth. Patients with mild disease (Hb 10 gms/dL) do not require splenectomy.

▲ **Clinical Warning:** Whenever possible, splenectomy should be postponed until the child is at least 5 years of age because of a higher risk of fatal post-splenectomy infections in infants and young children. All children should receive a pneumococcal vaccine several weeks before splenectomy, with a second dose 3 years later. Penicillin prophylaxis (125 mg twice daily for children younger than age 3 years; 250 mg twice daily for children age 3 years or older) must be continued for at least 5 years after splenectomy.

In the most recent series by Schilling and colleagues (1995), the risk of post-splenectomy sepsis was 0.073/100 patient-years. In this study, none of the patients who died had received pneumococcal vaccine, and none were taking prophylactic penicillin. Thus, the risk of fatal sepsis would be presumably lower for those who are immunized with pneumococcal vaccine and take prophylactic penicillin.

Hereditary Elliptocytosis (HE)

Hereditary elliptocytosis, an uncommon hemolytic anemia of varying severity, is characterized by a defect in the red cell membrane and a large number (15%) of elliptical erythrocytes on the blood smear. It is more common among individuals of West African origin. The disease has a wide spectrum of severity (see Display 42-9). The degree of elliptocytosis on the smear, however, is not predictive of the severity of hemolyis. The MCV ranges from 50 fl to normal. Mild cases do not require specific treatment. Splenectomy improves the hemoglobin levels significantly, and thus is beneficial in severe disease.

Hereditary Stomatocytosis

Hereditary stomatocytosis is a rare hemolytic anemia of varying severity in which the central pallor of the red cells is shaped as a slit or mouth-like opening. The osmotic fragility is increased. Peripheral blood smear shows 10% to 50% stomatocytes. MCV is increased (110–150 fl), and MCH is decreased (24–30). Hereditary stomatocytosis should be differentiated from acquired stomatocytosis seen in several conditions: thalassemia trait, spherocytosis, infectious mononucleosis, liver disease, acute alcoholism, and use of lipid-soluble drugs.

Red Cell Enzyme Disorders

G6PD Deficiency

Glucose-6-phosphate dehydrogenase (G6PD) is the first enzyme in the hexose monophosphate (HMP) shunt of the Embden Meyerhof glycolytic pathway, from which red cells derive most of their metabolic energy. The HMP shunt is concerned chiefly with the generation of reduced glutathione (GSH) through NADPH. GSH protects the red cells against injury by exogenous and endogenous oxidants, such as superoxide anion (O_2^-) and hydrogen peroxide (H_2O_2), which are produced by macrophages in infection and by red cells in the presence of certain drugs. Deficiency of G6PD sharply diminishes NADP synthesis, which leads to reduced levels of GSH and impaired resistance to oxidative stress.

History and Physical Exam

G6PD deficiency is an X-linked recessive disorder; thus, most affected individuals are males, although females can be affected. Most individuals with G6PD deficiency have episodes of acute intravascular hemolysis, which presents with dark-colored urine (hemoglobinuria), pallor, and jaundice. Infections or use of certain drugs often precipitate these hemolytic episodes. The symptoms begin acutely with an infection or within 1 to 3 days of exposure to the offending drug. Others may present with symptoms of acute severe anemia (dizziness, palpitation, and dyspnea), but without hemoglobinuria. The degree of hemolysis depends upon the amount of the inciting agent ingested or the severity of the triggering infection and the type of the enzyme deficiency.

● **Clinical Pearl:** In the A⁻ type of G6PD deficiency (occurring in 11% of African American males), the younger red cells have normal enzyme activity and thus are resistant to oxidant-induced hemolysis. Thus, hemolytic episodes may be self-limiting, and the patient may recover completely, even if the offending drug is continued. In the B⁻ type (Mediterranean), the hemolysis is more severe, and recovery from hemolytic episodes is slower, since even the young red cells are markedly deficient in G6PD.
Newborns with B⁻ type of deficiency may have severe hyperbilirubinemia. In A⁻ type deficiency, however, spontaneous hemolysis occurs only in premature babies. Some patients with B⁻ type of deficiency develop severe hemolysis following ingestion of fava beans (a Mediterranean dietary staple) because of their oxidative compounds. G6PD Canton is another common mutant enzyme with markedly reduced activity, occurring in about 5% of the Chinese population.

Diagnostic Criteria and Studies

The reticulocyte count is increased (5%–15%), and laboratory shows evidence of acute intravascular hemolysis (see Display 42-10). Blood smear reveals fragmented cells, a small number of spherocytes, *blister cells*, and *bite cells*. Supravital stains of the blood smear reveals Heinz bodies.

● **Clinical Pearl:** Direct quantitative G6PD assays show less than 10% activity in most patients. The enzyme levels, however, may be falsely normal during a hemolytic episode because of higher enzyme levels in the young red cells. Thus, it is necessary to repeat this assay after a few weeks.

Management

Treatment of underlying infection or removal of the offending drug will result in recovery for most patients. Supportive therapy including transfusion of red cells may be necessary if the anemia is severe. Males of high-risk ethnicity (eg, African American, Greek, southern Italian, Sephardic Jewish, Filipino, and southern Chinese) should be tested for the defect before receiving any of the known oxidant drugs (see Table 42-13).

Pyruvate Kinase Deficiency

Pyruvate kinase (PK) catalyzes one of the major reactions responsible for ATP production in the glycolytic pathway. Deficiency of this enzyme leads to decreased ATP synthesis. As a consequence of decreased ATP, red cells lose potassium and water, become rigid in the hypoxic splenic circulation, and are destroyed prematurely. The distal glycolytic block in PK deficiency increases the red cell 23-DPG, which minimizes the adverse effects of anemia by enhancing the release of oxygen from hemoglobin. The cause is an autosomal recessive genetic defect that results in marked reduction in red cell PK or production of an abnormal enzyme with decreased activity.

The severity of hemolytic anemia varies. Patients with mild disease are asymptomatic and may escape diagnosis until adulthood. Patients with severe disease present in the neonatal period with jaundice and require regular transfusions. Blood smear shows irregularly contracted and spiculated red cells, macrocytes, and rare acanthocytes. Demonstrating marked decrease in PK activity by quantitative assay confirms diagnosis. Splenectomy, although not curative, results in higher hemoglobin levels and strikingly high reticulocyte (30–70%) counts.

Immune Hemolytic Anemias

Warm Antibody Hemolytic Anemia

In most cases of warm antibody hemolytic anemia, no underlying cause (primary or idiopathic) can be defined. Rarely, an associated systemic disease (eg, systemic lupus erythematosus, lymphoid malignancy, immunodeficiency, or chronic inflammatory disease) can be recognized.

DISPLAY 42–10 • Laboratory Evidence of Acute Intravascular Hemolysis

- Hemoglobinuria (large amount of blood on dipstix; few or no red cells on microscopic examination)
- Increased LDH
- Increased indirect bilirubin
- Increased plasma hemoglobin
- Decreased serum haptoglobin

Table 42–13. FACTORS PRECIPITATING HEMOLYSIS IN GLUCOSE-6-PHOSPHATE DEHYDROGENASE DEFICIENCY

Medications		Illnesses
Antibacterials	*Others*	
Trimethoprim-Sulfamethoxazole	Acetophenitidin	Diabetic acidosis
	Vitamin K analogs	Hepatitis
Nalidixic acid	Methylene blue	
Chloramphenicol	Probenecid	
Nitrofurantoin	Acetyl salicylic acid	
	Phenazopyridine	
Antimalarials		
Primaquine	*Chemicals*	
Pamaquine	Phenylhydrazine	
Chloroquine	Benzene	
Quinacrine	Naphthalene	

History and Physical Exam

The onset may be sudden with hemoglobinuria, pallor, and jaundice or gradual with fatigue and pallor. Most cases (70%–80%) occur in children ages 2 to 12 years, have a relatively acute presentation, respond well to glucocorticoids, and recover completely within 3 to 6 months. Infants and children older than age 12 years frequently have chronic disease that lasts for many months or years. Response to steroid therapy in these patients may vary.

Diagnostic Criteria and Studies

Direct Coombs' test is positive in almost all patients; indirect Coombs' test is positive in some patients. Blood smear shows many spherocytes and nucleated red cells. Reticulocytes are markedly increased.

Management

Transfusion therapy is indicated only if the anemia is severe. Glucocorticoids are more effective than intravenous immune globulin (IVIG) in controlling the hemolytic process. Splenectomy should be considered only for patients with refractory disease.

Cold Agglutinin Disease

Cold agglutinin disease may be idiopathic (primary) or secondary to infections such as *Mycoplasma pneumoniae*, EBV or lymphoid malignancies. Patients often present with hemoglobinuria, which can be exaggerated when the patient is exposed to cold. The hemolysis is complement-mediated, mainly intravascular, and usually acute and self-limited. Patients should avoid exposure to cold. Glucocorticoids are much less effective in cold agglutinin disease than in warm antibody hemolytic anemia; splenectomy is not useful.

NEUTROPENIA

Neutropenia is defined as absolute neutrophil count (ANC) less than 1000/mm³ for infants and less than 1500/mm³ for older children. ANC is calculated by multiplying the total white blood cell (WBC) count by the percentage of segmented neutrophils + bands. African Americans have somewhat lower neutrophil counts. Compared to European Americans, the lower limits of normal can tentatively be considered 200 to 600/mm[3] lower (Dinauer, 1998).

Causes of neutropenia include the following:

Infections
Drugs
Autoimmune neutropenia of infancy
Neonatal alloimmune neutropenia
Congenital neutropenia syndromes: cyclic neutropenia, Kostmann syndrome (severe congenital neutropenia), Shwachman syndrome
Immune deficiency disorders
Metabolic disorders

Management of febrile neutropenic children on cancer chemotherapy is discussed in Chapter 31. This section will discuss some of the clinically important neutropenic disorders, such as autoimmune neutropenia of infancy and cyclic neutropenia

Clinical manifestations in neutropenic children include otitis media, cutaneous and subcutaneous infections, gingivitis, periodontitis, perirectal inflammation, pneumonia, and septicemia. In general, the risk of serious infections, such as sepsis or pneumonia, correlates with the severity and duration of the neutropenia. In febrile children on chemotherapy, an ANC less than 500/mm[3] is considered a clear indication for hospitalization. The presence of indwelling catheters, mucositis, and therapy-related hypogammaglobulinemia add to the risk of infections in children with cancer. Children with autoimmune neutropenia, however, rarely get serious infections because of their ability to mobilize adequate neutrophils from the bone marrow reserves to the peripheral blood during periods of infection.

Infection-Associated Neutropenia

● **Clinical Pearl:** By far, the most common cause of neutropenia seen in the primary care setting is viral. It is commonly seen with influenza, measles, rubella, varicella, roseola infantum, respiratory syncytial virus, and hepatitis A and B, although any virus may be implicated.

Viral neutropenia is usually not associated with anemia or thrombocytopenia, and it resolves within 1 to 3 weeks. If the child is otherwise well, the primary care provider can follow him or her with weekly blood counts.

▲ **Clinical Warning:** A pediatric hematology consultation is indicated if there is associated anemia or thrombocytopenia or if the neutropenia does not resolve in 2 to 3 weeks.

▲ **Clinical Warning:** In bacterial infections, severe neutropenia often indicates overwhelming sepsis.

Drug-Induced Neutropenia

Drugs may cause neutropenia by one of the following three mechanisms:

A direct toxic effect on the marrow microenvironment
Immune-mediated destruction of neutrophils
Excessive sensitivity of myeloid precursors to the drug

A partial list of drugs associated with neutropenia is given in Display 42-11. This list does not include cytotoxic drugs,

---

> **DISPLAY 42–11 • Drugs Associated With Neutropenia**
>
> - Ibuprofen, indomethacin, aminopyrine
> - Penicillins, sulfonamides, chloramphenicol
> - Phenytoin, carbamazepine
> - Propylthiouracil
> - Hydralazine, procainamide, quinidine
> - Chlorpropamide
> - Chlorpromazine, phenothiazines
> - Cimetidine, ranitidine, levamisole
>
> Adapted from: Dinauer, M.C. (1998). The phagocytic system and disorders of granulopoiesis and granulocyte function. In Nathan, D.G., & Orkin, S.H., (eds). *Nathan and Oski's hematology of infancy and childhood* (5th ed., p. 915). Philadelphia: WB Saunders.

which are used in cancer chemotherapy and predictably causes neutropenia in association with other cytopenias.

Drug-induced neutropenia usually begins 1 to 2 weeks after first exposure to the drug or soon after re-exposure. Neutropenia caused by an acute idiosyncratic reaction may last only for a few days, whereas immune-mediated neutropenia lasts for about a week. Once the neutropenia is severe (ANC <500/mm3), the offending drug must be immediately discontinued.

Autoimmune Neutropenia of Childhood

Autoimmune neutropenia is the most common cause of chronic neutropenia in childhood, with more than 95% of the cases occurring before age 3 years. The neutrophil count at diagnosis is usually between 150 and 250/mm[3] (Bux, Behrens, Jaeger, 1998). Almost all patients recover completely, and the median duration of neutropenia is 20 months. A pediatric hematologist should confirm clinical diagnosis of autoimmune neutropenia by careful exclusion of other causes of neutropenia. Once the diagnosis is established, the primary care provider can manage most patients' infections, usually in the outpatient setting. Granulocyte-colony stimulating factor (G-CSF) is effective in raising the neutrophil counts in these patients, and is indicated when the infection is severe enough to warrant hospitalization, IV antibiotics, or both.

Cyclic Neutropenia

Cyclic neutropenia is a rare disorder in which the patient develops severe neutropenia (absolute neutrophil count < 200/mm[3]) approximately every 21 days (range 14–35 days). The neutropenia lasts for 3 to 6 days. Common manifestations include recurrent mouth ulcers associated with fever, malaise, gingivitis, and periodontitis. Confirmation of diagnosis requires demonstrating the cyclic nature of neutrophil counts by serial blood counts—twice a week for 6 to 8 weeks. Treatment with G-CSF decreases the frequency of infections by reducing the severity and duration of the neutropenia.

Other Congenital Neutropenia Syndromes

Familial Benign Neutropenia

Familial benign neutropenia is an autosomal dominant disorder in which patients have mild neutropenia (ANC is between 1000 and 1500/mm[3]) but do not get frequent infections. Routine blood counts usually detect the presence of this condition, and family studies can confirm the diagnosis.

Kostmann Syndrome

In Kostmann syndrome, an autosomal recessive disorder, the infant suffers frequent and severe bacterial infections from birth due to severe neutropenia (ANC < 200/mm³). Bone marrow aspirate study shows a paucity of myeloid series beyond the promyelocyte and myelocyte stage. Most patients respond well to G-CSF therapy.

Shwachman Syndrome

Shwachman syndrome is a rare autosomal recessive disease of neutropenia, exocrine pancreatic deficiency, and metaphyseal chondrodysplasia. Affected infants usually present in the first 4 months of life with severe malabsorption. Neutropenia is often not severe, and there may be associated anemia and thrombocytopenia.

DISORDERS OF HEMOSTASIS

Normal hemostasis depends upon three factors: an intact vasculature, adequate numbers of functioning platelets, and normal levels of all coagulation factors. The first reaction to any trauma to the vascular bed is adhesion of platelets to the subendothelial collagen and microfibrils, a reaction requiring the presence of von Willebrand factor. These platelets change in shape and release ADP and thromboxane, which promote platelet-to-platelet interaction (aggregation) that leads to formation of the platelet plug. Platelets also participate in the coagulation pathway by releasing platelet factor 3, which absorbs factor VIII and IX to the platelet surface. Factor VIII and IX activate factor X. Factor X and V convert prothrombin to thrombin, which activates fibrinogen to fibrin. Factor XIII converts the fibrin to fibrin polymer, which is essential for stabilizing the clot formed by the platelet plug.

Classification of Bleeding Disorders

The following is a basic classification system of bleeding disorders:

I. Platelets
   A. Thrombocytopenias (eg, ITP, drug-induced, congenital)
   B. Platelet function disorders
      1. Inherited (eg, Glanzman's thrombasthenia, Wiscott Aldrich syndrome, Bernard Soulier syndrome)
      2. Acquired (eg, uremia, drugs)
II. Coagulation disorders
   A. Inherited (eg, Hemophilia A, B; von Willebrand disease; other coagulation factor deficiencies [XI, VII, II, V, X])
   B. Acquired: (eg, vitamin K deficiency, liver disease, disseminated intravascular coagulation)
III. Vascular disorders (eg, Henoch-Schönlein purpura, Ehlers-Danlos syndrome)

History and Physical Exam

Primary care providers often must determine if a child has a bleeding disorder because of symptoms or an abnormal result of a screening coagulation test. Symptoms that warrant investigation include repeated episodes of epistaxis, generalized bruises, subcutaneous hematomas, hemarthro-

sis, menorrhagia, rectal bleeding, delayed bleeding from surgical wounds, and intracranial bleeding with minimal or no trauma.

Epistaxis, generalized bruising, menorrhagia, and rectal bleeding are common in von Willebrand disease. Petechiae and purpuric lesions usually indicate thrombocytopenia, platelet dysfunction, or a vascular disorder (eg, Henoch-Schonlein purpura). Patients with hemophilia usually present with hemarthrosis, large subcutaneous or muscle hematomas, and occasionally intracranial hemorrhage. The provider should elicit a previous history of any surgery. Absence of any excessive bleeding after extraction of molar teeth, tonsillectomy, or other major surgery makes the diagnosis of an inherited bleeding disorder unlikely. On the other hand, absence of excessive bleeding after circumcision in the newborn does not rule out an inherited bleeding disorder. Although family history is usually positive in von Willebrand disease and hemophilia, its absence does not rule out diagnosis of a bleeding disorder.

Diagnostic Tests

A CBC should always be done first to rule out thrombocytopenia as the cause of the bleeding disorder. When thrombocytopenia is the cause, the platelet count is usually less than 20,000/mm³ and almost always less than 50,000/mm³. A prothrombin time (PT), a partial thromboplastin time (PTT), and a bleeding time (BT) are additional screening tests necessary to determine the nature of the bleeding disorder. A prolonged bleeding time in the presence of a normal platelet count indicates platelet function disorder. See Table 42-15 on page 510.

Thrombocytopenia

Normal platelet counts in children range from 150,000 to 400,000/mm³. Thrombocytopenia is defined as any platelet count less than 150,000/mm³. While ecchymoses caused by minor trauma are seen with platelet counts less than 50,000/mm³, serious spontaneous bleeding is seldom seen when the platelet count is greater than 20,000/mm³. Thrombocytopenia in an acutely ill child is usually secondary to infection, and may indicate disseminated intravascular coagulation. On the other hand, severe thrombocytopenia in a well-appearing child is most likely a case of immune thrombocytopenic purpura (ITP). Other causes of acquired thrombocytopenia include drug-induced thrombocytopenia, hemolytic uremic syndrome, and thrombotic thrombocytopenic purpura. Inherited thrombocytopenias are rare.

Immune Thrombocytopenic Purpura (ITP)

Immune Thrombocytopenic Purpura (ITP), one of the most common acquired bleeding disorders, occurs with a frequency of four to eight cases per 100,000 children per year (Medeiros, 1996). More than 80% of children with this disorder recover completely within 6 months, and they are considered to have acute ITP. When the condition persists for more than 6 months after diagnosis, it is considered chronic. Acute ITP affects both sexes equally and occurs most commonly between ages 2 and 5 years. Chronic ITP is seen mostly in children older than age 7 years and is more common in females.

About 90% of children younger than age 10 years recover completely within 6 months of diagnosis. Older children have a 10% to 30% risk of chronic disease. At the time of initial presentation, predicting the clinical course usually is difficult. Adolescent females with an insidious onset and an initial platelet count greater than 20,000/mm³ have a high risk for chronic ITP. Less than 5% of children have one or more recurrences of ITP, with normal platelet counts for more than 3 months between recurrences (Damshek, 1963).

Pathology

Viral infections or other unknown factors trigger production of antiplatelet antibodies (IgG), which coat the platelets. These platelet-associated IgG molecules attach to the Fc receptors on the reticuloendothelial cells of the spleen, which readily phagocytose the sensitized platelets.

History and Physical Exam

Most children have severe thrombocytopenia ($< 20,000/mm^3$) at diagnosis and present with sudden onset of generalized purpura. Epistaxis is seen in about 5% of children; gross hematuria and melena are less common. Physical exam reveals generalized purpura and petechiae.

Mucosal lesions can be recognized in the lips, buccal mucosa, and palate. There is no enlargement of lymph nodes, liver, or spleen. Intracranial hemorrhage (ICH) occurs in 0.5% of children with ITP (Woerner, 1981) and has a 46% mortality rate; it is almost never seen when the platelet count is greater than $20,000 mm^3$. Most reported cases of ICH have occurred spontaneously, without any precipitating factors (eg, trauma) and without any warning signs in the form of other bleeding (eg, epistaxis, gross hematuria, or melena).

Diagnostic Criteria and Studies

The provider can confidently make a clinical diagnosis of ITP if the child meets all the following criteria:

Sudden onset of generalized purpura
Otherwise well appearance
Negative physical examination except for purpura
Platelet count of less than $20,000/mm^3$
Normal WBC, neutrophil count, hemoglobin, MCV, and reticulocyte count

In the presence of fever, splenomegaly, anemia, neutropenia, a low reticulocyte count, or a high MCV, the provider should rule out a diagnosis of leukemia or aplastic anemia by a bone marrow aspirate and biopsy. Otherwise, if all other blood elements are normal, the patient requires no further diagnostic studies. Infants infected with HIV occasionally present with isolated thrombocytopenia; thus, the provider should perform HIV testing if the history is positive for HIV risk factors. Isolated thrombocytopenia may rarely be a presenting feature of systemic lupus erythematosus (SLE), especially in girls older than age 10 years; thus, a routine antinuclear antibody (ANA) test is helpful in older females. Rarely, inherited forms of thrombocytopenia can be misdiagnosed as ITP.

Management

Initial therapy does not affect the ultimate outcome of ITP. If the initial platelet count is greater than or equal to $20,000/mm^3$, no treatment is indicated.

Acute ITP

The goal of treatment in acute ITP is to rapidly raise the platelet count above $20,000/mm^3$, thus reducing the risk of ICH. Because children presenting with clinical bleeding (eg, epistaxis, gross hematuria, or melena) have a higher risk of ICH, clinicians should manage their illness aggressively

with intravenous immune globulin (IVIG), IV steroids, and even platelet transfusions if necessary. Most children with ITP, however, do not have any bleeding except purpura. They can be treated with one of the following three therapeutic regimens:

1. *Prednisone*: Patients treated with prednisone increase their platelet counts more rapidly compared to untreated patients. The conventional regimen is to continue 2 mg/kg/day for 21 days. Side effects include weight gain with cushingoid features, hypertension, impaired immunity, and mood changes. More recently, a regimen of 4 mg/kg/day for 7 days has been found to produce fewer side effects than the conventional regimen. Major advantages include low cost and outpatient treatment.
2. *Intravenous immune globulin (IVIG)* saturates the Fc receptor sites on the reticuloendothelial (RE) cells, making them unavailable for the sensitized platelets; thus, the platelets are spared from the phagocytic effects of the RE cells. The usual dose is 1 gm/kg given as 5% or 6% solution over 6 hours. (Recently, IVIG has become available as a 10% and 12% solution). In most patients, IVIG raises the platelet counts above $20,000/mm^3$ within 24 to 48 hours and to normal values within 1 week. The effects of IVIG usually last up to 4 weeks. Patients whose platelet counts drop below $20,000/mm^3$ after the effects of IVIG wane will need repeat doses of IVIG. Side effects of IVIG include high fever and chills during the early hours of administration. Headache and vomiting are seen in about 30% of patients, usually 24 hours after administration. Rarely, IVIG causes an aseptic meningitis syndrome with fever, neck stiffness, headache, and vomiting. Premedication with IV diphenhydramine or hydrocortisone is effective in preventing the early reactions; a 3 day course of oral prednisone started at the time of IVIG administration reduces the risk of developing delayed headache and vomiting.
3. *IV anti-D (RhO immune globulin-WinRho)* is a reasonable alternative to IVIG for Rh-positive patients with ITP. Its action is similar to IVIG, coating the Rh-positive red cells, which in turn attach to the Fc receptors of the reticuloendothelial cells. Eighty percent of children with ITP receiving IV anti-D increase their platelet count above $20,000/mm^3$ within 72 hours. The recommended dose is 50 mcg/kg body weight. Although IV anti-D is less effective than IVIG in raising the platelet count, it has two advantages over IVIG. It is administered as a rapid (5–10 minutes) IV bolus, thus preventing hospitalization in most cases. It costs half the price of the dose of IVIG.

Chronic ITP

Children with chronic ITP need treatment only if the platelet count drops below $20,000/mm^3$, or if the child has a special need for a higher platelet count, such as before surgery or participation in contact sports. The treatment choices are between IVIG and IV anti-D. Steroids are not suitable for the treatment of chronic ITP. Clinicians should instruct the child and parents how to recognize the appearance of petechiae, which usually indicate a platelet count less than $20,000/mm^3$. Ecchymoses on the extremities (without associated petechiae), especially following trauma, may occur with platelet counts in the range of $20,000$ to $50,000/mm^3$. Such knowledge will decrease the need for frequent blood counts to monitor the severity of the disease.

Splenectomy is curative in more than 70% of children with chronic ITP. Since 30% to 50% of children with chronic ITP eventually recover completely, providers should reserve splenectomy for children with severe chronic ITP, those with platelet counts less than 10,000/ mm^3 for more than 14 days in the absence of treatment, and children with recurrent and severe hemorrhage. The risk of mortality in splenectomized children (due to sepsis) is 1 per 300-1000. Because the risk of post-splenecomy sepsis is higher in young children, clinicians should postpone splenectomy whenever possible until the child is at least 5 years of age. Prior to splenectomy, the patient should receive pneumococcal vaccine, with repeat vaccines after 3 years.

▲ **Clinical Warning:** Following splenectomy, patients should be on penicillin prophylaxis until adulthood. More importantly, clinicians should instruct patients to seek immediate medical attention for any febrile illness with a temperature of 102°F or more. The provider should carefully evaluate such patients for sepsis and should administer IV antibiotics pending culture results.

Von Willebrand Disease (VWD)

VWD is the most common inherited bleeding disorder, affecting approximately 1% of the population. Type 1 and type 2A are the most common types, accounting for 80% and 15% of cases respectively. Type 3, the most severe form, is quite rare, with an incidence of 1 per million.

Pathology

A quantitative (Type 1, 3) or qualitative (Type 2) defect in von Willebrand Factor (VWF) results in impaired platelet adhesion and aggregation, leading to poor primary hemostasis (platelet plug formation), which is responsible for the bleeding episodes. Since VWF acts as a carrier protein for factor VIII, the level of factor VIII is also low in VWD. The decrease in factor VIII in patients with VWD, however, is usually not severe enough to cause prolonged PTT or clinical bleeding except in Type 3 VWD. The mode of inheritance is autosomal dominant for types 1, 2A, and 2B; other types follow an autosomal recessive pattern.

History and Physical Exam

Patients with VWD experience repeated episodes of skin and mucous membrane bleedings. These include generalized bruises, epistaxis, menorrhagia, gastrointestinal bleeding, and prolonged bleeding after dental extraction, surgery, or any accidental cuts and lacerations. At times, the bleeding can be severe enough to cause significant anemia or even acute hypovolemic shock.

Patients with Type 3 VWD have severe disease with symptoms similar to those of hemophilia—hemarthrosis and

hematomas of soft tissue and muscle. Patients with Type 2B VWD may have thrombocytopenia because of their unique feature of increased platelet aggregation, which may be mistaken for an inherited thrombocytopenia syndrome.

Diagnostic Criteria and Studies

Diagnostic tests necessary to confirm the diagnosis include platelet count, APTT, Factor VIII, (VWF Ag, VWF RCoF, and VWF multimers) (see Table 42-14). In the presence of abnormal tests, the provider can make a diagnosis even in the absence of bleeding episodes or a positive family history. If the laboratory tests are normal in the presence of strong personal and family history, however, the clinician should repeat the laboratory tests at least once before ruling out diagnosis of VWD. The provider can easily diagnose types 2 and 3 provided all the coagulation assays are done in a reliable laboratory. Diagnosis of type 1 is frequently difficult, because both Factor VIII and VWF act as acute phase reactants, and their levels increase by three- to five-fold during physiologic stress, resulting in falsely normal values.

Management

Desmopressin (DDAVP) by IV infusion or intranasal inhalation increases the levels of VWF and FVIII in plasma by two- to eight-fold, presumably by releasing VWF from the endothelial stores. Peak levels are achieved in 30 minutes and 90 minutes after IV and intranasal application, respectively. Thus, clinicians can manage most clinical situations in patients with Type 1 VWD with desmopressin infusion or inhalation. The recommended dose of the concentrated intranasal preparation (Stimate) is 150 μg for children less than 50 kg and 300 μg for children weighing 50 kg or more. The usual IV dose is 0.3 μg/kg given in 50 mL of normal saline over 30 to 60 minutes. More rapid infusion may cause headache and hypertension. Potentially serious side effects include hyponatremia and seizures; these are more likely to occur in children younger than age 2 years. Desmopressin is not useful in patients with type 3 VWD. In type 2B, the use of DDAVP is not recommended, since it can cause significant thrombocytopenia by increasing the platelet aggregation excessively. When DDAVP is not adequate for hemostasis, such as in major surgery, cryoprecipitate should be used.

Hemophilia

Both hemophilia A (FVIII deficiency) and hemophilia B (FIX deficiency) are rare X-linked recessive disorders with a prevalence of 1 per 10,000 males and 1 per 50,000 males, respectively. Depending upon the plasma factor level, hemo-

Table 42–14. CLASSIFICATION AND RESULTS OF LABORATORY STUDIES IN COMMON FORMS OF VON WILLEBRAND'S DISEASE

Study	Type 1	Type 2A	Type 2B	Type 2M	Type 2N	Type 3
VWF Ag	↓	↓	↓ or N	↓	↓ or N	Absent
VWF RCoF	↓	↓ ↓	↓	↓ ↓	↓	↓ ↓ (about 5%)
FVIII	↓	↓ or N	↓ or N	↓ ↓	↓ or N	Absent
RIPA	↓	↓ ↓	↑	↓ ↓	Normal	Absent
Multimers	Normal	Loss of intermediate and large multimers	Loss of large multimers	Normal	Normal	Absent

Reproduced from Lillicrap, D., Dean, L., Blanchette, V.S. (1999). von Willebrand disease. In Lilleyman, J.S., Hann, I.M., & Blanchette, V.S. (Eds.), *Pediatric hematology* (2nd Ed.). New York: Churchill Livingstone.

philia can be classified as severe (< 2%), moderate (2%–5%), or mild (5%–30%). Patients with severe or moderate hemophilia have spontaneous bleeding, whereas patients with mild hemophilia bleed only after a significant trauma. Sixty percent of all hemophilia A have severe disease compared to 44% of patients with hemophilia B.

History and Physical Exam

Both factors VIII and IX do not cross the placenta; thus, the newborn with hemophilia has low factor levels at birth. The newborn with hemophilia may develop large cephalohematomas or even intracranial hemorrhages after difficult vaginal deliveries. Intramuscular injections can result in large painful muscle hematomas. Circumcision in the hemophilic newborn does not always cause excessive bleeding. During the first year of life, soft tissue bruising can be striking and mistaken for child abuse. When the child begins to walk, subcutaneous hematomas and lacerations of the mouth and buccal mucosa can occur secondary to trauma.

Hemarthrosis, the hallmark of severe hemophilia, begins to manifest between ages 8 months to 3 years. The joints most commonly affected include ankles, knees, and elbows. The earliest sign of hemarthrosis is a feeling of stiffness followed by sharp pain and swelling of the joints. Hemarthrosis results in synovial inflammation. The increased vascularity of the synovial membrane makes the joint more prone to further episodes of joint bleeding, setting up a vicious cycle that leads to chronic damage to the joint surface. Prompt treatment of hemarthrosis is crucial for the prevention of such chronic hemophilic arthropathy.

Intracranial hemorrhage (ICH) is the most common cause of death in children with hemophilia. It may be subdural, subarachnoid, or intracerebral. Although trauma usually causes ICH, it also can occur spontaneously. Infants with ICH have vague symptoms of vomiting, lethargy, pallor, unequal pupils, tense fontanels, and neurologic deficits. A child with significant head trauma or symptoms of ICH should immediately receive factor infusion to raise the factor level to 100% before undergoing imaging studies.

Other forms of bleeding in the patient with hemophilia include hematuria, intraabdominal bleeding, ileopsoas bleeding, and compartment syndromes. Right-sided iliopsoas bleeding may mimic appendicitis. Bleeding into the forearms or calf muscles causes compartment syndrome. Due to the limited space, the hemorrhage into these spaces causes compression of nerves and vessels, resulting in significant neurologic deficits. Prompt replacement therapy with clotting factor is of paramount importance. Fasciotomy is indicated in severe cases.

Diagnostic Criteria and Studies

● **Clinical Pearl:** A significantly prolonged PTT with normal PT indicates a deficiency of one of the intrinsic clotting factors. Given these results, the provider should obtain assays of factor VIII and IX, since these are the most common intrinsic factor deficiencies.

A factor VIII level of less than 30% is diagnostic of hemophilia A, provided the clinician rules out the possibility of von Willebrand disease in patients with a negative family history of hemophilia. This diagnostic criteria applies to neonates also, since factor VIII levels in neonates are similar to older children and adults (50%–150%). A factor IX level less than 30% is diagnostic of hemophilia B in infants older than age 6 months. In newborns, factor IX levels can be phys-

iologically as low as 15%. In newborns, the provider can make the diagnosis based on factor assays from cord blood, since neither factor VIII nor factor IX crosses the placenta. Prenatal diagnosis can be made if necessary by chorionic villi sampling at 10 to 12 weeks of gestation.

Management

The goal of hemophilia treatment is to avoid chronic joint damage and to prevent or promptly treat any life-threatening hemorrhages. Thus, infusion of the factor at the earliest sign of hemarthrosis or any life-threatening hemorrhage is essential. Toward this goal, most parents of children with severe hemophilia receive instruction to administer the factor through a peripheral vein or a central venous access (Life-Port). Patients for whom such home care is not available rely upon emergency departments for episodic treatments. Thus, it is important for primary care providers to be familiar with the principles of hemophilia treatment.

Treatment of Bleeding Episodes

● **Clinical Pearl:** To achieve hemostasis in most bleeding episodes, providers need to increase the factor level to about 50%. In intracranial hemorrhage and in preparation for surgery, the factor level should be 100%. One unit of factor VIII/kg of body weight raises the plasma concentration of factor VIII by 2%. One unit of factor IX/kg of body weight increases the factor IX level by only 1%.

A child with a suspected ICH should receive 50 units of factor VIII/kg or 100 units/kg of factor IX to raise the levels to 100%. For the child with hemarthrosis or most other forms of bleeding, half of the above doses will be adequate.

Prophylactic Therapy

Recurrent hemarthroses of one or more joints are indications for prophylactic factor therapy. This will prevent further bleeding into the same joint, thereby promoting recovery of the affected joint. Patients who have had an episode of ICH also benefit from prophylactic therapy. Prophylaxis consists of regular administration of the needed factor (factor VIII on alternate days or factor IX twice a week) to maintain a minimum level of 5%. This level will prevent spontaneous bleeding in most patients.

Rare Inherited Bleeding Disorders

Deficiencies of other coagulation factors (XI, VII, II, V, X) are rare autosomal recessive disorders. Any of these deficiencies in the homozygous state can cause serious bleeding episodes, including ICH. The diagnostic screening profile is shown in Table 42-15. Confirmation of diagnosis depends upon assay of the specific coagulation factor. Deficiencies of factors II, V, VII, X, and XI can be treated with fresh frozen plasma (FFP), although commercial concentrates are available for factors VII, XI, and XIII. Deficiencies of factors II and X also can be treated with commercial prothrombin complex concentrates (which have factors II, VII, IX, and X).

Acquired Bleeding Disorders

Vitamin K deficiency in children may result from malabsorption syndromes, prolonged oral antibiotic therapy, and warfarin therapy. Since factor VII has the shortest half-life, in early stages of vitamin K deficiency only the PT is prolonged. In later stages, however, both PT and PTT are pro-

Table 42–15. DIFFERENTIAL DIAGNOSIS OF BLEEDING DISORDERS BASED ON LABORATORY DATA (ONLY ABNORMAL TESTS ARE SHOWN)

Disorder	Platelet count	Bleeding time[1]	APTT	PT	TCT
Thrombocytopenia	↓	*			
Platelet function disorder		↑			
Hemophilia (FVIII or FIX deficiency), FXI deficiency, F XII deficiency,[2] Antiphospholipid antibodies (Lupus anti-coagulant and anticardiolipin antibodies)[2]			↑		
Factor VII deficiency				↑	
Factor II, V, or X deficiency			↑	↑	
Vitamin K deficiency, Liver disease			↑	↑	
Disseminated intravascular coagulation (DIC)	↓		↑	↑	↑
von Willebrand disease[3]		↑ or N	N or ↑		
Hypofibrinogenemia/dysfibrinogenemia			↑	↑	↑
Factor XIII deficiency[3]					

Adapted from Hathaway, W.E. & Goodnight, S.H. Evaluation of bleeding tendency in outpatient child and adult (1993). In W.E. Hathaway & S.H. Goodnight (Eds.), *Disorders of hemostasis and thrombosis: A clinical guide.* New York: McGraw-Hill, Inc.

TCT (Thrombin clotting time) is not a routine screening test since afibrinogenemia and dysfibrinogenemia are extremely rare.

[1]The result of a bleeding time can be inaccurate due to technical reasons. The diagnosis of von Willebrand disease can not be ruled out on the basis of a normal bleeding time, if the other tests support the diagnosis.

*Bleeding time is generally not done in the thrombocytopenic patient, since it is expected to be prolonged.

[2]Factor XII deficiency and antiphospholipid antibodies cause in vitro prolongation of PTT; however, they do not cause bleeding. In fact, antiphospholipid antibodies are one of the important causes of thrombosis. Factor XII deficiency is rarely associated with thrombosis.

[3]If all the screening tests are normal in the presence of a definite history of bleeding disorder, von Willebrand disease and factor XIII deficiency should be ruled out by appropriate studies. Clot lysis time is the screening test for factor XIII deficency.
N=normal.

longed because of the fall in factors II, IX, and X, which are vitamin K-dependent. Clinically significant bleeding is uncommon. Vitamin K by subcutaneous route corrects the coagulation in abnormality in a few hours. If immediate correction is required, FFP or prothromin complex concentrates can be used.

Liver disease can cause a coagulopathy by secondary vitamin K deficiency or due to reduction in the synthesis of coagulation factors (except factor VIII and vWF). In advanced cases, both PT and PTT are prolonged, whereas in early stages, only PT is prolonged. Patients usually do not need corrective therapy except for bleeding episodes or diagnostic procedures. FFP in doses of 15 to 20 mL/kg can be given over 3 to 4 hours, which achieves hemostasis in most cases.

Disseminated Intravascular Coagulation (DIC) is diagnosed by the presence of thrombocytopenia, hypofibrinogenemia, and fibrin degradation products in addition to prolonged PT and PTT. Although DIC by itself can cause bleeding, thrombosis, or both, it is the underlying disorder that usually determines the prognosis. If purpuric lesions are seen in a febrile, ill-looking patient, the clinician should suspect meningococcemia and other infections that can cause purpura fulminans. Immediate heparin therapy may prevent the serious consequences of thrombotic complications.

REFERENCES

Beck, W. S., & Tepper, R. I. (1991). Hemolytic anemias III. Membrane disorders. In W. S. Beck (Ed.), *Hematology* (5th ed., p. 266). Cambridge: MIT Press.

Bux, J., Behrens, G., Jaeger, G., & Welte, K. (1998). Diagnosis and clinical course of autoimmune neutropenia in infancy: Analysis of 240 cases. *Blood, 91*(1),181–186.

Cherrick, I., Karayalcin, G., & Lanzkowsky, P. (1994). Transient erythroblastopenia of childhood. Prospective study of fifty patients. *American Journal of Pediatric Hematology and Oncology, 16*(4), 320–324.

Clinical Practice Guideline #6. Sickle cell disease: Screening, Diagnosis, Management and Counseling in Newborns and Infants. U.S. Department of Health and Human Services. Agency for Health Care Policy and Research (AHCPR) Rockville, Maryland. Publication No. 93-0562.

Daly, A., MacDonald, A., Aukett, A., et al. (1996). Prevention of anemia in inner city toddlers by an iron supplemented cow's milk formula. *Archives of Disease in Children, 75*, 9–16.

Damshek, W., & Ebbe, S. (1963). Recurrent acute idiopathic thrombocytopenic purpura. *New England Journal of Medicine, 269*, 647.

Dinauer, M. C. (1998). The phagocytic system and disorders of granulopoiesis and granulocyte function. In D. G. Nathan & S. H. Orkin (Eds.), *Nathan and Oski's hematology of infancy and childhood* (5th ed., p. 910). Philadelphia: W. B. Saunders.

Dozy, A. M., Kan, Y. W., Embury, S. H., et al. (1979). α-Globin gene organization in blacks precludes the severe form of α-thalassemia. *Nature, 280*, 605–607.

Edwards, C. R. W., Bouchier, I. A. D., Haslet, C., & Chilvers, E. R. (1995). *Davidson's principles and practice of medicine* (17th ed.). Edinburgh: Churchill Livingstone.

Embury, S. H., Hebbel, R., Mohandas, N., & Steinberg, M. H. (1994). *Sickle cell disease: Basic principles and practice.* New York: Raven Press.

Fuchs, G. J., Farris, R. P., DeWier, M., et al. (1993). Iron status with different feeding regimens: Relevance to screening and prevention of iron deficiency. *American Journal of Clinical Nutrition, 58*, 343–348.

Honig, G. R. (1996). Hemoglobin disorders. In R. E. Behrman, R. M. Kliegman, & A. M. Arvin (Eds.), *Nelson textbook of pediatrics* (15th ed., p. 1396). Philadelphia: W. B. Saunders Company.

Hughes-Jones, N. C., & Wickramasinghe, S. N. (1991). Macrocytosis and macrocytic anemias. In N. C. Hughes-Jones & S. N. Wickramasinghe (Eds.), *Lecture notes on haematology* (5th ed., p. 88). Boston: Blackwell Scientific Publications.

Jayabose, S., Giamelli, J., Levondoglu-Tugal, O., et al. (1999). Differentiating iron deficiency anemia from thalassemia minor by using an RDW-based index. *Journal of Pediatric Hematology and Oncology, 21*(4), 314.

Jayabose, S., Tugal, O., Sandoval, C., et al., (1996). Clinical and hematologic effects of hydroxyurea in children with sickle cell anemia. *Journal of Pediatrics, 129,* 559–565.

Kark, J. A., Posey, D. M., Schumacher, H. R., & Ruehle, C. J. (1987). Sickle cell trait as a risk factor for sudden death in physical training. *New England Journal of Medicine, 317,* 781–788.

Medeiros, D., & Buchanan, G. R. (1996). Current controversies in the management of idiopathic thrombocytopenic purpura during childhood. *Pediatric Clinics of North America, 43,* 757–772.

Pearson, H. A. (1989). Sickle cell trait and competitive athletics: Is there a risk? *Pediatrics, 83,* 613–614.

Schilling, R. S. (1995). Estimating the risk for sepsis after splenectomy in hereditary spherocytosis. *Annals of Internal Medicine, 122,* 187.

Schneider, R. G., Hightower, B., Hosty, T. S., et al. (1976). Abnormal hemoglobins in a quarter million people. *Blood, 48,* 629–637.

Schwartz, E. (1996). Anemias of inadequate production. In R. E. Berman, R. M. Kliegman, & A. M. Arvin (Eds.), *Nelson textbook of pediatrics* (15th ed., p. 1387). Philadelphia: W. B. Saunders Co.

Sears, D. A. (1994). Sickle cell trait. In S. H. Embury, R. Hebbel, N. Mohandas, & M. H. Steinberg (Eds.), *Sickle cell disease: Basic priciples and practice.* New York: Raven Press.

Segal, G. R. (1996). Hereditary spherocytosis. In R. E. Behrman, R. M. Kliegman, & A. M. Arvin (Eds.), *Nelson textbook of pediatrics* (15th ed., p. 1392). Philadelphia: W. B. Saunders Company.

Storb, R., Etzioni, R., Anasetti, C., et al. (1994). Cyclophosphamide combined with antithymocyte globulin in preparation for allogeneic marrow transplants in patients with aplastic anemia. *Blood, 84,* 941–949.

Woerner, S. J., Abilgard, C. F., & French, B. N. (1981). Intracranial hemorrhage in children with idiopathic thrombocytopenic purpura. *Pediatrics, 67,* 453.

Minor Trauma

• RICHARD BACHUR, MD

LACERATIONS AND ABRASIONS

Anatomy, Physiology, and Pathology

The three layers of skin include the epidermis, dermis, and subcutaneous layer. The epidermis, which has no blood vessels, protects the dermal layer from infection and desiccation. The dermis provides the tensile strength of the skin and contains capillary blood vessels. The subcutaneous layer contains loose connective tissue, fat, and the large vessels and nerves.

The term abrasion is used for superficial defects of the skin in which the outer layers have been scraped away. The most superficial abrasions involve loss of the epidermis, leading only to transudation of serous fluid but no bleeding. Deeper abrasions into the dermis will cause bleeding. Laceration implies a cut through the skin: superficial lacerations in the epidermis will not bleed, those into the dermis will have capillary bleeding, and lacerations into the subcutaneous layer will gape open and can have substantial bleeding.

Wound healing occurs in defined stages: coagulation, inflammation, proliferation, and maturation. Coagulation occurs immediately at the time of injury. First, the platelets adhere and form plugs. Second, the extrinsic clotting system is activated, leading to fibrin deposition. Inflammation, by polymorphonuclear cell migration, occurs within hours for defense against bacteria. As a result of chemotactic factors released by platelets, monocytes migrate to the area and, over days, clean up necrotic tissue and foreign material through phagocytosis. The macrophages also stimulate proliferation of surrounding fibroblasts. Myofibroblasts apply a collagen matrix that enables wound contraction. This proliferation phase is clinically seen as beefy red granulation tissue composed of macrophages, proliferating fibroblasts, and growing capillaries. As this process heals the dermal layer, reepithelialization of the epidermal layer occurs. Fibrin deposition and reorganization takes weeks to months to complete. During that time, the wound stays erythematous as a marker of ongoing healing.

Good nutrition, including adequate amounts of protein and vitamins A and C, optimizes wound healing. Several drugs interfere with healing: aspirin inhibits the coagulation phase, steroids inhibit cellular immunity and reepithelialization, and chemotherapeutic agents affect the number and function of white blood cells.

Management

Initial Approach to Lacerations

Providers should approach all lacerations in the context of the whole patient with regard to prioritizing the evaluation of other potentially more serious injuries. They can obtain hemostasis with direct pressure using a sterile dressing. Rarely will a patient require a tourniquet. The provider should question the patient about the details of the injury (time, mechanism), any pertinent past medical history, current medications, medication allergies and prior exposures to local anesthetics, tetanus status, possibility of foreign bodies in the wound, and paresthesias or weakness.

The clinician should inspect the wound for size and depth (this often requires the removal of dry blood on the skin), the condition of the skin edges, the presence of a foreign body, and the potential involvement of underlying structures including arteries, nerves, tendons, ligaments, and bones. Accurate inspection may require local anesthesia (with or without restraint or sedation); however, the provider needs to determine neurologic function and vascular status prior to anesthetic administration. He or she needs to do probing and deep inspection under sterile conditions. Proper inspection cannot occur without hemostasis and good lighting. In cases of suspected foreign body or injury of underlying bone, the provider should obtain a radiograph. When he or she cannot close wounds immediately, the clinician should apply saline-soaked gauze to prevent retraction and desiccation of the wound edges.

The clinician should clean surrounding skin with an antiseptic solution and irrigate the wound with sterile saline under pressure. Pressure irrigation is best achieved with a ready-made irrigation device or simply by connecting a 50 cc syringe to a 20 g intravenous (IV) catheter. The minimum volume for irrigation is 200 cc; considerably more is necessary for large or dirty wounds. The clinician should wear proper eye and face protection. After irrigation, he or she must carefully explore the wound, debride the edges, and formulate a strategy for closure. The provider must avoid extensive debridement, especially in cosmetic areas. If closure will be delayed, the clinician should apply a moist dressing and keep the wound elevated.

Wound Repair

Repair of lacerations is done to reduce the risk of infection and to hasten healing. Ideally, wounds are closed within 6 hours following the injury, although providers must give individual consideration to location, likelihood of contamination, and vascular supply of the area. Clinicians can treat most lacerations without subspecialty consultation but need to consider their own level of experience, the wound's location and complexity, and the patient's need for sedation. Providers should consider consultation under the following conditions:

Potential or definite injury to nerve, tendon, ligaments, or bone
Need for conscious sedation or general anesthesia to properly repair the wound
Stellate lacerations or other complicated wounds (because of jagged or complex edges or wound tension)
Highly cosmetic injuries (eg, flaps, vermilion border of the lips, animal bites to the face)

Many small wounds can be successfully anesthetized with local, topical anesthesia such as LET (lidocaine, epinephrine, and tetracaine) or TAC (tetracaine, adrenaline, and cocaine). The latter, however, requires refrigeration and management of a controlled substance. Larger wounds require injections of lidocaine locally or a nerve block. Providers should not inject epinephrine into areas of end circulation or cartilage.

▲ **Clinical Warning:** Clinicians should not use topical anesthesia with epinephrine near mucosal surfaces or areas of end circulation or cartilage (ie, digits, tip of nose, penis, and pinna).

The mechanics of suturing are beyond the scope of this text, but a few principles can be expressed. If deep ("buried") sutures can be placed, then they should be placed. Providers should close all cavities or dead space or place a drain to avoid infection created by fluid collecting in the space. All buried sutures should be absorbable suture materials. Cutaneous closure can be either absorbable or nonabsorbable; however, absorbable sutures cannot be used for skin closure in wounds under tension (such as those over joints). If absorbable sutures are to be used for cutaneous closure, clinicians should use the fast-absorbing variety to avoid prolonged inflammation and, therefore, increased scarring. The varieties of suture and their uses are presented in Table 43-1.

Removal of Sutures

The timing of removal of nonabsorbable sutures is based on wound condition, vascularity of the region and wound, presence of tension across the wound, and cosmetic importance. Sutures are typically removed after 5 days for the face, 7 days for the scalp, 7 to 10 days for the torso, and 10 to 14 days for the extremities. Wounds over joints or under tension may require skin tapes and prolonged immobilization after suture removal. In general, infection rates and scarring at the suture entry points increase with time. Additionally, providers may need to delay suture removal under conditions of poor perfusion or high tension (although they should watch the wound carefully for infection).

Table 43-1.   SUTURE MATERIAL AND USES

Type	Comments	Typical Use/Sizes
Nonabsorbable sutures Silk and cotton	• High infection risk over other materials • Strong tissue reaction	• Securing catheters to skin
Nylon (Ethilon and Dermalon) and polypropylene (Prolene)	• Synthetic • Low infection potential • Low tissue reactivity	• Suture material of choice for most skin closures • 6-0 face • 3-0, 4-0, 5-0 scalp • 4-0, 5-0 extremities • 5-0 hand • 4-0, 5-0 trunk
Polybutester (Novafil)	• Strong as nylon or polypropylene • Low tissue reactivity • Low infection potential • Stretches under low tension; therefore has advantage in wounds that tend to swell	
Absorbable sutures Plain gut	• Tension maintained for 7 days • High tissue reactivity • High infection risk	• 4-0 or 5-0 oral cavity
Chromic gut	• Tensile strength for 2–3 weeks • High tissue reactivity • High infection potential	• 4-0 or 5-0 oral cavity
Fast absorbing gut	• Tensile strength maintained for 5–7 days • Theoretical increased infection risk; therefore to be used in clean wounds with good perfusion • Suture material of choice for cutaneous closures requiring absorbable material	• 5-0 or 6-0 face • 4-0 or 5-0 trunk (low tension areas only) • 5-0 extremities (low tension areas only)
Polyglycolic acid (Dexon) and polyglactin (Vicryl)	• Synthetic • Less tissue reactivity compared to gut • Lower infection than plain or chromic gut • Braided, therefore more "drag" when pulled through tissue • Tensile strength 20%–50% at 30 days	• Deep sutures face: 5-0 • Deep sutures scalp: 2-0, 3-0, 4-0 • Deep sutures hand: 4-0, 5-0 • Deep sutures extremities: 4-0 • Deep sutures trunk: 4-0 • Oral mucosa 6-0
Polydioxanone	• Synthetic • Less tissue reactivity compared to gut • Lower infection than plain or chromic gut • Monofilament so easier to pull through tissues • Tensile strength 50% at 4 weeks	• As polyglycolic acid or polyglactin

Alternatives to Sutures

Skin Tape

Providers can use skin tapes (Steri-Strips, Shurstrips, and Clearon) to repair superficial lacerations or to provide skin closure on a wound approximated with deep sutures. Tape is not useful in areas under tension (eg, over joints), areas likely to get wet, or in young children who are more likely to remove them. Clinicians should use tape only after they have cleaned and explored the wound and the edges are dry. The tape will not adhere to moist skin. Applying benzoin can markedly approve its adherence. Providers must instruct parents to keep the wound dry and to allow the tape to self-detach.

Skin Staples

Staples are readily available in disposable units and are particularly good for small scalp lacerations. Providers can place staples much more rapidly than they can sutures. Certainly, staples require less equipment than sutures. Placement of staples can often be done with local, topical anesthesia. Because of the potential of scarring, providers should not apply staples to the face.

Tissue Adhesives

Adhesives have recently become available and are as good as sutures in small, simple, clean lacerations (Bruns, 1996). Adhesives are not only faster but also less painful. Evaluation and cleaning of the wound is still very important; therefore, the patient may still require local anesthesia for proper cleaning even if he or she does not need it for wound closure. Because it is fast drying, application around the eye and mouth must be done carefully. Clinicians should carefully read recommendations related to use, including time of drying, number of layers, avoidance of drips, and follow-up care. The manufacturer also offers techniques to undo mistakes. Providers should contact an ophthalmologist for eye exposures.

Follow-up Care

Following initial management of the wound, the provider must give the patient instructions related to wound care, dressing changes, follow-up (eg, suture removal), and reasons to return. In general, dressings should be changed daily unless otherwise specified by the person who cared for the wound. For small wounds, dressings may be unnecessary, or parents can simply apply a smear of antibiotic ointment. Larger wounds require a non-adherent dressing (Xeroform, Adaptic) against the wound, a layer of gauze to "sponge away" any drainage, and an outer wrap to guard against dirt and to secure the dressing.

● **Clinical Pearl:** Prophylactic antibiotics are not part of routine wound management but may be indicated in certain situations such as dirty wounds, wounds older than 12 hours prior to repair, punctures, bite wounds, exposure of bone, involvement of tendon sheaths, or host factors such as poor circulation or immunodeficiency.

BURNS

Most burns in pediatric patients occur at home and are accidental but preventable. Children younger than age 4 years are at greatest risk because of their curiosity and mobility. Only 3% to 5% of burns are life threatening (often secondary to house fires). Eighty percent are minor burns secondary to scalds.

Burn prevention is as important as the wearing of seatbelts and bike helmets. Simple interventions such as decreasing the temperature of water heaters to 120°F, installing smoke detectors and sprinklers, using flame retardant upholstery, and conducting anti-smoking campaigns can have a huge impact on public safety.

Children with burns may present directly to an emergency room or medical office. As described in the following section, providers can care for most minor burns in the office.

Pathology

The skin acts as a barrier to infection, regulates water loss and temperature, and provides sensory information. The outer, non-living layer is termed the epidermis, and the undersurface is termed the dermis. The dermis includes blood vessels, nerves, hair follicles, secretory glands, and sweat glands, all of which are necessary for repair of damaged skin.

History and Physical Exam

Superficial burns (first-degree) affect only the epidermis; typically, redness and pain are the only signs (sunburns are the most common example). They heal in 3 to 5 days with or without peeling. Partial-thickness or second-degree burns extend into the dermis. Superficial second-degree burns involve the epidermis and up to half of the dermis. Increased capillary permeability leads to a moist appearance, often with blister formation and edema. Healing occurs in about 2 weeks, and scarring is minimal. Deep second-degree burns extend through most of the dermis. They tend to be paler and drier compared to more superficial burns. Thrombosed blood vessels may give a speckled appearance to the skin. Pain may be less than with superficial burns secondary to injury to nerves. Healing may take weeks to months with risk of hypertrophic scars. Full-thickness or third-degree burns involve destruction of the epidermis and entire dermis. The burn may have a pale or charred color and a "leathery" appearance. Destruction of nerves in the dermis makes the area anesthetic. The edges may not be full-thickness and therefore may be a source of pain. With all the dermal elements gone, the skin cannot regenerate except at the edges. These burns often require skin grafting. Burns may be considered fourth-degree with the involvement of fascia, muscle, or bone.

The severity of the burn depends on the burn source (eg, radiation, thermal, chemical, electrical), the size of the burn area relative to the body size [percent body surface area (BSA)], the depth, and the location. The "rule of 9s" estimates the body surface area in adults: head and neck (9%), anterior trunk (18%), posterior trunk (18%), each leg (18%), each arm (9%), and anorectal area (1%). In children, the head is larger relative to the body and changes by age; therefore, providers cannot use simple rules (see Figure 43-1). In general, the size of a child's palm is roughly equivalent to 1% BSA.

Minor burns are defined as all first-degree burns, second-degree burns that cover less than 10% BSA in children younger than age 6 years, and second-degree burns that cover less than 15% BSA in older children and adults. Exceptions are burns that may cause loss of function or deformity (eg, burns over joints or circumferential burns), pose an infection risk, or involve the face, hands, feet, or perineum.

Moderate burns involve 10% to 20% BSA if second-degree and 2% to 10% if third-degree. Burns are classified as major

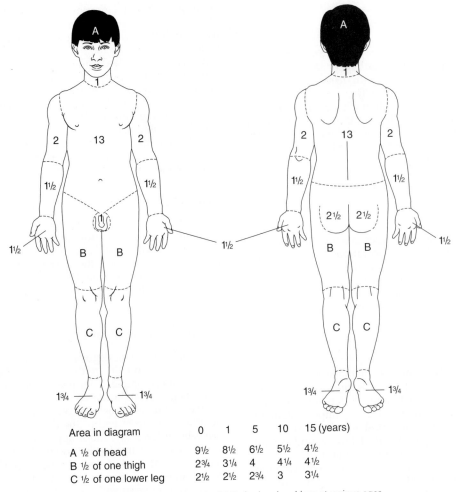

Area in diagram	0	1	5	10	15 (years)
A ½ of head	9½	8½	6½	5½	4½
B ½ of one thigh	2¾	3¼	4	4¼	4½
C ½ of one lower leg	2½	2½	2¾	3	3¼

Figure 43–1 ■ Percentage of BSA for head and legs at various ages.

if second-degree and involving greater than 20% BSA, third-degree and involving greater than 10% BSA, or second- or third-degree and circumferential or crossing flexor creases. Additionally, burns are considered major when associated with the following: inhalational injury, electrical burn (see below), fractures or other major trauma, in patients with significant pre-existing medical conditions, or with suspected child abuse.

Management

Providers can manage all minor burns on an outpatient basis. Moderate burns often require hospitalization and consultation with a burn specialist. The decision to hospitalize is determined by the need for IV fluid therapy, pain control, need for close observation, or suspicious circumstances. Second-degree burns covering more than 10% BSA in an infant or 20% BSA in a child may require IV fluids to prevent dehydration. A specialist (eg, plastic surgeon) should manage all full-thickness burns and partial-thickness burns that are circumferential, cross joints, or involve the face, perineum, hands, or feet.

Initial Management of Minor and Moderate Burns

First-degree burns do not need special attention other than pain control with over-the-counter pain relievers (topical

and oral). For partial-thickness and full-thickness burns, providers must prepare the wounds. They should remove clothing from the area. Initial care involves gentle irrigation with cool saline for pain control and to remove any dirt, debris, and dead skin. Clinicians must irrigate chemical burns extensively (they can place a small child in a sink or tub for this purpose). Pain control with narcotics may be necessary for adequate care. Providers also may use topical anesthetics such as viscous lidocaine for small burns (use in large burns can lead to toxicity). They can debride loose and necrotic skin, including flaccid blisters, with a forceps and scissors. Gentle wiping with saline-soaked gauze is quite effective for removing non-viable tissue. Providers should leave eschars, seen with deep partial-thickness and full-thickness burns, undisturbed. They should not try to remove any tar from wounds at the initial visit. They should leave blisters intact if fresh (less than 2 hours old). Large blisters (> 5 cm), flaccid or ruptured blisters, and any size blister crossing a joint are best debrided during the initial care. After debridement and irrigation, the provider should pat the wound dry with gauze.

Providers can manage burns in several different ways. The open method basically allows the burn to be its own dressing—whether it has a blister or eschar. A topical antibacterial ointment is applied to the open wound several times per day. Because children cannot be trusted to keep wounds clean, the open method is rarely used except in very small burns or in areas that are difficult to dress, such as the face. The closed method of care applies gauze dressing after the wound is prepared. Antibacterial cream, such as silver sulfadiazine (avoid if sulfa allergy, G6PD) or bacitracin/polymixin B, is applied to the thickness of a tongue blade then covered with gauze sponges loosely held by tape or some form of wrap. Alternatively, the antibacterial cream may be applied first to the gauze. For burns of the hands and feet, gauze may be placed between the digits, avoiding skin-skin contact.

Follow-up Care for Minor and Moderate Burns

After 24 hours, the provider should reinspect and further debride the burn as necessary. Thereafter, dressing changes should be once or twice daily; depending on the wound and the caregiver's abilities, these may be done at home with less frequent office visits. The frequency of follow-up visits will depend upon the extent of the burn, the need for ongoing debridement, and the ability, reliability, and comfort level of the primary caregiver. All caregivers must be vigilant for signs of infection that would necessitate aggressive treatment to avoid further complications and scarring. The deeper the wound, the more likely superinfection will occur. Standard tetanus prophylaxis is necessary with all second- and third-degree burns. Empiric antibiotics should not be used.

Management of Major Burns

For major burns, the patient should be managed in an emergency department and, immediately after stabilization, be referred to a pediatric burn center. Acute management must focus on the following complications:

   Direct smoke inhalation of particulate matter, toxins, and hot gases can cause airway inflammation and injury leading to compromise of upper and lower airways.
   Carbon monoxide poisoning should be suspected in all cases associated with enclosed fires or evidence of smoke inhalation.
   Dehydration and shock are possible from fluid losses through the burned skin.
   Renal failure is possible from myoglobinuria and dehydration.
   Risk of superinfection and sepsis is possible.
   Providers must give special attention to minimizing heat loss (exposure, cold IV fluids, wet dressings), providing sterile dressings, and adequately treating pain. Suspected carbon monoxide poisoning should be treated with maximal supplemental O_2, and any signs of respiratory distress may prompt early endotracheal intubation. Aggressive fluid resuscitation and monitoring are paramount.

Chemical Burns

Many household chemicals can cause burns. Acid burns tend to coagulate skin proteins, which in turn limit the depth, while alkali burns liquefy the skin and tend to penetrate deeper. Chemicals tend to cause burning for longer than thermal burns because the process continues until adequate neutralization or washing occurs, whereas thermal burns tend to be brief exposures or cool quickly. The burn may initially appear superficial despite deeper tissue destruction.

   Treatment of chemical burns (both acid and alkali) involves copious irrigation. Providers must protect surrounding normal skin and sensitive structures such as the eyes and mucosal membranes as they wash away the chemical. They should avoid attempts at neutralization unless

given specific instructions by a burn specialist. Providers can monitor the pH of the runoff to determine when to stop. Referral to an ophthalmologist for chemical burns of the eye is necessary after irrigation has begun.

Electrical Burns

Burns from electricity have some unusual characteristics. Most burns involve young children exposed to electrical appliances, damaged electrical cords, and electrical sockets. The thermal energy released depends on the tissue resistance, the voltage and type of current, and the duration of the exposure. For the scope of this text, only burns associated with low-voltage current will be discussed. Because electricity tends to find the path of least resistance, the current will typically follow blood vessels, nerves, and muscles, not skin. Therefore, "entrance wounds" may be less impressive, but clinicians must be suspicious for deep tissue injury.

   Although burns may occur from arcing of electricity instead of current literally passing through the body, the provider should thoroughly inspect the patient for exit wounds. For small fingertip injuries from household current, no additional testing need be done. If the history suggests prolonged contact, initial alteration in consciousness, or proximal pain or swelling, the provider should treat the burn as a major burn. For significant electrical burns, the provider should perform cardiac monitoring and an ECG for evidence of dysrhythmias. Elevated creatinine kinase or myoglobinuria suggest evidence of underlying muscle injury. In such cases, patients are admitted for monitoring, IV hydration, and alkalization (the latter if at risk for renal failure). A specific electrical injury to the lips occurs when a toddler bites an electrical cord. Providers should refer these burns to a specialist to minimize scarring and contracture. Bleeding from the labial artery 5 to 14 days after the injury may result in significant blood loss.

Inflicted Burns

Overall, approximately 10% of burns are inflicted, most of which are scalds. When an individual forcibly submerges a child's hands or feet into hot water, the burns tend to be deep with clear lines of demarcation and symmetric involvement of both extremities. Similarly, scald burns of the buttocks and posterior thighs can result from forcible submersion. Clinicians should carefully note the characteristics of the edges and splash marks to determine if the burn pattern fits the history. Small deep burns from cigarettes and distinctive patterns from heaters and irons should raise concern for abuse. The distinctive pattern of symmetrical depth (perfectly flat contact with a solid object) or multiple burns is not typical of accidents.

HEAD TRAUMA

Head trauma is the leading cause of morbidity in children older than age 1 year (Frankowski, 1985). Each year in the United States, 250,000 children younger than age 14 years are hospitalized and 25,000 die or are permanently disabled from head trauma (Kraus, 1990). Males suffer head injuries twice as often as females and have a fourfold increase in fatal head injury (Kraus, 1990; Frankowski, 1985). Interestingly, males have an increasing rate of head trauma from ages 5 to 25 years, whereas females have a steady decline throughout the first 15 years of life.

   The mechanism of head injury differs by age (Kraus, 1990). In infants and toddlers, head injury results from falls from furniture or from a caregiver's arms. In preschoolers, falls are still the major source of head injury, although motor vehicle collisions account for 25% of cases. In school-age children, falls, sports, and motor vehicles (sustained as a passenger, pedestrian, or bicyclist) equally account for head injuries. In adolescents, sports and motor vehicle accidents cause equal numbers of head injuries.

Anatomy, Physiology, and Pathology

The galea aponeurotics and the scalp cover the cranium. The galea is adherent to the scalp but only loosely connected to the cranium except at the margins. Inside the cranium, the dura is a fibrous membrane attached to the skull. Under the dura is the arachnoid. Finally the pia covers the brain. The space between the arachnoid and pia contains the cerebrospinal fluid.

The following factors make head injury common in pediatrics:

Poor judgement related to play activities and lack of safety with bicycles and crossing streets

Unfortunate dependence on adult supervision for seatbelt and helmet use

Relatively large head in proportion to the body, which makes head trauma likely during any form of injury

Brain injury can be divided into primary and secondary. Primary injury occurs from direct trauma to the brain either as a penetrating injury or by acceleration/deceleration injuries (as might occur with blunt trauma). Penetrating injury tends to produce focal injury, while acceleration/deceleration tends to produce a more diffuse injury. Blunt trauma occurs much more frequently than penetrating injuries in children. Secondary brain injury occurs from hypoventilation, hypoperfusion, or hypoxia either after isolated head injury or injury to other organ systems. The brain that has primary injury is much more susceptible to secondary injury.

The following is a classification of the different types of head injury:

Subgaleal hematoma. This represents bleeding beneath the galea aponeurotics. Because of the loose connection to the skull, blood loss in this space can be dramatic. Seemingly minor injuries, such as a tug on the hair, can cause dramatic bleeding. Despite the potential for large bleeds, complications such as orbital extension are rare.

Caput succedaneum. Scalp edema due to local pressure or suction may occur during labor and delivery. It is easily differentiated from cephalohematoma because the swelling is diffuse and not limited by the sutures.

Cephalohematoma. This is hemorrhage into the periosteum of the skull and therefore demarcated by the sutures. This finding is common in newborns from birth trauma.

Skull fractures. Skull fractures may present as focal swelling of the scalp, as a depression or crepitus to palpation, or on radiologic imaging of the brain following trauma. Fractures can be described as linear, depressed, or compound (ie, having multiple fragments). Basilar skull fractures should be considered in patients with epistaxis, hemotympanum, CSF rhinorrhea or otorrhea, or hemorrhage into the periorbital area (raccoon sign), postauricular skin (Battle's sign), mastoid air cells (as seen on CT scan), or nasopharynx.

Concussion. This is the most minor brain injury that has a clinical definition based on some alteration in brain functioning or mental status. Examples are loss of consciousness, amnesia, and sleepiness. The definition implies no gross structural injury to the brain. Patients do not need to have loss of consciousness at the time of the trauma, but often have retrograde amnesia for events recent to and antegrade amnesia for hours to days following the injury. Patients may appear alert or have somnolence for one to two days. Higher cognitive functions that require mental concentration may be the sole disability.

Contusion. Cerebral contusion is equivalent to a bruise of the brain and often results from blunt trauma. The contusion can be termed "coup" if immediately adjacent to the site of impact or "contracoup" if opposite the site of injury. CT scan is used to diagnose contusions. Patients with contusions may present with altered consciousness, persistent vomiting or headache (or irritability in an infant), or focal neurologic findings or seizures.

Subdural hematoma. As implied by the name, hemorrhage occurs between the dura and arachnoid membranes. Direct blunt trauma or shaking injuries result in tearing of the cortical veins. Skull fractures are found in a minority of cases. Often there is associated brain injury underlying the hemorrhage. Acute subdural hemorrhage can present as seizures or signs of increased intracranial pressure or simply as vomiting or headache.

Epidural hematoma. Bleeding occurs between the dura and the skull. Epidural hematomas are often associated with overlying skull fracture. Classically, the middle meningeal artery is lacerated, leading to a rapid deterioration of the patient after a "lucid interval" following the head injury. Epidural hematomas, however, also can be of venous origin, with a much more gradual deterioration, or present simply has headache, vomiting, or somnolence after a head injury.

Diffuse axonal injury. This refers to non-hemorrhagic brain injury with acute and diffuse brain swelling. These patients may present with coma or initially focal findings that progress to global neurologic deterioration over the following 18 to 48 hours, coinciding with peak intracranial pressure. Brain involvement often is extensive; therefore, prognosis generally is poor.

History and Physical Exam

Head injury can vary from simple laceration of the scalp to penetrating injury of the brain. The patient may present with any of the following findings alone or in combination: headache, dizziness, altered mental status (confused, somnolent, combative, irritable), or unconsciousness (coma or postictal state from seizure). Usually the presentation relates to the mechanism of injury; however, exact mechanisms are not always known. The head injury may appear to be isolated, but the mechanism of injury should dictate whether the provider needs to consider injuries to the cervical spine or other body areas. The patient with a minor head injury from a motor vehicle collision might have altered mental status from shock. Hopefully, patients with major mechanisms of injury will not present to the office or clinic setting. In such a circumstance, rapid triage to identify signs of significant injury should redirect the patient to an emergency department.

Important historical questions can provide an impression of the likelihood for brain injury (see Table 43-2). The provider should note the child's behavior immediately antecedent to the accident: is it possible the child first had a seizure and then fell off the bike? When the mechanism is unclear or seemingly inappropriate for the injury, the clinician must consider child abuse. Specific features in the history may raise suspicion of abuse: unexplained injury, discrepancy of the history between caregivers, mechanism of injury inconsistent with the injury or the developmental stage of the child, a delay in seeking medical care, or the presence of other injuries.

For patients who are unconscious or severely impaired, attention to airway, breathing, and circulation has priority. Patients who present with major alterations in consciousness after head injury require immediate transport to an emergency room after cervical spine immobilization. Medical personnel always must accompany the patient because of the potential for aspiration, airway obstruction in an unconscious state, and seizure. Providers always must consider other causes of altered mental status besides head injury (see Display 43-1).

For the more common scenario of a seemingly minor head injury, key historical points include the time of the injury; the behavior of the child since the injury; the presence of vomiting, somnolence, irritability (in the young child), or headache (in the older child); and disturbance of vision, speech, or gait.

● **Clinical Pearl:** On physical exam, the provider should assess overall alertness and appropriateness from across the room, before "bothering" an already frightened and stressed parent and child.

The provider should carefully inspect the scalp for abrasions, lacerations, and swellings. He or she should palpate the skull for bony "step-offs" that represent a depression of the skull. Hemorrhage can occur in the subgaleal space, making the swelling rapid and extensive. The clinician should examine the ears and nose for evidence of blood

---

DISPLAY 43–1 • Differential Diagnosis of Altered Mental Status

Central nervous system
Trauma
    Intracranial bleed
    Diffuse axonal injury
    Concussion
Hydrocephalus
Seizure
Stroke
Tumor

Cardiovascular
Arrhythmia
Shock

Metabolic
Hyponatremia
Hypoglycemia
Diabetic Ketoacidosis
Hyperammonemia
Severe metabolic acidosis
Uremia

Toxin/ingestion

Gastrointestinal
Intestinal catastrophe
Intussusception
Liver failure

(hemotympanum or in the external canal) or cerebrospinal fluid, both of which are associated with basilar skull fractures. He or she should note extraocular motions, pupil reactivity, symmetry, and fundoscopic exam in the older child. Ecchymoses under the eyes (raccoon eyes) or post-auricular (Battle's sign) are also signs of basilar skull fracture. A bulging fontanelle or separated sutures in a young infant may suggest increased intracranial pressure. Neck tenderness or decreased active range of motion may suggest a cervical spine injury. The provider should perform a careful neurologic examination as well as a general examination for other injuries.

Management

Management of severe head injuries (as defined by mechanism of injury, neurologic impairment, or both) is beyond the scope of this text. As stated earlier, such patients need rapid transport to an emergency department for stabilization and evaluation by a neurosurgeon. For patients with a minor or moderate head injury, the clinician needs to determine the likelihood for intracranial injury.

▲ **Clinical Warning:** The clinician should refer any patient with any neurological abnormalities including alterations in consciousness for head CT.

Providers should give special consideration to other coexisting injuries (such as cervical spine) in these patients. Patients with a penetrating injury (or potentially penetrating injury), a prolonged loss of consciousness (> 30 seconds), a full fontanel, obvious skull fracture, persistent vomiting, or progressive headache should also have a CT scan regardless of the neurologic examination. Clinicians should also have a lower threshold to obtain a CT on children younger than age

---

Table 43–2. ELEMENTS OF THE HISTORY IMPORTANT TO THE PATIENT WITH A HEAD INJURY

Type of Injury	Questions to Ask
All head injuries	Mechanism? (other injuries?) Somnolence? Any loss of consciousness? Any alteration in mental status? (dazed, somnolence, confused, inappropriately quiet) Seizure activity? Vomiting? Neck pain? Alteration in gait? Alteration in speech? Visual changes?
Falls	Height of fall? Impacting surface? Directly on head? Did caregiver fall on top of patient?
Pedestrian or bicycle (struck by car)	Speed of car? Damage to bumper? Was patient thrown by impact? Wearing a helmet?
Motor vehicle (passenger)	Restrained? How? Damage to car? Damage to interior? Windshield? Airbag? Were other occupants injured?
Direct blow	Mechanism (eg, ball, fist, bookcase)? Vector of force?

2 years with head injury and any symptoms. This age group is harder to assess and can be minimally symptomatic, even with significant intracranial injury.

● **Clinical Pearl:** Skull films have very limited utility: they only reveal fractures of the skull and offer no information about intracranial injury. In children, linear skull fractures have no prognostic significance.

Since depressed, compound, or basilar fractures are usually associated with either characteristic physical exam findings or neurological abnormalities, which would lead to a CT anyway, skull x-rays tend to be vastly overused. Skull films, however, have the advantage of being readily available and do not require sedation. A reasonable scheme may be to use skull films in infants younger than age 3 months with scalp findings who appear normal neurologically. If a fracture is detected, a CT scan can be performed to detect any associated intracranial injury.

Patients with neurologic impairment or any intracranial injury need neurosurgical evaluation. All patients with intracranial injury need hospitalization. For patients who have a normal CT scan but persistent vomiting, severe headache, or depressed mental status, hospitalization may be warranted for further observation and frequent neurologic evaluations. Patients who have a normal CT scan and are minimally symptomatic can be observed at home with strict discharge instructions regarding neurologic checks and reasons to return. Symptomatic infants younger than age 1 year and all infants younger than age 3 months with a skull fracture need admission for at least 24 hours. Patients with a suspicious history should be observed until the social situation is evaluated.

● **Clinical Pearl:** Patients with minor mechanisms of injury who did not sustain a loss of consciousness and who remain alert with a normal neurologic examination can be observed without any imaging.

Although evidence to support this practice is lacking, observation for 3 or more hours after the injury could be done in a medical setting. Thereafter, home observation can be safely done after the caregivers receive explicit instructions regarding reasons to seek care: persistent vomiting, progressive headache, increasing somnolence, or alterations in vision, gait, or speech.

Children frequently vomit even after relatively mild head injuries. One to two episodes of vomiting by itself, in an otherwise perfectly normal older child, should not prompt the need for imaging or admission. An algorithm describing the management of blunt head trauma in children is provided in Figure 43-2.

EYE INJURIES

History and Physical Exam

The provider should first ascertain the time and mechanism of injury. For penetrating injuries, the material, trajectory, and velocity can be important. Clinicians should ask about visual changes, foreign-body sensation, diplopia, pain, and photophobia.

Providers should carefully inspect the lids and surrounding orbit first. When inspecting the eye, they should note the sclera when testing extraocular motions. They should note

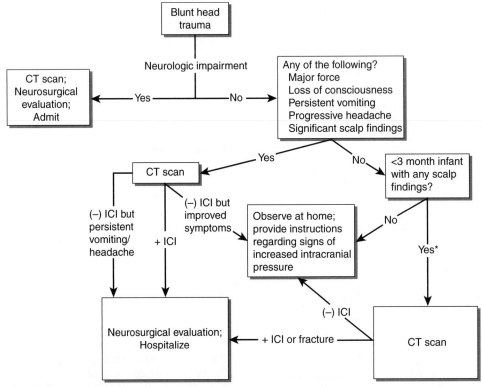

ICI = intracranial injury

*Skull films may be used at this step, and if a fracture is indentified, a CT scan should be performed.

Figure 43–2 ■ Management of blunt head trauma.

the size, symmetry, and reactivity of the pupil. Next, they should note the clarity of the cornea and anterior chamber, and examine the fundi for papilledema or vitreous or retinal hemorrhage. They may use fluoroscein staining to diagnose corneal or conjuctival abrasions, burns, or embedded foreign bodies. Clinicians should try to assess visual acuity in an age-appropriate manner. For patients who cannot open their eyelids secondary to pain, topical anesthetic may be necessary for adequate examination. Patients with a foreign-body sensation or those found to have multiple corneal abrasions need examination of the conjuctival surface of both the upper and lower lids due to the possibility of an imbedded foreign body and the potential for further corneal injury.

Subconjunctival Hemorrhage

Subconjuctival hemorrhage appears as a blood spot on the sclera and is relatively common after eye trauma or increased venous pressure associated with forceful coughing or vomiting. No therapy is required other than excluding other associated injury by examination. Circumferential subconjunctival hemorrhage after blunt trauma needs ophthalmology consultation to rule out posterior rupture of the globe.

Traumatic Iritis or Mydriasis

Following blunt injury to the eye, the patient may develop a traumatic iritis with symptoms of pain and photophobia. On examination, the pupil may be decreased in size with evidence of protein and cells in the anterior chamber (by slit-lamp examination). Administration of a topical mydriatic agent can give pain relief. The clinician should patch the eye and refer the patient to an ophthalmologist.

In traumatic mydriasis, the sphincter muscle has been injured, causing the pupil to be irregular, oval, dilated, and unresponsive. The provider should patch the eye and refer the child to an ophthalmologist.

Hyphema

Hyphema is blood in the anterior chamber. Initially, the only sign may be decreased clarity of the anterior chamber; as the blood settles over time, a blood/fluid level may appear. Providers should investigate associated injuries, such as scleral laceration. Major complications include ophthalmitis, glaucoma, and development of synechiae. Initial treatment includes mydriatics, elevation of the head 20 to 30 degrees, patching, rest, and immediate referral to an ophthalmologist.

Abrasions and Foreign Bodies

Corneal abrasions result in pain, photophobia, and tearing. On examination, the conjunctiva is injected, and the abrasion will be evident as a lesion of increased uptake with fluoroscein dye. The clinician should apply antibiotic ointment or drops. Controversy exists over the benefit of patching the eye. Most ophthalmologists now recommend against it, though it may provide comfort when pain is severe.

▲ **Clinical Warning:** Providers should never patch the eye when corneal injuries are associated with contact lenses.

If all symptoms disappear in 24 hours, the patient need not have specific follow-up but should continue using the topical antibiotic three times a day for 3 days. If the patient has any symptoms after 24 hours or if the abrasion was large or in the line of vision, the provider should reevaluate the patient for improvement. Patients should not wear contact lenses for a week. Although topical anesthetics provide dramatic relief and may be used to facilitate the examination, they should not be used in the outpatient setting secondary to toxicity to the corneal epithelium. An ophthalmologist should see any patient who lacks improvement after 48 hours.

Conjuctival and corneal foreign bodies are irritating, causing erythema and tearing. The patient's natural tendency to rub the eye may lead to corneal and conjunctival abrasions. Attempts to visualize the foreign body can be aided by the patient's localization of the foreign body, examination of the eyes with the lids inverted, and topical anesthetics. The disadvantages of topical anesthetics are the inability of the patient to feel if the foreign body is still present and the potential for abrasions, as the patient has no further apprehension about blinking or moving the eye. Most foreign bodies can be removed by rolling a cotton-tipped applicator on the eye surface. Embedded foreign bodies should be removed by someone skilled in removal techniques.

Chemical Burns

Providers should treat chemical injuries with immediate copious irrigation with normal saline (2 liters for 20 minutes). Alkali injuries tend to be more severe than acid burns. If both eyes are involved, clinicians should perform simultaneous irrigation rather than waiting to complete one eye. Once the eye has been fully irrigated, the provider should direct some irrigant under the upper lid. He or she can use a pH strip to assess the success of the irrigation (normal 6.5–7.5). The provider should consult an ophthalmologist during irrigation for any serious exposures. In cases of minor exposure to non-alkaline or weak acids in which the eyes are not injected, the clinician may defer consultation with an ophthalmologist. An ophthalmologist should immediately see any patient with opacification of the cornea or any ulceration.

Penetrating Injuries

Penetrating injuries must be considered when a patient suddenly exhibits eye pain after striking a rock or metal with a hammer or similar forceful collisions. Radiographs may reveal the object within the eye even when signs of trauma are not visible. Providers also should suspect penetration if the anterior chamber is shallow (iris is bowed toward the cornea), the pupil is distorted, or swelling of the conjunctiva is prominent. An ophthalmologist should see all suspected or obvious penetrating injuries immediately.

Orbital Trauma

Blunt trauma to the orbit can lead to orbital fractures. Palpation of the orbital rim for crepitis or a step-off can signal a fracture. Providers should obtain radiographs when they first suspect a fracture. They must consider co-existing injury to the eye. Blowout fractures of the orbit occur when an object larger than the orbit, such as a tennis ball or fist, strikes the eye. The sudden rise in orbital pressure leads to a fracture of the orbital floor (the roof of the maxillary sinus) or the nasal wall of the orbit into the ethmoid sinus. In such cases, enophthalmos and decreased sensation inferior to the orbit (infraorbital nerve) may be noted. Entrapment of the inferior rectus may lead to diplopia or limitation of upward gaze. An ophthalmologist, otorhinolaryngologist, or both should see any patient with orbital fractures.

NOSE INJURIES

Epistaxis

Local pressure usually can control epistaxis following nasal trauma. In more severe cases, providers can use topical vasoconstrictors or nasal packing. An otorhinolaryngologist (ORL surgeon) should see patients who may have posterior bleeding or history of bleeding diathesis.

Nasal Fractures and Septal Hematoma

Bruising and swelling over the bridge of the nose along with minor epistaxis is typical of nasal fractures. Providers also should consider associated injuries to the sinuses and orbit. Displacement or depression is often difficult to assess with significant swelling. Observing whether the nares are symmetrical may aid in assessing displacement.

▲ **Clinical Warning:** If deviation or depression is clinically evident, referral to an otorhinolaryngologist is necessary, since a displaced fracture is best treated in the first week after injury before fibrous connection stabilizes it.

● **Clinical Pearl:** Since a child's nose is primarily composed of cartilage, radiographs are very unreliable in the evaluation of nasal injuries and should not be obtained for routine management of suspected nasal fractures.

When swelling is present, repeat examination after the swelling subsides (3 days) should allow recognition of displacement or bony irregularity.

The provider always should examine the patient for a septal hematoma that presents as a soft, fluctuant mass protruding from the septum (unilateral or bilateral) and often blocking the nasal passage. Septal hematomas can be associated with necrosis and infection with resultant nasal deformity; therefore, providers should refer any cases to an ORL surgeon immediately for hematoma evacuation. Antibiotics (such as amoxicillin) are generally prescribed to prevent infectious complications of the invariably open fracture (open into the nasal cavity).

Foreign Body in the Nose

Foreign bodies of the nose present in two common ways: first is the parental report of insertion, and second is the presence of a unilateral, persistent, foul-smelling nasal discharge. Less common presentations include halitosis, chronic sinusitis, or epistaxis.

Adequate visualization is mandatory. Blind attempts with instruments rarely succeed. Visualization requires a strong light source and a nasal specula (either preformed plastic or adjustable). Useful equipment includes a right angle, alligator forceps and a rigid suction (eg, Yankauer). Use of a vasoconstrictor such as neosynephrine may improve visualization. Patients may require anesthesia in the form of topical preparations (ie, cocaine, lidocaine) and sedation; providers should consider anesthesia when a child is anxious or when the foreign body will be difficult to retrieve. Young children should be placed in a restraint device. Maximizing the environment and good preparation will limit initial failures that only make subsequent attempts more difficult.

The best technique depends on the location and type of foreign body. The right angle is useful for hard, round objects; the "hook" is simply placed behind the object and pulled out slowly. Providers always should insert instruments perpendicular to the plane of the face (straight in, not parallel to nasal bone) to avoid damage to the turbinates. The area superior and medial to the middle turbinate is in close proximity to the cribiform plate; therefore, clinicians should avoid instrumenting the medial wall. Providers may grasp soft objects with the forceps. Techniques employing "super glue" and Fogarty balloon catheters have been described but are not recommended. For shallow foreign bodies, the provider may instruct the patient to cover the opposite nostril and blow the nose; alternatively, he or she may apply a suction catheter. If after attempted removal significant bleeding occurs, the clinician can administer neosynephrine and apply pressure. The provider should never intentionally push the foreign body deeper because of the risk of aspiration. If the object appears to be going deeper or is impossible to reach, the clinician should refer the patient to an otolaryngologist for possible removal under anesthesia. After successful removal, providers should advise parents to return if there are any signs of a retained foreign body such as purulent discharge or epistaxis.

EAR TRAUMA

Pinna Hematoma

Hematoma of the pinna usually results from direct trauma and presents as a fluctuant swelling. Because pressure on the cartilage can cause ischemic necrosis, providers must evacuate hematomas. They can aspirate a fresh hematoma with a large bore needle, but older lesions (>24 hours) will require excision by a skilled surgeon. Providers need to apply a firm dressing to prevent reaccumulation of the hematoma.

External Canal Trauma

Trauma to the external canal from a child poking an object into the ear or suddenly moving while the parent is cleaning the ear is quite common. No specific therapy is needed to help the scratch heal, although the provider should assess the integrity of the tympanic membrane (visually or via tympanometry). Clinicians can treat large lacerations or those associated with considerable swelling with otic drops (neomycin, polymixin, and hydrocortisone). If the eardrum is not intact, providers should administer topical quinalones to avoid the potential of neomycin-induced ototoxicity.

Perforated Tympanic Membrane

Causes of acute traumatic perforation include a direct blow to the ear (even with an open hand), a nearby explosion, sudden change in pressure, or direct trauma as may occur while trying to clean the external canal. Providers should suspect dislocation or fracture of the middle ear ossicles in children who present with vertigo or hearing loss. An otorhinolaryngologist may need to see patients with vestibular symptoms or hearing loss. All others can be treated with analgesics. If the ear is draining, providers may prescribe topical quinalone otic drops for 10 days. Most perforations heal completely in 3 to 4 weeks, and this should be documented by the use of tympanometry. An ORL surgeon should examine perforations that do not heal within this time.

Foreign Body in the External Canal

Foreign bodies in the external ear canal are common. They often lodge at the narrow cartilage—bony junction of the canal. Unfortunately, the skin of the canal is thin and exquisitely sensitive. When a foreign body is large or mobile (such as a live insect), the patient may complain of excruciating pain. More often, patients are asymptomatic, and foreign bodies are only discovered on routine examination. Occasionally a child presents with decreased hearing.

Many techniques for foreign body removal have been described. The most common and universally accepted technique is to use alligator forceps under direct visualization with an operating head otoscope or a "miners cap" with direct lighting and magnifying lenses. Pulling the pinna superiorly and laterally will maximize visualization and provide the straightest route for extraction. For round smooth objects, the provider can pass a curette with a curved end behind the object. Blind attempts often will push the object in deeper. Proper patient position and restraint are paramount. A wrapped sheet and a papoose board are the best restraints for young children. In cases in which a live insect will not allow a child to calm down, mineral oil instilled in the ear will kill the insect prior to removal.

Another technique is irrigation, which works well for non-vegetable materials (which could swell) that the provider cannot reach with forceps. Irrigation is well tolerated, especially if the water is warmed to body temperature. Irrigation is best accomplished with 1.5 inch tubing of a butterfly needle (proximal end so hub can attach to syringe) or with a 20 gauge IV catheter attached to a 25 cc syringe. The clinician should direct the stream around the object and position the child such that gravity will help drainage during the procedure. In settings where suction is available, providers can use soft-tipped suction catheters to remove foreign bodies.

Providers should use tympanometry or pneumatic otoscopy to document an intact tympanic membrane after the procedure. They should prescribe a topical antibiotic/corticosteroid such as Cortisporin otic suspension for 3 to 5 days.

Acknowledging the fact that foreign body removal is difficult, 20% of cases require referral. If the provider cannot remove the foreign body after several attempts, he or she should refer the child to an otorhinolaryngologist who may have to perform removal under anesthesia.

DENTAL TRAUMA

When examining the teeth for injury or displacement, it is important to distinguish between a primary exfoliated tooth and a traumatic injury. See Table 43-3 for normal time of eruption and shedding. Clinicians must inspect in all four quadrants for missing, chipped, displaced, or fractured teeth. A socket with a clot or persistent or active bleeding is typical of traumatic injury. Exposed dentin appears yellow, and exposed pulp looks red. Bleeding from the tooth rather than the gum is a sign of pulp exposure. A cool or cold sensation when taking a fast inhalation is also a sign of pulp exposure. Involved parties should try their best to locate all missing teeth or pieces of a tooth; providers should palpate associated lip lacerations and explore for tooth fragments.

When evaluating patients with dental trauma, clinicians should consider associated fracture of the mandible and maxilla as well as cervical spine injuries. Patients who cannot open their mouths are suspect for mandibular fracture or temporomandibular joint injury. Additionally, patients with congenital heart disease, acquired heart disease, or immune compromise may need antibiotic prophylaxis for endocarditis. The following sections briefly describe the evaluation and management of various types of dental injury.

Table 43-3. CHRONOLOGICAL DEVELOPMENT OF NORMAL DENTITION

	Eruption (months)	Shedding (years)
Primary Teeth		
Central incisor	6–9	7–8
Lateral incisor	7–10	7–9
Canine	16–20	10–12
First molar	12–16	9–11
Second molar	20–30	11–12

	Eruption (years)	
	Lower	Upper
Secondary Teeth		
Central incisor	6–7	7–8
Lateral incisor	7–8	8–9
Canine	9–11	11–12
First premolar	10–12	10–11
Second premolar	11–12	10–12
First molar	6–7	6–7
Second molar	11–13	12–13
Third molar	17–25	17–25

Fracture

Clinically, the tooth may look jagged or "sharp" at the edge. All fractures require referral to a dentist, who can evaluate fractures that do not extend into the pulp (no bleeding from the core of the tooth) when convenient. Complicated fractures that extend into the pulp should be referred immediately. The prognosis of complicated fractures depends on the amount of exposed pulp, the position of the fracture, and the time elapsed prior to definitive treatment by the dentist.

Intrusion

Intruded teeth are displaced directly into the socket. Radiographs are often necessary to make the diagnosis, to distinguish the problem from an avulsion, and to evaluate its proximity to the developing permanent tooth bud. Intrusion injuries have a poor prognosis. Referral to the dentist should be within 24 hours.

Extrusion/Lateral Subluxation

Extruded and laterally displaced teeth present as teeth lifted from the socket in various directions. Luxated permanent teeth should be realigned and splinted as soon as possible. With early treatment, the prognosis is excellent. Primary teeth are usually extracted to avoid injury to the developing permanent tooth during realignment.

Subluxed

A child may describe a displaced and mobile tooth with the words, "My teeth do not feel right." This phrase probably refers to a change in alignment when the child closes the jaw. The tooth is often sensitive to percussion. Often blood is at the gum line secondary to damage of the periodontal ligament. Subluxed teeth, especially in permanent dentition, may require splinting and should be referred to a dentist. Primary teeth with minimal mobility (<15 degrees of motion) can be followed; teeth with larger degrees of mobility are usually extracted to avoid damage to the permanent tooth bud or risk of aspiration of the tooth.

Concussion

The term concussion is used for a tooth that is sensitive to percussion following trauma. As long as mobility or displacement is absent, the patient needs no immediate treatment. Most of these injuries require follow-up with a dentist to assess the need for radiographs.

Avulsions

Avulsion refers to a tooth displaced entirely from its socket. If the tooth is permanent and found, the provider should place it back in the socket after rinsing the tooth with water or saline. He or she should be careful not to hold the tooth by the root and not to scrub the root. For permanent teeth that cannot be immediately reimplanted, providers ideally should place them in a commercially available tooth-preserving solution. When such a solution is not available, they can use milk, saliva, or saline. Some practitioners have placed the tooth in the cheek or floor of the mouth, until the child reaches the dentist. It is best to avoid drying of the root surface. Avulsed teeth require immediate dental consultation. Avulsed primary teeth should not be reimplanted to avoid injuring the permanent tooth or the risk of possible aspiration in a very young child.

Maxilla and Mandible Injuries

Patients with orofacial trauma who have difficulty opening their mouths or have instability of the maxilla or mandible require referral to an oral or plastic surgeon.

SOFT TISSUE INJURIES OF OROPHARYNX AND PALATE

Bite Wounds

The most common oral injuries stem from biting the lips, cheek, or tongue during a fall.

● **Clinical Pearl:** Lacerations of the lips or cheek can initially bleed extensively, but most do not need repair.

Intraoral lacerations generally are not repaired unless large cavities are present or the defect could possibly interfere with swallowing or speech, such as with a forked tongue. For persistent bleeding or large lacerations, absorbable sutures are usually placed.

▲ **Clinical Warning:** Lip lacerations involving the vermilion border and those that are full thickness need repair.

Prophylactic antibiotics generally are not prescribed for mouth or lip lacerations.

Mouth Punctures

Another common intraoral injury occurs when children fall with an object in their mouth. When the puncture involves the central portion of the palate, there is little risk of complicated injury. Therefore, these children can often be sent home on oral antibiotics that cover oral flora such as amoxicillin for 5 to 7 days with follow-up.

Trauma to the lateral palate or the posterior pharyngeal wall raises the concern of vascular injuries to the carotid artery and jugular vein, which may manifest as expanding hematomas and persistent bleeding. Simple lacerations in these areas may require observation in a hospital; deeper lacerations may require angiography and surgical exploration. Antibiotics are generally prescribed for 5 to 7 days. In treating puncture wounds of the oropharynx, exploration of the wound or radiograph may be necessary to determine the presence of a retained foreign body.

ACQUIRED TORTICOLLIS

Torticollis refers to a contracture of one sternocleidomastoid muscle leading to pain and tilting of the head toward the affected muscle with the chin rotated away from the contracted side. Distinct from congenital or neonatal torticollis, acquired torticollis can be associated with minor upper respiratory infections, bacterial infections of the para- and retropharyngeal tissues, or from minor muscular neck trauma. When associated with upper respiratory infections, inflammation of cervical spine ligaments at the atlanto-axial level leads to rotatory subluxation. When associated with trauma, the provider should obtain cervical spine films. Otherwise, initial treatment consists of a soft collar and nonsteroidal anti-inflammatory medications.

Any patient with neurological complaints associated with a torticollis requires immobilization, detailed imaging of the cervical spine, and neurosurgical evaluation. Other conditions such as discitis, vertebral osteomyelitis, retropharyngeal infections, and adenitis can also cause torticollis, but these are usually accompanied by other physical findings (eg, fever, cervical spine pain, extraordinary throat pain, posterior pharyngeal swelling).

SKIN ABSCESS INCISION AND DRAINAGE

Cutaneous abscess is usually the result of a break in the skin with subsequent local infection. An abscess may be primary from a deep inoculation (such as a puncture) or secondary to a localized cellulitis that progresses to infection of the deeper tissues. Bacterial enzymes contribute to necrosis, and the white cell response adds further enzymatic activity, liquefaction, and formation of pus.

A cellulitis will often resolve with antibacterial therapy alone, whereas abscesses require drainage. Without drainage, infection may spread deeper and involve underlying structures. Percutaneous needle aspiration does not adequately drain an abscess and leads to persistent or recurrent abscesses. Incision and drainage is a simple, and mostly curative, procedure.

Factors contributing to abscess formation include open skin, punctures or bites, foreign bodies, poor circulation, and poor immunity. Skin areas with extra secretory glands are also prone to abscesses from obstruction of the glands—axilla, groin, and breast. The bacterial agents represent the skin flora of the area. Staphylococcus and Group A Streptococcus are most common, although enteric organisms may be found in abscesses around the anus or perineum, and oral flora in abscesses associated with repeated contact with the mouth such as the fingers of infants. Axillary abscesses often contain gram-negative aerobic organisms.

An abscess may be difficult to distinguish from cellulitis; both have pain, erythema, warmth, swelling, and induration. Fluctuance on examination indicates the presence of an abscess, although when not obvious, needle aspiration of pus will confirm the diagnosis.

Contraindications to incision and drainage include highly cosmetic areas, possible involvement of deeper structures (joint, nerve, blood vessel, tendon, bone), possible congenital cyst or fistula, or the inability to provide adequate local or regional anesthesia. Additionally, a kerion in association with tinea capitis, adenitis secondary to Mycobacterium, or a herpetic Whitlow should not be incised. Chronic or recurrent abscesses often require resection of the outer walls, and therefore are difficult to accomplish without surgical consultation.

After careful positioning and immobilization, the provider can prep the abscess and surrounding skin with an antiseptic solution. He or she can anesthetize the surrounding noninfected skin with 1% lidocaine by local infiltration or regional block. He or she can then anesthetize the top of the abscess with intradermal injections. For purposes of culture, needle aspiration of the abscess prior to incision may be necessary. The clinician should incise the abscess cavity with a scalpel blade in a linear fashion parallel to the skin folds. The incision needs to extend to the edges of the cavity (not edge of erythema) for drainage. The provider can then place a blunt tip instrument into the cavity to break up any loculations and facilitate complete drainage. Milking the skin is important to remove all pus. Larger wounds require irrigation to remove all the necrotic tissue and plasma.

Small wounds that completely drain and collapse the cavity need warm soaks several times a day to keep the incision open during healing. Abscesses with a residual cavity after drainage require packing with gauze packing strips. The provider should not tensely pack the wound, but careful placement of the gauze into all edges of the wound is necessary. The provider should leave at least ½ inch of gauze external to the wound to prevent closure of the incision and to facilitate removal of the packing. For wounds that are packed with gauze, daily unpacking and repacking are necessary. Providers can tape layers of gauze over the wound for protection and to absorb any drainage. In particular situations, clinicians can teach family members how to pack and dress the wound; the discomfort associated with subsequent dressing changes diminishes after the first few days. Although abscess drainage may be curative, providers should consider antibiotics for deep wounds, for those with surrounding cellulitis or lymphangitis, or for any patient with systemic symptoms associated with the abscess. They need to consider parenteral antibiotics for wounds involving deeper structures (tendon, fascial planes, muscle, or near bone) and those patients with high fever, immunocompromise (including diabetes), poor circulation, or very young age. For small abscesses, topical spray refrigerants may provide adequate anesthesia for incision (but are not adequate for probing, breaking loculations, or packing).

Paronychia

A paronychia is an infection of the tissue surrounding a fingernail or toenail. When a localized area of pus develops, proper and complete drainage is necessary. Management of the common paronychia should be performed in a pediatric office or clinic.

Pathology

Typically, paronychias are secondary to invasion of skin flora into the soft tissues that surround the nail plate. Many infections have a mix of pathogens, and oral flora may be present among young children who suck their fingers or older children who bite their nails. In infancy, toe paronychias are common from tight-fitting clothes, and finger or toe paronychias from cutting the nails too short. Most adolescents develop paronychias from minor trauma. Paronychias can also be complicated by deeper extension to bone or finger joints or destruction of the germinal matrix that is responsible for nail growth.

Management

A paronychia may begin as a cellulitis around the nail edge. Warm soaks and oral antibiotics are sufficient at this point. Once the surrounding skin becomes swollen or fluctuant, drainage is necessary. Most paronychia are simply drained by lifting up the cuticle edge of skin (the eponychium) between the nail plate and skin using a Number 11 surgical blade. The provider should keep the blade parallel to the nail plate. If the paronychia is localized to one side and has little proximal swelling, he or she may do so without anesthesia or with some refrigerant spray. When the infection involves the whole base or one of the lateral margins, a digital block (1% lidocaine, no epinephrine) or skin refrigerant is necessary for adequate drainage. For extensive paronychia or recurrent infections, the nail may need to be partially removed because it acts as a nidus; referral to a specialist may be necessary. Once the drainage is complete, a dry dressing is temporarily placed. Warm soaks with water or diluted hydrogen peroxide will aid healing. Oral antibiotics are often prescribed for 5 to 7 days; antibiotics typically used include cephalexin, dicloxacillin, and amoxicillin-clavulanate.

TRAUMA TO NAILS

Subungual Hematoma

Trauma to the tip of a digit may lead to blood between the nail plate and the nail bed. Besides the pain associated with the injury, the expanding hematoma builds pressure under the nail that intensifies the pain. Large subungual hematomas (> 50% of the nail) may be associated with underlying fracture, and thus providers should obtain a radiograph; likewise, decreased range of motion of the distal joint or remarkable swelling (even in the absence of a large subungual hematoma) warrants a radiograph. If soft tissue injury is extensive or the underlying bone is fractured, the provider should refer the patient to have the nail removed and the nail bed repaired.

The pain associated with the subungual hematoma can be relieved in two fashions: if the hematoma is very distal near the edge, lifting the nail plate should allow drainage. If the hematoma is proximal, then the drainage is best accomplished by making a hole in the nail with a cautery device. The provider should avoid being sprayed by blood as he or she makes the hole. The finger should be soaked three times per day to avoid infection. Providers should warn parents about complications of subungual hematomas including onycholysis, nail deformity, and infection.

Subungual Foreign Body

Occasionally, children will acquire a foreign body, often a splinter, directly under the nail plate. If the foreign body extends to the fingertip, a hemostat or forceps may be sufficient for removal. Deeper foreign bodies can be removed in one of two ways. Multiple foreign bodies or those complicated by infection or large subungual hematomas are best removed by partial or complete nail removal after a digital nerve block. For simple, uncomplicated foreign bodies, the nail can be shaved with the edge of a Number 11 scalpel blade until the foreign body can be reached. The provider should hold the blade perpendicular to the foreign body and 90° to the horizontal plane. He or she should always shave the nail in a proximal to distal direction to promote distal migration of the foreign body. Once exposed, he or she should remove the splinter with hemostats or forceps. The patient should soak the finger in an antiseptic solution three times per day to prevent infection.

FINGERTIP AVULSIONS AND AMPUTATIONS

Partial avulsions of the fingertip should be repaired by someone capable of inspecting the integrity of the nailbed and underlying bone. Tip amputations without bone exposure and intact nailbeds can be managed conservatively by cleaning the wound, applying a nonadherent dressing, and splinting for protection. The provider should schedule routine wound care. He or she should approach fingertip amputations based on whether the amputated segment is proximal or distal to the distal interphalangeal joint (DIP) and whether bone is exposed. All amputations proximal to the DIP require referral to a hand surgeon for reimplantation. The amputated segment should be kept cold and moist by wrapping in saline-soaked gauze and placing in plastic next to ice. Providers should avoid direct contact with ice or drying.

PLANTAR PUNCTURE WOUNDS

Plantar punctures are commonly caused by nails and occur mostly in the summer. These wounds are always at high risk for serious complications such as cellulitis, abscess, foreign body granulomas, pyoarthritis, and osteomyelitis.

Pathology

Because of the proximity of underlying structures and the potential for deeper penetration, the forefoot has the highest rate of infectious complications, followed by the arch and the heel. Most acute infections are caused by to Staphylococcus and Group A Streptococcus, whereas pyoarthritis and osteomyelitis are often due to *Pseudomonas aeruginosa*. Infections occur in approximately 15% of plantar punctures despite proper initial management.

Management

A complete history should include when the injury happened, the estimated penetration, and the integrity of the puncturing device after the injury. Providers must seriously consider the possibility of a retained foreign body in all puncture wounds. They should obtain radiographs in all grossly contaminated wounds, in all deep punctures that may extend near bone, and in those in which the history cannot exactly determine the offending item's appearance after the injury. If the patient presents late with signs of infection, a radiograph also is necessary.

Providers can cleanse minor and clean puncture wounds with local antiseptics to the surrounding skin. Soaking the foot in antiseptic solution has never been shown to decrease rates of infection. The provider should perform pressure irrigation using a 20 gauge angiocath with a 25 (or greater) cc syringe or a commercial irrigation device. In cases of contaminated wounds or known deep punctures, "coring" of the puncture site is necessary. Local anesthesia, either by local infiltration or peroneal nerve block at the ankle, also is required. This procedure is very difficult in young children, because providing local anesthesia to the plantar surface is so challenging. Once anesthesia has been achieved, the provider must remove a 2mm to 3 mm circular rim of tissue (near-full or full thickness) with a blade or iris scissors. He or she must then copiously irrigate the wound with at least 200 cc of sterile irrigant. For large puncture wounds, the clinician should insert a wick. Puncture wounds are best dressed with bulky gauze for pain relief and to keep the wound clean. The patient may need to use crutches for comfort. Daily dressing changes should be done for the first 48 hours to watch for infection. Controversy exists whether wounds which were not cored should be soaked daily to prevent closure of the skin.

Prophylactic antibiotics have not been shown to be effective in preventing infection. If prescribed, however, they should only be directed against gram-positive organisms (staph and strep), and not against pseudomonas, even if the puncture occurred through a sneaker. First-generation cephalosporins are usually good choices. The provider must address tetanus status and mention explicit risks of infection to the soft tissues and bone to the patient and family. He or she should make special note of the delayed appearance of infections to reinforce the need for follow-up if any pain or local signs of infection develop. If the patient presents or returns with an infected puncture wound, surgical consultation is advised.

INGROWN TOENAIL REPAIR

Ingrown toenails during the first year of life are common and usually result in mild tenderness and erythema. In this age group, simply avoiding restrictive clothing, cutting the nail straight instead of curved at the edges, and pulling the skin away from the nail after baths should suffice. Management in older children with thicker and harder nails is more challenging. Ingrown nails can lead to local cellulitis, abscess formation, or chronic irritation with granuloma formation. Mild cases may require trimming the nail, soaking the toe, topical antibiotics, and avoidance of tight-toe shoes. Cases associated with cellulitis, extreme pain, or granuloma formation require removal of the edge of the nail. Adequate removal of the nail section (to its base) is best accomplished after digital block.

GENITAL TRAUMA

Straddle Injuries

Straddle injuries in females often lead to vulvar hematomas and rarely to lacerations of the labia or vagina. Most hematomas are successfully managed with rest and ice packs. Mild urinary retention can be managed by voiding in a tub of warm water. Absolute urinary retention requires gynecological evaluation. Lacerations or punctures of the perineum, labia, or vagina require thorough inspection and exploration. Providers always must consider sexual abuse in cases of genital injury.

Straddle injuries in males can lead to scrotal hematomas, testicular hematomas, testicular rupture, testicular dislocation (into canal), or torsion. When pain or swelling limits the exam, the provider should use ultrasound to assess testicular integrity and blood flow. Providers can manage patients without evidence of testicular injury conservatively with icepacks and scrotal support. A urological surgeon should evaluate patients with evidence of testicular injury. Lacerations that are full thickness as well as puncture wounds also require surgical consultation.

Perineal Lacerations

Providers can manage superficial lacerations of the perineum with sitz baths and local care. Deep lacerations can extend into the rectum, vagina or urethra, and therefore require surgical consultation.

Zipper Injury to the Penis

Entrapment in the zipper mechanism can injure the skin of the penis. Prompt and painless extrication of the entrapped skin is easy to perform and greatly appreciated by all concerned. In general, extrication procedures are simple and can be done in the office with the right equipment.

Quick dressing and undressing in boys not wearing underwear predisposes for zipper injuries. Typically, the foreskin or ventral skin is entrapped. All zippers are composed of two opposing rows of interlocking teeth; a fastening mechanism (composed of two plates separated by a median bar at the bottom) aligns the teeth in a single plane.

Because prolonged entrapment may make management more difficult secondary to swelling, providers should see all zipper injuries promptly. Three approaches to skin extrication have been described.

The median bar can be cut with a wire cutter or bone cutter. Once cut, the fastening mechanism will separate, and the provider can easily pull apart the zipper. The provider also can open the zipper by cutting the surrounding pant material with bandage or trauma scissors. He or she can use the scissors to completely cut through the zipper above and below the entrapped skin, thereby effectively removing the fastener mechanism that was holding the zipper together. Alternatively, if the scissors cannot transect the zipper, cutting the cloth up to the edges of the zipper should facilitate separation of the zipper. The clinician must exercise special care to avoid cutting the penis, which is hidden by the pants. Cutting the median bar is easier and faster given the right tools. The provider also can apply mineral oil to the tissues, following with gentle traction on the tissue until it slides out the zipper.

Although not necessary, ice to the involved tissue may minimize swelling. Providers always should use antiseptic solutions on the involved skin. They should give consideration to conscious sedation or local anesthesia. If using anesthesia, regional blocks are necessary, since local infiltration will lead to further swelling. Providers should not use local anesthetic containing epinephrine on the penis. Following successful removal, standard wound care is required.

A urologist should be involved when standard maneuvers cannot easily free the skin, or when there is involvement of the urethra, full thickness lacerations to the scrotum, blood at the urethral meatus, or hematuria.

UPPER EXTREMITY INJURIES

Clavicular Fractures

History and Physical Exam

Difficult deliveries often cause clavicle fractures in newborns. In older children, they often result from falling on an outstretched arm or directly on the shoulder. Fractures from direct force to the clavicle may be associated with pulmonary or neurovascular injuries. Fractures in newborns are often detected during the routine newborn exam as crepitus or swelling over the clavicle. Occasionally the infant may be noted to have pseudo-paralysis; the provider must distinguish fracture from brachial plexus injury or traumatic separation of the proximal humeral epiphysis.

Experienced clinicians will make the diagnosis on clinical grounds alone; in most cases x-rays are not necessary. If any uncertainty surrounds the physical findings, radiographs should confirm the diagnosis.

Management

● **Clinical Pearl:** Clavicular fractures heal remarkably well, even in the presence of angulation or overlapping ends. As such, most cases are very amenable to treatment by the primary care provider and do not require orthopedic referral. Patients with open fractures, tenting of the overlying skin, or associated neurovascular injury, however, do need orthopedic referral.

For children younger than age 2 years, a swath to bind the arm to the trunk can be done for 3 to 7 days; thereafter, no treatment is necessary other than warning caregivers to be careful when lifting the child. Children ages 2 to 12 years usually are more comfortable if the arm is immobilized with a figure-of-eight harness or an arm sling. Union should be present in 2 to 4 weeks, and immobilization can be discontinued after 3 weeks. Children older than age 12 years usually have complete fractures. Here, a figure-of-eight provides the most support (realignment) and comfort. A figure-of-eight is usually better treatment in all age groups if the clinician suspects angulation or displacement. The sling can be discontinued after 3 to 4 weeks. The patient should avoid contact sports for 3 months.

Shoulder

Clavicle Dislocations

These rare dislocations in children involve the acromioclavicular (AC) joint and are associated with a tear of the coraco-clavicular ligaments or a distal clavicle fracture. The typical history is a teenager who has a fall directly on the tip of the shoulder. On examination, point tenderness of the AC joint and limitation of range of motion secondary to pain are common. The clinician should obtain AP and lateral radiographs of the shoulder to note any displacement of the clavicle and to reveal associated fractures. Initial management for patients with normal radiographs is an arm sling and follow-up. Patients with abnormal radiographs require placement in a sling and referral to an orthopedist when convenient.

Glenohumeral Dislocations

Glenohumeral dislocations are rare prior to physeal close; when they do occur, they tend to be anteriorly displaced. This injury is often due to falling on the elbow or hand with the arm abducted and externally rotated. Patients often protect the injured arm; therefore, cutting off the clothing is often necessary to get an appropriate exam. On examination, patients are very uncomfortable, and the contour of the shoulder will be altered with a prominent acromion and a depression under it. The shoulder appears to "sag." The clinician should test both sensory function of the axillary nerve (deltoid area) and distal neurovascular function. Immobilizing the arm with a sling or swathe-like wrap is a comfort measure. The provider should obtain radiographs (AP, lateral, and Y scapular views) prior to reduction attempts.

Several techniques for reduction are usable, but only experienced clinicians should perform these maneuvers. Narcotic analgesics or benzodiazepines can facilitate reductions. Following reduction, clinicians should retest axillary nerve function and place patients in a sling and swathe. Follow-up with an orthopedist is necessary to monitor healing and to guide physical therapy.

Pulled Shoulder

Forceful traction of the shoulder in a young child can result in a partial tear of the joint capsule without dislocation. Patients complain of shoulder pain and have no deformity or swelling, but manifest decreased mobility secondary to pain. Radiographs will be normal. The patient requires placement in an arm sling. If the pain persists more than one week, repeat radiographs may reveal a Salter I fracture of the proximal humerus. In such case, orthopedic follow-up is needed.

Rotator Cuff Injury

The rotator cuff consists of three muscles that stabilize the shoulder in the glenoid fossa: the teres minor, supraspinatus, and infraspinatus. These muscles abduct and externally rotate the shoulder. Direct falls on the shoulder, dislocations, or strenuous throws or lifting can injure these muscles. On physical exam, passive range of motion may be normal. Pain at the insertion point of the muscles (greater tubercle of the humerus) and weakness with abduction or external rotation often are noted. The clinician should obtain radiographs of the shoulder to identify any other bony injury. They should place patients in a sling and suggest orthopedic follow-up when convenient.

Fractures of the Humerus

Proximal Humerus

Fractures may occur through the growth plate or metaphysis from a fall on an outstretched arm or by direct force. On exam, the clinician will note tenderness, swelling, and decreased range of motion. Radiographs will demonstrate the fracture. The provider should obtain scapular Y views if he or she suspects an associated dislocation. He or she should refer the patient to the orthopedist, although the usual treatment is a sling and swathe.

Humeral Shaft

Transverse fractures are usually due to direct blows, whereas spiral fractures result from twisting injuries. Predictably,

findings include swelling, tenderness, and limited motion. Providers should note distal neurovascular function. Radiographs will demonstrate the fracture. Clinicians can place patients with incomplete fractures in a sling, swathe, and refer them to an orthopedist in the next 48 hours. They should refer patients with complete fractures immediately to an orthopedist. Providers should suspect child abuse in children younger than age 3 years with spiral fractures.

Elbow

Radial Head Subluxation

Pathology

Radial head subluxation or "nursemaid's elbow" results from excessive axial traction of an extended elbow in a child younger than age 5 years. The typical story is the toddler who, while walking with Mommy and being held by the hand, suddenly decides to become dead weight and fall to the ground. An overly playful father, swinging a child around by the outstretched arms, is also a common precipitant. Child abuse is usually not a concern in cases of nursemaid's elbow.

History and Physical Exam

On exam, the child holds the arm in a slightly flexed position with the forearm pronated. The child may be quiet when still but will meet any attempt to examine the arm with significant resistance. Providers should carefully palpate the clavicle and wrist and examine them for injury. They should obtain radiographs if the history is atypical or examination reveals any swelling, deformity, or point tenderness away from the radial head. The diagnosis is considered based on a consistent history and physical exam and will be confirmed upon successful reduction.

Management

All clinicians who care for young children should be familiar and comfortable with reducing a subluxed radial head.

● **Clinical Pearl:** Reduction is accomplished by supinating the forearm completely, by gentle traction, extending the elbow maximally, and then fully flexing the elbow while maintaining supination.

The reduction is usually palpable. Even after a successful reduction, most toddlers will refrain from moving the affected arm because of anticipated pain, and providers must fully explain this fact to the caretaker. Commonly, the practitioner or parent can successfully demonstrate full voluntary range of motion by offering a treat or little toy. Clinicians should instruct parents that if the child does not use the arm normally within a few hours, they should consider radiographs. If the x-rays are normal and a repeat maneuver does not result in normal motor function, the arm should remain in a sling. The toddler should take non-steroidal anti-inflammatory drugs (eg, ibuprofen), and then return for re-evaluation in 24 hours. Providers can refer cases of recurrent subluxations to an orthopedist.

Fractures and Dislocations

These usually result from falls on outstretched arms and only rarely from direct force. A non-displaced supracondylar fracture is the most common fracture of the elbow and results from hyperextension after even minor falls. On exam, swelling, tenderness, and limited motion are noted. Neurovascular injury often complicates elbow fractures; therefore, the provider should assess distal function. Radiographs will often reveal the fracture. In the absence of an obvious fracture, a posterior fat pad sign suggests an intra-articular fracture. The provider should splint and elevate the elbow to reduce or minimize swelling. Elbow fractures require immediate orthopedic consultation.

Fractures of the Radius and Ulna

These are typically the result of a fall on an outstretched hand. The type of fracture depends on the exact mechanism of injury and age of the child. As expected, swelling and tenderness are invariably present at the fracture site. The clinician should assess neurovascular function, especially with large deformities. He or she should obtain AP and lateral radiographs of the forearm including the elbow. Radiographs will demonstrate the fracture and point tenderness over the physis. In the face of strong clinical findings, negative radiographs can suggest a Salter I fracture. The provider should apply a splint for fractures or suspected fractures. Displaced fractures require immediate orthopedic consultation. Clinicians can splint non-displaced fractures, including buckle fractures, and delay orthopedic consultation for up to 48 hours.

Hand and Wrist

Scaphoid Fractures

These result from forceful hyperextension of the wrist, typically in adolescents. Because of the potential for poor healing if undiagnosed, clinicians should maintain high suspicion for this injury when examining patients with wrist pain.

● **Clinical Pearl:** On examination, tenderness in the anatomic snuffbox and pain with supination against resistance or with axial compression of the thumb are present.

Swelling is usually absent, but range of motion and strength may be diminished. Clinicians should obtain radiographs of the wrist (AP, lateral, and oblique views). If these are negative but suspicion is still high, they should obtain special scaphoid views or CT scan images. Orthopedic consultation is necessary for all scaphoid fractures. For non-displaced fractures, a thumb-spica splint/cast is placed for 6 to 10 weeks. Displaced fractures may require open fixation. When the provider suspects a fracture but it is not radiographically apparent, he or she should apply a thumb spica and repeat examination and radiographs in 2 weeks.

Metacarpal Fractures

Metacarpal fractures result from crush injuries or from direct impact along the axis, as when hitting something with a fist. Distal fractures are more common than shaft or proximal injuries. Swelling, tenderness, and deformity are often present. Pain limits active motion, and most distal fractures will have a rotational defect (as assessed with the fingers in flexion). Radiographs will define the fracture. Any displaced, intra-articular, or open fracture requires reduction by an orthopedist. Closed reduction is necessary if angulation exceeds 30°. Non-displaced fractures can be put in a gutter splint with the wrist neutral and the metacarpophalangeal joints at 70°. Orthopedic follow-up is recommended.

Phalangeal Fractures and Dislocations

Primary care practitioners are frequently consulted for finger injuries. Since most sprains and fractures are managed the same (by splinting or buddy-taping), most cases do not require radiographs.

● **Clinical Pearl:** Whether or not to x-ray finger injuries depends on the provider's clinical ability to differentiate between an uncomplicated and complicated fracture.

An uncomplicated phalangeal fracture is one with minimal angulation, no rotational deformity or displacement, and no joint involvement. If the fracture meets these conditions and the provider can assure follow-up in 3 to 5 days, then the patient does not need x-rays and treatment can proceed by splinting. At follow-up, if no angulation or rotational deformity exists and passive range of motion is full though somewhat tender, further splinting is all that is required. If the fracture fails to meet these conditions, the clinician should obtain x-rays and consult an orthopedist, especially to identify an intra-articular fracture that might require pinning.

Distal phalangeal fractures usually result from crush injuries and are often accompanied by nailbed lacerations. Avulsion fractures of the distal phalanx also can occur from hyperflexion (dorsal avulsion, mallet finger) or hyperextension (volar avulsion). Distal phalangeal fractures are rarely displaced, and splinting or buddy taping is usually sufficient.

Middle phalangeal fractures are often caused by direct force. Uncomplicated fractures (minimal angulation, no rotational deformity, not intraarticular) can be managed by finger splint or buddy-taping. Complicated fractures require orthopedic referral.

An orthopedist needs to see proximal phalangeal fractures that, as with other hand fractures, involve the joint, have rotational deformity, or are displaced. The most common childhood fracture is a Salter II injury of the base of the little finger. This fracture often has some ulnar deviation (valgus). Immobilization to the adjacent finger and referral to an orthopedist is necessary. The splint for proximal phalangeal fractures should place the wrist in mild extension (30°), the metacarpophalangeal joint at 70°, and the interphalangeal joint at 15° (best accomplished with a gutter or trouser splint). Neck fractures of the proximal phalanx often are associated with distal segment displacement. Because successful reductions are difficult to perform and maintain with splinting, the clinician should consult an orthopedist.

Metacarpophalagneal (MP) and Interphalangeal (IP) Joint Sprains and Dislocations

With sprains, swelling, tenderness, ecchymosis, and decreased range of motion will be present after the injury. Providers should obtain radiographs to eliminate fracture. Joint laxity is difficult to assess secondary to pain. Buddy-taping or immobilization are sufficient unless the joint is unstable, in which case orthopedic consultation is necessary.

Dislocations of MP joints most often result from hyperextension and may be associated with fractures. In simple dislocations, the proximal phalanx remains hyperextended with the carpal head displaced volarly into the palm. In complex dislocations, the dorsal phalanx and volar metacarpal are parallel ("bayonet" relationship). The clinician should assess neurovascular status and obtain AP and lateral radiographs prior to reduction attempts. They should attempt closed reduction only for simple dislocations. Reduction can be performed by flexion of the digit after applying longitudinal traction. If reduction is successful, the finger can be buddy-taped for 3 weeks. Complex dislocations involve entrapment of the volar plate with the joint and therefore require surgical reduction.

Dislocations of the IP joint also result from hyperextension; therefore, most are dorsally dislocated. Clinicians should obtain AP and lateral views prior to the reduction. After digital block anesthesia, applying longitudinal traction and then flexing the distal segment into position can reduce the dislocation. Providers should obtain post-reduction films. After the reduction, they should test the joint for lateral stability. If lateral instability exists, the provider should splint the finger for 3 weeks in consultation with an orthopedist. If stable, he or she can buddy-tape the finger for 7 to 10 days. The provider should refer volar dislocations to an orthopedist for presumed tendon and ligamentous injury.

LOWER EXTREMITY INJURIES

Femur

● **Clinical Pearl:** Femoral shaft fractures in children younger than age 2 years usually result from a twisting or direct blow. Providers should always consider child abuse in such cases.

Fractures in children older than age 2 years are usually from high-energy accidents; therefore, providers should seek concomitant injuries. On examination, proximal shaft or neck fractures may present as immobility, shortening of the leg, and external rotation. Shaft fractures often have deformity and massive swelling. Clinicians should assess distal neurovascular function. All such fractures require immediate orthopedic involvement.

Knee

Dislocation of the Patella

This usually occurs with extreme valgus stress on the knee, as when doing "splits." On physical exam, the deformity will be obvious unless it self-reduced. A dislocated patella is displaced laterally, and the medial edge will be "flipped up." After spontaneous or active reduction of an acute traumatic dislocation, knee effusion and medial joint line pain will be present. The patient may be anxious with lateral displacement of the patella (administer apprehension test). Radiographs of the knee may show the upturned patella, fragments of the lateral femoral condyle, or a shallow patella groove. Or they may be normal. With normal radiographs, the provider can make a presumptive diagnosis based on a typical history and physical exam. Reduction of the knee is accomplished by extension of the knee and medial pressure on the patella. Post reduction films are required to exclude a fracture of the lateral femoral condyle or the medial patella facet. The knee should be splinted for 2 weeks followed by orthopedic consultation.

Ligamentous Injuries of the Knee

- *Medial collateral ligament (MCL).* Injury to this ligament often results from a lateral blow to the knee or a twisting motion. Pain will be present over the MCL, and the provider may note laxity by applying a valgus stress. A joint effusion and limitation of motion often coexist.
- *Anterior cruciate ligament (ACL).* The ACL is injured secondary to hyperextension of the knee or sudden deceleration with the foot planted, causing abduction and external rotation of the leg. Often a hemarthrosis is present, and a Lachman and anterior drawer tests will be positive.
- *Posterior cruciate ligament.* These tend to result from a direct blow to the tibia while the knee is flexed, thereby forcing the proximal tibia posteriorly. On exam, the posterior knee will be tender, and a small effusion will be present.

For all suspected ligamentous injuries, the provider should obtain AP and lateral radiographs to exclude any concomitant fractures. Often the provider cannot make a diagnosis of ligamentous injury until all swelling and tenderness subside. ACL injuries associated with avulsion fractures (tibial spine) require immediate orthopedic evaluation. For all other suspected ligamentous injuries, initial management should include ice, elevation, compression, nonsteroidal anti-inflammatory medications, and rest (no weight bearing). The provider should refer the patient to an orthopedist once swelling and tenderness subside (often after several days). In cases of large hemarthroses, joint aspiration can relieve excess pain.

Meniscal Injury

This usually results from twisting or bending with the knee flexed and the foot planted. Meniscal injuries are more common in adolescents than children and involve the medial meniscus five times more often than the lateral meniscus. The patient may present having heard a "pop" or "snap" with a buckling of the knee. A limp, decreased range of motion, and occasionally swelling then follows. After the acute episode, the patient may experience symptoms of impingement: a sensation of locking or "giving out," or recurrent swelling with activity. On physical exam, the knee will be tender along the medial or lateral joint line that corresponds to the meniscus that was injured. The knee may lock in flexion or be unable to fully extend. The provider should obtain radiographs to exclude fractures. He or she should use immobilization, crutches, elevation, and compression after acute injuries. Referral to orthopedist is indicated several days after the acute injury.

Toddler's Fracture

This classically refers to an oblique non-displaced fracture of the distal tibia without a fibular fracture. The child typically presents with an acute antalgic gait or refusal to weight-bear after a seemingly minor fall. Physical exam is often unrevealing except for tenderness and possibly mild swelling. The provider should obtain AP and lateral radiographs of the tibia. If x-rays are negative but the patient has focal tenderness, the clinician should order oblique views. Once the fracture has been identified, long leg casts are needed to adequately immobilize a toddler. In the presence of a spiral fracture in a non-walking child, the provider also must consider child abuse. In general, fractures of the tibia from abuse tend to be midshaft, whereas toddler's fractures tend to be more distal.

Ankle and Foot

Ankle Sprains

Most ankle sprains are due to inversion injury, especially during plantar flexion. Varying amounts of tenderness, swelling, and ecchymosis may be present. The clinician should note any tenderness over the growth plates. The talofibular ligaments are most commonly disrupted and lead to tenderness, just anterior to the lateral malleolus. Ankle sprains are graded as I (stretched, minimal laxity, ability to bear weight), II (tear, obvious laxity, diffuse swelling, difficulty bearing weight), and III (complete disruption with instability, marked swelling, and inability to bear weight). Providers should obtain radiographs to exclude fracture. Acute injuries without radiographic abnormalities are considered sprains; however, physeal injuries are more common than ligamentous injuries. Therefore, it is impossible to exclude Salter I fractures in a young child. For any tenderness or swelling over the growth plate, the provider must treat the injury as presumed Salter I fracture with splinting (or casting), elevation, crutches, and orthopedic follow-up in one week. Grade I sprains are immobilized with an elastic wrap or air splint and treated with ice, elevation, and crutches for 3 days or until weight-bearing without pain can be achieved. Grade II and III sprains require immobilization with a cast or posterior splint and crutches for 3 weeks with slow resumption of activities. The provider must carefully plan rehabilitation of the ankle to avoid recurrent sprains.

Metatarsal and Phalangeal Fractures

Fractures of these bones usually result from direct force or hyperextension/flexion injuries of the forefoot. Focal swelling or tenderness will be present, and radiographs will demonstrate the fracture. For metatarsal and phalangeal fractures with minimal displacement or angulation, a splint and crutches will suffice. Simple fractures of the toes, excluding the large toe, can be managed with buddy-taping and hard-soled shoes. Large toe fractures require splinting or casting (in the 48 hours after injury) and non–weight-bearing. The clinician should consult an orthopedist for all intraarticular fractures, significantly displaced fractures, and physeal fractures.

REFERENCES

Bruns, T., Simon, H., & McLario, D. (1996). Laceration repair using tissue adhesive in a children's emergency department. *Pediatrics, 98*, 673–675.

Fleisher, G., & Ludwig, S. (Eds.) (2000). Textbook of pediatric emergency medicine (4th ed.). Philadelphia: Lippincott Williams & Wilkins.

Frankowski, R. F., Annengers, J. F., & Whitman, S. (1985). The descriptive epidemiology of head trauma in the United States. *Central Nervous System Trauma, 1*(33).

Kraus, J. F., Rock, A., & Hemyari, P. (1990). Brain injuries among infants, children, adolescents, and young adults. *American Journal of Diseases in Children, 144*(6), 684–691.

Common Orthopedic Complaints

• KEITH P. MANKIN, MD, and JENNIFER GRISWOLD, RN, MSN, PNP

INTRODUCTION: THE LIMPING CHILD

The presentation of a limp in the growing child is a frequent cause of concern. Although most limps are benign and transient, causes of limps range from minor trauma to serious illness.

● **Clinical Pearl:** Clinicians must take any limp seriously, since children complain of pain frequently but limp only in the context of true organicity.

An understanding of the entities that can cause a limp may help the provider to determine the severity and prognosis, as well as to assist the parents in dealing with the child's problem. As with all medical problems, a careful and complete history and physical exam is essential. Radiographs are frequently recommended, since the likelihood of underlying pathology is higher in children than in adults. More specialized studies such as Technetium Bone Scan or Magnetic Resonance Imaging (MRI) may add information but are costly and may require sedation or anesthesia. Routine screening bloodwork (eg, complete blood count [CBC], cell differential, erythrocyte sedimentation rate [ESR]) is often useful to help rule out underlying infection.

The differential for a limping child should include the following:

Acute fracture
Septic joint, bone infection, or toxic synovitis ("irritable hip syndrome")
Acute apophysitis (Osgood-Schlatter disease or Sever's disease) and other "growing pains"
Slipped capital femoral epiphysis (SCFE)
Acute back disorder (spondylolysis, infection, tumor, or disk)
Legg-Calvé-Perthes disease (LCPD) (osteonecrosis of the hip)
Rheumatoid or other arthritides, including Lyme disease in endemic areas
Other bone or systemic pathology (primary tumors, leukemia, lymphoma, etc.)

Providers may suspect acute injury based on history and plain radiographs (see Chapter 43). The limb requires stabilization (brace or splint), and the clinician should refer the child to an orthopedic specialist as soon as possible for definitive care.

SEPTIC JOINT, OSTEOMYELITIS, AND TOXIC SYNOVITIS

Musculoskeletal infection is very common in younger children, and providers should always suspect it in the face of an acute gait disturbance.

● **Clinical Pearl:** A septic joint (septic arthritis) is a true surgical emergency that providers need to rule out first and foremost in any child with a limp.

Osteomyelitis or infection of the bone may have a more indolent presentation, but it is frequently associated with severe systemic signs and symptoms and requires aggressive treatment.

● **Clinical Pearl:** Benign transient or toxic synovitis is the most common cause of hip pain that clinicians treat. It is a diagnosis of exclusion, however, and the clinician should only consider it when he or she has comfortably ruled out the much less common but more dangerous conditions of septic arthritis and osteomyelitis.

Anatomy, Physiology, and Pathology

In growing children, increased circulation to the joint and the growing ends of the bone facilitates seeding of these areas with bacteria. Thus, most cases of osteomyelitis and septic joint are from hematogenous spread. Direct penetration of the joint or bone also may lead to infection. Finally, contiguous spread of infection from the bone to the joint has been documented, so providers should consider concomitant orthopedic infections in all cases. Children with blood disorders or other chronic constitutional illnesses will have a higher incidence of infection with more atypical bacteria.

Toxic synovitis probably represents a response by the joint mounted against a non-specific irritant such as blood-borne virus. The joint produces an abundance of fluid (effusion) and may show signs of inflammation (eg, pain, swelling, erythema), which may mimic acute infection. The fluid, however, is sterile. Aspiration of the fluid may be delayed if the examination is relatively benign (ie, no systemic toxicity, minimal pain on joint range of motion) and the child can be closely observed over a short period (from 4 to 6 days) for worsening symptoms.

Epidemiology

Orthopedic infections demonstrate a bimodal incidence, with peak occurrence in the young and the very old or immunocompromised patients. The most frequently involved skeletal areas are those of most rapid growth: knee, elbow, hip, and heel. Slower growing bones such as the clavicle, scapula, and spine are less frequently involved (Dagan, 1993). The most frequent infective agent varies somewhat by age and clinical setting (see Table 44-1).

Toxic synovitis tends to occur in young boys between ages 3 and 6 years and usually in association with or closely following a viral infection. This self-limited illness tends to resolve completely without sequelae in 1 week. The etiology of this very common condition remains unknown.

Table 44–1.   COMMON ORGANISMS INFECTING BONES AND JOINTS (MORRISSEY, 1996)

Age or Clinical Setting	Most Common Organism	Comments
Neonate	Group B strep	
1–5 Years	Staph and strep spp. (H flu)	Incidence of H flu has decreased with vaccine
5 Years on	Staph and strep spp.	
Sexually active	Gonococcus	Most common cause of single joint involvement; clinical course more indolent
Sickle cell anemia	Salmonella	
Direct penetration foot	Pseudomonas	Requires urgent drainage

History and Physical Exam

Common history and physical findings are shown in Table 44-2.

Diagnostic Criteria

Infection

The diagnosis requires positive blood or regional cultures. Up to 40% of joint aspirates in clinically septic joints, however, may be culture-negative (Dagan, 1993).

Toxic Synovitis

A diagnosis toxic synovitis is established by excluding infection and observing the typical clinical course of gradual improvement over several days.

Diagnostic Studies

In joint infection, radiographs may show effusion and in extreme cases, subluxation of a joint. The reader is referred to Figure 44-1. In neonates, apparent joint disruption may be the only clue to a septic arthritis. Ultrasound may be useful to confirm fluid in the joint. For osteomyelitis, specific radiographic changes include periosteal reaction and bone destruction. Please see Figure 44-2 for osteomyelitis in a 2-year old child.

● **Clinical Pearl:** Radiography findings may lag up to 4 weeks after the onset of clinical infection.

Technetium Bone Scan will be positive with 90+% sensitivity in osteomyelitis but may be less sensitive for a septic joint (Morrissey, 1996). Because of the association between septic arthritis and bone infection, a bone scan is recommended even when joint infection is proven on aspiration.

CBC and differential will show increased white blood cell counts in most infections of the bone and joint but will be normal in toxic synovitis. ESR is generally elevated for infection, but is non-specific. Both CBC and ESR may be falsely negative in very young children. C-Reactive Protein may be more specific for orthopedic infections (Unkila-Kallio, 1994), but it is costly and not readily available in all settings. In the toxic child, blood cultures are mandatory and may have a high yield of identifying the infective organism. Depending on the child's age and clinical condition, the clinician may need to perform a complete septic work-up.

In the face of high clinical suspicion of joint infection, aspiration of the joint fluid is essential. The provider must culture the fluid, perform Gram staining, and test for white blood cells. A white blood cell (WBC) count greater than 100,000 is felt to be diagnostic for a true bacterial infection. A WBC count between 50,000 to 75,000 may indicate arthritis, sympathetic effusion from an osteomyelitis, or possibly a less virulent joint infection. Lowered lactic acid and glucose in the joint fluid (compared to serum levels) are also indicative of infection.

Management

The most important step in treatment is recognition of a potentially limb-threatening situation. Basic treatment strategies are described in Table 44-3. Since gram-positive organisms (staph and strep) predominate, currently recom-

Table 44–2.   HISTORY AND PHYSICAL FOR INFECTIOUS PROCESSES OF BONE AND JOINT

Joint sepsis	Systemically ill with high fevers; unable to bear weight; pain on motion of joint. "Splinting" in comfortable position
Osteomyelitis	May be more indolent, but spiking fevers and acute toxicity common. Point tender over infected bone with localized inflammation.
Toxic synovitis	More mild clinical signs, often with pre-existing viral symptoms. Pain on hip abduction may be exquisite, but there tends to be less splinting.

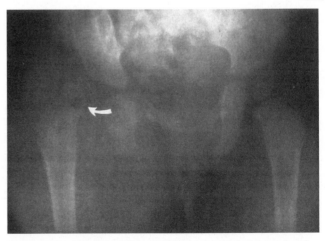

Figure 44–1 ■ Dislocation of the hip from joint sepsis in a 6-month-old infant. (From Tolo, V.T., & Wood, B. [eds.]. [1993]. *Pediatric Orthopedics in Primary Care*. Baltimore: Williams & Wilkins.)

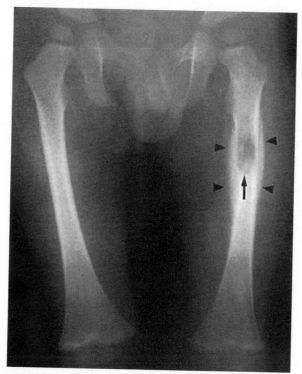

Figure 44–2 ■ Late radiographic changes of osteomyelitis in a 2-year-old child. Note new bone around the cortex (arrowheads) and the central lytic area (arrow). (From Tolo, V.T., & Wood, B. [eds.]. [1993]. *Pediatric orthopedics in primary care.* Baltimore: Williams & Wilkins.)

mended antibiotic regimens are 2 weeks of intravenous (IV) treatment with 150 mg/kg/day of Oxacillin or Nafcillin divided every 6 hours, followed by 100 mg/kg/day of high-dose, oral Cephalexin divided every 6 hours for 4 weeks (Morrissey, 1996). Although quinolones such as ciprofloxacin may be more effective orally, these antibiotics are not used in children because of concern about growth arrest (Menschik, Neumuller, Steiner, et al., 1997). Joint arthritis is treated with 2 weeks of IV antibiotics alone. Clinicians should adjust all antibiotics according to cultures and sensitivities and response to treatment, as evidenced by symptom improvement and decreasing ESR. The treatment of toxic synovitis includes rest, reassurance, non-steroidal anti-inflammatory drugs (NSAIDs), and close daily follow-up, to ensure that the clinical course is one of gradual improvement.

● **Clinical Pearl:** Urgent or emergent referral is recommended for all children who have leg pain and any systemic toxicity. Clinicians may follow milder cases with less toxic presentations and normal lab work, including a normal CBC and ESR, with frequent follow-up and the close cooperation of the child's parents.

Children with bone infections may have a prolonged hospitalization or home restriction during the treatment process. Home-nursing services may be necessary to assist with long-term antibiotics and wound care. Tutoring programs are often necessary if the infection occurs during the school year.

GROWING PAINS AND APOPHYSITIS

Specialized centers known as "growth plates" or "physes" control growth in the bone. Muscle tissue has no growth center but grows in response to the stretch that the elongating bone provides.

● **Clinical Pearl:** At times of rapid growth, the bone length may outstrip the compensatory stretch of the muscle, leading to a period of relative muscle tightness. At these times, increased force and resulting irritation occur at the muscle insertions. If the insertion is a wide area, the irritation leads to growing pains. If the muscle inserts onto a growth plate (or apophysis), the increased stretch causes growth plate irritation or apophysitis.

Apophysitis involves specific sites. The most common site is the anterior shin or tibial tubercle, called Osgood-Schlatter's disease (OSD). Involvement of the lower pole of the patella is termed "jumper's knee" or Sindig-Larsen-Johannson's disease. The back of the heel bone may develop apophysitis from pull of the Achilles tendon (gastroc-soleus complex) and is called Sever's disease.

Epidemiology

Growing pains are seen in children between ages 3 and 6. The incidence is difficult to assess since parents often do not bring their children to providers for evaluation when symptoms appear too mild.

Apophysitis tends to occur in older children (ages 11 years and older), although Sever's may occur in younger children at the first major spurt in shoe size. Boys are affected for all apophysitides more frequently than girls (2:1). The most common type is OSD. One apophysitis may coexist with another (Tolo, 1996).

History and Physical Exam

Growing pains will present as vague pain, usually poorly localized around both knees. Rarely, the child may voluntarily limit activities. The pain will often respond to massage and analgesics such as NSAIDs or acetaminophen. Constitutional symptoms should always be absent. Physical exam generally is non-focal, with no point tenderness, joint dis-

Table 44–3.   TREATMENT OF ORTHOPAEDIC INFECTIONS

Type	Treatment	Comment
Joint infection	Emergent surgical drainage. IV/oral* antibiotics 2–4 weeks.	High risk of late arthritis.
Bone infection	IV/oral antibiotics for 4–6 weeks. Surgery if no clinical response.	Late sequelae (chronic osteo, bone deformity); now rare.
Toxic synovitis	Observation, non-steroidal anti-inflammatory drugs	Rule out other infection. May recur within 6 mo.

ruption, or gait disturbance. Any positive findings should point to another diagnosis.

● **Clinical Pearl:** The classical picture of growing pains is that of a normally active child during the day who runs around nonstop, without interruption of activity or limp, but who often complains bitterly at night.

The clinical picture of apophysitis is that of pain that worsens with activity, although pain may be present at rest if inflammation is significant. The pain may respond to NSAIDs and ice or heat, but relief is generally limited and short. Apophysitis always features point tenderness over the inflamed portion of the limb. In OSD the anterior shin will be markedly tender and prominent with mild erythema and swelling. There may be a limp, and range of motion of the knee will be painful, especially with extension and extension against resistance. "Jumper's knee" can be differentiated by tenderness over the lower pole of the patella, with no significant swelling or bony prominence. Knee straightening may be painless, but resisted bending will often elicit symptoms. Sever's disease involves tenderness over the back of the foot, directly at the end of the heel bone. There may be a reddened, prominent area with increased warmth locally as in OSD. Children will have difficulty standing on their toes but complain of most pain when duck or heel walking.

Diagnostic Studies

If the clinical picture is classic for either growing pains or true apophysis, extensive laboratory or radiographic testing may not be necessary. If there is a history of trauma or any systemic illness, providers should obtain x-rays of the limb (or limbs) to rule out fracture, infection, or another less common entity.

For growing pains, x-rays and laboratory studies are by definition negative and unnecessary unless the pain persists for an extended period. Radiographs of the painful area in OSD or other apophysitis will show elevation and widening of the growth plate and possibly fragmentation of the bone. It may be difficult to differentiate OSD from acute fracture of the tibial tubercle.

Management

Growing pains will almost always respond to gentle massage, ice or heat, and occasionally analgesics. Gentle stretching may be useful, particularly in long-standing cases. Episodes will typically be of limited duration, lasting no more than 6 to 9 months, and recurrence is extremely unusual. If the pain is persistent, or if it worsens in the face of other clinical findings, the provider should evaluate the child with a complete work-up including x-rays, bone scan, and screening labs. The clinician should evaluate the child with persistent episodes of waking from sleep for possibly non-orthopedic etiology, such as night terrors or recurrent muscular spasm.

Treatment of apophysitis includes anti-inflammatory doses of NSAIDs, gentle stretching, and short-term activity modification. Bracing can be helpful, with a patellar-stabilizing ("donut hole") sleeve knee brace for OSD or "jumper's knee" and heel wedges for Sever's disease. In severe cases, the child may need short-term casting to allow the inflammation to completely resolve. Although by definition all apophysitis will resolve at the cessation of growth, early aggressive treatment is advocated to minimize the painful course and to allow as quick a return to normal activity as possible. As with growing pains, recurrence is highly unusual.

Although most cases of apophysitis and growing pains can be treated at the primary care level, clinicians should refer recalcitrant cases for further evaluation and possibly more aggressive therapy. Providers should reassure parents and children that the pain is self-limited and will resolve with conservative care, but that any bony deformity is permanent.

SLIPPED CAPITAL FEMORAL EPIPHYSIS (SCFE)

Providers should suspect slipped capital femoral epiphysis (SCFE), another surgical emergency, in all adolescents with groin or thigh pain. SCFE also may present as knee pain. In severe cases, the pain may mimic an acute fracture of the hip and may progress to long-standing problems such as bone collapse or arthritis.

Pathology

Loss of the constraining rim of the upper growth plate of the thighbone allows slow migration of the femoral head off its neck. If the migration is slow enough ("stable"), the growth plate may stretch and remodel. The growth plate can be unstable, however, and may slip more rapidly ("unstable"), leading to more severe symptoms (Kallio, 1995). The process may be hormonally mediated, although the actual mechanism of the slip is unclear. Obesity and endocrine disorders, such as hypothyroidism, renal disease, or growth hormone usage, may predispose children (Kehl, 1996). Children with SCFE will have delayed bone age.

Epidemiology

SCFE occurs most frequently in adolescents ages 12 to 15 years, with a slightly higher incidence in males. Incidence of clinically significant slips is approximately 1:50,000, although there also may be subacute or silent slips (Kehl, 1996). SCFE occurs bilaterally in up to 50% of cases, so providers should assess the non-painful side as well. There is no clearly defined familial trait, aside from predisposing endocrine diseases.

History and Physical Exam

The child with SCFE will present with a painful limp and pain that may be localized to the groin, thigh, or anterior and medial knee. The child may recall acute trauma, although far less significant than the symptoms would indicate. Frequently, the pain will have been long-standing with an acute exacerbation.

● **Clinical Pearl:** The most important point on history is the child's ability to bear weight, with or without pain. Inability to bear weight indicates unstable SCFE and may determine the acuity of care and eventual outcome (see Table 44-4).

On physical exam, range of motion of the hip will be significantly limited, particularly internal rotation both with the hip flexed and fully straight. Flexion of the hip leads to "obligate" external rotation and abduction of the hip. Table 44-4 reviews the clinical picture and treatment recommendations for stable and unstable SCFE.

▲ **Clinical Warning:** The provider should test range of motion very gently since aggressive movement of the hip can

Table 44–4. CLASSIFICATION OF SLIPPED CAPITAL FEMORAL EPIPHYSIS WITH REFERRAL AND TREATMENT CONSIDERATIONS

	Clinical Picture	Referral and Treatment Considerations
Unstable	Marked severe pain; inability to bear weight.	X-ray and refer emergently. May require emergent surgical fixation.
Stable	Pain more indolent. Able to bear weight, although may be painful.	X-ray. Refer urgently (within 1–2 days). Crutches for ambulation until then

further displace the SCFE and may disrupt the hip's blood supply.

Diagnostic Studies

Providers should obtain x-rays (AP and "frog lateral" or true lateral) in all suspected cases. X-rays will show a classic pattern of slip with the femoral head rotated posteriorly and medially with respect to the femoral neck. See Figure 44-3.

● **Clinical Pearl:** SCFE may be bilateral in up to 50% of cases, so the contralateral side should also be imaged.

Laboratory work is generally negative and is not recommended as a routine screen. Providers should obtain endocrine studies (thyroid function tests, calcium, phosphate, alkaline phosphatase, renal or liver function tests) when SCFE occurs in an unusual clinical setting, particu-larly in a thin-framed child or a child younger than age 10 years.

Management

Treatment of SCFE is always an urgent or emergent surgical stabilization of the growth plate. Providers should treat unstable slips with pin fixation at the earliest possible time. The child should remain on strict bed rest until surgery. Stable SCFE can be referred and treated on a semi-elective basis (within 6 or 7 days of diagnosis) if the patient can be reliably protected with a two-crutch gait and limited weight-bearing on the affected side.

Clinicians should inform children and parents that there may be some long-term disability depending on the amount of slip and the functional loss at presentation. The child will be on crutches for an extended period (up to 1 month) and may require physical therapy. Recurrence even after surgical

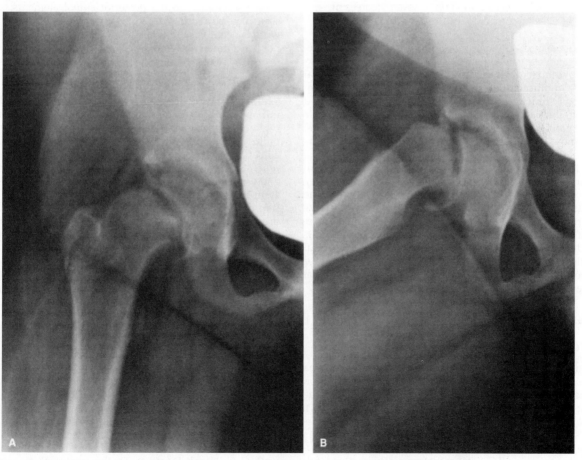

Figure 44–3 ■ Slipped capital femoral epiphysis in a 12-year-old child. Note that the displacement is more apparent on the frog lateral (B) than on the AP x-ray. (From Morrissy, R.T., & Weinstein, S. L.. [eds.]. [1996]. *Lovell and Winter's pediatric orthopaedics* [4th ed.] Philadelphia: Lippincott-Raven.)

fixation is possible (5% to 10% of cases), as are late problems such as arthritis. Because of the high risk of bilateral involvement, the clinician should encourage child and parent to report any further hip or leg pain as early as possible in its course.

ACUTE BACK DISORDERS

Back pain can frequently lead to disruption of gait and other activities in children. The most frequent disorders leading to back pain in children include the following:

Stress fractures (spondylolysis)
Infection — either localized to the bone or originating in another organ, such as kidney or base of the lung
Tumors

▲ **Clinical Warning:** Unlike adults, true "muscular" back pain is very unusual in children (Ginsberg, 1997). Therefore the work-up of a child complaining of back pain should be aggressive, with x-rays recommended for all but the mildest cases.

Acute trauma leading to spinal fracture is generally the result of high-level injury and probably will not present primarily in the out-patient setting. Disc disease, such as herniation, is relatively uncommon, but providers should suspect it in a child with unilateral back and leg pain.

● **Clinical Pearl:** Scoliosis, even up to severe degrees of curvature, does not ordinarily lead to pain.

With increased activity levels, athletic training and expectations, and especially increased weight of school book-bags, pediatric orthopedists are seeing an anecdotal increase in muscular strain in children. The clinical examination is similar for all disorders: the provider should examine the back upright and with forward bend to rule out curvature or other asymmetry. He or she can palpate the spinous processes over the entire extent of the spine and note any point tenderness. In addition, the clinician should check the paravertebral muscles for spasm. With the patient lying down, the provider tests a straight leg raise on both sides. The test is considered positive if the patient experiences pain under 40°. This sign of nerve root irritation may indicate discogenic pain. The "figure-4" test, with pain when one leg is bent across the other, is considered highly indicative of sacroiliac pain. A careful neurological exam focusing on the sensory and motor systems as well as the deep tendon reflexes is essential whenever providers suspect back pain.

Stress Fracture (Spondylolysis)

Pathology

The lower back stress injury typically occurs in an area where there is a defect of the normal bony connection between distinct embryological areas, typically between the lowest lumbar vertebra (L5) and the sacrum or pelvis (S1). As the body grows, this area may stretch, leading to a forward slip of the upper vertebral body ("spondylolisthesis") or to an acute fracture ("spondylolysis"). The lowest articular level of the spine (L5–S1) is most frequently involved, followed closely by L4 to L5.

Epidemiology

Symptomatic spondylolysis may occur at any age but is most frequent in early adolescence. It is most common in young athletes who participate in flexibility-type activities such as ballet, gymnastics, or skating (Lonstein, 1996). Wrestlers and football players also have a higher incidence.

History and Physical Exam

The history may reveal some activity producing flexion stress to the spine. The child presents with focal low back pain either acutely or chronically. Even in acute pain, there is often a history of "backaches."

● **Clinical Pearl:** In spondylolysis, the pain is worse when the child sits in one position for an extended period, such as in class. Although it is unusual to report night pain, the child may complain of pain when first awakening.

Physical examination demonstrates point tenderness over the posterior elements of the lower spine, usually at the junction of the lumbar and sacral spines. Bending is usually exquisitely painful, and muscular spasm will occur around the lower spine. Although the straight leg test is negative, tightness of the back of the knees and some pain in the hamstrings may occur when the leg is flexed to 90°.

Diagnostic Studies

Although the x-ray is frequently diagnostic, demonstrating a classic separation in the posterior spinal elements, a bone scan may be required to rule out an acute process. Blood work is negative, and unless there are systemic signs, should not be routinely ordered.

Management

Children may be treated with short-term rest and anti-inflammatory medicines, but usually also require a bracing regimen in the acute stages. A molded lumbar brace is recommended, although a commercially available flexible corset with a posterior bolster may provide some pain relief. The child should wear the brace all through the day and especially for sleeping, generally for 4 to 8 weeks until symptoms subside. Children may infrequently have recurrent episodes, although these are most likely muscular in origin and of shorter duration. Surgical intervention is rarely needed, unless pain is disabling or chronic or if there is progressive forward slip of the vertebra. If a true vertebral slip is documented, the clinician should refer the patient urgently for orthopedic evaluation. The slip will need to be closely followed to rule out progression into adulthood.

Infection

Pathology

The intervertebral disc, vertebral body, or sacroiliac joint may all be potential sites for infection. As with other orthopedic infections, the etiology is usually hematogenous from blood-borne bacteria, with mostly the same infective organisms as long bone infections (Ring, 1995). There is usually a significant inflammatory component as well as the frank infection, so the treatment may include anti-inflammatory doses of NSAIDs as well as antibiotics.

Lower spinal segments (lumbar, sacral) account for nearly 90% of all cases.

Epidemiology

Discitis is up to two times more common than true vertebral osteomyelitis, although the two entities overlap (Ring, 1995). Boys and girls are equally affected, with a common age range of early to late teens.

History and Physical Exam

The clinical picture of spine infection is impressive, with pain severe enough that even slight movement leads to marked distress. Fevers, sweats, weight loss, and other constitutional symptoms may be present. In addition to pain on motion and rigid splinting of the spine, examination will demonstrate acute, severe muscle spasm and point tenderness over the infected region. There may be nerve route irritation or sciatic-type pain into the back of the legs, most likely from muscle spasm. Neurologic examination will be intact unless there is a spinal abscess.

▲ **Clinical Warning:** The provider also must perform a careful chest and abdominal examination, since infections in the lower bases of the lung or in the kidneys (pyelonephritis) may mimic spinal pain.

Diagnostic Studies

An x-ray may show loss of disc height or destruction of the vertebral body. In the case of sacroiliitis, the sacral wing may show, but these changes occur late in the course and are notoriously non-specific. Bone scan or even MRI is generally more sensitive, and most sources recommend a screening MRI if osteomyelitis is suspected to rule out any spread to the dural space. Blood cultures, CBC, and ESR should be sent for diagnosis and to follow response to treatment. The role of biopsy for organism identification is controversial, since spinal biopsy has a high morbidity. Empiric therapy may be followed unless there is worsening or a lack of initial response.

Management

Except in the case of documented abscess, the initial line of treatment is medical, not surgical. Current recommendations are the same as for osteomyelitis and consist of 2 weeks of Nafcillin or Oxacillin (150 mg/kg/day divided every 6 hours) or a first-generation cephalosporin (100mg/kg/day divided every 6 hours) followed by 4 weeks of high dose oral antibiotics (Cefalexin, 100 mg/kg/day divided every 6 hours). Pro-viders should always prescribe anti-inflammatory doses of NSAIDs if the child can tolerate them. Acute acting NSAIDs such as Ketorolac (30–60 mg IM or IV every 6 hours for 48 hours) may have high success. Initial bedrest may be followed by a course of rigid bracing as there is clinical response to the medication. The bracing should continue for at least 4 weeks. If no clinical response occurs within 48 hours or the ESR shows no improvement by 2 weeks after treatment begins, surgical debridement may be indicated.

If the child has true sacroiliitis, the initial course of treatment should be anti-inflammatory doses of NSAIDs in addition to the antibiotics mentioned above (Morrissey, 1996). If the pain persists, cross-sectional imaging such as CT or MRI can rule out an abscess. Aspiration of the joint is a high-risk, low-yield procedure and is seldom indicated, although surgical debridement may be necessary in severe cases.

A child with spinal or S-I infection can often be treated definitively with non-surgical modalities. Consultation with orthopedics is indicated in a child who has limited response to medical therapy or for any child whose clinical picture or neurologic signs and symptoms are worsening.

Tumors
Pathology

Because of its rich blood supply, the spine is a relatively common site for primary bone tumors. The most common benign tumors are osteoblastoma in the posterior elements, hemangiomas, and aneurysmal bone cysts (ABC), both in the vertebral body itself (Springfield, 1996). In children younger than age 10 years, Langerhan's histiocytosis, otherwise known as eosinophilic granuloma, may cause vertebral collapse and pain (Floman, 1997). Primary malignancies of the spine are extremely uncommon, although metastatic small cell tumors such as Wilm's or Retinoblastoma have been described (Freiberg, 1993). In unusual cases, tumors in adjacent tissues in the abdomen may cause pressure that can mimic back pain.

History and Physical Exam

● **Clinical Pearl:** The most specific complaint in children with spinal tumors is night pain that wakes the child from sleep.

Osteoblastoma and ABC will have a marked (although temporary) im-provement with anti-inflammatory doses of NSAIDs which may be diagnostic. Examination will frequently show point tenderness over the affected level with no focal neurologic signs.

Diagnostic Studies

X-rays may show erosions or bony reaction in the posterior elements or the body of a vertebra. Bone scan is usually positive and confirmatory by the location of the lesion. The provider should obtain an MRI to determine the extent of bone involvement and to rule out spread into the spinal canal.

Management

Although many benign tumors will "burn out" with time and conservative treatment (eg, anti-inflammatory doses of NSAIDs), the duration of symptoms may be long enough to warrant interventional therapies. Excisional biopsy of a tumor can be curative, and most authors recommend excisional biopsy or heat ablation of the tumor. Recurrence is extremely rare.

Since the treatment of spinal tumors is most frequently surgical, urgent referral to a pediatric orthopedist or tumor specialist is necessary for all children with a suspected spinal lesion.

LEGG-CALVÉ-PERTHES DISEASE

Legg-Calvé-Perthes disease (LCPD) is defined as idiopathic necrosis of the femoral head, which can lead to bone collapse or deformity. The early inflammatory stage can also involve pain and hip stiffness. Although relatively uncommon, long-term disability may be severe enough to make this disorder a catastrophic event in the life of a child.

● **Clinical Pearl:** Children may present with a limp, but no pain. As with other hip problems (such as infection or SCFE), the pain from LCPD may be referred to the thigh or even around the knee.

Pathology

The actual event leading to LCPD is unknown, but it is theorized that an acute vascular insult leads to loss of the blood supply to the femoral head and subsequent bone death (osteonecrosis). The bone attempts revascularization, which can lead to weakening and collapse. The reader is referred to Figure 44-4. The ultimate recovery depends on the condition of the cartilage overlying the bone and on the child's remodeling potential. This is why younger children with the disease have a much better prognosis.

There is a strong family tendency, leading some to believe that a familial anatomic abnormality in the blood supply or possibly thickening of the blood components leads to the initial insult (Glueck, Crawford, Roy, et al., 1996). Early stage LCPD mimics toxic synovitis (see above), so there may be some relationship with infectious processes.

Epidemiology

LCPD has been reported in children ages 4 to 10 years, with the highest incidence in children ages 5 to 9 years. Boys have a five times higher incidence (Weistein, 1996). Children with LCPD tend to be of small stature and have delayed bone age. Bilateral involvement is unusual; if present, the provider should suspect a systemic developmental or growth disorder.

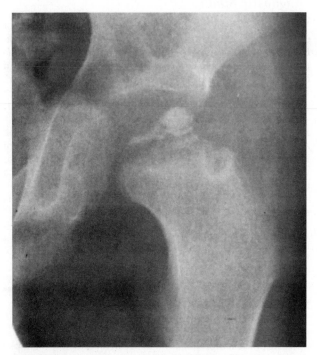

Figure 44–4 ■ Advanced stage Legg-Calvé-Perthes disease in a 6-year-old child. Note the collapse and fragmentation of the femoral head epiphysis. (From Morrissy, R. T. and Weinstein, S. L. [eds.]. [1996]. *Lovell and Winter's pediatric orthopaedics* (4th ed.). Philadelphia: Lippincott-Raven.)

History and Physical Exam

The history, examination, and laboratory findings depend on the clinical stage. The timing of each stage depends on the child's own growth rate and therefore cannot be generalized. Table 44-5 describes the clinical features of each major stage.

Management

In general, the treatment of LCPD is directed at containing the hip in its socket and allowing as much remodeling as possible. This may include bracing, traction, surgical releases, or bone reconstruction.

● **Clinical Pearl:** Although the extent of radiologic changes is an important prognostic factor, the most important determinant of outcome is the child's age at presentation. The younger the age of presentation, the more favorable is the prognosis (Herring, 1994).

Children under age 6 years do uniformly well despite the appearance of the x-rays. Children older than age 8 years do very poorly.

Any child with positive x-rays should be referred urgently for evaluation and treatment. A young child with persistent limp and limited motion may be referred for MRI to rule out early stage LCPD if x-rays are negative.

Providers should make parents aware of the seriousness of the disorder. Discussion of long-term outcome should be very guarded until a full evaluation is completed.

INFLAMMATORY DISORDERS

In unusual cases, the limp may be due to an inflammatory disease such as rheumatoid arthritis (RA), collagen vascular disease, or a reactive disorder such as post-streptococcal or psoriatic arthritis. In endemic areas, Lyme disease may be the most common etiology (see Chapter 48). The presentation of all these disorders may be similar and, except in very florid cases, the pain and the limping may be present for some time before the child complains. As with other processes, chronic leg pain is very concerning and needs close attention to rule out such a disorder.

Pathology

The causes and mechanism of inflammatory joint disease remain uncertain but are felt to be immune system modulated. A biologic trigger (protein or infectious) may cause the joint to produce destructive inflammatory compounds. RA and other types of arthritis tend to run in families; specific gene sites have been identified in more severe types of arthritis.

Epidemiology

The true incidence of juvenile arthritis is uncertain, since many of the milder forms may be underreported (Sherry, 1996). In its more florid form, arthritis has an overall incidence of less than 1 in 100,000 children. The forms may range from a mild, single-joint disease to a more severe condition involving other organ systems. Skin, kidneys, and eyes may be involved, and all children with suspected rheumatic dis-

Table 44–5   CLINICAL EXAMINATION AND LABORATORY FINDINGS IN LEGG-CALVÉ PERTHES DISEASE.

Stage	Exam	Labs
Early or inflammatory stage	Painful limp; Pain on ROM. No fevers or systemic illness.	X-rays may show consolidation of bone. ± fluid in hip. CBC, ESR negative.
Revascularization stage	Pain resolves. Progressive loss of ROM.	Collapse of bone, fragmentation (see 44-4)
Remodeling stage	Loss of ROM. Leg length difference. Trunk tilt on gait. Muscle weakness and atrophy.	Change in shape of bone; hip uncovered in socket.

ease require a complete multi-organ evaluation, including slit-lamp examination of the eyes.

● **Clinical Pearl:** Pauciarticular RA is the most common type of inflammatory arthritis in children comprising roughly 60% of all cases.

Pauciarticular RA is defined as the asymmetric involvement of a few joints without severe systemic disease (Sherry, 1996). Eye inflammation is a common component. The joint disease presents as low level pain and swelling, with some redness and increased warmth. The joints may be involved all at once or may arise serially, and the pain will be episodic.

Other forms of RA include monoarticular, hand-and-foot involvement, or global severe oligoarticular, or multiple-joint disease. It is difficult to distinguish true RA from other rheumatic disorders (eg, systemic lupus erythematosis (SLE), Reiter's syndrome, Lyme disease) on a clinical basis. Accompanying rashes or skin conditions are frequently helpful in establishing a diagnosis.

Non-rheumatoid types of arthritis such as Lyme disease, psoriatic, or Reiter's syndrome may be more frequent as a whole. There will most often be associated illness, and the disease seldom presents as an isolated limp or leg pain. Systemic symptoms such as fevers or weight loss may accompany the early onset of inflammatory arthritis.

Diagnostic Studies

Serum laboratory evaluation is one of the diagnostic criteria for inflammatory arthritis. The CBC will frequently show elevation in chronic inflammatory type cells (lymphocytes or monocytes). ESR is usually elevated.

● **Clinical Pearl:** Specialized tests such as Rheumatioid Factor (RF) and ANA are rarely positive in children and are of uncertain clinical significance.

Lyme titers and other immunologic screening should be ordered to rule out a treatable arthropathy. Specific gene patterns may be helpful in diagnosis (specifically HLA-B27), but are not screening tests.

X-rays may not show specific joint space changes until late in the course and, therefore, may not be helpful in establishing the diagnosis. Because of a high association of cervical spine involvement, x-rays of the neck are routinely done in patients with known arthritis, especially before procedures.

Management

Treatment will vary according to the extent of symptoms. Anti-inflammatory doses of NSAIDs, steroids, gold injections, and even anti-cancer agents such as methotrexate have all shown some effectiveness in limiting symptoms, but unfortunately do not alter the course of the disease (More-

land, 1997). Further genetic research may ultimately enable gene therapy as a more effective and specific means of diagnosis and treatment.

Inflammatory arthritis is uncommon, but should be suspected in any recurring or chronic joint disturbance. Any child with long-standing non-specific joint pain, systemic symptoms, and especially a family history of arthritis should be referred for orthopedic or rheumatologic evaluation.

OTHER SYSTEMIC DISEASES

Infrequently, the work-up of leg pain will demonstrate a destructive tumor in the leg bones. Figure 44-5 shows a proximal femur with a large unicameral bone cyst in the femoral neck. Although most skeletal tumors in children are incidental and benign, malignancies can occur. Like infections, tumors such as osteosarcoma or Ewing's disease have a predilection for rapidly growing bone, with peak incidence at ages 12 to 20 years. The presence of any destructive or suspicious lesion on an x-ray is indicative of urgent referral to an orthopedist.

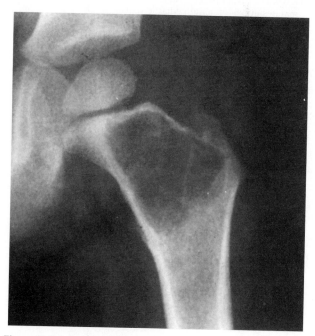

Figure 44–5 ■ Proximal femur with a large unicameral bone cyst in the femoral neck. Although a benign tumor, it may weaken the bone enough to lead to fracture. Treatment may involve bone grafting and pinning. (From Morrissy, R. T. and Weinstein, S. L. [eds.]. [1996]. *Lovell and Winter's Pediatric Orthopaedics* [4th ed.]. Philadelphia: Lippincott-Raven.)

The presentation of childhood leukemia as leg pain without other constitutional symptoms has been reported in anecdotal case reports, but fortunately the numbers are small enough to still represent a curiosity (Gallagher, 1996). The presence of other symptoms (weight loss, bleeding problems, excessive tiredness) may require a more complete hematologic work-up.

▲ **Clinical Warning:** Although cases are exceedingly rare, any child with limb pain that does not resolve or have a clearly defined underlying cause should be evaluated for an unusual presentation of leukemia or other malignancies.

Other blood abnormalities may present with severe acute leg pain. Hemophiliac children may have bleeding into the joints or muscles if their clotting levels become critically low (Rodriguez-Merchan, 1997). The presentation may be similar to acute septic arthritis. Children with sickle cell disease may present with an acute "painful crisis," probably caused by collection of the byproducts of destruction of their abnormal red cells (Smith, 1996). These children will have severe symmetric leg pain often requiring admission for intravenous pain medication. The clinical and laboratory presentation may be very similar to osteomyelitis, so careful evaluation may be necessary to rule out underlying infection. The reader is referred to Chapter 42 for a more detailed discussion of sickle cell disease.

REFERENCES

Dagan, R. (1993). Management of acute hematogenous osteomyelitis and septic arthritis in the pediatric patient. *Pediatric Infectious Disease Journal, 12,* 88–92.

Floman, Y., Bar-On, E., Mosheiff, R., et al. (1997). Eosinophilic granuloma of the spine. *Journal of Pediatric Orthopaedics, 17,* 260–265.

Freiberg, A. A., Graziano, G. P., Pritchard, D. J., et al. (1993). Metastatic vertebral disease in children. *Journal of Pediatric Orthopaedics, 13,* 148–153.

Gallagher, D. J., Dhillips, D. J., & Heinrich, S. D. (1996). orthopaedic manifestations of acute pediatric leukemia. *Orthopaedic Clinics of North America, 27,* 635–644.

Ginsberg, G. M., & Bassett, G. S. (1997). Back pain in children and adolescents: Evaluation and differential diagnosis. *Journal of the American Academy of Orthopaedic Surgery, 5,* 67–78.

Glueck, C. J., Crawford, A., Roy, D., et al. (1996). Association of antithrombotic factor deficiencies and hypofibinolysis with Legg-Perthes disease. *Journal of Bone and Joint Surgery, 78A,* 3–13.

Herring, J. A. (1994). The treatment of Legg-Calve-Perthes disease: A critical review of the literature. *Journal of Bone and Joint Surgery, 76A,* 448–458.

Kallio, P. E., Mah, E. T., Foster, B. K., et al. (1995). Slipped capital femoral epiphysis: Incidence and clinical assessment of physical instability. *Journal of Bone and Joint Surgery, 77B,* 752–755.

Kehl, D. K. (1996). Slipped capital femoral epiphysis. In R. T. Morrissey & S. L. Weinstein (Eds.), *Lovell and Winter's pediatric orthopaedics* (4th ed.). Philadelphia: Lippincott-Raven.

Lonstein, J. E. (1996). Spondylolysis and sponsylolisthesis. In R. T. Morrissey & S. L. Weinstein (Eds.), *Lovell and Winter's pediatric orthopaedics* (4th ed.). Philadelphia: Lippincott-Raven.

Menschik, M., Neumuller, J., Steiner, C. W., et al. (1997). Effects of ciprofloxacin and ofloxacin on adult human cartilage in vitro. *Antimicrobial Agents and Chemotherapeutics, 41,* 2562–2565.

Moreland, L. W., Heck, L. W., Jr., & Koopman, W. J. (1997). Biologic agents for treating rheumatoid arthritis: Concepts and progress. *Arthritis and Rheumatism, 40,* 397–409.

Morrissey, R. T. (1996). Bone and joint infection. In R. T. Morrissey & S. L. Weinstein (Eds.), *Lovell and Winter's pediatric orthopaedics* (4th ed.). Philadelphia: Lippincott-Raven.

Ring, D., Johnston, C. E., II, & Wenger, D. R. (1995). Pyogenic infectious spondylolitis in children. *Journal of Pediatric Orthopaedics, 15,* 652–660.

Rodriguez-Merchan, E. C. (1997). Pathogenesis, early diagnosis, and prophylaxis for chronic hemophilic synovitis. *Clinical Orthopaedics, 343,* 6–11.

Sherry, D. D., & Mosca, V. S. (1996). Juvenile rheumatoid arthritis and seronegative spondyloarthropathies. In R. T. Morrissey & S. L. Weinstein (Eds.), *Lovell and Winter's pediatric orthopaedics* (4th ed.). Philadelphia: Lippincott-Raven.

Smith, J. A. (1996). Bone disorders in sickle cell disease. *Hematology and Oncology Clinics of North America, 10,* 1345–1356.

Springfield, D. S. (1996). Bone and soft tissue tumors. In R. T. Morrissey & S. L. Weinstein. (Eds.), *Lovell and Winter's pediatric orthopaedics* (4th ed.). Philadelphia: Lippincott-Raven.

Tolo, V. T. (1996). The lower extremity. In R. T. Morrissey & S. L. Weinstein (Eds.), *Lovell and Winter's pediatric orthopaedics* (4th ed.). Philadelphia: Lippincott-Raven.

Unkila-Kallio, L., Kallio, M. J., Eskola, J., et al. (1994). Serum C-reactive protein, erythrocyte sedimentation rate, and white blood cell count in acute hematogenous osteomyelitis of children. *Pediatrics, 93,* 59–62.

Weinstein, S. L. (1996). Legg-Calve-Perthes disease. In R. T. Morrissey & S. L. Weinstein (Eds.), *Lovell and Winter's pediatric orthopaedics* (4th ed.). Philadelphia: Lippincott-Raven.

Acute Dermatologic Complaints

• HERSCHEL R. LESSIN, MD, FAAP, and PRADEEP SHARMA, MD

Urticaria and Angioedema

INTRODUCTION

Urticaria, commonly known as hives, consists of episodic pruritis with swelling of the skin as a result of histamine release from mast cells in the epidermis. In angioedema, the mast cells involved lie in the dermis. In this instance, histamine release leads to a more localized swelling, which is not itchy or only mildly itchy.

PATHOPHYSIOLOGY

The pathology of urticaria and angioedema varies with etiology. Urticaria is an acute vasodilatory response to an insult. The characteristic wheal arises from the increased vascular permeability of this vasodilatory event. When swelling is more diffuse, widespread, and accompanied by deeper tissue involvement, the process is described as angioedema. Histamine release from mast cells underlies the swelling.

In allergic urticaria, histamine (and, to some extent, bradykinin) is activated by an IgE-mediated degranulation of mast cells. This degranulation is an allergic response to an antigen to which the child has been previously sensitized (Friedmann, 1999).

Urticaria can also occur without antigenic stimulation. In these cases, mast cells will release histamine spontaneously (twitchy mast cell syndrome), as seen in patients with physical urticaria. Inflammatory cells, including eosinophils, monocytes, and neutrophils, are not prominent in acute urticaria. These cells can be seen in patients with chronic urticaria who may also exhibit signs of vasculitis.

Immunogenic Urticaria

Hives caused by immunologic reactions can be further classified using the traditional Bell and Combs method for classification of allergic reactions.

- *Type 1 hypersensitivity reaction*. This involves the IgE antibody. When exposed to antigens to which they were previously sensitized, allergic individuals may develop urticaria of varying intensity. Type 1 reaction is often associated with other signs of an acute allergic reaction, including wheezing, sneezing, and acute anaphylaxis. The most common etiology in pediatrics is an allergic reaction to hymenoptera, foods, drugs, or exposure to animal dander or saliva. See Chapter 48, Environmental Hazards, for further discussion on the diagnosis and management of anaphylaxis.

- *Type II hypersensitivity reaction*. Rarely seen in children, type II reactions occur as urticaria resulting from blood transfusion reactions involving IgG and IgM cytotoxic antibodies.
- *Type III hypersensitivity reaction*. In this condition, antigen-antibody complexes trigger a serum-sickness type of reaction which may include urticaria, arthralgia, and fever.
- *Hereditary angioedema*. This is a very rare but potentially life-threatening condition that presents as acute angioedema of the upper airway, face, and the gastrointestinal tract. This condition is caused by either an absent or dysfunctional C1 esterase inhibitor. This leads to a cascade of the complement system as a result of trauma, infection, or stress.
- Aspirin and nonsteroidal anti-inflammatory drug (NSAID) use. Unlike most drug allergies, aspirin sensitivity does not involve IgE antibody but, rather, the prostaglandin pathway. This trigger to urticaria and angioedema is seen mostly in adults who have chronic urticaria.

Nonimmunogenic Urticaria

Causes not mediated by the immune system include the following:

- *Direct histamine releasing agents*. Certain drugs (such as codeine and morphine), foods, and radiocontrast materials may cause direct release of histamine from mast cells, with consequent and prompt development of pruritus and urticaria.
- *Physical response*. This is a major cause of urticaria and may be a result of twitchy mast cell syndrome (where mast cells release contents with minimal provocation).
- *Cold urticaria*. Exposure to cold is the trigger. Children and young adults will present with urticaria after swimming in cold water, or with outdoor winter activities. Cold exposure can lead to massive release of histamine in these individuals, resulting in urticaria. Although rare, shock, and drowning (for swimmers), can occur.

  The most common form of cold urticaria is the acquired idiopathic type. Diagnosis can be established by placing an ice cube on the forearm, which will lead to development of localized urticaria with itching. The familial variety is very rare and transmitted as an autosomal dominant trait. These individuals develop urticaria after prolonged exposure to cold. Fever, arthralgia, and headaches may accompany.
- *Cholinergic urticaria*. Exposure to a hot environment or heat as a result of physical activity can cause cholinergic urticaria in affected individuals. This is a fairly common form of urticaria. The lesions tend to be wheals, which are 2 to 3 mm in diameter and extremely pruritic. This condition is occasionally associated with

exercise-induced anaphylaxis, wherein intense exercise can lead to pruritus, cholinergic urticaria, and anaphylaxis.

- *Dermatographia*. One of the leading causes of physical urticaria, dermatographia is seen in 20% of in-patients with chronic urticaria (Tharpe, 1996). Urticarial lesions are seen over friction- and trauma-prone areas of the body, such as the waist. Simply stroking the skin with pressure can provoke hives.
- *Solar*. This variant occurs because of histamine release from mast cells due to sunlight. The lesions develop over exposed skin upon exposure to sunlight.
- *Papular urticaria*. Children who have been bitten by mosquitoes, black flies, fleas, or other biting insects may present with papular urticaria. The lesions, seen mostly over the lower limbs, consist of pruritic wheals. The reaction may involve IgE antibody to the saliva of the biting insect. Occasionally, a delayed type 4 component may also be present.
- *Bacterial and viral infections*. One of the leading causes of acute urticaria may be bacterial and viral infections. It may also be seen with infectious mononucleosis.

● **Clinical Pearl:** In this instance: Group A β-hemolytic streptococcal infections may be associated with a treatable form of acute urticaria.

- *Vasculitis*. Urticaria associated with vasculitis is seen in a small number of patients with chronic urticaria. The urticarial lesions here tend to persist for 1 to 2 days and may be associated with signs of autoimmune diseases such as arthralgia and arthritis.
- *Urticaria pigmentosa*. When local mast cells infiltrate the dermis, small, hyperpigmented lesions develop which may urticate upon stroking (Darrier's sign). Urticaria pigmentosa is a rarer and milder condition in children than in adults.
- *Psychogenic urticaria*. This can be a chronic form. Stress is a cause, but more so in adults than in children.

EPIDEMIOLOGY

Urticaria and angioedema affect approximately 10% of the population. Often seen in children, it is usually a transient acute phenomenon. Chronic urticaria, which is a vexing problem in adults, fortunately is only rarely seen in children (Tharpe, 1996).

HISTORY, PHYSICAL EXAM, AND DIAGNOSTIC CRITERIA

A history of lesions establishes the diagnosis of urticaria. However, parents bring their children to the provider wanting to know what precisely is causing these hives. This question can rarely be answered. A detailed history may help to establish an etiology, especially using the classification as outlined.

Physical urticaria can be confirmed by history. Dermatographia can be established by stroking the skin. Cold urticaria can be proven by the ice cube test. Cholinergic urticaria can be diagnosed by a good history. Exercising a patient on a treadmill is not necessary.

DIAGNOSTIC STUDIES

Because urticaria is usually an acute, transient problem, a laboratory or allergy work-up is not generally necessary.

▲ **Clinical Warning:** Work-up is necessary only in those patients who have evidence of chronic urticaria (hives three or more times a week for about 4 to 6 weeks).

Acute urticaria due to type I reaction (acute allergic/anaphylaxis) can be diagnosed by history. Hives may be associated with signs of anaphylaxis. There will often be history of antigen exposure (usually an ingestant such as medication, drugs, or food) or by injection via hymenoptera sting. In this situation, an allergy work-up or laboratory work-up may be necessary immediately, not because of urticaria but because of the anaphylaxis which may be associated with it.

Chronic urticaria is occasionally associated with an autoimmune phenomenon. Hence, an erythrocyte sedimentation rate (ESR), antinuclear antibody (ANA), and rheumatoid factors should be obtained. In suspected hereditary angioedema, C2, C4, and C1 esterase inhibitor levels should be obtained. These will be low in patients with active disease.

● **Clinical Pearl:** In cases in which the diagnosis is in doubt, a skin biopsy may be considered by a dermatologist.

MANAGEMENT

Treatment is based on etiology. In cases of urticaria due to type I reactions, avoidance of the allergen, when known, is most important. Allergen-specific immunotherapy may be necessary in type I urticaria associated with life-threatening anaphylaxis, if appropriate antigens are available. These include hymenoptera venoms.

PHARMACOTHERAPY

In patients with active lesions, antihistamines (H_1-blockers) are the mainstay of treatment. Nonsedating antihistamines should be used, especially in school-aged or older children. Ceterizine (Zyrtec) and loratadine (Claritin) are available in a syrup form. Syrup formulation is a big advantage for children unable to swallow pills or capsules. A dosage of 5 to 10 mg once daily may be sufficient. Diphenhydramine may be added as a rescue medication at a dose of 25 to 50 mg, and repeated every 4 to 6 hours if necessary.

In urticaria not responding to H_1-blockers, the addition of H_2-blockers such as ranitidine can be helpful. Tricyclic antidepressants such as doxepin are reported to be about 80 times more potent than diphenhydramine and, hence, may be used in children with urticaria not responding to H_1- and H_2-blockers. However, sedation can be a problem with doxepin.

▲ **Clinical Warning:** The use of tricyclic medication in children and adolescents remains controversial. Before considering prescribing a tricyclic, the provider is advised to consult with a pediatric neurologist as well as with an allergist.

Corticosteroids may be necessary in acute urticaria, especially for angioedema that does not respond to H_1- and H_2-

blockers. Sympathomimetics such as epinephrine are useful in the emergency treatment of acute, severe urticaria, or associated angioedema or anaphylaxis.

Cromolyn sodium can help the itching of mastocytosis, but its effect on urticaria appears to be minimal.

Because urticaria can sometimes be unresponsive to the aforementioned medications, newer drugs are being looked into. These include the LTD4 receptor antagonists Singulair and Accolate. These plus the calcium channel blocker nifedipine have shown promise when used in conjunction with H_1-blockers (Tharpe, 1996).

Referral Point

The majority of patients with urticaria respond to H_1 receptor antagonists promptly and require no work-up or referral. The provider should consider referral if the urticaria occurs as part of an acute anaphylactic event. The clinician should also refer the child to a pediatric allergist if the urticaria is a chronic problem (lasting more than 4–6 weeks), if it does not respond to H_1- and/or H_2-blockers, if it is associated with systemic disease, or if the diagnosis of urticaria is in doubt.

Bacterial Infections

INTRODUCTION

Although the skin has many built-in defenses, bacterial skin infections are quite common in children. Children are prone to breaks in the mechanical barriers of the skin, and their often notorious lack of concern for hygiene predisposes to invasion by the countless numbers of organisms to which they are exposed on a daily basis.

Although bacterial skin infections can be caused by a broad array of pathogens, the most common causative organisms are group A β-hemolytic streptococci (GABHS) and *Staphylococcus aureus*. The different clinical presentations depend on the depth of the infection and its location on the body. Impetigo, ecthema, folliculitis, furuncles, carbuncles, and cellulitis are the clinical manifestations of bacterial infections progressing from the most superficial to the deeper layers of the skin.

PATHOPHYSIOLOGY AND PHYSICAL EXAM

Impetigo

Impetigo is a superficial, highly contagious skin infection. It occurs in all ages, but most frequently in younger children. Lesions can involve any skin surface but are most common on exposed areas. The causal organisms are streptococci and *S. aureus*. In the past, a distinction was made between impetigo with a bullous presentation and other forms, because it was felt that staphylococcus was the etiologic agent in bullous lesions, as opposed to the classic variety in which streptococci predominated. Today the term bullous impetigo is purely descriptive, because in reality, staphylococci are the most common cause in all lesions of impetigo.

Impetigo usually begins with a small break in the skin, which soon becomes infected. The lesions start with small erythematous macules or bullae surrounded by a thin erythematous ring. The lesions go on to enlarge and often develop the classic golden yellow crusts but can also have a smooth, red, "weepy" appearance or appear simply as enlarging bullae. The weepy exudate from the lesions or from broken bullae can be spread by contact to the patient or to others, creating the spread of new lesions.

Ecthyma

Ecthyma typically begins similarly to impetigo and has the same etiology. Bacterial penetration, however, goes deeper through the epidermis, resulting in a punched-out, ulcerative-appearing lesion. The initial lesion can start as a bulla, which eventually produces a thick crust. When this crust is removed, the shallow ulcer remains. Ecthymal lesions are most common on the lower extremities and often occur at the site of insect bites. They tend to have a more chronic course than the lesions of impetigo and can be quite painful.

Folliculitis

Folliculitis is a superficial infection of the hair follicle, usually caused by *S. aureus*. The lesions appear as small papules or pustules that are associated with hair follicles. They often occur in crops and are usually painless. In increasingly common subset is the so-called hot tub folliculitis, which is noted after bathing in an infected hot tub. The follicular lesions will often be more prominent in areas covered by bathing suits and are nodular or pustular. The causative organism is not staph, but pseudomonas.

Furuncles and Carbuncles

Furuncles, better known as boils, are superficial abscesses with central necrosis and suppuration. They are usually caused by *S. aureus*. They are more common in older children. They can be secondary to other, more superficial lesions such as impetigo and folliculitis, but they may also develop as a primary infection. Clinically, they are enlarging, red, painful nodules that are deeper in the skin. Over time, they become fluctuant and may drain purulent material.

Carbuncles are larger aggregations of furuncles that are more deeply seated abscesses. They can have multiple superficial lesions connected to the primary lesion that may drain. They are larger than furuncles, slower to develop and suppurate, and may cause systemic symptoms (eg, fever, chills) as well as local symptoms.

Cellulitis

Cellulitis is an infection involving the dermis and the subcutaneous tissues. The etiology is usually staph and GABHS with invasion via a break in the skin. Most cellulitis occurs on the extremities. A special case is facial cellulitis, particularly in infants. This often represents hematogenously spread infection and is much more serious, with systemic symptoms and complications. Prior to mass vaccination, the etiology of facial cellulitis was *Hemophilus influenzae* type B (HIB), an invasive organism with severe complications, including meningitis and septic arthritis. Since the introduction of the HIB vaccine, this etiology has all but disappeared. Staph, GABHS, pneumococcus, and nontypable *H. influenzae* species can also cause facial cellulitis.

All forms of cellulitis appear as areas of erythema and swelling that are quite tender. The overlying skin often has a thin, shiny appearance. The borders are not generally well demarcated, with the exception of erysipelas, a superficial cellulitis caused by GABHS, which has a very sharply demarcated border. A specific variant of erysipelas that should be recognized is perianal strep. This presents as a sharply demarcated erythema located around the anus and often the vagina that can easily be mistaken for a contact diaper rash. There is often pain on defecation with these lesions. Sometimes a rectal swab will test positive on rapid strep tests.

Staphylococcal Scalded Skin Syndrome

An exfoliative toxin produced by a staphylococcal infection causes this distinctive syndrome. Symptoms begin with systemic symptoms of fever, malaise, and irritability. Soon, generalized erythema begins, which can be quite tender. It usually starts in the skin folds and then spreads, sparing hairy skin. Next, exudate appears around the mouth and often the eyes, and the skin begins to appear wrinkled. The epidermis begins to separate and will come off with light touch (Nikolsky sign). Bullae can develop with generalized exfoliation, leaving the scalded appearance that gives the syndrome its name. This is a serious, often life-threatening illness.

Necrotizing Fasciitis

Necrotizing fasciitis (NF), sensationalized in the lay press as "flesh-eating bacteria," is also a serious, life-threatening illness. It presents as diffuse swelling of an extremity, followed by bullae that become violaceous in color. There are marked systemic symptoms with fever and toxicity, and the infection may progress to cutaneous gangrene, myonecrosis, and shock. There are two types of NF, one caused by anaerobes, gram-negative organisms, and enterococci, and another caused by GABHS. Early NF can look like cellulitis, but it requires much more aggressive treatment. Predisposing factors include varicella, breaks in the skin, particularly penetrating injuries, burns, and surgery.

▲ **Clinical Warning:** Varicella today may well be the leading cause of NF in children. Recently, there has been concern about ibuprofen use in varicella and the possibility of an increased incidence of NF. Studies are ongoing, but at present, most authorities caution that ibuprofen should not be used for symptomatic relief of varicella symptoms.

MANAGEMENT

Impetigo

The lesions of impetigo can be isolated or widespread. Small isolated lesions can be treated topically with mupiricin cream or ointment applied three times daily for 7 days. Over-the-counter antibiotic ointments penetrate the skin poorly and are not very effective. Crusts should be removed with warm water and the lesions kept covered to minimize spread. Good hand-washing is a must. The patient's fingernails should be trimmed in an attempt to reduce autoinoculation through scratching. For more widespread lesions, systemic antibiotics are indicated. Any antibiotic chosen must have good coverage for gram-positive organisms, including strep and staph. First-generation cephalosporins such as cephalexin and cefadroxil are good choices, as is erythromycin for community-acquired infection. Dicloxacillin is very effective, but the liquid form is highly unpalatable. Newer macrolides and cephalosporins as well as amoxicillin clavulinate may be used but are too broad in coverage and expensive. Penicillin or amoxicillin alone is usually ineffective owing to poor staph coverage.

Impetigo is generally uncomplicated, but there is a small yet significant risk of poststreptococcal glomerulonephritis. Certain nephritogenic strains of streptococci can produce glomerulonephritis in a significant percentage of those infected. Although treatment can eliminate the organisms, it does not appear to reduce the risk of nephritis.

Ecthyma

Treatment of ecthyma is similar to that of impetigo. Local care is even more important because the lesions are somewhat deeper. Systemic antibiotics should be used with or without topical mupiricin.

Folliculitis

For limited areas, gentle cleansing and topical mupiricin will suffice. Oral antibiotics are indicated for widespread or resistant lesions. Avoidance of external precipitating factors is helpful to prevent recurrence. Hot tub folliculitis due to pseudomonas is usually self-limiting and requires only local cleansing; the affected hot tub should be drained and cleaned. In severe cases, ciprofloxacin can be used, but only in older adolescents. Recurrent disease is often caused by nasal carriage of the organism. This can be treated by mupiricin to the nares three times daily for 5 to 7 days.

Furuncles and Carbuncles

Local care and warm soaks along with antistaphylococcal antibiotics are the treatment of choice. As with many abscesses, incision and drainage (I&D) is often the key to resolution. If lesions do not spontaneously drain with other measures, I&D may be needed. Carbuncles almost always require such I&D. Recurrent disease should elicit nasal cultures looking for carriage, and treatment if found.

Cellulitis

The treatment of cellulitis is dependent on its location and severity. Most limited cellulitis of the trunk or extremities can be treated with oral antistaphylococcal antibiotics, such as first-generation cephalosporins or dicloxacillin. Given the greater possibility of systemic or deep tissue spread of cellulitis, the use of erythromycin is rarely indicated owing to possible resistance. Use of newer macrolides such as clarithromycin may be considered in penicillin- or cephalosporin-allergic patients. It should be noted, however, that the molecular structure of the various cephalosporins is sufficiently different that an allergic reaction to one does not necessarily predict a reaction to another. In this light, many clinicians will not hesitate to prescribe a different cephalosporin.

▲ **Clinical Warning:** Outpatient management of cellulitis should be reserved for those cases in which systemic symptoms are absent or mild, the infection is clearly localized, and close clinical follow-up can be ensured. In cases in which there is high fever, an elevated white blood cell count, or clinical evidence of spread, such as lymphangitis, the clinician would be prudent to initiate hospitalization and intravenous (IV) antibiotic therapy after appropriate tissue and blood cultures are obtained.

Empiric IV therapy for cellulitis should consist of a semi-synthetic penicillin, such as nafcillin or oxacillin, or a first-generation cephalosporin to ensure good strep and staph coverage. In severe cases, IV clindamycin should be considered (see section on management of necrotizing fasciitis).

Facial cellulitis should usually be treated with systemic broad-spectrum antibiotics. In the past, hospitalization has always been indicated, although recently, outpatient treatment with intramuscular (IM) ceftriaxone has been used in selected cases. Given the frequent hematogenous source of facial cellulitis, the risk of spread to deep tissues such as joints, bone, or the central nervous system (CNS) must be a consideration. Chosen antibiotics must cover not only staph and GABHS but also hemophilus species. Parenteral third-generation cephalosporins with an antistaph agent are the drugs of choice. In all cases of cellulitis with systemic symptoms, the primary care provider must consider resistant staphylococci as potential etiological agents. If the local incidence of such organisms is high or if there is poor clinical response to initial empiric therapy, the use of vancomycin must be entertained.

Erysipelas and perianal strep are best treated with oral penicillin. Parenteral treatment is rarely indicated for perianal strep but may be necessary for erysipelas if located on the face or if the patient has significant systemic illness.

Staphylococcal Scalded Skin Syndrome

If limited in area, this illness can be treated in a nontoxic older child with the same oral antistaph agents discussed previously, assuming close clinical follow-up. In young infants or children with systemic toxicity or widespread skin involvement, hospitalization with parenteral antistaph agents is indicated. Close attention to fluid management in such cases is a must, because larger amounts of fluid can be lost through the denuded skin.

Necrotizing Fasciitis

Hospitalization is mandatory for patient with this illness, because tissue necrosis, systemic sepsis, and shock are common sequelae. In addition to parenteral broad-spectrum antibiotics, surgical debridement and decompression of the involved areas are almost always necessary. IV clindamycin, which has excellent tissue penetration, should be used along with other antimicrobials. Because some GABHS strains are resistant to clindamycin, it should not be used alone until culture and sensitivity results are known. Antibiotic therapy alone will rarely suffice. Again, close attention to fluid management and hemodynamic support is critical to outcome, because NF can be life-threatening. The management of NF requires a multidisciplinary team approach, usually necessitating the combination of skills and technology typically found in a pediatric intensive care unit.

Fungal Infections

INTRODUCTION

Superficial fungal infections of the skin occur frequently in children. The three most common etiologies are *Candida albicans*, commonly known as yeast infections; tinea versicolor, caused by another yeast called *Malassezia furfur*; and the dermatophytes, commonly known as ringworm. There are three genera of dermatophytes: Trichophyton, Epidermophyton, and Microsporum. All have multiple species capable of causing pathology in children, but the most common cause in children is *Trichophyton tonsurans*.

The clinical presentation of superficial fungal infections depends largely on the age of the child and the location of the infection. Dermatophyte infections are named "tinea" followed by the Latin word for the involved anatomic site. The use of the term "tinea versicolor" for a condition caused by a yeast lends confusion to this classification.

PATHOPHYSIOLOGY

Superficial fungal infections are just that: superficial. They affect the outermost layers of the skin (the stratum corneum), mucus membranes, hair shaft, and nails. Most reproduce via spores, which are contagious. When spores come in contact with the skin, their ability to cause disease depends on various factors such as adherence to the skin, ability to invade the keratinized outermost layers, and various host defense factors (Elewski, 1996). The latter are the most important. They include the age of the child, the integrity of the skin (eg, breaks in the epidermis or moist environment), the location of the infections (eg, diaper area, mucosal surface, nails, hair follicles), concomitant skin or systemic diseases (eg, seborrhea, diabetes), and the competence of the host immune system.

The host response to the infection can be highly variable. The immunologically mediated, inflammatory id reaction can be more impressive and extensive than the original causative agent, particularly in the diaper area and the scalp.

PHYSICAL EXAM

Candida

Candida has three distinct presentations, depending on the age of the child and the location of the infection.

Oral Candidiasis

Oral candidiasis, or thrush, occurs primarily in the mouths of young infants, although it can occur at any age if there is immunologic compromise. It is characterized by cheesy, thick, whitish plaques usually on the buccal mucosa and tongue. Unlike milk or formula, the plaques are adherent to the mucosa, which is often red and eroded beneath it. It is most common in the first few months of life. Some infants exhibit various degrees of irritability with thrush; others do not appear to be bothered. If it occurs outside of infancy, a search for an underlying predisposing condition (eg, diabetes, immunodeficiency states) should be considered.

Cutaneous Candidiasis

Cutaneous candidiasis is also most common in infants and toddlers who are still in diapers. Because the organism prefers warm, moist environments, this predilection is not surprising. In addition to diaper dermatitis (monilia), Candida can cause infection in intertriginous areas, particularly in obese individuals (intertrigo). In the diaper area, the lesions are often fiery red and show a preference for skin fold areas. There is a sharp demarcation between normal and abnormal skin, and there are often characteristic satellite lesions, which can be macular, papular, or even pustular, around areas of confluent erythema. Clinicians have likened it to a relief map depicting the coast of Maine, with islands off the coast. The rash typically looks worse than it appears to feel, because most infants do not appear to be affected by it. Most contact diaper dermatitides, if present for more than several days, become infected with Candida as well. Intertrigo in older children has a moist, almost eroded look in areas of skin folds and skin-on-skin areas in obese children.

Vulvovaginal Candidiasis

Vulvovaginal candidiasis is an illness of postpubertal females. It is more common with diabetes and with the use of systemic antibiotics. The labia are often edematous and erythematous. There are white patches on the mucosal surfaces associated with painful itching and burning. There may be dysuria as well. A thick, white discharge may also be present.

Tinea Versicolor

Despite the use of the term "tinea," tinea versicolor is a superficial infection caused not by a dermatophyte, but by a yeast. It occurs primarily in adolescents and is rare in young children. It is characterized by oval macular lesions on the shoulders, back, and upper torso. These can be erythematous and slightly scaly. A more common presentation is that of hypopigmented macules that become prominent in the summer when surrounding normal skin becomes tanned. Lesions can also be hyperpigmented, particularly in the winter, the presentation varies by the color of the skin.

Dermatophytes

The clinical appearance of dermatophyte infection is entirely dependent on the location of the process.

Tinea Capitis

Tinea capitis denotes a fungal infection of the scalp and its hair follicles. Clinically, infected areas appear as areas of hair loss, often with broken-off hairs a few millimeters above the scalp. It can also present as diffuse areas of scaliness, appearing seborrheic in appearance. Another distinctive form is "black dot" tinea capitis, with hairs broken off right at the scalp line. It is generally a disease of prepubertal children and is much more common in boys than in girls (Hurwitz, 1993). A common complication is a kerion, which is an inflammatory reaction resulting in a boggy, edematous, often oozing mass. This is commonly mistaken for a bacterial infection by the uninitiated, but it is inflammatory in nature and does not respond to antibiotics.

Tinea Corporis

Tinea corporis occurs on the nonhairy skin of the trunk, face, or extremities. The lesions start as red papules, then progress to the classic lesion of tinea corporis: an annular erythema with raised, slightly scaly borders and central clearing. This appearance resulted in the misnomer "ringworm" for this fungal infection. The ring will slowly enlarge with time if untreated. The lesions are occasionally pruritic. The lesions are contagious person to person, and exposure to infected domestic animals is also a cause of spread to children. Lesions can be single or multiple and may occasionally have a polymorphous or unusual appearance which complicates diagnosis. It can easily be confused with erythema chron-

icum migrans of Lyme disease, nummular eczema, psoriasis, granuloma annulare, and the herald patch of pityriasis rosea.

Tinea Pedis

Tinea pedis, or athlete's foot, is a dermatophyte infection of the skin of the toes and feet. It occurs almost exclusively in postpubertal children. It is very rare in younger children.

● **Clinical Pearl:** When lesions that resemble athlete's foot appear in healthy prepubertal children, they more likely represent a form of dyshydrosis or eczema.

Tinea pedis classically occurs in the interdigital webs but can spread to the plantar and dorsal foot surfaces. It can range in appearance from vesiculopustular to diffusely scaly. There is usually a large inflammatory component with painful itching and burning.

Tinea Manuum

Tinea manuum, or ringworm of the hand, is rare in children and occurs mostly in adolescents and young adults. It occurs primarily on the palms and can have a varied appearance, from diffusely scaling to a more inflammatory vesicular reaction. It can be mistaken for psoriasis, eczema, and contact dermatitis. It is often seen involving one hand, with tinea pedis on both feet.

Tinea Unguium

Tinea unguium (onychomycosis) is a dermatophyte infection of the nails. It occurs most commonly on toenails but can affect fingernails as well. Clinically, the infection starts with whitish or yellowish discoloration at the lateral and distal nail. Debris collects under the nail, and as the invasion worsens, the nail becomes more discolored and thickened. This infection is rare in children and occurs primarily in older adolescents and young adults.

DIAGNOSTIC CRITERIA AND STUDIES

Some superficial fungal infections are clinically distinctive enough to be definitively diagnosed by their appearance and location. This is particularly true of candidal infections such as monilial diaper dermatitis, thrush, and vaginal candidiasis. It is somewhat true of tinea versicolor and the classic presentation of tinea corporis as well. Although the Wood's lamp has been used to diagnose some fungi that fluoresce (eg, *Microsporum audouinii*—green-blue), this is rare. Tinea versicolor will sometimes fluoresce yellow.

The key to the diagnosis of superficial fungal infections is the KOH (potassium hydroxide) preparation. Because the clinical presentation of many fungi is so protean, identification of fungal elements is of utmost importance in order to come to the correct diagnosis and treatment. The lesion must be scraped aggressively enough to get superficial cells containing fungi. This is usually done at the periphery of advancing lesions, under the roof of vesicles or under the nail as proximal as possible. The scrapings should be placed on a microscope slide and a few drops of 10% to 20% KOH added. The slide can be left to sit for a few minutes, or better, heated gently to dissolve the cells, revealing the fungal elements. Care must be taken not to boil the KOH because this will cause crystalization, which by itself might be confused with groups of fungal hyphae. Alternatively, KOH mixed with DMSO will rapidly dissolve cells without heating. A KOH preparation is positive if fungal hyphae or spores are visualized.

In addition to microscopy, fungal cultures can be done in an office setting using dermatophyte test medium (DTM). Scrapings should be inoculated into the tube, and the lid should be loosened to provide air. A positive test result is denoted by a color change in the medium. Fungal cultures should be left to grow for at least 2 weeks. This test is of limited initial clinical utility because most experienced practitioners will have initiated therapy on clinical grounds.

MANAGEMENT

Candida

Oral Candidiasis

Oral thrush can be treated with nystatin oral suspension, which acts topically on the oral mucosa and is not systemically absorbed. This is sometimes a very stubborn infection that can take a few weeks to resolve. Providing the parents with detailed instructions on administration techniques may often spell the difference between therapeutic success and failure. Caretakers should be instructed to use a cotton swab to apply the suspension directly to the white patches, followed by instilling the drops on each side of the mouth between the gums and the buccal mucosa four times per day. Mouth objects such as pacifiers and bottle nipples should be boiled once a day. Nursing mothers should be instructed to apply the suspension to their nipples and areolae after each feeding. Treatment should be continued until the white patches are no longer visible to the naked eye and then for a few additional days. An oral preparation of fluconazole drops that works systemically is also available but, it is very expensive and should be reserved for those cases resistant to topical nystatin.

Cutaneous Candidiasis

Monilial dermatitis is best treated topically. The area should be kept as dry as possible. Cornstarch, which does not promote candidal growth, can be used as a drying agent, but talc should never be used, owing to the risk of aspiration to the infant. Keeping the diaper off for a while is also helpful. Any of the older topical antifungals can be used (nystatin, miconazole, clotrimazole). These are generally less expensive, and some of them are available over the counter. Some experts prefer newer topicals (econazole, ketoconazole) because they have some anti-inflammatory and antibacterial effects, but they are considerably more expensive. All should be applied twice daily. Topical terbinafine is not indicated for Candida infection. Mild topical steroids (1% hydrocortisone) can be used if inflammation is severe.

▲ **Clinical Warning:** Fluorinated steroids and combination products containing such steroids (Lotrisone) should never be used on diaper areas owing to the risk of developing dermal atrophy.

Vulvovaginal Candidiasis

Vulvovaginal candidiasis is best treated with over-the-counter vaginal suppositories, available as many of the same azoles previously mentioned, in a single dose or 3-day course. In addition, oral fluconazole tablets can be used systemically as a single dose of 150 mg.

Tinea Versicolor

In most cases, tinea versicolor can be treated topically. The most economical choice is selenium sulfide shampoo 2.5% (prescription strength). This should be applied to the entire skin surface from the neck down to the knees and wrists, with vigorous scrubbing or use of an abrasive sponge. The medication should be applied at bedtime, left on overnight, and washed off in the morning. This treatment should be done once weekly for 4 weeks and then once monthly for another 3 months. Alternatively, topical azoles can be used twice daily, but because of the extensive areas to be covered, this is quite expensive. Some dermatologists use ketoconazole shampoo 2% once daily for 3 days.

For severe or resistant cases, systemic therapy is an option as well. Several different regimens exist, but griseofulvin and terbinafine are ineffective and should not be used. Ketoconazole can be given in a dose of 400 mg and repeated in 1 week. Fluconazole can be given as a single 400-mg dose. Itraconazole and ketoconazole can also be used daily for 5 to 10 days at 200 mg per day. These drugs can be hepatotoxic, and liver function tests may need to be monitored.

Preventative treatment is sometimes needed. Monthly applications of selenium sulfide or monthly 3-day pulses of ketoconazole 200 mg have been used.

Patients should be warned that the pigmentary changes will not resolve immediately with treatment and are not an indication of treatment failure. The lesions will gradually repigment over a period of months.

Dermatophytes

Tinea Capitis

▲ **Clinical Warning:** Topical therapy alone is ineffective for tinea capitis and should not be used, no matter how mild the case appears initially. In children, oral griseofulvin remains the treatment of choice.

The dose is 10 to 20 mg/kg per day for 4 to 6 weeks. Treatment should continue for 2 weeks after cure is documented by fungal culture on DTM. Topical therapy with antifungal shampoos or azoles is useful in decreasing spread and hastening resolution. If a kerion is present, a short course of systemic steroids may be necessary to reduce the intense inflammation that accompanies these lesions. Although kerions look as though they are infected, antibiotics are of no benefit.

Patients should be instructed to look for sources of infection such as combs, brushes, and pets. Infected objects should be boiled or replaced, and pets should be treated.

Tinea Corporis

Any of the topical azoles (clotrimazole, miconazole, oxiconazole, sulconazole, etc) or topical terbinafine is effective. Lesions should be treated for at least 2 weeks and often should be treated for a week or more after clinical "cure." Combination products with potent steroids should not be used, owing to the potential of dermal atrophy.

For widespread lesions, oral therapy is also an option. Terbinafine 250 mg daily for 2 weeks, itraconazole 400 mg daily for 1 week, or fluconazole 300 mg as one dose with a second dose in 1 week are some options.

Patients should keep lesions covered and use good hand-washing to prevent person-to-person spread.

Tinea Pedis

For limited disease without nail involvement, any of the topical creams previously described can be used for 1 to 4 weeks. Topical powders such as Zeasorb can be a useful adjunct to reduce the moisture in the area. Systemic therapy for severe infection can also be used; dosages are given in Table 45-1. Teenagers live in sneakers and sweat socks, making for hot, moist, sweaty feet, which are the perfect incubating grounds for fungi. Counseling patients to take off their sneakers at home and to wear leather shoes on occasion is good adjunctive management.

Tinea Manuum

A trial of topical agents should be instituted. If this is unsuccessful, or if there is poor response, systemic agents can be added until the patient is clinically clear.

Tinea Unguium

Given the slow growth of the nails, long treatment times are needed for this condition.

▲ **Clinical Warning:** In cases of tinea unguium, topical therapy is ineffective. Given the potential for hepatotoxicity with long courses of systemic therapy, baseline liver function tests should be obtained and followed at least monthly during therapy.

Because of its poor bioavailability, griseofulvin has limited usefulness, and newer agents are preferred.

For all drugs, toenail infections require longer treatment courses than fingernails. Terbinafine seems to be the drug of choice, although other regimens have similar cure rates. Table 45-2 shows treatment regimens for fingernails and toenails.

Table 45–1. SYSTEMIC THERAPY FOR SEVERE TINEA PEDIS

Drug	Dose	Duration
Terbinafine	250 mg daily	2–6 weeks
Griseofulvin microsize	500 mg daily	4–8 weeks
Itraconazole	400 mg daily	1 week
	200 mg daily	2 weeks
Fluconazole	300 mg once weekly	2–4 weeks

Table 45–2. SYSTEMIC THERAPY FOR TINEA UNGUIUM

Drug	Dose	Duration Fingernails	Duration Toenails
Terbinafine	250 mg daily	6 weeks	12 weeks
Itraconazole	200 to 400 mg daily		12 weeks
	Pulse therapy: 200 mg twice daily for 1 week per month	2–3 months	3–4 months
Fluconazole	300 mg once a week	3 months	6 months

COMMUNITY RESOURCES

American Academy of Dermatology
930 N. Meacham Road
Schaumburg, IL 60173
Telephone: (847) 330-0230
Toll-free: (888) 462-DERM (3376)
Internet address: *http://www.aad.org*
Web site Patient Information section provides patient education and links to support organizations.

Dermatology Internet Service (DermIS)
Internet address: *http://www.dermis.net*
Project of the University Erlangen. Provider-oriented Web site is offered in English and German and features links to international institutions, organizations, and journals. Features the Dermatology Online Atlas (DOIA), an on-line image bank of dermatologic conditions, available at: *http://www.dermis.net/bilddb/INDEX-E.HTM.*

BIBLIOGRAPHY

American Academy of Pediatrics. (1997). *Red book: report of the committee on infectious diseases,* 24th edition. Evanston, IL: Author.
Degree, H.J., & Dedocker, P.R. (1994). Current therapy of dermatophytosis. *J Am Acad Dermatology* 31, S25–S30.
Elewski, B.E. (1996). The dermatophytoses. In K.A. Arndt, P.E. LeBoit, J.K. Robinson, and B.U. Wintroub (Eds.). *Cutaneous medicine and surgery,* vol. 2., pp.1043–1055. Philadelphia: W.B. Saunders.
Friedmann, P.S. (1999). Assessment of urticaria and angio-oedema. *Clin Exp Allergy* 29 (Suppl 3), 109–115.
Goldstein, B.G., Goldstein, A.O. (1997). *Practical dermatology,* 2nd edition. St. Louis: Mosby.
Hurwitz, S. (1993). *Clinical pediatric dermatology,* 2nd ed. Philadelphia: W.B. Saunders.
Tharpe, M.D. (1996). Chronic urticaria: Pathophysiology and treatment approaches. *Journal of Allergy and Clinical Immunology* 98, 6.

CHAPTER 46

Acute Neurological Complaints

• RONALD I. JACOBSON, MD, and MARTIN L. KUTSCHER, MD

INTRODUCTION

Paroxysmal events include any sudden, unexpected change in body position or mental state that may be any duration in length. These events typically last seconds or minutes and may be simple or complex, recurrent, and stereotyped. They may stem from a neurological process and represent seizures, a movement disorder, or a normal mannerism or habit. Nonneurological causes may mimic these events as well, such as nonepileptic seizures or a response to pain in an infant. Display 46-1 demonstrates the varied differential diagnoses that must be considered.

Seizure Disorders

INTRODUCTION

● **Clinical Pearl:** A seizure is an involuntary, sudden, and usually temporary alteration in neurological function that is produced from an abnormal electrical discharge from a localized or generalized neuronal source in the central nervous system.

Faced with a paroxysmal neurological event(s), the practitioner must first decide whether the event is a seizure, because this is the most significant clinical problem. Once an event has been determined to be a seizure, it must be further classified as to seizure type or seizure syndrome to determine appropriate work-up, prognosis, and treatment.

EPIDEMIOLOGY AND CLASSIFICATION

Seizures occur in about 8% of all people over a lifetime; however, the prevalence rate of epilepsy is between 0.5% and 1% of the population. Epilepsy begins before age 20 years in approximately 75% of patients (Holmes, 1987). Two different schemes are used in the classification of epileptiform events: classification by type of seizure and classification by epilepsy syndrome. The term *seizure* refers to the specific neurological event, such as an absence seizure or a tonic-clonic seizure, while the term *epilepsy* represents the chronic vulnerability or manifestation of seizure events. The term *epilepsy syndrome* refers to a full syndrome consisting of the type(s) of seizures seen in that syndrome, electroencephalogram (EEG) findings, typical age of patient, and typical prognosis. For example, absence seizure refers to the specific event of staring for several seconds; whereas absence epilepsy refers to the syndrome of a young, neurologically normal child whose EEG shows 3/second spike-wave discharges and whose seizures eventually remit in 90% of

patients. The seizures and their corresponding epilepsy syndromes are divided into two broad categories: generalized and partial. By definition, primary generalized seizures are those that start simultaneously from both hemispheres. Partial seizures start from one location within a hemisphere (localization-related epilepsy). When a seizure focus spreads or generalizes to both hemispheres, the seizure and process is termed secondarily generalized seizures. The epilepsy syndromes are similarly divided into the generalized and partial epilepsies. The classification of seizures and the major childhood epilepsies is summarized in Table 46-1.

HISTORY AND PHYSICAL EXAM

● **Clinical Pearl:** The distinction between generalized and partial seizures is important for several reasons and affects the history, work-up, and treatment of a child with seizures.

During the history, one must determine if the seizure has any features of a focal onset event: Did the seizure start or affect one part of the body more than the others? Was there an aura? The latter question is important because a well-defined aura certainly means that the seizure began focally. The aura of a seizure is actually just its focal onset. During an aura, the rest of the brain is "watching" that part of the brain have its seizure. In contrast, a generalized seizure does not have a well-defined aura. Consciousness requires one working cerebral hemisphere and an intact brainstem. A generalized seizure, however, affects the entire brain at its onset and thus leaves "no one there" to be aware of the spell. Determination of an aura, then, is extremely useful. Remember to ask both the observer and the child about the specific onset of the seizure. Young children may be unable to verbalize an aura and may just demonstrate unusual behavior or run to their parent to get help. Also, the aura or focal onset of a seizure may be so brief that it is not noticed before secondary generalization of the seizure occurs. Thus, a focal seizure does not necessarily have an identifiable aura.

● **Clinical Pearl:** Because focal seizures are more likely to have underlying focal structural abnormalities, classification of focal versus generalized seizures may affect the child's evaluation as well. In addition, different anticonvulsants are chosen based on the type of epilepsy classification.

Generalized Seizures

Generalized seizures include absence, tonic-clonic, and minor motor seizures.

Absence Seizures

Typical absence seizures can be subtle or distinct, and they always recur during the course of several hours or days. Absence seizures typically begin in young school-aged chil-

DISPLAY 46–1 • Differential Diagnosis
of Paroxysmal Events: Epileptic Versus
Nonepileptic

Epileptic Events
- Typical seizure is easy to differentiate
- For atypical types, note pattern and frequency, effect of sleep, mental status change, postictal state, and electroencephalogram
- Do not overlook focal seizures, simple partial seizures, myoclonic jolts, tics if single type, and repetitive sleep events

Nonepileptic Paroxysmal Events
- Apnea
- Benign paroxysmal vertigo
- Breath-holding spells: pallid and cyanotic
- Cardiac arrhythmias
- Cataplexy
- Colic (beware infantile spasms)
- Daydreaming and microsleep
- Episodic dyscontrol (rage)
- Gastroesophageal reflux
- Hyperexplexia (startle disease—may cause apnea and sudden infant death syndrome)
- Hyperventilation syndrome (carpal-pedal spasm)
- Hypoglycemia
- Jittery or tremulous baby (postanoxia, hypocalcemia, hyponatremia, hypoglycemia)
- Migraine
- Moro reflex
- Narcolepsy
- Night terrors and other sleep disorders (exaggerated sleep myoclonus in infants)
- Pediatric autoimmune neuropsychiatric disorders associated with streptococcal infections (PANDAS)
- Paroxysmal choreoathetosis
- Nonepileptic seizures (pseudoseizures or psychogenic seizures)
- Sandifer's syndrome (dystonic dyspepsia)
- Shuddering attacks or benign shuddering of infancy
- Spasmus nutans
- Syncope
- Tics and Tourette syndrome
- Transient ischemic attacks

dren. As with all generalized seizures, there is no aura. They consist of brief (3-30 seconds) staring spells, accompanied by a cessation of activity. Sometimes eye fluttering, mild lip movements, or twitches occur. There is no postictal state after a typical absence seizure.

Tonic-Clonic Seizures

Tonic refers to continuous stiffening of the extremities. *Clonic* refers to the rhythmic alternating contraction and relaxation of the muscles. A tonic-clonic seizure is one that starts with continuous tonic stiffening and is then followed by a clonic phase of rhythmic jerks. Most tonic-clonic seizures are accompanied by loss of bladder control and are followed by a postictal state characterized by confusion, fatigue, headaches, muscle aches, and no memory of the seizure event. Note that partial seizures may have such rapid secondary generalization that they may be clinically indistinguishable from true primary generalized tonic-clonic seizures.

Minor Motor Seizures

There are two basic types of minor motor seizures. Myoclonic seizures are brief body jerks, often occurring in irregular flurries. Atonic (akinetic) seizures are drop attacks. They are so brief that consciousness has been regained by the time the child strikes the floor.

Partial Seizures

Partial seizures are classified into three types: simple partial, complex partial, and partial seizures with secondary generalization. Simple and complex partial seizures may be quite subtle with little noticeable change in appearance, or they may be readily apparent to any observer. Do not neglect to take a careful history from teachers, school nurses, and even the young child, who may be able to draw a picture or enact the event.

Simple Partial Seizures

Simple partial seizures begin focally in one hemisphere and do not impair the level of consciousness. They may consist of virtually any task of which the brain is capable, such as jerking of just one extremity or abnormal sensation of one part of the body.

Complex Partial Seizures

Complex partial seizures begin focally in one hemisphere and do impair the level of consciousness. There is usually a well-defined aura followed by confusion, which is accompanied by lip smacking, fumbling, twisting or turning, neck motion, eye deviation, or eyelid fluttering. Unlike absence seizures, these spells tend to last several minutes and are accompanied by an aura and postictal state.

Partial Seizures with Secondary Generalization

Although the secondary generalization may be the most striking feature to the family, it is the partial onset of these seizures that matters most to the clinician. A *Jacksonian march* is the label given to a seizure that spreads through the cortex of one hemisphere with resultant spread of the clinical seizure. The child may be aware of this focal march along one side of the body, and then lose consciousness as the seizure spreads to the other hemisphere during secondary generalization.

Selected Epilepsy Syndromes

Comprehensive discussion of the specific epilepsy syndromes is beyond the scope of this chapter. Although a few comments will be given here about some prototypical epilepsies, the reader is referred to standard texts such as those by Swaiman and Ashwal, 1999, and Wylie, 1997. Children with these conditions are typically managed by their primary care giver in conjunction with a neurologist with special competency in child neurology.

Benign Rolandic Epilepsy

Benign rolandic epilepsy is the most common type of focal epilepsy in school-aged children. Seizures are often focal, such as just a rhythmic twitch of the mouth. A clue to the diagnosis is their predominance during sleep, especially during the later part of sleep just prior to waking. The EEG

Table 46–1   CLASSIFICATION OF SEIZURES AND THE EPILEPSIES

Generalized (start in both hemispheres)

Seizure Class	Infantile Spasms (EEG: hypsarrhythmia)	Lennox-Gastaut (EEG: slow spike/wave)	Classic Absence Epilepsy (EEG: 3/sec spike/wave)	Juvenile Myoclonic Epilepsy	Grand Mal Epilepsy	Febrile Seizures (EEG: normal)
Absence Seizure		+	++	+		
Tonic-Clonic Seizure						
Tonic Seizure		+	+/−	+	++	+
Clonic Seizure						
Atonic Seizure		++				
Myoclonic Seizure	++	+		++		

Partial (start in part of one hemisphere)

Seizure Class	Rolandic Epilepsy (EEG: stereotyped noctural spikes)	Lennox-Gastaut with Partial Seizure	Simple Partial Epilepsy	Complex Partial Epilepsy
Partial Simple	+	+	+	
Partial Complex		+		+
Partial Seizure with secondary generalization	+	+	+	+

EEG = electroencephalogram.

may be normal during wakefulness, yet sleep records show prominent stereotyped and simplified central-temporal spikes. The word "benign" is built into the name of this epilepsy syndrome because there is no serious underlying structural brain disorder. The response rate to anticonvulsant medication is excellent, and the remission rate is close to 100%. When treatment is indicated, carbamazepine (Tegretol) or the newest anticonvulsant agent oxycarbamazepine (Trileptal) is the appropriate anticonvulsant choice.

Absence (Petit Mal) Epilepsy

Absence epilepsy has commonly been referred to as petit mal seizures, but this is no longer the current terminology. This epilepsy syndrome usually occurs in neurologically normal preschool- and school-aged children who have absence seizures. These appear as brief staring spells during which the children stop their activity and are unresponsive to even strong stimuli. The EEG shows 3/second spike-wave activity, especially during hyperventilation.

● **Clinical Pearl:** Hyperventilation is an office maneuver that may precipitate absence seizures and is an important, simple, and quick diagnostic test. To perform an adequate hyperventilation test, the patient is requested to breathe in and out deeply for up to 3 minutes. Some younger patients need an aid, such as a piece of paper to blow with each breath. The patient is observed carefully during hyperventilation for any lapses in rhythmic breathing or staring. At the completion of hyperventilation, the patient is asked to count to 30—this is most revealing as the stream of speech and content is interrupted by an absence seizure.

The parent and physician together witness the clinical seizure during a hyperventilation maneuver, which allows precise confirmation that the parent's observations at home correlate with the actual seizure event. Parents should be reassured that the increased respiratory rate during physical exercise does not induce seizures and is physiologically very different from static hyperventilation. About 10% of children with absence epilepsy will develop tonic-clonic seizures. Prognosis for remission occurring within 2 to 4 years after the onset of the seizures is excellent. Treatment is usually valproate or ethosuximide.

Infantile Spasms

Infantile spasms, also known as West syndrome, is an epilepsy syndrome of infants beginning at 6 months and rarely commencing after age 3 years. Typical features include myoclonic seizures and an EEG finding of hypsarrhythmia (a triad of high-voltage multifocal spikes, disorganized background, and burst-suppression). These spasms usually cluster in bouts of 3 to 6 myoclonic jerks, momentary loss of tone, or as clusters of forceful extension or flexion of the head, legs, and trunk. The features distinguishing myoclonic seizures from the normal Moro response are given in Table 46-2. However, the distinction is not always clear.

▲ **Clinical Warning:** Because early treatment (typically adrenocorticotropic hormone [ACTH] injections) appears to be critically important in an attempt to maintain neurologic function, prompt referral should be made to a pediatric neurologist whenever this diagnosis is considered.

Table 46–2. MORO RESPONSE VERSUS
MYOCLONIC SEIZURES

	Normal Moro Response	Myoclonic Seizure
Age of child	Maximal frequency at birth	Rare at birth
	Stop by 4–5 months of age	Begin from several months of age to 2 years
Induced by stimulus such as load noise	Yes	No
Repetition	No, one Moro per stimulus	Yes, tend to occur in clusters over several minutes

Children with an identifiable underlying neurologic abnormality have a worse prognosis in regards to both developmental outcome and tendency to develop more complex or recurrent seizures (typically Lennox-Gastaut syndrome).

DIAGNOSTIC CRITERIA AND STUDIES

As an initial step, nonepileptiform conditions such as those in Display 46-1 need to be considered and evaluated as appropriate for conditions such as cardiac arrhythmias, prolonged QT interval, etc. Evaluation of seizures per se usually includes obtaining a complete blood count (CBC), SMA20, EEG (preferentially containing sleep), and magnetic resonance imaging (MRI) scan. A noncontrast computed tomography (CT) scan is frequently used as an initial screen in the emergency department but is not by itself generally a sufficient neuroimaging technique when evaluating seizures. It should be followed by a contrast CT scan or, quite preferentially, a MRI scan. Lumbar puncture should be performed if meningitis or encephalitis is a consideration. Toxicology screen may also be appropriate.

The diagnosis of an epileptiform event is established by carefully considering the history and correlating the EEG findings.

MANAGEMENT

The family needs to know that it is unlikely—although certainly not impossible—to be hurt or die from a seizure. The decision to treat with anticonvulsants is often made jointly by the family, the primary practitioner, and the neurologist. Factors in the decision include the type of seizures (including focality and duration), type of epilepsy syndrome, age of the child, family concerns, and EEG and MRI results.

● **Clinical Pearl:** In general, most neurologists do not prescribe anticonvulsants to children after a first, generalized, brief seizure in the setting of a normal EEG and MRI. In such a setting, the risk of a recurrent seizure is only about 30% (Swaiman & Ashwal, 1999).

The decision for each child must be individualized, taking into account the risks of seizures versus the risks of medication.

Anticonvulsant Therapy

An appropriate anticonvulsant is chosen based on safety, side-effects profile, and the type of epilepsy. The patient's age, gender, presence of other medical problems, and use of other medications are significant factors to consider when selecting which anticonvulsant to prescribe. As demonstrated in Table 46-3, certain anticonvulsants are more effective for particular seizure types or syndromes. Carbamazepine, oxycarbamazepine, phenytoin, and phenobarbital are indicated mainly for the partial seizures, but they also work well for tonic-clonic seizures. When possible, carbamazepine or oxycarbamazipine is usually chosen first in order to avoid the hyperactivity frequently seen with phenobarbital and the gum hypertrophy and facial hirsutism of phenytoin. However, phenobarbital is usually used first in children younger than a few years. Valproate works particularly well for generalized seizures, including primarily generalized tonic-clonic and absence seizures. Valproate is effective for partial seizures as well. Risk factors for valproate hepatic failure include young age, neurologic impairment, and concomitant use of other anticonvulsants. Ethosuximide use is limited to absence seizures. The newer anticonvulsants such as gabapentin (Neurontin), topiramate (Topamax), tiagabine (Gabatril), and lamotrigine (Lamictal) are currently indicated as add-on therapy for partial seizures in children older than 12 years.

▲ **Clinical Warning:** The use of Lamictal in children below 16 years is limited by the increased incidence of Stevens-Johnson syndrome.

Oxycarbamazipine (Trileptal) is very similar to carbamazipine, which it may replace in selected patients because it has a broader anticonvulsant effect and has fewer potential side effects. Oxycarbamazipine was released in the United States market in February 2000 and is an approved anticonvulsant medication for add-on use in children and for add-on therapy and monotherapy in adults. These new medications are described in detail in several review articles and standard texts (Pellock, et al., 1998; Wyllie, 1997).

Laboratory testing for patients taking anticonvulsants needs to be individualized. In general, a CBC, differential, liver function tests, and drug levels (when available or indicated) are monitored 1 month into treatment, then monthly for several months, and then every 6 months.

Discontinuation of Anticonvulsants

Typically, children are treated with anticonvulsant agents for a period of 2 years without seizures. At that point, the EEG is repeated, and the possibility of tapering the medication is discussed with the family and child, as appropriate for the patient's developmental or chronological age. After the complete clinical picture is considered, including the child's seizure history, presence of side effects to continuing medical treatment, and personal lifestyle, the anticonvulsant may be tapered over a 2- or 3-month period. Risk factors for a relapse include initial difficulty in obtaining seizure control, partial seizures, an abnormal neurological examination, and an abnormal EEG.

First Aid and Accident Precautions

For any child with episodes of altered levels of consciousness, whether due to seizures or not, it is appropriate to counsel families regarding first aid and reasonable accident precautions (see Display 46-2). These precautions apply particularly until the child has been symptom-free for 1 year from the

Table 46–3   ANTICONVULSANT SPECTRUMS

Seizure Type	PARTIAL — Partial (simple & complex)	GENERALIZED — Tonic-Clonic	Absence	Minor Motor (myoclonic & atonic)
Carbamazepine (Tegretol) Phenytoin (Dilantin) Phenobarbital	✓ ✓ ✓ ✓	✓ ✓ ✓ ✓		
Valproic Acid (Depakote) (Depakene)	✓ ✓ ✓	✓ ✓ ✓ ✓	✓ ✓ ✓ ✓	✓ ✓ ✓ ✓
Ethosuximide (Zarontin)			✓ ✓ ✓ ✓	
Benzodiazepine (Klonopin) (Ativan) (Tranxene)	✓ ✓	✓ ✓ ✓	✓ ✓ ✓	✓ ✓ ✓ ✓
Gabapentin (Neurontin)	✓ ✓ ✓	✓ ✓ ✓		
Lamotrigine (Lamictal)	✓ ✓ ✓	✓ ✓ ✓	✓ ✓ ✓	✓ ✓ ✓
Vigabatrin	✓ ✓ ✓	✓ ✓ ✓		✓ ✓
Tiagabine (Gabatril)	✓ ✓ ✓	✓ ✓ ✓		

DISPLAY 46–2 • First Aid and Accident Precautions for Seizure Patients

First Aid
- Stay calm
- Lay the child down with head to the side
- Loosen tight clothing
- Place something soft under the head
- Clear the airway of food, debris, or vomit
- Do not place anything in the child's mouth
- If the seizure persists for more than a few minutes, is followed by a prolonged postictal state, or is atypical, the child should be taken to the emergency room
- All first seizures require prompt medical attention

Accident Precautions
- No driving, or biking around cars
- No climbing higher than the child's height
- 1:1 supervision around water, including the bathtub and especially near or in shallow water when less caution is often exhibited (showers are usually left unsupervised)
- Set hot water temperature in the house to lower than scalding temperature
- Routine sports are allowed

---

beginning of diagnosis or after significant changes in anticonvulsant regimens. Practitioners should be familiar with their state's driving laws for patients with seizures and/or loss of consciousness. Most states require that the patient be free from loss of consciousness episodes for 1 year prior to driving. If this degree of seizure control is met, the ongoing use of anticonvulsants does not preclude obtaining a driver's license.

● **Clinical Pearl:** The general principle in caring for patients with epilepsy is to encourage an independent lifestyle and to promote self-esteem whenever possible and to the fullest extent appropriate to their condition.

■ *Status Epilepticus*

DIAGNOSTIC CRITERIA

Status epilepticus is defined as either continuous seizure activity lasting at least 15 to 20 minutes or intermittent seizure activity over at least a 15- to 20-minute period, during which time the patient does not regain consciousness. Status epilepticus is a neurological emergency, although long-term neurological damage is unusual. A study by Shinnar (Maytal, Shinnar, Moshe, et al., 1989) showed that most of the neurological damage seen after status epilepticus can be traced to the underlying etiology, and that 98% of children presenting in status epilepticus due to either idiopathic epilepsy or fever had a normal neurological outcome. There are several recent reviews on the treatment of status epilepticus in children (Pellock, 1998; Sabo-Graham, et al., 1998; Tasker, 1998). The most practical points are discussed in the following section.

MANAGEMENT

Supportive Treatment

It is a mistake to even consider anticonvulsant therapy until basic vital functions are evaluated and supported. As in any acute situation, attention should be first focused on the ABCs—airway, breathing, and circulation.

During the initial phase of treatment, a focused history and physical examination should be performed. The entire stabilization and seizure control process should occur during a 30-minute timeline. Particular historical points include previous history of seizures; medications prescribed and medication compliance; the state of the child before the seizure; presence of fever, trauma, and possible ingestion. During examination, remember to look for evidence of infection and other organ system problems, particularly in the neck and abdomen. Careful fundoscopic examination is important, searching for papilledema and retinal hemorrhages.

Initial laboratory investigations should include blood for electrolytes, glucose, calcium, liver function tests, CBC, and lead level in selected patients. When appropriate, also obtain drug levels, arterial blood gases, and blood culture.

● **Clinical Pearl:** Always run an immediate fingerstick glucose test on any patient with an unexplained acute alteration of neurological function to assess the possibility of hypoglycemia.

The finding of hypothermia in a patient with or without an environmental exposure or infection may indicate the presence of hypoglycemia.

Anticonvulsant Therapy

The dosages for medications used in the treatment of status epilepticus are given in Table 46-4. Notice that recommended pediatric dosages and rates of administration tend to vary among the different medications and may depend on the medical condition of the patient and previously prescribed medications. For example, the sequential administration of intravenous (IV) phenobarbital and a benzodiazepam in a compromised patient will increase the possibility of respiratory depression; the rate of administration may need to be lowered to prevent the subsequent need for intubation. The administration of medications used to treat status epilepticus should not exceed adult maximum doses. Because these are potentially dangerous medications being used in a critical life-threatening circumstance, they should be used appropriately by an experienced health care team including the medical, nursing, and pharmacy staff members. The recommended sequence of supportive therapies and anticonvulsants is illustrated in Display 46-3.

Anticonvulsant therapy usually begins with a benzodiazepam. Lorazepam (Ativan) is the preferred medication because its anticonvulsant effect lasts 4 to 12 hours, compared with only 20 minutes for diazepam. Thus, lorazepam protects against seizures much longer than diazepam, yet it

Table 46–4.   IV ANTICONVULSANTS FOR STATUS EPILEPTICUS

Drug	IV Load (Pediatric) NOT TO EXCEED ADULT DOSES!	IV Load (Adult)	Side Effects
Ativan (lorazepam) 2 mg/mL IV First-line drug in status. Anticonvulsant effects last 4–12 hours.	DOSE: 0.05 to 0.1 mg/kg (ie, 1/2 of Valium dose) RATE: over several minutes. May repeat every 5–10 minutes. Do not use PR (absorbs too slowly).	DOSE: 2–4 mg (ie, 1/2 of Valium dose) RATE: over several minutes. May repeat every 5–10 minutes. Do not use PR (absorbes too slowly).	Respiratory depression (especially if used *after* phenobarbital). Hypotension.
Valium (diazepam) 5 mg/mL IV or Diastat Gel (2.5, 5, 10, 20 mg) Anticonvulsant effects last 1/2 hour.	DOSE: 0.1 to 0.2 mg/kg RATE: over several minutes. May repeat every 5–10 minutes. May use PR (0.2–0.5 mg/kg/dose; we usually use 0.2 mg/kg). Remove needle!	DOSE: 5–10 mg RATE: over several minutes. May repeat every 5–10 minutes. May use PR (5–10 mg; usually ≤ 5 mg)	Respiratory depression (especially if used *after* phenobarbital).
Cerebyx (fosphenytoin) 50 mg PE/mL IV, IM Loading without sedation. Not for febrile seizures. Use same dosages as Dilantin, but can give 3 times faster than DPH because metabolized by body first, and less toxic diluent than DPH.	DOSE: 18 mg PE/kg if needs total load RATE IN STATUS: maximum 3 mg PE/kg/min (ie, load in 6 min) OTHERWISE: maximum 1.5 mg PE/kg/min (ie, load in 12 min) Note: In any IV fluid; Follow EKG and BP. Flush slowly at end. USE CAUTION. NOT FOR CARDIAC PTS!	USUAL ADULT DOSE = 1000 mg PE RATE IN STATUS: maximum 150 mg PE/min OTHERWISE: maximum 75 mg PE/min Note: see Pediatric.	Less likely hypotension and arrhythmias than Dilantin Also, parasthesias indicating need to slow infusion. No IV/IM site reaction.
Dilantin (diphenylhydantoin) 50 mg/mL IV (not IM!) Loading without sedation. Not for febrile seizures.	DOSE: 18 mg/kg if needs total load RATE IN STATUS: maximum 1 mg/kg/min OTHERWISE: maximum 0.5 mg/kg/min Note: In normal saline; Follow EKG and BP. Flush slowly at end. USE CAUTION. NOT FOR CARDIAC PTS!	USUAL ADULT DOSE = 1000 mg RATE IN STATUS: maximum 50 mg/min OTHERWISE: maximum 25 mg/min Note: see Pediatric.	Allergic reaction. Hypotension. Arrhythmias. Severe burns if IV infiltrates.
Phenobarbital	FULL LOADING DOSE: 15–20 mg/kg. Often use less, ie, 10 mg/kg to start. RATE: maximum 1 mg/kg/min	Usual adult dose given in 120 to 240 mg slow boluses	Respiratory depression. Hypotension.

BP = blood pressure; DPH = diphenylhydantoin; EKG = electrocardiogram; IM = intramuscular; IV = intravenous; PR = per return.

DISPLAY 46–3 • Status Epilepticus: Summary of Treatment During the First 30 Minutes

1. Take control of the ABCs (ie, airway, breathing, and circulation). Intubate when in doubt. Cardiopulmonary monitor. IV glucose.
2. Perform a focused history and physical examination, including fundoscopic examination.
3. Obtain stat fingerstick glucose, blood for electrolytes, blood urea nitrogen, glucose, calcium, liver function tests, and complete blood count. When appropriate, also obtain drug levels, arterial blood gases, and blood culture.
4. Give lorazepam (Ativan) or diazepam (Valium) bolus. May repeat every 5 minutes, usually up to three doses as needed.
5. Give fosphenytoin (Cerebyx) or phenytoin (Dilantin) IV load.
6. If the seizure continues, intubation should be very strongly considered.
7. If the seizure continues, give IV phenobarbital bolus.
8. If seizures persist, intubate if not already done, and check patency of IV lines.
9. Additional options include:
   • Further phenobarbital boluses (usually at 5 mg/kg bolus) until a serum level of 50 mcg/mL.
   • Further boluses of benzodiazepams.
   • Further phenytoin boluses to push the *total* loading dose to 25 mg/kg.
   • Benzodiazepam drips or general anesthesia.
10. See text for further evaluation such as computed tomography and lumbar puncture.

IV = intravenous.

---

ogist may allow IV use of either phenytoin or fosphenytoin with certain forms of arrhythmias, because these medications also have an antiarrhythmic action.

If the seizure continues, intubation should be very strongly considered at this point. If needed, phenobarbital is usually added next. As indicated in Table 46-4, start with less than the full loading dosage owing to the respiratory, hypotensive, and sedative effects of phenobarbital boluses, particularly if combined with a benzodiazepam drug. If seizures persist, the patient should certainly be intubated if this has not already done. Patency of IV lines should be checked. Further options include further phenobarbital boluses (usually at 5 mg/kg per bolus) until a serum level of 50 is achieved. Consider further boluses of a benzodiazepam. Further phenytoin boluses can push the *total* loading dose to 25 mg/kg. Finally, benzodiazepam drips or general anesthesia may be used.

Another relevant treatment paradigm is to consider treatment options for status epilepticus based on the location of the patient at the time of seizure. These measures may be started at home by the family or caregivers in a patient at risk for seizures, or in the ambulance by the emergency medical technician team, or in an office setting by the medical and nursing staff. Display 46-4 summarizes these options and may serve as the basis for instruction for knowledgeable caregivers of susceptible children who may benefit from home treatment protocols.

Management After Obtaining Seizure Control

After seizure control is achieved, a complete history and physical can be performed. In addition, a noncontrast CT scan should usually be obtained after the seizure is controlled, unless the history would indicate that this is unnecessary. A lumbar puncture should be strongly considered after the CT, especially if the patient has a fever.

is just as effective and is neither safer nor more dangerous. Doses may be repeated every 5 minutes as needed, usually up to three doses.

A phenytoin preparation is usually given next, if necessary. Even if seizure control has already been achieved, this medication may be needed to prevent seizure recurrence. If available, IV fosphenytoin (Cerebyx) should be used instead of IV phenytoin (Dilantin). Phenytoin contains high levels of propylene glycol (a cardiac suppressant), which may cause hypotension, and has a pH of 12, which may produce skin irritation. In contrast, fosphenytoin is a neutral phosphorylated formulation of phenytoin and is less likely than IV phenytoin to cause cardiac suppression. Phosphenytoin also does not have the potential of skin sloughs at an IV site infiltration. IV fosphenytoin can be given in any IV solution (unlike phenytoin, which cannot be given with glucose-containing solutions which precipitate the medication). The other main benefit is that fosphenytoin may be administered intramuscularly in a patient with no IV access. Phenytoin should never be administered intramuscularly. Although IV fosphenytoin can be given three times faster than phenytoin, its time to onset of action remains unchanged compared with phenytoin, because it is a prodrug and requires the action of a phosphorylase in the circulation to convert the inactive prodrug into phenytoin with its typical anticonvulsant properties in vivo. Cardiac arrhythmias remain the major risk of either preparation, especially in children with a history of cardiac disease or heart block. In fact, a prior allergic history or a history of heart block is a contraindication to using either phenytoin or fosphenytoin. Note that a cardiol-

---

DISPLAY 46–4 • Emergency Treatment of Prolonged Seizures Before Arrival in the Emergency Department

• Turn the patient on the side; clear the airway of saliva, vomit, food, or debris.
• Clear the surrounding area of sharp or intrusive objects.
• Loosen tight-fitting garments to protect the patient from physical harm and to allow better observation of the rate of breathing.

For those seizures not stopping spontaneously within about 3 minutes after onset:

• Call 911 or appropriate sources for emergency medical services.
• If available easily, get another person to help.
• If appropriate, administer rectal diazepam using the intravenous preparation via a 1 cc syringe without the needle (0.2 mg/kg) or Diastat to attempt to terminate the seizure.
• Some emergency medical technicians are trained to administer intravenous anticonvulsants on site and will follow emergency department management protocols including communication with emergency department personnel to individualize the treatment plan.

▲ **Clinical Warning:** Encephalitis can cause seizures without fever or meningeal signs. In such a case, the best clues would be altered mental status before or after the seizure or focal neurological findings during or after the seizure. Meningeal signs are also not reliable in patients with altered mental states.

Sometimes it is most expedient to give antibiotics and/or antiviral medication during the treatment phase and later perform the CT scan and lumbar puncture.

Hospitalization should be in a setting where careful monitoring and further intervention are possible, most likely in a pediatric intensive care unit setting. An EEG and MRI are usually obtained during this time. Maintenance anticonvulsant therapy is usually required, to be decided in consultation with a neurologist with competence in child neurology.

■ *Febrile Seizures*

Febrile seizures are quite common and occur in about 4% of all children. The average age of onset is 24 months; they are rare in children younger than 6 months or older than 5 to 6 years. They usually occur within the first 24 hours of a febrile illness at the point of a rapid increase in temperature commonly above 102°F.

Febrile seizures can be classified as simple, complex, or atypical (Hirtz, 1997).

- Simple febrile seizures last less than 15 minutes, are generalized, and occur only once per 24 hours.
- Complex febrile seizures last longer than 15 minutes, have a focal nature or occur more than once per 24 hours.
- Atypical febrile seizures differ in some other way from the preceding, such as a lower temperature than usual or unusual age of the child.

The more the seizure manifestations diverge from the classical syndrome, the better it is to call the events *seizures with fever*. Such a label is a good reminder that the diagnosis is not yet final or certain. Febrile seizures should rarely be diagnosed simultaneously in children who also have a diagnosis of afebrile seizures or epilepsy. This combination implies two separate diagnoses in one patient; the more likely conclusion is that the child has epilepsy that is occasionally precipitated by a febrile episode.

Although usually benign, febrile seizures are very frightening to the parents. They may not seem so significant to experienced health care providers, but most parents witnessing the first febrile seizure in their child are convinced that they just observed a near death. Reassurance is key, both with careful medical evaluation and with patient, compassionate, and detailed explanations.

DIAGNOSTIC STUDIES

Lumbar Puncture

According to the American Academy of Physicians (AAP) practice parameter, about 15% of children with meningitis present with seizures, and in one third of these children (primarily those younger than 18 months), meningeal signs and symptoms may be absent (AAP Practice Parameter, 1996). In

---

> **DISPLAY 46–5** • Risk Factors for Meningitis in Seizures With Fever
>
> - Suspicious physical or neurological findings
> - Complex febrile seizure (recurrent in 24 hours, focal or any seizure longer than 15 minutes)
> - Prior physician visits for fever within 48 hours before the seizure
> - Seizures on arrival at the emergency department
> - Prolonged postictal state
> - Initial seizures in a child older than 3 years

contrast, another study found a low incidence of clinically unsuspected meningitis in patients with seizures and fever (Green, 1993). It should be additionally noted that a recognized source of fever does not exclude meningitis (nor does a previous febrile seizure). Meningitis may be missed in cases in which the children are younger than 18 months, or when adequate medical care is not available. Risk factors for meningitis in a child with fever and seizures are listed in Display 46-5.

Although some physicians suggest a lumbar puncture for all first febrile seizures, the authors recommend it more selectively in the context of the entire clinical situation and taking into account the past and family history of febrile seizures. Indications for lumbar puncture in the setting of seizures with fever are listed in Display 46-6.

Laboratory Evaluation

CBC and routine chemistries are not indicated for simple febrile seizures unless suggested by the patient's history, physical examination, or the need for evaluation of the fever itself (AAP Practice Parameter, 1996).

● **Clinical Pearl:** EEGs, CTs, and MRIs are not recommended in a neurologically healthy child with a first simple febrile seizure.

> **DISPLAY 46–6** • Indications for Lumbar Puncture in Febrile Seizures
>
> - Lumbar puncture is recommended in a child younger than 12 months.
> - Lumbar puncture is necessary if the history, physical examination, or laboratory data suggest an intracranial infection or sepsis.
> - Lumbar puncture should be strongly considered for children who were previously on antibiotics, or when antibiotics will be started for systemic infections.
> - Lumbar puncture should be strongly considered if the patient will be sedated with anticonvulsants.
> - Lumbar puncture should be considered for children ages 12 to 24 months.
> - Children with atypical or complex febrile seizures are at a higher risk of serious pathology and generally need CT scan, lumbar puncture, and admission.
> - Lumbar puncture is not needed in a well or healthy-appearing older child after a simple febrile seizure unless other risk factors are present.

EEGs and MRIs are usually obtained if the seizures are complex or atypical, the child is neurologically abnormal, or if there are multiple febrile seizures. Even so, studies fail to show the usefulness of EEGs of predicting epilepsy in these cases.

MANAGEMENT

For the vast majority of simple febrile seizures, management should be directed toward reassuring and educating the family.

● **Clinical Pearl:** The clinician must stress that as frightening as the seizure appears, it causes no damage to the child (AAP, 1999). Parental fear and anxiety are the only sequelae.

There is no evidence that simple febrile seizures cause structural central nervous system (CNS) damage or promote the development of mental retardation. Recurrence, however, is distinctly probable, and the possibility of recurrence should be discussed openly and honestly. Children younger than 1 year with their first simple febrile seizure have a 50% risk of developing a recurrence. After 1 year of age, the risk drops to 30% after one episode but is 50% after the second. Parents should be reassured that the risk of developing epilepsy is very small, approximating 1% for a simple febrile seizure. Even for patients at greatest risk (multiple simple febrile seizures beginning at age younger than 1 year), the risk is only 2.4% (AAP, 1999).

Hospitalization

Children with typical simple febrile seizures are usually not hospitalized—assuming they look well, do not need hospitalization for other reasons, have been observed for several hours, and have reliable caretakers who are comfortable watching the child at home. Atypical or complex features indicate a risk of underlying CNS pathology and usually indicate the need for in-patient observation or treatment.

Risks and Treatment Options

Because the risk of developing epilepsy after febrile seizures is low and maintenance anticonvulsant medication does not reduce this risk, long-term anticonvulsant therapy is not recommended for the vast majority of children with febrile seizures.

▲ **Clinical Warning:** The AAP in its 1999 Practice Parameter states categorically that "neither continuous nor intermittent anticonvulsant therapy is recommended for children with one or more simple febrile seizures."

Children with frequent recurrence of complex (prolonged) febrile seizures, those who have underlying neurological abnormalities, or those extreme cases in which parental anxiety colors the entire family's ability to function normally may benefit from some form of pharmacological intervention.

▲ **Clinical Warning:** It should be stressed that anticonvulsant therapy for febrile seizures should never be a substitute for parental education and counseling.

Options include rectal diazepam for intermittent use to control prolonged seizures and continuous daily phenobarbital prophylaxis. The known side effects of hyperactivity and potential learning difficulties make daily phenobarbital prophylaxis a far less desirable option.

In 1997, the U.S. Food and Drug Administration (FDA) approved a rectal diazepam gel preparation called Diastat, the first at-home FDA-approved alternative for the IV form of the drug diazepam, already used by emergency departments to stop a seizure. Designed specifically for patients affected by multiple, frequent, and prolonged seizures, Diastat starts to reach the bloodstream in about 2 minutes.

Valproic acid (Depakene, Depakote) treatment is also effective for febrile seizure prophylaxis but is rarely used in this setting because of the potential hepatotoxicity in this age range. Phenytoin (Dilantin) is not effective in the treatment of febrile seizures. In the setting of a prolonged febrile seizure approaching the duration definition of status epilepticus, phenobarbital should probably be used for follow-up after the benzodiazepam. Treatment options are illustrated in Displays 46-7 and 46-8.

DISPLAY 46–7 • Rectal Diazepam for Treatment of Febrile Seizures

Commonly Used Indications:
- Children with prolonged febrile seizures
- Children with multiple febrile seizures
- Children with high risk of recurrent seizures

Dosage:
- Diazepam 0.2 mg/kg per rectum (usual maximum 5 mg) for a seizure longer than 3 minutes. Some authors recommend 0.3 to 0.5 mg/kg (not to exceed 10 mg) per rectum.
- Diastat dose is 0.5 mg/kg because it is absorbed more slowly. Pediatric-sized rectal dispensers are prefilled at 2.5 mg, 5 mg, and 10 mg syringes.
- In children with high risk of recurrence, the use of rectal diazepam as needed for fever itself may be appropriate.

Important Points:
- Parents must be carefully instructed on the use of rectal diazepam.
- Lorazepam (Ativan) is not recommended rectally for status because it may take 45 minutes to be absorbed.
- Diastat brand of rectal diazepam suppositories is FDA-approved, although the intravenous preparation of diazepam is often used "off label" via a TB syringe with the needle off.
- Sedation and rare instances of respiratory depression are possible side effects.

FDA = Food and Drug Administration.

DISPLAY 46–8 • Phenobarbital Prophylaxis for Febrile Seizures

Usual Indications:
- Neurologically abnormal children with prolonged febrile seizures.
- Rarely, some practitioners treat neurologically normal children with prolonged or frequent febrile seizures for several weeks to several months (see text).

Dosage:
- Phenobarbital 5 mg/kg per day divided into two doses (starting dose not to exceed 90 mg total per day).

Important Points:
- Phenobarbital given orally only at the time of fever to prevent seizures is **not** effective.
- Most common side effects are hyperactivity, sedation, learning difficulty, or rash.

Movement Disorders

INTRODUCTION

Display 46-1 reviewed the nonepileptic conditions that are considered in the differential diagnosis of paroxysmal disorders. These nonepileptic conditions comprise a diverse group of neurological, cardiac, systemic, and metabolic processes that need to be foremost on the clinician's mind, since many are common and are frequently mistaken for seizures. Conversely, seizures may be misdiagnosed as one of these paroxysmal events. This section focuses on movement disorders, with particular emphasis on recognizing the relevant clinical observations of the symptoms and signs that form the basis for proper diagnosis, treatment, and appropriate referral to a pediatric neurologist. For more detailed information, the reader should consult such standard textbooks as Fenichel (1997) and Swaiman and Ashwal (1999).

PATHOPHYSIOLOGY

Movement disorders are traditionally understood via the model of Parkinson's disease and Huntington's chorea. The concepts derived from these two historic movement disorders—the first to be well-understood—place the locus of abnormal involuntary movements within the basal ganglia. Yet, the relationship between abnormal movements and dysfunction of the neurochemical and neuroanatomic systems within the basal ganglia is not as clear for many movement disorders that are important in pediatric medicine, such as tics, tremors, dystonia, myoclonus, and some forms of chorea. Notwithstanding this comment, it is useful to consider the disorders of involuntary movement conceptually linked in one well-organized chapter.

HISTORY AND PHYSICAL EXAM

The recognition of the abnormal movement provides the basis for diagnosis. Experience and good visual observational skills are critical.

● **Clinical Pearl:** The key clinical features that distinguish the types of abnormal movements include location in the body, rhythm, regularity, frequency, speed, stereotypic nature, and associated symptoms.

For example, a postural tremor is described as a distal extremity, rhythmic, regular, repetitive movement. Tics are described as complex, sudden, brief, purposeless, stereotypic movements or utterances, which can be suppressed. Because most tics began around the head region, the location in the body serves as a useful associated feature that helps to confirm the diagnosis. Finally, the descriptive terms used represent the symptom, not the disorder or final diagnosis. To illustrate the difference between the symptom and the disorder, consider dystonia as a symptom versus Dystonia, a genetic disease with a known DNA mutation. Display 46-9 summarizes these features, which may be applied to daily observations of patients and their complaints. Experience with a visual representation of these movements is necessary to appreciate the descriptive terms, which at best only approximate the actual movement.

● **Clinical Pearl:** The availability of home video recordings of patients has facilitated the solution to many diagnostic problems, because many normal or abnormal movements may not be apparent during an office visit. When parents express concern about a questionable abnormal movement, the practitioner should ask them to try to videotape the disturbing activity. A video recording also allows easy access for second opinions from colleagues or specialists.

Once the abnormal movements are appropriately categorized, the clinician needs to formulate a differential diagnosis regarding the actual cause or etiology. Display 46-10 summarizes some of the more common or important causes of pediatric movement disorders. The remainder of this section will describe in detail the more common or important movement disorders and their differential diagnosis.

■ Tics, Tourette Syndrome, Obsessive-Compulsive Disorder, and PANDAS

Tics typically begin in young school-aged children and may resolve spontaneously over several months, progress to the same or new tic, or most commonly remit and exacerbate each time with new features. Single transient tics are called simple motor tics. The course of the symptoms is reflected in the descriptive terms chronic or complex motor tic. Vocalizations or phonic tics represent another component of tic disorders.

Tourette syndrome is a term used for patients with a chronic and complex motor-vocal tic disorder greater than 1 year in duration. Tourette syndrome is commonly associated with obsessive-compulsive disorder (OCD), attention deficit disorder, and learning disabilities.

● **Clinical Pearl:** Tourette syndrome per se does not denote that the disorder is permanent or that the tic disorder is severe.

DISPLAY 46-9 • Classification and Definition of Abnormal Movement Disorders

Athetosis: slow, writhing movement of limbs often with chorea.

Ballismus (hemiballismus, hemichorea): rapid violent flinging of a limb.

Bobble-head Doll Syndrome: rhythmic up and down movement of head.

Chorea: rapid, migrating, nonrhythmic, nonstereotyped movements of face, tongue, and limbs often associated with restlessness; may be focal or diffuse.

Dyskinesia (tartive dyskinesia): buccolingual masticatory, lip smacking, puckering and chewing movement.

Dystonia (blepharospasm, dystonic tic, torticollis, retrocollis, antereocollis, writers cramp, trismus, oculogyric crisis, vocal cord, nocturnal): simultaneous contraction of agonist and antagonist muscles in a writhing posture; may be uncomfortable, focal, segmental, unilateral, or generalized, and/or movement induced; may lead to fixed deformities or postural changes.

Miscellaneous Paroxysmal Disorders: (astasia-abasia, ataxia, vestibular dysfunction, narcolepsy, cataplexy, micro sleep, restless legs syndrome, fasiculations, myokymia, myotonia, carpal-pedal spasm, neuromyotonia, hemifacial spasm, gratification phenomena, paroxysmal dystonic choreoathetosis): less common or rare entities

Myoclonus (opsoclonus-myoclonus, palatal): rapid muscle jerks; may be focal, multifocal, generalized, rhythmic or nonrhythmic, or activated by movement or sensory stimulation.

Rigidity (akathesia, hypokinesia, bradykinesia, malignant hyperthermia, neuroleptic malignant syndrome): "Lead pipe" resistance to *both* flexion and extension.

Shuddering Attacks: brief bodily shiver or quiver lasting 2 to 5 seconds.

Spasmus Nutans: triad of nystagmus, torticollis, and head bobbing horizontal or vertical.

Spasticity: "Clasp knife" more resistance to either extension or flexion, but not both.

Tremor (postural, resting, intention; called titubation when head is involved): involuntary oscillating movement of distal extremities with fixed frequency.

Tics and Tourette Syndrome (often with ADD, OCD, occasional PANDAS): complex, sudden, brief, purposeless, stereotypic movements or utterances, which can be suppressed. Head region common including blinking, eye deviation, headshake, retrocollis, grimace, eye opening or jaw widening, nose wiggling, shoulder shrug, abdominal thrusting, copropraxia, or joint subluxation. Phonic tics include throat clearing, cough, bark, inhalation noises, sniffing, snorting, grunting, subvocalization, coprolalia.

DISPLAY 46-10 • Differential Diagnosis of Selected Movement Disorders

Tics and Tourette Syndrome
- Drug-induced (Adderal, Dexadrine, levodopa, Ritalin, Risperidal, Tegretol)
- Genetic
- Poststreptococcal (PANDAS)

Tremor (postural tremor)
- Benign shuddering of infancy (Bactrim, Septra, monosodium glutamate)
- Drug-induced (β-adrenergic agonists, caffeine, carbamazapine, lithium, phenytoin, thyroid hormone excess, valproate, epinephrine)
- Hyperthryoid state
- Pheochromocytoma
- Wilson's disease ("wing-beating" tremor)

Torticollis
- Benign paroxysmal torticollis
- Cervical cord syringomyelia
- Cervical cord tumors
- Cervicomedullary infections, malformations, and tumors
- Cervical spine subluxation (C1–C2)
- Diplopia
- Dystonia—genetic, acquired, drug-induced
- Familial paroxysmal choreoathetosis
- Juvenile rheumatoid arthritis
- Sandifer syndrome
- Spasmus nutans
- Stenocleidomastoid infections or injuries, congenital or acquired
- Tics and Tourette syndrome

Ballismus (hemiballismus, hemichorea)
- Subthalamic nucleus contralateral injury, bleed, or stroke
- Meningitis
- Associated with Sydenham's chorea

Chorea
- Burn encephalopathy
- Drug induced (estrogens, INH, lithium, stimulants, tricyclic antidepressants, valproic acid)
- Encephalitis (tongue chorea)
- Endocrinopathies (hyperthyroidism, hypernatremia, hypocalcemia, adrenal insufficiency)
- Genetic diseases
- Postpump after cardiopulmonary bypass
- Poststreptococcal rheumatic fever
- Pregnancy
- Systemic lupus erythematosus
- Tumors

Athetosis
- Often associated with chorea
- Perinatal brain injury with hypotonic cerebral palsy
- Kernicterus

Dystonia (blepharospasm, dystonic tic, torticollis, retrocollis, antereocollis, writer's cramp, trismus, oculogyric crisis, vocal cord, bradykinesia, rigidity, opisthotonos, nocturnal)
- Dopa-responsive
- Drug-induced (dopamine receptor antagonists)
- Familial and genetic
- Tumors

Myoclonus (opsoclonus-myoclonus, segmental, palatal)
- Drug-induced (levodopa, Tegretol, tricyclic antidepressants)
- Epileptic
- Metabolic—dialysis, renal or hepatic failure, electrolyte disturbance
- Neuroblastoma
- Palatal (brain stem segmental cause dentato-olivary pathways)
- Physiologic—anxiety, exercise, sleep, nocturnal
- Posthypoxia, trauma, stroke
- Postvacination
- Spinal cord tumor (segmental)

It may impact some individuals, but most patients have mild to moderate symptoms that eventually improve or resolve.

PANDAS (pediatric autoimmune neuropsychiatric disorders associated with streptococcal infections) is a recently described syndrome associated with group A β-hemolytic streptococcal (GABHS) infection, probably related to Sydenham's chorea (SC) (Swedo, Leonard, Garvey, et al., 1999).

PATHOPHYSIOLOGY

Most cases of tics or Tourette syndrome have a genetic basis, but no specific gene has yet been identified. Some cases are caused by or exacerbated by medications including Adderal, Dexadrine, levodopa, Ritalin, Risperidal, and Tegretol. In those cases, the medication should be eliminated if possible. There are instances when the underlying problem necessitates that the medication be continued, particularly if the drug-induced tic is mild. A specialist such as a pediatric neurologist or child psychiatrist usually manages these patients.

OCD may occur with carbon monoxide poisoning, tumors, allergic reactions to wasp sting, postviral encephalitis, Prader-Willi syndrome, traumatic brain injury, and Sydenham's chorea (SC).

Basal ganglia involvement in SC is well described pathologically, and there is neurological imaging evidence of similar involvement in both SC and OCD. Additionally, antineuronal antibodies have been demonstrated in both SC and OCD.

Presumably, PANDAS represents a group of disorders in a spectrum of autoimmune phenomenon related to infection with GABHS, which includes SC and OCD. Exacerbation of PANDAS symptoms seem to occur with GABHS infections, even if they are promptly treated. Whether successful and prompt treatment of an initial GABHS infection can prevent the development of PANDAS, as it does with acute rheumatic fever, remains to be seen (Swedo, et al., 1998).

HISTORY AND PHYSICAL EXAM

Tics

Tics are described as complex, sudden, brief, purposeless, stereotypic movements or utterances, that can be suppressed. Tics are more common within the head region including blinking, eye deviation, headshake, retrocollis, grimace, eye opening or jaw widening, nose wiggling, or shoulder shrug. Bodily tics include abdominal thrusting, copropraxia, or joint subluxation. Phonic tics include throat clearing, cough, bark, inhalation noises, sniffing, snorting, grunting, subvocalizations, and coprolalia. Although it is a common worry among patients and families with Tourette syndrome, coprolalia (frequent nondirected swearing) is not at all common.

For most practitioners, tics will present as mild disorders, increasing in severity during times of childhood stress. September and early October usually bring a number of these cases to the office, coinciding with the beginning of school. Parents may be reassured that these tics will usually calm down once acclimation to the routine of school is achieved.

OCD

The DSM-IV criteria for OCD requires the presence of obsessions or compulsions that cause impairment in terms of marked distress, time consumed (more than 1 hour per day), or significant interference with daily routine, academic or social functioning. The most common symptoms of OCD in childhood are obsessive contamination fears, often accompanied by protracted washing or avoidance of contaminated objects and compulsive repetitive checking. Other common compulsions include repetitive counting, arranging, or touching in patterns. Although some compulsions may be tied to a specific worry, many consist of actions repeated until they feel "just right." The elusive sense of closure or completion may require symmetry (eg, repeating with the left hand actions done with the right, or evening up shoe lace length and tension) or repeating actions odd or even numbers of times. Compulsive rereading or rewriting of school assignments may interfere with academic performance. Mental rituals may consist of silent praying, repetition, counting, or having to think about or look at something in a particular way until it feels "just right." Simple compulsions, such as repetitive or symmetrical touching, may lack a discernible ideational component and may be phenomenologically indistinguishable from complex tics. Preoccupation with multiple mental rituals may interfere with normal activities. Trichotillomania, persistent hair pulling to the point of alopecia, is a unique symptom that may occur associated with tics and OCD or may present as an isolated compulsion.

PANDAS

The abrupt onset of OCD and/or tic disorder or a dramatic acute exacerbation of such symptoms after a group A β-hemolytic streptococcal infection is called PANDAS. Associated symptoms include irritability, emotional lability, and separation anxiety.

DIAGNOSTIC CRITERIA AND STUDIES

The diagnosis of tics or OCD is based on the patient's history and physical examination.

● **Clinical Pearl:** Children who present with an abrupt onset of symptoms of tics or OCD should be evaluated for recent or past GABHS infections with throat cultures or rapid strep antigen test. Serological evidence of antibodies to GABHS should also be pursued.

MANAGEMENT

The treatment of tics and Tourette syndrome is a rather complex endeavor because the disorder encompasses so many factors of the child's life, including school, family, friends, self-esteem, and even vocational choice.

The vast majority of patients seen by the primary care provider will have mild symptoms. After an accurate diagnosis, reassurance and information concerning the condition are the only treatments necessary.

● **Clinical Pearl:** The child and family should be reassured that the problem is mild, but that exacerbations may occur with stressors such as starting school, sports or dance tryouts, performances, exams, a move, or a new sibling. Parents need to understand that for the vast majority of tics, only the parent is bothered. The child, the child's friends, and the child's teachers are commonly unaware and unconcerned.

The more a parent tries to modify the tic by reminding the child of it, the more repetitive and intensified it becomes. Parents should not call attention to tics.

The Tourette Syndrome Association is a wonderful resource for the complete spectrum of simple tics to the more complicated cases involving Tourette syndrome and OCD with attention deficit disorder (*http://www.tsa.mgh.harvard.edu*).

The clinician needs to determine in concert with the patient and family whether the tics interfere with normal childhood functioning.

▲ **Clinical Warning:** It is a mistake to treat a child with medication if the child is functioning normally in school and with friends, because the medications used for these disorders have significant side effects.

More complex disorders that do interfere with normal functioning may require referral to a specialist familiar with the full range of management decisions including pharmacological, psychological, and educational treatments or therapies. The standard pharmacological agents include clonidine or dopamine receptor antagonists such as haloperidol to suppress the tics and selective serotonin reuptake inhibitors (SSRIs) to treat the OCD component. There is an overlap in many patients between what is a tic versus an OCD manifestation, and both agents may be used separately or in combination.

If PANDAS is suspected based on serological evidence of recent GABHS infection, an antibiotic trial may be appropriate as well. A recent study—attempting to determine whether antibiotic prophylaxis, similar to what is used in acute rheumatic fever, could prevent PANDAS re-exacerbations—was flawed. The methodology employed oral penicillin prophylaxis and, not surprisingly, was ineffective in reducing recurrent GABHS infections; therefore, no conclusions could be reached (Garvey, Perlmutter, & Allen, 1999).

■ *Tremor*

Tremors are classified as either postural, resting, or intention tremors. A resting tremor is typical in Parkinson's disease as a pill-rolling tremor at rest. Intention tremors manifest at the point of touch to the desired or intended target. Cerebellar and brainstem disease produce intention tremors.

■ *Postural Tremor*

Postural tremors begin in childhood but are more common in teenagers. They are best observed with the patient at rest with the arms extended. The patient and clinician observe an involuntary oscillating movement of the distal extremities with a fixed frequency. If the head is affected, the movement is termed titubation. Younger children may have poor handwriting, and teenagers may worry about their appearance in that tremors may produce the false impression that a patient is anxious or using drugs. Recording the child's handwriting samples will preserve a visual record to monitor progress or response to treatment. Most cases are autosomal dominant with incomplete penetrance—observing the parents is an important component of a complete examination.

In severe cases, the tremor progresses to a point that poor coordination degrades a patient's fine motor performance. This usually prompts pharmacological intervention. β-adrenergic blockers such as propanolol and other agents such as primidone usually reduce the tremor to satisfactory levels. Most patients are satisfied with the reassurance that

the condition is not serious or progressive. Treatment also involves avoiding or reducing medications that produce or exacerbate a tremor. These include adrenergic agonists, epinephrine, caffeine, carbamazapine, lithium, phenytoin, thyroid hormone excess, and valproate.

■ *Benign Shuddering of Infancy*

Young infants exhibit a variant of childhood tremors called shuddering attacks or benign shuddering of infancy. Most cases truly represent an infantile tremor, and one or both parents may exhibit a postural tremor confirming the genetic tendency. Occasionally patients have an identifiable medical etiology, including exposure to Bactrim or Septra; occult ureteral obstruction; and occult gastroenterological disease, such as malrotation or superior mesenteric artery syndrome. Typical shuddering attacks begin at 6 months of age and resolve over the course of 12 months. The events are brief, lasting up to 3 seconds, and consist of bodily shivers or shudders that do not affect consciousness. If the condition is not correctly observed, the health care provider should consider whether a more complete evaluation is needed to exclude the differential consideration of myoclonic seizures. An experienced clinician can usually diagnose benign shuddering spells without the need for a laboratory evaluation.

■ *Torticollis*

Torticollis, or head tilt, represents a symptom complex that spans several categories described here, and in total comprises a frequent pediatric condition.

● **Clinical Pearl:** The importance of torticollis is that a significant number of diverse conditions begin with a head tilt as the initial symptom.

The typical movement disorder categories include torticollis as a symptom of a drug-induced dystonic reaction and other forms of dystonia. Some patients with a tic disorder may have a head tilt component or a so-called dystonic tic, which is actually a variant of a tic rather than a feature of dystonia. A head tilt or torticollis may be the initial feature of tumors of the neck, cervical cord, brainstem, or infections. Diplopia from any cause, as part of the above neurological conditions or as an isolated ophthalmologic problem, may first come to the family's attention as a head tilt. Sandifer syndrome (dystonic dyspepsia) is the unusual occurrence of a head tilt caused by gastroesophageal reflux. The torticollis resolves when the underlying gastroesophageal reflux is treated.

Spasmus nutans occurs in infants 6 months to 3 years of age. The symptom complex is variable but includes a triad of head tilt, head bob, and nystagmus. This benign condition is self-limiting. An MRI scan is obtained to exclude the rare chance of a third ventricular tumor.

The most common of all cases of torticollis are those infants with congenital torticollis from intrauterine restriction or injury to the sternocleidomastoid muscle. The condition is detected in these infants in the first few months of life. In addition to the head tilt, the infant shows facial and skull asymmetry and restriction of full head rotation and lateral flexion due to tightening of the stenocleidomastoid muscle. Physical therapy consisting of range of motion exercises reduces the burden of the head tilt as well as skull and facial asymmetry for most children. Cervical spine subluxation should be excluded before starting physical therapy.

■ Athetosis

Athetosis often accompanies chorea and is a rare, isolated finding. The most common setting for athetosis is in a child with perinatal brain injury and associated hypotonic cerebral palsy. The slow writhing and twisting movement may increase the caloric needs and prevent smooth coordinated movement. There is no specific treatment for athetosis.

■ Ballismus

Although considered rare, ballismus may actually be a variant of chorea and presents as part of post streptococcal SC. The rapid violent flinging limb movements sometimes also occur during the initial treatment phases of bacterial meningitis. When that occurs it may be confused with a focal seizure. Dopamine receptor antagonists such as haloperidol significantly reduce the movements.

■ Chorea

SC or poststreptococcal chorea is less common but remains an important childhood disorder that is often misdiagnosed in its early stages. The typical patient may not have a recognized prior streptococcal infection. The initial clinical features include mood change, emotional lability, and decline in schoolwork, attention, and handwriting. Parents describe a clumsy, restless, emotional child with irregular, rapid, migrating movements. The face, tongue, and distal limbs are common locations. The symptoms begin gradually and may persist, regress, or progress to completely debilitate the child to a state where walking, eating, and talking are quite difficult. The clinical signs associated with chorea include milk-maid's grip, darting tongue, pronator sign, spoon hand, hypotonia, hung-up reflexes, and dysarthria. Twenty percent of patients relapse within 2 years.

▲ **Clinical Warning:** A cardiac work-up is necessary in all patients suspected of poststreptococcal chorea because carditis can recur even if not initially present. Continuous treatment with prophylactic antibiotics to prevent rheumatic fever recurrences is also necessary.

Treatment for the chorea includes supportive care, diazepam, haloperidol, and steroids, among others. Most patients recover completely.

■ Dystonia

Many forms of dystonia are rare and do not constitute an emergency. In contrast, the many faces of drug-induced dystonia are common, require urgent recognition, are often not diagnosed, and are amazingly easy to treat.

● **Clinical Pearl:** The clinical features of drug-induced dystonia include trismus, torticollis, bradykinesia, rigidity, oculogyric crisis, and opisthotonos. Forceful twisting of the head and neck, either intermittent or continuous, is the most typical manifestation of drug-induced dystonic reactions.

Stiffness of the jaw progressing to complete forced closure of the jaw and inability to drink or speak describes trismus. Perhaps the most unusual dystonic reactions include oculogyric crisis. This may begin as forced upward eye deviation—either intermittent or persistent—and it may then progress to retrocollis with the eyes elevated and forced extension of the head, neck, and upper torso. Not only is this frightening to the patient as well as family, caregivers, and health care professionals; but it can also be uncomfortable or painful.

Dopamine receptor antagonists are responsible for these dystonic reactions. Rapid dosing titration and larger doses predispose to this side effect. Despite the careful use of these medications, some patients are particularly sensitive and develop side effects even at low doses. Nonpsychiatric and nonneurological use of mild dopamine receptor blockers is most common in postoperative patients or others with nausea and vomiting treated with Compazine or Phenergan.

Treatment with intravenous Benadryl is effective within 1 minute. To prevent the occurrence of dystonic reactions, some clinicians prescribe Cogentin before initiating treatment or after the onset of a dystonic reaction if ongoing drug treatment is necessary.

MANAGEMENT OF MOVEMENT DISORDERS

● **Clinical Pearl:** A lesson that all clinicians eventually learn is to resist the temptation to infer a psychogenic cause based solely on the appearance of unusual or bizarre movements that are exacerbated by stress and appear to be under voluntary control.

Patients typically counter the abnormal movement and may voluntarily suppress the movement or convert it to some "normal"-appearing action, leading to further erroneous conclusions that the movements represent a psychiatric disorder. Indeed these more complex responses to the abnormal movements are typical features inherent to movement disorders.

Referral Considerations

Movement disorders are often challenging to diagnose and treat. Referral to a pediatric neurologist for diagnosis and management in collaboration with the primary care practitioner may be required. Movement disorders such as poststreptococcal chorea, acute-onset tics, or those without a clear clinical diagnosis require prompt referral.

Typical chronic movement disorders, such as a mild tic disorder or a nonprogressive postural tremor, that do not affect the patient's daily lifestyle should be managed by the primary care provider.

It is important for the practitioner to provide lifestyle advice and information that will assist patients to live in harmony with their movement disorders because many are told or feel that they must be responsible for suppressing the abnormal movement. Family- and patient-centered resources and medical information are more widely available today and provide an important component of clinical management.

COMMUNITY RESOURCES

Seizures and Epilepsy

A variety of resources are available to help patients, their families, and health care providers manage the medical, socioeconomic, legal, and lifestyle ramifications connected with a diagnosis of a seizure or epilepsy. Several useful organizations and their Web sites are summarized below.

Epilepsy Foundation of America (EFA)
4351 Garden City Drive
Landover, MD 20785
Telephone: (301) 459-3700
Toll Free: (800) EFA-1000
Fax: (301) 577-4941
Internet address: *http://www.efa.org*

The EFA represents the interests of people with epilepsy. The web site includes education, news, programs, and services, as well as information on research and advocacy groups.

International Epilepsy Foundation
Internet address: *http://www.epilepsy-international.com*

This web site, offered in English and Spanish, provides global news and information specifically for people with epilepsy and their caregivers and medical team.

Epilepsia
Internet address: *http://www.epilepsia.com*

Web site of the official journal of the International League Against Epilepsy.

American Academy of Neurology (AAN)
1080 Montreal Avenue
St. Paul, MN 55116
Telephone: (651) 695-1940
Internet address: *http://www.aan.com*

The AAN is the official organization for physicians and health care professionals who specialize in neurology. The web site provides abstracts from past issues of Neurology as well as useful links.

Neuroscience for Kids
Internet address:
http://faculty.washington.edu/chudler/neurok.html

Information specifically designed to help school-aged children understand the brain.

Movement Disorders

Tourette Syndrome Association
42-40 Bell Boulevard
Bayside, New York 11361-2874
Telephone: (718) 224-2999
Fax: (718) 279-9596
Internet address: *http://www.TSA.mgh.harvard.edu*

A national, nonprofit organization providing a crisis hotline, physician referral listings, and patient advocacy. Web site has listings of recommended books and movies (*http://tsa.mgh.harvard.edu/allourstuff/toreadandview.html*)

Pediatric Neurology

A Pediatric Neurology Center
Internet address: *http://www.pediatricneurology.com*

Resources and selected links for a wide range of children's neurological problems.

REFERENCES

American Academy of Physicians. (1996). Practice parameter: the neurodiagnostic evaluation of the child with a first simple febrile seizure. *Pediatrics, 97,* 769–775.

American Academy of Physicians. (1999). Practice parameter: long term treatment of the child with simple febrile seizures. *Pediatrics, 103,* 1307–1309.

Berg, A.T. (1996). Complex febrile seizures. *Epilepsia 37,* 126–133.

Fenichel, G.M. (1997). *Clinical pediatric neurology,* 3rd edition. Philadelphia: W.B. Saunders.

Garvey, M.A., Perlmutter, S.J., Allen, A.J. (1999). A pilot study of penicillin prophylaxis for neuropsychiatric exacerbations triggered by streptococcal infections. *Biol Psychiatry, 45,* 1564–1571.

Green, S. (1993). Can seizures be the sole manifestation of meningitis in febrile children? *Pediatrics, 92,* 527–534.

Hirtz, D.G. (1997). Febrile seizures. *Pediatrics in Review, 18,* 5–8.

Holmes, G.L. (1987). Diagnosis and management of seizures in children. W.B. Saunders.

Maytal, J, Shinnar, S, Moshe, SL, & Alvarez, LA. (1989). Low morbidity and mortality of status epilepticus in children. *Pediatrics, 83,* 323–331.

Nelson, K. (1978). Prognosis in children with febrile seizures. *Pediatrics, 61,* 720–726.

Pellock, J.M. (1998). Management of acute seizures in children. *Journal of Child Neurology, 13*(Suppl 1).

Pellock, J.M., Morton, L.D., Watemberg, N. (1998). New antiepileptic drug therapy for children. *The Neurologist, 4*(Supplement), S16–S22.

Sabo-Graham, T., & Seay, A.R. (1998). Management of status epilepticus in children. *Pediatric Review, 19*(9), 306–310.

Swaiman, K.F., & Ashwal, S. (1999). *Pediatric neurology: principles and practice,* (3rd Ed.). St. Louis: Mosby.

Swedo, S.E., Leonard, H.L., Garvey, M., et al. (1998). Pediatric autoimmune neuropsychiatric disorders associated with streptococcal infections: clinical description of the first 50 cases. *American Journal of Psychiatry, 155,* 264–271.

Tasker, R.C. (1998). Emergency treatment of acute seizures and status epilepticus. *Arch Dis Child, 79,* 78–83.

Wyllie E. (1997). *The treatment of epilepsy: principles and practice,* (2nd Ed.). Baltimore: Williams & Wilkins.

Acute Endocrine Complaints

• PAVEL FORT, MD, and PHYLLIS W. SPEISER, MD

P A R T 1 ▲

Adrenal Insufficiency and Crisis

• PHYLLIS W. SPEISER, MD

INTRODUCTION

Adrenal insufficiency is important to recognize because of its potentially life-threatening implications. Symptoms and signs of this disorder are varied and nonspecific. In infancy, these include lethargy, vomiting, poor appetite, and failure to thrive. Clinicians may mistake these problems for formula intolerance or inadequate lactation, or alternatively, primary infectious or gastrointestinal disorders. In older children, chronic fatigue, headache, gastrointestinal symptoms, salt craving and hyperpigmentation may be noted. Patients may undergo extensive evaluation before a diagnosis is made.

ANATOMY, PHYSIOLOGY, AND PATHOLOGY

The adrenal glands, located at the upper pole of each kidney with a combined weight of 10 g in the adult, are composed of cortex and medulla. The adrenal cortex is the primary site of cortisol and aldosterone synthesis and a secondary site of sex hormone synthesis. The adrenal medulla is responsible for catecholamine synthesis, epinephrine, and norepinephrine, important in nervous system regulation. This section is restricted to discussion of adrenal cortical disease.

Glucocorticoids, such as cortisol, are essential for survival, mediating myriad developmental and physiologic processes. Some actions of cortisol include stimulating gluconeogenesis and glycogenolysis. By increasing cellular breakdown of sugars, protein, and fat, more substrate is provided for gluconeogenesis. Glucocorticoids also increase cellular resistance to insulin, thereby decreasing glucose uptake and use in peripheral tissues. The overall effect is to raise and maintain blood glucose levels, especially during stress (Pilkis & Granner, 1992). Thus, glucocorticoid deficiency may cause hypoglycemia.

Glucocorticoids also increase cardiac output and enhance vascular sensitivity to pressor hormones (Kelly, Mangos, Williamson, & Whitworth, 1998). Hence, glucocorticoid defi-ciency reduces cardiac output and may predispose the patient to heart failure and shock.

These problems are exacerbated by concomitant aldosterone deficiency. Aldosterone is essential for normal sodium homeostasis; deficiency of this hormone results in sodium loss through the kidney, colon, and sweat glands (Bonvalet, 1998).

Cortisol and aldosterone are synthesized from cholesterol in the adrenal cortex in several enzymatic steps (see Figure 47-1). Aldosterone synthesis differs from cortisol synthesis in that a specific 11β-hydroxylase isozyme (enzyme), termed *aldosterone synthase*, is used at the terminal step. Aldosterone synthesis is separately regulated, principally by the renin-angiotensin system. Cortisol synthesis is regulated primarily by pituitary adrenocorticotropic hormone (ACTH) and hypothalamic corticotropin-releasing hormone (CRH). Insufficient production of these tropic hormones or unresponsiveness to their actions results in select adrenocortical hormone deficiencies. Enzymatic blocks impairing cortisol synthesis or resistance to cortisol's actions also presents as adrenal insufficiency (Speiser & White, 1998). Excessive ACTH secretion is a consequence of cortisol deficiency, causing both adrenal hyperplasia and hyperpigmentation. If aldosterone synthesis is blocked or if there is selective resistance to aldosterone action, sodium wasting and failure to thrive will result without complete adrenocortical insufficiency.

Secondary Adrenal Insufficiency

This refers to an externally induced alteration in pituitary structure or function preventing normal ACTH secretion and thus causing adrenal insufficiency. A frequent cause of iatrogenic secondary adrenal insufficiency, both acute and chronic, is withdrawal of exogenous glucocorticoid therapy. Table 47-1 shows the most commonly used glucocorticoids, their relative potencies, equivalent doses, and mineralocorticoid actions.

▲ **Clinical Warning:** Administration of hydrocortisone, prednisone, or dexamethasone in supraphysiologic doses (eg, prednisone = 10 mg daily) for periods of greater than 2 to 3 weeks requires gradual tapering to allow the hypothalamic-pituitary-adrenal (HPA) axis time to recover from suppression.

● **Clinical Pearl:** Short courses of steroids (eg, asthma treatment with oral steroids over 5–7 days) do not require long-term tapering (Orth & Kovacs, 1998).

Steroid tapering should be individualized because each patient tolerates reduction of treatment differently; this will depend on the total dosage, dose schedule, and duration of steroid treatment. Usually, a high therapeutic dose may be reduced in a serial, step-wise fashion over a period of about 1 week to a level typically used in treating adrenal insufficiency in periods of crisis or stress, termed the *stress physio-*

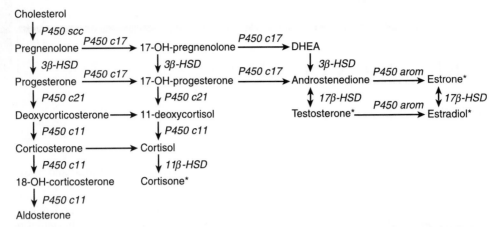

Figure 47–1 ■ Diagram of the pathways of corticosteroid synthesis. Cholesterol is converted in several steps to aldosterone, cortisol, or sex steroids. Hormones marked by an asterisk (*) are produced largely outside the adrenal cortex. Deficiency of a given enzyme causes accumulation of hormonal precursors and a deficiency of products. DHEA = dehydroepiandrosterone; HSD = hydroxysteroid dehydrogenase. Adapted with permission from Speiser, P.W. (1995). Congenital adrenal hyperplasia. In K.L. Becker (ed.). *Principles and practice of endocrinology and metabolism, 2nd ed.* Philadelphia: J.B. Lippincott.

logic dose. Further tapering may then proceed during the next week, until a maintenance level is achieved at the presumed physiologic dose (basal levels that the body produces). Final tapering leading to discontinuation of therapy should then proceed slowly so that the duration of tapering approximates the total length of treatment, up to 6 to 9 months (Orth & Kovacs, 1998). Intercurrent febrile illness or surgical procedures demand a temporary increase in steroid dose for several days (Lamberts, Bruining, & de Jong, 1997).

Documentation of an intact HPA axis should be obtained before subjecting a patient to surgery who has a known history of prior high-dose, long-term glucocorticoid treatment. This may be done by documenting an 0800 plasma cortisol greater than 10 µg/dL or by performing low-dose cosyntropin challenge (see following section). If such documentation cannot be obtained in time, it is safest to treat with supplemental stress physiologic steroid coverage in the perioperative period for any patient within 1 year of withdrawal of steroid therapy (Oelkers, 1996). Figure 47-2

illustrates an algorithm for the tapering of long-term steroids.

Although theoretically possible, adrenal insufficiency is uncommon in infants born to mothers treated with glucocorticoids during pregnancy. Only dexamethasone crosses the placenta to an appreciable degree.

Adrenal insufficiency is a common cause of mortality in the postoperative period for patients after pituitary surgery (Bates, Van't Hoff, Jones, & Clayton, 1996). Patients who have been subjected to pituitary surgery should be covered with stress doses of glucocorticoids during and immediately after surgery. Several months after steroid tapering has been completed, such patients should be tested to determine whether the HPA axis is intact.

Congenital Adrenal Hyperplasia

Congenital adrenal hyperplasia (CAH) should be considered in the differential diagnosis of adrenal insufficiency, especially

---

Table 47–1.   COMMONLY USED GLUCOCORTICOIDS

Duration of Action*	Glucocorticoid Potency†	Equivalent Glucocorticoid Dose (mg)	Mineralocorticoid Activity
Short Acting			
Cortisol (hydrocortisone)	1	20	Yes‡
Cortisone	0.8	25	Yes‡
Prednisone	4	5	No
Prednisolone	4	5	No
Methylprednisolone	5	4	No
Intermediate Acting			
Triamcinolone	5	4	No
Long Acting			
Betamethasone	25	0.60	No
Dexamethasone	30	0.75	No

*The classification by duration of action is based on Harter JG. Corticosteroids. N Y State J Med 1966;66:827.
   †The values given for glucocorticoid potency are relative. Cortisol is arbitrarily assigned a value of 1.
   ‡Mineralocorticoid effects are dose related. At doses close to or within the basal physiologic range for glucocorticoid activity, no such effect may be detectable.
   Adapted with permission from Axelrod, L. (1995). Corticosteroid therapy. In K. L. Becker (ed.), *Principles and practice of endocrinology and metabolism* (2nd ed.). Philadelphia: J.B. Lippincott.

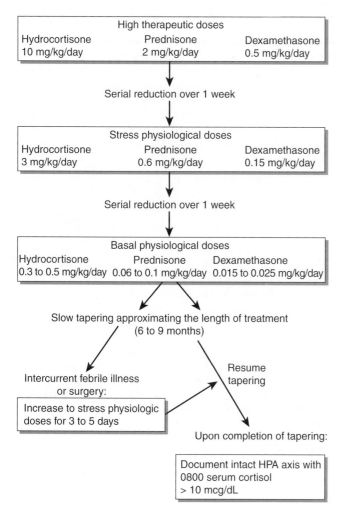

Figure 47–2 ■ Tapering of long-term steroids.

in the infant. Patients with CAH due to 21-hydroxylase deficiency (90%–95% of all CAH) cannot adequately synthesize cortisol. Inefficient cortisol synthesis causes the hypothalamus and pituitary to increase CRH and corticotropin (ACTH), respectively, and causes the adrenal glands to become hyperplastic. Instead of producing cortisol, the adrenals of CAH patients produce excess sex hormone precursors, which do not require 21-hydroxylation for their synthesis. Once secreted, these hormones are further metabolized to testosterone and dihydrotestosterone, active androgens, and to a lesser extent, estrogens, estrone, and estradiol. The net effect is prenatal virilization of the female fetus, producing a newborn girl with ambiguous genitalia. Males with CAH have no genital ambiguity. Rapid somatic growth with early epiphyseal fusion occurs in both sexes if the disease is not recognized and treated (Speiser & White, 1998).

About 75% of patients also have insufficient aldosterone to maintain sodium balance and are termed *salt wasters*. These patients usually are diagnosed at 1 to 4 weeks of age with severe illness characterized by hyponatremia (serum sodium often < 120 mEq/L), hyperkalemia (serum potassium often > 7 mEq/L), acidosis, and hypovolemic shock. These adrenal crises may prove fatal if proper medical care is not delivered.

▲ **Clinical Warning:** This problem is particularly critical in infant boys, who have no genital ambiguity to alert providers to the diagnosis of CAH prior to the onset of dehydration and shock.

Clinical clues to the diagnosis of salt-wasting CAH include lethargy, weak feeding pattern, vomiting, poor weight gain, pallor, or gray color with possible hyperpigmented scrotum and nipples.

Electrolytes should be measured in any infant with these features. The mortality rate for CAH remains high in such patients, suggested by the discrepancy in the number of male patients identified in case reports versus newborn screening. For this reason, many localities and several westernized foreign countries have included hormonal testing for CAH in the mandatory newborn disease screen (Pang & Shook, 1997).

Addison's Disease

The most common cause of Addison's disease is autoimmune (Laureti, Vecchi, Santeusanio, & Falorni, 1999). Type I polyglandular autoimmune syndrome, also termed Schmidt's disease, has a mean age of presentation of 12 years. Hypoparathyroidism and adrenal insufficiency are the most frequent presenting signs, found in 79% and 72% of cases, respectively (Kong & Jeffcoate, 1994). Candidiasis, due to a defect in T cells' handling of fungi, is the presenting sign of the disease in 60% of patients and is eventually detected in long-term follow-up of all patients. Antibodies can be detected to the adrenocortical steroidogenic enzymes, frequently to steroid 21-hydroxylase (Yu et al., 1999). Hypogonadism is seen more often in affected females than males. Other associated glandular defects include hypothyroidism and diabetes mellitus. Vitiligo is another cutaneous manifestation, while pernicious anemia and chronic active hepatitis are other systemic manifestations of this potentially fatal disease (Betterle, Greggio, & Volpato, 1998).

Tuberculosis and human immunodeficiency virus infection remain prominent causes of adrenocortical failure in children. Additional rare causes of adrenal insufficiency are listed in Table 47-2.

Adrenal Hemorrhage

Unilateral adrenal hemorrhage is often asymptomatic; however, bilateral adrenal hemorrhage presents with shock due to subcapsular blood loss and adrenal insufficiency. Neonates may suffer adrenal hemorrhage after long labor and traumatic delivery with attendant hypoxemia. Acute and overwhelming infection due to meningococcemia (Waterhouse-Friderichsen syndrome), *Haemophilus influenzae* type B (no longer prevalent due to vaccination), group A β-hemolytic *Streptococcus*, or *Pneumococcus* may also be associated with bilateral adrenal hemorrhage and adrenal crisis. Prompt glucocorticoid administration can improve the outlook for these patients. Adrenal hemorrhage should be considered in blunt abdominal injury; in adrenal tumors, such as neuroblastoma and pheochromocytoma; and in patients with congenital or acquired bleeding diatheses or coagulation defects (Rao, 1995).

EPIDEMIOLOGY

The exact overall incidence of adrenal insufficiency in childhood is unknown because of its multifactorial etiology. Secondary adrenal insufficiency due to pituitary failure is probably the most common cause and is a frequent cause of morbidity and mortality in children who have undergone treatment with cranial radiation, surgery, or exogenous glucocorticoids for extended periods. No data are available on

Table 47–2.   CAUSES OF ADRENAL INSUFFICIENCY

Disease	Mode of Inheritance	Most Common Gene Defect
Primary Adrenal Diseases		
Addison's disease	Autosomal recessive	Polyglandular autoimmune syndrome due to autoimmune regulator, AIRE
Adrenal hemorrhage	NA	—
Congenital adrenal hyperplasia	Autosomal recessive	21-hydroxylase, CYP21
Adrenoleukodystrophy	X-linked	Peroxisomal ATP-binding transporter
Adrenal hypoplasia congenita X-linked		DAX1
Wolman's disease	Autosomal recessive	Lysosomal acid lipase
Secondary Adrenal Diseases		
Hypopituitarism	—	—
Withdrawal of glucocortiocoid therapy	—	—
End-Organ Unresponsiveness		
ACTH resistance	Autosomal recessive	ACTH receptor
Cortisol resistance	Autosomal dominant	Glucocorticoid receptor
Pseudohypoaldosteronism	Autosomal recessive	Sodium channel (ENaC)
	Autosomal dominant	Mineralocorticoid receptor

the prevalence and incidence of pituitary-induced adrenal failure. The epidemiology of classic CAH due to 21-hydroxylase deficiency (21-OHD) is approximately 1 in 10,000 to 1 in 15,000 live births (Pang & Shook, 1997). Primary adrenal insufficiency, Addison's disease, is relatively rare in the pediatric population. The prevalence in Great Britain is 110 per million population of all ages, with more than 90% of cases attributed to autoimmune destruction of the adrenal cortex. A similar prevalence was found in Umbria, Italy (Laureti et al., 1999). The calculated incidence is approximately 5 to 6 per million population per year (Kong & Jeffcoate, 1994).

HISTORY AND PHYSICAL EXAMINATION

▲ **Clinical Warning:** Clinical clues to the diagnosis of adrenal insufficiency are extremely nonspecific. Infants may be jittery or have convulsions due to hypoglycemia. Chronic adrenal insufficiency will result in failure to thrive. Older children may exhibit fatigue, malaise, muscle aches, headache, abdominal pain, nausea, vomiting, salt craving, and weight loss with glucocorticoid or mineralocorticoid deficiencies.

Physical examination can provide important clues that direct the clinician to appropriate laboratory diagnosis. In suspected adrenal insufficiency, as in the evaluation of any chronic childhood illness, careful review of linear growth and weight gain is critical to understanding the nature and chronicity of the problem.

● **Clinical Pearls:**

- Orthostatic hypotension and pulse changes are sensitive bedside indications of mineralocorticoid deficiency or volume depletion.
- In untreated primary adrenal insufficiency, physical examination often shows hyperpigmentation, especially of non–sun-exposed areas, such as palms, soles, and oral mucosa.

This is a direct result of cosecretion of melanocyte-stimulating hormone with pro-opiomelanocortin, the precursor of

ACTH. In the case of adrenal hemorrhage or tumor, a flank mass may be palpated on careful abdominal examination. Patients with global adrenocortical insufficiency chronically lacking adrenal androgens will often have sparse pubic and axillary hair. On the other hand, CAH patients produce excess androgens.

● **Clinical Pearls:**

- Females with CAH will show genital ambiguity as neonates, and girls with CAH not detected in infancy often have an enlarged clitoris without true genital ambiguity.
- Males with CAH are much more difficult to identify clinically. They may show an enlarged penis and pubic hair and a hyperpigmented scrotum with small testes.

DIAGNOSTIC CRITERIA AND STUDIES

Relevant basic laboratory studies to confirm adrenal insufficiency include serum and urine electrolytes, glucose, early morning cortisol, ACTH, and plasma renin activity. One expects to find low serum (and high urine) sodium, high serum (and low urine) potassium with metabolic acidosis. There is an inappropriately low cortisol for the degree of ACTH elevation and high plasma renin activity. One should not attempt to restrict sodium intake in a patient with adrenal insufficiency, except under direct medical supervision, because this can provoke adrenal crisis. If central adrenal insufficiency is suspected, a low-dose cosyntropin stimulation test (1 μg intravenous [IV] bolus of ACTH 1-24) is the best way to assess the intactness of the HPA axis. Cortisol should rise after 30 to 60 minutes to a level greater than 15 to 20 μg/dL (Oelkers, 1996).

● **Clinical Pearl:** If CAH is suspected, the primary care provider should at least obtain a rapid measurement of basal serum 17-hydroxyprogesterone by radioimmunoassay.

Classic, severely affected CAH patients usually have markedly elevated random basal serum 17-hydroxyprogesterones in the range of greater than 10,000 to 20,000 ng/dL (New et al., 1983). Newborn screening programs are in effect in several states and rely primarily on filter paper determinations of blood 17-hydroxyprogesterone. The cost, sensitivity, specificity, and predictive values of these screening tests vary depending on the assay, the number of tests, and the established cut-off levels. Premature infants tend to have higher levels of 17-OHP than term infants and generate many false-positive results. Suggested weight-adjusted cut-offs range from 165 ng/mL in blood collected on filter paper for infants under 1300 g to 40 ng/mL for infants over 2200 g in Wisconsin (Allen et al., 1997); in Texas, cut-offs of 40 and 65 ng/mL are used for infants greater or less than 2500 g, respectively (Therrell et al., 1998). Because some radioimmunoassays cross-react with other steroids, positive screens should be confirmed. A more specific diagnostic test involving a complete profile of adrenocortical hormones before and 1 hour after high-dose cosyntropin stimulation (250 μg IV bolus) is obtained to distinguish CAH due to 21-hydroxylase deficiency from other forms of adrenal disease.

Radiographic imaging can be a helpful adjunct to biochemical testing in some types of adrenal insufficiency. Ultrasound is used in neonates with suspected adrenal hemorrhage; adrenal enlargement and inferior renal displacement may be detected. If done at 5-day intervals, ultrasound imaging may document changes in the lesion from solid to cystic to final calcification about a month later. Computed tomographic (CT) scan or magnetic resonance imaging is most sensitive for imaging adrenal pathology in older patients (Brant, 1999).

MANAGEMENT

Prompt recognition of adrenal insufficiency is the key to a good outcome. Timely initiation of glucocorticoid replacement therapy is the most important factor.

● **Clinical Pearl:** When acute adrenal failure is recognized, an initial bolus of parenteral hydrocortisone (25 mg for infants, 50 mg for children, or 100 mg for adolescents and adults) of hydrocortisone sodium succinate (Solu-Cortef) either IV or intramuscular [IM]) can be life-saving.

Hydrocortisone has mineralocorticoid properties, and thus additional mineralocorticoid treatment is not immediately necessary. Drugs such as prednisone and dexamethasone do not possess significant mineralocorticoid activity and are not first-choice drugs for acute treatment (see Table 47-1). Because all patients in adrenal crisis and many with chronic adrenal insufficiency are dehydrated, isotonic fluid administration, in the form of a 20 mL/kg bolus of IV normal saline or lactated Ringer's solution, is also required. Subsequent fluid replacement should be tailored to the individual patient's needs, based on blood pressure, heart rate, mental status, and capillary refill.

Continued steroid treatment should be ordered for the acutely ill patient as IV hydrocortisone every 6 hours, at 3 mg/kg per day for the first 24 hours, representing a stress physiologic dose. Subsequently, the dose can be tapered until a reasonable maintenance dose is achieved. In children, the preferred maintenance cortisol replacement is hydrocortisone (which is the same as cortisol) in two or three divided doses totaling 0.3 mg/kg per day (or about 10 mg/m² per day), the basal physiologic dose. CAH patients often require higher doses of glucocorticoids, not to exceed 0.6 mg/kg per

day (or about 20 mg/m² per day). A minimum dose of 6 mg/d of hydrocortisone (oral hydrocortisone cypionate, Cortef, suspension 10 mg/5 mL) in three divided doses is usually administered to infants with CAH.

The short half-life of hydrocortisone minimizes growth suppression and other adverse side effects of longer acting, more potent glucocorticoids, such as prednisone and dexamethasone. However, a single daily dose of a short-acting glucocorticoid is insufficient as replacement therapy and therefore a longer-acting steroid may be used in patients who cannot comply with a drug regimen requiring frequent dosing.

Efficacy of Treatment

Treatment efficacy for Addison's disease cannot be assessed by measuring plasma cortisol, because only exogenous hydrocortisone would be measured. Plasma ACTH is also not a reliable measure of treatment efficacy, because this rather labile hormone has circadian variability. Rather, the patient's sense of well-being is most important. Symptoms such as chronic headache, dizziness, and fatigue would suggest insufficient treatment.

Treatment efficacy for CAH (ie, suppression of adrenal sex hormones) is monitored by 17-OHP and androstenedione levels. Testosterone can also be a useful parameter in females and prepubertal males. The target 17-OHP range is usually 100 to 1000 ng/dL, depending on age and sex. Hormones should be measured consistently at the same time in relation to medication dosing. Plasma renin activity, blood pressure, and pulse are useful measures of sodium and fluid repletion.

Side Effects

▲ **Clinical Warning:** Overtreatment with glucocorticoids reduces linear growth and promotes centripetal obesity, hyperglycemia, hypertension, and bone mineral loss, as well as psychologic sequelae ranging from depression to psychosis. It is therefore advisable to evaluate steroid-treated children three to four times annually to assess linear growth, weight gain, and blood pressure.

Adults should be monitored at least yearly. As noninvasive techniques for measuring bone density become more widely available, these tests may eventually become standard for such patients.

What to Tell Parents

There are both transient and permanent forms of adrenal insufficiency. In either case, it is important to stress that steroid treatment and hydration are vital to support the patient at risk for adrenal crisis during surgery or other potentially life-threatening periods. Individuals diagnosed with permanent forms of adrenal insufficiency (Addison's disease and CAH) should wear a medallion indicating their diagnosis and medications. Primary care practitioners and school health personnel should be informed of necessary measures in case of shock. A home kit with injectable hydrocortisone sodium succinate should be supplied, and parents or caregivers instructed in its proper use. A person with adrenal insufficiency who is either lethargic or unresponsive outside the hospital setting should be given an IM injection of hydrocortisone sodium succinate (25 mg infant, 50 mg child, 100 mg adult). An IV line with isotonic fluids should be established and the patient brought promptly to an acute care facility. If the individual is conscious, clear electrolyte fluids should be provided (sports drinks, such as Gatorade or Powerade, are ideal).

Addison's disease and CAH are unremitting conditions requiring lifelong treatment. Nevertheless, most patients lead unrestricted and productive lives. Patients receiving low-dose maintenance glucocorticoid therapy are not at risk for immunosuppression. There are no significant interactions between these medications and other commonly used pediatric drugs.

Referral

Most primary care providers will request consultation from an endocrinologist to help care for patients with known or suspected adrenal insufficiency. The clinician should be familiar with signs and symptoms of these disorders, and should perhaps discuss basic laboratory evaluation before referring the patient to the specialist. It is particularly important to recognize signs of systemic progression of polyglandular endocrinopathy, and such patients should undergo annual screening for other glandular malfunctions specified above.

COMMUNITY RESOURCES

The following organizations provide information and support to patients and families with various adrenal disorders.

Magic Foundation
1327 N. Harlem Avenue
Oak Park, IL 60302
Telephone: (708) 383-0808
Fax: (708) 383-0899
Internet address: *http://www.magicfoundation.org*

This foundation for children and adults with growth disorders offers educational brochures, a networking system for parents, newsletters for adults and children, and divisions on specific disorders.

National Adrenal Diseases Foundation
505 Northern Boulevard
Great Neck, NY 11021
Telephone: (516) 487-4992
Internet address: *http://www.medhelp.org/nadf*

National Institutes of Health
Internet address:
http://www.niddk.nih.gov/health/endo/pubs/addison/addison.htm

Pituitary Tumor Network Association
Telephone: (805) 499-2262,
Internet address: *http://www.pituitary.com*

REFERENCES

Allen, D. B., Hoffmann, G. L., Fitzpatrick, P., Laessig, R., Maby, S., & Slyper, A. (1997). Improved precision of newborn screening for congenital adrenal hyperplasia using weight-adjusted criteria for 17-hydroxyprogesterone levels. *Journal of Pediatrics, 130*, 128–133.

Bates, A. S., Van't Hoff, W., Jones, P. J., & Clayton, R. N. (1996). The effect of hypopituitarism on life expectancy. *Journal of Clinical Endocrinology and Metabolism, 81*, 1169–1172.

Betterle, C., Greggio, N. A., & Volpato, M. (1998). Clinical review 93: Autoimmune polyglandular syndrome type 1. *Journal of Clinical Endocrinology and Metabolism, 83*, 1049–1055.

Bonvalet, J. P. (1998). Regulation of sodium transport by steroid hormones. *Kidney International Supplement, 65*, S49–56.

Brant, W. E. (1999). Adrenal glands and kidneys. In W. E. Brant & C. A. Helms (Eds.), *Fundamentals of diagnostic radiology* (2nd ed.) (pp. 769–792). Philadelphia: Lippincott Williams & Wilkins.

Brosnan, C. A., Brosnan, P., Therrell, B. L., Slater, C. H., Swint, J. M., Annegers, J. F., & Riley, W. J. (1998). A comparative cost analysis of newborn screening for classic congenital adrenal hyperplasia in Texas. *Public Health Reports, 113*, 170–178.

Kelly, J. J., Mangos, G., Williamson, P. M., & Whitworth, J. A. (1998). Cortisol and hypertension. *Clinical and Experimental Pharmacology and Physiology Supplement, 25*, S51–56.

Kong, M., & Jeffcoate, W. (1994). Eighty-six cases of Addison's disease. *Clinical Endocrinology (Oxf), 41*(6), 757–761.

Lamberts, S. W., Bruining, H. A., & de Jong, F. H. (1997). Corticosteroid therapy in severe illness. *New England Journal of Medicine, 337*, 1285–1292.

Laureti, S., Vecchi, L., Santeusanio, F., & Falorni, A. (1999). Is the prevalence of Addison's disease underestimated? *Journal of Clinical Endocrinology and Metabolism, 84*, 1762.

New, M. I., Lorenzen, F., Lerner, A. J., Kohn, B., Oberfield, S. E., et al. (1983). Genotyping steroid 21-hydroxylase deficiency: Hormonal reference data. *Journal of Clinical Endocrinology and Metabolism, 57*, 320–326.

Oelkers, W. (1996). Adrenal insufficiency [see comments]. *New England Journal of Medicine, 335*, 1206–1212.

Orth, D. N., & Kovacs, W. J. (1998). The adrenal cortex. In J. D. Wilson, D. W. Foster, H. M. Kronenberg, & P. R. Larsen (Eds.), *Williams textbook of endocrinology* (9th ed.) (pp. 605–610). Philadelphia: W.B. Saunders.

Pang, S., & Shook, M. K. (1997). Current status of neonatal screening for congenital adrenal hyperplasia [see comments]. *Current Opinion in Pediatrics, 9*, 419–423.

Pilkis, S. J., & Granner, D. K. (1992). Molecular physiology of the regulation of hepatic gluconeogenesis and glycolysis. *Annual Review of Physiology, 54*, 885–909.

Rao, R. H. (1995). Bilateral massive adrenal hemorrhage. *Medical Clinics of North America, 79*(1), 107–129.

Speiser, P. W., & White, P. C. (1998). Congenital adrenal hyperplasia due to steroid 21-hydroxylase deficiency. *Clinical Endocrinology (Oxf), 49*, 411–417.

Therrell, B. L. J., Berenbaum, S. A., Manter-Kapanke, V., Simmank, J., Korman, K., et al. (1998). Results of screening 1.9 million Texas newborns for 21-hydroxylase-deficient congenital adrenal hyperplasia. *Pediatrics, 101*, 583–590.

Yu, L., Brewer, K. W., Gates, S., Wu, A., Wang, T., et al. (1999). DRB1*04 and DQ alleles: Expression of 21-hydroxylase autoantibodies and risk of progression to Addison's disease. *Journal of Clinical Endocrinology and Metabolism, 84*(1), 328–335.

P A R T   2   ▲

Thyrotoxicosis

• PAVEL FORT, MD

INTRODUCTION

Thyrotoxicosis is a rare disease in prepubescent children, but its frequency increases in adolescents and young adults. The most common cause of thyrotoxicosis is Graves' disease, which accounts for over 95% of cases in the pediatric age group.

Other much less common causes of thyrotoxicosis include hyperfunctioning thyroid nodules, thyrotropin (thyroid-stimulating hormone [TSH])-induced hyperthyrodism, autoimmune thyroiditis, subacute thyroiditis, administration of thyroid hormones, iodine-induced hyperthyroidism in iodine-deficient areas, certain tumors producing thyroid stimulators, and mutation in the TSH receptor gene (Dallas & Foley, 1996; Zimmerman & Lteif, 1998).

Because the onset of the disease is often insidious, accurate diagnosis is often delayed. Untreated, thyrotoxicosis has a high degree of morbidity and can, in severe cases, be fatal. Therefore, it is the clinician's responsibility to make the diagnosis promptly and institute early treatment in cooperation with a pediatric endocrinologist. This is especially important in patients with neonatal thyrotoxicosis, because proper levels of circulating thyroid hormones are essential for brain maturation.

PATHOPHYSIOLOGY

Thyrotoxicosis is characterized by excessive levels of unbound circulating thyroid hormones. Mechanisms producing thyrotoxicosis include the following:

- Thyroid follicular cell hyperplasia with increased synthesis and secretion of thyroxine (T_4) and triiodothyronine (T_3)
- Thyroid follicular cell destruction with release of preformed T_4 and T_3 into the circulation
- Ingestion of thyroid hormones

Hyperfunction of thyroid cells can be either autonomous or mediated through stimulation of TSH receptors. These mediators include thyrotropin receptor antibodies (TRAb), TSH, or human choriogonadotropin. Autonomous hyperfunction of thyroid follicular cells, which is represented by toxic adenoma, is rare in children.

Graves' disease is an immunogenetic disorder characterized by hyperthyroidism, thyromegaly, and infiltrative ophthalmopathy. Genetic studies have shown that Graves' disease is a polygenic disorder with most genes to be involved in immunoregulation associated with specific HLA types (A1, B8, DR3). A family history of thyroid disease is present in up to 60% of patients. Because the concordance rate between monozygotic twins is no more than 50%, it is believed that environmental factors, such as chemicals, drugs, infections, and perhaps stress, play an important role in the development of Graves' disease. However, the extent to which environmental factors can alter immunoregulatory genes is not known. Several hypotheses trying to explain the production and control of TRAb have been proposed. These include a deficiency of specific suppressor of T-cell function and a defect in the immunoregulation of B lymphocytes (Dallas & Foley, 1996).

HISTORY AND PHYSICAL EXAMINATION

The majority of children with thyrotoxicosis present with insidious development of classic symptoms and signs of a hypermetabolic state, such as increased fatigue, decreased attention span, nervousness, disturbances of sleep, poor weight gain (or weight loss despite increased appetite), increased frequency of bowel movements, heat intolerance, and tremor. A decline in school performance is often observed.

▲ **Clinical Warning:** In thyrotoxicosis, unless there is an obvious goiter or eye changes, psychologic or behavioral problems are often suspected as underlying etiologies. This often results in an inaccurate or delayed diagnosis (Clayton, 1982).

On physical examination, more than 90% of patients have thyromegaly (goiter). The gland is usually diffusely enlarged, smooth, and nontender on palpation. Other physical findings include tachycardia, increased pulse pressure, hyperreflexia of deep tendon reflexes, and tremor.

● **Clinical Pearl:** Eye changes, such as proptosis, lid lag, stare, and periorbital edema, are often seen but are usually much less severe than those in adults, and consequently, the diagnosis of Graves' disease may be missed.

In a growing child, there is an acceleration of growth velocity with advanced skeletal maturation. Other autoimmune disorders can coexist with Graves' disease, such as type 1 diabetes mellitus, rheumatoid arthritis, vitiligo, nephritis, autoimmune hepatitis, and myasthenia gravis. Rarely, patients may present with a suprasternal mass representing enlargement of the thymus.

DIAGNOSTIC CRITERIA AND STUDIES

The laboratory evaluation of Graves' disease and other conditions presenting as thyrotoxicosis is rather simple and straightforward. In most cases, the measurement of T_4, T_3, and TSH will be adequate for making the diagnosis of a hyperthyroid state. Both serum T_4 and T_3 levels will be elevated, while TSH is suppressed.

TRAb measurements should always be obtained, because their presence will confirm the diagnosis of Graves' disease. Currently, two major types of assays are used to measure TRAb:

1. The receptor assay measures the ability of the patient's immunoglobulin G to inhibit TSH binding to a thyroid membrane-thyrotropin-binding inhibitory immunoglobulin.

2. The bioassay measures the ability of the patient's immunoglobulins to stimulate the thyroid cell production of cAMP-thyroid-stimulating immunoglobulins (Dallas & Foley, 1996; Burman & Pandian, 1998).

TRAb will be detected in more than 90% of children with Graves' disease and less often in other autoimmune thyroid diseases, such as Hashimoto's thyroiditis. Antithyroid antibodies can also be detected in many patients with the disease.

An I123 thyroid uptake (both at 6 and 24 hours) and scan should be obtained in all patients presenting with thyrotoxicosis, because it can help differentiate Graves' disease from other causes of hyperthyroidism, such as subacute thyroiditis. Other tests include complete blood count with differential, sedimentation rate, liver function tests, serum calcium and phosphorus, electrocardiogram, and chest radiograph.

MANAGEMENT

The aim of treatment is to restore both clinical and chemical euthyroidism as quickly as possible. Treatment is best carried out with close consultation by a pediatric endocrinologist.

Presently, there is some controversy as to what the ideal treatment of hyperthyroidism in children should be. The issue specifically involves treatment with antithyroid drugs versus radioactive ablation of the gland. Surgical management, involving subtotal thyroidectomy, is performed much less frequently today. In the initial stages, most pediatric endocrinologists prefer the use of drugs as opposed to radioactive treatment. This is based on the observation that there is up to a 50% remission rate for every 2 years of disease duration (Lippe, Landaw, & Kaplan, 1987).

Initial Treatment

Propylthiouracil (PTU) and methimazole (MTZ) are the drugs recommended and currently used in the United States (Zimmerman & Lteif, 1998). Both drugs inhibit the incorporation of iodine into tyrosine residues of thyroglobulin and block the formation of T_4 and T_3. Unlike MTZ, PTU also inhibits the peripheral conversion of T_4 to T_3. Whether these drugs also exert immunosuppressive activity remains controversial (Tamai et al., 1995). The usual starting dose of PTU is between 300 and 600 mg/d (5–7 mg/kg) divided into three equal doses every 8 hours. The dose of MTZ is 10 times less (0.5–0.7 mg/kg per day) divided into two equal doses every 12 hours.

Because the effects of drugs will not take place immediately, the addition of β-adrenergic blockers, such as propranolol 10 to 20 mg three to four times a day, will be beneficial to patients with significant tachycardia. The drug also impedes the peripheral conversion of T_4 to T_3, which is an additional benefit. Rarely, patients will need diazepam (Valium) to ameliorate their agitation.

Maintenance Treatment

After 2 to 3 weeks, once clinical and chemical euthyroidism is achieved, either the dose of antithyroid drugs must be cut by approximately one third or more, or levothyroxine (Synthroid) must be added to avoid hypothyroidism. Both methods have their pluses and minuses.

● **Clinical Pearl:** In adolescents, it is preferable to treat patients with maintenance dosages of MTZ, because there is a great degree of noncompliance with the treatment regimen, especially when using the combination of high doses of PTU and levothyroxine.

▲ **Clinical Warning:** The use of PTU has been associated with liver damage, occasionally progressing to irreversible liver failure (Williams et al., 1997).

Both drugs have adverse side effects, such as agranulocytosis, collagen vascular disease, skin reactions, arthritis, and nephrotic syndrome, in addition to the aforementioned liver damage. The onset of agranulocytosis can be very rapid, and it is the clinician's responsibility to advise patients and their families to have white blood cells checked immediately when the child is ill with a sore throat or fever.

The use of radioactive iodine for the treatment of pediatric Graves' disease remains controversial because most patients will become hypothyroid, requiring lifelong treatment with thyroid hormone supplements (Rivkees, Sklar, & Freemark, 1998). To the contrary, there has not been any increased incidence of adverse genetic effects and neoplastic disorders either in patients or their offspring. Radioactive treatment of Graves' disease has even been used in young children (Clark, Gelfand, & Elgazzar, 1995). Both hyperparathyroidism and hypoparathyroidism have also been reported in patients treated with radioactive iodine. Theoretically, it remains unclear whether such treatment could worsen ongoing autoimmune processes.

Subtotal thyroidectomy is usually reserved for patients with large goiters and for those who are not amenable to drug or radiation therapy. Apart from permanent hypothyroidism, subtotal thyroidectomy carries a risk of hypoparathyroidism and laryngeal nerve damage as well.

Prognosis

The remission rate can be estimated at about 25% to 50% for every 2 years of disease duration. Many patients will not go into spontaneous remission and must be maintained on antithyroid drug treatment indefinitely. This is true especially in those with large goiters, initial serum T_4 levels above 20 mcg/dL (257.4 nmol/L), T_3 toxicosis, opthalmopathy, and persistence of TRAb. These patients may be better suited for radioactive iodine therapy. On the other hand, patients with rapidly diminishing size of the goiter and disappearance of TRAb from the circulation have a good chance of going into remission (Dallas & Foley, 1996; Zimmerman & Lteif, 1998, Lippe et al., 1987).

P A R T   3   ▲

Neonatal Thyrotoxicosis

● PAVEL FORT, MD

INTRODUCTION

Although extremely rare, occurring once in every 25,000 pregnancies (Fisher, 1986), untreated neonatal hyperthyroidism can lead to mental retardation (Fisher, 1986; Clayton, 1982). Most such patients are born to mothers with active Graves' disease.

▲ **Clinical Warning:** The clinician must realize that both the clinical and biochemical symptoms of neonatal thyrotoxicosis can be masked for several days due to maternal antithyroid therapy.

In most infants, thyrotoxicosis is transient as the maternal thyroid-stimulating antibodies are cleared from the circulation. Rarely is the disease long-lasting. Untreated severe neonatal thyrotoxicosis can be fatal and carries a high risk of severe brain damage as a result of the hypermetabolic state, premature closure of the cranial bones, and the direct effect of excess thyroid hormones on brain maturation (Daneman & Howard, 1980).

PATHOPHYSIOLOGY

The neonatal form of Graves' disease is thought to be caused by the transplacental passage of TRAb, which mimics the action of TSH in stimulating thyroid growth and function (McKenzie & Zakaria, 1992). Fortunately, only 2% to 3% of mothers with Graves' disease have affected babies, as neonatal thyrotoxicosis is usually seen only in children whose mothers have the most potent TRAb. Since TRAb can also exert a blocking rather than stimulating effect, some babies can present with hypothyroidism rather than hyperthyroidism (Yoshida et al., 1992). In addition, TRAb can have a biphasic effect, whereby large amounts can suppress the thyroid gland, and small amounts can stimulate the gland (Yoshida et al., 1992).

HISTORY AND PHYSICAL EXAMINATION

Patients with neonatal Graves' disease are often born before term (Howard & Hayles, 1978). If the mother has received antithyroid drugs, which readily cross the placenta, the baby may be asymptomatic for several days until the drug has been cleared from the circulation. Unlike the case in older children with Graves' disease, goiter and exophthalmos are infrequent features of neonatal thyrotoxicosis, although large goiters sufficient to cause respiratory impairment may occur secondary to large dosages of antithyroid drugs in the mother.

More often, such patients have tachycardia and respiratory distress. Hypermetabolic symptoms may eventually lead to heart failure. Other features include hyperkinesis, restlessness, diarrhea, and poor weight gain despite increased calorie intake (Howard & Hayles, 1978). Bone maturation is accelerated and may result in premature craniosynostosis (Daneman & Howard, 1980). Other features of neonatal thyrotoxicosis include jaundice, pitting edema, hepatosplenomegaly, thrombocytopenia, enlargement of the reticuloendothelial system, hyperviscosity syndrome, and ventricular extrasystoles (Singer, 1977).

DIAGNOSTIC CRITERIA AND STUDIES

As in older children with thyrotoxicosis, there is an elevation of T_4 and T_3 levels with suppression of TSH. Apart from thyroid hormone levels and TRAb, no other tests are usually necessary for diagnosis and management.

Not all infants with elevated T_4 and T_3 levels have thyrotoxicosis. As shown in Table 47-3, several other conditions manifested by hyperthyroxinemia must be taken into consideration, especially when an infant is clinically euthyroid. In these cases, TSH is not suppressed. These include alterations of binding proteins and thyroid hormone resistance.

Table 47–3.   DIFFERENTIAL DIAGNOSIS OF INCREASED T_4 LEVELS IN INFANTS

Syndrome	Total T_4	RT_3U[a]	TBG[b]	FT_4I[c]	Free T_4	Total T_3	Free T_3
Thyrotoxicosis	↑	↑	N	↑	↑	↑	↑
TBG excess	↑	↓	↑	N	N	↑	N
Increased T_4 binding to albumin	↑	N	N	↑	N	N	N
Increased T_4 binding to prealbumin	↑	↓ (N)	N	↑	N	N	N
T_4 resistance	↑	↓	N	↑	↑	↑	↑
I_2 contamination	±	N	N	N	N	↑	N

↑ = Increased; ↓ = Decreased; N = normal; [a]RTB = T_3 resin uptake; [b]TBG = thyroxine-binding globulin; [c]FT_4I = free thyroxine index.

MANAGEMENT

An infant with clinical and biochemical symptoms and signs of hyperthyroidism represents a medical emergency (Howard & Hayles, 1978). Consultation with a pediatric endocrinologist is mandatory.

The first important aspect of treatment is to combat the overstimulation of the cardiovascular system by administering beta-adrenergic blockers, such as propranolol, 1 to 2 mg/kg per day in three divided doses. The next step is to suppress the hypersecretion of thyroid hormones using a saturated solution of potassium iodide and thioamides, such as PTU. Iodides may be administered as 10% potassium iodide solution, 1 drop every 8 hours. If necessary, PTU, in a total daily dose of 5 to 10 mg/kg divided into three equal doses, can be added but will not be effective for several days. Severely affected infants may also benefit from glucocorticoids. It is important to realize that the treatment of the hyperthyroid state may result in hypothyroidism very quickly. Therefore, frequent measurements of thyroid function are necessary. Levothyroxine should be added as needed. There have been several reports of the successful use of sodium ipodate in infants with thyrotoxicosis without the consequence of hypothyroidism (Transue, Chan, & Kaplan, 1992). Because thyroid hormones have a profound effect on brain maturation, infants with neonatal thyrotoxicosis should have a complete neurologic assessment.

COMMUNITY RESOURCES

The following organizations provide information and support to patients and families with various thyroid disorders.

National Graves' Disease Foundation
P.O. Box 1969
Brevard, NC 28712
Telephone: (828) 877-5251
Internet address: *http://www.ngdf.org*

Thyroid Society
7515 South Main Street, Suite 545
Houston, TX 77030
Telephone: (713) 799-9909
Toll-free: (800) THYROID/(800) 849-7643
Internet address: *http://www.the-thyroid-society.org*

REFERENCES

Burman, K. D., & Pandian, R. (1998). Clinical utility of assays for TSH receptor antibodies. *The Endocrinologist, 8*, 284–290.

Clark, J. D., Gelfand, M. J., & Elgazzar, A. H. (1995). Iodine-131 therapy of hyperthyroidism in pediatric patients. *Journal of Nuclear Medicine, 36*, 442–445.

Clayton, G. W. (1982). Thyrotoxicosis in children. In S. A. Kaplan (Ed.), *Clinical pediatric and adolescent endocrinology* (pp. 110–117). Philadelphia: W.B. Saunders.

Dallas, J. S., & Foley, T. P., Jr. (1996). Hyperthyroidism. In F. Lifshitz (Ed.), *Pediatric endocrinology* (pp. 401–414). New York: Marcel Dekker.

Daneman, D., & Howard, N. J. (1980). Neonatal thyrotoxicosis: Intellectual impairment and craniosynostosis in later years. *Journal of Pediatrics, 97*, 257–259.

Fisher, D. A. (1986). Neonatal thyroid disease in the offspring of women with autoimmune thyroid disease. *Thyroid Today, 9(4)*, 1 to 7.

Howard, C. P., & Hayles, A. B. (1978). Neonatal Graves' disease. *Clinics in Endocrinology and Metabolism, 7*, 131–134.

Lippe, B. M., Landaw, E. M., & Kaplan, S. A. (1987). Hyperthyroidism in children treated with long term medical therapy: Twenty-five percent remission rate every two years. *Journal of Clinical Endocrinology and Metabolism, 64*, 1241–1245.

McKanzie, J. M., & Zakoria, M. (1992). Fetal and neonatal hyperthyroidism due to maternal TSH receptor antibodies. *Thyroid, 2*, 155–159.

Rivkees, S. A., Sklar, C., & Freemark, M. (1998). The management of Graves' disease in children, with special emphasis on radioiodine treatment. *Journal of Clinical Endocrinology and Metabolism, 83*, 1367–1376.

Singer, J. (1977). Neonatal thyrotoxicosis. *Journal of Pediatrics, 91*, 749–751.

Tamai, H., Hayaki, I., Kawai, K., et al. (1995). Lack of effect of thyroxine administration on elevated thyroid stimulating hormone receptor antibody levels in treated Graves' disease patients. *Journal of Clinical Endocrinology and Metabolism, 80*, 1481–1484.

Transue, D., Chan, J., & Kaplan, M. (1992). Management of neonatal Graves' disease with iopanoic acid. *Journal of Pediatrics, 121*, 472–474.

Williams, K. V., Nayak, S., Becker, D., et al. (1997). Fifty years of experience with propylthiouracil-associated hepatotoxicity: What have we learned? *Journal of Clinical Endocrinology and Metabolism, 82*, 1727–1733.

Yoshida, S., Takamatsu, J., Kuma, K., et al. (1992). Thyroid-stimulating antibodies and thyroid-stimulation-blocking antibodies during the pregnancy and postpartum period: a case report. *Thyroid, 2(1)*, 27–29.

Zimmerman, D., & Lteif, A. N. (1998). Thyrotoxicosis in children. *Endocrinology and Metabolism Clinics of North America, 27*, 109–126.

P A R T   4   ▲

Diabetic Ketoacidosis

• PAVEL FORT, MD

INTRODUCTION

Diabetic ketoacidosis (DKA) is a major medical emergency that a clinician may face. With proper treatment, the majority of children with DKA will recover uneventfully; however, severe metabolic acidosis or hyperglycemic hyperosmolar coma can be life-threatening. Therefore, the management of children with DKA should be carried out in an appropriate clinical setting, preferably in a pediatric intensive care unit, where close supervision and frequent monitoring of a patient's clinical status and biochemical parameters are readily available.

DKA can present itself in a child with newly diagnosed, usually type I insulin-dependent diabetes mellitus (IDDM), or it can develop in a child with existing diabetes mellitus. It is the clinician's responsibility to investigate all possible events that could precipitate the development of DKA. These include a failure to recognize symptoms of a new-onset diabetes mellitus or a failure to monitor diabetes mellitus properly and take necessary action when diabetes mellitus is out of control.

When faced with a child in DKA, a clinician must ask the following questions:

- Is the child known to have diabetes mellitus?
- Does the child have diseases other than diabetes mellitus?
- Have there been similar episodes in the past, and if yes, under what circumstances?
- What was the child's last dose of insulin?
- How rapidly did the symptoms of DKA develop?

The answers to these questions will not only allow for the better management of DKA, but can also help prevent similar episodes in the future.

PATHOPHYSIOLOGY

The hallmark of metabolic derangement in DKA is a lack of insulin with concomitant increase of anti-insulin stress hormones, such as glucagon, epinephrine, cortisol, and growth hormone. The metabolism of glucose, protein, and fat is severely compromised in DKA (Fleckman, 1993).

Hyperglycemia is the result of both insulin deficiency (decreased glucose utilization) and excessive production of anti-insulin hormones promoting neoglucogenesis and glycogenolysis (increased glucose production). Hyperglycemia causes an osmotic diuresis and dehydration.

Lack of insulin leads to decreased uptake of amino acids by muscle, causing diminished protein synthesis and muscle wasting. Under normal circumstances, insulin inhibits lipolysis and promotes lipogenesis. In insulin deficiency states, increased lipolysis will result in an excess of circulating free fatty acids, which serve as substrate for ketogenesis. The flux of free fatty acids to ketogenesis is further enhanced by the reduction of lipogenesis from both insulin deficiency and excess glucagon. Epinephrine, cortisol, and growth hormone act in a similar manner (ie, they promote neoglucogenesis, proteolysis, and lipolysis).

These metabolic alterations lead to overproduction and decreased peripheral use of glucose and free fatty acids, resulting in hyperglycemia and ketonemia. Unless this vicious cycle is broken by providing insulin and fluids, DKA will invariably lead to coma and death.

EPIDEMIOLOGY

The exact incidence of DKA among children is not known. Fortunately, the majority of children with new-onset IDDM are now diagnosed early before the development of DKA. Fewer than 20% of children with newly diagnosed diabetes mellitus develop DKA.

▲ **Clinical Warning:** Parents and clinicians may not recognize the new onset of diabetes mellitus in very young children whose symptoms are not typical of diabetes mellitus. Such patients are especially vulnerable to the detrimental effects of severe hyperglycemia and acidosis. Therefore, it is imperative to consider diabetes mellitus in the differential diagnosis of a sick, young child.

Because of the ever-increasing emphasis on education of patients with IDDM and their families, including frequent home blood glucose monitoring with proper and timely adjustments of the insulin dose, severe DKA in an established patient with IDDM is becoming less frequent. There are, however, patients whose suboptimal participation with the therapeutic regimen puts them at risk of DKA. It is the clinician's responsibility to identify such patients early and to develop frequent and effective communication with the patient's family.

▲ **Clinical Warning:** In the case of recurrent episodes of DKA due to poor participation with the therapeutic regimen or adverse home situations, the temporary placement of the child in a chronic care facility should be considered.

HISTORY AND PHYSICAL EXAMINATION

Most patients will have symptoms of diabetes mellitus, such as polyuria and polydipsia, well before the onset of DKA. In an established patient with diabetes mellitus, the worsening glycemic control with the presence of urinary ketones will often be noticed and brought to a clinician's attention. Stress may be present, such as infection or psychological stress. Children, especially the young ones, often develop nocturnal enuresis. There may be a tendency to lose body weight despite increased appetite and food intake. As a result of diminished protein synthesis and increased protein degradation, patients will experience fatigue due to muscle weakness. Once the patient is unable to compensate for fluid losses through increased fluid intake, progressively worsening dehydration will develop, followed by metabolic acidosis. Initially, an increased respiratory rate (Kussmaul breathing) will compensate for the metabolic acidosis. Later, especially in young children, respiratory compensation may fail because of increasing exhaustion, and when acidosis becomes severe, the respiratory center will be suppressed rather than stimulated. The combination of both metabolic and respiratory acidosis will lead to a rapid deterioration of vital functions.

The history of incipient DKA in a small child is less clear. Such children can show irritability, poor appetite, soaked diapers, and diaper rash. They may be temporarily consoled by extra fluids, which are often juices and which can only compound the severity of hyperglycemia. Unlike older children, they may progress to coma rather quickly.

In uncomplicated mild to moderately severe DKA, the physical examination is often unremarkable and the variable degree of dehydration is often the only positive physical sign. In most severe cases of DKA, hyperventilation (Kussmaul's breathing) with various levels of obtunded consciousness can be seen. Such patients may be restless with flushed cheeks, diminished skin turgor, and smell of acetone on the breath. Patients in DKA will often complain of nonspecific abdominal and back pain. Despite the dehydration, patients in DKA will continue to have good urinary output, violating common homeostatic rules. Rarely, a patient with DKA presents in coma or renal shutdown, which usually results from morbid hyperosmolality, the management of which is discussed later in this section.

DKA must be differentiated from acidosis and coma from other causes, such as salicylate or other poisonings; lactic acidosis; various metabolic diseases affecting glucose, protein, and fat metabolism; central nervous system (CNS) infections and lesions; severe gastroenteritis; uremia; and drug overdose. In a patient with known diabetes mellitus, hypoglycemia must be ruled out. Displays 47-1 and 47-2 highlight the pertinent features of the history and physical examination in DKA.

DIAGNOSTIC CRITERIA

The diagnosis of DKA is usually easy to make. It can be defined as hyperglycemia (glucose > 300 mg/dL; > 16.6 mOsm/L), ketonemia (serum ketones positive at greater than 1:2 dilution), acidosis (pH < 7.30 and HCO_3 < 15 mEq/L), glycosuria, and ketonuria, in addition to classical symptoms and signs of uncontrolled diabetes mellitus (Display 47-3) (Sperling, 1996).

DIAGNOSTIC STUDIES

The majority of children with DKA will be first evaluated in an emergency department setting. The Dextrostix/Chemstrip should be obtained immediately to ascertain hyperglycemia. This will also help to rule out hypoglycemia, which could present as a coma. The following laboratory

---

DISPLAY 47-1 • History

Polyuria, polydipsia, polyphagia
Nocturnal enuresis
Physical/emotional stress
Increased fatigue
Worsening dehydration
Increased respiratory rate (Kussmaul's breathing)
Deterioration of vital functions

DISPLAY 47-2 • Physical Examination

Usually stable vital signs
Variable degree of dehydration
Flushed cheeks
Smell of acetone on breath
Hyperventilation (Kussmaul's breathing)
Nonspecific back and abdominal pains

---

evaluations will be necessary to guide the clinician in managing the patient in DKA and are listed in Display 47-4.

Serum Glucose

The measurement of serum glucose will assess the degree of hyperglycemia. In the majority of patients in DKA, the serum glucose will be between 300 and 1000 mg/dL (16.6 and 55.5 mmol/L). In patients presenting with serum glucose greater than 1000 mg/dL (> 55.5 mmol/L), the treatment should be modified because such patients are usually in a severe hyperosmolar state (see the section on morbid hyperosmolality).

Serum Ketones

The presence of serum ketones, primarily beta hydroxybutyrate, indicates ketosis, which is the main cause of acidosis in patients with DKA. It is important to realize that the beta hydroxybutyrate will not be detected on usual Acetest tablet assays, and the direct measurement of beta hydroxybutyrate may be requested. During recovery, beta hydroxybutyrate is converted to acetoacetate, which is detectable on Acetest tablet assays, resulting in a temporary rise of ketone bodies in the serum.

pH and Serum Bicarbonate

The measurement of blood pH and serum bicarbonate will assess the severity of acidosis.

▲ Clinical Warning: Unless the acidosis is severe (pH < 7.10), there is often no need for bicarbonate replacement therapy, because the administration of insulin together with IV fluids leads to the rapid correction of acidosis. In fact, the overzealous use of bicarbonate can be disadvantageous because it may precipitate metabolic alkalosis with adverse effects on serum potassium and the CNS.

In addition, most patients with DKA are able to compensate for metabolic acidosis by hyperventilating. However, small children and those with concurrent pneumonia or myopathic states do not effectively hyperventilate. The lack of hyperventilation in the face of severe metabolic acidosis can be an ominous sign indicating the life-threatening combination of metabolic and respiratory acidosis. The measurement of an arterial pH is usually not necessary unless there is a concern about respiratory status or oxygenation.

DISPLAY 47-3 • Diagnostic Criteria

Blood glucose greater than 300 mg/dL (16.6 mmol/L)
Serum ketones positive at greater than 1:2 dilution
Blood pH less than 7.30 and HCO_3 less than 15 mEq/L
Glycosuria and ketonuria

DISPLAY 47–4 • Diagnostic Studies

Immediate
Serum glucose
Serum ketones
Blood pH
Blood bicarbonate
Serum electrolytes
Serum osmolality
Complete blood count
Serum amylase
Urine analysis
Electrocardiogram
Appropriate cultures
Serum insulin and C-peptide (in patients with new onset
   of diabetes)

Later
Markers of an autoimmune process (best obtained prior to
   the initiation of insulin therapy)
Glycosylated hemoglobins (HbA1c)
Thyroid function tests
Serum lipids

Serum Electrolytes

The most important serum electrolyte to follow is potassium. Patients with DKA often have severely depleted total body potassium stores, and dangerous hypokalemia may develop after the introduction of insulin therapy and correction of acidosis.

●**Clinical Pearl:** The clinician must remember that a normal serum potassium level in the face of severe metabolic acidosis should not be reassuring, because potassium is primarily an intracellular ion. To compensate for the excess hydrogen ions seen in metabolic acidosis, hydrogen enters the cell in exchange for potassium. What appears to be a normal serum level is actually a depleted total body potassium.

Serum sodium is often low because of increased blood glucose and lipids (pseudohyponatremia). The sodium is falsely depressed at a level of 1.6 mEq/dL for each 100 mg/dL that the blood sugar is above normal. In addition, patients with DKA are often sodium depleted because of urinary losses of electrolytes secondary to osmotic diuresis and decreased food intake with or without vomiting.

Blood urea nitrogen (BUN) will be elevated in dehydrated patients. Serum calcium and especially serum phosphorus are often diminished. Severe, clinically significant hypophosphatemia may develop during the correction of hyperglycemia with insulin unless phosphate supplements are administered.

Serum Osmolality

The determination of serum osmolality, preferably by direct measurement, is essential. Although all patients with DKA will have elevated serum osmolality, usually in the 310 to 240 mOsm/L range, in some, serum osmolality may be over 375 mOsm/L, indicating a morbid hyperosmolality state with a high risk for intracranial bleeding, cerebral edema, and renal shutdown (refer to the section on morbid hyperosmolality). If direct measurement of serum osmolality is not available, the following formula can be used to estimate the serum osmolality:

$$2(Na + K) + glucose{:}18 \text{ plus } BUN{:}2.6.$$

Complete Blood Count

The complete blood count values will help the clinician to assess for evidence of bacterial or viral infection. However, in DKA there is often an elevated white cell count in the absence of an infectious process due to bone marrow demargination as a result of physiologic stress.

Serum Amylase

Many patients in DKA will complain of midabdominal pain, nausea, and vomiting. The measurement of serum amylase may help to rule out the possibility of pancreatitis. However, even in uncomplicated DKA, there is often some degree of elevated serum amylase, probably of salivary origin.

Urine Analysis

The presence of glucose and ketones in the urine is the hallmark of uncontrolled diabetes mellitus. In some patients, there may be a small amount of proteinuria present.

Electrocardiogram

The electrocardiogram will allow for a rapid, bedside assessment of the physiologic levels of body potassium and cardiac function.

Other Tests

In the presence of fever or other signs of infection, cultures of blood, urine, throat, and, if present, the wound should be obtained. A spinal tap to rule out infection of the CNS should also be considered if the clinical history and examination suggest a CNS infection.

Later Studies

The following studies will be needed but are not necessary for the acute management of DKA. These include the measurement of glycosylated hemoglobins (HgbA1c), thyroid function, insulin/C-peptide level, serum lipids, and various markers of an autoimmune process, such as islet cell antibodies, anti-insulin antibodies, and anti-GAD (glutamic acid decarboxylase) antibodies.

MANAGEMENT

The effective treatment of DKA consists of simultaneous administration of IV fluids with insulin and, when necessary (only in severe acidosis), correction with sodium bicarbonate. This is summarized in Display 47-5. During the acute phase of treatment, blood glucose and electrolytes must be monitored on an hourly basis. The patient must be kept NPO (Zangen & Levitsky, 1996). A flow sheet should be available for every patient (Fig. 47-3).

Correction of Fluid and Electrolyte Deficit

Rapid Restoration of Circulating Fluid Volume

An initial loading dose of 20 mL/kg of normal saline (NS) or Ringer's lactate (RL) should be given within the first hour of treatment. The use of RL is equally effective as NS; however, the lactate content will hamper the measurement of lactic acid in

DISPLAY 47–5 • Treatment of Diabetic Ketoacidosis

Monitor

Vital signs, mental status, input and output, serum glucose, hourly during the initial period of treatment

Serum osmolality, serum electrolytes, and blood pH every 2 to 4 hours

Fluids

Give bolus 20 mL/kg of normal saline or Ringer's lactate to restore circulating fluid volume.

Infuse maintenance fluids plus calculated deficit evenly over 24 to 36 hours.

Change initial solution to 0.45% saline with added potassium, 40 mEq/L after 1 to 2 hours (half given as KCl, half as KPO_4).

Adjust electrolyte composition of fluids as needed.

When blood sugar falls below 300 mg/dL, add dextrose in the form of D5% or D2/12% to IV solutions.

Insulin

Provide continuous intravenous infusion of regular (human) insulin at a rate of 0.1 U/kg/h (0.05 U/kg/h in children younger than 4 years).

Once acidosis is corrected (serum pH > 7.30), decrease infusion rate by 50%.

Acidosis

Blood pH > 7.10	No $NaHCO_3$ is needed.
Blood pH 7.10–7.00	Correct the bicarbonate deficit slowly over an hour or more. Deficit = (15 − serum HCO_3) × kg body weight × 0.6
Blood pH < 7.00	Administer 1 mEq of $NaHCO_3$ per kg by slow intravenous push (monitor heart rhythm).

Continue IV insulin and IV fluids until serum pH and blood sugar have normalized.

---

the serum. Prolonged administration of NS should be avoided, especially in small children, because it may result in hypernatremia. Therefore, the electrolyte status must be quickly determined to allow for the proper selection of IV fluids.

Amount of Intravenous Fluids

The total amount of fluids given to a patient with DKA consists of maintenance fluids and correction of deficit. Mainte-nance fluid therapy should be given in a uniform manner throughout the day (24 hours). Among many techniques for calculating maintenance fluids, the one based on giving 1500 mL of water per square meter of body surface area per day is commonly used.

Deficit fluid therapy is based on the assessment of dehy-dration using the usual clinical criteria and, when possible, supported by obtaining the recent change in body weight. In DKA, acute weight loss is mainly water. It is preferable to administer water deficit over 24 to 36 hours at a constant rate. This will minimize rapid fluid shifts between the extra-cellular and intracellular space.

▲ **Clinical Warning:** In order to minimize the likelihood of potentially fatal cerebral edema, total fluids given should not exceed 4 L/m²/day.

Unusual losses of fluids, such as nasogastric aspirate, succus entericus, or diarrhea, usually do not have to be replaced. Similarly, during the initial stages of treatment, the patient may continue to have significant urinary losses due to osmotic diuresis. Again, it is not recommended that these losses be replaced to avoid dangerous fluid overload. The correction of hyperglycemia will lead to diminished osmotic diuresis rather quickly.

Composition of Intravenous Fluids

After the initial administration of NS, the fluids are usually changed to 0.45% saline with added potassium 20 to 40 mEq/L given as half KCL and half KPO_4. The amount of sodium and potassium in the fluids may need to be adjusted depending on serum electrolytes.

▲ **Clinical Warning:** The persistence of hyponatremia despite the correction of hyperglycemia can be due to inappropriate secretion of antidiuretic hormone and a warning sign of CNS complications. In such an event, the amount of fluids should be decreased and the composition of fluids made relatively more hyperosmolar.

Insulin Administration

The most physiologic and preferable route of insulin admin-istration is the continuous intravenous infusion of regular insulin (Humulin) at a rate of 0.1 U/kg per hour. In children younger than 4 years, half of the dose, or 0.05 U/kg of regu-lar insulin per hour, should be used. An initial loading bolus of insulin is rarely needed. The insulin solutions are usually prepared by diluting regular insulin in NS so that the result-

---

DKA Flow sheet   **Patient name:**   MR#

Date & Time	Serum Glucose	Serum Osmolality	Serum Sodium	Serum Potassium	BUN	pH	HCO_3	pCO_2	Insulin u/kg/h	Fluid intake	Fluid output	Body weight	Level of consciousness	Others

Figure 47–3 ■ Flow sheet for patients with diabetic ketoacidosis.

ant solution contains 1 U of insulin per 1 mL. This is piggy-backed by pump into the IV line. Hourly monitoring of blood glucose is essential while the child is receiving the continuous insulin drip.

When the blood glucose falls below 300 mg/dL (16.6 mmol/L), 5% dextrose should be added to the IV fluids. As long as the patient remains acidotic (blood pH < 7.30), the dose of insulin infusion should remain constant. If the blood glucose continues to fall, the concentration of glucose in the infusate should be increased. Once the acidosis is corrected (blood pH > 7.30), it is preferable to decrease the insulin infusion rate (usually by 50%) over the increased glucose concentration in the IV fluids.

The insulin drip and IV hydration should be maintained until both hyperglycemia and acidosis have been corrected.

Among other routes of insulin administration to patients with DKA, the IM administration of 0.1 U of regular insulin (0.05 U in children younger than 4 years) per kg every hour can be quite effective.

▲ **Clinical Warning:** It is important to keep in mind that dehydration will preclude the efficient absorption of subcutaneously administered insulin.

Correction of Acidosis

Metabolic acidosis in DKA is primarily due to ketoacidosis and less to lactic acidosis. The lactic acidosis will respond to vascular volume replenishment and reinstitution of adequate capillary infusion. Ketoacidosis will respond to insulin administration.

● **Clinical Pearl:** The combination of fluid and insulin therapy will effectively correct mild to moderate acidosis, and no bicarbonate replacement is necessary.

In severe acidosis (blood pH < 7.10), which could be life-threatening, sodium bicarbonate should be administered as follows:

- pH between 7.10 and 7.00—Correct the bicarbonate deficit slowly over an hour or more. The bicarbonate deficit is calculated as follows:

$$\text{deficit} = (15 - \text{serum HCO}_3) \times \text{kg body weight} \times 0.6$$

- pH less than 7.00—Give 1 mEq/kg NaHCO$_3$ by slow IV push while carefully monitoring heart rhythm.

▲ **Clinical Warning:** The overuse of sodium bicarbonate can lead to hypernatremia. Furthermore, because the equilibrium across the respiratory center of the brain is slow for bicarbonate but rapid for carbon dioxide, quick correction of metabolic acidosis can lead to retention of carbon dioxide and paradoxical CNS acidosis. Finally, rapid correction of metabolic acidosis can precipitate hypokalemia, because alkalosis promotes the influx of potassium into cells.

Follow-up Care

During the acute phase of DKA, the typical patient is unable to tolerate oral feedings. When the acute phase of DKA is over, the patient will be ready to eat and will need insulin to cover the food intake.

Patients with preexisting diabetes mellitus can resume their usual insulin regimen. In patients with newly diagnosed type 1 diabetes mellitus, the dose of insulin will need to be calculated. One approach has been to start all newly diagnosed patients on a combination of Humulin NPH or

LENTE and the new extremely fast-acting Humalog (lispro insulin) given before breakfast and before dinner. Most patients will require between 0.5 and 1.0 U/kg per 24 hours. The total dose of insulin per day is divided into two thirds in the morning (to be given before breakfast) and one third in the evening (to be given before dinner). Both the morning and the evening doses of insulin are further broken down into NPH or LENTE and Humalog in a 3:1 ratio. The dose of Humalog insulin can be adjusted up or down according to blood glucose levels (sliding scale). The goal is to maintain blood glucose levels in the 90 to 140 mg/dL range in older children and in the 100 to 200 mg/dL range in preschool children. When Humalog insulin is used, the patient should eat immediately after the injection of insulin.

Patient Education

After recovery from DKA, patients with new-onset diabetes mellitus and their families must receive an intensive education about the basics of diabetes management. In patients with preexisting diabetes mellitus, knowledge about diabetes and its proper management should be reviewed.

Diabetes self-management education of the child and parents is the key to achieving and maintaining the best possible metabolic control of diabetes mellitus. The management of diabetes is complex; therefore, the combined effort of the provider, a pediatric endocrinologist, a diabetes educator, a nutritionist, an exercise physiologist and a psychologist can add great support to developing a successful treatment plan and managing this complex disease.

MORBID HYPEROSMOLALITY

Morbid hyperosmolality (MH) is loosely defined as serum osmolality greater than 375 mOsm/L (Pugliese et al., 1990). Such patients usually present with severe hyperglycemia well over 1000 mg/dL (55.5 mmol/L) and only mild ketosis. Patients with MH have some residual insulin excretion; however, they are unable to maintain adequate fluid intake in the face of rising blood sugar. In adults, there is often a preexisting condition, such as sepsis or use of various drugs, whereas in children, MH is usually seen in younger children with undiagnosed diabetes mellitus. MH represents a serious condition with high mortality and morbidity. MH can be seen in children who are preverbal or have preexisting neurologic damage. Failure to consider diabetes mellitus in the differential diagnosis of an irritable, dehydrated, and lethargic child can delay proper treatment.

The disorder can precipitate disseminated intravascular coagulation (DIC), acute renal failure, and CNS hemorrhage. Overzealous and rapid correction of severe hypertonicity can, on the other hand, lead to cerebral edema with all its negative consequences. These patients must not be managed single-handedly, and a team consisting of a pediatric endocrinologist, intensivist, neurologist, and nephrologist should be available.

The hallmark of appropriate management of MH is to correct dehydration and hyperglycemia slowly over 48 to 72 hours. The rapid correction of dehydration and hyperglycemia may lead to fluid overload and dangerous cerebral edema.

Monitoring the Patient

Patients with MH often present with markedly diminished sensorium or in frank coma. The attendant severe cellular dehydration can cause intracranial bleeding by tearing bridging meningeal vessels. The bleeding can further be aggravated by DIC and the formation of arterial and venous thrombi owing to the hyperviscosity. Rapid rehydration, especially with hypotonic solutions, will result in cerebral edema. To discern which lesion is present, CT of the brain may be required. Intracranial pressure monitoring will allow rising pressures to be diagnosed early before the development of clinical signs of cerebral edema.

During resuscitation of the hyperosmolar patient, careful attention must be paid to the amount of infused fluids: Too much fluid will cause cerebral edema, whereas too slow repletion of blood volume can cause renal shutdown and worsen acidosis. Therefore, central venous and arterial lines should be placed early. They will allow for proper monitoring of hydration status, blood pressure, and cardiovascular tone.

Fluid and Electrolyte Therapy

The two major goals of fluid and electrolyte therapy are as follows:

1. Resuscitation of the patient from shock and maintenance of an adequate perfusion of vital organs
2. Gradual reduction of the serum hyperosmolality

By carefully monitoring the interplay of the arterial pressure, central venous pressure, and fluid intake and output, the clinician should be able to accomplish the above goals. When too much fluid results in increased intracranial pressure, various methods to lower the pressure, such as hyperventilation, barbiturate coma, and head elevation should be used.

Either isotonic or hypertonic solutions should be used to dilute the hyperosmolality. Most cases of fatal cerebral edema documented in the literature occurred in the presence of serum hyponatremia from the use of hypotonic solutions. Therefore, the infused fluids should be only 30 to 40 mOsm/L lower than the patient's osmolality. This can be easily achieved with normal saline and potassium salts. It has been agreed that cerebral edema is unlikely to occur if total fluid restitution is held below 4 L/m^2 per 24 hours.

Insulin Therapy

Insulin should always be given to these patients. However, because it is undesirable to drop blood glucose too quickly, there is some controversy about the dosage of insulin required. One approach has been to give only half of the usual dose of insulin (ie, 0.05 U of regular insulin per kg per hour by constant insulin infusion). In children younger than 4 years, even less insulin (0.02 U/kg per hour) is often needed. This may be decreased even further if there is a rapid drop in blood glucose. The goal is to maintain blood glucose levels around 250 mg/dL (13.9 mmol/L) because cerebral edema usually occurs when the blood glucose is forced below 250 mg/dL (13.9 mmol/L) by insulin.

COMMUNITY RESOURCES

Juvenile Diabetes Foundation
120 Wall Street
New York, NY 10005
Telephone: (212) 785-9500
Toll-free: (800) JDF-CURE
Fax: (212) 785-9595
Internet address: *http://www.jdf.org*

REFERENCES

Fleckman, A. M. (1993). Diabetic ketoacidosis. *Endocrinology and Metabolism Clinics of North America, 22*, 181–207.
Pugliese, M. T., Fort, P., Lifschitz, F. (1990). Treatment of diabetic ketoacidosis. In F. Lifshitz (Ed.), *Pediatric endocrinology* (2nd ed.) (pp. 745–766). New York: Marcel Dekker.
Sperling, M. A. (1996). *Pediatric endocrinology* (pp. 229–263). Philadelphia: W.B. Saunders.
Zangen, D., & Levitsky, L. L. (1996). Diabetes ketoacidosis. In F. Lifshitz (Ed.), *Pediatric endocrinology* (3rd ed.) (pp. 631–643). New York: Marcel Dekker.

Environmental Hazards

DANIEL ARONZON, MD, FAAP; PRADEEP SHARMA, MD; RICHARD BACHUR, MD;
SUNIL K. SOOD, MD; and VINCENT P. BELTRANI, MD

P A R T   I   ▲

Lead Poisoning

• DANIEL ARONZON, MD

INTRODUCTION

In the early 1970s, lead poisoning was viewed as an environmental hazard limited to large, urban pediatric inpatient services, where occasionally children with encephalopathy were diagnosed and treated. It was falsely assumed that only such high-level exposures caused permanent damage, and studies focused on the effects of chelation therapy for very high blood lead levels (BLLs) in excess of 45 mcg/dL and its ability to reverse deleterious neurologic effects (Silbergeld, 1997).

Newer studies raised the very disturbing concern that lead could cause irreversible damage at much lower BLLs than previously imagined. A landmark article by Needleman and Gatsonis (1990) proved that exposure to lead had significant effects on the behavior and cognition of children. Clearly, chelation therapy can lower BLLs and total body lead, and in doing so, it can prevent acute neurotoxicity, such as seizures. What is unclear is whether postexposure chelation can reverse the long-term neurologic sequelae of lead poisoning (Silbergeld, 1997).

These concerns have led to a new public health strategy focusing on eliminating lead exposure from the environment and recognizing that toxicity may be associated with a BLL above 10 mcg/dL. National initiatives in the United States have eliminated lead from gasoline and indoor paints. The variables of income, race, and residence, however, and the fact that lead poisoning is not evenly distributed among all children in the United States continue to raise obstacles to its universal prevention (Silbergeld, 1997).

PATHOLOGY

The classic markers of lead toxicity, encephalopathy, and red blood cell basophilic stippling are rarely seen in this era (American Academy of Pediatrics [AAP], 1995). Numerous studies have demonstrated the relationship between BLLs and cognitive defects. The 1998 AAP Policy Statement lists cognitive deficits, attention problems, and aggressive, antisocial, and delinquent behaviors as possi-

ble sequelae of low-level lead poisoning. It also provides an excellent bibliography.

▲ **Clinical Warning:** For every 10 mcg/dL increase in BLL, there is an estimated decrease of two IQ points (Glotzer & Weitzman, 1995).

Diet affects lead toxicity. Iron deficiency increases the absorption of lead from the gastrointestinal (GI) tract, while adequate iron intake decreases absorption. Calcium deficiency increases lead retention in bone.

Knowledge of lead pharmacokinetics is very primitive. Elimination from bone is measured in years. BLLs represent only a fraction of the total body lead, the majority of which is in bone. Chelation therapy temporarily lowers BLLs until equilibration with bone takes place. If any reduction in total body lead is to occur, it may require long-term chronic chelation therapy, the effects of which are unknown (AAP, 1995).

EPIDEMIOLOGY

The mean BBL in the United States has decreased from 12.8 mcg/dL in 1980 to 2.3 mcg/dL in 1994. In 1994, 2.2% of the population had BLLs greater than 10 mcg/dL. From 1980 to 1994, the percentage of children with BLLs greater than 10 mcg/dL decreased from 88.2% to 4.4%. Figures are much higher, however, among African American, poor, and urban children. These declines are attributed to the removal of lead from gasoline, paint, and food cans. Lead in paint was banned in 1970, and lead-containing gasoline was gradually phased out and finally banned in 1990 (AAP, 1998; Needleman, 1998).

Lead poisoning is not just a problem for the urban poor. Seventy-four percent of privately owned homes contain lead paint, with age and condition of housing, not location, as prime risk factors (AAP, 1998). Lead-based paint in the form of paint chips and house dust are the prime sources. Other sources include soil (contaminated from gasoline for decades), water (from lead pipes), household renovations, occupational exposures, and lead-containing pottery, folk medicines, and cosmetics.

HISTORY AND PHYSICAL EXAMINATION

Low-level chronic lead poisoning may not be associated with any specific clinical findings other than a history of older housing. It is associated with a hypochromic microcytic anemia, and lead exposure should be considered in that differential.

Acute intoxication may result in abdominal pain, constipation, headaches, vomiting, and in severe cases, changes in the level of consciousness or seizures.

DIAGNOSTIC CRITERIA AND STUDIES

The diagnosis is commonly established from the results of screening tests. Risks for lead intoxication are determined from patient questionnaires and actual measurement of BLL.

MANAGEMENT

Management falls into four basic categories: identification through screening; patient education; abatement; and chelation for those with elevated levels. Screening and chelation are discussed in the following sections.

Screening

In 1991, the Centers for Disease Control and Prevention (CDC) recommended and the AAP endorsed universal screening between ages 9 and 12 months and then again at age 2 years. They revised these guidelines in 1998, because in certain geographic areas, the incidence of abnormal BLLs was so low that it did not justify the cost. The CDC felt that targeted screenings would be more appropriate than universal screenings. The AAP endorsed and justified this measure to reduce unnecessary testing of children unlikely to be at risk.

The new guidelines appear complex and difficult to interpret and implement. In communities where the prevalence of elevated BLL (>10 mcg/dL) is unknown and where older housing predominates (more than 27% built before 1950), universal screening is still recommended. Targeted screening based on the answers to a questionnaire (Display 48-1) is recommended for locales where less than 12% of children have BLLs greater than 10 mcg/dL or where less than 27% of the homes were built before 1950. The burden for determining which communities will have targeted or universal screening falls to local and state public health officials (AAP, 1998). It is not surprising that this apparent backslide in policy has

raised controversy, particularly among public health officials (Needleman, 1998; Silbergeld, 1997).

Patient education is recommended as part of anticipatory guidance for all. The AAP in its 1998 policy statement identifies risk factors and prevention strategies that are listed in Table 48-1. Management of elevated BLLs identified during screening, as recommended by the AAP, including education and abatement, is outlined in Table 48-2.

▲ **Clinical Warning:** Fingerstick lead results may be falsely high due to dust contamination. No treatment decisions can be made without first obtaining a confirmatory venous sample.

Chelation

The 1995 AAP policy statement provides an excellent review of the classic chelation modalities, dimercaprol (BAL in oil) and calcium disodium EDTA. Parenteral administration for each is required. Penicillamine is also discussed as an oral chelator.

Most clinicians who treat lead poisoning now use succimer (an oral analog of dimercaprol). As an oral agent, it may be used on an outpatient basis but only after environmental safety is guaranteed. There is no evidence that with BLLs between 25 and 45 mcg/dL, chelation avoids or reverses neurotoxicity (Berlin, 1997); however, if elevated levels persist in this range, despite all efforts at abatement, succimer may be indicated after consultation with an expert. Succimer is definitely indicated for children with BLLs greater than 45 mcg/dL who have no symptoms of encephalopathy. Hospi-

---

DISPLAY 48-1 • A Basic Personal-Risk Questionnaire*

____Yes   ____No   1. Does your child live in or regularly visit a house or child care facility built before 1950?

____Yes   ____No   2. Does your child live in or regularly visit a house or child care facility built before 1978 that is being or has recently been renovated or remodeled (within the last 6 months)?

____Yes   ____No   3. Does your child have a sibling or playmate who has or did have lead poisoning?

The state or local health department may recommend alternative or additional questions based on local conditions. If the answers to the questions are "no," a screening test is not required, although the provider should explain why the questions were asked to reinforce anticipatory guidance. If the answer to any question is "yes" or "not sure," a screening test should be considered.

From American Academy of Pediatrics. (1998). Screening for elevated blood lead levels. *Pediatrics, 101,* 1072–1078.

Table 48–1. RISK FACTORS FOR LEAD EXPOSURE AND PREVENTION STRATEGIES

Risk Factor	Prevention Strategy
Environmental	
Paint	Identify and abate
Dust	Wet mop, frequent handwashing
Soil	Restrict play in area, ground cover, frequent handwashing
Drinking water	2-min flush of morning water; use of cold water for cooking, drinking
Folk remedies	Avoid use
Old ceramic or pewter cookware, old urns/kettles	Avoid use
Some imported cosmetics, toys, crayons	Avoid use
Parental occupations	Remove work clothing at work
Hobbies	Proper use, storage, and ventilation
Home renovation	Proper containment, ventilation
Buying or renting a new home	Inquire about lead hazards
Host	
Hand-to-mouth activity (or pica)	Frequent handwashing
Inadequate nutrition	High iron and calcium, low-fat diet; frequent small meals
Developmental disabilities	Frequent screening

From American Academy of Pediatrics. (1998). Screening for elevated blood lead levels. *Pediatrics, 101,* 1072–1078.

Table 48–2. RECOMMENDED FOLLOW-UP SERVICES, ACCORDING TO DIAGNOSTIC BLOOD LEAD LEVELS (BLL)

BLL (mcg/dL)	Action
< 10	No action required.
10–14	Obtain a confirmatory venous BLL within 1 mo; if still within this range, do the following:
	Provide education to decrease blood lead exposure.
	Repeat BLL test within 3 mo.
15–19	Obtain a confirmatory venous BLL within 1 mo; if still within this range, do the following:
	Take a careful environmental history.
	Provide education to decrease blood lead exposure and to decrease lead absorption.
	Repeat BLL test within 2 mo.
20–44	Obtain a confirmatory venous BLL within 1 wk; if still within this range, do the following:
	Conduct a complete medical history (including an environmental evaluation and nutritional assessment) and physical examination.
	Provide education to decrease blood lead exposure and to decrease lead absorption.
	Either refer the patient to the local health department or provide case management that should include a detailed environmental investigation with lead hazard reduction and appropriate referrals for support services.
	If BLL is > 25 mcg/dL, consider chelation (not currently recommended for BLLs < 45 mcg/dL), after consultation with clinicians experienced in lead toxicity treatment.
45–69	Obtain a confirmatory venous BLL within 2 d; if still within this range, do the following:
	Conduct a complete medical history (including an environmental evaluation and nutritional assessment) and a physical examination.
	Provide education to decrease blood lead exposure and to decrease lead absorption.
	Either refer the patient to the local health department or provide case management that should include a detailed environmental investigation with lead hazard reduction and appropriate referrals for support services.
	Begin chelation therapy in consultation with clinicians experienced in lead toxicity therapy.
≥ 70	Hospitalize the patient, and begin medical treatment immediately in consultation with clinicians experienced in lead toxicity therapy.
	Obtain a confirmatory BLL immediately.
	The rest of the management should be as noted for management of children with BLLs between 45 and 69 mcg/dL.

From American Academy of Pediatrics. (1998). Screening for elevated blood lead levels. *Pediatrics, 101,* 1072–1078.

talization is usually recommended, initially to monitor for side effects and then either to abate the current housing or to find new safe housing. The dose is 30 mg/kg/d for 5 days followed by 20 mg/kg/d for 14 days. Some children report GI discomfort and malaise. There have been case reports of reversible neutropenia and anemia; therefore, hematologic surveillance is recommended during therapy (AAP, 1995).

For cases of encephalopathy manifested by changes in the level of consciousness, headache, or vomiting or those with BLLs greater than 70 mcg/dL, parenteral chelation combining BAL and EDTA is advised. Only professionals experienced in treating lead toxicity should undertake this type of treatment.

● **Clinical Pearl:** After completion of chelation therapy, the provider should obtain a repeat venous lead level after 14 days to allow for reequilibration. Further management as outlined in Table 48-2 will be predicated on the repeat level.

REFERENCES

American Academy of Pediatrics Policy Statement. (1998). Screening for elevated blood lead levels. *Pediatrics, 101,* 1072–1078.

American Academy of Pediatrics Policy Statement. (1995). Treatment guidelines for lead exposure in children. *Pediatrics, 96,* 155–160.

Berlin, C. M. (1997). Lead poisoning in children. *Current Opinion in Pediatrics, 9,* 173–177.

Glotzer, T. E., & Weitzman, M. (1995). Commonly asked questions about childhood lead poisoning. *Pediatric Annals, 24,* 630–639.

Needleman, H. L., & Gatsonis, G. A. (1990). Low level lead exposure and the IQ of children: A meta-analysis of modern studies. *Journal of the American Medical Association, 263,* 673–678.

Needleman, H. L. (1998). Childhood lead poisoning: The promise and abandonment of primary prevention. *American Journal of Public Health, 88,* 1871–1877.

Silbergeld, E. K. (1997). Preventing lead poisoning in children. *Annual Review Public Health, 18,* 187–210.

PART II ▲

Allergies, Anaphylaxis, Stinging Insects (Hymenoptera), and Drug Allergies

• PRADEEP SHARMA, MD, and RICHARD BACHUR, MD

ALLERGIES

Allergic diseases affect approximately 25% of all children. The economic implications are enormous, with direct medical costs approaching $1.2 billion and indirect costs estimated to be the same. Inclusion of diseases such as asthma, chronic sinusitis, otitis media with effusion, and nasal polyps, all associated with allergic rhinitis, bring the cost close to a staggering $10 billion. The incidence of allergic diseases, especially asthma, is rising; the exact causes for this increase are unknown. The exact incidence of anaphylaxis and acute allergic reactions is also unknown.

Upon presentation of an antigen, the immunologic response can proceed along two pathways: TH1 pathway (T helper cell 1) in the nonatopic individual and TH2 pathway in the atopic. In the nonatopic individual, exposure to antigens leads to the division of the helper T cells. The immune response then proceeds along the TH1 cell pathway, which, under influence of interluekin 2 and inteleukin 6, causes the B cell and plasma cells to produce immunoglobulin G (IgG) antibodies. These antibodies are protective and do not lead to an allergic reaction. In the atopic individual, however, the TH2 cell is involved, which secretes interleukin 4 (IL4), causing the B cell and plasma cells to secrete primarily IgE antibody. The IgE antibody then can affix to receptors on the mast cells.

Repeated exposure to antigens to which the host previously has been sensitized will then lead to degranulation of the mast cell, resulting in the release of preformed mediators of allergy, primarily histamine and heparin. The result is an immediate type 1 allergic reaction with clinical symptoms that can culminate in anaphylaxis. Also, mast cell degranulation releases several chemotactic factors that lead to a migration of inflammatory cells (eosinophils, neutrophils), leading to chronic airway inflammation and tissue injury, which are hallmarks of the late-phase reaction. The result may be chronic inflammation, such as seen in bronchial asthma and allergic rhinitis. The mast cell also is involved in activation of phospholipase A_2, leading to activation of the arachidonic acid into leukotreines and prostaglandins.

One of the many approaches in treating allergic diseases includes drugs that lower IL4. Such drugs would reduce production of IgE antibodies and modify the immune response so that it proceeds along the TH1 pathway. Recent evidence has shown that one of the mechanisms by which allergy immunotherapy works may be by reduction in IL4 (Ebner, 1998).

ANAPHYLAXIS

Anaphylaxis is the acute onset of potentially life-threatening, multiorgan symptoms due to the release of mediators from mast cells and basophils. It occurs in individuals who are exposed to an antigen to which they were previously sensitized.

Pathology

The bridging of two adjacent IgE antibodies by an antigen leads to a release of preformed mediators of allergy, resulting in the early phase of the type 1 reaction and, in severe cases, anaphylaxis.

Reactions Based on the Immune System

IgE mediated (type 1) reactions are responsible for most cases of anaphylaxis that involve immune mechanisms. Common responsible agents are foods such as peanuts, milk, eggs, chocolate, and shellfish. Reactions to insect stings from Hymenoptera, vaccines, and allergy immunotherapy are also seen in children.

The following can cause anaphylaxis by IgE mediated immune mechanisms:

- Antibiotics (haptens): penicillin, cephalosporins
- Venomous (Hymenoptera): yellow jackets, white face hornets, yellow hornets, honey bee, and wasps
- Foods: milk, peanuts, eggs, shellfish, chocolate
- Vaccines: allergen extracts, tetanus
- Hormones: insulin
- Miscellaneous: latex
- Antiserum: tetanus

Anaphylaxis by way of the immune system but not involving the IgE antibody would include anaphylaxis following a blood transfusion, which is usually a result of IgG-based immune complex mechanism. A complement-mediated anaphylaxis reaction can result from blood transfusion reaction associated with IgA deficiency.

Anaphylaxis from Nonimmune Mechanisms (Anaphylactoid)

The following are examples of anyphylaxis caused by nonimmune mechanisms:

- Direct histamine-releasing agents: radiologic contrast media, succinylcholine, and ciprofloxin
- Arachidonate-mediated: aspirin and nonsteroidal anti-inflammatory drugs (NSAIDs)
- Unknown mechanisms: exercise-induced anaphylaxis, cold urticaria, and mastocytosis

Epidemiology

The exact incidence of anaphylaxis in children is unknown; however, data suggest that the incidence of anaphylaxis may be 0.25% in patients receiving allergy immunotherapy. Anaphylaxis to Hymenoptera occurs in about 1% to 2% of the general population, and fatalities (mostly in adults) from Hymenoptera stings total approximately 25 to 50 per year in the United States. Fatal reactions to penicillin also have been reported but are extremely rare and occur mostly due to parenteral administration at a rate of 0.002%. Anaphylaxis is much less likely if penicillin is administered orally. The incidence of fatal anaphylaxis appears to be twice as high in patients with asthma. Patients on beta-blockers also may be at high risk for anaphylaxis (Lang, 1995).

Risk factors for anaphylaxis include the following:

- Asthma
- Female sex
- Nature of specific antigens; some allergens, such as those found in peanuts, shellfish, and penicillin, are much more likely to cause anaphylaxis than others.
- Route of entry of allergen; intramuscular or intravenous (IV) route of entry is more likely to lead to anaphylaxis than the oral route.
- Use of beta-blockers

History and Physical Examination

Quick recognition of clinical symptoms listed in Table 48-3 is key to establishing a diagnosis of anaphylaxis. Key features include rapid onset of generalized itching, urticaria, angioedema, flush, erythema, headache, sneezing, rhinorrhea, wheezing, difficulty swallowing, abdominal cramping, diarrhea, sensation of impending doom, respiratory arrest, and sometimes cardiovascular collapse. The presentation varies, and not all organ systems are involved in all patients. Nonetheless, in this potentially life-threatening situation, symptoms can start within seconds, reaching a peak severity from 5 to 30 minutes after exposure to the offending agent. Late-phase reaction also may occur 6 to 12 hours later, with symptoms lasting up to as much as 24 hours despite treatment. Most children have cutaneous symptoms, which may progress to involve the respiratory system and a feeling of anxiety. Only rarely, however, do symptoms progress to respiratory failure or cardiovascular collapse.

Diagnostic Criteria

The diagnosis is based on obtaining a history of exposure to an offending agent or recognition of the classic signs and symptoms. The presence of cutaneous symptoms and signs (ie, pruritus, urticaria, angioedema) makes the diagnosis more obvious.

Anaphylaxis can be confused with vasovagal syncope. Distinguishing features are that vasovagal reactions occur during stressful conditions, such as venipuncture, vaccinations, and allergy skin tests. Patients appear pale and sweaty and may have bradycardia. Unlike with anaphylaxis, patients with vasovagal episodes maintain normal blood pressure and have no pruritus, urticaria, angioedema, or bronchospasm. They also recover spontaneously within minutes.

Diagnostic Studies

Laboratory tests are generally not necessary to establish a diagnosis of anaphylaxis; however, tryptase levels are elevated in most cases. Providers may draw a level if diagnosis of anaphylaxis is in doubt. The window in which tryptase levels may accurately reflect anaphylaxis is about 2 hours after onset of symptoms (Schwart et al., 1989). After the event, if the etiology is in doubt, allergy skin testing may be indicated if a clinician suspects an ingestant (food), Hymenoptera sting, or inhalant as the culprit.

Management

Prompt recognition and treatment of anaphylaxis are important, because anaphylaxis can be life threatening. The reader is referred to the algorithm in Figure 48-1, which describes the treatment of an acute allergic reaction in the office or clinic setting. Epinephrine is the drug of choice in anaphylaxis. It reduces mediator release and may reverse the physiologic effects of many mediators. Because most providers in private practice are not experienced in advanced life support, which may be needed in management of anaphylaxis, they must know when to call for help for patients who fail to respond to the administration of epinephrine and antihistamines. Providers can encounter anaphylaxis at any time; therefore, mock drills practicing management of anaphylaxis may be helpful. An emergency cart accessible to all personnel also is essential. All health care providers should maintain basic cardiopulmonary resuscitation certification. Display 48-2 presents the basic supplies and equipment recommended for management of anaphylaxis in an office setting.

Instructions to School Personnel

Families should provide detailed written instructions to school personnel regarding management of anaphylaxis in individuals in whom anaphylaxis is likely. These instructions can be created from the contents presented in Display 48-3.

Reactions to Egg-Based Vaccines

Clinicians often are confronted with a patient due to receive an egg-based vaccine (eg, measles, mumps, rubella (MMR); influenza; yellow fever) but is also allergic to eggs. Most reactions to MMR and other egg-based vaccines are not due to sensitivity to egg protein but to other vaccine constituents. In the case of MMR, when immediate allergic reactions do occur, most appear to be due to the gelatin or neomycin also present in the vaccine.

Table 48–3.   CLINICAL SYMPTOMS OF ANAPHYLAXIS

Organ System	Symptoms
Cutaneous	Generalized pruritus, erythema, flush, urticaria, angioedema
Respiratory	Sneezing, rhinorrhoea, lump in throat, hoarseness, difficulty swallowing, coughing, wheezing, "can't breathe," progressive breathing difficulty, apnea, asphyxia, respiratory failure
Cardiovascular	Tachycardia, hypotension, vascular collapse, dysrhythmia, and cardiac arrest
Gastrointestinal	Nausea, vomiting, abdominal cramps, diarrhea
Genital	Uterine cramps
Neurologic	Anxiety, feelings of impending doom, seizures.

Adapted from Friday and Fireman Atlas of Allergies

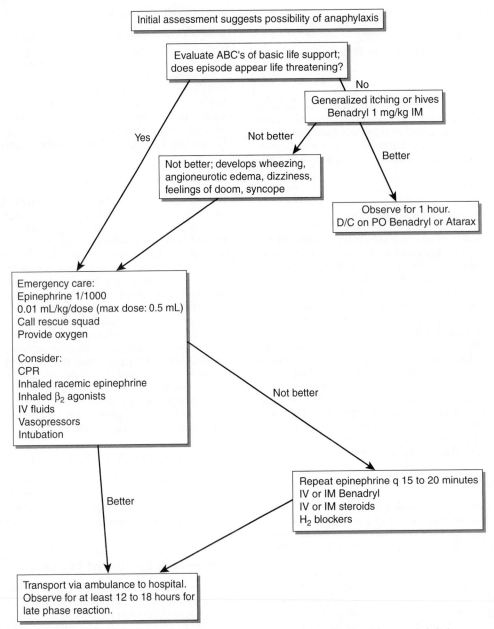

Figure 48–1 ■ Office or clinic management of the child with acute allergic reaction or anaphylaxis.

DISPLAY 48–2 • Basic Office Equipment for Managing Anaphylaxis

1. Stethoscope and sphygmomanometer
2. Tourniquets, syringes, hyperdermic needles, and a large-bore (14 gauge) needle
3. Aqueous epinephrine 1:1000
4. Equipment for administering oxygen by mask; make sure pediatric sizes are available
5. Equipment for administering intravenous fluids
6. Oral airway
7. Diphenhydramine or similar antihistamine
8. Coticosteroids for intravenous injections
9. Vasopressors

The MMR vaccine is a highly refined product prepared in chick embryo fibroblast cells, decreasing the amount of protein that could react with ovalbumin to a level unlikely to cause anaphylaxis. The influenza and yellow fever vaccines are prepared in embryonated cells and hence may contain higher amounts of egg protein.

Numerous studies have established the safety of MMR vaccine in egg-sensitive subjects. In reviewing 17 studies, MMR vaccine was safely administered to 1209 patients who were egg sensitive on skin test. Studies show that 99.75% of egg-sensitive patients with positive skin test to eggs received MMR vaccine without having an anaphylactic reaction.

● **Clinical Pearl:** The latest AAP recommendations in the 1997 Red Book state that children with a history of egg allergy or sensitivity may be given MMR without prior skin

---

DISPLAY 48–3 • Emergency Health Care Plan

Place
Child's
Picture
Here

ALLERGY TO:_____

Student's
name: _____ D.O.B.:_____ Teacher:_____

Asthmatic   Yes ❏   No ❏   *High risk for severe reaction

SIGNS OF AN ALLERGIC REACTION INCLUDE:

Systems:	Symptoms:
*MOUTH	itching and swelling of the lips, tongue, or mouth
THROAT	itching and/or a sense of tightness in the throat, hoarseness, and hacking cough
*SKIN	hives, itchy rash, and/or swelling about the face or extremities
*GUT	nausea, abdominal cramps, vomiting, and/or diarrhea
LUNG	shortness of breath, repetitive coughing, and/or wheezing
HEART	"thready" pulse, "passing-out"

The severity of symptoms can quickly change. *All above symptoms can potentially progress to a life-threatening situation!

ACTION:

1. If ingestion is suspected, give_____
                                                    medication/dose/route
   and_____immediately!
2. CALL RESCUE SQUAD:_____
3. CALL: Mother _____Father _____or emergency contacts
4. CALL: Dr._____ at_____

DO NOT HESITATE TO ADMINISTER MEDICATION OR CALL RESCUE SQUAD EVEN IF PARENTS OR DOCTOR CANNOT BE REACHED!

_____   _____   _____M.D.   _____
Parent's signature   Date   Doctor's signature   Date

EMERGENCY CONTACTS	TRAINED STAFF MEMBERS
1._____ Relation:_____Phone:_____	1. _____Room_____
2._____ Relation: _____Phone:_____	2. _____Room_____
3._____ Relation:_____ Phone:_____	3. _____Room_____

For children with multiple food allergies, use one form for each food. 5/95

testing, because skin testing is not predictive of a vaccine-allergic reaction.

Egg-sensitive patients also have been given yellow fever vaccine safely. The data for influenza vaccine, however, are incomplete. Providers should use caution when administering influenza vaccine to egg-sensitive patients (Fasano, Wood, Cook, & Samoson, 1992).

The following are recommendations for administering yellow fever or influenza vaccines to egg-sensitive patients:

- Take a detailed history. Does the child have a history of anaphylactic reaction to eggs, or was the reaction mild and localized to the skin?
- Children or adolescents with less severe reactions to eggs may receive influenza or yellow fever vaccines and do not warrant skin testing.
- Children with severe or anaphylactic reactions to eggs should not receive influenza vaccine, given the availability of chemoprophylaxis.
- A trained allergist should perform skin testing on children with severe or anaphylactic reactions to eggs before administration of yellow fever vaccine.

HYMENOPTERA STINGS

The incidence of Hymenoptera sensitivity is about 2% to 3% of the general population. Young males tend to be stung more often, but most fatalities occur in the elderly. Fatal reactions also have been reported in the pediatric population.

History and Physical Examination

Most children report a painful sting, although they are unable to identify the insect that stung them. In the United States, the most common culprits are insects from the hornet family, with yellow jackets being most common, followed by other hornets, wasps, and finally honeybees. The various presentations consist of local and systemic reactions. At the least, there is usually redness, pain, and some degree of swelling at the site of the sting, due to irritation from the venom. Allergic reactions to Hymenoptera are sometimes confused with large local reactions, which are raised, red, painful, and at times itchy at the site of the sting. The differential point is that these reactions are limited to the bite site, and no systemic signs of generalized pruritus, urticaria, or airway difficulty are present. Local reactions do not involve the IgE antibody. Evidence has shown that about 50% of individuals with history of a systemic reaction give a history of progressively increasing large local reactions before occurrence of the first systemic reaction. Some individuals with large local reactions may have higher than normal IgE antibodies against the class of stinging insect responsible for the sting. The symptoms of more systemic reactions and anaphylaxis to a Hymenoptera sting are the same as for other causes, and the reader is referred to Table 48-3.

Diagnostic Criteria

The history of a sting immediately preceding a local, systemic, or anaphylactic reaction establishes the diagnosis. As recurrent allergic reactions to Hymenoptera insects can be life threatening, the provider needs to identify the stinging insect responsible. To do so, a consultation with an allergist for appropriate skin testing for Hymenoptera may be necessary.

Management

Acute Management

Bees tend to deposit a barbed stinger in the skin, whereas wasps can sting multiple times. If the stinger is present in the skin, removal should be as soon as possible. Although "scraping" the stinger was previously felt to be advantageous over using a forceps (which may squeeze more venom into the skin), a recent study did not find a difference related to removal method (Visscher, Veller, & Camazine, 1996).

Further treatment is based on the severity of the allergic reaction. Providers may treat local irritation or local hives initially with cold compresses. Patients exhibiting generalized itching or hives should receive diphenhydramine (Benadryl) 1 mg/kg (maximum 50 mg). They require observation for at least 1 hour. These patients can then be discharged on diphenhydramine or hydroxyzine (Atarax) for the next 24 hours. Patients with any other systemic reactions, including wheezing, angioneurotic edema, dizziness, vomiting, or syncope, should receive epinephrine 1:1000 (0.01 mL/kg, maximum 0.5 mL) subcutaneously. They then require transport by emergency personnel to an emergency room.

Patients with a previous history of anaphylaxis should be empirically treated with diphenhydramine 1 mg/kg and transported immediately to an emergency room by emergency personnel. These individuals should receive epinephrine (as above) for any signs of allergic reaction.

Follow-up Management

Local reactions require no follow up. If the reaction was systemic, the clinician should prescribe an antihistamine and epinephrine (an Epipen) for emergency use in the event of another sting and provide the patient or parents with specific written instructions regarding their use. For systemic reactions, the provider also should refer the child to an allergist. Following consultation with an allergist, if the history and workup (allergy skin tests for Hymenoptera) confirm allergy, then the provider, patient, and family should take the following measures:

- Reduce sting possibility by avoiding bright-colored clothing, perfumes, colognes, and areas where Hymenoptera are common.
- Manage accidental field stings by administration of oral diphenhydramine and use of epinephrine (Epipen or Epipen Jr.) as described in the module on anaphylaxis.
- Use venom immunotherapy as appropriate. Venom immunotherapy for Hymenoptera is highly effective, with treatment failures occurring in less than 5% of patients. Data also suggest that protection from Hymenoptera stings may last for a long time after cessation of immunotherapy (Golden, Kwiterovich, Kagey-Sobotka, Valentine, & Lichtenstein, 1996). An experienced allergist should perform venom inmmunotherapy. It is indicated for children who have suffered from a life-threatening reaction, such as symptoms involving the airway or cardiovascular system. Children with strictly a systemic cutaneous reaction, such as urticaria, may be managed without venom immunotherapy. Exceptions may be made if the family desires the added protection provided by immunotherapy or if the patient is at a high risk for future stings because of special situations. Examples are a child allergic to honey bees whose parents are beekeepers or children who spend an unusual amount of time outdoors camping and hiking.

DRUG ALLERGY

Drug allergy is defined as an adverse event following administration of a drug due to a specific immunologic sensitization that usually involves the IgE antibody. This reaction must be distinguished from nonimmunologic events, such as side effects, toxic reactions, and drug-to-drug interactions.

Epidemiology

The exact incidence of drug allergy in children is unknown; however, about 5% to 15% of the general population will give a history of an adverse drug reaction as a result of penicillin. A controlled study suggests an actual incidence of 3.2%. Allergic reactions to second- or third-generation cephalosporins are rare (1%–3%). Cross-reactivity with patients who are allergic to penicillin is about 2%. The vast majority of parents confuse side effects and idiosyncratic reactions with true allergic reactions.

● **Clinical Pearl:** Only a small fraction of patients in whom a history of penicillin allergy is elicited actually have a true penicillin allergy.

History and Physical Examination

A meticulous history is most important and must include a detailed drug history. What medications was the child taking at the time of the reaction? Was the reaction urticarial? Was the rash pruritic? Were there signs of anaphylaxis? Unfortunately, in children, the history may not be reliable. Many parents or children do not remember the name of the antibiotic or type of reaction. Because the actual incidence of drug allergy is usually lower than what parents relate, labeling a patient allergic to drugs (especially the beta lactams) may lead to use of alternate, less effective, more toxic, more broad spectrum, and commonly more expensive drugs. Hence, a proper diagnosis of drug allergy is most important.

In true drug allergies, typical symptoms, such as itching, sneezing, and wheezing, will be present. Urticaria and angioedema are seen frequently. Classic anaphylaxis is rare but is obviously the most serious manifestation.

Symptoms of true drug allergy may include the following:

- Pruritus
- Pruritic rashes, such as urticaria
- Abdominal cramping and diarrhea (as an isolated symptom, probably not due to allergy)
- Wheezing
- Symptoms of anaphylaxis (described elsewhere in this chapter)

Common nonallergic symptoms that many parents falsely perceive to be allergic include the following:

- A nonitchy maculopapular exanthem, especially with amoxicillin
- Loose bowel movements, seen with many antibiotics
- Stomach upset or vomiting, seen with erythromycin

Diagnostic Criteria

The provider can narrow down the possibility of drug allergy by reviewing a detailed and careful history. If suspicion for true allergy is low, such as a nonpruritic, nonurticarial rash after amoxicillin, then he or she can give an oral challenge in the office and observe the patient carefully for an hour. (The office should be equipped and personnel trained to handle anaphylaxis.)

In situations in which suspicion is high and the suspected drug is indeed the treatment of choice, then the provider should consider consultation with an allergist. He or she should consider skin testing for drug allergy in these patients. Skin tests, however, are hindered by the fact that, for most drugs, appropriate antigens are not available. Even for penicillin allergy, all necessary testing reagents (especially the minor determinants of penicillin allergy) are not yet commercially available, making the task of proper diagnosis difficult. Physicians experienced with these procedures, such as allergists, should perform skin testing and graded oral challenges.

Providers can use the following steps when diagnosing drug allergy:

- A detailed history
- Skin testing if available, such as with penicillin
- RAST testing if skin testing is not possible
- Oral drug challenge
- Patch testing in cases in which the route of entry is contact through skin in drugs used topically

Management

Acute reactions are treated based on symptoms. Mild pruritic reactions are best treated with antihistamines. Bronchodilators may be necessary for wheezing. Anaphylaxis will require adrenaline, as discussed in the module on anaphylaxis. Once the diagnosis is established, avoidance is advised.

▲ **Clinical Warning:** Clinicians commonly face the problem of the development of true allergic symptoms, such as hives, in the middle of a course of treatment. Unless the underlying illness is life threatening, the clinician should not initiate another antibiotic for at least 72 hours, because ongoing hives to the first prescription may be confused for an allergic reaction to the second.

Common drug allergy problems encountered by providers are discussed below.

Penicillins

In case of penicillin allergy, if an alternate drug is not available, then providers should initiate oral or parenteral desensitization.

● **Clinical Pearl:** Nonpruritic, macular papular rashes seen with amoxicillin are common. They are not IgE mediated and do not represent penicillin allergy. If the rash is urticarial and pruritic, then the provider should suspect allergy.

Newer studies suggest that the incidence of reactions to a cephalosporin is no greater in patients with true penicillin allergy than for the general population (Matloff, 1999). This contradicts the conclusions of older studies, in which cross-reactivity was felt to be as high as 10% to 15%. This new information has led to oral cephalosporins being used routinely, albeit cautiously, in penicillin-allergic patients. Recent studies have concluded that most children will "outgrow" penicillin allergy (Mendelson, 1998).

Cephalosporins

The molecular structures of second- and third-generation cephalosporins are sufficiently distinct so that when a patient has an allergic reaction to one member of the class an alternative cephalosporin with a different side chain will probably be well tolerated. The serum sickness-like reactions seen with cefaclor are extremely common and have led to a marked decrease in its use. They are non-IgE mediated, and the provider can safely prescribe another cephalosporin.

Sulfonamides

Reactions may vary from mild rashes to severe life-threatening eruptions, such as Stevens-Johnson syndrome. For this reason, any reaction to a drug in this class should lead to prompt discontinuation and avoidance of future use of any sulfa drug.

Aspirin and Nonsteroidal Anti-inflammatory Drugs

Aspirin and NSAID reactions are not IgE mediated but nonetheless can be life threatening. Avoidance of all aspirin and NSAIDs is advised. Acetaminophen would be the alternative drug of choice. The patient may tolerate trisalicylate and salsalate.

Radiocontrast Agents

Radiocontrast agent reactions, though involving histamine and other mediators released from mast cells, are not IgE mediated but can lead to life-threatening reactions. Prophylactic treatment consists of using low osmolar nonionic radiocontrast agents. Pretreatment with antihistamines and steroids may prevent reactions from occurring.

REFERENCES

Chips, B. E., Valentine, M. D., Kagey-Sabotka, A., Schuberth, K. C., & Lichtenstein, L. M. (1980). Diagnosis and treatment of anaphylactic reactions to hymenoptera stings in children. *Journal of Pediatrics, 97*, 177–184.

Kwiterovich, K. A., Kagey-Sobotka, A., Valentine, M. D., & Lichtenstein, D., Golden, B. K., et al. (1997). Natural history of Hymenoptera venom sensitivity in adults. *The Journal of Allergy and Clinical Immunology, 100*, 760–766.

Ebner, C. (1998). Immunological mechanisms operative in allergen specific immunotherapy: The diagnosis and management of anaphylaxis. *The Journal of Allergy and Clinical Immunology, 101* (6 Part 2).

Fasano, M. B., Wood, R. A., Cook, S. A., & Samoson, H. A. (1992). Egg hypersensitivity and adverse reactions to measles mumps and rubella vaccine. *Journal of Pediatrics, 120*, 878–881.

Fireman, P., & Slavin, G. *Atlas of allergies*. (2nd ed.).

Golden, D. B. K., Kwiterovich, K. A., Kagey-Sobotka, A., Valentine, M. D., & Lichtenstein, L. M. (1996). Discontinuing venom immunotherapy: Outcome after 5 years. *Journal of Allergy and Clinical Immunology, 97*, 579–587.

Hendrik, K., Van Halteren, et al. (1997). Discontinuation of yellow jacket venom immunotherapy: Follow up of 75 patients by means of deliberate sting challenge. *The Journal of Allergy and Clinical Immunology, 100*, 767–770.

Lang, D. M. (1995). Hazards of beta-blockers. Anaphylactoid and anaphylactic reactions. *Drug Safety, 12*(5), 299–304.

Marquart, D., & Wasserman, S. (1993). Anaphylaxis. In Middleton et al. (Eds.), *Allergy: Principles and practice* (pp. 1525–1536). St. Louis: Mosby.

Matloff, S. M. (1999). In R. A. Dershowitz (Ed.). *Ambulatory pediatric care*. Philadelphia: Lippincott-Raven.

Mendelson, L. M. (1998). Adverse reactions to beta lactam antibiotics. *Immunology and Allergy Clinics of North America*, 745–757.

Middleton, Reed, & Ellis. (1996). *Allergy principles and practice* (4th Ed.).

Schwartz, L. B., et al. (1989). Time course of appearance and disappearance of human mast cell tryptase in the circulation after anaphylaxis. *Journal of Clinical Investigation, 83*(5), 1551–1555.

Valentine, M. D., Schuberth, K. C., Kagey-Sobotka, A., Graft, D. F., et al. (1990). The value of immunotherapy with venom in children with allergy to insect stings. *New England Journal of Medicine, 323*, 160–163.

Visscher, P., Veller, R., & Camazine, S. (1996). Removing bee stings. *Lancet, 348*, 301.

PART III

Tick-Borne Infections ▲

• SUNIL K. SOOD, MD

INTRODUCTION

Tick-borne diseases are common causes of morbidity in children in the United States. An inordinate degree of fear exists in the public, as well as some confusion about prevention and treatment among health care providers. This chapter summarizes current knowledge and provides practical guidelines appropriate for primary care clinicians to implement.

LYME DISEASE

Lyme disease, an infectious disorder caused by the spirochete *Borrelia burgdorferi* sensu lato, is the most common vector-borne infection in the United States. When the term sensu lato ("in a broad sense") is used, it includes strains not present in the United States, especially *Borrelia afzelii* and *Borrelia garinii*, which cause Lyme disease in Europe. The vectors in North America are black-legged ticks of the genus *Ixodes*. These ticks are widely distributed throughout the United States, yet only a few areas are considered endemic for Lyme disease. The following states have the highest incidence rates and account for more than 90% of cases: Connecticut, Rhode Island, New York, New Jersey, Pennsylvania, Maryland, Wisconsin, and Minnesota (Dennis, 1998). In the northeastern and north-central regions, high populations of deer and mice sustain transmission of the spirochete, resulting in a higher infection rate in the deer tick variety of *Ixodes*. Because small mammals, such as the white-footed mouse (*Peromyscus leucopus*) can bring ticks into parks and around homes and can nest in backyard debris, children can be exposed in the "peridomestic" environment.

The number of cases of Lyme disease is still increasing and underreported. Primary care clinicians must continue to report new cases to local health authorities so that they can maintain accurate statistics. They can use these statistics to plan environmental measures and immunization strategies.

● **Clinical Pearl:** Most children (89% in a prospective series) present with single or multiple forms of erythema migrans (EM). This finding should greatly help correct the mistaken perception that Lyme disease is unrecognizable until it is too late to be easily treated.

Arthritis (7%), facial palsy (3%), aseptic meningitis (1%), and carditis (0.5%) are less common symptoms (Gerber, Shapiro, Burke, Parcells, & Bell, 1996). The original classification of clinical manifestations into stages I to III has been replaced by early (generally within 8 weeks after the tick bite) and late Lyme disease. Providers should recognize that extracutaneous involvement can manifest within days of the tick bite.

Pathology

Early-Localized and Early-Disseminated Lyme Disease

Erythema Migrans

Early-localized Lyme disease manifests as a single lesion at the site of inoculation called EM. Mild systemic symptoms may accompany the rash: In one study, 24% of children had fever, 33% had arthralgia, 42% complained of headache, and 58% complained of fatigue (Gerber et al., 1996). It is presumed that at this stage of the infection, spirochetal invasion is restricted to the skin in most patients, but dissemination to the central nervous system (CNS) is occasionally subclinical (Kuiper et al., 1994). A recent discovery is that *B. burgdorferi* strains vary in their ability to disseminate and cause systemic disease depending on their outer surface protein C (OspC) type.

The incubation period after the tick bite is up to 1 month. Typically, EM is somewhat circular and enlarges gradually. It is hardly evanescent, expanding and lasting for 1 to 2 weeks.

● **Clinical Pearl:** Central clearing, thought previously to be the hallmark of the lesion, is absent in two thirds of cases.

Clearing is a function of the time the rash has been present. Thus, the rash may present as a red plaque, which could be confused with cellulitis. It is painless and nonpruritic, but the patient may experience mild stinging. Figure 48-2 illustrates EM with central clearing.

● **Clinical Pearl:** An EM diameter of at least 5 cm is an important diagnostic consideration, even in children.

Vesicular, urticarial, scaling, purpuric, and linear-shaped variants occur. A careful examination of the scalp is important because all or part of the rash may occur above the hairline (EM occurs on the head or neck in about 25% of children). As part of the differential diagnosis, smaller ringlike lesions may represent a local allergic reaction to an insect bite, a small area of nummular eczema, tinea corporis, or a reaction to tick saliva that usually fades without expansion. The important consideration is that these lesions do not expand, as does EM.

● **Clinical Pearl:** A common fear is that Lyme disease will be undetected because not all patients develop the rash;

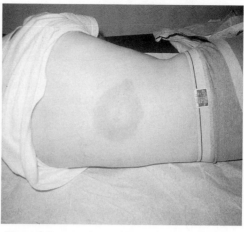

Figure 48–2 ■ Erythema migrans with central clearing.

however, 89% of affected individuals do develop the rash either in single or multiple form. Its expanding nature, large size, and continued presence for 1 to 2 weeks leads to early detection in the vast majority of cases in endemic areas (Gerber et al., 1996).

Multiple Erythema Migrans

Multiple EM, a consequence of hematogenous spread of the infection, may be confused with erythema multiforme. The main distinction is that EM lesions are circular and not raised, though varying in size, whereas erythema multiforme consists of lesions of varying morphology, including some urticarial lesions.

Neurologic Infection

Peripheral neuropathy (usually VII nerve palsy) and lymphocytic meningitis are common neurologic manifestations of early-disseminated Lyme disease. Even in an endemic area, most Bell's palsy is idiopathic, but providers should always obtain serology for Lyme disease. Positive serology is usually an indication for antibiotic treatment, whereas there is no established treatment modality for Bell's palsy (Jain et al., 1996).

Controversy exists about the necessity to perform a lumbar puncture in every child with facial palsy due to Lyme disease (Sood, 1998). Most experts believe that it is unnecessary in the absence of clinical signs of meningeal irritation or headache. A long-term study of untreated facial palsy in Swedish children, including some with cerebrospinal fluid (CSF) pleocytosis, revealed no long-term sequelae (Niemann et al., 1997). Still, it is important to assess the need for lumbar puncture carefully, because in the presence of meningitis, the treatment of choice will be an IV antibiotic. Lyme meningitis is a lymphocytic meningitis with elevated protein levels. Several cases complicated by pseudotumor cerebri have been reported (Kan, Sood, & Maytal, 1998).

Other cranial neuropathies very rarely are due to Lyme disease, but providers should investigate any unexplained palsy for Lyme disease. Bannwarth's syndrome of radiculoneuritis, typically nerve pain parasthesia or weakness originating in the cervical or thoracic nerve roots, is uncommon in North American Lyme disease and is rarely encountered in U.S. children. Nevertheless, providers should consider Lyme disease in the differential diagnosis of limb paresthesias, motor or sensory deficits, or neuralgia, especially in the cervical and thoracic dermatomes.

Other Manifestations

Migratory arthralgia, periarticular pain, or frank arthritis may present as early manifestations. Partial or complete atrioventricular conduction or bundle branch block may be asymptomatic or cause bradycardia. Hence, obtaining an electrocardiogram (EKG) in a child who has any other clinical manifestation of disseminated Lyme disease (eg, facial palsy, meningitis, and multiple EM) is important, because presence of heart block may require IV antibiotic treatment.

Acute Constitutional Illness Without Focal Manifestations

This is also inaccurately termed, viral-type illness or "flu-like" illness, and is known to occur in children as a manifestation of early *B. burgdorferi* infection. Thus, providers should consider early Lyme disease in the differential diagnosis of fever and fatigue, which may be accompanied by headache or neck pain, especially during the summer in an endemic area (Nadelman & Wormser, 1998). The diagnosis is made by demonstration of seroconversion on paired acute and convalescent serum specimens. Antibiotic treatment is as for EM.

Late Lyme Disease

Most children with late Lyme disease seen by the primary care clinician have arthritis. Late neurologic manifestations are very rare in children, although several neuropsychological conditions may be erroneously ascribed to CNS Lyme disease.

Arthritis

The mean time to onset of Lyme arthritis is about 4 months, with a range of 2 days to 20 months after the initial manifestation of early Lyme disease (Gerber, Zemel, & Shapiro, 1998). Lyme arthritis can be the first manifestation of the disease in children who have no history of a tick bite or rash. In some patients, there is a history of migratory arthralgias and periarticular inflammation in the weeks leading up to frank arthritis.

● **Clinical Pearl:** Lyme arthritis is an oligoarticular arthritis, which involves one or both knees in 90% of cases. The arthritis is painful but less than one would expect given the degree of swelling and redness. In this respect, Lyme arthritis resembles juvenile rheumatoid arthritis more than septic arthritis.

Lyme arthritis is very apparent on physical examination, even to an inexperienced observer. The arthralgias that may precede it are differentiated from common "growing pains" by the fact that the arthralgias interrupt the child's normal activities. Lyme arthritis is generally less severe in young children than it is in adolescents and adults.

Late Neurologic Disease

Reports have described behavioral and sleep changes, auditory and visual sequential processing deficits, high signal areas in the white matter on magnetic resonance brain imaging, and periventricular focal necrosis, in association with serologic evidence of the infection (Sood, 1999). Association of neurologic abnormalities with Lyme disease, however, is usually difficult to establish because culture of the CSF is negative at this stage, and DNA, antibody, and antigen detection tests have poor specificity and sensitivity. It is known that late neurologic disease is very uncommon in children, because extensive experience in endemic areas demonstrates that the long-term neuropsychological outcome in children who have had Lyme disease is excellent. It is incorrect to assume that conditions such as attention deficit hyperactivity disorder or poor school performance are due to Lyme disease in endemic areas.

▲ **Clinical Warning:** When neuropsychological or emotional problems are diagnosed in children who are seropositive for *B. burgdorferi* infection, these are more likely to be preexisting conditions than complications of previous Lyme disease.

If a provider suspects late CNS Lyme disease, he or she should not initiate treatment with an IV antibiotic unless the child meets the following minimum criteria:

- The provider can find no other identifiable cause of the symptoms.
- Prior Lyme disease is proven by immunoblot, with recognition that positive serology may also reflect past resolved infection unrelated to present complaints.
- CSF analysis demonstrates an elevated CSF/serum antibody index by enzyme-linked immunosorbent assay (ELISA), or a positive polymerase chain reaction (PCR) assay, performed preferably in a Lyme disease research laboratory.

Asymptomatic Seroconversion

It is common for infection to occur asymptomatically after a tick bite (Steere et al., 1998). Presumably, such subclinical infection resolves without sequelae in most instances. Generally, obtaining acute and convalescent-paired serum specimens after tick bites is not recommended. Consequently, the diagnosis of asymptomatic infection usually will not be made in primary practice.

Perinatal Transmission

Congenital infection with *B. burgdorferi* has been described but is very rare. No congenital syndrome is recognized (Sood, 1999). In fact not all case reports have documented evidence of infection in the mother, and identification of spirochetes in the fetus or infant often was based on immunofluorescent staining, which can yield false-positive results. Studies of series of women with Lyme disease during pregnancy revealed no increased fetal risk attributable to *B. burgdorferi* infection (Markowitz, Steere, Benach, Slade, & Broome, 1986; Maraspin et al., 1996; Strobino, Williams, Abid, Chalson, & Spierling, 1993). Evaluation of an infant born to a mother with untreated Lyme disease should consist of serology for IgM and IgG antibodies with positive results confirmed by immunoblot. Antibiotic treatment is not indicated in the absence of serologic evidence of infection.

Coinfection with Other Deer Tick-Borne Pathogens

The deer tick in the northeast can concomitantly transmit *B. burgdorferi*, the human granulocytic ehrlichiosis agent, and *Babesia microti* (Nadelman et al., 1997; Krause et al., 1996). Coinfection may increase the severity of Lyme disease. Providers should use doxycycline to treat dual infection due to *B. burgdorferi* and *Ehrlichia* species.

Diagnostic Criteria

Lyme disease that presents as EM or multiple EM is diagnosed purely on the basis of the physical examination. Serologic testing often will not be positive in cases in which the rash was not present for more than 1 week (Table 48-4) and treatment should be initiated while observing the classical rash. In endemic areas, the clinical findings of Bell's palsy or knee arthritis are suggestive of Lyme disease but will require serologic confirmation.

Diagnostic Studies

Isolation of *B. burgdorferi* on culture is confirmatory and has a high yield from skin aspirate or biopsy but is not feasible in most primary practice settings. In practical terms, the detection of antibodies to multiple *B. burgdorferi* antigens confirms the diagnosis (Sood, 1999). Providers should use serologic assays to confirm suspected Lyme disease, unless a pathognomonic EM rash is present. Clinicians should not order them to rule out the diagnosis in patients with nonspecific symptoms. If the provider has a strong clinical suspicion of Lyme disease and the initial serology is negative, he or she should draw a second specimen 2 to 4 weeks later.

▲ **Clinical Warning:** Overdiagnosis of Lyme disease based on false-positive and equivocal results of ELISA tests is still very common, and leads to anxiety and unnecessary antibiotic treatment.

● **Clinical Pearl:** Providers should only suspect Lyme disease (on the basis of characteristic physical signs) if in a patient who has at least a reasonable possibility of exposure to ticks.

Practitioners should follow the "two-step" approach recommended by the CDC-consensus panel for serologic confirmation of Lyme disease (Second National Conference on Serologic Diagnosis of Lyme Disease, 1995). Providers can use any commercially available ELISA test (in common parlance a "Lyme titer") to detect serum antibodies that bind to *B. burgdorferi* antigens. The intensity of a positive reaction does not predict how likely it is that the patient has Lyme disease, and false-positives occur due to cross-reacting antibodies present from other conditions (eg, Epstein-Barr virus infection). The second-step test, immunoblot (western blot), identifies whether the antibodies are specific.

● **Clinical Pearl:** The provider should instruct the laboratory to automatically run an immunoblot on the serum sample if the ELISA result is positive or equivocal.

The adoption of consensus criteria, which are different for IgM and IgG immunoblots, has facilitated the interpretation of an immunoblot. The IgM immunoblot is only useful for diagnosis of early Lyme disease, and results are considered valid during the first 4 weeks of infection. It is positive if two or more of the following bands are present: 23, 39, or 41 Kd. Unfortunately, no antibody is completely specific for *B. burgdorferi* infection and because only two are required for a

TABLE 48–4. Serologic Findings in Lyme Disease

Clinical Manifestation	Test	Expected Serologic Findings	
		At Presentation	2 to 4 Weeks Later
Early-localized (EM)			
Rash present < 1 wk	EIA	Negative	Positive in ½ to ⅔
	IgM immunoblot	Negative	Positive in ½
	IgG immunoblot	Negative	Usually negative
Rash present > 1 wk	EIA	Positive in ⅓	Positive in ⅓ to ⅔
	IgM immunoblot	Positive in ½	Positive
	IgG immunoblot	Usually negative	Positive in ⅓
Early-disseminated Multiple EM			
Rash present < 1 wk	EIA	Negative	Positive
	IgM immunoblot	Positive in ⅓	Positive
	IgG immunoblot	Negative	Negative
Rash present > 1 wk	EIA	Positive	Positive
	IgM immunoblot	Positive	Positive
	IgG immunoblot	Positive in ½	Positive in ⅔
Facial palsy or meningitis	EIA	Positive or negative	Positive
	IgM immunoblot	Positive	Positive
	IgG immunoblot	Negative	Positive
Late			
Arthritis or neurologic	EIA	Positive	Positive
	IgM immunoblot	Often positive but not relevant	
	IgG immunoblot	Positive	
Other			
Asymptomatic seroconversion or acute constitutional illness	EIA	Negative	Positive
	IgM immunoblot	Negative	Positive
	IgG immunoblot	Negative	Positive

EIA, enzyme immunoassay for total IgG and IgM antibodies to *B. burgdorferi,* also called enzyme-linked immunosorbent assay (Sood, 1999).

positive IgM immunoblot, false-positives are common. A positive IgG immunoblot, usually presents 2 to 4 weeks after onset of infection, provides seroconfirmation.

An IgG immunoblot is positive if five or more of the following bands are present: 18, 23 (aka 24 or OspC), 28, 30, 39, 41, 45, 60, 66, or 93 kD. If the clinical likelihood of Lyme disease is strong and the initial serology is negative, a second specimen should be drawn 2 to 4 weeks later. There is no reason to obtain follow-up samples because antibodies generally persist after treatment and lack any prognostic value. A guide to the interpretation of serology in the different manifestations of Lyme disease is presented in Table 48-4.

▲ **Clinical Warning:** The persistence of a positive ELISA or IgG immunoblot is not a reliable measure of treatment efficacy because IgG antibodies will persist for years. Even IGM antibodies can persist for several months.

The use of PCR to detect DNA has the potential to be a valuable diagnostic aid, but technical hurdles, such as contamination, currently limit its practical application. Synovial fluid PCR may be used to help decide whether to administer repeated courses of antibiotics in Lyme arthritis (Nocton et al., 1994). Providers should consider all other diagnostic tests investigational. Importantly, the Food and Drug Administration has not approved urine antigen tests to detect *B. burgdorferi*, and clinicians should not use them to diagnose Lyme disease.

Management

Both early and late Lyme disease respond well to antibiotic treatment, and the prognosis is excellent, despite the public misperception that the disease is difficult to treat and that relapses are common. Clinical improvement occurs within days, irrespective of the duration of symptoms. Occasionally, children with arthritis experience persistence of musculoskeletal symptoms for weeks, which can be treated with anti-inflammatory agents. Arthritis can relapse after treatment but usually responds well to retreatment, either with an oral or parenteral antibiotic regimen.

True treatment resistance is rare. In these patients, frequency of the HLA-DRB1*0401 allele is increased, and the arthritis resembles a reactive arthritis. Infection may no longer be present, and the mechanism of inflammation appears to be autoimmune (Gross et al., 1998). Therapeutic measures, such as intra-articular steroids and synovectomy, may be necessary in these rare cases.

Children who have had Lyme disease do very well in the long term, whether they experienced EM, neurologic infection, or arthritis (Wang et al., 1999). Behavioral and emotional problems, musculoskeletal or neurologic symptoms, and EKG abnormalities are not more common than in controls when assessed several years later. Immunity is not long lasting, however, and reinfections do occur due to new tick bites. These respond equally well to treatment.

Antibiotic Treatment

Regimens currently preferred for the treatment of Lyme disease in children are shown in Table 48-5. Oral courses of treatment are efficacious in cases of EM, disseminated EM, facial palsy, and acute Lyme arthritis. Doxycycline may be preferable over amoxicillin in certain clinical situations. These include patients with possible coinfection with ehrlichiosis and children who are allergic to penicillin or cephalosporins especially because erythromycin has inferior efficacy. Because of its excellent CNS penetration, doxycycline has a theoretical advantage over amoxicillin because of the possibility of subclinical CNS infection in early Lyme disease. Experience with its use in children younger than 8 years is expanding, especially because the risk of tooth staining appears to be less than with older tetracyclines. If both beta-lactam and tetracycline allergy are present, providers may consider the use of clarithromycin, but this is based on very limited efficacy data in the treatment of EM (Dattwyler, Grunwaldt, & Luft, 1996). Clinicians should not use azithromycin to treat Lyme disease, because data on its efficacy are lacking. Providers should treat neurologic disease, except isolated facial palsy, and most recurrences of arthritis with an IV antibiotic.

▲ **Clinical Warning:** Prolonged courses of treatment for chronic arthritis or for suspected chronic CNS disease are inappropriate, because they are no more effective than 4-week regimens. It is inappropriate to treat patients as having Lyme disease if they have a positive ELISA test but are asymptomatic or have symptoms unrelated to Lyme disease.

As in other spirochetal diseases, some children experience a Jarisch-Herxheimer reaction consisting of fever, chills, and sweats shortly after initiation of antibiotic treatment. This is the result of toxin release from dead spirochetes, and providers should not misinterpret it as a treatment complication or failure. Clinicians should counsel parents about the possibility of this occurrence whenever they prescribe antibiotic treatment for Lyme disease.

Prevention of Tick Bites

Some practical environmental measures that a family can use to reduce the likelihood of tick bites include clearing woodpiles and leaf heaps from domestic yards and applying acaricides, such as cyfluthrin and fluvalinate. The primary preventive measures against Lyme disease, however, are personal protection and, with its anticipated availability for use in children, immunization with the Lyme disease vaccine. Children should stay on trails in wooded areas, avoid playing in potentially infested vegetation, wear long-sleeved clothing, and use tick repellents. Parents should consider the toxicity of chemical repellents. They should avoid using permethrin on skin, and should use N,N-diethyl-m-toluamide (DEET) sparingly and in low concentration formulations because the skin absorbs it and it is neurotoxic, especially in young infants (Fradin, 1998). For this reason, many clinicians oppose the use of any tick repellant on bare skin. Parents and older children can apply repellants more liberally to clothing and still maintain some efficacy. They should wash off repellents at the end of the day.

● **Clinical Pearl:** In endemic areas, the best protection against Lyme disease is to perform a careful and complete "tick check" using bright illumination every night before bed.

If families perform tick checks daily, then any tick found at night could only have been acquired during the day. Thus, the tick could only have been attached for a maximum of 8 to 16 hours, making disease transmission extremely unlikely.

TABLE 48–5. Treatment of Lyme Disease in Children

Manifestation	First-Line Drugs*	Equivalent Alternative Drugs	Second-Line Drugs
Early localized (EM)	**Amoxicillin** PO **10–21** d or doxycycline PO **10–21** d	Cefuroxime axetil† PO 10–21 d	Erythromycin PO 10–21 d or **clarithromycin** 10–**21** d
Early disseminated Multiple EM	Amoxicillin PO 21–**28 d** or **doxycycline** PO 21–28 d	**Cefuroxime axetil** PO† 21–**28 d** or ceftriaxone 14 d or cefotaxime 14 d	Erythromycin PO 21–**28** d or **clarithromycin** 21–**28 d**
Facial palsy	Amoxicillin PO 21–28 d or **doxycycline** PO 21–**28 d**	**Ceftriaxone** IV **14**–28 d or cefotaxime IV **14**–28 d	Erythromycin PO 21–28 d or **clarithromycin** PO 21–28 d
Meningitis OR facial palsy with meningitis OR polyneuropathy	**Ceftriaxone IV 14**–28 d or cefotaxime IV **14**–28 d	Doxycycline PO 28 d	Penicillin IV **14**–28 d
Cardiac‡	Amoxicillin PO 21 d or **doxycycline PO** 21 d OR **ceftriaxone IV** or cefotaxime IV initially		Erythromycin PO 21 d or **clarithromycin** PO 21 d or penicillin IV 14 d
Late Arthritis	**Amoxicillin** PO 28 d or doxycycline PO 28 d	**Ceftriaxone§** IV **14**–**28 d** or cefotaxime‡ IV **14**–**28 d**	Penicillin IV 14–28 d
Neurologic	**Ceftriaxone** IV **14**–**28 d** or cefotaxime IV **14**–**28 d**	Doxycycline PO **28 d**	Penicillin IV **14**–28 d
Other Asymptomatic seroconversion OR Acute constitutional illness	Amoxicillin PO 21 d or **doxycycline** PO 21 d	Cefuroxime axetil PO† 21 d	Erythromycin PO 21 d or **clarithromycin** PO 21 d
Tick bite prophylaxis¶	**Amoxicillin** PO 10 d or doxycycline PO 10 d		

From Sood, S.K. (1999). Lyme disease. *Pediatric Infectious Disease Journal, 18*(10), 913-915.

*Doses: doxycycline PO 2–4 mg/kg/d divided into two doses, up to adult dose of 100 mg b.i.d.; amoxicillin PO 40–50 mg/kg/d divided into three doses, up to adult dose of 2 g/d; cefuroxime axetil PO 30 mg/kg/d divided into two doses, up to adult dose of 500 mg b.i.d.; erythromycin PO 30–40 mg/kg/d divided into four doses, up to adult dose of 250 four times a day; clarithromycin PO 15 mg/kg/d divided into two doses, up to adult dose of 500 mg twice a day; ceftriaxone IV 100 mg/kg/d once daily, up to 2 g once daily; cefotaxime IV 180 mg/kg/d, up to 2 g every 8 h; penicillin IV 200,000–400,000 U/kg/d, divided into four doses, up to 24 million U/d. Duration: Pediatric clinical study data on which to base recommendations are limited. **The author's preferences are indicated in bold type.**

†Cefuroxime axetil was tested in children 12 y and older but is expected to be efficacious in all children, given its satisfactory pharmacokinetics in young children.

‡First-degree block with PR interval <0.3 s PO therapy; PR >0.3 s or higher grade, IV initially, then PO if responds rapidly.

§For oral therapy failures only.

¶Only if *identified* deer tick with *measured* attachment ≥72 h.

EM = erythema migrans.

Tick Removal

Use of a washcloth while showering will dislodge most ticks. A simple pair of tweezers is all that is needed to pull off an attached tick; no chemicals should be applied. Timely removal decreases the risk of transmission of the spirochete, which requires time to migrate from the tick's midgut to its salivary gland. The risk of transmission is increased 20-fold after an attachment of 72 or more hours in humans (Sood et al., 1997). Because examination of the tick can influence how the primary care clinician manages the bite, parents should save ticks in a dry container rather than destroying them.

Management of a Deer Tick Bite

Finding a tick on their child causes considerable anxiety to parents. A tick bite is not an emergency, and providers can handle it during routine office hours. Many bites are from dog ticks or Lone Star ticks, which do not transmit *B. burgdorferi*. In the event of a deer tick bite, parental reassurance is extremely important given the great amount of misinformation (approaching hysteria) that accompanies this disease.

● **Clinical Pearl:** The incidence of Lyme disease following a deer tick bite is very low, usually 1% to 2%, even in endemic areas (Shapiro et al., 1992).

Several variables affect the risk, and it is helpful for the clinician to review these with the family. Not all deer ticks are infected with *B. burgdorferi*, and the infection rate varies considerably from one location to another. Nymphal stage ticks, in the spring and summer, are more likely to transmit the spirochete than are ticks of other stages. The duration of attachment (DOA) is probably the most important variable.

The second step in counseling involves discussion of the fact that antibiotic prophylaxis generally is not indicated. If Lyme disease occurs, it can be easily and effectively treated.

● **Clinical Pearl:** Watchful waiting is the preferred management of tick bites; antibiotic prophylaxis is usually not recommended.

Parents and provider should watch the site of the bite carefully for the development of EM. Nevertheless, parents usually remain anxious despite hearing these reassurances. Practitioners frequently but erroneously take the path of least resistance and prescribe an antibiotic, even without confirmation of the tick's identity.

To refine this practice, we have proposed an algorithmic approach to antibiotic management of a tick bite based on a prospective study of risk (Sood et al., 1997). The risk of human infection after a documented deer tick bite was 1.1% if the tick was attached less than 72 hours, and 18% to 25% for attachment more than 72 hours. PCR assay for *B. burgdorferi* DNA in the tick was not predictive of risk. The high risk of infection after attachment for more than 72 hours should justify antibiotic prophylaxis.

The DOA can be accurately measured by an index of engorgement called the scutal index, which requires some expertise but can be learned in any laboratory that identifies ticks. Often patients and practitioners can recognize engorged ticks with no more than a hand lens. This approach requires the primary care clinician to attempt or request tick identification and a measurement of engorgement and discourages the practice of sending the tick for detection of spirochete. This method enables selection of a small subgroup of bitten individuals who are candidates for prophylaxis. Ten days of amoxicillin or doxycycline (see Table 48-5) may be an adequate course of prophylactic therapy.

● **Clinical Pearl:** Agreement is almost universal that tick bites in which the DOA was short (less than 24 hours) pose a very small risk, and watchful waiting is the management of choice. Some experts feel that antibiotic prophylaxis is justified if the DOA was more than 72 hours.

Controversy remains, however, about the management of tick bites with unknown or intermediate length DOA. Many times, the removal process either destroys or mutilates the offending tick, and practitioners are not willing or able to measure engorgement with any degree of accuracy. In these cases, routine prophylaxis is still discouraged. Watchful waiting is still the treatment of choice.

Use of serologic testing may have a place, however, in situations in which the DOA is unknown and parental anxiety is high. Comparing baseline (within a day or two of the tick bite) and convalescent (4–6 weeks later) antibodies to *B. burgdorferi* by ELISA and immunoblot and finding no seroconversion can be reassuring to parents and practitioners alike. This approach is imperfect but is a better alternative than antibiotic prophylaxis, because children in endemic areas may experience several bites of this nature every summer.

Immunization

The recent licensure of a vaccine for immunization of adolescents and adults provides the primary care clinician with an additional preventive measure to use in endemic areas. Two vaccines were studied; one has been licensed so far. The antigen in both is an outer surface protein called outer surface protein A (OspA). This is the only vaccine that works by killing the offending microbe outside the human body. During its blood meal, the deer tick ingests antibody to OspA, produced in the vaccinee. The spirochetes are killed in the tick's midgut before they can enter the human body (Fikrig et al., 1992).

● **Clinical Pearl:** People who receive the Lyme disease vaccine will develop positive serology. Because the molecular weight of the vaccine OspA is 31 kD, visualization of a 31-kD band on immunoblot can distinguish due to vaccine from natural disease.

Two vaccine formulations, manufactured by recombinant DNA technology, have been evaluated for efficacy in prevention of Lyme disease in endemic areas, and one is currently licensed for those ages 15 years and older (Sigal et al., 1998; Steere et al., 1998). This vaccine, manufactured and distributed by SmithKline Beecham Pharmaceuticals, has a high efficacy (76%) after administration of three doses on a 0, 1, and 12-month schedule.

The vaccines are considered safe in that no unusual or severe adverse effects were observed. A theoretical concern is whether OspA vaccine could cause arthritis. The speculation owes its origin to the fact that rarely individuals develop treatment-resistant Lyme arthritis, and these individuals frequently have detectable antibody to OspA, an antibody not detected in the serum in early infection. OspA has molecular mimicry with at least one human leukocyte antigen, leading to concern that antibody to this protein could cause synovial inflammation. It is reassuring that late (30 days or more postvaccine) musculoskeletal symptoms occurred no more frequently in vaccinees than in controls in the study of the currently licensed vaccine that included about 10,000 subjects. This vaccine also proved to be highly efficacious in prevention of asymptomatic infection as assessed by seroconversion. This suggests that vaccination will not place recipients at risk for latent subclinical infection.

As currently recommended for use, three doses of vaccine are administered over 1 year, but accelerated schedules have been found equivalent and may be allowed in the future. Antibody levels to OspA wane significantly over one year, and periodic boosters will most probably be recommended, based on analysis of ongoing studies.

▲ **Clinical Warning:** Considering the focal distribution of Lyme disease within endemic regions, this vaccine should not be universally administered to children or adults living in these regions.

However, there are many people at high risk of infection because of occupational or recreational exposure or whose homes are in tick-infested wooded areas. Primary care clinicians should offer immunization to these people (Recommendations of the Advisory Committee on Immunization Practices, 1999). A study to confirm the vaccine's safety in children ages 4 to 18 years is underway. At present, the vaccine should be considered for adolescents age 15 years and older who are at risk for tick bites by virtue of their work or recreation in wooded environments in endemic areas.

ROCKY MOUNTAIN SPOTTED FEVER

Rocky Mountain spotted fever (RMSF) is a tick-borne rickettsial illness caused by *Rickettsia rickettsii*, an obligate intracellular gram-negative organism. It is the most prevalent rickettsial disease in the United States. The infection is acquired from the bite of the wood tick in the western United States or the American dog tick in the eastern and southern United States. It is prevalent in many areas of the country, but most cases currently occur in a broad geographic band from Virginia and the Carolinas to Texas, Oklahoma, and Kansas (Thorner, Walker, & Petri, 1998). The name, therefore, derived from outbreaks investigated by Dr. Howard Ricketts in Montana, is not very descriptive of its current epidemiology.

History and Physical Examination

When a history of tick bite is uncertain, a history of a visit to the woods may be a clue. The incubation period is 14 days. The peak incidence is between ages 5 and 9 years (Dalton et al., 1995). The illness begins as fever with a severe headache in the absence of signs of meningeal irritation. The characteristic rash may appear several (usually within 3–5) days into the illness and is a blanching maculopapular eruption that evolves into petechial or hemorrhagic lesions. The distribution of the rash is classic, starting peripherally on the hands and feet or wrists and ankles and then spreading to the arms, legs, and finally the trunk (centripetal). By contrast, in meningococcemia, the rash has no characteristic pattern, appearing in several locations simultaneously. In rare cases, the disease may present as purpura fulminans or septic shock mimicking meningococcemia. Meningitis occurs in a small percentage of cases. The other characteristic feature is severe myalgia, present in more than 70% of cases. Other physical signs include edema of the extremities and nonexudative conjuctivitis.

Diagnostic Criteria and Studies

● **Clinical Pearl:** A low or normal total white blood cell (WBC) count with an elevated percentage of band forms is a key laboratory finding in RMSF, especially if accompanied by thrombocytopenia and hyponatremia. This pattern is quite uncharacteristic of viral or bacterial infections.

The diagnosis is based on the history and physical examination findings; laboratory evidence is only supportive. The diagnosis can be confirmed with specific serologic assays to detect a rise in titer of four-fold or more to *R. rickettsii* antigens, but the results usually are not available until after the illness has resolved. The traditional Weil-Felix reaction (antibodies to *Proteus* antigens) is considered nonspecific and has no current role in diagnostic confirmation.

Management

The first 3 to 5 days provide a "therapeutic window" during which the primary care clinician can observe the febrile child for emergence of a rash before initiating antibiotic treatment, as long as he or she agrees to daily follow-up. The drug of choice is doxycycline, and the provider should institute treatment based on clinical grounds. Providers should temper fear of using a tetracycline in young children with the knowledge that a single course of doxycycline is unlikely to produce tooth staining. A week of therapy or until the child is afebrile for 2 or more days is sufficient. A child who maintains adequate oral intake and is stable hemodynamically does not require hospitalization for treatment. Prophylactic antibiotic therapy for a tick bite is not recommended, especially as it may delay the diagnosis by partially masking the symptoms.

EHRLICHIOSIS

Ehrlichiae are intraleukocytic rickettsia-like organisms that cause febrile illnesses. At least two tick-borne ehrlichioses are in the United States: human monocytic ehrlichiosis (HME) caused by *Ehrlichia chaffeensis* and human granulocytic ehrlichiosis (HGE) caused by the still unnamed species referred to as the HGE agent. The former pathogen is believed to be mainly transmitted by *Amblyomma americanum*, the Lone Star tick, and is endemic to several southeastern and south central states (Spach et al., 1993). The HGE agent is transmitted by the same vector tick that transmits *B. burgdorferi*, *Ixodes scapularis*; it is unclear if the common dog tick, *Dermacentor variabilis*, can also transmit it. Up to 25% of adult deer ticks were found to be coinfected with *B. burgdorferi* and the HGE agent in Westchester County, New York, and cotransmission with *B. burgdorferi* has caused dual infection (Nadelman et al., 1997).

HGE is primarily encountered in Minnesota, Wisconsin, several mid-Atlantic states, and southern New England. Very few cases are known to have occurred in children, so information about HGE is mostly inferred from adult studies.

Pathology

Providers must consider the diagnosis of ehrlichiosis in any patient who presents with an acute febrile constitutional illness during the spring and summer months without an identifiable cause. If the patient reports a known tick bite, the incubation period most often is less than a week. Because the geographic distribution has not yet been clearly defined and additional vectors may be implicated in transmission, the ehrlichioses are potentially more widely distributed than Lyme disease and babesiosis. Also, no clinical sign is pathognomonic, and providers frequently will miss the diagnosis in the absence of a high index of suspicion. The practical implication is that treatment delay can occur in patients with severe illness. Although ehrlichiosis can rarely be fatal, mild or unrecognized infections are far more common (Magnarelli et al., 1995).

● **Clinical Pearl:** The clinical profile of ehrlichiosis consists of fever, often with chills, in an ill-appearing person with laboratory evidence of bone marrow suppression.

Headache, arthralgia, malaise, and myalgia are common symptoms, and aseptic meningitis is frequently part of the illness. Leukopenia, thrombocytopenia, or both occur in about 80% of cases (Aguero-Rosenfeld et al., 1996). Most patients have elevated liver enzymes. The lowered WBC count is attributable to lymphopenia or neutropenia, with the degree of each being correlated with the duration of illness. Atypical lymphocytosis is observed in most patients.

Diagnostic Criteria

An early diagnosis can be made by visualization of *Ehrlichia morulae*, which are aggregates of dividing organisms, on a Wright-stained smear of WBCs from the buffy coat of a peripheral blood sample. These are present inside monocytes and granulocytes respectively in human monocytic ehrlichiosis (HME) and HGE. Detection of *E. morulae* is not a sensitive diagnostic method, nor is it practical for the busy clinician. PCR assay for detection of DNA is the most sensitive early diagnostic method but is not universally available at present.

▲ **Clinical Warning:** Because of the limitations of early diagnostic modalities, providers should initiate treatment based on clinical suspicion alone. They should suspect coinfection with the HGE agent in a patient with Lyme disease and moderate or severe constitutional symptoms, in particular those who manifest leukopenia or thrombocytopenia.

Serologic testing can confirm the diagnosis. The current serologic assays in use detect rising titers of antibodies by immunofluorescent assay to *Ehrlichia* antigens: *Ehrlichia equi,* a species believed to be closely related to the HGE agent for diagnosis of HGE, and *E. chaffeensis* for diagnosis of HME. The serologic assays are limited by the fact that there is cross-reactivity between *E. chaffeensis* and *E. equi,* rendering precise seroconfirmation of either infection difficult.

Management

The antibiotic of choice for both ehrlichioses is doxycycline. Providers should temper fear of using tetracycline in young children with the knowledge that a single course of doxycycline is unlikely to produce tooth staining. Rapid and complete resolution of the illness results in 24 to 48 hours (Dumler, 1998). Some patients, mostly adults, are ill enough to require hospitalization and supportive care. Hemodynamic and renal functions need to be monitored in these patients.

BABESIOSIS

Babesiosis is a parasitic infection of red blood cells caused by unicellular tick-borne organisms of the genus *Babesia.* They are called piroplasms because of the pear-like shape of the intraerythrocytic stage. In the northeast and Great Lakes region of the midwestern United States, *B. microti* is the causative species and is transmitted by the bite of *I. scapularis,* the same vector that transmits *B. burgdorferi.* In the northeastern United States, it is most prevalent on the southern coasts of Massachusetts, Rhode Island, Connecticut, and New York (especially Long Island) (Spach et al., 1993). The distribution appears to be more focal than that of Lyme disease. In coastal northeast United States, the main mammalian reservoir, *Peromyscus leucopus* is the same as that for *B. burgdorferi. B. burgdorferi* and *Babesia* spp. have been concurrently recovered from 18.6% of nymphal *Ixodes* ticks from Nantucket Island, and concurrent human infection has been reported (Krause et al., 1996). Infections from related species have been identified in California, Washington, and Missouri. In Europe, babesiosis is caused by *Babesia divergens* and is usually a more fulminant disease. Transfusion-acquired and transplacental infections have been reported rarely.

History and Physical Examination

The organism parasitizes erythrocytes and results in a spectrum of illness ranging from asymptomatic infection to fulminant disease resembling blackwater fever of malaria with fever, hemolysis, and hemoglobinuria. The disease is often mild in children and in those who are immunocompetent, making the disease indistinguishable from an acute viral infection (Krause et al., 1992). Providers should be aware, however, of the uncommon scenario of fatal infection in asplenic, immunocompromised, or elderly patients. Babesiosis should be in the differential diagnosis in a child with fever of uncertain origin with anemia, thrombocytopenia, or both. Persistent infection for up to 2 years, with clinical recrudescence, has been described (Krause et al., 1998).

Diagnostic Criteria

Providers should consider the diagnosis in patients with fever of uncertain origin during the transmission season (May to October) in an endemic area. Most cases occur during the summer. Diagnosis is made by examination of a blood smear for the intraerythrocytic parasites. An inexperienced microscopist can mistake the ring forms for malarial parasites. If the parasite is visualized as tetrads, which is uncommon, this is pathognomonic. Serum antibody assays can be used after the infection has been present for 2 to 4 weeks and are useful when ordered as part of the workup for prolonged fever. The current serologic test of choice is an indirect immunofluorescent assay for IgM and IgG antibodies. Confirmatory tests are small animal inoculation and a commercially available PCR but are not recommended for routine use.

Management

Treatment of babesiosis is with clindamycin and quinine. This is somewhat problematic because of the high incidence of side effects (Krause et al., 1998). Quinine is poorly tolerated in about half of treated patients, who experience hearing loss, tinnitus, GI symptoms, and occasionally hypotension. In the future, combination treatment with azithromycin and atovaquone may become the therapy of choice. Antibiotic regimens for babesiosis are listed in Table 48-6.

TULAREMIA

This bacterial infection caused by *Francisella tularensis* also can be transmitted by ticks, most commonly the wood and Lone Star ticks. Almost every state has reported tularemia, with Arkansas, Tennessee, Texas, Oklahoma, and Missouri accounting for nearly 50% of cases (Spach et al., 1993).

Pathology

Infection can occur through skin or mucosal contact. Tularemia can present in many ways, including fever without other signs, but ulceroglandular tularemia, due to an infected tick bite, characterized by lymphadenitis with or without cutaneous ulcers, is the most common presentation. Other forms include the oculoglandular, oropharyngeal, and GI varieties from conjunctival contact or ingestion of this highly infectious bacterium (Shapiro, 1998).

Diagnostic Criteria

A hemagglutination assay to detect antibodies to the causative bacterium is available through most commercial laboratory services and is a sensitive means of detecting evidence of recent or current infection. Typically, IgM and IgG titers of hemagglutinating antibody are markedly elevated.

Management

Mild cases, especially those presenting with unifocal lymphadenitis, are self-limited. Severe disease may require treatment with intramuscular gentamicin, because oral antibiotics, except perhaps the quinolones, are usually ineffective (Limaye & Hooper, 1999).

TABLE 48–6. Treatment of Other Tickborne Diseases in Children

Disease	Drugs of Choice	Alternate Drugs	Duration
Rocky Mountain spotted fever	doxycycline	chloramphenicol	7–10 d
Babesiosis	clindamycin PO plus quinine PO	atovaquone PO plus azithromycin PO	7–10 d
Ehrlichiosis, monocytic or granulocytic	doxycycline PO		10 d
Tularemia	gentamicin IM	ciprofloxacin PO	10–14 d
Doses: Clindamycin 30 mg/kg/d			
Quinine 25 mg/kg/d			
Doxycycline 2–4 mg/kg/d			
Gentamicin 7.5 mg/kg/d			

REFERENCES

Aguero-Rosenfeld, M. E., Horowitz, H. W., Wormser, G. P., McKenna, D. F., Nowakowski, J., Munoz, J., et al. (1996). Human granulocytic ehrlichiosis: A case series from a medical center in New York State. *Annals of Internal Medicine, 125*(11), 904–908.

Dalton, M. J., Clarke, M. J., Holman, R. C., Krebs, J. W., Fishbein, D. B., Olson, J. G., et al. (1995). National surveillance for Rocky Mountain spotted fever, 1981-1992: Epidemiologic summary and evaluation of risk factors for fatal outcome. *American Journal of Tropical Medicine and Hygiene, 52*(5), 405–413.

Dattwyler, R. J., Grunwaldt, E., & Luft, B. J. (1996). Clarithromycin in treatment of early Lyme disease: A pilot study. *Antimicrobial Agents and Chemotherapeutics, 40*(2), 468–469.

Dennis, D. T. (1998). Epidemiology, ecology and prevention of Lyme disease. In D. T. Rahn & J. Evans (Eds.), *Lyme disease* (pp. 7–34). Philadelphia: American College of Physicians.

Fikrig, E., Telford, S. R., Barthold, S. W., Kantor, F. S., Spielman, A., & Flavell, R. A. (1992). Elimination of Borrelia burgdorferi from vector ticks feeding on OspA-immunized mice. *Proceedings of the National Academy of Science United States of America, 89*(12), 5418–5421.

Fradin, M. S. (1998). Mosquitoes and mosquito repellents: A clinician's guide. *Annals of Internal Medicine, 128*(11), 931–940.

Gerber, M. A., Shapiro, E. D., Burke, G. S., Parcells, V. J., & Bell, G. L. (1996). Lyme disease in children in southeastern Connecticut. Pediatric Lyme Disease Study Group [see comments]. *New England Journal of Medicine, 335*(17), 1270–1274.

Gerber, M. A., Zemel, L. S., & Shapiro, E. D. (1998). Lyme arthritis in children: Clinical epidemiology and long-term outcomes. *Pediatrics, 102*(4 Pt 1), 905–908.

Gross, D. M., Forsthuber, T., Tary Lehmann, M., Etling, C., Ito, K., Nagy, Z. A., et al. (1998). Identification of LFA-1 as a candidate autoantigen in treatment- resistant Lyme arthritis [see comments]. *Science, 281*(5377), 703–706.

Jain, V. K., Hilton, E., Maytal, J., Dorante, G., Ilowite, N. T., & Sood, S. K. (1996). Immunoglobulin M immunoblot for diagnosis of Borrelia burgdorferi infection in patients with acute facial palsy. *Journal of Clinical Microbiology, 34*(8), 2033–2035.

Kan, L., Sood, S. K., & Maytal, J. (1998). Pseudotumor cerebri in Lyme disease: A case report and literature review. *Pediatric Neurology, 18*(5), 439–441.

Krause, P. J., Telford, S. R., Pollack, R. J., Ryan, R., Brassard, P., Zemel, L., et al. (1992). Babesiosis: An underdiagnosed disease of children. *Pediatrics, 89*(6 Pt 1), 1045–1048.

Krause, P. J., Spielman, A., Telford, S. R., Sikand, V. K., McKay, K., Christianson, D., et al. (1998). Persistent parasitemia after acute babesiosis. *New England Journal of Medicine, 339*(3), 160–165.

Krause, P. J., Telford, S. R., Spielman, A., Sikand, V., Ryan, R., Christianson, D., et al. (1996). Concurrent Lyme disease and babesiosis. Evidence for increased severity and duration of illness. *Journal of the American Medical Association, 275*(21), 1657–1660.

Kuiper, H., de Jongh, B. M., van Dam, A. P., Dodge, D. E., Ramselaar, A. C., Spanjaard, L., et al. (1994). Evaluation of central nervous system involvement in Lyme borreliosis patients with a solitary erythema migrans lesion. *European Journal of Clinical Microbiology and Infectious Diseases, 13*(5), 379–387.

Limaye, A. P., & Hooper, C. J. (1999). Treatment of tularemia with fluoroquinolones: Two cases and review. *Clinical Infectious Disease, 29*(4), 922–924.

Magnarelli, L. A., Dumler, J. S., Anderson, J. F., et al. (1995). Coexistence of antibodies to tick borne pathogens of babesiosis, ehrlichiosis, and Lyme borreliosis in human sera. *Journal of Clinical Microbiology, 33*, 3054–3057.

Maraspin, V., Cimperman, J., Lotric Furlan, S., Pleterski Rigler, D., & Strle, F. (1996). Treatment of erythema migrans in pregnancy. *Clinical Infectious Diseases, 22*(5), 788–793.

Markowitz, L. E., Steere, A. C., Benach, J. L., Slade, J. D., & Broome, C. V. (1986). Lyme disease during pregnancy. *Journal of the American Medical Association, 255*(24), 3394–3396.

Nadelman, R. B., & Wormser, G. P. (1998). Management of tick bites and early Lyme disease. In D. T. Rahn & J. Evans (Eds.), *Lyme disease* (pp. 49–76) Philadelphia: American College of Physicians.

Nadelman, R. B., Horowitz, H. W., Hsieh, T. C., Wu, J. M., Aguero Rosenfeld, M. E., Schwartz, I., et al. (1997). Simultaneous human granulocytic ehrlichiosis and Lyme borreliosis. *New England Journal of Medicine, 337*(1), 27–30.

Niemann, G., Koksal, M. A., Oberle, A., & Michaelis, R. (1997). Facial palsy and Lyme borreliosis: Long-term follow-up of children with antibiotically untreated "idiopathic" facial palsy. *Klinische Padiatrie, 209*(3), 95–99.

Nocton, J. J., Dressler, F., Rutledge, B. J., Rys, P. N., Persing, D. H., & Steere, A. C. (1994). Detection of Borrelia burgdorferi DNA by polymerase chain reaction in synovial fluid from patients with Lyme arthritis [see comments]. *New England Journal of Medicine, 330*(4), 229–234.

Recommendations of the Advisory Committee on Immunization Practices (ACIP). (1999). Recommendations for the use of Lyme disease vaccine. *Morbidity and Mortality Weekly Report,* 48(RR-7), 1-5.

Recommendations of the Advisory Committee on Immunization Practices (ACIP). (1999). Published erratum to Recommendations for the use of Lyme disease vaccine. *Morbidity and Mortality Weekly Report,* 48(37), 833.

Second National Conference on Serologic Diagnosis of Lyme Disease. (1995). Recommendations for test performance and interpretation. *Morbidity and Mortality Weekly Report,* 44(31), 590–591.

Shapiro, E. D. (1998). Tick-borne infections. In S. L. Katz, A. A. Gershon, & P. J. Hotez (Eds.), *Krugman's infectious diseases of children.* St. Louis: Mosby-Year Book.

Shapiro, E. D., Gerber, M. A., Holabird, N. B., et al. (1992). A controlled trial of antimicrobial prophylaxis for Lyme Disease after deer-tick bites. *New England Journal of Medicine, 327*, 1769–1773.

Sigal, L. H., Zahradnik, J. M., Lavin, P., Patella, S. J., Bryant, G., Haselby, R., et al. (1998). A vaccine consisting of recombinant Borrelia burgdorferi outer-surface protein A to prevent Lyme disease. Recombinant Outer-Surface Protein A Lyme Disease Vaccine Study Consortium. *New England Journal of Medicine, 339*(4), 216–222.

Sood, S. K. (1998). Facial palsy in Lyme disease [letter]. *Archives of Pediatric and Adolescent Medicine, 152*(9), 928–929.

Sood, S. K. (1999). Lyme disease. *Pediatric Infectious Disease Journal, 18*(10), 913–925.

Sood, S. K., Salzman, M. B., Johnson, B. J., Happ, C. M., Feig, K., Carmody, L., et al. (1997). Duration of tick attachment as a predictor of the risk of Lyme disease in an area in which Lyme disease is endemic. *Journal of Infectious Diseases, 175*(4), 996–999.

Spach, D. H., Liles, W. C., Campbell, G. L., Quick, R. E., Anderson, D. E., Jr., & Fritsche, T. R. (1993). Tick-borne diseases in the United States [see comments]. *New England Journal of Medicine, 329*(13), 936–947.

Steere, A. C., Sikand, V. K., Meurice, F., Parenti, D. L., Fikrig, E., Schoen, R. T., et al. (1998). Vaccination against Lyme disease with recombinant Borrelia burgdorferi outer-surface lipoprotein A with adjuvant. Lyme Disease Vaccine Study Group [see comments]. *New England Journal of Medicine, 339*(4), 209–215.

Strobino, B. A., Williams, C. L., Abid, S., Chalson, R., & Spierling, P. (1993). Lyme disease and pregnancy outcome: A prospective study of two thousand prenatal patients. *American Journal of Obstetrics and Gynecology, 169*(2 Pt 1), 367–374.

Thorner, A. R., Walker, D. H., & Petri, W. A., Jr. (1998). Rocky Mountain spotted fever. *Clinical Infectious Diseases, 27*(6), 1353–1359.

Wang, T. J., Sangha, O., Phillips, C. B., Wright, E. A., Lew, R. A., Fossel, A. H., et al. (1999). Outcomes of children treated for Lyme disease. *Journal of Rheumatology, 25*(11), 2249–2253.

P A R T   I V　▲

Scabies, Lice, and Sun

● VINCENT P. BELTRANI, MD

SCABIES AND LICE

Whether six-legged insects or eight-legged arachnids, arthropods plague human skin with itchy or toxic bites, annoying infestations, and infectious inoculations. Clinicians must clearly understand basic "bug biology" and the pathogenesis of related human disease to care adequately for affected hosts. Unfortunately, writing a prescription for "the right cream" is rarely sufficient.

Examples of arthropods' vast repertoire are seen daily in many primary care practices. The immediate swollen urticarial plaque of a hymenoptera (ie, wasp, hornet, bee) sting represents the classic type 1 IgE-mediated allergic reaction that can eventuate into full-blown anaphylaxis, due largely to the effects of histamine. The annoying itchy bumps of mosquito bites, however, occur as a result of type 4 delayed hypersensitivity and, while developing hours to days after a bite, can persist for weeks due to the impressive cellular inflammatory response at the skin site. Many arthropods act as vectors of infectious disease, such as Lyme disease and leishmaniasis. The brown recluse spider and other arthropods cause disease by direct inoculation of various toxins. Finally, scabies and lice are obligate human parasites. These arthropods do not bite and run, but live and multiply on human skin cells or blood. When evaluating patients with arthropod-induced disease, the clinician must consider the type and number of arthropods causing the symptoms, the period over which the insult takes place, the pathogenesis of the reaction, the epidemiology and potential spread of disease, and finally the appropriate tests, treatments, and prognosis.

SCABIES

Sarcoptes scabiei var. *hominis* is an obligate human parasite belonging to the arachnid class of arthropods. A rather fat little mite with eight short legs, the adult female measures approximately 0.4 by 0.3 mm; the male is about half that size (Elgart, 1990). The fertilized female can burrow through the epidermis at a rate of 2 to 5 mm/day and can lay anywhere from 10 to 25 eggs over 5 to 10 days before dying. Less than 10% of the six-legged larvae survive to adulthood. Mature adults copulate in shallow pockets in the stratum corneum, continuing the life cycle.

Pathology

Close personal contact of 15 minutes or more can transmit the infestation. Clearly, hand-holding is the most common route of exposure and may well explain the prevalence of burrows on the fingers. Mites also favor breasts and genitals. They are very rarely found elsewhere. Interestingly, the total mite population usually stabilizes at 10 to 20, often peaking after 2 to 3 months of infestation before gradually declining. Spontaneous resolution of the infestation is rare.

The eruption that results from sarcoptic infestation depends on a type 4 delayed hypersensitivity reaction, and the intensity of the response reflects the host's sensitivity to various mite antigens (McDonald, Stites, & Bunton, 1997). Hence, "nonallergic" hosts will have rather asymptomatic burrows containing live mites and essentially no other symptoms. Consistent with type 4 immunology, the rash and pruritus occur after a 2- to 4-week incubation period and sooner if prior infection has sensitized the patient.

● **Clinical Pearl:** The major reason for the impressive rash seen in most individuals is a hypersensitivity reaction to the 10 to 20 mites.

Epidemiology

Scabies infestation strikes people of all ages and races regardless of personal hygiene. The mites are uniquely adapted to survive on human skin. Any venture off human skin by an intrepid mite ensures rapid death. In addition to being blind, these arthropods have short legs that are incapable of walking on flat surfaces. They have no protective suit of armor, as do other "free-living" mites. Because they cannot survive more than a few hours off human skin, the issue of scabies spreading through clothing, bedding, and other inanimate fomites remains controversial (Elgart, 1990; Maunder, 1998).

History and Physical Examination

● **Clinical Pearl:** The hallmark of scabies infestation is the presence of burrows on the wrists, hands, web spaces of the fingers, waistline, breasts, and genitals. In older children and adults, the face and scalp are spared. In infants, the lesions are commonly seen in the scalp, axillae, palms, and insteps of the feet (Metry & Hebert, 2000).

Sarcoptic burrows may be hard to identify in infants but have been described as gray threadlike trails of scale on the skin (Metry & Hebert, 2000). Practice and experience will enable astute practitioners to see a tiny black dot at the end of a burrow, which represents the 0.3 to 0.4 mm female mite. With increasing expertise, providers generally can confirm the diagnosis by physical examination of the hands alone. An additional helpful finding in male patients is the presence of erythematous 4- to 6-mm nodules on the scrotum. These inflammatory nodules, which contain live mites, are occasionally found elsewhere and may last for months, even after effective treatment.

Surprisingly, the impressive and intensely pruritic generalized rash that often warrants a visit to the provider is the least helpful and most distracting feature of scabies. Most patients present with a generalized eczematous (red and scaly) rash with excoriations. Others present with urticarial papules and plaques. Rarely, pustules and impetiginous crusts develop due to secondary infection, though the use of antibiotics has made bacteremia and secondary glomerulonephritis rare (Elgart, 1990). The differential diagnosis includes contact dermatitis, atopic dermatitis, impetigo, and arthropod bites.

Diagnostic Criteria and Studies

Confirmation of the diagnosis of scabies requires the isolation of the mite, eggs, or feces. The simplest technique requires scraping the skin over the burrow with a #15 scalpel blade, smearing the scrapings on a glass slide, and applying a drop of mineral oil to the debris. After applying a cover slip, the clinician can usually identify diagnostic findings of mites, eggs, or mite feces with ease. Some clinicians prefer to apply mineral oil to the burrow directly, making it easier to identify. Other methods to assist detection include the application of ink to the skin around the burrow, then wiping the skin with alcohol and allowing the burrow to remain inked. With practice, the provider should be able to identify diagnostic evidence in 100% of suspected patients. Skin biopsies may be diagnostic if specimens contain actual mites; otherwise, the histologic features are nonspecific but often include findings of eczema with impressive eosinophilia. Blood tests generally are not useful because no specific abnormalities are diagnostic for scabies.

Norwegian or "crusted" scabies is a rare variant occurring in institutionalized patients with mental retardation or severe underlying diseases like leukemia, acquired immunodeficiency syndrome, and other immunosuppressive illnesses. Patients present with grotesque verrucous or hyperkeratotic crusts on the hands, feet, scalp, and nails. Many progress to an erythroderma with adenopathy and eosinophilia. These patients are highly contagious and harbor thousands of mites. As a consequence in this particular situation, fomites are likely to be an important source of transmission.

A final variation of scabies is "animal scabies" or sarcoptic mange. Given that sarcoptic mites are species specific, *S. scabiei* var. *canis* naturally affects dogs (mange). Close animal contact can produce generalized nonspecific itchy rashes in humans with a distinct absence of burrows and mites. Therapy requires concomitant treatment of the affected pet.

Management

● **Clinical Pearl:** Successful therapy of scabies requires the understanding that treatment will kill the mites but will not suppress the symptomatic immunologic reaction.

Scabies is an epidemiologic challenge, and all close contacts must be treated or reinfection is likely. The most common treatments are permethrin 5% cream (Elimite) and lindane 1% lotion (Kwell).

Permethrin cream is the newest topical therapy for scabies. There are no significant side effects, and it can be used in infants older than 2 months. The provider should instruct the parent to apply the lotion before bed, generally from the neck down but also to the head and scalp in prepubertal children. The following morning, after 8 to 12 hours, parents should wash it off. Providers must emphasize that parents must treat every square inch of skin, paying special attention to hands, fingers, under the nails, and genitals. All close family contacts should be treated simultaneously to avoid reinfestation (AAP, 1997). Many clinicians recommend a second course of treatment 7 to 10 days later, but the evidence supporting this practice is lacking. The current *Red Book* recommends that providers should instruct patients that, after showering, they should launder any bedclothes, clothing, linens, and towels they used in the past 24 to 48 hours. This statement is controversial, however, as entomologists will argue that the sarcoptic mite has virtually no chance of surviving very long off the human host (Maunder, 1998). The exception may be Norwegian scabies, as mentioned previously, in which the sarcoptic burden is high enough to allow survival of some mites. Permethrin offers more than 90% cure rates with only one application, and its use is not limited by any systemic toxicity (Taplin, Meinking, & Porcelain, 1986). Thirty grams of cream (half of a tube) generally suffices for an adult or child.

Lindane, an older therapy, is applied in two sessions 1 week apart. It is recommended to apply it to dry skin, because freshly bathed skin will increase absorption of the drug, increasing the risk of CNS toxicity. While effectively curing patients 60% to 90% of the time, there is a potential for CNS toxicity, which may include dizziness and convulsions (Chouela et al., 1999; Taplin et al., 1986). Lindane resistance has been reported (Purvis & Tyring, 1991). Lindane should not be used in infants and is pregnancy category B (not recommended). Because of its potential for toxicity and since the advent of permethrin, lindane usage has greatly diminished for pediatric patients.

Oral ivermectin, a drug initially used in humans to control outbreaks of onchocerciasis in Africa and Latin America, is a recently reported therapy for scabies that appears promising due to its single oral dosing and remarkable safety (Chouela et al., 1999; Meinking et al., 1995). In a recent study, healthy patients with scabies were cured with a single dose of 200 mcg/kg, and the treatment was also very effective in human immunodeficiency virus-infected patients with scabies (Meinking et al., 1995). Cure rates are similar to that of lindane, though resolution of symptoms may be more rapid (Chouela et al., 1999). The potential for control of community outbreaks of scabies with a single oral dose of ivermectin offers many potential advantages over topical therapies. While not yet approved for the treatment of scabies in both pediatric and adult populations, ivermectin may certainly revolutionize the treatment of scabies if further research confirms its efficacy and safety in children (Jaramillo-Ayerbe & Berrio-Munoz, 1998).

Because of the safety and efficacy of these therapies, older treatments, such as crotamiton 10% lotion and sulfur ointment, are essentially of historic interest. The exception is treatment for the infant younger than 2 months. In this group, 6% precipitated sulfur in petrolatum applied on three successive nights is recommended (Metry & Hebert, 2000).

● **Clinical Pearl:** No matter what treatment a provider selects, the pruritic eruption will gradually fade over weeks, and persistent pruritus is not a reflection of treatment failure.

In some cases, small inflammatory nodules may persist for months. It is not uncommon for itching to last for up to 6 weeks after successful treatment, due to the patient's continued hypersensitivity to the mite carcasses.

▲ **Clinical Warning:** Development of new lesions more than 2 to 3 weeks after initial treatment is indicative of treatment failure, misdiagnosis, or reinfection.

Some patients need topical or systemic steroids to suppress the persistent pruritic inflammation. Oral antihistamines may help control pruritus if the patient presents with an urticarial dermatitis. Prophylactic treatment of close family contacts and in the case of day care epidemics, prophylaxis of those individuals with prolonged skin-to-skin contact, can reduce rates of reinfection (AAP, 1997). Children can return to school after completing a course of treatment.

LICE

Lice are blood-sucking, wingless arthropods belonging to the class *Insecta*. Two species are specific human ectoparasites: *Pediculus humanus* and *Phthirus pubis*. Both of these six-legged creatures are clearly visible to the naked eye. As obligate human parasites, lice are unable to survive off the human host for longer than 1 to 2 days (Maunder, 1998). Head lice (pediculosis capitis) and body lice (pediculosis corporis) are due to infestation with the slender louse *P. humanus*, whereas pubic lice (crabs) results from the shorter, wider, hairier, and clawed louse, *Phthirus pubis*.

History and Physical Examination

Head Lice

In pediculosis capitis, lice and nits (egg cases) live on the hair shaft. Adults jump to the scalp for their blood meal. The adult female lays eggs at the base of the hair and may lay three eggs per day. Hair grows about 1 cm per month, so the duration of infestation can be determined by measuring the distance of the nits from the scalp. Viable nits are brown, while empty nits are white. Pruritus can be intense and excoriation with secondary infection can lead to cervical adenopathy.

Clinical examination requires careful examination of the scalp, often staring while still to observe the lice in motion. Nits can be seen as hard casings on the hair shaft, though if they are more than 1.5 cm from the scalp, it is unlikely that a viable egg remains (Elgart, 1990). No age, sex, or socioeconomic group is immune to the plague of head lice, because transmission commonly occurs by fomites, such as shared combs, brushes, hats, and pillows.

Body Lice

Unlike head lice, body lice (pediculosis corporis) are found in the seams of clothing rather than on the patient. Intense pruritus is still the rule, often with excoriation or urticaria. The incidence of body lice dwindles with affluence and better hygiene. Body lice are the only lice that can be vectors for other infectious diseases, such as typhus and trench fever.

Pubic Lice

The crab louse that causes pubic lice is a dramatically different bug, clinging tenaciously to the pubic hair with its large lobster-like claws. While sexually transmitted in most instances, the lice can ultimately be found on any body hair, including scalp, axillae, and eyelashes. Occasionally small blue marks called maculae cerulea occur at the base of hairs and can be a helpful finding. As always, careful examination with the help of a magnifying glass or microscope is essential.

Management

Treatment of head lice and pubic lice most commonly involves a 1% permethrin cream rinse (NIX) (Metry & Hebert, 2000). Careful attention to proper usage is important. The hair should be shampooed with any commercial product, rinsed, and towel dried. The permethrin rinse is then applied liberally, left on for 20 minutes, and rinsed off. In localities where there has been resistance to therapy or if live lice are seen more than 3 hours after treatment, then the 1% permethrin rinse should remain for 60 minutes.

Alternate treatment involves over-the-counter RID, a pyrethrin-based product available as a shampoo. It is applied as above except that the hair is shampooed after application. It is less ovacidal than permethrin and does not have residual activity; therefore, a repeat application is mandatory after 7 days (Metry & Hebert, 2000). Prescription 1% lindane shampoo is also available. Alternatively, lindane lotion can be applied overnight. As in scabies, lindane therapy is contraindicated in infants and carries a risk of CNS toxicity.

The prolonged residual and highly ovacidal activity of permethrin results in a cure rate of up to 90% after a single application. No repeat treatment is routinely recommended; however, most experts recommend that treatments with pyrethrin shampoos and lindane should be repeated after a week to ensure the killing of any newly hatched nymphs that survived the original application. After successful therapy, patients can remove empty nits with nit combs for cosmetic reasons.

● **Clinical Pearl:** Children should not be isolated and may return to school after their first treatment despite the presence of residual nits. No-nit policies are inappropriate, because nits are not indicative of active infection.

Pubic lice on the eyelid are best treated with simple occlusive petrolatum ointment. Body lice are effectively eradicated by attention to hygiene. Frequent showering or bathing and clean clothes usually suffice.

SUN

Ultraviolet radiation from the sun is implicated in acute sunburns and the vast majority of skin cancers. Cumulative ultraviolet exposure has been blamed for nonmelanoma skin cancers (ie, basal cell and squamous cell carcinomas), while sudden intense sun exposures and blistering burns may be more related to melanoma formation. UVB (ulraviolet energy with a wavelength of 290–320 nm) penetrates superficially into the epidermis but is most effective at producing sunburn and stimulating melanin production. Window glass blocks 100% of UVB radiation and 50% of UVA radiation. An intact ozone layer can block up to 90% of incident UVB. The ozone does not affect UVA energy, which is therefore far more abundant. This wavelength (320–400 nm) that penetrates deeper into the dermis may be implicated in premature aging.

Many studies have suggested that childhood sun exposure is a significant risk for later development of skin cancers. In addition, sun exposure to unprotected eyes is also a major risk for later cataracts. Given that up to 80% of lifetime UV exposure occurs before age 18 years, sun protection in childhood is of paramount importance (Wiss et al., 1990).

It is strongly advised that parents shield children younger than 6 months from any excess sun with hats, clothing, umbrellas, and shade. In older age groups, children should apply sunscreens heavily 30 minutes before exposure. They should use sunscreens with a sun protection factor (SPF) of 15 or greater. (If a person normally burns in 1 hour, an SPF of 15 will protect them from a burn for 15 hours. Similarly, people who burn in 10 minutes will only obtain 150 minutes of protection with the same sunscreen). Children with light eyes and lighter complexions would do better with an SPF of 30. Reapplication after water immersion or sweating is also advocated. Still, a sunscreen's protection is not perfect, and hats, long sleeves, and pants are extremely helpful, especially during the peak hours of 11 AM to 2 PM, when children should avoid sun exposure. Several manufacturers make clothing with exceptionally high SPFs. Providers should make parents aware that children need these sun protection measures on cloudy days and especially when near reflective surfaces, such as water and snow.

Concerns about the relationships between sunscreens and vitamin D deficiency and potential carcinogenicity appear unfounded. At this time, studies support the belief that normal childhood diets provide adequate vitamin D, and sunscreen use is unlikely to promote deficiency (Wiss et al., 1990).

REFERENCES

Chouela, E. N., et al. (1999). Equivalent therapeutic efficacy and safety of ivermectin and lindane in the treatment of human scabies. *Archives of Dermatology, 135,* 651–655.
American Academy of Pediatrics. (1997). *1997 Red book: Report of the Committee on Infectious Diseases.* : Author.
Elgart, M. L. (1990). Scabies. *Dermatologic Clinics, 8*(2), 253–263.
Jaramillo-Ayerbe, F., & Berrio-Munoz, J. (1998). Ivermectin for crusted Norwegian scabies induced by use of topical steroids. *Archives of Dermatology, 134,* 143–145.
Maunder, J. W. (1998). Lice and scabies: Myths and reality. *Dermatologic Clinics, 16*(4), 843–846.
McDonald, L. L., Stites, P. C., & Bunton, D. M. (1997). Sexually transmitted diseases update. *Dermatologic Clinics, 15*(2), 221–232.
Meinking, T. L., Taplin, D., Hermida, J. L., et al. (1995). The treatment of scabies with ivermectin. *New England Journal of Medicine, 333,* 26–30.
Metry, D. W., & Hebert, A. A. (2000). Insect and arachnid stings, bites, infestations, and repellants. *Pediatric Annals, 29,* 39–48.
Purvis, R. S., & Tyring, S. K. (1991). An outbreak of lindane-resistant scabies treated successfully with permethrin 5% Cream. *Journal of the American Academy of Dermatology, 25,* 1015–1016.
Taplin, D., Meinking, T. L., & Porcelain, S. L. (1986). Permethrin 5% dermal cream: A new treatment for scabies. *Journal of the American Academy of Dermatology, 15,* 995–1001.
Wiss, K., et al. (1990). Lasers, tissue expansion and sun protection in pediatric dermatology. *Cutis, 45,* 331–334.

PART V ▲

Contact Dermatitis: Poison Ivy, Oak, and Sumac

• PRADEEP SHARMA, MD

CONTACT DERMATITIS

Contact dermatitis is most often associated with contact with poison ivy, poison oak, or poison sumac. These plants are widespread throughout North America. A vast majority of the population is capable of sensitization following exposure. The incidence of contact dermatitis in children due to exposure to other causes is unknown (Mortz & Andersen, 1999).

Pathology

Contact dermatitis is a type 4 reaction under the Gell and Coombs definition of immunologic reactions. There is no IgE antibody involvement, which explains why antihistamines and allergy immunotherapy are ineffective in treating or

preventing this condition. The leaves, stems, and roots of these plants contain a mixture of chemicals called urushiol. Urushiol is derived from catechols, the major catechol being pentadecylcatechol. When urushiol is deposited on the skin, it is metabolized to quinone derivatives. Quinone derivatives then bind to proteins such as keratin, leading to a delayed hypersensitivity (type 4) reaction involving T lymphocytes. The T lymphocytes release cytokines, leading to inflammation along with cellular damage (Juckett, 1996). The resulting clinical picture is one of contact dermatitis.

Once a person has washed off the offending chemicals, poison ivy, oak, or sumac is not contagious. When the urushiol is freshly acquired (before washing), potential spread exists by either scratching or close skin-to-skin contact. A fairly common mode of transmission, however, is from the fur of domestic animals.

History and Physical Examination

Inflammation of skin is the hallmark of contact dermatitis. In poison ivy, poison oak, or poison sumac, the lesions tend to be over exposed areas, such as the limbs or face. The inflammation is linear in character and consists of a papular eruption with intense itching. In severe cases, considerable erythema with blistering and oozing can occur.

Management

Providers should teach parents and children how to recognize and avoid these plants. Plenty of educational pictures are available in books and on the Internet for reference.

Avoidance can be further enhanced if children dress in a way that helps them to avoid contact. In sensitive individuals, barrier creams, such as Dermashield, may be helpful if applied over exposed skin. If a child is playing outdoors in areas where poison ivy, oak, or sumac abound, a prompt change of clothes and shower to wash off the urushiols before they metabolize to quinones (which may take a few minutes) may prevent or reduce development of contact dermatitis (Fisher, 1990).

In most cases, the contact dermatitis rash is mild and will clear up spontaneously within 2 weeks. For mild cases, non-halogenated corticosteroid creams, such as hydrocortisone 1% to 2.5% or mometasone (Elocon) 0.1%, may be sufficient. Though they have no effect on the type 4 immune response, antihistamines may provide some relief from itching. This effect is probably due to medication-induced somnolence. Calamine lotion may help significant oozing.

In more severe cases, oral corticosteroids may be necessary for 1 to 2 weeks. Prednisone is preferred over medrol dose packs. The dose recommended is 2 mg/kg/day. A larger loading dose up to 2 mg/kg may be given if the rash and attendant symptoms are severe. There is no need to taper prednisone if the total duration of treatment is less than 2 weeks.

▲ **Clinical Warning:** In children or adolescents who are not immune to varicella, the clinician must be cautious in prescribing systemic steroids.

Proivders must weigh the risk of the child acquiring varicella against any therapeutic benefit, especially in mild or moderate disease. If the child has recently been exposed to chickenpox, the provider should prescribe neither topical nor systemic steroids.

Anecdotal reports have been found regarding successful immunization against poison ivy by allergen immunotherapy using crude poison ivy extracts. Some allergists are still using these extracts as a form of immunotherapy. Because contact dermatitis is a delayed sensitivity phenomenon (type 4), it is not surprising that scientific evidence for successful immunotherapy is lacking. For this reason, immunotherapy is not recommended and should not be used (Fisher, 1996).

REFERENCES

Fisher, A. A. (1990). Efficiency of topical barrier creams in prevention of poison ivy dermatitis. *American Journal of Contact Dermatitis*, *1*, 208.

Fisher, A. A. (1996). Poison ivy/oak dermatitis. Part I: Prevention—soap and water, topical barriers, hyposensitization. *Cutis*, *57*(6), 384–386.

Juckett, G. (1996). Plant dermatitis. Possible culprits go far beyond poison ivy. *Postgraduate Medicine*, *100*(3), 159–163, 167–171. Review.

Mortz, C. G., & Andersen, K. E. (1999). Allergic contact dermatitis in children and adolescents. *Contact Dermatitis*, *41*(3), 121–130.

P A R T   V I   ▲

Animal and Human Bites, Thermal Disease, Insect Bites, and Toxicology

• RICHARD BACHUR, MD

ANIMAL AND HUMAN BITES

Epidemiology

Bites by animals and humans are quite common, with a cumulative lifetime incidence reaching nearly 50%. Mammalian bites have very high infection rates; therefore, they need immediate care and close follow-up. Wounds that pose a particularly high risk for infection include human, dog, and cat bites as compared with other mammalian bites; puncture wounds; bites to hands, wrists, feet, and ankles; wounds older than 12 hours; and bites in immunocompromised hosts or those with impaired circulation.

Management

The treatment of significant bites must include local wound care, surgical closure, antibiotic and tetanus prophylaxis, and consideration of rabies prophylaxis. Bites that are already infected require aggressive pharmacologic and surgical management.

Local Wound Care

For fresh wounds, clinicians must assess the type and extent of the injury: body area, depth, puncture versus laceration, and possible involvement of underlying tendons, nerves, vascular structures, or bone. Providers should obtain radiographs if they suspect associated fractures, joint injuries, or foreign bodies. All wounds require aggressive irrigation. Effective irrigation of puncture wounds includes flushing saline through an IV catheter placed directly into the wound. Providers should give local anesthesia if the patient's pain is limiting effective irrigation. They should débride any devitalized tissue.

Closure

▲ **Clinical Warning:** Clinicians should not close any wound older than 24 hours or with evidence of infection.

For large wounds, providers should loosely approximate the skin after thorough irrigation (they should consider drains when anatomically feasible). A plastic surgeon should repair facial lacerations. Generally, puncture wounds are not closed. For extremity injuries, especially hand injuries, elevation and splinting are important.

Pharmacologic Management

● **Clinical Pearl:** Providers should prescribe prophylactic antibiotics for all bites other than abrasions.

Mammalian bites have a combination of gram-positive and gram-negative bacteria, both aerobic and anaerobic (Table 48-7). No antibiotic covers all possible bacteria, but amoxicillin plus clavulanate (Augmentin) covers most common organisms. Alternatives include second-generation cephalosporins (eg, cefuroxime), erythromycin, or a fluoroquinolone plus clindamycin (in older children). Clinicians must determine the patient's tetanus status and

TABLE 48–7. Microorganisms Associated With Bites

Human Bites	Dog and Cat Bites
Staphylococcus aureus	*S. aureus*
Haemophilus species	*Bacteriodes* species
Bacteroides species	*Haemophilus* species
Streptococci	*Pasteurella* multocida
Eikenella corrodens	*Capnocytophaga canimorsus*

take appropriate action if the child is not adequately immunized.

● **Clinical Pearl:** Because cats lick their paws frequently, providers need to consider cat scratches within the same category as bites requiring antibiotic prophylaxis.

Providers also must consider rabies prophylaxis. In the United States, wild animals, such as raccoons, skunks, woodchucks, and bats, carry the greatest risk of rabies exposure. Wild rodents, such as rats, mice, chipmunks, squirrels, and hares, almost never carry rabies. Similarly, domesticated rodents, gerbils, hamsters, ferrets, and pet rabbits pose little risk. If in doubt, providers should contact the local health departments or state authorities for help.

Human bites can be associated with transmission of some blood-borne infections. No guidelines, however, have been universally adopted to handle these situations.

Infected Bites

For infected wounds, providers should perform careful débridement and drainage. They should obtain radiographs to exclude signs of osteomyelitis or gas in the wound. They should obtain cultures from the base of the wound or aspirate from the cellulitis. Patients with large areas of cellulitis, deep infections, rapidly progressive infections, and any systemic signs require IV therapy and hospital admission.

What to Tell Parents

Providers should caution parents that the risk of infection is very high. They should arrange follow-up so that they can inspect all wounds after 24 to 48 hours for signs of infection. They should give patients and parents strict instructions to seek evaluation for any signs of local or systemic infection.

THERMAL ILLNESS

Heat Illness

Three types of heat illness are recognized: heat cramps, heat exhaustion, and heat stroke. Heat cramps are sudden, intermittent, and painful muscle spasms often related to physical activity. Typically, the patient sweats profusely. Fluid replacement has been adequate, but insufficient salt replacement and electrolyte depletion is thought to be the primary etiology of the cramps.

The patient with heat exhaustion has suffered large water and electrolyte losses by working or playing in hot conditions. The presentation includes severe thirst, lethargy, vomiting, weakness, altered sensorium, tachycardia, and, in extreme cases, hypotension. Body temperature can rise above 102°F (39°C), and laboratory measures will exhibit hypernatremia, hemoconcentration, concentrated urine, and low urinary sodium.

Heat stroke is a life-threatening emergency. It manifests as hyperpyrexia (≥41°C), hot and dry skin, and severe CNS dysfunction. Sweating is no longer possible. Although the CNS dysfunction can be sudden, symptoms will progress over hours. Symptoms may vary from euphoria, combativeness, confusion, headache, dizziness, or gait disturbance. Seizures, coma, and posturing may occur. Circulatory collapse, rhabdomyolysis, and renal failure can complicate heat stroke.

Most cases of heat cramps are mild and require no specific therapy. Providers should instruct patients to rest in a cool environment and to consume salt-containing fluids and solids. For those with severe or prolonged cramps, IV administration of saline is effective.

For all but the mildest cases, the best treatment for heat exhaustion is rest and IV fluids. In alert children with minimal symptoms, providers may treat heat exhaustion with oral fluids and salt. In more severe cases, however, patients require an IV saline bolus (room temperature, 10–20 mL/kg) and electrolyte measurement. Providers may accomplish cooling by removing the child's clothing and using fans and sponge baths. Ice bags and ice baths are not recommended for heat exhaustion. Persistent symptoms or considerable electrolyte derangement need correction over 24 hours.

All patients with heat stroke need emergency fluid resuscitation, cooling measures, and intensive monitoring. These interventions are best accomplished in an intensive care facility.

Frostbite

Cold injury typically occurs in the ears, nose, fingers, hands, toes, and feet. Signs include pallor, mottling, numbness, and, when severe, a waxing texture. When treating, providers should remove all clothing and constrictive articles from the patient. They should avoid rubbing or exposing the patient to dry heat. Treatment of affected body parts is immersion in a warm water bath (40°C) for 20 to 30 minutes. Warming can be painful; therefore, appropriate pain relief should be available. When completely thawed, the skin often will appear flushed. Providers should then wrap the affected part in dry warm gauze, elevate it, and refer the patient to a plastic surgeon for possible débridement and follow-up. Providers cannot accurately predict tissue viability in the first few hours of treatment; therefore, patients will require observation for at least that period.

INSECT BITES AND STINGS

Spiders

More than 100,000 species of spiders are known, all of which have fangs and venom to immobilize and kill their prey. Most species do not have fangs large or strong enough to penetrate human skin. Typical spider bites either go unnoticed or may show transient signs of local irritation. Larger spiders may cause a more severe local reaction with pain and blistering of the skin. Two species can cause severe reactions: the brown recluse spider and the black widow spider.

Brown Recluse Spiders

Brown recluse spiders are found predominantly in the southern and midwestern states. They are generally small (½–¾ in), with a brown, violin-shaped patch on the dorsum of the thorax. Initial symptoms after a bite by a brown recluse spider are minimal, but over the next 24 hours, the surrounding skin becomes progressively discolored, and a central pustule or blister forms. Over the next 3 days, the lesion enlarges up to 15 cm with varying degrees of central necrosis. Systemic symptoms, such as fever, vomiting, hemolysis, and joint pains, have been reported but are uncommon. No specific therapy is recommended other than local care. In the past, dapsone, steroids, and hyperbaric oxygen have been tried, but none has shown consistent benefit. Because of the risk of methemoglobinemia, dapsone is not recommended in children. Providers should refer patients with necrotic lesions to a plastic surgeon. Patients with systemic manifestations require hospitalization for close monitoring.

Black Widow Spiders

Black widow spiders are the number one cause of spider-related deaths in the United States. These shiny black spiders have a red hourglass marking on their abdomens. Their venom is a neurotoxin that typically leads to muscle rigidity 1 to 8 hours after the bite. The bite itself causes no local signs or symptoms. The patient may report nausea, vomiting, and chills along with muscle cramps. Severe abdominal muscle rigidity may actually mimic a surgical abdomen. The key differential is the hypertension associated with the spider bite.

The overall mortality is 5%, with death resulting from cardiovascular collapse; young children have mortality rates approaching 50% (Fleisher, 2000). An antivenin has been developed from horse antibodies. For children who weigh less than 40 kg, providers should administer the antivenin as soon as possible after confirmation of such a bite. For those children weighing more than 40 kg, the situation is less urgent, and providers can delay antivenin therapy until signs of respiratory difficulty or hypertension develop.

Tick Bite Paralysis

Ticks can transmit a variety of infectious agents, including viruses, spirochetes, rickettsiae, bacteria, and protozoa. Examples include Lyme disease, babesiosis, ehrlichiosis, RMSF, tularemia, and Colorado tick fever. The reader is referred to the section on tick-borne infections for a complete discussion of these entities.

Ticks also are responsible for tick paralysis, a syndrome of cerebellar dysfunction and ascending weakness that can progress to death. Tick paralysis has been associated with the wood tick, dog tick, and deer tick, and providers should consider it as a diagnostic possibility in any acute nontraumatic paralysis. Removal of the tick affords a dramatic and complete recovery. Other than transmission of disease and tick paralysis, tick bites themselves are not harmful. Providers can remove ticks by gently grabbing them close to the skin and lifting vertically with steady pressure. They should take care to avoid squeezing the body of the tick and thereby potentially increasing the risk of disease transmission.

Centipedes and Millipedes

Centipedes have pincer jaws with venom. Bites often are extremely painful but otherwise innocent with minimal local reaction. Millipedes are harmless.

TOXICOLOGIC PROBLEMS

Poisonings are a common cause of pediatric emergency room visits. Some poisonings are unintentional, as in tod-dlers tasting household products; some occur intentionally, as in adolescents with suicidal ideation. Management of pediatric poisonings is beyond the scope and intent of this text; the reader is referred to reference works on pediatric emergency medicine and toxicology for more complete discussions. Common poisoning and toxicologic issues are addressed below.

Use of Ipecac

Ipecac should only be used after the ingestant has been identified. Use of ipecac is primarily reserved for relatively nontoxic or minimally toxic ingestions in the home. In most instances, it will induce vomiting within 20 minutes. Administration can be repeated safely once.

▲ **Clinical Warning:** Ipecac should not be used in children younger than 6 months, those with depressed levels of consciousness, or those who have ingested hydrocarbons or caustic agents.

Use of ipecac must be very early in the course of tricyclic antidepressant ingestions. Because tricyclics lead to rapid obtundation, many authorities instead move quickly to the use of activated charcoal.

The usual dosage of ipecac is 5 mL for children ages 6 to 9 months, 10 mL for children ages 9 to 12 months, 15 mL for children ages 1 to 12 years, and 30 mL for children ages 12 years and older. Providers should follow ipecac administration with oral fluid (5 mL/kg, max 300 mL). Ipecac is available over the counter.

● **Clinical Pearl:** At the 6-month well child visit, all pediatric primary care providers should counsel parents to purchase ipecac and keep it available.

Common Ingestants

Because of the vast number of commercially produced products, the potential for exposure is great. Fortunately, most products have ingredients listed on the packaging, and most localities have a poison control center that can identify the contents and determine the seriousness of exposure. Many common nontoxic household items are listed in Display 48-4. Common pharmaceutical agents and household products that are very harmful to toddlers are listed in Table 48-8.

Common Overdoses

With most pediatric poisonings, knowing exactly how much of the potentially toxic substance the child actually ingested is extremely rare. The typical situation is that the medicine container was "about half full, and a lot was spilled." The results of the initial evaluation (serum levels) will determine further evaluation and treatment.

▲ **Clinical Warning:** Clinicians must proceed with the initial evaluation of potentially toxic ingestions based on the maximum possible dose ingested, not the estimated dose. In most instances, this means calculating a per-kilogram dose based on the entire potential contents of the medicine or pill bottle.

Salicylate Overdose

The incidence of salicylate intoxication has decreased, because aspirin is now contraindicated for fever control in children. A large number of products contain salicylates,

DISPLAY 48–4 • Frequently Ingested Products That are Relatively Nontoxic

Abrasives
Adhesives
Antacids
Antibiotics
Baby-product cosmetics
Ballpoint pen inks
Bath oil
Bleach (< 5% sodium hypochlorite)
Body conditioners
Bubble bath
Calamine
Candles (beeswax or paraffin)
Caps (toy guns, potassium chlorite)
Chalk
Cigarettes (< one whole or three butts)
Clay
Colognes
Contraceptive products
Corticosteroids
Crayons (marked AP, CP)
Dehumidifying products (silica or charcoal)
Detergents
Deodorants
Deodorizers (spray and refrigerator)
Elmer's glue

Etch-A-Sketch
Eye makeup
Fabric softener
Fertilizer (if no pesticides or herbicides added)
Glues and pastes
Golf ball
Grease
Hair spray
Hair dyes
Hand lotions and creams
Hydrogen peroxide (≤ 3%)
Incense
Indelible markers
Ink
Laxatives
Lipstick
Lubricants
Lysol brand disinfectant (not toilet bowl cleaner)
Magic markers
Matches
Mineral
Newspaper
Paint (latex)
Pencils (graphite, coloring)

Perfume
Petroleum jelly
Phenolphthalein laxative (Ex-Lax)
Play-Doh
Porous tip marking pens
Putty (< 2 oz.)
Rubber cement
Sachets (essential oils, powder)
Shampoos
Shaving creams and lotions
Soaps
Spackles
Suntan preparations
Sweeteners (saccharin, cyclamates, Nutrasweet)
Teething ring liquids
Thermometers (mercury)
Toothpaste
Vitamins without iron
Warfarin (rat poisons, excludes "superwarfarins")
Watercolors
Zinc oxide (desitin)
Zirconium

Adapted from Mofenson H. C., Greensheer, J., & Caraccio, T. R. (1984). Ingestions considered nontoxic. *Emergency Medical Clinics of North America,* 2, 159.

TABLE 48–8.   Common Products With High Toxicity for Toddlers

Name	Where found
Acetonitrile	Artificial nail products; used as a nail primer; not to be confused with nail polish remover (acetone, low toxicity)
Ammonium fluoride	Glass etching, de-rusting, wheel cleaners
Benzocaine	Local anesthetic for teething gels, intra-oral rinses, hemorrhoidal creams, first aid creams
Brodifacoum	Superwarfarins, rodenticides
Butyrolactone	Paint removers, solvent for some "super" glues
Camphor	Rubefacient, chest cold inhalant, topical anesthetic
Chloroquine	Pharmaceutical preparations for treatment of malaria, rheumatoid arthritis, lupus
Chlorpromazine/ thioridazine	Pharmaceutical preparations
Clozapine	Pharmaceutical preparations
Desipramine/tricyclics	Pharmaceutical preparations
Diphenoxylate	Diarrheal products
Hydrocarbons	Household cleaning products, solvents, gasoline, kerosene, naphtha
Hyoscyamine	Antimotility agents, including infant antispasmotics
Imidazoline	Over-the-counter and prescription ocular and nasal decongestants
Lindane	Pharmaceutical and commercial insecticide
Methadone	Pharmaceutical preparations
Methanol	Glass cleaners, paint stripper, windshield deicers
Methyl salicylate	Over-the-counter linaments, lotions, and food-flavoring additives, oil-of-wintergreen
Pennyroyal oil	Health food stores—sold to remedy respiratory complaints, induce menses, and as a digestive aid
Quinine	Pharmaceutical preparations
Salt	Salt for foods, ice-melting
Selenious acid	Gun-blueing compounds, craft stores
Theophylline	Pharmaceutical preparations

however, and an acute single ingestion of 250 mg/kg can produce toxicity. Oil of wintergreen (methyl salicylate) is highly toxic because it is so concentrated, with 700 mg of salicylate/mL. A salicylate level drawn at 2 to 4 hours correlates with toxicity, as depicted in the widely published Done diagram (Figure 48-3). Chronic ingestions exhibit more severe toxicity at even lower levels. Therapeutic levels in rheumatoid arthritis are 15 to 30 mg/dL.

Patients with significant ingestions present with hyperpnea, tachypnea, vomiting, tinnitus, and hyperthermia. Patients also may show CNS signs with lethargy, confusion, seizures, and coma. Providers should refer patients with signs of toxicity or predicted toxicity to an emergency room. Along with supportive care, alkalization, correction of electrolyte abnormalities, and maintenance of urine output are primary goals in salicylate overdose. Patients with levels greater than 60 mg/dL at 6 hours, who have ingested methyl salicylates, or those with chronic ingestion should be hospitalized.

Acetaminophen Overdose

The toxic dose for acute ingestion is roughly 150 mg/kg. Toxicity occurs in stages: Stage 1 occurs in the first several hours after ingestion. The patient may have diaphoresis, nausea, and vomiting. Stage 2 is the latent phase lasting 24 to 48 hours after ingestion. The GI symptoms resolve, and the patient appears well. Stage 3 is from 72 to 96 hours after ingestion, when hepatic toxicity is peaking as manifested by elevated transaminases, prolonged prothrombin time, elevated bilirubin, and in severe cases, hepatic encephalopathy, oliguria, jaundice, and possibly death.

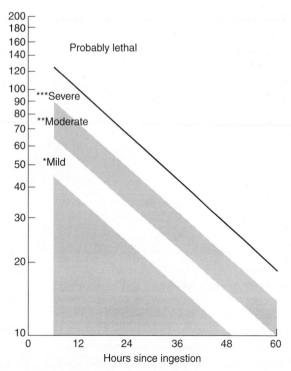

Figure 48–3 ■ Nomogram relating serum salicylate level to severity of intoxication at varying intervals after acute ingestion of single doses of aspirin. (Adapted from Done. (1978). Aspirin overdose: Incidence, diagnosis and management. *Pediatrics, 62*(suppl.), 895. Reproduced by permission of Pediatrics.)

Management is based on estimation of the amount ingested and the time since the ingestion. When the history provides absolute certainty that ingestion was less than 100 mg/kg, the patient needs no specific therapy, although charcoal and a cathartic can be used. Absolute certainty about the exact amount ingested is rare in most poisonings, however.

● **Clinical Pearl:** For any possibility of an acetaminophen ingestion greater than 100 mg/kg (including when the amount cannot be accurately determined), the provider should give activated charcoal and obtain an acetaminophen level at least 4 hours after the ingestion.

Providers can use a widely available Rumack-Matthew nomogram to predict hepatic toxicity (Figure 48-4). Only levels obtained after 4 hours are predictive. Clinicians should base further therapeutic decisions on the acetaminophen level. They should treat levels in the toxic range with a full course of the antidote, N-acetylcysteine (NAC). NAC prevents hepatotoxicity when given within 8 hours postingestion, and it decreases the degree of hepatotoxicity when given in the first 16 hours.

● **Clinical Pearl:** When a patient presents beyond 6 hours postingestion with even the possibility of toxicity, the clinician should give the initial dose of NAC while waiting for the serum level.

For patients with levels in the toxic range, hospitalization for a full course of NAC and monitoring of liver function is necessary. For the newer extended-release preparations of acetaminophen, providers also can plot a second level drawn at 8 hours postingestion on the nomogram. If either level is toxic, they should give NAC.

Iron Overdose

Providers should use the elemental iron content, not the iron salt content, of an ingested substance to determine the potential for toxicity. Ferrous sulfate contains 20% elemental iron; ferrous gluconate, 12%; and ferrous fumarate, 33%. Normally, serum iron is 50 to 100 μL/dL, and the total iron binding capacity (TIBC) is 300 to 400 μL/dL. Serum iron in excess of the TIBC leads to toxicity. An ingestion of 60 mg/kg of elemental iron or higher will often lead to toxicity, whereas ingestions less than 20 mg/kg are almost always nontoxic.

Most toxicity involves the GI and cardiovascular systems. GI symptoms predominate in the first stage (0.5–6 hours) with diarrhea, abdominal pain, vomiting, and GI bleeding. During the second stage (6–24 hours), termed the latent period, the patient will seem to improve. Persistent symptoms during this stage imply severe toxicity. In stage 3 (12–30 hours), the patient exhibits severe systemic toxicity with metabolic acidosis, shock, fever, hyperglycemia, and GI bleeding. Stage 4 (48–96 hours) is characterized by seizures, coma, and hepatic failure.

Providers should refer patients who ingested more than 20 mg/kg to the emergency room for blood studies, gastric decontamination, and monitoring. Radiographs of the abdomen may show unabsorbed tablets. Clinicians should institute chelation therapy with deferoxamine for the following patients:

- Those with a probable toxic ingestion and for whom providers cannot readily obtain iron levels (provocation test dose)
- Patients with serum iron levels greater than the TIBC

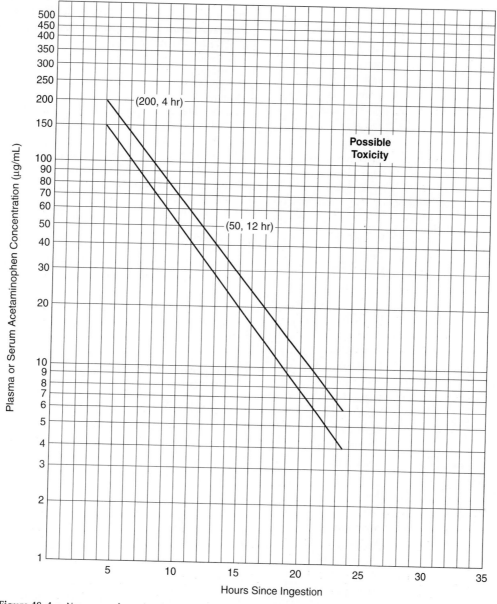

Figure 48–4 ■ Nomogram for estimating severity of acute acetaminophen poisoning. (Modified with permission from Rumack, B.H., & Marrhew, H. *Pediatrics, 55,* 871–876. Copyright, American Academy of Pediatrics, 1975.)

- Those with serum iron levels above 350 mcL/dL and whose TIBC is unobtainable
- Cases in which serum iron is greater than 500 mcL/dL regardless of TIBC

Caustic Ingestions

Commonly ingested caustic agents include lyes, strong cleaning agents (eg, toilet, oven, and swimming pool cleaners), dishwasher and laundry powders, and drain treatments. Drooling, stridor, oropharyngeal swelling, respiratory distress, and dysphagia are signs of severe toxicity. Examination of the lips, mouth, and throat may be dramatic, revealing ulcerations, burns, or edema. It may be remarkably unrevealing, even when severe esophageal burns are present. Providers should refer patients with definite exposures or any symptoms or signs for endoscopy. In the face of a reasonable history of caustic ingestion, the absence of oral findings should not preclude endoscopic evaluation. Patients

with any respiratory distress require immediate transport to a pediatric emergency room.

Alcohol Intoxication

Ethanol is the most commonly ingested alcohol. Other alcohols, such as methanol, ethylene glycol, and isopropyl alcohol, also cause severe toxicity. Ethanol ingestion typically leads to nausea, vomiting, ataxia, and stupor in children. Infants and toddlers who ingest alcohol have a very different clinical course with a triad of coma, hypothermia, and hypoglycemia, even with levels below 100 mg/dL. The ingested volume of ethanol necessary to cause intoxication depends on its concentration. In general, 1 g/kg of ethanol will raise blood levels to 100 mg/dL. For beer (5% alcohol) this amount would be 10 to 15 mL/kg; for 80-proof liquor (40% alcohol) the amount would be 1 to 2 mL/kg. If a patient presents less than 1 hour from the time of ingestion, the provider should decontaminate the stomach. He or she should

TABLE 48–9. Common Nontoxic Plants

Abelia	Eugenia
African daisy	Gardenia
African palm	Grape ivy
African violet	Hedge apples
Airplane plant	Hens and chicks
Aluminum plant	Honeysuckle
Aralia	Hoya
Asparagus fern (may cause dermatitis)	Impatiens
Aspidistra (cast iron plant)	Jade plant
Aster	Kalanchoe
Baby tears	Lily (day, Easter, tiger)
Bachelor buttons	Lipstick plant
Begonia	Magnolia
Birds nest fern	Marigold
Blood leaf plant	Monkey plant
Boston ferns	Mother-in-law tongue
Bougainvillea	Norfolk island pine
Cactus	Peperomia
California holly	Petunia
California poppy	Prayer plant
Camelia	Purple passion
Christmas cactus	Pyracantha
Coleus	Rose
Corn plant	Sanservieria
Crab apples	Schefflera
Creeping charlie	Sensitive plant
Creeping jennie, moneywort, lysima	Spider plant
Croton (house version)	Swedish ivy
Dahlia	Umbrella
Daisies	Violets
Dandelion	Wandering jew
Dogwood	Weeping fig
Donkey tail	Weeping willow
Dracaena	Wild onion
Easter lily	Zebra plant
Echevaria	

Adapted from K. C., Osterhoudt, M., Shannon, & F. M., Henretig, (2000). Toxicologic emergencies. In Fleisher, G. R., & Ludwig, S., (Eds.), *Textbook of pediatric emergency medicine* (4th ed.). Philadelphia: Lippincott Williams & Wilkins.

DISPLAY 48–5 • Toxic Plants When Ingested

Gastrointestinal Irritants
Philodendron
Diffenbachia
Pokeweed
Wisteria
Spurge laurel
Buttercup
Daffodil
Rosary pea
Castor bean

Cyanogenic Effects*
Pear (seeds)
Apple (seeds)
Crab apple seeds
Hydrangea
Elderberry
Prunus species (chokecherry, wild black cherry, plum, peach, apricot, bitter almond)

Digitalis Effects†
Lily of the valley
Foxglove
Oleander
Yew

Epileptogenic Effects
Water hemlock

Nicotinic Effects**
Wild tobacco
Golden chain tree
Poison hemlock

Atropinic Effects‡
Jimsonweed (thorn apple)
Deadly nightshade

---

*Cyanide poisoning; cellular hypoxia leads to multisystem dysfunction. Treat with supportive care and specific antidotes (amyl nitrate, sodium nitrite, sodium thiosulfate).
†Digitalis poisoning; leads to conduction defects and serious arrhythmias. Treat with supportive care and digoxin-specific antibodies.
**Nicotinic poisoning leads to vomiting within 1 hour, followed by salivation, headache, fever, mental confusion, muscular weakness, convulsions, coma. Treatment is charcoal and supportive care.
‡Atropinic poisoning, blurred vision, dilated pupils, dry mouth, hot and dry skin, fever, delirium, psychosis, and convulsions. Treatment is supportive and possibly physostigmine.

---

promptly refer the patient to an emergency room if symptomatic or predicted to be symptomatic based on the amount ingested.

Hydrocarbon Ingestion

Hydrocarbons are toxic when aspirated or inhaled. Most toxicity is due to pulmonary aspiration or inhalation of the vapors. Volatile hydrocarbons (eg, ether, turpentine, gasoline, mineral spirits, and kerosene) are more likely to be aspirated. Signs of aspiration include choking, gagging, and tachypnea. Within 6 hours, respiratory distress and pulmonary findings by examination and radiography are apparent. CNS toxicity is generally mild with somnolence, dizziness, and headache.

Providers should obtain a chest radiograph and oxygen saturation in any patient with possible hydrocarbon ingestion. Gastric decontamination is contraindicated. When the vital signs, examination, and radiograph are normal, clinicians can observe the child for 4 to 6 hours and obtain a repeat chest radiograph. They should admit any child with any respiratory or CNS symptoms.

Poisonous Plants

Plant ingestions are common; fortunately, most house and garden plants are nontoxic (Table 48-9). If providers cannot identify an ingested plant as nontoxic, they should consider administering ipecac. Activated charcoal also can be used to absorb plant toxins. If clinicians cannot recognize or identify the plant, they may need to observe the child for 2 to 3 hours for the appearance of symptoms. Both children who have ingested toxic plants and those who develop symptoms should be admitted for observation and specific or supportive treatment. Toxic plants and their effects are listed in Display 48-5.

REFERENCES

Fleisher, G., & Ludwig, S., (Eds.) (2000). *Textbook of pediatric emergency medicine* (4th ed.). Philadelphia: Lippincott Williams & Wilkins.

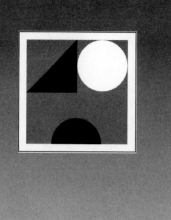

PRIMARY CARE OF CHRONIC DISEASE

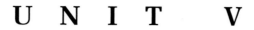

CHAPTER 49

The Child With Chronic Illness

• JOSEPH P. DAMORE, JR., MD

INTRODUCTION

Estimates are that between 10 and 20 million children and adolescents in the United States suffer from some type of chronic physical illness or dysfunction: a condition or impairment that is expected to last for an extended period and requires substantial medical attention, extensive hospitalization, or in-home health services (Committee on Children with Disabilities and Committee on Psychosocial Aspects of Child and Family Health, 1993). Chronic conditions can be described in terms of their duration and severity. Though each condition varies significantly in terms of its course, a chronic condition tends to last 3 months or longer (Perrin et al., 1993). Similarly, severity of a condition refers to the effects of the disorder on a child's physical, educational, emotional, or social functioning (Stein et al., 1987). Examples of typical chronic conditions in children include the following:

- Asthma
- Diabetes
- Seizure disorders
- Neuromuscular disease
- Acquired immunodeficiency syndrome
- Solid tumors
- Chronic hematologic disorders (especially leukemia, lymphoma, sickle cell anemia, the thalassemias, and hemophilia)
- Juvenile rheumatoid arthritis
- Cystic fibrosis
- Congenital heart disease
- Cancer

Chronic illnesses are associated with the potential for long-term sequellae and, in most cases, death. Their life-threatening quality tends to drive the psychological reactions seen in affected children and their families. Estimates vary about the incidence of psychiatric disorders in children and adolescents affected by chronic illness. It has long been posited that children with chronic physical illness or impairment are at an increased risk for psychiatric and psychosocial morbidity. While some evidence suggests that the rate of psychiatric comorbidity in such children may be as high as twice that of their healthy counterparts, other research suggests that the psychiatric impact of such conditions is small (Canning, Canning, & Boyce, 1992). At Memorial Sloan-Kettering Cancer Center, the Pediatric Psychiatry Service conducted 74 new consultations in a 1-year period. The treatment of patients with chronic illness accounted for more than 420 visits to the Psychiatry Service in that year alone (Damore, 1998). Reports also have shown that such conditions create significant disturbances in the quality of life in at least 10% of such children (Committee on Children with Disabilities and Committee on Psychosocial Aspects of Child and Family Health, 1993). Furthermore, these illnesses can

and often do disrupt relationships between family members (Jessop, Reissman, & Stein, 1988; Hoore & Kerley, 1991). Regardless of discrepancies reported in the literature, such statistics obtained in a naturalistic clinical setting are difficult to ignore.

▲ **Clinical Warning:** Chronic physical conditions have been demonstrated to be a major risk factor for grade repetition and for placement in special education programs (Gortmaker, Walker, Weitzman, & Sobol, 1990).

This chapter is meant to provide the pediatric primary care provider with an overview of common psychosocial sequellae to most chronic illnesses seen in children. The first section presents usual, nonpathologic responses encountered when children and families face chronic illness. The second section discusses problematic behaviors providers may encounter in children with chronic illness and explores possible interventions.

NORMAL RESPONSES TO CHRONIC ILLNESS

As a result of advances in medical technology, many childhood illnesses that once were rapidly fatal can now be managed and do not necessarily result in a child's death. Though the death of an affected child may be forestalled or even prevented, the shock and disbelief that accompany the diagnosis and the uncertainty associated with treatment and follow-up normally create ripples of sadness and fear.

Diagnostic Phase

In her book *Armfuls of Time*, Barbara Sourkes shares the following description of a colorful drawing made by an 8-year-old child recently diagnosed with cancer:

> "When I heard that I had leukemia, I turned pale with *shock*. That's why I chose yellow—, it's a pale color. *Scared* is red—for blood. I was scared of needles, of seeing all the doctors, of what was going to happen to me. I was *MAD* [black] about lots of things: staying in the hospital, taking medicines, bone marrows, spinal taps, IVs, being awakened in the middle of the night. I was *sad* [purple] that I didn't have my toys, and that I was missing out on everything. I chose blue for *lonely* because I was crying about not going home and not being able to go outside. Green is *hope:* getting better, going home, eating food from home, and seeing my friends" (1995, p. 31).

The feelings that children associate with the diagnosis of a chronic, potentially life-threatening illness are clearly evident in this description. Other feelings children report during and immediately following diagnosis include terror, pain, embarrassment, and shame. Clearly, the family's world is no longer the same. The diagnosis stands as a partition between health and illness. The family finds itself in the middle of an experience that often includes painful procedures and scary tests. Children and parents are forced to cope with the uncertainty of illness that threatens the need for consistency and its implied safety. Because of the frightening impact of such news, providers must be candid and reassuring, while presenting realistic hope (Sourkes, 1995). Chapters 17, Part 2 of 19, and Part 2 of 55 present views and opinions about what it feels like to receive such news, while also emphasizing the importance of realistic hope.

The initial shock of the diagnosis may last days to weeks. Responses to such bad news are idiosyncratic, and families cope using a wide spectrum of emotions. Tears, anger, bargaining, blame, and shame all may be encountered during this time. Because each family demonstrates different levels of resilience to such trauma, predicting when such emotions will cool is difficult. Providers working with this population must be aware of the range of emotions, allowing children and parents to grieve and mourn in their own way. There is no "right" or "wrong" way. If the need to mourn is understood and the process is given time and support, most children and families progress to the next level of coping without psychological sequelae.

Chronic Phase

For most children and their families, the initial shock of diagnosis eventually gives way to a re-equilibration of functioning. The family develops a routine involving trips to the clinic, follow-up tests, and at-home monitoring, procedures, and management. Emotionally, a pattern develops as well. Sourkes reports that "fluidity is the hallmark of the child's response to diagnosis: different emotions surge to the forefront or recede into the background at different times. In addition, anticipatory grief—grief associated with the potential for loss—begins with diagnosis, and waxes and wanes throughout the illness experience" (1995, p. 34).

In this chronic phase, children and their families may attempt to cope with the illness in a variety of ways. Some opt for a "business as usual" approach, attempting to maintain activities enjoyed prior to diagnosis as much as possible. Denial of the severity of the illness and its consequences often is encountered in families who follow this approach.

● **Clinical Pearl:** The provider should remember that denial is not necessarily pathologic. Provided that the family keeps clinic appointments, follows instructions about care, and has realistic expectations of treatment, the clinician may reasonably support such a coping style.

Other families attempt to cope with an illness through cognitive mastery. Such attempts at mastery are associated with both factual and distorted information regarding treatment and prognosis. Sometimes providers misinterpret attempts at mastery on the part of the parents as second-guessing or challenging the clinician.

● **Clinical Pearl:** Providers might misinterpret a parent's practice of writing down everything said, including blood count results, as overcontrolling and evidence of mistrust. Only when providers understand the importance of a parent's need for intellectual mastery over the illness will they be able to address adequately the family's inquiries and emotional needs.

It is not unusual during this phase to find that children, and occasionally parents, view the illness as punishment for previous bad acts. Children, who use concrete, cause-and-

effect systems of thought, may conceptualize their illness as punishment in an attempt to make sense of it. Such a conceptualization can sometimes lead to the development of overcompliance or oppositionality (Sourkes, 1995). Work with these children involves challenging their misconceptions and facilitating an understanding of illness as "nobody's fault." During this phase, chronically ill children and their families most often long for a return to the time before diagnosis. Sourkes writes: "For the child, facets of 'normal' include being regular (not special), ordinary (not exceptional), and fitting in (not being different). From looking to feeling to being normal, the concept has implications for the child's sense of competence and self esteem" (1995, p. 82).

● **Clinical Pearl:** Continuing to treat their child as normal is a formidable task for parents, especially regarding discipline. However, their ability to do so sends a critical message to their child that the illness may be abnormal, but the child—as a person—is normal (Sourkes, 1995).

ABNORMAL RESPONSES TO CHRONIC ILLNESS

As time passes, most children return to a level of functioning that closely resembles their life before the illness. In many cases, however, the emotional demands of illness and its treatment overwhelm the psychological defenses of children and their families. In these situations, significant psychiatric disorders are noticed most often.

A discussion of all possible psychiatric disorders encountered in chronically ill children is beyond the scope of this chapter. The following section presents disorders that are most commonly encountered in chronic illness and the point at which a provider is likely to see each. The clinician should expect that patients may present with either an adjustment disorder, mood disorder, anxiety disorder, or exacerbation of a preexisting psychiatric disorder. The timing of psychiatric consultation and the psychiatric diagnosis given usually occur according to the following guidelines:

- Almost invariably, adjustment disorders are diagnosed during the diagnostic phase.
- Mood disorders are most often diagnosed in the chronic phase.
- Anxiety disorders appear to be diagnosed equally in both the diagnostic and chronic phases.
- Diagnoses such as delirium, parent–child relational problem, and oppositional defiant disorder (ODD) can be diagnosed at any point (Damore, 1998).

Adjustment Disorders

One of the most common psychiatric diagnoses encountered in the diagnosis phase and seen by providers is adjustment disorder. By definition, an adjustment disorder refers to the development of clinically significant emotional or behavioral symptoms in response to an identifiable psychosocial stressor or stressors.

Overview

Symptoms of an adjustment disorder must develop within 3 months after the onset of the stressor. The clinical significance of the reaction is indicated either by marked distress in excess of what would be expected given the nature of the stressor or by a significant impairment in social or occupational (academic) functioning. The American Psychiatric Association (1994) stipulates that such a disorder dissipates within 6 months of the ending of the stressor or its results. For the purpose of evaluating children who experience chronic illness, "the symptoms may persist for a prolonged period (longer that 6 months) if they occur in response to a chronic stressor (eg, a chronic, disabling general medical condition) or to a stressor that has enduring consequences (eg, the financial and emotional difficulties resulting from a divorce)" (American Psychiatric Association, 1994, p. 623). The stressor may be a single event, or there may be multiple stressors. Stressors may be recurrent or continuous. Adjustment disorders are not diagnosed in situations of bereavement (American Psychiatric Association, 1994).

There are several subtypes of adjustment disorders. These are specified according to their predominant symptomatology:

- *Adjustment disorder with depressed mood*: Patient may appear sad, forlorn, or hopeless and may cry often.
- *Adjustment disorder with anxiety*: Patient displays excessive noninvasive restlessness or fear of separation from major attachment figures.
- *Adjustment disorder with anxiety and depressed mood*: Patient exhibits features of both of the above.
- *Adjustment disorder with disturbance of conduct*: In this subtype, the patient shows a violation of age-appropriate societal norms or the rights of others. This subtype often is seen in teenagers with chronic illness and can be manifested by noncompliance with medication regimens (such as in diabetes), missed clinic appointments, or increased fighting with peers.
- *Adjustment disorder with mixed disturbance of emotions and conduct*: The patient displays conduct and emotional symptoms.
- *Adjustment disorder, unspecified*: These patients have maladaptive reactions, such as physical ailments, social withdrawal, or school problems (American Psychiatric Association, 1994).

Reports of the prevalence rate of adjustment disorder in other pediatric settings ranges from 25% to 65% (Jacobson et al., 1980). As is typical of the disorder, the condition arises almost immediately after the diagnosis of chronic disease, thus prompting the referral, and may last for the duration of the stressor. Once the stressor abates, the adjustment disorder usually abates as well.

Management

Treatment of an adjustment disorder works best when it is implemented quickly. The goals of such intervention are to decrease the stress experienced by the child and to firm up the coping defenses of both child and family. In addition, counseling aimed at helping parents understand their child's experience can empower the entire family. Each child's experience of illness is different, and there is no substitute for discussion with an affected child. Unfortunately, the constraints of clinical practice and managed care often make labor-intensive therapeutic contact unreasonable for providers. When features of an adjustment disorder arise, especially if they are severe, it is appropriate to arrange referral to a child mental health specialist. Ideally, a specialist with expertise in both the physical and emotional ailments is in the best position to help.

Usually, a referral to a child psychiatrist is the best first step. Such referrals often are met with stiff resistance from parents who want to avoid the stigma associated with psychiatric illness. The clinician does the family a great service by explaining that the child psychiatrist is part of the health care team and is interested only in helping the child to feel

better. It also should be mentioned that psychiatric treatment of adjustment disorder tends to be time-limited (6–12 months of weekly sessions) and that medications are hardly ever prescribed. If medication is needed, it typically is used for a short period (Cunningham & Enzer, 1997).

Mood Disorders

In a 1-year period, approximately one third of patients referred from a pediatric oncology service met the criteria for a mood disorder, usually either major depression or a mood disorder secondary to the medical condition. The course of mood disorders in chronically ill children has not been well studied, although the progression seems quite variable. In one study, depressive symptoms tended to correlate well with psychosocial life events, such as the number of hospitalizations. Depressive symptoms, however, appeared to be unrelated to the course of the illness (Kaplan, Busner, Weinhold, & Lenon, 1987). In addition, adaptive style has been reported to influence both the medical and psychological outcome of ill children and may account for the variance in depression over that explained by the severity of their illness (Canning et al., 1992). Clearly, more research is necessary to determine the long-term manifestations of mood disorders in physically ill children and adolescents.

Overview

Major Depression

The diagnostic criteria for major depression are as follows:

A. Five (or more) of the following symptoms, which have been present during the same 2-week period and represent a change from previous functioning. At least one of the symptoms is either (1) depressed mood or (2) loss of interest or pleasure. Symptoms are not included if they clearly are due to a general medical condition or mood-incongruent delusions or hallucinations.
  (1) Depressed mood most of the day, nearly every day, as indicated by either subjective report (eg, feels sad or empty) or observation made by others (eg, appears tearful)

▲ **Clinical Warning:** In children and adolescents, depressed mood can present as irritability.

  (2) Markedly diminished interest or pleasure in all, or almost all, activities most of the day, nearly every day (as indicated either by subjective account or observation made by others)
  (3) Significant weight loss when not dieting or weight gain (eg, a change of more than 5% of body weight in a month) or a decrease or increase in appetite nearly every day

● **Clinical Pearl:** In infants and young children, failure to make expected weight gains should be considered in the differential for depressed mood.

  (4) Insomnia or hypersomnia nearly every day
  (5) Psychomotor agitation or retardation nearly every day (observation by others, not merely subjective feelings of restlessness or being slowed down)
  (6) Fatigue or loss of energy nearly every day
  (7) Feelings of worthlessness or excessive or inappropriate guilt (which may be delusional) nearly every day (not merely self-reproach or guilt about being sick)

(8) Diminished ability to think or concentrate or indecisiveness nearly every day (either by subjective
account or as observed by others)

(9) Recurrent thoughts of death (not just fear of
dying), recurrent suicidal ideation without a specific plan, or a suicide attempt or a specific plan for
committing suicide

B. The symptoms do not meet criteria for a mixed
episode.

C. The symptoms cause clinically significant distress or
impairment in social, occupational, or other important
areas of functioning.

D. The symptoms are not due to the direct physiologic
effect of a substance (eg, a drug of abuse, a medication)
or a general medical condition (eg, hypothyroidism).

E. The symptoms are not better accounted for by bereavement (ie, after the loss of a loved one), persist for longer
than 2 months, or are characterized by marked functional impairment, morbid preoccupation with worthlessness, suicidal ideation, psychotic symptoms, or
psychomotor retardation (American Psychiatric Association, 1994, p. 327).

A careful interview is necessary to determine the presence
of major depressive symptoms. In children and adolescents
with chronic illnesses, this diagnosis can be particularly difficult to make, because symptoms of the illness (such as
weight loss) may mimic the symptoms of major depression.

● **Clinical Pearl:** Symptoms that are common to both the
chronic illness and depression should count toward the
diagnosis of major depression, unless the symptoms can be
directly attributed to the chronic illness. For example, weight
loss secondary to ulcerative colitis and inability to eat should
not be counted toward major depression (American
Psychiatric Association, 1994).

Mood Disorder Secondary to a General Medical Condition

In this situation, the mood disturbance is considered directly
attributable to a physical condition. The mood can be
depressed, elevated, or irritable. For example, certain malignancies (such as carcinoma of the pancreas) and illnesses
(such as systemic lupus erythematosus) are associated with
mood changes as part of their constellation of symptoms
(American Psychiatric Association, 1994).

In contrast to major depression, mood disorders due to a
general medical condition are characterized as follows:

A. A prominent and persistent disturbance in mood predominates in the clinical picture and is characterized
by either (or both) of the following:
1. Depressed mood or marked diminished interest or
pleasure in all, or almost all, activities
2. Elevated, expansive, or irritable mood

B. Evidence from the history, physical examination, or
laboratory findings shows that the disturbance is the
direct physiologic consequence of a general medical
condition.

C. The disturbance is not better accounted for by another
mental disorder (eg, adjustment disorder with
depressed mood, in response to the stress of having a
general medical condition).

D. The disturbance does not occur exclusively during the
course of delirium or dementia.

E. The symptoms cause clinically significant distress or
impairment in social, occupational, or other important

areas of functioning (American Psychiatric Association,
1994, pp. 369–370).

The type is specified as follows:

- *With depressive features*: The predominant mood is
depressed, but the full criteria are not met for a major
depressive episode.
- *With major depressive-like episode*: The full criteria are met
(except criterion D) for a major depressive episode.
- *With manic features:* The predominant mood is elevated,
euphoric, or irritable.
- *With mixed features*: Symptoms of both mania and
depression are present, and neither predominates
(American Psychiatric Association, 1994, pp. 369–370).

Management

Recognition of mood disorders in physically ill children and
adolescents is the first step toward proper treatment.
Providers must be diligent in their inquiry about changes in
sleep, interest, concentration, appetite, and energy level. In
addition, it is vital to remember that mood disorders carry
with them an increased risk of suicide. Parents and
providers alike often worry that frank discussion about suicide will "put ideas into a patient's head." This does not
appear at all true. In fact, such frank discussion often allows
a child or adolescent to express feelings that he or she previously considered taboo.

▲ **Clinical Warning:** When a mood disorder is suspected,
the provider must address the risk for suicide directly by
asking the patient the following:

- Do you sometimes wish you had never been born?
- Do you sometimes think it would be okay if you died
today?
- Have you ever felt so sad or so bad about your situation
that you thought of killing yourself?

An answer of "yes" to any of the above questions should
prompt the provider to obtain an immediate psychiatric
referral and to establish the child's safety until such a referral
is obtained.

Once a mood disorder is suspected, a referral to a child
mental health specialist usually is appropriate. A referral to
a clinician acquainted with the child's physical and emotional condition often is best prepared to provide the child
with needed care. Usually this person is a child psychiatrist.
Most mood disorders in chronically ill children will respond
to a combination of antidepressant medication, particularly
selective serotonin reuptake inhibitors (SSRIs), and psychotherapy. Because dosing of these medications and monitoring of clinical conditions in therapy can be complicated, a
referral makes very good clinical sense. Refer to Chapter 28
for a discussion of antidepressants and the challenge surrounding their usage in pediatrics.

Anxiety Disorders

At Memorial Sloan-Kettering, the most commonly encountered anxiety disorder is anxiety disorder not otherwise
specified (NOS) (Damore, 1998). This category includes disorders with prominent anxiety and avoidance that do not
meet criteria for either a specific mood disorder, like major
depression, or an anxiety disorder, like panic disorder. Anxiety Disorder NOS includes conditions with the following:

- A mixed anxiety or depressed disorder
- Clinically significant social phobic symptoms that are related to the social impact of having a chronic medical condition
- Situations in which the clinician has concluded an anxiety disorder exists but is unable to determine if it is primary or due to a medical condition or is substance-induced (American Psychiatry Association, 1994)

Overview

Children with an anxiety disorder may present in a number of ways. They may become fearful of previously tolerated experiences, such as going to see their provider. They may develop fears of separation from their parents, especially when active treatment ends and they must return to school. Finally, it is quite common for a child with an anxiety disorder to manifest the problem somatically. The youngster may demonstrate panic attacks, with associated tachycardia, shortness of breath, choking, nausea, vomiting, and derealization. Other children and adolescents may demonstrate fatigue, teariness, or difficulty with sleep or concentration. It is helpful to ask parents about the child's activities of daily living and about school.

● **Clinical Pearl:** Often changes in behavior at home and school are the first signs of an anxiety disorder.

Management

As with mood disorders, diagnosis of anxiety disorders is the first step toward proper treatment. Once such a disorder is suspected, a referral to a pediatric mental health professional is warranted. Again, a clinician acquainted with the child's physical and emotional condition, usually a child psychiatrist, is the best-prepared professional to provide the patient with the care needed. The therapist becomes for the child "a consistent and abiding presence" (Sourkes, 1995, p. 169). It is this relationship that seems to assist the patient in the daily struggle with illness.

Most anxiety disorders can be treated rapidly and successfully through a combination of medication and psychotherapy. Interestingly, SSRI antidepressants have been used for this indication and are well tolerated. The course of anxiety disorders in children and teenagers with chronic illnesses varies. In this author's experience, exacerbation of anxiety correlates with exacerbation of illness.

Exacerbation of a Preexisting Psychosocial Disorder

In general, a child or adolescent with a preexisting psychological disorder, such as attention deficit hyperactivity disorder (ADHD) or ODD, may create a management problem when a chronic illness develops. In the same way, chronic illness can exacerbate long-term parent–child relational problems. When such disorders are known at the onset of the chronic illness, the clinician does well to ensure that treatment for the psychological disorders continues during the diagnosis and treatment of chronic illness. Proper medication for ADHD and proper family therapy for ODD can go a long way toward making chronic illness more manageable for patients and their families.

COMMUNITY RESOURCES

For the name of a child and adolescent psychiatrist in the reader's geographic area, contact the following:

The American Academy of Child and Adolescent Psychiatry
3615 Wisconsin Avenue, NW
Washington, D.C. 02216-3007
Internet address: *http://www.aacap.org*

The Academy of Psychosomatic Medicine
5824 North Magnolia
Chicago, IL 60660
email address: ApsychMed@aol.com
Internet address: *http://www.apm.org*

The following books are recommended reading for parents and the provider:

- *Armfuls of Time* by Barbara Sourkes, 1995, University of Pittsburgh Press.
- *The Deepening Shade* by Barbara Sourkes, 1982, University of Pittsburgh Press.

REFERENCES

American Psychiatric Association. (1994). *Diagnostic and statistical manual of mental* disorders (DSM-IV) (4th ed.). Washington, D.C.: Author.
Canning, E. H., Canning, R. D., & Boyce, W. T. (1992). Depressive symptoms and adaptive style in children with cancer. *Journal of the American Academy of Child and Adolescent Psychiatry, 31,* 1120–1124.
Committee on Children with Disabilities & Committee on Psychosocial Aspects of Child and Family Health. (1993). Psychosocial risks of chronic health conditions in childhood and adolescence. *Pediatrics, 92,* 876–877.
Cunningham, S. D., & Enzer, N. (1997). Adjustment and reactive disorders. In J. M. Weiner (Ed.), *Textbook of child and adolescent psychiatry* (2nd ed.) (pp. 682–683). Washington, D.C.: American Psychiatric Press.
Damore, J. P. (1998). New York, NY: Memorial Sloan-Kettering Hospital. Unpublished Data.
Gortmaker, S. L., Walker, D. K., Weitzman, M., & Sobol, A. M. (1990). Chronic conditions, social economic risks, and behavioral problems in children and adolescents. *Pediatrics, 85,* 267–276.
Hoore, P., & Kerley, S. (1991). Psychosocial adjustment of children with chronic epilepsy and their families. *Developmental Medicine and Child Neurology, 33,* 201–215.
Jacobson, A. M., Goldberg, I. D., Burns, B. J., Hoeper, E. W., Hankin, J. R., & Hewitt, K. (1980). Diagnosed mental disorder in children and use of health services in four organized health care settings. *American Journal of Psychiatry, 127,* 559–565.
Jessop, D. J., Reissman, C. K., & Stein, R. E. (1988). Chronic childhood illness and maternal mental health. *Developmental and Behavior Pediatrics, 9,* 147–156.
Kaplan, S. L., Busner, J., Weinhold, C., & Lenon, P. (1987). Depressive symptoms in children and adolescents with cancer: A longitudinal study. *Journal of American Academy of Child and Adolescent Psychiatry, 26*(5), 782–787.
Perrin, E. C., Newacheck, P. W., Pless, I. B., et al. (1993). Issues involved in the definition and classification of chronic health conditions. *Pediatrics, 91,* 787–793.
Sourkes, B. (1995). *Armfuls of time.* Pittsburgh: University of Pittsburgh Press.
Stein, R. E., Gortmaker, S. L., Perrin, E. C., et al. (1987). Severity of illness: Concepts and Measurements. *Lancet, 2,* 1506–1509.

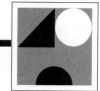

The Interdisciplinary Team: The Social Worker as a Key Player in the Care of a Chronically Ill Child

• GOLDIE MULAK, CSW, ACSW

INTRODUCTION

Optimal health care for children involves participation from patients, families, and health care professionals. Children's health and well-being depend greatly on the care they receive from their families and communities (Szilagy & Schor, 1998). The needs of children and their families often include unresolved, and sometimes unidentified, social and emotional problems. Such psychosocial problems often impede access to health care delivery and create distress for children, family members, and health care providers.

Primary care providers are often the first professionals to whom families turn for psychosocial care. Providers are the first contact for as many as 85% of typical psychosocial problems (Gross, Rabinowitz, Feldman, & Boerma, 1996). As the first line of contact with patients, these providers often have the best opportunity to recognize patients with mental health problems and to treat them or refer them to specialists (Glied, 1998). For this reason, primary care clinicians need a strong awareness of the role played by social workers as well as the ability to work with these professionals. The chronic illness of a child forever changes the life of the child and the entire family. Professional social workers can work closely with pediatric health care providers to identify and treat the stresses that a chronic illness produces. This chapter provides an overview of the psychosocial issues affecting chronically ill children and their families and the roles that social workers play in providing assistance.

THE ROLE OF SOCIAL WORK

Social work and primary care orientations are alike in that they emphasize both continuity and comprehensiveness of care (Badger, Ackerson, Buttell, & Rand, 1997). The National Association of Social Workers maintains in its code of ethics that the primary mission of social work is "to enhance human well-being and help meet the basic needs of all people, with particular attention to the needs and empowerment of people who are vulnerable, oppressed, and living in poverty" (1996). Consistent access to social workers is a challenge, however, because no government mandate exists to provide social work services to families in need. Hospital and ambulatory care clinic settings usually employ social workers who specialize in health care. Child welfare prevention service agencies, nonprofit social service agencies, and federal and state programs also employ social workers. School districts and school health projects also use professional social workers on behalf of children. Professional social workers are those who have received a master's degree in social work from an accredited university. Each state has individual requirements to practice, with some states requiring a license and some offering state certifications. Many trained social workers, like child psychologists and child psychiatrists, are also employed in private practice settings, and sessions can be reimbursed through insurance coverage. Professional social workers are also on panels of health maintenance organizations for mental health service coverage.

Some organizations use professional social workers as counselors to help people with chronic illnesses deal with the emotional impact of their illness. These organizations also provide information on self-help groups and political advocacy initiatives related to the illness.

COLLABORATION: WORKING TOGETHER AS A TEAM

As professionals, social workers provide a knowledge base in defining and handling social problems on an individual and community level, often working with others to solve problems. An interdisciplinary team is a functioning unit, composed of individuals with various and specialized training, who coordinate their activities to provide services to a client or group of clients (Ducanis & Golin, 1979). The social work assessment helps the team to gather facts and impressions about the economic, psychological, religious, and sociocultural functioning of the patient and family. Because social workers intersperse facts with a value orientation and what appears to be a subjective assessment (Mizrahi & Abramson, 1985), primary care providers may be concerned about a lack of "hard data." The social worker incorporates the points of view of other disciplines while developing a treatment plan.

Many of the most useful skills that social workers use in a team are drawn from group training. These skills include assessing the team as a group, contracting, monitoring the team process as it occurs, dealing with conflict, and understanding professional differences (Abramson, 1990). The social worker can be an essential member of the interdisciplinary team that provides services to patients and families.

Case Management

Case management services have become a method that agencies, hospitals, and insurance companies use to provide direct case contact and to improve coordination of needed services for clients. The primary focus is a coordinated dialogue between providers and patients to help guide patients through a continuum of services, rather than to "compartmentalize" their care (Fox & Fama, 1996). Managed care companies often employ case managers to review the medical needs of people with chronic illnesses to provide services in a timely manner and reduce costs. Because clients have multiple and complex needs, a case manager can assist in promoting independence and foster optimum social functioning. Professional social workers and nurses are often case managers, with their training in identifying health care, home, and school needs for children with chronic illnesses. Other professionals in health care also may be designated as case managers.

Social Functioning and the Psychosocial Focus

As people who work with children know, the child is part of both a family and a larger society. The recognition of the psychological and social underpinnings of many current child health problems raises questions about whether some health concerns are best defined in medical or social terms (Palfrey, 1997). At the time of the diagnosis of a chronic illness, it is important to know what the family functioning was prior to the onset of the illness.

Evaluation of Problems in Social Functioning

Because an initial appointment provides the opportunity for gathering information about developmental milestones and current social information, the provider can use baseline information as a screening tool for further reference as a relationship develops with the family. When a particular problem arises, it is also important to find out if any "precipitant factor" has occurred. A precipitant factor is a recent episode in psychosocial functioning that has set off severe enough behavior or stress to warrant professional attention. The provider must consider this in addition to the stress of coping with a new diagnosis. Other chapters in this book detail the issues in the psychological disorders and behaviors of childhood.

Primary care providers differ in their personal levels of comfort in terms of probing into the lives of their patients, especially the personal lives of parents. Clinicians seeking information about emotional issues need to use a sensitive, open-ended approach with empathy and patience, listening for the underlying feelings and themes that a parent communicates.

Some factors in the context of a child's world have both a direct and indirect influence on emotional and social development (Display 50-1). Children who are having emotional or behavioral difficulties need a full assessment of what is happening in the world around them. At the same time, providers must avoid simplistic judgments. Providers also must consider variables related to the parents (Display 50-2).

Assessment of High Social Risk Situations

Primary care providers are becoming increasingly aware of situations of child abuse and domestic violence. Even if a provider has never discovered physical signs of abuse in any child, he or she has probably been in contact with at least one parent who has been harsh, restrictive, or emotionally unavailable with a child. Every state has laws mandating health care professionals to report suspected or identified abuse and neglect.

Although primary care providers may be able to identify initial signs of physical abuse, such as unexplained bruises, burns, lacerations, or fractures, signs of physical and emotional neglect often are more difficult to determine. Physical

---

DISPLAY 50–1 • **What Variables Characterize the Child's World?**

Emotional
Behavioral
Peer
School
Parent relationships
Developmental issues
Language
Ethnic identity development
Religious training
Family values

---

neglect can include hunger or poor hygiene, while emotional neglect often includes little supervision or lack of parental interest. Neglect does not equate with poverty or child abuse. Many parents who have few resources struggle to maintain a sense of home and family.

● **Clinical Pearl:** Because they may not want to lose an already established relationship with a family, practitioners may have a difficult time making a decision about filing a child abuse report. Consultation with a hospital or county child protection committee can be very useful. Preventive social service agencies are organized to provide homemakers, find food resources, and teach parental guidance to families to minimize neglect. Providers can contact social work colleagues in local hospitals and schools for assistance in referring families to social service agency resources. They also can use church organizations in finding assistance for families.

Sexual abuse is a highly complex issue. Providers should ask children directly if they have ever been touched in an area that is a "private part." They should encourage children to learn how to say no and to confide in an adult they trust. If no signs of physical penetration in a child appear but a provider is still suspicious, he or she should perform further evaluation and individual counseling. Children may not reveal anything because of their own shame or fear.

● **Clinical Pearl:** Encouragement of the development of trust with an outside counselor can be a way for children to have the opportunity for help. The primary goal of child protection work is to protect the child.

DISPLAY 50–2 • **What Variables Characterize the Parent's World?**

Personal-emotional
Stage of identity
Relationships with one's own parents
Single or two parents
Alternative parenting issues
Work
Extended family issues
Beliefs about the cause and cure of illness
Cultural-ethnic identity
Religious identity
Assimilation and immigration status
Health insurance status

Pediatric primary care providers may suspect domestic violence when they see a parent who is wearing sunglasses, looks bruised or worn, or appears to have a domineering, aggressive partner. Support is critical in these situations. If a parent acknowledges any battering, remember that he or she can file police charges, have orders of protection filed against the partner, or move into a shelter. Hospital emergency rooms are effective in helping adults through the crisis of an episode of domestic violence.

Entitlement and Social Services

Social workers usually are knowledgeable about state and federal entitlement to services and are familiar with the process of advocacy for families. They can guide a family to appropriate agencies for help with particular problems. The financial cost of a child's chronic illness can be devastating. Health care bills can prove overwhelming, and insurance forms are often confusing, with implied threats to a family's financial security if bills are not promptly paid. Often a working parent has to take time off to care for a child or attend frequent medical appointments. Parents are sometimes also dealing with the financial and health issues of their own elderly parents. These families need information, assistance, and sometimes referrals for financial or legal help. The following case demonstrates how a social worker can effectively support the primary care team.

> A mother who was divorced from her husband and had a difficult relationship with her sister, her only support, had a 4-year-old son, whose disability application for Social Security's Supplemental Security Income was denied. The mother had missed several appointments while she was busy caring for her disabled son. The social worker in the family medicine clinic facilitated the follow-up process of appeals and accompanied the mother to her appointments. The child was accepted after a successful review. To encourage the child's independent functioning, the social worker arranged for the child to receive a motorized wheelchair and to attend a preschool program that specialized in working with children with physical impairments.

Assisting Families to Participate in Health Care Regimens

When a family does not follow up with adherence to a health care plan, team members must examine multiple possible causes for the proper intervention. Many factors are associated with noncompliance, including demographic factors, lack of health insurance, poor family supports, and lack of a trusting relationship between provider and patient. Understanding the beliefs of parents about illness, such as social and religious beliefs that may interfere with adherence, and sensing the family's ability to adapt to changes can be important to the development of realistic plans for following through on recommendations and treatments. Religious beliefs may dictate food choices, clothing styles, customs of birthing and dying, etiquette in the sick room, use of modern conveniences, invasive procedures, organ donation, use of blood products, spiritual influences on or control of sickness and healing, wearing of protective devices or tattoos, and need for prayers and rituals performed by various religious specialists (Ratcliff, 1996). A family may lack access to medical care or have difficulties in transportation or child care arrangements that prevent them from keeping medical appointments. When education or behavioral regimen changes are needed, it is useful to have more than one professional focus on the problem, as in the following scenario:

> A 10-year-old boy stopped taking his medication during a long-term illness. He was not interested in talking with his primary care provider about this. When medical staff felt frustrated by the child's mother's initial passivity in letting this happen, they formed a multidisciplinary plan. The social worker sought out the child in an individual session, in which he told her that he was afraid of dying of this illness, no matter what he did. She worked with his provider in arranging for a public health nurse who visited him and his family at home, overseeing the actual administration of the medicine, providing education and support for both him and his parents.

Dealing With Chronic Illness

Accepting and Understanding a Diagnosis

The nature of problems that confront children and their families in the diagnosis, course, and outcome of a chronic illness varies, depending on factors related to the illness. A child's personal characteristics and a family's particular way of adapting and organizing itself also play a role. The illness may be chronic or have either progressive or episodic manifestations. The family needs to understand the seriousness of the illness and be able to communicate it to the child in a way that allows expression of feelings. An illness with a genetic component may produce feelings of guilt and responsibility that parents need to understand and express. It is important to "give permission" to families to express feelings of loss, anxiety, or uncertainty. Children need to understand in their own language what the illness means while also maintaining emotional stability. The ability to maintain emotional balance will depend on the child's developmental level and coping mechanisms. Siblings need to be included in explanations of the meaning of an illness and treatment implications. Family meetings can be very valuable in uncovering misunderstandings and untapped feelings, as in the following scenario:

> A mother was very harsh with her 9-year-old son who developed diabetes, being overprotective with him at home and disapproving of his wanting to spend a lot of time with his friends. The primary care provider was able to convince the mother that "everyone needs someone to talk to sometimes." The mother entered counseling with a social worker and learned improved ways of handling her growing son as she gained insight into her own parenting responses better. The father was also engaged in this experience and was able to understand his child's medical needs in a family session with the whole family, the primary care provider, and the social worker. The meeting enabled the parents to improve their own communication and allowed the son to take more responsibility for his own care.

Living With an Illness

Each illness has its own issues surrounding treatment regimens. Children often do not want to look or feel different from their friends. They may deny or minimize their illness. Exploration and supportive counseling can be useful in helping a child express anger and sadness. Social workers who work with children with chronic illness often develop groups and programs to facilitate children with similar diagnoses meeting one another in normalized, social settings. Special summer camps for children with illnesses include those for children with asthma, diabetes, cancer, or acquired immunodeficiency syndrome. They provide recreational fun in a safe environment. Parent support groups encourage networking, parental guidance, and mutual support for parents who feel they are isolated. Many books geared to helping families cope with chronic illness are found in libraries and bookstores and through disease-specific foundations and organizations.

Bereavement

Chronic illness can produce a constant sense of loss as the body fights to maintain control. In a progressive disease, children and parents struggle with feelings of grief over physical loss and maintaing self-esteem in the anxiety of an unpredictable future.

The terminal phase of a child's illness and the child's death become times that can bring a family closer or drive them apart through dysfunctional patterns, unresolved emotional issues, and inability to deal with the reality of an overwhelming situation. Health care personnel are closely drawn to families at these times, and primary care providers need to deal with their own feelings of loss and failure at not curing the child.

To deal with grief openly, the primary care provider has to be honest with the family. Families need to decide how direct to be with their child, balancing the reality involved against the need to maintain a sense of hope. Children who are terminally ill need opportunities for expression of their feelings through play and talking without being immediately cut off if they make comments about death and dying.

Developmental levels affect how a child understands death. The preschool child will think that death is temporary and reversible, while a school-age child can internalize the universality of death, its permanence, and the belief of an afterlife. Adolescents, who understand death as a natural process, may have a more difficult time because they are busy shaping their own lives and find it easier to talk to peers than parents (Goldman, 1994). Chapter 49 provides a more in-depth exploration of the psychological and emotional needs of children with chronic illness.

If a parent can be honest, sad, or angry in front of a child, the child can have the permission to express himself or herself. A parent needs to allow a dying child to have periods of angry outbursts and temper tantrums, sometimes directed at the parent. Siblings also need to participate in the process of dealing with their own feelings.

Parents, even those who are separated or divorced, need to be able to communicate. Because individuals have different coping styles, the stress of a dying child can increase tensions. Parents may differ in how many medical treatments should be offered. Overwork, substance use, avoidance, or anger can become methods of avoiding intimacy. Parents need to find adult supports through peers, families, religious contacts, and counselors. Opportunities for expression of feelings and grief need to be encouraged.

Bereavement also occurs when a parent is sick, chronically ill, or dying. The child experiences grief. If the child has not encountered death before through the loss of a pet or grandparent, the emotions can be very confusing. Children need to make sure that they do not feel the loss is their fault. Explanations, using age-appropriate language and concepts, are important. Children are sometimes shielded from a parent's illness or funeral without enough direct discussion. Families should ask them if they want to attend the funeral.

Grief work, for both parent and child, involves resolving the loss over time by exploring its meaning. Professionals trained in grief counseling and religious leaders are available for additional support.

SUMMARY

Pediatric primary care providers can use the assistance of social workers to identify, evaluate, and intervene in the emotional and social needs of chronically ill children and their family members. Hospital social workers can be initial contacts for finding the right professional social workers or community agency that can benefit chronically ill children and their families.

Referrals to professional social workers should be made in the following situations:

- A family has a child with a new diagnosis of a chronic illness. The social worker can provide information on organizations and services available to the family and child and assess their coping skills and style. The social worker can also assist them in talking with other families who are undergoing the same situation. Not every parent is interested in support groups, but the social worker can provide families with information about these mutual support resources.
- A family expresses anxiety about the financial impact of the illness. A social worker can provide assistance in identifying financial resources and assisting in advocacy in complex medical health care costs.
- A child or sibling suddenly displays a change in behavior. Warning signs include not wanting to go to school, failing grades, not wanting to socialize with friends, or becoming physically harmful to children or animals. These problems may or may not be related to the child's coping with the disease.
- An ill child or sibling threatens to hurt himself or herself.
- An ill child or sibling has recent severe changes in sleeping or eating habits.
- An ill child or sibling starts continual use of drugs or alcohol.
- An ill child has lost a parent and shows no signs of grief. This may be normal grief, but if a family member becomes worried, a consultation can be useful.
- An ill child or sibling shows signs of neglect or abuse.

Social workers can also provide referrals for children or parents with emotional and behavioral problems. Primary care providers who are physicians may prefer referring child behavior problems to a child psychiatrist for an initial evaluation and treatment. Child psychiatrists have graduated from medical school and are trained in medical and psychiatric settings They can prescribe medication and admit acutely emotionally ill children to child psychiatry inpatient settings for evaluation. Professional guidance counselors and school social workers can also provide counseling. Because children spend most of their daytime hours in school, providing intervention in the school setting can be efficient and effective.

Maintenance of health involves the work of primary care providers and the need to understand stress reduction, nutrition, and health. Relaxation training and complementary therapies need continued attention, and it is critical for providers to understand parents' beliefs and practice in these areas. Providers need to be educated about these methods while making their own judgment about the benefits of referring patients. Professionally trained social workers, child psychologists, counselors, family and marital therapists, and child development specialists can be resources for families who need counseling. Many families may also find spiritual guidance and comfort in turning to their local church pastor or religious leader.

The following are some common presenting psychosocial problems seen by pediatric providers. Although they are covered in depth in several other chapters, they are summarized here:

- *Parental guidance issues, including discipline, bedwetting, and toilet training.* Any developmental challenge for a child is a stressful time for a parent. The primary care provider has the primary relationship with the parent and should consult a professional if he or she feels that the parent is not dealing appropriately with the stress of normal, age-appropriate developmental issues or if the parent needs additional individual guidance. The parent may also benefit from educational and support groups.
- *Acting out of the child at home.* The primary care provider may judge that the child is in need of counseling. A consultation with a social worker, child psychologist, or professionally trained counselor is indicated.
- *Acting out at school.* School guidance counselors, school social workers, and school psychologists are all useful resources. The child may need an educational evaluation. The primary care provider should initiate discussion with the parent about the services available through the school or school district. Problems in school may also be a symptom of other emotional problems or family stresses at home.
- *Adolescence.* Often during this period problems at home erupt. Rebelliousness, possible substance use, lack of interest in school, and risk-taking behavior can all be "red flags." Weathering this period is a challenging time for all. Family or individual counseling can provide support and strategies for minimizing problems. A mental health professional should evaluate as soon as possible serious emotional symptoms, such as suicidal thoughts or gestures.
- *Sibling issues, including rivalry and the birth of a sibling.* The primary care provider can consult with a mental health professional or family therapist if the child and family can benefit from counseling sessions.
- *Bereavement issues.* The primary care provider, a mental health professional, and a religious leader can all provide guidance and counseling.
- *Adult issues.* Overt signs of adult depression, substance abuse, or the risk of violence can all impact the child. Mental health providers can provide counseling and

referrals. Inpatient treatment programs are available for acute issues, including severe depression, and suicidal gestures or attempts. Inpatient alcohol detoxification programs and Alcoholics Anonymous groups are very valuable.
- *Divorce.* Mental health professionals can provide counseling to both children and parents during this conflict-ridden period.

Pediatric primary care providers are in a key role to find social resources that can help families. As part of the multidisciplinary team, social workers can intervene in meeting the needs of children and the families and communities in which they live.

BIBLIOGRAPHY

Abramson, J. (1990). Making teams work. *Social Work with Groups, 12*(4), 45–63.

Badger, L. W., Ackerson, B., Buttell, F., & Rand, E. H. (1997). The case for integration of social work psychosocial services into rural primary care practice. *Health and Social Work, 22*(1), 20–30.

Ducanis, A., & Golin, A. (1979). *The interdisciplinary health team—A handbook.* Germantown, MD: Aspen Systems Corp.

Fox, P. D., & Fama, T. (1996). *Managed care and chronic illness.* Gaithersburg, MD: Aspen Pubishers.

Glied, S. (1998). Too little time? The recognition and treatment of mental health problems in primary care. *Health Services Research, 33*(4), 891–909.

Goldman, L. (1994). *Life and loss: A guide to help grieving children.* Muncie, IN: Accelerated Development.

Gross, R., Rabinowitz, J., Feldman, D., & Boerma, W. (1996). Primary health care physicians' treatment of psychosocial problems: Implications for social work. *Health and Social Work, 21*(2), 89–95.

Mizrahi, T., & Abramson, J. (1985). Sources of strain between physicians and social workers: Implications for social workers in health care settings. *Social Work in Health Care, 10*(3), 33–51.

National Association of Social Workers. (1996). *Code of ethics.* Washington, D.C.: Author.

Palfrey, J. (1997). Tensions in delivering care to children. In R. Stein (Ed.), *Health care for children: What's right, what's wrong, what's next.* New York: United Hospital Fund.

Poole, D. L., & Van Hook, M. (1997). Retooling for community health partnerships in primary care and prevention. *Health and Social Work, 22*(1), 1–3.

Ratcliff, S. S. (1996). The multicultural challenge to health care. In M. C. Julia (Ed.), *Multicultural awareness in the health care professions.* Boston, MA: Allyn and Bacon.

Szilagy, P. G., & Schor, E. L. (1998). The health of children. *Health Services Research, 33*(4), 1001–1039.

CHAPTER 51

Headaches

• JAY E. SELMAN, MD

INTRODUCTION

By age 15 years, 50% of children will have experienced at least one headache (Scheller, 1995). Effective management requires recognition and classification of the headache type, appropriate evaluation, selection and monitoring of therapeutic interventions, and family support. When the headaches do not follow the expected course, neurologic consultation is necessary. This chapter provides a framework for the diagnosis and management of both migraine and nonmigraine headaches in children and adolescents.

ANATOMY, PHYSIOLOGY, AND PATHOLOGY

Understanding the anatomic sites from which pain can emanate is important in the evaluation and treatment of headaches. The major anatomic structures with pain receptors include the cranium; musculoskeletal attachments; and ophthalmologic, otorhinolaryngologic, and dental structures. Cranial structures include the scalp, periosteum, meninges, and large arteries and veins.

Major ophthalmologic pathologic processes involved in headaches include infection and inflammation of the globe, conjunctivae, sclerae, and adnexa, as well as glaucoma (increased intraocular pressure). Refractive errors seldom cause headaches. Screening with the Snellen chart can reassure the family.

Otorhinolaryngologic etiologies include sinusitis, otitis media, pharyngeal irritation and infection, peritonsillar abscess, and glossopharyngeal nerve irritation (Bordley & Bosley, 1973). Dental causes include temporomandibular joint (TMJ) dysfunction and pathologic processes within the tooth, including the pulp, dentin, cementum, and the periodontal structures. Dental pain is usually identifiable by inspection, application of heat, local pressure, or percussion. TMJ syndrome occurs in children and adolescents. Dental consultation can provide additional help.

Pathophysiologic theories of migraine etiology include the vascular, neurogenic, unified or neurovascular, and serotonergic. The vascular hypothesis postulates that neurologic symptoms, such as aura, result from intracranial vasoconstriction, whereas pain follows extracranial vasodilation. The neurogenic hypothesis attempts to explain the spreading wave of reduction in cerebral blood flow (oligemia), which has been documented in special studies of patients having actual migraine headaches. This pattern typically begins over the occipital area and spreads anteriorly. The current hypothesis states that the altered neuronal function results in oligemia.

The unified, or neurovascular, hypothesis unifies these two mechanisms and relates a complex interaction between the trigeminal-vascular complex, intracranial vessels, brain-

stem, and cortical structures and events. Individuals who are susceptible to migraine may have a "central neuronal hyperexcitability," which reduces the threshold for headaches. Certain factors (eg, dietary, hormonal, hereditary) may trigger the release of serotonin and norepinephrine from neurons in the locus ceruleus and the dorsal raphe of the brainstem. This cascade of events leads to the manifestations of the migraine headache. Once activated, the neurons release vasoactive peptides, such as calcium gene related protein, substance P, and acetylcholine, which cause a "sterile" inflammatory response and vasodilation (Waeber, 1998; Sarhan, 1998). The trigeminal nerve, which innervates many cranial vessels, carries impulses to the remainder of the brain, which interprets the signals as pain.

The serotonergic (5-hydroxytriptamine [5-HT] or serotonin) hypothesis builds on the preceding model, because the nerve cells of the dorsal raphe are serotonergic. Possible explanations of serotonergic imbalance, which appears to play a key role in migraine headaches, include suboptimal 5-HT synthesis, unstable 5-HT complexes, excessive metabolism of 5-HT, and defects in 5-HT receptor function. The 5-HT1 receptor agonists, such as rizatriptan, sumatriptan, and ergotamine, ameliorate or abort the migraine attacks, while the 5-HT2 receptor antagonists, including the tricyclic antidepressants and methysergide, are prophylactic agents. The much-improved efficacy and side-effect profile of the triptan drugs (eg, sumatriptan, rizatriptan, naratriptan) probably reflect their specificity as compared with other drugs, such as the tricyclics, β-blockers, and methysergide, which affect many other neurotransmitter systems.

Some researchers believe that all headaches, including tension type and migraine, belong to a single clinical spectrum related to the same basic etiology but differing in clinical manifestations. However, clinical management requires consideration of the epidemiology and management of each type separately.

HEADACHE TYPES

Display 51-1 delineates the major headache types and categories, as defined in the *International Statistical Classification of Diseases and Related Health Problems*, 10th revision (ICD-10) and by the International Headache Society (IHS, 1997). The headache types reviewed here are the most relevant for children and adolescents.

Migraine Headaches

Twenty three million Americans have migraine headaches (IHS, 1997). Migraine headache can occur with or without an aura. Table 51-1 outlines the diagnostic criteria for these two most common forms of migraine headaches.

Many clinicians have suggested various modifications because they believe that the criteria delineated in Table 51-1

DISPLAY 51–1 • Headache Types

Migraine
  Without aura
  With aura
  Complicated
  Basilar artery
  Equivalents
    Abdominal
    Cyclic vomiting
    Benign positional vertigo
    Acute confusional state
Tension type
  Episodic
  Chronic
Headache caused by mass lesion
  Neoplasm
  Subdural hematoma
  Chiari I malformation
  Arteriovenous malformation
  Aneurysm
Headache from other causes
  Exertional
  Post-shunt
  Benign intracranial hypertension
  Cervicogenic
  Temperomandibular joint syndrome
  Sinus
  Post–lumbar puncture
  Altitude sickness

---

there is visual distortion, with either micropsia or macropsia (Emergy, 1977).

Types of Migraine Headaches

Complicated migraine requires fulfilling the criteria for migraine per Table 51-1 and the presence of focal neurologic deficits for 7 days or the demonstration of ischemic infarction in an anatomically appropriate area by neuroimaging. Other causes of infarction must be excluded (IHS, 1997). Although often familial, complicated migraine requires a very thorough evaluation for vascular, inflammatory, and metabolic problems (Arroyo et al., 1990). Magnetic resonance imaging (MRI) is the preferred imaging test. MRI can reveal periventricular white matter changes that may not correlate well with neurologic deficits. However, cortical abnormalities, which can occur alone or with the periventricular changes, have a greater correspondence with clinical findings.

Patients who have had cranial irradiation for leukemia or other neoplasms (especially when accompanied by chemotherapy) may develop a migraine-like syndrome or a stroke many years later. However, the mechanism is probably different, resulting from radiation damage to the endothelium of the cranial vessels (Shuper et al., 1995).

Basilar artery migraine is a special subtype of migraine that begins in early childhood, often before 4 years of age (Barlow, 1994). Most striking is the dramatic, precipitous, and often recurrent presentation of multiple neurologic deficits, all of which are attributable to transient disturbances in the posterior circulation (vertebro-basilar artery). Symptoms include transient ataxia, vertigo, diplopia, alternating hemiparesis, facial paresis, tinnitus, hearing impairment, ataxia, vomiting, paresthesias, and depressed level of consciousness. Attacks tend to be more severe with increasing age of onset. Many children with vestibular symptoms will have labyrinthine dysfunction on electronystagmographic testing, especially if the episodes are moderate or severe (Eviator, 1981). A strong female preponderance and a very striking family history of migraine are commonly present in up to 86% of families studied, usually among female members on the maternal side.

Differential diagnoses include stroke, arteriovenous malformations (AVMs), toxic-metabolic encephalopathies, and neoplasms. Fortunately, most patients recover completely.

exclude many children and some adolescents who actually have migraine. These include reducing the duration to 1 hour and including either unilateral or bilateral localization, abdominal pain, and a family history of migraine as diagnostic criteria (Raieli et al., 1995; Scheller, 1995; Winner et al., 1995; Sweeting & West, 1998). In clinical practice most neurologists do not adhere rigidly to the criteria of the ICD-10 classification.

Although migraine auras usually precede the migraine, they may occur with the headache itself. One unusual aura variant is the "Alice in Wonderland" syndrome, in which

---

Table 51–1.   DIAGNOSTIC CRITERIA FOR MIGRAINE HEADACHES

Migraine Without Aura: Diagnostic Criteria	Migraine With Aura: Diagnostic Criteria
A. At least five attacks fulfilling criteria B–D	A. At least two attacks fulfilling criterion B
B. Headache attack lasting 4–72 h (< 15 y old: 2–48 h)	B. At least three of the following:
C. At least two of the following:	1. One or more fully reversible aura symptoms (see criterion C)
1. Unilateral	2. At least one aura developing gradually over more than 4 min or two or more symptoms occurring in succession
2. Pulsating	3. No auras lasting more than 60 min
3. Moderate-to-severe intensity	4. Headache in less than 60 min
4. Aggravated by routine physical activity, climbing stairs, walking	C. Typical auras include
D. During headache at least one of the following:	1. Homonymous visual field disturbance
1. Nausea or vomiting	2. Unilateral paresthesias
2. Phonophobia and photophobia	3. Unilateral weakness
E. Exclusion of other headaches, conditions	

Adapted from International Headache Society. (1997). ICD-10 guide for headaches. *Cephalalgia, 17*(Suppl. 19), 18–19.

Although basilar artery migraines usually cease in adolescence, many patients will later develop more typical migraines.

▲ **Clinical Warning:** Children and adolescents presenting with possible basilar artery migraine require a thorough neurologic assessment, MRI scan, and appropriate laboratory screening.

Abdominal migraine presents with episodic abdominal pain, with or without vomiting and headaches. In a large epidemiologic survey, Abu-Arafeh and Russell (1995b) found that about 10% of a community-based sample of 1754 children ages 5 to 15 years had migraine headaches, while 4% had abdominal migraine. The clinical patterns and provoking and ameliorating factors were virtually identical in the two groups. Nevertheless, this diagnosis requires a thorough evaluation to exclude other causes of abdominal pain. A recent open-label study of 36 children with abdominal migraine revealed a 75% "excellent" response to propranolol (Inderal) and a 33% response to cyproheptadine (Worawattanakul, Rhoads, Lichtman, & Ulshen, 1999). Refer to Chapters 38 and 57 for more information about differential diagnosis of abdominal pain. Chapters 21, 23, 40, and 62 may contribute to the formulation of the differential diagnosis.

Cyclic vomiting is an uncommon "periodic" (or recurrent) syndrome in children and adolescents (Cavazzuti, 1982). The clinical characteristics are fairly stereotyped in the individual patient. Discrete episodes of vomiting, which occur without apparent triggering events, last from 1 day to several weeks, usually averaging 2 to 3 days. Withers and colleagues (1998), who studied 32 children and adolescents, reported an average of about nine attacks of cyclic vomiting per year, with two thirds of the patients missing more than 10 days of school annually. At times, the vomiting was severe enough to require hospitalization. Precipitating events included intercurrent infections and stress. In some patients, other neurologic phenomena occurred, including headaches, vertigo, hypotonia, auras, and drowsiness resembling those seen in basilar artery migraines. Although many children with cyclic vomiting later develop typical migraine syndromes, there is also an increased incidence of psychological problems.

A thorough evaluation to exclude structural disease of the central nervous system; gastrointestinal lesion disorders; metabolic encephalopathies, such as maple syrup urine disease; porphyria; and hyperammonia-related syndromes is essential (Withers et al., 1998). Butalbital and propranolol have produced equivocal responses. Gokhale and colleagues (1997) reported that using phenobarbital 30 to 120 mg at bedtime led to significant improvement. The main adverse reaction to barbiturates is hyperactivity, known to occur in up to 30% of children.

Benign positional vertigo (BPV), a periodic syndrome occurring in about 2.5% of children, causes recurrent, discrete episodes of vertigo lasting from seconds to several minutes (Britton, 1988). Nausea, vomiting, anxiety, nystagmus, vasomotor changes, and sometimes headache may accompany the episodes, although the neurologic examination and electroencephalogram (EEG) are normal (IHS, 1997). Among children with BPV, there is a 2.5-fold increase in migraine headaches, abdominal pain, and motion sickness (Abu-Arafeh & Russell, 1995a).

A careful history and examination are critical in making the diagnosis of BPV. Initial episodes or persistent neurologic deficits require a neurologic evaluation, including MRI scanning. Although rare, other conditions, such as neoplasms (medulloblastoma, meningioma), cerebellar proc-

esses, and inner ear pathology (perilymphatic fistula, Meniere's disease), may cause similar symptoms.

Acute confusional state with disorientation occurs infrequently in children after mild head injury and may recur with subsequent trauma (Gascon, 1970). As the child matures, typical migraine headaches may develop. Some cases may represent episodes of transient global amnesia that may be related to brief vasoconstriction of the arteries supplying the hippocampus (Jensen, 1980).

Epidemiology

Infancy

Although headaches can begin in infancy, the family often does not recognize such episodes as migraines (Barlow, 1994). Manifestations in infancy include vomiting, pallor, crying, and behavioral changes. As children develop the ability to communicate, parents become increasingly aware of the headaches. By 3 to 4 years of age, the child can indicate head pain.

Childhood

Epidemiologic studies from many countries and cultures confirm clinical experience that headaches occur frequently in childhood. Although the incidence is equal in both sexes in the preadolescent period, headaches occur more frequently in girls than boys in adolescence. In a general population survey of 5-year-old Finnish children, 50% had had a headache in the previous 6 months; the prevalence of migraine was 7% (Sillanpaa & Anttila, 1996). This 50% figure represents an increase in headache incidence in the intervening decades since Bille's work in 1962. Bille's classic study found that 2.5% of 9000 Swedish children studied had frequent headaches, with 14% having frequent migraine headaches (Bille, 1962). Psychosocial stress seems to have contributed to this increase. Other behavioral problems, including temper tantrums and stomach aches, occurred much more often in children with headaches, but the explanation of this association is unclear (Sillanpaa & Anttila, 1996).

Adolescence

A general population survey of 13-year-old Finnish children conducted in 1992 demonstrated that 51% had had a headache in the previous 6 months. Ten percent of these subjects had had a migraine in the same period (Sillanpaa & Anttila, 1996). Again, these figures suggest a significant increase in the incidence of migraine headache in the years since Bille (1962) conducted his research, finding that 16% of his Swedish subjects had recurrent headaches, with 5% having frequent migraines.

Tension-Type Headaches

Two types of tension-type headaches (TTH) occur: episodic and chronic. Episodic TTH is a very common disorder that may or may not be associated with tenderness of the pericranial muscles. Children and adolescents may have both migraine headaches and TTH. However, most TTHs are relatively mild and respond to simple analgesic treatment. Display 51-2 presents diagnostic criteria for episodic TTH.

When chronic TTH exists, a careful search for possible stressors is extremely important. Because TTH can occur with migraine headaches, the clinician should evaluate both conditions. Wober-Bingol and colleagues (1996) found that

---

DISPLAY 51–2 • Diagnostic Criteria for Episodic Tension-Type Headaches

---

A. At least 10 episodes fulfilling criteria B–D with fewer than 15 headache-days per month for at least 6 months, but fewer than 180 headache-days per year
B. Duration from 30 minutes to 7 days
C. Two or more of the following:
  1. Pressing/tightening (nonpulsatile) quality
  2. Mild-to-moderate intensity that may inhibit but not prohibit activities
  3. Bilateral location
  4. Not aggravated by routine activity
D. Both of the following:
  1. No nausea or vomiting
  2. Phonophobia or photophobia may be present, but not both
E. Absence of other specific headache disorders (eg, chronic post-traumatic)

Adapted with permission from International Headache Society. (1997). ICD-10 Guide for Headaches. *Cephalalgia, 17*(Suppl. 19), 14–16.

---

the major differentiating factors between migraine and TTH were the intensity of the headaches and the presence of nausea and vomiting. Children with TTH often report more trigger factors than those with migraine, but there is an increase in associated musculoskeletal symptoms in children with headaches, regardless of the type. Children with migraines or TTH have more somatic complaints and school absences than children without headache, especially if they have both types (Carlsson, 1996). Many adults with chronic TTH (previously known as chronic daily headaches) actually began having them in childhood or adolescence. Episodic TTH may "transform" into chronic TTH. Precipitating factors can include head, neck, or back trauma; viral illnesses; sinusitis; and surgical procedures (Marcus, Scharff, Mercer, & Turk, 1999). Display 51-3 presents the diagnostic criteria for chronic TTH.

DISPLAY 51–3 • Diagnostic Criteria for Chronic Tension-Type Headaches

---

A. History of headaches occurring more than 15 days per month for at least 6 months, or at least 180 days per year, and criteria B–D
B. Must have two of the following:
  1. Pressing/tightening pain, must be nonthrobbing
  2. Mild-to-moderate intensity may inhibit but does not prohibit activities
  3. Bilateral location
  4. Not aggravated by routine physical activity
C. Both of the following:
  1. No vomiting present
  2. None or only one of the following is present:
    a. Nausea
    b. Photophobia
    c. Phonophobia
D. Absence of other specific headache disorders (eg, chronic post-traumatic)

Adapted with permission from International Headache Society. (1997). ICD-10 Guide for Headaches. *Cephalalgia, 17*(Suppl. 19), 16–17.

Headache Caused by Mass Lesions

Commonly occurring lesions associated with increased intracranial pressure and headaches include neoplasms, subdural and epidural hematomas, empyemas, Chiari I malformations, AVMs, and aneurysms. The common characteristics of intracranial mass lesions include distortion and destruction of anatomic structures, obstruction of the flow of cerebrospinal fluid (CSF), and changes in the compliance of brain tissues. The rapidity of presentation is proportional to the rate of change of the mass, brain compliance, and intracranial pressure (ie, the slower the onset of the pathologic process, the later the presentation).

Intracranial neoplasms are the second most common tumor seen in children. Cohen and Duffner report the prevalence at 2.4 per 100,000 (Swaiman, 1994). Risk factors include genetic conditions, such as neurofibromatosis, ataxia-telangiectasia, immunosuppression, and exposure to x-rays and other toxins.

Intracranial lesions develop in the supratentorial or infratentorial compartments or in the midline. Supratentorial lesions present with focal neurologic deficits, headaches, or seizures, which may be localized or generalized. Infratentorial lesions present with headaches and signs of increased intracranial pressure, visual symptoms, dyscoordination (lateral cerebellum), gait ataxia (midline or lateral cerebellum), and cranial nerve abnormalities (diplopia, facial weakness, dysphagia, dysarthria). Midline tumors typically have associated visual problems, endocrine dysfunction (eg, appetite, thirst, and growth disorders), headaches, and emotional disturbances. Acute obstruction of the aqueduct of Sylvius, which connects the third and fourth ventricles in the midline, results in rapid dilation of the frontal horns and lateral ventricles, thereby causing lethargy, vomiting, and diplopia.

A choroid cyst of the third ventricle can act as a ball-valve, causing intermittent obstruction of the CSF pathways and therefore very positionally dependent symptoms. Infratentorial neoplasms account for approximately 50% of tumors in children younger than 12 years but decrease significantly through adolescence toward the adult pattern of 80% to 90% supratentorial and 10% to 20% infratentorial. The most typical presentation is a gradual but progressive onset of minor symptoms, such as mild headaches that will respond initially to simple analgesics.

● **Clinical Pearl:** Headaches associated with mass lesions increase in frequency and severity; they may be present upon awakening or will awaken the child from sleep at night or occur with exertion. As this pattern evolves, vomiting, diplopia, lethargy, and loss of neurologic function may accompany the headache. Any suspicion of an intracranial mass requires an urgent neurologic assessment.

With either subdural or epidural hematomas, the history of head trauma, albeit mild, is almost always elicitable. Typically, focal headaches begin gradually, followed by an altered level of consciousness. Focal neurologic deficits and seizures can also occur. The interval between the head trauma and the presentation of symptoms can vary significantly with subdural hematomas, which result from tearing of the bridging veins across the calvarium.

● **Clinical Pearl:** Young infants are particularly prone to subdural hematomas because of the large ratio between the mass of the brain and that of the body. This results in disproportionately large shearing forces being applied to the brain in traumatic injuries, whether accidental or intentional.

Epidural hematomas result from trauma in which lateral head injury causes shearing of the middle meningeal artery. About 70% of epidural hematomas are associated with skull fractures. Hemorrhage in the epidural space can occur immediately or after a brief period (minutes to a few hours) of relative normalcy, the "lucid period." Once present, symptoms of increased intracranial pressure can develop very rapidly because the bleeding occurs under arterial pressure. The mortality rate approaches 25%.

▲ Clinical Warnings

- When the primary care provider suspects either a subdural or epidural hematoma, an emergency computed tomography (CT) scan of the brain without contrast is mandatory. The clinician should contact both a neurologist and a neurosurgeon immediately if the CT scan confirms the diagnosis or if the child has any abnormalities on neurologic examination.
- Occasionally an empyema may form in the subdural space, either directly from nearby infected sinuses or indirectly from hematogenous seeding. Headaches and fever often occur early in the process. Because these infections can rapidly cause severe disability or death, emergency neurologic, neurosurgical, and ear, nose, and throat consultations are imperative.

Chiari I malformation is a congenital anomaly, leading to displacement of the cerebellar tonsils into the spinal canal at the craniocervical junction. Although often asymptomatic for decades, some patients present with headaches in childhood or adolescence. Typically occipital or frontal, the headaches are often accompanied by neck pain, gait ataxia, dysphagia, nystagmus, and even respiratory distress. The presence of the latter is an ominous finding because rarely, Chiari I malformations can affect the brainstem respiratory centers and cause traction on the lower spinal nerves, resulting in respiratory failure and death.

An AVM is a congenital malformation that usually presents as seizures or focal neurologic deficits as a result of local ischemia or hemorrhages. However, associated headaches may resemble migraine headaches or TTH.

▲ **Clinical Warning:** Any patient with a persistent, unilateral headache always confined to the **same** side of the head may have an AVM that is leaking intermittently.

An aneurysm, a congenital malformation in the medial or muscular layer of medium and large arteries, weakens the arterial wall at the bifurcation. As individuals age, the defect tends to enlarge, thereby increasing the probability of rupture. The aneurysm can leak without rupturing completely, producing the "sentinel" or warning headache caused by blood in the subarachnoid space or a pressure effect. Meningeal symptoms can accompany these headaches. A family history of aneurysms should increase the clinician's index of suspicion.

Headache From Other Causes

Children and adolescents experience other headaches with which the primary care provider should be familiar, including exertional, post-shunt, benign intracranial hypertension, TMJ, cervicogenic, sinus, post–lumbar puncture, and altitude sickness headaches.

Exertional headaches occur rarely in children and occasionally in adolescents. They typically develop with sudden vigorous physical exertion without warming up and with sudden physiologic activities, such as coughing, sneezing, or even yawning. Adolescents report similar headaches with sexual activity. Some patients with typical migraines note exertion as a triggering event. The differential diagnosis should include posterior fossa lesions, subdural hematoma, Chiari I malformation, congenital lesions of the craniocervical junction, and pheochromocytoma. The quality of the headache is variable but often has a throbbing or pulsatile character. Other patterns include sharp or stabbing pain that is unilateral or bilateral.

Management of exertional headaches requires an accurate diagnosis. Adequate hydration and warm-up prior to strenuous physical activity are needed to increase the cardiac output slowly. If these measures fail, then indomethacin, isometheptene (Midrin), or ergotamine tartrate can be used about 30 to 60 minutes before the activity. Propranolol is a useful prophylactic agent.

Post-shunt headaches are potentially ominous. Immediately after the procedure for obstructive hydrocephalus, usually a ventriculo-peritoneal shunt, the headaches may result from failure of the shunt apparatus (valve, tubing, connections, or obstruction of the proximal or distal ends). Subdural hematomas may result from rapid decompression of the ventricles, inward movement of the brain, and shearing of the extradural veins. After the perioperative period, the main concerns are shunt failure and infection. The latter usually presents with fever, headache, irritability, vomiting, and change in mental status. Shunt failure can cause a rapid increase in intracranial pressure, obtundation, and even death. After the shunt has been in place for several months, the brain compliance is often significantly reduced. Therefore, a small increase in the volume of CSF, caused by shunt malfunction, will result in a disproportionate elevation in intracranial pressure.

▲ **Clinical Warning:** Any suspicion of shunt failure or malfunction requires an emergency pediatric neurosurgical consultation. Depending on scope of practice, the provider should know how to tap the commonly used reservoirs, because this can always be done emergently if no surgical help is available.

Benign intracranial hypertension occurs more often in adolescent females with obesity and menstrual irregularities. Potential provoking factors include the use of steroids, macrodantins, tetracyclines, fat-soluble vitamins, isoretinoin compounds (Bigby, 1988), chronic otitis media, and Lyme disease. Patients present with headaches, diplopia from sixth nerve palsy, papilledema, and vomiting. The greatest danger is sudden blindness, which can evolve rapidly in the absence of other symptoms. Treatment consists of lumbar puncture(s), acetazolamide (Diamox), steroids, and a neurologic and possibly an ophthamologic consultation. Long-term management includes a weight-loss program in obese children. In severe cases, especially when visual function is threatened, a lumboperitoneal shunt or optic nerve fenestration may be required.

Uncommon in children and adolescents, *cervicogenic headaches* arise in the neck region. The pain may radiate fairly widely to the temporal and frontal areas. Typically, tenderness of the cervical paraspinous muscles and loss of range of motion are the clinical highlights of this entity (Sjaastad et al., 1989). Conservative treatment with reduction of the weight of book bags, application of heat, anti-inflammatory medications, and physical therapy may be helpful.

Headaches related to TMJ dysfunction have been found in up to 80% of children, adolescents, and adults presenting to a specialized clinic for facial and myofascial pain disorders, including TMJ (Pilley et al., 1992). Other symptoms include ear pain, throat symptoms, dizziness, muffling, jaw clicking and clenching or locking, popping in and around the ear, loss of range of movement, or clicking sensation (Cooper & Cooper, 1993; Capurso et al., 1997). Examination reveals tenderness over the preauricular area. Palpation of the pterygoid muscles in the hypopharynx often identifies areas of tenderness. Many patients also complain of neck pain. More severe problems require a comprehensive dental examination, which may entail special radiographs, scintigraphic scans, or MRI scans.

Although patients and families often attribute headaches to sinus disease, the condition accounts for a low percentage of headaches. Burton's 1997 study of an urban emergency department found that 1.3% of children ages 2 to 18 years had a primary complaint of headache; of these, 16% had sinusitis (Burton et al., 1997). Until the sinus becomes aerated, it cannot be inflamed or infected and therefore cannot cause pain. Table 51-2 delineates the maturation of the sinuses and the patterns of pain referral.

The IHS (1997) has established criteria to be used for the diagnosis of sinus headache. These criteria include the following:

- Purulent discharge in the nasal passage.
- Pathologic findings on one or more of the following examinations:
  - Radiograph
  - CT scan
  - Transillumination
- Simultaneous onset of the headache and sinusitis
- Headache located according to the affected sinus, often described as aching and aggravated by direct percussion or Valsalva maneuver:
  - Frontal: directly over the sinus with radiation to the vertex or retro-orbital area
  - Maxillary: over the antral area with radiation to the upper teeth or forehead
  - Ethmoid: between and behind the eyes, radiating to the temporal areas
  - Sphenoid: occipital, vertex, frontal or retro-orbital
- Headache resolution with treatment of the sinusitis

A persistent leak of CSF from the thecal sac after lumbar puncture can cause a post–lumbar puncture headache, especially with the use of larger-bore lumbar puncture needles and, perhaps, in thinner individuals. However, there is no relationship between the occurrence and the site of the lumbar puncture, the amount of fluid withdrawn, or the time the patient remains flat after the procedure. Sitting and standing worsen the headache, whereas reclining alleviates it. Con-servative treatment consists of bed rest for 1 to 2 days, increased fluid intake, and caffeine.

● **Clinical Pearl:** Persistent headaches often respond to an epidural blood patch to seal the leak. Using a small-bore, specially tapered needle (eg, Sprotte or Whittaker) significantly reduces the incidence of these headaches.

Altitude sickness headache occurs in children and adolescents who have an upper respiratory illness when they ascend rapidly to about 8000 ft. Symptoms include headache, nausea, shortness of breath, fatigue, tachycardia, and even pulmonary edema that present at night because of pulmonary hypoventilation. Development of visual changes or confusion usually signals high-altitude cerebral edema, requiring emergent transport to a lower altitude. Patients typically describe the headaches as bilateral and throbbing.

Acute treatment consists of oxygen, fluids, and rest. Prophylaxis consists of gradual ascent to the destination, pretreatment with acetazolamide 5 mg/kg per day in two divided doses (use with caution in the presence of allergy to sulfa; some patients experience paresthesias in the toes and fingers), and increased hydration. Acute treatment includes fluids, rest, dexamethasone for headache at 0.6 mg/kg per dose to a maximum of 10 mg/d for 2 days, and oxygen at night. If headache is severe, the patient will require transport to a lower altitude. The patient should avoid all strenuous activity for the first 24 to 48 hours after arriving at the high altitude and should absolutely refrain from alcohol to prevent the condition (Freedman, 1999).

HISTORY AND PHYSICAL EXAMINATION

Headache evaluation must include a thorough history, pediatric and neurologic examinations, and appropriate laboratory and imaging studies. The history is critical in identifying the headache type, severity, and underlying psychosocial factors. Historic data can assist the clinician in formulating an evaluation and treatment plan.

● **Clinical Pearl:** Interview the patient alone during the assessment process; this will reveal information not available in any other way. Ask the patient why he or she has the headache and about school and peer issues, symptoms of depression, abuse, familial problems, alcohol and drug use (patient, family, peers), sexual activity, and eating patterns.

History

Ask about the number of different headache types. Children and teens often have more than one headache type, most typically migraine and TTH. Having the patient and

Table 51–2. DEVELOPMENT OF PARANASAL SINUSES

Sinus	Onset of Aeration	Completion of Aeration	Pain Referred to
Maxillary	Infancy	Early adulthood	Cheek, forehead, retro-orbital
Ethmoid	2 y old	Late puberty	Vertex, temples, retro-orbital
Sphenoid	4 y old	Late puberty	Vertex, occipital, frontal, neck, or shoulder
Frontal	6–8 y old	Late puberty	Frontal, vertex, retro-orbital
Mastoid	Infancy	Adolescence	Ear, neck

parents assess the different types separately will facilitate management. However, sometimes the patient who reports multiple headache types has, in reality, only one type with varying manifestations. Clarifying this for the patient is important.

● **Clinical Pearl:** Suspect significant emotional problems in the patient who truly appears to have more than two different headache types.

Antecedent event(s) for the first headache of each type must be understood. Head trauma, a serious illness, a medication reaction, envenomation (Lyme, ehrlichiosis, babesiosis, Rocky Mountain spotted fever), or unusual stress may accompany the onset of headaches.

Determine if there has been a change in pattern in the recent past. Changes in the patient's typical headache pattern, including the frequency, duration, severity, or symptoms (depending on when the headaches began), can alert the clinician to a more serious underlying process such as an evolving mass lesion or new stresses in the patient's life.

Understanding provoking factors for each headache type can help the patient and family avoid or modify them. These include sleep deprivation, change in sleep times (eg, going to bed or arising earlier or later than usual), skipping meals, specific foods (see Appendix 51-1), stress, other medications, Valsalva maneuver (coughing, sneezing, or straining at defecation), position (supine, sitting, or standing), posture (bending over), weather change, odors (tobacco, soaps, perfumes), and menses. Appendix 51-1 provides a compilation of potential triggers for patients with migraine headache.

In addition, the provider should ask about the following:

- *Prodrome:* Ask the patient about description, duration, and localization of the warning phase before the aura. Some patients or their families can recognize a stereotyped change in mood, appearance, or activity level for hours to a day or so before the onset of the headache.
- *Aura:* Determine the type (visual, auditory, olfactory), description (scintillation, scotomata, fortifications), localization, duration, relation to the onset of headache, associated symptoms.
- *Onset:* Include the following factors:
  - *Diurnal pattern:* Does the headache begin at a consistent time of day? If the headache begins during the night on a consistent or increasing basis, consider an intracranial mass lesion. If the headache is present upon awakening, also consider the possibility of a sleep disorder. If the headache occurs only on school days, then social or academic stress(es) require further exploration. Headaches occurring only around a parental visitation in a divided family should likewise lead to further questioning about psychosocial issues.
  - *Localization:* If the headache begins only on the same side, then consider an intracranial process. Migraine headaches can have a very strongly lateralized pattern; but if the patient never recalls having had a headache that began on the opposite side or bifrontally, then consider an intracranial process (mass, aneurysm, AVM, hemorrhage).
  - *Onset time:* A headache that reaches its maximum intensity almost immediately warrants increased concern, because the differential diagnosis includes the vascular etiologies (aneurysm, AVMs), structural lesions, and the more benign exertional headache.

- *Radiation:* Where does the headache pain go? This can suggest other etiologies, such as TMJ dysfunction, cervical strain, or sinus disease.
- *Pain descriptor:* Is the pain sharp, dull, aching, throbbing, squeezing? Encourage the patient to use his or her own terms. Because young children are often unable to do this, the clinician will need to provide some choices.

● **Clinical Pearl:** Migraine headaches typically have a throbbing quality; TTHs cause more pressure or have a squeezing character.

- Severity and rating scales (eg, 1–10 maximum; mild-moderate-severe): Ask about the headaches in general and how often the patient has severe headaches. Clinicians should note any discrepancy between their own assessment of the patient's affect, appearance, activity level, and degree of discomfort and the assessments of the patient and parents. If the patient looks much better than the self-rating or the parent's assessment, then the provider should explore carefully for secondary gain. On the other hand, if the child appears more ill than the parent's rating, consider other familial issues.

● **Clinical Pearl:** If the patient has a headache during the evaluation, ask him or her and the parent(s) to rate the severity.

- *Duration:* Ask about duration of the average headache and the more severe ones.
- *Frequency:* The frequency of the headaches helps quantify the problem.
- *Associated symptoms:* Ask about nausea, vomiting, photophobia, phonophobia, aggravation with movement, pallor, paresthesias, focal motor or sensory deficits (weakness or numbness on one side of the body), anorexia, diarrhea, ataxia, and vertigo.
- *Aggravating factors:* Aggravating factors may include movement, light, noise, eating, stress, position, posture (with the latter two, suspect an intracranial lesion).
- *Ameliorating factors:* What helps the patient (eg, dark room, sleeping, ice or heat)?
- *Treatment:* Include the following factors:
  - *Nonpharmacologic:* Inquire how the family and patient manage the headache, and evaluate their emotional reactions to the treatment and their level of concern.
  - *Pharmacologic:* Note all current and past prescription, over-the-counter, and alternative medications used and the number per day. If the number of analgesic units (ie, total number of all pills/teaspoons of medication taken for headache) exceeds about five per day for more than 3 days per week, then the patient is at risk for rebound headaches. Note all previous medications tried for headache management with doses used, if possible. Also note all medica-tions taken for other conditions. Ask about all over-the-counter, herbal, and complementary (ie, alternative) medications because some of these can cause headaches. If an eating disorder is suspected, ask specifically about laxatives, emetics, and diet preparations.

● **Clinical Pearl:** Failure to detect excessive medication use significantly increases the probability of a poor response to treatment.

- *Lifestyle:* This plays a critical role in modulating the severity of the headaches and how the patient and family are dealing with the problem.

- *Diet:* Inquire about specific dietary patterns, especially caffeine intake, eating patterns, and the possibility of eating disorders.
- *Stress:* Stress at home, at school, and with peers plays a tremendous role in aggravating headaches. Repeated inquiry is essential because the patient may not provide complete information on the first or even subsequent visits. Watch for any identification by the patient with other family members who have or had headaches.
- *Sleep history:* This reveals information about insomnia, frequent nocturnal awakening, snoring, bruxism, early morning awakening, or daytime somnolence. Although uncommon in children, sleep apnea can cause significant headaches. Functional sleep disorders (ie, not related to apnea) should suggest underlying depression. Nocturnal seizures can also present with early morning headaches. Refer to Chapters 28 and 46 for more information on these topics.
- *School or work attendance:* Information about school or work missed is critical because this reflects both the severity of the process and the coping mechanisms of the patient and family. Ask about the number of days missed because of headaches and other medical problems. Also, ask how often the child misses part of the school day. Ask about the patient's activities during school absences. Ask about the work missed by the parent(s) because of the child's medical or headache problems. This will provide additional insight about the impact on the family. The change in pattern of school absences is a critical indicator of the success of the treatment program.
- *Academic performance:* The presence of learning disabilities, attentional problems, or behavioral difficulties may aggravate headaches because of the associated stress or because of medications such as psychostimulant drugs. Note carefully a decline in grades. Refer to Chapter 21 for more information about prescribed medications in attention deficit disorder.
- *Life impact:* How does the child's problem affect the family? Does the child receive disproportionate attention? Is the headache the only or major way that the child receives attention? Refer to Chapter 49 for more insight on family-centered management of the patient with a chronic problem.
- *Exercise:* How active is the child? Too much time spent watching television, playing video games, or sitting at the computer may reflect social withdrawal or depression. Exercise and play allow the child and adolescent to release tension and stimulate endorphin secretion, which may help alleviate pain.
- *Social:* This encompasses some of the previous points but includes the child's interpersonal relations with peers. Headaches may signal difficulties in this area.
- *Current medical problems:* These require careful assessment with a review of symptoms, systems, medication use, allergies, and immunization status. If the child has two or more other serious conditions, such as asthma or gastrointestinal symptoms, look very carefully for underlying stress factors.
- *Medical history:* Past medical history should be explored, as with any patient.
- *Family history:* This should include careful attention to members with headaches. Explore briefly the actual headache patterns of other family members because people's self-descriptions are notoriously inaccurate. Ask about depression, postpartum depression, bipolar disorder, substance dependencies, attentional disorders, or serious medical problems, because this information can yield valuable clues about comorbid issues that can affect management.

Physical and Neurologic Examinations

After the history, the most important part of the evaluation is the physical examination, which should include a general pediatric medical component and a neurologic assessment. The approach to the patient depends on the clinical presentation, the duration and severity of the complaints, and the appearance of the child. The clinician may use the screening examination in a nonurgent assessment when the patient appears well. A comprehensive examination is essential with the ill-appearing child or with more complex presentations. With practice, the clinician should be able to complete a normal screening examination in about 5 to 7 minutes in a cooperative child.

● **Clinical Pearl:** The sensory examination is the most difficult, time-consuming, and least rewarding, especially in the younger child. If the remainder of the examination is normal, the provider need not spend much time with this part of the examination.

● **Clinical Pearl:** For almost any child with headaches, reevaluate in 1 to 6 weeks, depending on the clinical circumstances. This permits a prospective review of the headache diary (Appendix 51-2). The reassessment also provides for an evaluation of the patient's participation in any lifestyle changes or medication regimen, noting response to treatment recommendations. These data also help exclude a more serious, progressive disorder (Pollack, 1999).

When the headaches are severe or chronic, the patient will require a comprehensive evaluation and usually a pediatric neurologic assessment. Table 51-3 presents an approach for both screening and comprehensive neurologic examinations of the child with headache.

DIAGNOSTIC STUDIES

Self-Study: The Headache Diary

Teaching the patient and family how to keep a headache diary provides valuable information about the headache pattern(s). The clinician gains additional insight into the patient's and family's motivation and their interactions by their consistency in recording data and bringing the diary to clinic appointments. Appendix 51-2 presents a sample format for a headache diary.

Laboratory and Imaging Studies

The primary care provider should order only laboratory and imaging tests necessary to evaluate specific diagnoses related to the patient's clinical problems (eg, infectious, inflammatory, or toxic-metabolic etiologies). Appendix 51-3 presents *possible* laboratory studies for use in diagnosing headache etiology.

● **Clinical Pearl:** For uncomplicated TTH or typical migraine, laboratory and imaging studies are usually not necessary.

Occasionally, a lumbar puncture may be an important part of the headache evaluation. The three primary indications

Table 51–3. SCREENING AND COMPREHENSIVE EXAMINATION OF THE PATIENT WITH HEADACHE

Component	Screening Examination	Comprehensive Examination
Vital signs	Blood pressure, pulse, temperature, weight, height, head circumference	Same
Mental status	Level of consciousness, communication appropriate for age	Plus detailed testing of naming, praxis, memory, calculations as indicated
Cranial nerves	II: Funduscopic examination: Disk margins, presence of spontaneous venous pulsations, absence of hemorrhages III, IV, VI: Pupillary responses (equal and reactive), extraocular movements, absence of ptosis VII: Facial movements should be symmetrical XII: Tongue protrusion should be in the midline	Plus (where indicated) I: Sense of smell II: Optikokinetic reflexes; visual field tests V: Corneal reflexes and strength of pterygoid muscles (lateral jaw deviation) VII: Facial symmetry at rest and with volitional activity; strength of eye and lip closure, symmetry of forehead elevation VIII: Auditory screening; whispering numbers in each ear IX, X: Swallowing function and palatal movement XI: Lateral neck rotation and shoulder elevation (sternocleidomastoid and trapezei)
Motor	Drift (arms held extended in supination and should remain at the same level without rising or falling) Symmetrical use and strength of deltoid, triceps, extensor carpi radialis (wrist extension), iliopsoas (hip flexion), anterior tibialis (ankle extensors)	Same
Muscle stretch reflexes	Biceps, brachioradialis, triceps, patella, Achilles	Same
Pathologic reflexes	Babinski, plantar (Stroking outer aspect of sole of foot from the heel to base of toes and then moving medially over the skin overlying the heads of the metatarsal bones; stimulus should be irritative but not painful. If the great toe moves to an extensor position with fanning or abduction of the other toes, the response is labeled a Babinski response [ie, pathologic])	Hoffman (Extend wrist and fingers, flick middle digit. Normal: no flexion of thumb or other fingers. Abnormal: flexion of thumb or other fingers.)
Coordination	Rapid alternating movements, finger to nose, finger-nose-finger	Heel-knee-shin, past pointing, Romberg
Cervical range of motion	Flexion to exclude meningismus, lateral rotation, extension, palpation of cervical paraspinous muscles	Same
Auscultation	Carotid arteries, closed eyes, and cranium for bruits	Same
Sensation		Light touch, pin prick, vibration, joint position sense, higher cortical function

for a lumbar puncture include (1) evaluation of an infectious process, such as meningitis, encephalitis, or Lyme disease; (2) measurement of intracranial pressure in suspected cases of benign intracranial pressure; and (3) detection of subarachnoid hemorrhage associated with an aneurysm.

▲ **Clinical Warning:** Lumbar punctures are contraindicated when intracranial masses may be present, when the patient is anticoagulated, or when the skin overlying the lumbar spine is broken or infected.

Imaging studies can also assist in diagnosing headache in specific instances. The three primary imaging modalities of skull radiographs, CT scans, and MRI scans can assist in the evaluation of selected patients with headaches; namely, those in whom the clinician has concerns about a structural lesion or, rarely, a degenerative process. Skull radiographs

have a very limited use in the management of headaches. Table 51-4 provides a comparison between CT and MRI scanning as a diagnostic tool.

● **Clinical Pearl:** Skull radiographs may be obtained after head trauma with an open wound or with suspicion of a depressed skull fracture. However, CT of the head without contrast is the test of choice in head trauma. Always evaluate the patient for possible cervical spine trauma and obtain cervical spine radiographs when indicated.

Obtain a CT scan when there is a history of significant acute head trauma. Otherwise, an MRI scan will provide the maximum information. When the differential diagnosis includes a neoplastic process or vascular malformation (aneurysm, AVM), intravenous gadolinium enhancement is usually necessary. If a child requires sedation, the neurolo-

Table 51–4.   COMPUTED TOMOGRAPHIC SCANNING VERSUS MAGNETIC RESONANCE IMAGING

Factor	CT Scan	MRI
Acute/subacute trauma	Yes	No
Chronic process	No	Yes
Neoplasm	Fair	Preferred
Sedation necessary	Usually not	Often in young child
Radiation exposure	Yes	None
Contrast enhancement	Usually not	Often
Time	3–10 min	40–60 min
Resolution	Moderate to excellent	Excellent
Posterior fossa visualization (cerebellum, brainstem)	Poor to fair	Excellent
Calcium-containing lesions	Excellent	Fair
Vascular abnormalities	Good (with contrast)	Excellent (with MRA)
Cost	$200–$500	$500–$1,200

CT = computed tomography; MRA = magnetic resonance angiography; MRI = magnetic resonance imaging.

gist will often order the MRI with contrast enhancement to avoid a second procedure and resedation.

Magnetic resonance angiography (MRA) provides noninvasive visualization of the vascular structures, especially the arteries of the neck and the brain. The MRA is a screening, but not definitive, test for diagnosing aneurysms because lesions smaller than 3 mm can be easily missed. The definitive test is an angiogram.

Magnetic resonance venography permits noninvasive visualization of the venous structures (veins and sinuses), which is especially important when venous or sinus thrombosis is suspected (eg, trauma, infection, or hypercoaguable states). Some patients with benign intracranial hypertension or pseudotumor cerebri have sinus thrombosis.

▲ **Clinical Warnings:**
- Imaging studies are essential when the presentation suggests increased intracranial pressure, possible structural lesions, or a degenerative process. If the clinician suspects any of these etiologies, a neurologic consultation is usually advisable.
- The provider should consider an EEG only when the differential diagnosis includes a seizure disorder or progressive cognitive impairment and, possibly, unexplained altered mental status. If there is a significant change in mental status associated with the headache, then the neurologist may order an EEG to assess the organization and quality of the background activity and the presence of abnormal patterns. An EEG is almost never an initial procedure. Although patients with migraine headaches often have EEG abnormalities, few neurologists use the EEG for establishing the diagnosis.

MANAGEMENT

The management of headaches in the child or adolescent includes the following steps:

- Diagnosis: Identify the type(s) of headaches.
- Examination: Perform a pediatric and neurologic examination.
- Psychosocial assessment: Assess patient, family, and peers.

- Treatment plan:
  - Establish therapeutic goals.
  - Determine nonpharmacologic treatment.
  - Discuss pharmacologic treatment.
    - Abortive
    - Prophylactic
  - Monitor response to treatment and adjust interventions.

Because nonpharmacologic treatments of headache are the initial therapies, these are discussed first.

Nonpharmacologic Treatment

Helping the child and family recognize and modify specific stressors, such as school, homework, presentations, peer relations, or family dynamics, may yield significant improvement in the headaches. If significant emotional problems exist, consultation with a mental health specialist is essential.

Other simple, inexpensive measures can improve headache symptoms. For example, ice therapy for 10 to 15 minutes every hour for 2 to 3 hours (if necessary) may help ameliorate the headaches. Resting in a darkened room and sleep are often effective, although they may not be convenient or feasible if the headache occurs during school hours.

Lifestyle adjustments reduce the frequency and severity of headaches. Simple adjustments include sleep regulation, which involves developing routines for going to bed and arising and ensuring that the child or teenager has adequate sleep. Similarly, dietary interventions can sometimes prove efficacious. The provider should discuss the importance of regular mealtimes, including eating breakfast to avoid relative hypoglycemia, which may trigger headaches in some children and adolescents. Appendix 51-1 provides a list delineating the most commonly suspected dietary agents that may provoke migraine.

● **Clinical Pearl:** The response to elimination diets is highly variable and unpredictable in the absence of specific factors elicited in the history. Only a small percentage of patients respond to elimination diets. Because the relationship between diet and migraine headaches is at least partially anecdotal, families should understand that not every person has headaches triggered by specific foods each time they are consumed. In some patients, there seems to be a threshold effect, requiring a certain amount or combination. When trying an elimination diet, select the three or four items that the patient may consume excessively or to which the child may be susceptible. Have the patient refrain from these for 3 to 4 weeks and return for reevaluation. Enlist the assistance of the patient in the experiment, explaining that together, provider, child, and parents will reevaluate the response at the next visit in 3 to 4 weeks. If there is no change, try another three to four items in a similar trial.

Pharmacologic Treatment

Pharmacologic management includes treatment of individual headaches and prophylactic medications. The major drug classes used for the treatment of individual headaches include the following:

- Analgesics, useful for both episodic TTH and migraine headaches
- Antiemetics, for migraine
- Abortives, for migraine

Analgesic Medications

Analgesics play an important role in the treatment of both episodic TTH and migraine headaches. Always begin with the simplest and safest therapy. Analgesics fall into four categories:

1. Simple analgesics
   Acetaminophen
   Aspirin (not to be used in children or when the risk of Reye syndrome exists)
   Nonsteroidal anti-inflammatory drugs (NSAIDs; risk of peptic ulcer disease)
   COX-2 inhibitors (role in headache unclear; very useful in patients with a history of gastritis, gastroesophageal reflux, or ulcers)
   Caffeine
2. Simple analgesics with alternate routes of administration
   Indomethacin PR (not for young children)
   Ketorolac (Toradol) IM, IV
3. Combination analgesics
   Aspirin and/or acetaminophen in combination with a barbiturate and/or caffeine (eg, butalbital [Fiorinal], butalbital APAP [Fioricet, Axocet], Excedrin Migraine)
   Acetaminophen with codeine

Isometheptene (Midrin)—a sympathomimetic with acetaminophen and dichloalphenazone, a choral hydrate derivative (not approved for young children)
4. High-potency analgesics—almost never used in children except with postoperative pain or terminal illnesses

Table 51-5 lists the doses and formulations of the common analgesic medications.

Antiemetic Medications for Migraine Headaches

Because nausea and vomiting virtually never occur in TTH, antiemetics play a role only in migraine headaches. They often work well together with an analgesic agent. Table 51-6 lists antiemetic medications and their dosages.

▲ **Clinical Warnings:**
- The antiemetic medications can cause extrapyramidal side effects, which usually respond to diphenhydramine (Benadryl).
- Because the medium- and high-potency analgesics and the antiemetics can cause drowsiness, adolescent patients must be warned to avoid driving and using dangerous equipment.

Abortive Treatment of Migraine Headaches

Abortive treatment of individual migraine headaches, using either of the two major classes, the triptans and ergot derivatives, is a cornerstone of management when simple or moderate analgesics have failed. Because most neurologists begin with a triptan and because most primary care providers will not use the ergots, the ergotamine preparations are summarized in Appendix 51-4. Table 51-7 details the major triptan preparations.

Although the use of triptan agents in children is not FDA approved, some companies did post-marketing studies with sumatriptan. Many pediatric neurologists do use these medications in children older than 6 years when analgesics and antiemetics are ineffective.

Contraindications to triptan medications include the following:

- Do not use ergotamines within 24 hours of using a triptan drug, and vice versa.

Table 51-5. ANALGESIC MEDICATIONS IN THE MANAGEMENT OF MIGRAINE

Medication	Dose	Formulation
Acetaminophen (Tylenol)	10–15 mg/kg per dose every 4 h	Tablet: 80, 325, 500 mg Syrup: 160 mg/tsp
Ibuprofen (Advil)	5–10 mg/kg per dose q.i.d.	Tablet: 200, 400, 600, 800 mg Syrup: 100 mg/tsp
Naproxen sodium (Naprosyn)	10–20 mg/kg per dose b.i.d.	Tablet: 250, 375 mg Oral suspension: 25 mg/mL
Butalbital APAP (Fioricet)	1 every 3–4 h, maximum of 3 per day or 6 per wk in teenagers	Tablet
Codeine	0.5–1.0 mg/kg per dose every 4–6 h	Tablet: 15, 30, 60 mg Elixir terpine hydrate with codeine: 10 mg/5 mL
Isometheptene (Midrin)	1 or 2 at onset, then 1 every 4 h; maximum of 2 per day, 6 per week; use in adolescents only	Capsule

Table 51–6. ANTIEMETIC MEDICATIONS IN THE MANAGEMENT OF MIGRAINE

Medication	Dose	Formulation
Promethazine (Phenergan)	0.25–0.5 mg/kg per dose	Tablet: 12.5, 25, 50 mg
		Syrup: 6.25, 12.5 mg/tsp
Prochlorperazine (Compazine)	2.5–5.0 mg b.i.d.	Tablet: 10, 15 mg
	2.5 mg b.i.d. (9–13 kg)	Syrup: 5 mg/tsp
	2.5 mg b.i.d.–t.i.d. (14–18 kg)	Suppository: 2.5, 5, 25 mg (write 2.5 as 2½ mg to prevent
	15 mg max (over 19 kg)	confusion with 25 mg suppository)
Chlorpromazine (Thorazine)	0.5–1.0 mg/kg PO,	Tablet: 10, 25, 50 mg
	IV q6h	Syrup: 10 mg/5 mL
		Ampule: 25 mg/mL
Trimethobenzamide (Tigan)	100–200 mg b.i.d.–t.i.d.	Tablet: 100, 250 mg
	15-20 mg 1 kg 1d PO	Suppository: 100, 200 mg
Metoclopramide (Reglan)	1–2 mg/kg; max 10 mg	Tablet: 5, 10 mg
		Syrup: 5 mg/tsp

b.i.d. = twice daily; t.i.d. = three times per day.

- Do not use a second (different) triptan within 24 hours of using the first.
- Avoid in hemiplegic and basilar artery migraine.
- Avoid in patients with significant cardiac disease, including angina, ischemic heart disease, and uncontrolled hypertension.
- Rizatriptan only: Use only 5-mg tablet for patients on β-blockers.

Side effects of triptans include chest tightness and pressure, paresthesias, dry mouth, nausea, and dizziness (usually seen with the nasal spray and subcutaneous forms); rarely, aggravation of the headaches may occur.

With the exception of Tfelt-Hansen's study (1998), which showed a minimal advantage for zolmitriptan over sumatriptan, there does not appear to be any consistent, significant difference among the different triptans. However, some patients may experience more complete relief or fewer side effects with one particular preparation. At present, the triptans are the treatment of choice for migraine headaches that do not respond to analgesic medication either alone or with an antiemetic.

Although the triptans are all closely related, there is some difference in the onset of action and duration, which can help the clinician select a medication. If the headache tends to last from several hours to all day, then start with naratriptan (Amerge). If the patient has significant nausea or vomiting that is present at or soon after the onset of the headache, try the sublingual form of rizatriptan (Maxalt MLT) or the sumatriptan nasal spray. Adding an NSAID to the initial dose of the triptan may increase the efficacy in some patients. If the headaches begin to return after a few hours, try repeating the dose of the NSAID first. If this does not consistently provide relief, then a second dose of the triptan or a change to a longer acting triptan (naratriptan) may improve the response.

Prophylactic Treatment

Placing a child or adolescent on daily prophylactic medication requires a careful assessment and thorough counseling with the patient and family. The following are indications for prophylaxis for both TTH and migraine headaches:

Table 51–7. TRIPTAN MEDICATIONS FOR THE MANAGEMENT OF MIGRAINE

Name	Formulation	Doses per Attack	Time to Onset (Minutes)
Sumatriptan* (Imitrex)	Tab: 25, 50 mg	100 mg	30–60
	Nasal spray:[†] 5,[‡] 20** mg	2	15–45
	Injection: 6 mg SC	2	10
Zolmitriptan (Zomig)	Tab: 2.5, 5.0 mg	2 in 24 h	30–60
Rizatriptan (Maxalt)	Tab: 5, 10 mg	3 in 24 h	30
	Sublingual: 10 mg (MLT)		
Naratriptan (Amerge)	Tablet: 1, 2.5 mg	3 in 24 h	60–90

b.i.d. = twice daily; t.i.d. = three times per day.
*Maximum dosage: 0.6 mg/kg
[†]All Sumatriptan nasal sprays: take one or two sour candies just before using (eg, Sour Patch or Warheads) to mask taste of spray.
[‡]Sumatriptan nasal spray 5 mg: patient < 50 lb (22 kg): 1 spray (= 5 mg); > 50 lb (22 kg) but < 100 lb (44 kg): 1 spray; if headache present in 20–30 min, then repeat 1 spray.
**Sumatriptan nasal spray 20 mg: patient > 100 lb (44 kg): use 1 spray; if headache present in 20–30 min, repeat 1 spray.
Winner, P. K. (1997). Treating headache in children. *Seminars in Headache Management*, 2(4), 12–13.
Linder, S. L. (1994). Treatment of childhood headache with dihydroergotamine mesylate. *Headache, 34*, 578–580.

- Headache frequency is about once per week.
- Headache frequency is twice monthly with prolonged duration of attacks (greater than 24–48 hours).
- Headaches become incapacitating, interfering significantly with school and activities.
- Abortive therapy is needed two or more times per week.
- Patient is unable to tolerate abortive medication or overuses analgesics and abortive agents.
- Abortive medication(s) cease to work.
- Special headache types occur (eg, severely incapacitating headaches, even if infrequent, or hemiplegic migraine with significant morbidity).

● **Clinical Pearl:** Always begin treatment with a single prophylactic agent. Reserve the use of polypharmacy for unusual situations in which specific problems exist. Abortive treatments for individual headaches should be continued when prophylactic medications are used.

Prophylactic Treatment of Migraine Headaches

The efficacy of the medications in Table 51-8 has been established in one or more controlled studies. Although they are FDA approved for migraine prophylaxis in adults, they have not been approved for use in children; nevertheless, they are commonly used by pediatric neurologists.

● **Clinical Pearl:** In routine clinical practice and in the absence of asthma, propranolol, of which use in children is supported by valid research, would usually be the initial drug of choice for migraine prophylaxis.

▲ **Clinical Warning:** The use of methysergide (Sansert) in children younger than 12 years should be considered only under the most unusual circumstances and only under the care of a headache specialist. The use of divalproex sodium (Depakote) especially in combination with other medications, has been associated with an increased incidence of severe or even fatal hepatic failure.

Table 51-9 lists non–FDA-approved medications that are accepted and frequently used by headache specialists. In some cases, one member of a pharmacologic family will have been approved (Battistella et al., 1990; Solomon, 1995). Many of these are commonly used by headache specialists, albeit in an "off-label" manner.

In addition to the information provided in Table 51-9, note the following:

- *Nadolol:* The main advantage is the ability to give a single daily dose. All the β-blockers have similar side effects and contraindication profiles.
- *Verapamil:* Calcium channel blockers have an equivocal role in the management of headaches. This would be a second-order medication in children and teenagers.
- *Cyproheptadine:* The advantage of this medication is its availability in a liquid form (elixir: 2 mg/5 mL), which facilitates its use in the younger pediatric population. Increase the dose slowly to avoid sedation.
- *Amitriptyline/nortriptyline:* The tricyclic antidepressants have long been used in the management of migraine. The major disadvantage of amitriptyline—sedation—may be useful when there is associated insomnia. Nortriptyline, one of the metabolic by-products of amitriptyline, seems to cause less sedation than amitryptyline. Start with a single bedtime dose.

▲ **Clinical Warning:** Current recommendations for amitriptyline/nortriptyline include obtaining a baseline electrocardiogram prior to initiating therapy and then periodically as the dose increases or if the patient experiences any significant side effects, such as dizziness, exertional symptoms, or chest pain.

- Riboflavin: Very limited research supports this treatment. In a study of adults, 15% of subjects taking placebo and 59% taking 400 mg of riboflavin had 50% improvement when treated for 3 months (Schoenen et al., 1998). Although the mechanism of action is unknown, headache is not a manifestation of riboflavin deficiency.

Table 51–8. FDA-APPROVED PROPHYLACTIC MEDICATIONS FOR MANAGEMENT OF MIGRAINE HEADACHES

Medication	Starting Dose	Maximum Dose	Formulation	Side Effects	Contraindications
Propranolol (Inderal)	10	0.6–2 mg/kg/d	Tablet: 10, 20, 40 mg	Asthma, cardiac conduction defect, nausea, shortness of breath, hair loss	Asthma, diabetes, A-V conduction defects (bradyarrhythmias), depression
			Long acting (LA) capsule: 60, 80, 120 mg	Same as propranolol	Same as propranolol
Timolol (Blocadren)	5	30 mg total	Tablet: 5, 10 mg		
Divalproex Na (Depakote)	125 mg	20–40 mg/kg	Sprinkle: 125 mg Capsule: 125, 250, 500 mg	Nausea, GI pain, hepatic dysfunction, pancytopenia, hair loss	Liver disease, thrombocytopenia
Methysergide (Sansert; adolescents only)	2 mg	8 mg total	Tablet: 2 mg	Systemic fibrosis, cramps, nausea, sedation	Peptic ulcer disease, hypertension, cardiovascular disease, familial fibrotic diseases

FDA = Food and Drug Administration; GI = gastrointestinal.

TABLE 51–9. NON–FDA-APPROVED PROPHYLACTIC MEDICATIONS FOR MANAGEMENT OF MIGRAINE HEADACHES

Medication	Starting Dose	Maximum Dose	Dosage	Side Effects	Contraindications
Nadolol (Corgard) β-blocker Advantage: can be given on a q.d. dosing basis	10 mg	240 mg	Tablet: 20, 40, 80 mg	Asthma, cardiac conduction defect, nausea, shortness of breath, hair loss, depression, fatigue	Asthma, diabetes, A-V conduction defects (bradyarrhythmias); depression is uncommon but would also be a contraindication if it occurred
Verapamil (Calan) Calcium channel blocker	40 mg	480 mg	Tablet: 40, 80, 120 mg	Constipation, peripheral edema	Bradycardia, hypotension, A-V conduction defects
Cyproheptadine (Periactin) Serotonin antagonist	2 mg	0.25–1.5 mg/kg/d	Syrup: 2 mg/5 mL Tablet: 4 mg	Drowsiness, constipation	Asthma, respiratory disease
Amitriptyline (Elavil)	10 mg	0.1–2.0 mg/kg/d	Tablet: 10, 25, 50 mg	Drowsiness, dry mouth, weight gain	Cardiac disease, glaucoma, MAOIs
Nortriptyline (Pamelor)	10 mg	0.1–2.0/ mg/kg/d	Capsule: 10, 25, 50 mg	Drowsiness, dry mouth, weight gain	Cardiac disease, glaucoma, MAOIs
Riboflavin	200 mg	400 mg	Tablet: 50, 100 mg	None known	
Gabapentin (Neurontin)	100 mg	2400 mg	Tablet: 100, 300 mg	Somnolence, dizziness, fatigue	Renal failure
Carbamazepine (Tegretol)	50–100 mg	20–40 mg/kg	Suspension: 100 mg/5 mL Tablet: 100 mg chewable, 200 mg	Sedation, GI, pancytopenia, hyponatremia	Liver abnormality
Magnesium (elemental)	300 mg	400 mg		Diarrhea, abdominal cramps	

FDA = Food and Drug Administration; GI = gastrointestinal; MAOIs = monoamine oxidase inhibitors.

- Magnesium: Magnesium's role in migraine and TTH is only partially understood. Magnesium may have an effect on central neuronal excitability and may be related to the spreading depression of neuronal activity. Several studies in adolescents and adults have documented depressed ionized magnesium levels in patients with migraine and TTH, even when total magnesium levels are normal (Mauskop et al., 1996; Peikert et al., 1996; Aloisi et al., 1997). Mauskop reports the most impressive results, using intravenous magnesium for the management of migraine and TTH. The individuals with the lowest serum ionized magnesium levels had the most dramatic responses to an infusion of magnesium. Serum ionized magnesium levels are difficult and expensive to measure. The recommended daily allowance for children and teens is 270 mg/d (elemental). Results with oral supplementation require up to 3 months to reach maximum benefit.
- Baclofen (Lioresal): An open-label study in older teenagers and adults reported substantial improvement in the frequency, duration, and severity of migraines with the use of baclofen (Hering-Hanit, 1999).

Prophylactic Treatment of Tension-Type Headaches

Chronic TTH often responds to the following medications:

- Tricyclic antidepressants
- Selective serotonin reuptake inhibitors (SSRIs) such as paroxetine (Paxil) or sertraline (Zoloft), beginning with low doses (5 mg and 12.5 mg, respectively) and slowly increasing as necessary
- Neurontin, beginning with a dose of about of 100 mg once or twice daily and increasing every 3 to 5 days as necessary
- Divalproex sodium, beginning at 5 mg/kg per day and increasing slowly

● **Clinical Pearl:** Do not neglect active exploration and treatment of psychosocial factors.

Polypharmacy

Modern prescribing practices discourage the use of polypharmacy, because the incidence of side effects increases significantly. However, there are situations in which such treatment can be quite helpful. Treatment should always begin with a single medication that has a minimal side-effect profile. For example, a child with migraine with symptoms of depression could be started with nortriptyline. If headache control were suboptimal and if the depression were well controlled, then one could add a small dose of an β-blocker, such as propranolol. Divalproex sodium would be a good alternative, except that its side-effect profile is less advantageous.

Other possible combination therapies for treatment of migraine headache are described in Table 51-10.

▲ **Clinical Warning:** Combinations to avoid include (1) β-blocker with calcium channel blockers or SSRIs, because of the risk of hypotension, and (2) divalproex sodium with barbiturates, because of the resulting increased levels of both drugs.

Table 51-10. POSSIBLE COMBINATION THERAPIES FOR THE MANAGEMENT OF MIGRAINE HEADACHES

Primary Drug	Possible Secondary Drug
β-Blocker	Tricyclic antidepressant, divalproex Na
Tricyclic antidepressant	β-Blocker, divalproex Na, calcium channel blocker, SSRI
Divalproex Na	β-Blocker, calcium channel blocker, tricyclic antidepressant, SSRI

SSRI = selective serotonin reuptake inhibitor.

Management of Special Headache Conditions

Patient who Cannot Swallow Solid Medications

The child who cannot swallow solid medications presents real management problems. As noted in Tables 51-5, 51-6, 51-7, and 51-9, only a few medications are available in a liquid form. For abortive therapy, acetaminophen and ibuprofen are available in liquid form. Sumatriptan (Imitrex) is available in a nasal spray form (5 mg and 20 mg), which can be used in cooperative children and in adolescents. Rizatriptan is available in a sublingual (MLT) form. Some pharmacists can formulate DHE as a lozenge, and it is now also available as a nasal spray; both of these may be useful for the older child or adolescent. For prophylactic therapy, neurontin (Gabapentin) capsules can be opened and the contents of the capsule dissolved in liquids or put directly in the mouth, followed by a drink of water; cyproheptadine (Periactin), divalproex, and carbamazepine (Tegretol) are all available in liquid form.

Rebound Headaches

Rebound headaches occur in patients with TTH or migraine headaches. As the headache frequency increases, the patient takes more and larger doses of medication(s), which become progressively less effective. Recognition of this pattern is critical, because all headache treatments will be futile until the patient undergoes "detoxification" from the overused medication. This requires neurologic and often psychological or psychiatric support.

▲ **Clinical Warning:** Rebound headaches can occur with the overuse of any class of medication for headaches (eg, simple analgesics, such as aspirin, acetaminophen, NSAIDs, and, especially, caffeine-containing preparations). Overuse of barbiturate, narcotic, ergotamine, and probably even triptan medications can also lead to rebound headaches (Lewis, 1995).

Incapacitating Migraine Headaches

The clinician will occasionally encounter a child with a severe or incapacitating migraine headache. If the child has had a thorough evaluation or is also under the care of a pediatric neurologist, then the information provided in Display 51-4 and Table 51-11 may provide guidance for the management of the acute, incapacitating headache in the emergency department or well-equipped clinic.

Menstrual Headaches

A substantial number of female adolescent patients with migraines will have some or all of their headaches in the peri-

---

DISPLAY 51-4 • Management of Acute, Incapacitating Migraine

History

Physical examination

Neurologic examination

Imaging study, if indicated (new headache, significant change in existing pattern)

Primary Medications
- Triptan SC or intranasal (cannot use ergotamine within 24 hours)

or
- Metoclopramide, 1–2 mg/kg to max 10 mg, alone or followed by DHE 0.25–1.0 mg, per age and weight (cannot use triptan within 14 hours) (see Table 51-11)

Adjunctive Medications
- Ketorolac, 15–60 mg IM depending on weight and age, (adolescents only)

and/or
- Magnesium sulfate, up to 1000 mg, given by slow IV push
- Compazine, 5–10 mg, slow IV

or
- Thorazine: mix 10 or 20 mg in total volume of 10 mL of normal saline (ie, 1–2 mg/mL of solution) and give at rate of 1–2 mg slowly over every 4–6 minutes. Almost all individuals respond, usually with 10–15 mg total. Must have IV hydration running briskly and observe for orthostatic hypotension for 20–30 minutes afterwards.

Patient should be started on some type of prophylactic medication before discharge from the emergency department.
Arrange for follow-up soon after discharge (2–5 days).
or
Admit patient for observation if there is any concern about underlying pathology, failure to respond to treatment, or the social situation.

DHE = dihydroergotamine; IM = intramuscular; IV = intravenous; SC = subcutaneous.

---

menstrual part of the cycle. Recognition of this pattern can lead to special treatment approaches, including the following:

- Explain the relationship to the patient and her family.
- Modify lifestyle during the time of increased susceptibility, including the following:
  - Avoiding chocolate, caffeine, simple sugars (candy), salty foods, cheese, nitrate- and nitrite-preserved foods, alcohol, or any of the patient's specific triggers
  - Maintaining adequate and regular sleep habits
  - Getting regular exercise (preferably at least 25 minutes per day of moderate activity, 5 days per week)
- Suggest that the patient take a B-vitamin supplement and vitamin E 400 IU.
- Suggest NSAIDs, such as naproxyn, on a twice-daily dose for 4 to 6 days prior to and continuing through the second or third day of the menses, if there is no medical contraindication.

Table 51–11. MANAGEMENT OF ACUTE, INCAPACITATING HEADACHE

Age	DHE (SC or IV)	DHE and Metoclopramide (PO or IV)
6–9 y	0.1 mg/dose	0.15 mg DHE, 30 min after 2 mg metoclopramide
9–12 y	0.15 mg/dose	0.15 mg DHE, 30 min after 5 mg metoclopramide
12–16 y	0.2 mg/dose	0.2 mg DHE, 30 min after 5–10 mg metoclopramide
	OR	

Age		Sumatriptan (Imitrex) SC
≥ 6 y		0.06 mg/kg, maximum = 6 mg

▲ **Clinical Warning:** No triptan can be used within 24 hours of any ergotamine, and vice versa.

DHE = dihydroergotamine; IM = intramuscular; IV = intravenous; PO = oral; SC = subcutaneous.
Winner, P. K. (1997). Treating headache in children. *Seminars in Headache Management, 2*(4), 12–13.
Linder, S. L. (1994). Treatment of childhood headache with dihydroergotamine mesylate. *Headache, 34,* 578–580.

- Plan and explain a treatment program for the headaches if they occur, as outlined in the section on treatment of the individual or episodic migraine headache.
- Monitor the response, and adjust accordingly.

Complementary Medications for Migraine

Many patients express interest in "natural," herbal, or alternative therapies for headaches. The most consistently cited herb is feverfew (Tanacetum parthenium), a daisy-like perennial. O'Hara, Kiefer, Farrell, and Kemper (1998) reviewed three double-blind placebo-controlled studies. Two studies confirmed feverfew's efficacy while the third did not. Feverfew causes vasodilation, reduces inflammation, and inhibits platelet aggregation, phagocytosis, and the secretion of inflammatory mediators, such as arachidonic acid and serotonin. It may also down-regulate cerebrovascular biogenic amines, which may explain why continued use for several months is necessary to obtain optimal results. Side effects include the development of aphthous ulcers and gastrointestinal irritation and rebound headaches with sudden discontinuation. Refer to Chapter 4 for more information on feverfew's actions.

▲ **Clinical Warning:** Because the safety and efficacy of feverfew in children are unknown, it cannot be recommended.

Clinicians should be aware that some herbal products (eg, ma huang [ephedra], evening primrose oil, gingko biloba, saw palmetto berry) may actually cause headaches. A complete history of all allopathic and complementary medications should be sought in each patient. Indiscriminate use of herbal medications could cause significant side effects either directly or by interacting with allopathic medications.

▲ **Clinical Warning:** Ephedra, a component of many preparations used for treating a wide variety of ailments, can cause arrhythmias, myocardial infarction, seizures, renal stones, tremor, hypertension, stroke, and even death (Cupp, 1999).

What to Tell Parents

Discuss the diagnosis with the patient in an age-appropriate manner and with the parents. Acknowledge the pain and the headache. Discuss the treatment goals and plan, which should include the following:

- Headache diary (see Appendix 51-2): If the patients are sufficiently mature, they should be able to keep the log with minimal assistance from parents. The practitioner should review the log at each visit.
- List of potential trigger factors (see Appendix 51-1): Emphasize that these are only guidelines, especially the lists of specific foods.
- Modification of specific or general stressors, including the following:
  - School is by far the major stressor for most children and adolescents. Sometimes, helping the child deal with issues such as procrastination in preparing assignments and projects will indirectly help the headaches. If learning disabilities are present, specific intervention may be very helpful.
  - Self-image issues (eg, issues arising from acne) can affect social adjustment in school and act as general stressors.
  - Family issues are often significant, especially when marital problems, substance abuse, and siblings with significant medical or psychological problems are present. Addressing these issues is essential in the treatment of the child with headaches.
  - Establish regular sleep habits, avoiding significant changes in time of retiring and awakening in the morning.
  - Establish regular mealtimes and avoid skipping meals.
  - Consider relaxation therapy. Biofeedback techniques, which can be used in some children as young as 6 years, involve the patient's learning to modify specific physiologic functions, which have been associated empirically with a reduction in pain. Typically, a psychologist or biofeedback therapist teaches the technique(s). Unfortunately, most managed care plans do not cover such services. Other relaxation techniques, such as visualization, breathing, meditation, and massage, may play a useful adjunctive role in headache management.

Educate parents about the treatment plan for managing individual headaches, incorporating the following:

- Indications for specific medications and directions for use
- Review of side-effect profile
- Indications requiring parents to contact the clinician
- Day care/school treatment:
  - Child who is attending day care or school should continue in class, if at all possible.

- Discuss with the patient and the family that minimizing missed school or coming home from school will help avoid issues of secondary gain.
- Communicate with school nurse/personnel to facilitate headache management and keep the child in school.
- Clearly write instructions for administration of medication and other treatments in school; see Appendix 51-5 for a sample form.
- Activity restrictions:
  - Mild headaches: Modifications may not be necessary.
  - Moderate or severe headaches: The patient should be excused from gym or physical education activities on the day of the headache and occasionally on the following day.
- Imaging studies: Imaging studies are not mandatory for every child with headache. See guidelines for ordering imaging studies described earlier in this chapter. The decision not to order imaging studies should be discussed with the parents.
- Call back: Parents should be instructed to call the provider if either of the following develops:
  - Any questions about medications or instructions
  - Any change in the headache pattern or the emergence of new symptoms
- Reevaluation: Headache of recent origin or in a young child requires a reevaluation within 4 to 6 weeks. Display 51-5 lists conditions and situations that should serve as red flags to the provider. Warning signs and symptoms of increased intracranial pressure should be reviewed with the family and specific instructions given to contact the clinician immediately if any of the following develop:
  - Increasing frequency of headaches
  - Increasing severity of headaches
  - Emergence of new symptoms, especially vomiting or change in level of alertness, gait, coordination, visual (especially diplopia), or cognitive function
  - Nocturnal awakening
  - Headaches upon awakening in the morning
  - Increased difficulty in awakening the child in the morning

The child who develops a severe, acute headache with alteration of level of consciousness, vomiting, or focal symptoms requires emergent evaluation in an emergency room setting.

DISPLAY 51-5 • Red Flag Headaches

Patient younger than 6 years
New onset of headaches
Progressive symptoms, especially if change is rapid
Nocturnal awakening
Headache on awakening
Vomiting
Loss of cognitive/neurologic functioning
Significant change in existing headache pattern
Focal neurologic signs
Papilledema
Head trauma with loss of consciousness lasting more than 10 minutes
Inability to control the headaches
Emergence of significant psychosocial problems

COMMUNITY RESOURCES

The provider and patients should be especially careful to evaluate the source and credibility of any information gleaned from the World Wide Web.

Pediatric neurologists can be located through local medical societies, medical schools, or the Child Neurology Society.

Child Neurology Society
3900 Northwoods Drive, Suite 175
St. Paul, MN 55112.
Telephone: (651) 486-9447
Fax: (651) 486-9436
Internet address: *http://www.umn.edu*

New York Online Access to Health (NOAH)
Ask NOAH About: Headache
Internet address:
http://www.noah.cuny.edu/headache/headache.html

Journal of the American Medical Association
Migraine Information Center
Internet address:
http://www.ama-assn.org/special/migraine/migraine.htm
Children and Migraines
Internet Address:
http://www.ama-assn.org/special/migraine/support/educate/child.htm

American Council for Headache Education
19 Mantua Road
Mt. Royal, NJ 08061
Telephone: (856) 423-0043
Fax: (856) 423-0082
Internet address: http://www.ahsnet.org

REFERENCES

Abu-Arafeh, I., & Russell, G. (1995a). Paroxysmal vertigo as a migraine equivalent in children: A population-based study. *Cephalalgia, 15*, 22–25.

Abu-Arafeh, I., & Russell, G. (1995b). Prevalence and clinical features of abdominal migraine compared with those of migraine headache. *Arch Dis Child, 72*, 413–417.

Aloisi, P., Marrelli, A., Porto, C., Tozzi, E., & Cerone, G. (1997). Visual evoked potentials and serum magnesium levels in juvenile migraine patients. *Headache, 37*, 383–385.

Arroyo, S., Sanchez-Portocarrero, J., Barquero, S., Garcia Urra, D., & Varela de Seijas, E. (1990). Complicated migraine: A study of 7 cases. *Neurologia, 5*(4), 125–129.

Barlow, C. F. (1994). Migraine in the infant and toddler. *J Child Neurol, 9*, 92–94.

Battistella, P. A., Ruffilli, R., Moro, R., Fabiani, H., Berton, S., Antolini, A., & Zacchello, F. (1990). A placebo-controlled crossover trial of nimodipine in pediatric migraine. *Headache, 30*, 264–268.

Bigby, M., Stern, R.S. (1988). Adverse reactions to isotretinoin. A report from the Adverse Drug Reaction Reporting System. *Journal of the American Academy of Dermatology, 18*, 543–552.

Bille, B. (1962). Migraine in school children. *Acta Paediatr Scand, 51*(Suppl 136), 1–151.

Bordley, J. E., & Bosley, W. R. (1973). Mucoceles of the frontal sinus: Causes and treatment. *Ann Otol Rhinol Laryngol, 82*, 696–702.

Britton, B. H., & Block, L. D. (1988). Vertigo in the pediatric and adolescent age group. *Laryngoscope, 98*, 139–146.

Burton, L. J., Quinn, B., Pratt-Cheyney, J.L., & Pourani, M. (1997). Headache etiology in a pediatric emergency department. *Pedi-*

atr Emerg Care, 13, 1–4.

Capurso, U., Marini, I., Vecchiet, F., Bonetti, G.A. (1997). Headache and cranio-mandibular disorders during adolescence. *J Clin Pediatr Dent, 21,* 117–123.

Carlsson, J. (1996). Prevalence of headache in schoolchildren: Relation to family and school factors. *Acta Paediatr, 85,* 692–696.

Cavazzuti, G. B., & Ferrari, P. (1982). Childhood periodic syndromes and their long-term development. *Pediatria Medica E Chirurgia, 4,* 593–600.

Cooper, B. C., & Cooper, D. L. (1993). Recognizing otolaryngologic symptoms in patients with temporomandibular disorders. *Cranio, 11,* 260–267.

Cupp, M. J. (1999). Herbal remedies: Adverse effects and drug interactions. *American Family Physician, 59,* 1239–1245.

Emergy, E. S. (1977). Acute confusional state in children with migraine. *Pediatrics, 60,* 111–114.

Eviatar, L. (1981). Vestibular testing in basilar artery migraine. *Annals of Neurology, 9,* 126–130.

Freedman, P. (1999). Management of altitude sickness. Personal communication.

Gascon, G., & Barlow, C. (1970). Juvenile migraine, presenting as an acute confusional state. *Pediatrics, 45,* 628–635.

Gokhale, R., Huttenlocher, P. R., Brady, L., & Kirschner, B.S. (1997). Use of barbiturates in the treatment of cyclic vomiting during childhood [Published erratum appears in 1997, J Pediatr Gastroenterol Nutr, 25, 559.] *J Pediatr Gastroenterol Nutr, 25,* 64–67.

Hering-Hanit, R. (1999). Baclofen for prevention of migraine. *Cephalalgia, 19,* 589–591.

International Headache Society (1997). ICD-10 guide for headaches. *Cephalalgia, 17*(Suppl. 19), 1–82.

Jensen, T. S. (1980). Transient global amnesia in childhood. *Dev Med Child Neurol, 22,* 654–658.

Lewis, D. W. (1995). Migraine and migraine variants in childhood and adolescence. *Semin Pediatr Neurol, 2,* 127–143.

Linder, S. L. (1994). Treatment of childhood headache with dihydroergotamine mesylate. *Headache, 34,* 578–580.

Marcus, D., Scharff, L., Mercer, S., & Turk, D. (1999). Musculoskeletal abnormalities in chronic headache: A controlled comparison of headache diagnostic groups. *Headache, 39,* 21–27.

Mauskop, A., Altura, B. T., Cracco, R.Q., & Altura, B.H. (1996). Intravenous magnesium sulfate rapidly alleviates headaches of various types. *Headache, 36,* 154–160.

O'Hara, M., Kiefer, D., Farrell, K., & Kemper, K. (1998). A review of 12 commonly used medicinal herbs. *Archives of Family Medicine, 7,* 523–536.

Peikert, A., Wilimzig, C., Kohne-Volland, R. (1996). Prophylaxis of migraine with oral magnesium: results from a prospective, multi-center, placebo-controlled and double-blind randomized study. *Cephalalgia, 16,* 257–263.

Pilley, J. R., Mohlin, B., Shaw, W.C., & Kingdon, A. (1992). A survey of craniomandibular disorders in 800 15-year-olds. A follow-up study of children with malocclusion. *Eur J Orthod, 14,* 152–161.

Pollack, M. A. (1999). Commentary on pediatric headaches. Personal communication.

Raieli, V., Raimondo, D., Cammalleri, R., & Camarda, R. (1995). Migraine headaches in adolescents: A student population-based study in Monreale. *Cephalalgia 15,* 5–12, discussion 4.

Sarhan, H. (1998). The therapeutic potential of 5-HT 1B autoreceptors and heteroreceptors and 5-HT Moduline in CNS disorders. *CNS Spectrums, 3*(8), 50–58.

Scheller, J. M. (1995). The history, epidemiology, and classification of headaches in childhood. *Semin Pediatr Neurol, 2,* 102–108.

Schoenen, J., Jacquy, J., & Lenaerls, M. (1998). Effectiveness of high-dose riboflavin in migraine prophylaxis. A randomized controlled trial [see comments]. *Neurology, 50,* 466–470.

Shuper, A., Packer, R. J., Vezina, L.G., Nicholson, H.S., & Laford, D. (1995). "Complicated migraine-like episodes" in children following cranial irradiation and chemotherapy. *Neurology, 45,* 1837–1840.

Sillanpaa, M., & Anttila, P. (1996). Increasing prevalence of headache in 7-year-old schoolchildren. *Headache, 36,* 466–470.

Sjaastad, O., Fredriksen, T. A., et al. (1989). The localization of the initial pain of attack. A comparison between classic migraine and cervicogenic headache. *Funct Neurol, 4,* 73–78.

Solomon, G. D. (1995). Pharmacology of medications used in treating headache. *Seminars in Pediatric Neurology, 2,* 165–177.

Swaiman, K. (1994). *Pediatric neurology: Principles and practice* (pp. 661–714). St. Louis: Mosby.

Sweeting, H., & West, P. (1998). Health at age 11: Reports from schoolchildren and their parents. *Arch Dis Child, 78,* 427–434.

Tfelt-Hansen, P. (1998). Oral rizatriptan versus oral sumatriptan: A direct comparative study in the acute treatment of migraine. *Headache, 38,* 748–755.

Waeber, C. (1998). The role of 5-HT 1B/1D receptors in the treatment of migraine. *CNS Spectrums, 3*(8), 30–39.

Winner, P., Martinez, W., Mate, L., & Bello, L. (1995). Classification of pediatric migraine: Proposed revisions to the IHS criteria. *Headache, 35,* 407–410.

Winner, P. K. (1997). Treating headache in children. *Seminars in Headache Management, 2*(4), 12–13.

Withers, G. D., Silburn, S. R., & Forbes, D.A. (1998). Precipitants and aetiology of cyclic vomiting syndrome. *Acta Paediatr, 87,* 272–277.

Wober-Bingol, C., Wober, C., Wagner-Ennsgraber, C., Karwautz, A., Vesely, C., Zebenhoizer, K., Geldner, J. (1996). IHS criteria for migraine and tension-type headache in children and adolescents. *Headache, 36,* 231–238.

Worawattanakul M., Rhoads, J. M., Lichtman, S. N., & Ulshen, M. H. (1999). Abdominal migraine: Prophylactic treatment and follow-up. *J Pediatr Gastroenterol Nutr, 28,* 37–40.

A P P E N D I X   5 1 – 1

Potential Trigger Factors in Patients With Migraine Headaches

Potential Triggers for Migraine Headaches

Emotional tension or relaxation after tension
Lack of sleep or oversleeping
High humidity, heat, sunbathing
Intense light, glare, flickering lights
Physical exertion or fatigue
High altitudes, airplanes
Pungent odors from perfumes, smoke, solvents

Head injury
Hunger or fasting
Weather changes
Menstruation
Birth control pills, estrogen
Pregnancy and postdelivery
Overuse of pain medications

Foods That May Produce Headaches

Food Class	Avoid	Acceptable
Dairy	Aged, strongly flavored cheeses	American cheese
	Yogurt	Cottage cheese
	Sour cream	Velveeta
Beverages	Coffee, colas, other caffeine-containing drinks, tea, chocolate	Noncaffeinated beverages
	Alcohol: wine and liquor	
Meats and fish	Canned, salted, dried meats and fish	Broiled, baked, roasted meats
	Pickled meats and fish	
	Nitrate- and nitrite-containing meats	
	Aged game, fermented sausage	
	Luncheon meats (eg, bologna, salami, pastrami, hot dogs)	
	Fried foods	
Fruits and vegetables	Avocados, bananas, citrus fruits, figs, onions, papayas, raspberries, red plums	
Beans and grains	Broad beans, fava beans, lima beans, lentils, soy beans, wheat	
Miscellaneous	Chocolate, vanilla, licorice, molasses	
	Yeast extracts and homemade yeast breads	
	Various nuts, peanut butter	
	Soy sauce, soup cubes, monosodium glutamate (MSG)	
	Occasionally ice cream and other cold foods	
	Metabisulfite in wines and salad bars, vinegar	
	Coffee-flavored foods	
	Aspartame (Nutrasweet)	

A P P E N D I X   5 1 – 2

Patient Headache Log

A log is an excellent tool to help patients increase their awareness of their headaches, potential triggers, aggravating and ameliorating factors, and other patterns. The following is an example of a log that can be given to patients:

HEADACHE LOG

Date	Pain Severity (Mild, Moderate, Severe)	Time of Onset	Duration of Pain	Name, Number of Pills Taken	Comments (provocative factors; what you were thinking, doing, feeling; responses to treatments)

A P P E N D I X 5 1 – 3

Possible Laboratory Studies in Patients With Headaches

Order laboratory tests specifically to answer clinical questions or to monitor therapeutic interventions.

Basic Laboratory Assessment

Complete blood count (CBC)
Fasting biochemical profile
Thyroid-stimulating hormone level
Sedimentation rate
Antinuclear antibodies (ANA)
Lyme titer (depending on geographic factors)

Comprehensive Laboratory Assessment

Basic profile
Vasculitic profile: double-stranded DNA, anticardiolipin assay, lupus anticoagulant, prothrombin time/partial thromboplastin time (PT/PTT), antithrombin III, protein S, protein C, VDRL
Amino acid screen
Lactic acid
Infection: Lyme disease, Ehrlichiosis, infectious mononucleosis
Tumor profile: 24-hour vanillylmandelic acid (VMA), catecholamines, epinephrine, cortisol levels, serum protein electrophoresis
Cryoglobulin

A P P E N D I X   5 1 – 4

Ergotamine Preparations

Preparation	Formulation	Doses per Attack	Maximum Dosage (adolescents)
Ergotamine tartrate			
Oral	1 mg plus caffeine 100 mg	2–4 tab	2–4 tab/d; 7–10 tab/wk
Sublingual	2 mg	1–3 tab	2 tab/d; 5 tab/wk
Suppository	2 mg plus caffeine 100 mg	½–2 sup	2 sup/d; 5 sup/wk
Dihydroergotamine			
Intranasal	4 mg/mL	0.5 mg per nostril, repeating in 15 min	2 mg/d
Intramuscular	1 mg/mL	0.25–1 mg	3 mg/d
Intravenous	1 mg/mL	0.25–1 mg	3 mg/d

sup = suppository; tab = tablet.

Treatment of Migraine Headaches: Specific Agents

Ergotamine and Dihydroergotamine (DHE)
Action
   More nonspecific activator of 5-HT receptors
   Vasoconstrictors
Advantages
   Efficacy
   Intravenous form (DHE)
Disadvantages
   Limited use in children except in inpatient/emergency setting
   Potential for rebound
   Risk of ergotism from excessive use and protracted vasoconstriction
   Risk of ischemia to muscles, myocardium
   Nausea, vomiting, muscle cramps, encephalopathy
Role in migraine treatment in children and adolescents
   Limited use in children older than about 7 years as secondary agent
   Limited use in children with intractable migraine when given in an inpatient setting
   As a detoxifying agent in adolescents with chronic rebound headaches from overuse of analgesic agents
Cannot use within 24 hours of taking any triptan medication.

Triptans
5-HT receptor agonists, mainly at 1B/1D sites
Highly effective
Reasonable side-effect profile
Cannot use within 24 hours of taking any ergotamine/DHE medication.

APPENDIX 51 – 5

Information and Instruction Sheet for the School

Name: _____ Age: ____ Grade: _____ Date: _____

_____ (name) is under my care for _____ (type) headaches.

Allergies: _____ none. _____

If he/she has a headache, please follow these guidelines. If you have any concerns or questions about the child's condition or this headache in particular, please contact the family at _____ or my office at _____ .

_____ Allow the child to go to the nurse's office.

_____ Assess the child's condition and complaints: precipitating factors, location of pain, quality and severity of pain, aggravating factors, ameliorating factors.

_____ If this is a "typical" headache, please do the following:

• Allow the child to rest in a darkened room.

• Reassure the child that you are there and you will help him/her feel better.

• Ice pack for the head for 10 to 15 minutes at a time; repeat every 15 to 30 minutes as necessary.

• When the child feels better, he/she should return to class.

_____ No physical education class for remainder of day if child has _____ any, _____ moderate, _____ severe headache.

_____ **Medication for mild headache:** _____

_____ Acetaminophen mg at onset of the headache; you may repeat _____ mg in _____ hours

_____ Ibuprofen _____ mg at the onset of the headache; you may repeat ___ mg in _____ hours

_____ **Medication for moderate to severe headache:** _____

_____ Ibuprofen _____ at the onset of the headache; you may repeat _____ mg in _____ hours

_____ Butalbital APAP: 1 at the onset of the headache; you may repeat _____ in _____ hours

_____ (Triptan) mg via _____ po or _____ sublingual at the onset of the headache; you may repeat _____ mg in _____ hours

_____ **Medication for nausea and or vomiting:** _____

_____ (name) _____ mg by _____ (route: po, pr) at onset of _____ headache, _____ nausea, _____ vomiting

If you have any concerns about this headache or the recommendations for medications, please contact the parent or our office.

_____ (your signature)

Congenital and Acquired Vision Disorders

• MORTON A. ALTERMAN, MD

INTRODUCTION

Education programs in primary care usually allow little time for exposure to ocular disease, despite vision being considered the dearest of senses. The effort to evaluate the eyes systematically as part of each examination is important. The eyes are exposed organs, and a great deal may be learned from their examination without needing the specialized equipment found in the eye clinic. The ophthalmoscope may be helpful for external and internal examination. If additional instruction in its use is necessary, the provider may find a short time with a friendly ophthalmologist or optometrist beneficial. This chapter provides content related to the assessment of visual acuity, as well as the diagnosis and primary care management of visual disorders commonly seen in pediatrics. Information related to rare eye diseases and serious complications of disease is presented briefly, because serious disease falls within the purview of the ophthalmologist.

VISUAL ACUITY

Testing of visual acuity or screening for potential vision problems can and should begin shortly after birth, when the red reflex may be evaluated and obvious structural abnormalities noted (American Academy of Ophthalmology [AAO], 1997). Table 52-1 guides the provider in the timing of screening examinations. It also provides criteria for ophthalmology referral.

Strabismus

The term "strabismus" is from a Greek root alluding to ocular misalignment. This cosmetic blemish may disturb a parent's early attitudes toward a child and the child's later relations with peers. Amblyopia is defined as diminished vision despite an anatomically normal eye. It is a frequent but usually reversible sequella of ocular misalignment if treatment starts in infancy or early childhood. Providers should encourage parents to seek early treatment and to continue regular follow-up. Amblyopia is unlikely to recur after age 9 or 10 years.

Epidemiology

Esotropia is a convergence of the ocular axes. It may be hereditary and is the most common form of strabismus. It occurs in 1% to 2% of births (Nelson, 1998). Infantile esotropia is categorized as being evident within the first 6 months of life. The degree of esotropia is usually quite marked. The infant may use the right eye to visualize objects to the left and the left eye to visualize objects to the right (crossed fixation). Esotropia may simulate bilateral sixth cranial nerve palsy, a much rarer cause of esotropia.

Acquired esotropia is most frequent between ages 1 and 3 years and commonly is related to hyperopia (farsightedness). Acquired esotropia has a marked propensity to cause amblyopia.

▲ **Clinical Warning:** A complaint of double vision or a tendency to close one eye to avoid double vision indicates recent onset or intermittent symptoms and warrants urgent referral.

Pseudoesotropia is characterized by a wide nasal root and prominent but normal epicanthal folds. Little sclera shows medial to the corneas. The turn therefore seems most marked on gaze left or right, although the ocular axes are aligned.

Exotropia, or outward ocular deviation, is much less frequent in early infancy. At its outset, exotropia is usually intermittent, occurring with fatigue, fever, illness, or on first awakening. It may be difficult to elicit on casual examination.

● **Clinical Pearl:** Parents who report having observed a transient exotropia almost always are correct. Because it is intermittent, amblyopia is less likely to occur than constant misalignment. Delayed referral has no benefit.

Hypertropia or vertical misalignment occurs less frequently than horizontal misalignment. These two forms will frequently coexist. Most common is overaction on one or both inferior oblique muscles, resulting in an upward deviation of the adducted eye (toward the nose) in lateral gaze. Tilting of the head may correct the diplopia, in this instance simulating primary torticollis.

▲ **Clinical Warning:** The provider must rule out ocular torticollis before considering any surgical intervention for torticollis.

● **Clinical Pearl:** Associated neurologic conditions, including myasthenia gravis, are more common with vertical strabismus than purely horizontal misalignment.

History and Physical Examination

The light reflex test (Hirshberg's test) is helpful if strabismus is moderate to severe. To perform it properly, the child must gaze directly at the examiner's light. The reflection should be in the same position in each pupil. If clearly lateral in one eye, that eye is esotropic. If clearly medial, that eye is exotropic. When in doubt, the provider should assume that misalignment exists. The clinician should then refer the child to an ophthalmologist who specializes in infants and children. Diagnosis is made by physical examination.

Table 52–1.   RECOMMENDED AGE, SCREENING METHODS, AND CRITERIA FOR REFERRAL IN EYE EXAMINATION*

Recommended Age for Screening	Screening Method	Criteria for Referral to an Ophthalmologist
Newborn–3 mo	Red reflex	Abnormal or asymmetric
	Inspection	Structural abnormality
6 mo–1 yr	As above, plus fix and follow with each eye	Failure to fix and follow in cooperative infant
	Alternate occlusion	Failure to object equally to covering each eye
	Corneal light reflex	Asymmetric
	Red reflex	Abnormal or asymmetric
	Inspection	Structural abnormality
3 y (approximately)	Visual acuity*	20/50 or worse, or two lines of difference between the eyes
	Corneal light reflex/cover-uncover†	Asymmetric/ocular refixation movements
	Red reflex*	Abnormal or asymmetric
	Inspection	Structural abnormality
5 y (approximately)	As above plus visual acuity*	20/40 or worse or two lines of difference between the eyes
	Stereo acuity**	Failure to appreciate stereopsis
Older than 5 y	As above but visual acuity*	20/30 or worse or two lines of difference between the eyes

*Figures, letters, "tumbling E," or optotypes. Standard eye charts include 20/20, 20/25, 20/30, 20/40, 20/50, and 20/70 lines at a minimum. Care must be taken that the occluded eye is actually occluded.

†One eye is covered while the child is looking at an object of interest. If normal binocularity is present, the uncovered eye will not move, because it is already being fixed on the object of interest. The test is then repeated covering the opposite eye. Movement of the uncovered eye to gain fixation indicates strabismus.

**Optional: Random Dot E (RDE) game, Titmus Stereograms (Titmus Optical Inc., Petersburg, Virginia), Randot™ Stereograms (Stereo Optical Company, Inc. Chicago, IL)

Management

Goals of management for strabismus include achieving the following:
- Normal and equal vision
- Cosmetically straight eyes
- The highest achievable binocular cooperation

▲ **Clinical Warning:** Despite anecdotal reports from patients or families, it is rare for a child to outgrow an evident eye turn. Newborns or infants may have occasional transient misalignment without concern, but any strabismus that is constant or frequent beyond ages 3 to 6 months warrants referral to an ophthalmologist.

Amblyopia

Pathology

Amblyopia is a unilateral or bilateral decrease in vision for which no cause is found on physical examination. It occurs when there is interference with sensory stimuli required for the development of normal binocular vision. This interference may result from blurring of an image, as for example from a transient corneal or lens opacity, a large refractive error, or strabismus. In the latter case, amblyopia derives from the adaptive adjustment made in the brain to avoid diplopia.

● **Clinical Pearl:** The younger the child with amblyopia is recognized and referred, the more likely corrective measures will successfully overcome the amblyopia. After age 3 or 4 years, the rate of treatment success diminishes with each passing year. By late childhood, amblyopia treatment is only rarely effective.

Management

Treatment modalities include the following:

- Correction of any refractive error
- Full-time or part-time occlusion of the normally fixing eye
- Penalization or blurring of vision in the normally preferred or fixing eye to the point where the amblyopic eye has the better acuity. Penalization may be accomplished with spectacles, atropine or other accommodation blocking drops, or a blurring film applied to a spectacle lens.

▲ **Clinical Warning:** Because early treatment may be successful in the vast majority of cases, early recognition of amblyopia and referral for initiation of therapy are critical. An eye injury, optic neuritis, or vascular occlusion later in life is devastating if the remaining eye is amblyopic.

NYSTAGMUS

Bilateral rhythmic oscillations of one or both eyes are termed nystagmus. When the movements are slow and sweeping, a retinal abnormality or other pathology causing diminished vision is more likely than when movements are rapid and jerky. Congenital nystagmus is often hereditary and may diminish with time and maturity. Most patients with congenital nystagmus are able to achieve 20/20 to 20/80 vision, with no visual consequences for school performance.

Acquired nystagmus is more frequently associated with significant neurologic abnormality. Imaging studies usually will be needed. Thorough pediatric ophthalmologic evaluation is indicated in all cases of nystagmus; pediatric neurologic and otolaryngologist (ENT) consultation will be helpful in some instances.

LEARNING DISABILITY

A comprehensive eye examination by an ophthalmologist who is skilled in assessing a child with learning disability is a necessary part of evaluation of children who appear to have specific learning or reading problems. Occasionally, an oculomotor or visual impairment is present that spectacles can correct. Refer to the Chapter 21 for further discussion on the diagnosis and management of learning disability.

● **Clinical Pearl:** Almost universally, ophthalmologists believe that visual training is not helpful and may delay more effective educational strategies (AAP, 1998a). Defects in ocular function do not cause the neurologic problem of learning disability (Romanchuk, 1995; Silver, 1995).

▲ **Clinical Warning:** The AAP shares this view and has stated so categorically based on scientific evidence (AAP, 1998a). Some optometric practitioners hold the opposite view, but their experience is anecdotal and not based on evidence.

ORBITAL PROBLEMS

Composed of processes of the cranial bones, the orbit may be malformed when premature closure of cranial sutures or other structural anomalies are noted. Neurologic and systemic abnormalities may coexist. Associated strabismus should be treated early to prevent irreversible amblyopia.

Exophthalmos and Proptosis

Exophthalmos and proptosis both describe forward protrusion of the eye. Benign dermoid tumors are a commonly encountered cause of orbital swelling in the pediatric population. They occasionally will cause proptosis but usually are found as discreet, rubbery, nontender lesions of the upper lid, more common temporally than medially. Growth may occur intermittently. Excision is generally elective. Small lesions require a small incision and therefore a smaller scar.

Hyperthyroidism can cause exophthalmos, especially in girls. Exophthalmos, however, occurs less frequently than in adulthood. Eyelid retraction is seen more typically and is an early indicator of the hyperthyroid state. Eyelid retraction can best be appreciated when examining the eye in the downward gaze component of examining the six cardinal fields of gaze. Refer to Chapter 60 for more information about assessing for exophthalmos.

Non–thyroid-related inflammation can cause the appearance of tumor. This type of presentation, also called orbital pseudotumor, may be unilateral or bilateral. Whether benign or malignant, orbital tumors are rare but do occur. They generally are of an acute or subacute onset. An acute onset of a pseudotumor can suggest cellulitis. An extension of sinusitis also may be part of the differential diagnosis.

The provider must closely question the patient presenting with orbital swelling as to duration of the presentation. Refer to Chapter 32 for information about the diagnosis and management of acute onset orbital swelling. For the child whose orbital swelling began more insidiously, the examiner should consider whether the swelling is unilateral or bilateral. He or she should note the presence or absence of edema to the eyelid, as well as erythema, proptosis, chemosis, and pain to the orbit itself. The provider should assess intraocular tissues for signs of inflammation.

The most common tumor of the orbit is a capillary hemangioma, which can present as a superficial tumor involving the lids and orbit of the eye. A strawberry nevus is a common presentation of a superficial nevus, which is confined to the skin itself. Such a lesion will appear to be red or purple. Referral to a pediatric ophthalmologist and a plastic surgeon may prove helpful in assessing and managing options for treatment.

Malignant causes of orbital tumor include rhabdomyosarcoma, which is the most common type of orbital cancer in the pediatric population, and myeloid leukemia. In the instance of rhabdomyosarcoma, physical examination reveals a massed lesion that is palpable in the eyelid tissue or conjunctiva itself. This tumor can be congenital, appearing around age 7 years. Myeloid leukemia also is known as granulocytic sarcoma and chloroma. This malignancy presents localized symptoms. Age of onset is about 7 years. Cytologic analysis of orbital cells demonstrates the presence of neoplastic cells.

Neuroblastoma can lead to orbital metastasis and, in some instances, can be the initial presentation of the disease. Physical examination reveals proptosis and often some degree of orbital inflammation. The differential diagnosis must therefore include orbital cellulitis.

● **Clinical Pearl:** Providers must evaluate any child with a history of neuroblastoma presenting with nontraumatic ecchymosis of both eyelids for metastatic neuroblastoma.

When he or she cannot find a cause for orbital swelling and associated sequellae, the provider should consider other less frequent differential diagnoses. These more rare causes of orbital swelling include the following:

- Optic nerve glioma
- Optic nerve meningioma
- Lymphangioma
- Fibro-osseous tumors
- Teratoma
- Thrombosis of a cavernous sinus
- Histiocytosis X
- Mengioencephaloceles
- Cyst associated with microopthalmos
- Juvenile xanthogranuloma
- Metastatic Ewing's sarcoma

Diagnostic Studies

Providers should promptly evaluate all patients with proptosis. Imaging studies almost always are indicated.

Management

The provider should refer any orbital swelling for which a clear diagnosis is not apparent for ophthalmologic evaluation and management. If the proptosis is acute, treatment of any associated cellulitis may be necessary. Refer to Chapters 32 and 33 for more information about acute and orbital cellulitis. Should the clinician's findings indicate that the proptosis is due to exophthalmos, Chapter 60 will provide information on the diagnosis and management of hyperthyroidism.

LIDS AND LACRIMAL SYSTEM

Lid Ptosis

Most blepharoptosis is congenital, and cases more often are unilateral than bilateral. If the lid obscures the pupil, prompt referral for evaluation and correction is indicated so measures can be taken to avoid ambylopia. Astigmatism often is associated with ptosis, so early referral is indicated in all cases. Surgical correction, when necessary, is best postponed until age 4 or 5.

Acquired ptosis always demands a search for an etiology. Horner's syndrome will have ipsilateral miosis. The pupil will be smaller because of the absence of adrenergic innervation. Asymmetry will be greatest in diminished illumination. Congenital Horner's does not require neurologic evaluation, while the suspicion of acquired Horner's necessitates that the provider refer the patient to a pediatric neurologist immediately for evaluation.

● **Clinical Pearl:** When available, photographs will help establish the date of onset of acquired ptosis.

Blinking and Blepharospasm

Frequent blinking is most commonly an attention getting device or a nervous tic that will pass but may indicate corneal or palpebral conjunctival foreign body or inflammation of glands on the lid margin. The cause may be bacterial or due to seborrheic dermatitis. Crab louse infestation occasionally is the cause. Refer to Chapter 54 for information about the diagnosis and treatment of seborrheic dermatitis and to Chapter 48 for content on louse infestation.

Blepharitis can have an anterior and a posterior component. Chronic inflammation of the lid margin secondary to ongoing staphyloccal infection characterizes the anterior type of belpharitis. The conjunctiva may appear hyperemic. The eyelashes will present with scaling, exudative clumping at the bases. Severe conjunctivitis can be an acute exacerbative outcome of the exotoxins that the staphylococci release.

The posterior variant of blepharitis occurs in response to chronic meibomian gland dysfunction. Oil accumulates on the lid margins at the opening of the glands and can be plainly seen on the lid margins. In some instances, so much oil has accumulated that when the child cries, tears appear foamy along the lower lids. The school-age and older patient can present with both oily and dry-type atopic dermatitis, with blepharitis as part of the presentation. The reader should refer to Chapter 32 for information on correcting the underlying bacterial infection in blephorism. It also presents content on controlling for recurrence through lid hygiene.

Tearing

Tearing results when ocular irritation causes excessive tear production or impairment in tear drainage. Injection, itching, or burning usually attends excess production. The most frequent cause of tearing in infancy results from incomplete canalization of one or both nasolacrimal ducts. The provider should refer to Chapter 32 for management.

Sturge-Weber Disease

Port wine stain of the skin of the face is associated with intracranial angiomas and frequently epilepsy. The provider should refer the patient with such a presentation to a pediatric neurologist for initial evaluation and possible comanagement. Because a significant percentage of these patients also will develop glaucoma, an ophthalmologist should follow any child with Sturge-Weber.

CONJUNCTIVA

The conjunctiva is a mucous membrane covering the anterior part of the eye, beginning at the limbus (juncture of cornea and sclera) and extending to the inner lids. It encompasses a blind pouch above and below, called the inferior and superior fornices. Any noxious stimulus, infectious or not, will cause dilation of blood vessels as a prominent sequella.

Allergy, persisting blepharitis, or irritation from local or airborne agents may cause chronic conjunctival injection. Careful questioning usually is more helpful in diagnosis than examination.

Localized conjunctival areas of thickening, discoloration, or both are rarely sinister. Rapid growth and increasing vascularity are signs of possible malignancy. Conjunctival tumors are extremely unusual in children.

Pinguecula are focal, adjacent to the limbus, age-related, and rarely cosmetically significant. They represent thickening of subepithelial connective tissue, probably in response to ultraviolet exposure. When the lesion extends to the cornea, it is termed a pterygium. If progressive, pterygia may require excision.

Conjunctival nevi may be pigmented or salmon-colored. Pigment will frequently increase at puberty, and small cystic structures are often embodied. Unsightliness is the prime indication for excision. Malignant melanoma may occur but is extremely rare.

In darkly pigmented individuals, 0.5- to 1-mm pigment spots may be found several millimeters from the limbus at sites where nerves or vessels perforating the sclera carry them from underlying choroidal layers. The provider should reassure the child and parents that these pigmented spots are benign and have no sequellae.

▲ **Clinical Warning:** Extensive areas of slate gray pigmentation encompassing a centimeter or more represent ocular melanosis or, when there is associated abnormal skin pigmentation, oculodermal melanocytosis. In either condition, there is a unilateral surfeit of melanocytes. These conditions may affect iris color and structure. Any patient with either of these findings has a higher than usual incidence of choroidal melanoma and should have regular dilated ophthalmoscopy.

● **Clinical Pearl:** Providers may reassure parents that almost all discolorations and elevated conjunctival lesions are benign. Referral is indicated for lesions that appear unfamiliar or uncharacteristic to the practitioner.

CORNEA

The cornea is avascular and depends on nutrient and oxygen supply from air, tears, limbal vessels, and the aqueous humor that bathes its posterior surface.

Most corneal problems in children are acquired and related to injury or infection. Because of corneal clarity and exposure, congenital and hereditary abnormalities are evident on inspection. Any unusual shape, size, or appearance of the cornea warrants prompt evaluation by an ophthalmologist because of the profound effect of any corneal abnormality on vision.

A large corneal diameter at birth may be an isolated finding, but the provider needs to consider this presentation as glaucoma until proven otherwise. Corneal opacities may be the result of aberrations in corneal development alone or part of systemic metabolic disease, such as Hurler's disease or Lowe syndrome. Familial dysautonomia is associated with diminished tear production, which may cause chronic ocular irritation and corneal ulcers. Dermoid tumors can present at birth and may involve the cornea. Bilateral dermoid tumors are part of Goldenhar's syndrome, which also includes auditory and vertebral anomalies. There are rare corneal dystrophies in which, subsequently, painless corneal opacification develops, generally in late childhood. Keratoconus is a central thinning and distortion that may develop in late childhood or adolescence but would be diagnosed on ophthalmologic or optometric examination for diminished vision.

● **Clinical Pearl:** The fitting professional generally deals with contact lens problems. Except in rare circumstances, youngsters must be sufficiently responsible to carry out proper lens care regimens without parental intervention if they are to be fitted. Young patients sometimes are concerned that lost or broken lenses might lodge behind the eye. Anatomy precludes that possibility. Everting the upper lid may disclose a lens or fragment in the upper conjunctival fornix. In the case of a soft lens (90% of wearers), fluorescein dye will stain the lens and increase visibility.

CATARACT AND LEUKOCORIA

Opacification of the lens, which is a cataract, or of the vitreous or retina will result in the loss of the red reflex and a white pupil termed leukocoria. The incidence of visually significant congenital cataract has been estimated at 0.35% in the United States (American Academy of Ophthalmology, 1996). Cataract may be unilateral or bilateral, congenital or acquired, isolated or one of multiple abnormalities. Chronic systemic or topical steroid use may result in cataract formation and in some patients, increased intraocular pressure.

▲ **Clinical Warning:** In patients on long-term steroids, providers should check the red reflex and intraocular pressure regularly.

Providers must rule out tumors, particularly retinoblastoma. A number of hereditary or inflammatory conditions may present with leukocoria. Ophthalmologic examination under anesthesia frequently will be necessary to establish a diagnosis.

Surgical intervention sometimes is indicated for cataracts in early infancy, particularly in unilateral cases. The clinician should refer the patient to a pediatric ophthalmologist immediately for evaluation.

GLAUCOMA

Congenital glaucoma is rare, occurring in 1 in 10,000 births (American Academy of Ophthalmology, 1997b). In its severe form, corneal opacification and enlargement of the corneal diameter are evident. There may be associated structural abnormalities of the cornea and iris. Less advanced disease may present only with tearing, light sensitivity, and forced lid closure, called blepharospasm. Most cases are evident in the first year, and many present in the newborn period. High pressure enlarges the eye in infancy and early childhood. One or both corneal diameters may be increased. Glaucoma also may develop later in childhood, sometimes as an isolated condition.

UVEA

The iris, ciliary body, and choroid together are termed the uvea. All are pigmented and derive from the same embryologic layer. A coloboma is a sectorial absence of structure. This problem may be limited to the iris or may extend posteriorly to include structures all the way back to the optic nerve. Variance from a round, reactive pupil requires explanation. The provider must refer the patient who presents with this finding to an ophthalmologist.

Congenital toxoplasmosis occurs after maternal infection during gestation. It may be associated with jaundice, hepatosplenomegaly, and hydrocephalus. Severe visual loss frequently occurs because of destruction of the macula. The clinician should refer the child who he or she suspects of having congenital toxoplasmosis to an ophthalmologist for evaluation and management of macular function.

Iritis, also called anterior uveitis, has a high association with juvenile rheumatoid arthritis (JRA). Iritis frequently is attended by injection most marked around the cornea, photophobia, and tenderness of the globe to palpation. These signs are frequently absent or very subtle in JRA. Pauciarticular JRA most often is attended by uveitis. Other causes of visual degeneration seen in children with JRA can include those that arise from chronic inflammation of the iris. These complications include adhesions to the lens, cataract, and calcium deposits in the cornea. It is important that the primary care provider refer any patient with JRA to an ophthalmologist for evaluation and for ongoing, regular examination using a slit lamp.

The frequency of iritis is higher in the pauciarticular form and with a positive antinuclear antibody (ANA). When systemic symptoms of rheumatoid arthritis (RA), multiple joint involvement, fever, and anemia are present, the likelihood of iritis is diminished (Wright, 1995).

▲ **Clinical Warning:** Asymptomatic chronic iridocyclitis is a much greater risk for children with JRA than are long-term joint deformities. Asymptomatic chronic iridocyclitis must be diagnosed early by slit lamp examination if it is to be treated successfully. Therefore, the clinician must refer any patient with suspected JRA to an ophthalmologist for slit lamp examination, even in the presence of a negative antinuclear antibody test. Early diagnosis and treatment may prevent the visually devastating complications of uveitis, intraocular scarring, cataract, and glaucoma (Dana et al., 1997).

Table 52-2 lists current recommendations for ophthalmologic examination, depending on ANA and JRA status.

Pars planitis, also called chronic cyclitis or peripheral uveitis, is a chronic, smoldering inflammation that usually begins in late childhood or early teenage years. The inflammation creates vitreous opacities appreciated as debris or "floaters." Swelling in the macular area of the retina and partial cataract may diminish vision. No specific cause is recognized, but suppression of inflammation and its consequences may be accomplished with judicious steroid use, prescribed by an ophthalmologist.

Table 52–2. CURRENT RECOMMENDATIONS FOR OPHTHALMOLOGIC EXAMINATION, DEPENDING ON ANA AND RA STATUS

Age	ANA/RA Status	Examination Frequency
Younger than 7 y	ANA positive	Every 3–4 mo
Older than 7 y	or ANA negative	Every 6 mo
Systemic RA		Every 12 mo

ANA = antinuclear antibody; RA = rheumatoid arthritis.
Depending on ANA and RA Status. Source: AAP, 1993

▲ **Clinical Warning:** A child who complains of hazy vision or "floaters" should be referred to an ophthalmologist for evaluation and possible treatment.

RETINA AND OPTIC NERVE

The following discussion is meant to provide the clinician with a brief understanding of rare disorders of the retina and optic nerve that require referral to and management by a pediatric ophthalmologist. It does not include a full discussion of diagnostic criteria and management. Primary care providers who desire more information are referred to any current, standard pediatric ophthalmology text.

Retina

Retinal and optic nerve abnormalities frequently have profound effects on vision. A host of familial metabolic abnormalities are associated with retinal changes, the best known of which is retinitis pigmentosa (RP). Initially, RP is associated with diminished night vision. It may progress to profound visual loss. A neonatal analog is Leber's amaurosis, a fortunately rare autosomal recessive, inherited condition that causes effective blindness in the first years of life.

Albinism is associated with abnormal development of the macula, resulting in diminished vision. In many patients with these and similar conditions, a family history is present. Providers may help to diminish parental anxiety by thorough examination, discussion of findings, and assistance with options for management. Few therapeutic options are available in this group of diseases. Support groups and low vision aids, when indicated, will be very helpful to parents.

Diabetic retinopathy is rare during the first 3 to 5 years of disease. After that time, regular dilated ophthalmoscopic examination by an optometric professional skilled in performing and interpreting findings is indicated in children older than age 10 years (American Diabetes Association, 2000). Refer to Chapter 61 for more information on retinopathy, including prevention strategies.

Optic Nerve

Malformations of the optic nerve may be isolated anomalies or associated with structural abnormalities of the brain and with diminished vision. Profound abnormality of the optic nerve will diminish the pupillary response to light.

● **Clinical Pearl:** In most patients, spontaneous pulsation of the main branches of the central retinal vein is present and can be recognized with the ophthalmoscope. This may provide comfort and reassurance when providers see patients with head injury or headache.

Primary care providers can benefit their patients remarkably from a moderate investment in time and interest through examination of children's eyes and vision. A group of age-appropriate acuity charts, a stereopsis test booklet, a small flashlight, and an ophthalmoscope are all readily available. With regular use, the clinician will gain increasing confidence and accuracy in diagnosis.

COMMUNITY RESOURCES

The following resources are for both clinician and patient:

American Academy of Ophthalmology
http://www.eyenet.org./
American Academy of Optometry
Executive Blvd, Suite 506
Rockville, MD 20852
http://www.oaopt.org/

American Association of Pediatric Opthalmology and Strabismus
http://www.aapos.bu.edu/

Lighthouse International
111 East 59th St
New York, NY 10022
http://www.lighthouse.org

   Information for blind and visually handicapped patients and their families.

National Center for Learning Disabilities
381 Park Ave. S, Ste.1401
New York, NY, 10016
http://www.ncld.org

   A resource that may support patients and their families who are dealing with learning disabilities

REFERENCES

American Academy of Ophthalmology. (1996). Childhood cataracts. *Focal Points, 14*(1).
American Academy of Ophthalmology. (1997a). *Preferred practice patterns: Pediatric eye evaluations.* San Francisco: Author.
American Academy of Ophthalmology. (1997b). *Focal Points, 15*(5).
American Academy of Pediatrics. (1993). Sections on Rheumatology and Ophthalmology: Guidelines for Screening. *Pediatrics, 92,* 295-6.
American Academy of Pediatrics. (1998a). Committee on Learning Disabilities. Learning Disabilities, Dyslexia, and Vision: A subject review (RE9825). *Pediatrics, 102*(5), 1217–1219.
American Academy of Pediatrics. (1998b). Committee on Practice and Ambulatory Medicine and Section on Ophthalmology. Eye examination and vision screening in infants, children, and young adults. *Pediatrics, 98,* 153–157.
American Diabetes Association. (2000). Standards for medical care for patients with diabetes mellitus. *Diabetes Care, 23,* Supplement 1.
Dana, M. R., Merayo-Lloves, Schaumberg, D.A., & Foster, C.S. (1997). Visual outcome prognosticators in juvenile rheumatoid arthritis associated uveitis. *Ophthalmology, 104,* 236–244.
Nelson, L. B. (1998). *Harley's pediatric ophthalmology.* Philadelphia: W.B. Saunders.
Romanchuk, K. G. (1995). Skepticism about Irlen filters to treat learning disabilities. *Canadian Medical Association Journal, 153,* 397.
Silver, L. B. (1995). Controversial therapies. *Journal of Child Neurology, 10*(suppl 1), S96–S100.
Wright, K. W. (1995). *Pediatric ophthalmology and strabismus.* St. Louis: Mosby-Yearbook.

Hearing Impairment and Disorders

• STELLA C. LAUFER TURK, MS, CCC-A, FAAA, and ANNE C. BALANT, PhD, CCC-A

INTRODUCTION

Communication is the most fundamental component of human interaction and learning. Sound production, perception, and understanding are prerequisite to spoken language learning, and, ultimately the attainment of higher level cognitive skills. The healthy neonate is prepared to begin the process of language development and can perceive sounds at birth, although responses such as the ability to localize to the direction of a sound source continue to mature during infancy. Assessment of hearing may be performed within hours after birth through behavioral observation by a trained examiner and by tests such as the auditory brainstem response or otoacoustic emissions.

Without intervention, hearing impairment has a calamitous effect on the speech and language development of a child. Impairment may also cause significant deficits in educational and psychosocial development. Even minimal, unilateral, and transient hearing loss from otitis media has been shown to have a detrimental impact (Bess, Dodd-Murphy, & Parker, 1998). Children who receive intervention for hearing loss within the first 6 months of life have significantly better language outcomes and improved overall development in a number of areas, compared with those who receive later intervention (Yoshinaga-Itano, 1998; Yoshinaga-Itano & Apuzzo, 1998).

Diagnosis and intervention must take place during the first year of life, ideally within the first 6 months. At present, the age of identification of hearing loss in the United States still averages 12 to 25 months, with an additional delay of up to 1 year prior to intervention. These averages are far from the U.S. Department of Health and Human Services' Healthy People 2010 goal of increasing "to 100 percent the proportion of newborns who are screened for hearing loss by 1 month of age, have diagnostic follow-up by 3 months and are enrolled in appropriate intervention services by 6 months" (1999, section 12, objective 33). Delays in identification and intervention have been attributed to the following three factors:

- Universal infant hearing screening is not yet widespread.
- Many parents are unaware of the indicators of hearing loss.
- Primary care providers often respond to parental concerns with a "wait and see" attitude instead of a referral for audiologic evaluation (U.S. Department of Health and Human Services, 1999).

Established screening programs have documented success in reducing the age of identification and intervention for hearing loss, and their performance improves with time. For example, the Rhode Island Hearing Assessment Program decreased its initial mean ages of confirmation (8.7 months) and intervention (13.3 months) to 3.5 months and 5.7 months

respectively from 1993 to 1996 (Vohr, Carty, Moore, & Letourneau, 1998). Universal infant hearing screening programs, such as the Rhode Island initiative, are highly sensitive, specific, and cost effective.

● **Clinical Pearl:** Problems associated with delay could be reduced through more widespread implementation of universal infant hearing screening.

Infant hearing screening is inexpensive compared with other forms of disease screening, with a cost ranging from about $10.00 to $30.00 per infant screened or about $5000.00 to $10,000.00 per hearing loss identified (Maxon, White, Behrens, & Vohr, 1995; Mehl & Thomson, 1998). The cost of screening plus intervention for those with hearing loss has been shown to compare favorably with the cost of special education and language services that would otherwise be required (Mehl & Thomson, 1998). Useful guidelines for infant hearing screening programs have been published by a task force of the American Academy of Pediatrics (Erenberg, Lemons, Sia, Trunkel, & Ziring, 1999). A model of a typical hospital-based infant hearing screening program can be found in Appendix 53-1.

Even when infants receive hospital-based hearing screening, there is always the possibility of a later onset or progressive hearing impairment. For these infants, parental concern is often the chief means of identification. Typically, such concerns are initially addressed with the child's primary care provider. Therefore, the primary care provider forms a crucial link between children who have or are at risk for hearing loss and the wide range of services available to meet their needs. One of the objectives of the draft of Healthy People 2010 guidelines (1999) is to "increase the proportion of primary care providers who routinely refer or screen infants and children for impairments of vision, hearing, speech, and language . . . as part of well-child care" (U.S. Department of Health and Human Services, Section 12, objective 38). Early identification of hearing loss, frequent monitoring, appropriate medical and rehabilitative intervention, and realistic parental counseling continue to be the best means to reduce the devastating impact of hearing loss.

ANATOMY, PHYSIOLOGY, AND PATHOLOGY

When an airborne sound wave enters the ear canal, it is amplified, filtered, and converted by the intricate structures of the auditory system from acoustic to mechanical to electrochemical energy and ultimately to neural impulses. These neural impulses are organized by their timing and place within the auditory system, from cochlea to auditory cortex. Understanding the anatomy and physiology of the auditory system is essential to understanding how its different sections are affected by pathologies.

The system is often divided into the peripheral (outer, middle, and inner ear) and central auditory systems. To facilitate the understanding of the interrelationship between anatomy, physiology, and pathology, the divisions that are used here are related to possible sites of lesions, including the following:

- Conductive system (outer and middle ears)
- Sensorineural system (cochlea including the distal ends of the cochlear nerve fibers)
- Central auditory pathways (remainder of cranial nerve VIII through the auditory cortex)

Conductive System

The conductive system transfers the acoustic signal to the inner ear and protects the ear's more delicate structures. Pathology, owing to obstructions or improperly functioning structures, may reduce the sound available to the normally functioning inner ear. The loss may range from mild to moderate-severe, and it may be temporary or permanent. Most conductive hearing losses are treatable with medication or surgery. Figure 53-1 presents the peripheral auditory system.

Outer Ear

The auricle, or pinna, and external auditory meatus comprise the outer ear. The pinna has minimal effect on hearing sensitivity, but its irregular shape aids in sound source localization (ie, directional hearing). The shape and length of the meatus provide a resonant effect by amplifying sound in the range of 2000 to 5000 Hz in adults. These are important frequencies for speech perception. Higher-frequency resonances are observed in infants and children. The ear canal directs sound waves to the tympanic membrane (TM), or eardrum.

Disorders of the outer ear include the following (conditions marked with an asterisk are associated with hearing impairment):

- Congenital structural anomalies* (microtia, aplasia, aural stenosis)
- Impacted cerumen*
- Foreign bodies
- Growths and tumors
- Otitis externa
- Necrotizing external otitis
- Herpes zoster oticus* (associated with sensorineural hearing loss, vertigo, and facial palsy)

Middle Ear

The middle ear, or tympanic cavity, is an air-filled cavity medial to the external auditory meatus. It includes the TM, ossicular chain, middle ear muscles, eustachian tube, and the oval and round windows. The healthy TM appears pearly gray, translucent, and concave through the otoscope. The cone of light, a triangular reflection of light from the otoscope, is usually evident. At birth, the TM is obliquely angled so that it almost lies on the floor of the canal. As the canal grows and lengthens, the TM becomes more upright and hence more visible on otoscopic examination.

The ossicular chain is made up of the three smallest bones in the human body: the malleus, incus, and stapes. They are fully developed at birth. The structures of the middle ear help to overcome the difference in mechanical impedance between the air in the ear canal and the fluids of the cochlea by approximately 30 decibels (dB). The eustachian tube opens into the anterior wall of the middle ear at one end and the nasopharynx at the other, allowing equalization of the middle ear with ambient air pressure and drainage of middle ear secretions into the nasopharynx. In children, the tube is shorter, wider, more horizontal, and more flexible than in adults. This leads to a greater susceptibility to spread of upper respiratory infections. Abnormal patency, intrinsic closure, and extrinsic closure of the tube can lead to atelectasis, negative middle ear pressure, and effusion.

The tensor tympani and the stapedius muscles are the smallest striated muscles in the body. They contract reflex-

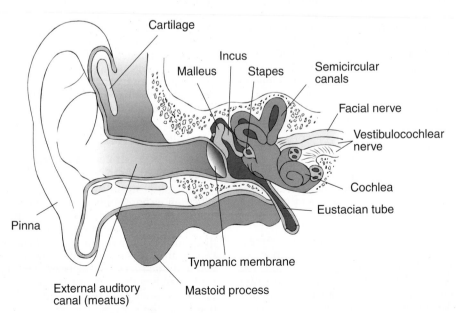

Figure 53–1 ■ Peripheral auditory system.

ively and stiffen the ossicular chain to protect the inner ear against some types of high-level acoustic signals. This acoustic reflex can be elicited by an acoustic signal 80 to 90 dB above an individual's auditory threshold. Because the onset of the acoustic reflex is not immediate, it cannot protect the ear against explosive sounds. The audiologist tests the integrity of the auditory nerve, cranial nerve VIII (afferent supply), and the facial nerve, cranial nerve VII (efferent supply), by eliciting an acoustic reflex as part of an acoustic immittance test battery (American Speech-Language Hearing Association, 1990).

Disorders of the middle ear include the following (conditions marked with an asterisk are associated with hearing impairment):

- Congenital structural anomalies*
- Acoustic trauma and barotrauma*
- TM perforation*
- Eustachian tube dysfunction
- Ossicular discontinuity or fixation*
- Glomus tympanicum and glomus jugular tumors*
- Otitis media*
- Cholesteatoma*

Sensorineural System

The sensorineural system consists of the inner ear, or cochlea, and the distal ends of the cochlear nerve fibers. In some types of hearing loss (eg, due to aging), both the cochlear and the cochlea nerve are affected, so a cochlear hearing loss is referred to collectively as a sensorineural hearing loss. This is sometimes mistakenly termed a nerve loss. Sensorineural hearing loss typically reduces the overall dynamic range of the auditory system, in that soft sounds are not perceived well but loud sounds are perceived almost normally. The loss may be stable or progressive, but it usually is irreversible.

The sensory organ for hearing is the organ of Corti. It is housed within a snail-shaped continuation of the osseous labyrinth called the cochlea. The cochlea is 35 mm in length, coiling approximately 2½ times around a bony core, the modiolus. The outer hair cells actively modify the properties of the cochlea, increasing its sensitivity and its ability to resolve individual frequencies of sound and generating otoacoustic emissions. The inner hair cells deliver auditory information in an organized fashion to the fibers of cranial nerve VIII. Damage to hair cells or associated structures leads to sensorineural hearing loss.

Disorders associated with sensorineural hearing impairment include the following:

- Congenital inner ear anomalies or dysplasias
- Perilymphatic fistulas
- Trauma
- Noise-induced hearing loss
- Ototoxicity-induced hearing loss
- Congenital perinatal infections

Other etiologies for hearing loss are discussed in the section History and Physical Examination.

▲ Clinical Warnings:

- Children with congenital diaphragmatic hernia who present with severe neonatal respiratory failure are at high risk of developing sensorineural hearing loss within the first 2 to 5 years of life (Robertson, Cheung, Haluschak, Elliot, & Leonard, 1998). Infants and children

with this or any of the other risk factors for progressive hearing loss listed in Table 53-1 require periodic audiologic monitoring.
- Infants and children are more vulnerable to the effects of hazardous noise at lower levels than are adults. Some commercially available toys may produce hazardous noise levels if held too close to the ear.
- Children and teens must be monitored to keep volume down on televisions, personal stereo headsets, and car stereo systems. Use of hearing protection is essential for children or teens who are exposed to firearms, snowmobiles, power tools, and other sources of potentially hazardous noise.

Central Auditory Pathways

The central auditory nervous system consists of complex, interwoven neural pathways extending from the cochlea through the brainstem and midbrain to the auditory areas of the cortex. Specific sites along these pathways may be affected by retrocochlear disorders, such as neurofibromatosis. In contrast, central auditory processing disorders (CAPD) in children are not usually linked to an identifiable lesion in these pathways. Central auditory processing is defined as "what we do with what we hear." Hence, CAPD is a disorder in the mechanisms or processes that are responsible for the following (adapted from ASHA, 1996):

- Sound localization and lateralization
- Auditory discrimination and pattern recognition
- Temporal aspects of audition, including temporal resolution, masking, integration, and ordering
- Auditory performance decrements with competing or degraded acoustic signals

Diagnosis of CAPD is based on history and performance on diagnostic tests.

● Clinical Pearl: CAPD should be considered when a child is having academic difficulties and hearing loss or developmental disabilities have been ruled out. Referral to a speech-language pathologist and audiologist is indicated. Children with CAPD may be effectively managed with various strategies, including assistive devices recommended by an audiologist. These devices improve intelligibility of speech in the classroom.

Disorders of the central auditory pathways that can affect hearing include the following (conditions marked with an asterisk are associated with hearing impairment):

- Retrocochlear lesions* (acoustic neuromas [eg, neurofibromatosis type 2])
- Hydrocephalus*

Associated conditions include the following:

- Chronic otitis media with conductive hearing loss*
- Attention deficit disorder/attention deficit-hyperactivity disorder
- Language learning disability

▲ Clinical Warning: Children with a history of recurrent middle ear pathology who demonstrate speech and language deficits or other educational delays should not be expected to recover these skills spontaneously when hearing returns to the normal range.

Table 53–1. RISK FACTORS FOR PERIPHERAL HEARING LOSS/CENTRAL AUDITORY PROCESSING DISORDERS

Risk Factors	Neonatal 0–28 Days	Infancy 29 Days–24 Months	Childhood	Progressive Sensorineural
Family history*	X	X		X
In utero infection associated with sensorineural hearing loss (toxoplasmosis, syphilis, rubella, cytomegalovirus, herpes)	X	X		X
Neurofibromatosis type 2				X
Craniofacial anomalies	X	X		
Low birth weight (< 1500 g)	X	X		
Hyperbilirubinemia requiring exchange transfusion	X	X		
Stigmata or other findings associated with syndromes involving sensorineural or conductive hearing loss	X	X		
Ototoxic medications in multiple courses or combined with loop diuretics	X	X	X	X
Low apgar scores: 0–4 at 1 min or 0–6 at 5 min	X	X		
Mechanical ventilation for > 5 d	X	X		
Bacterial meningitis	X	X	X	
Respiratory distress syndrome (Kountakis et al., 1997)	X			
Prolonged stay in NICU (Kountakis et al., 1997; Fortnum & Davis, 1997)	X			
Retrolental fibroplasia (Kountakis et al., 1997)	X			
Congenital diaphragmatic hernia (Robertson et al., 1998)				X
Concern about hearing, speech-language, or developmental delay by parent or caregiver		X		
Neurodegenerative disorder or demyelinating disease		X	X	
Head trauma associated with skull fracture or loss of consciousness		X	X	
Persistent or recurrent otitis media with effusion lasting > 3 mo (may also be a risk factor for CAPD)		X	X	
Verbal IQ lower than performance scores (CAPD)			X	
Need for highly structured classroom setting (CAPD)			X	
Academic/behavior problems (Gravel & Wallace, 1998)			X	
Complaint of hearing difficulty			X	
Excessive noise exposure			X	
Tinnitus			X	
Vertigo			X	

CAPD = central auditory processing disorders; NICU = neonatal intensive care unit.
*Specific questions have been designed to screen for syndromes including Waardenburg's syndrome, Stickler syndrome, brachio-oto-renal syndrome, Alport's syndrome, onychodystrophy, otosclerosis, neurofibromatosis, osteogenesis imperfecta, Usher's syndrome, and Jervell and Lange-Nielson syndrome (Smith et al., 1998).
Adapted with permission from American Academy of Pediatrics Joint Committee on Infant Hearing: Joint Committee on Infant Hearing 1994 Position Statement. *Pediatrics, 95,* 152–156.

● **Clinical Pearl:** Refer any child with recurrent otitis media for an audiologic evaluation. A clear picture of the degree of communication handicap is extremely helpful in documenting the need for additional referrals, such as otolaryngology, speech-language pathology, and educational evaluation.

EPIDEMIOLOGY

The reported prevalence rates of peripheral hearing loss among children are quite variable. These values depend both on age and on the type and severity of the hearing loss (ie, unilateral versus bilateral, conductive versus sensorineural).

Newborns and Infants

The prevalence rates of peripheral hearing loss in newborns and infants include the following:

- 1 to 2 per 1000 have a permanent bilateral hearing loss (Vohr et al., 1998; Fortnum & Davis, 1997).
- About 6 per 1000 infants exhibit all types of losses, including unilateral and conductive.
- Among infants who are "at risk," 30 to 50 per 1000 have such a loss (Kittrell & Arjmand, 1997).
- A higher incidence of hearing loss may be operant among male children of African American heritage (Van Naarden, Decoufle, & Caldwell, 1999). The age of diag-

nosis has been reported to be later in non-Caucasian than Caucasian children, regardless of socioeconomic status (Kittrell & Arjmand, 1997; Kountakis, Psifidas, Chang, & Stiernberg, 1997).

About one half of all congenital hearing impairment is associated with the neonatal risk factors originally identified by the Joint Committee on Infant Hearing (Mehl & Thomson, 1998; Yoshinaga-Itano & Apuzzo, 1998). These and additional neonatal risk factors recently mentioned in the literature are listed in Table 53-1.

Any other remaining hearing impairments result from genetic factors, environmental factors, or both. About one third of these impairments are associated with well-characterized genetic syndromes (Jacobson, 1995; Fortnum & Davis, 1997). The prevalence of hearing loss among children with these syndromes may be much higher than in the general population. For example, conductive, sensorineural, and mixed hearing losses are common in children with Down syndrome, with an overall prevalence of greater than 70% (Diefendorf, Bull, Casey-Harvey, 1995).

Preschoolers

The prevalence of hearing loss increases during the preschool years. This is due to conductive hearing loss secondary to otitis media, which peaks around age 2 years (Northern & Downs, 1991). Some of the risk factors for otitis media are environmental and controllable (eg, the type of child care situation, the presence of passive smoking, and whether the baby is breastfed or bottle fed). There is a strong genetic predisposition that appears to be related to the anatomy of the eustachian tube (Bluestone, 1998).

School-Age Children

The prevalence rate for hearing loss in school-age youngsters varies depending on the dB threshold affected. At thresholds of greater than 25 dB HL (hearing level), the rate is 5% to 6% for hearing loss. This figure may be viewed as a low estimate because it has been reported that in a group of children in whom hearing loss was not suspected, about 3% had hearing thresholds exceeding 25 dB HL (Sorri et al., 1997).

Prevalence of unilateral hearing loss at thresholds of greater than 25 dB HL is 1 to 2 children per 1000. A recent decline in prevalence is attributed to reductions in the incidence of mumps and measles and improved management of otitis media. At thresholds of greater than 15 dB HL, the prevalence of hearing loss, including unilateral losses, approaches 10% to 11% (Bess et al., 1998; Niskar et al., 1998; Vatianene & Karjalainen, 1998). The prevalence of CAPD has not been definitively established (Singer, Hurley, & Preece, 1998).

● Clinical Pearl: About one out of three children with serious hearing impairment (moderate through profound) also has one or more developmental disabilities (Fortnum & Davis, 1997; Van Naarden et al., 1999).

Prevalence of hearing loss, including minimal hearing losses, may be lower in non-Hispanic Caucasian and African American children than in Puerto Rican or Cuban American children (Lee, Gomez-Martin, & Lee, 1996). Prevalence of unilateral losses is reported to be lowest among Mexican American children and highest among Cuban American children (Lee, Gomez-Martin, & Lee, 1998).

HISTORY AND PHYSICAL EXAMINATION

History

For information related to screening for and management of hearing loss in prematurity, the reader is referred to Chapter 16. For all other patients and as indicated in Table 53-1, the primary care provider should routinely inquire about family history and other known risk factors for hearing loss. It is also important to ask about attainment of speech-language milestones. Typical speech-language developmental milestones are provided in Table 53-2. The corresponding development in auditory behavior is included to aid the primary care provider in interpreting diagnostic tests provided by audiologists.

● Clinical Pearl: The presence of risk factors for progressive hearing loss necessitates periodic monitoring. This monitoring should occur every 6 months through age 3 years and periodically thereafter even if a hearing screening was passed at birth or if hearing is within normal limits on initial evaluation.

Health records should be checked for results of an in-hospital universal newborn hearing screening. If the infant was missed or referred, parents should be urged to follow up with their hospital's audiology service. Although parents' perceptions have not been shown to be predictive of the degree of hearing loss in cases of otitis media, suspicion on the part of informed parents is an accurate indicator of the presence of hearing loss (Borgstein & Raglan, 1998; Rosenfeld, Goldsmith, & Madell, 1998; Stewart et al., 1999).

● Clinical Pearl: The suspicion of a hearing loss on the part of the parents or provider is grounds for audiologic referral.

▲ Clinical Warnings:

- Primary care providers and parents should avoid attempting to test the hearing of an infant or child with uncalibrated noisemakers or nonvalidated techniques.
- Because not all parents suspect hearing loss even when it is present, case history, screening, and observation of behavior by the primary care provider are vital in detecting hearing loss.

Physical Examination

Table 53-3 presents the procedures that are recommended for otologic evaluation by the primary care provider. Referral to an audiologist should be made if any of the following are noted:

- The parent or primary care provider suspects hearing loss.
- There are significant risk factors for hearing loss (see Table 53-1).
- The child demonstrates delays in speech-language development (see Table 53-2).
- The child fails the air-conduction hearing screening at any test frequency (1000 Hz, 2000 Hz, 4000 Hz at 20 dB HL) in either ear.
- The child fails tympanometry screening (see manufacturer's pass/refer criteria) on three sequential office screenings.
- The child suffers from repeated episodes of otitis media.
- CAPD is suspected.

Table 53–2.   DEVELOPMENTAL MILESTONES FOR AUDITORY BEHAVIOR AND SPEECH-LANGUAGE

Developmental Age	Auditory Behavior	Speech-Language Milestones
Birth–3 mo	Startles to loud sounds	
	Awakens to loud sounds	
3–4 mo	Rudimentary head; turn toward sounds may develop by 4 mo	
	Quiets to mother's voice	
6–9 mo	Localizes sounds at ear level by 7 mo	Coos and gurgles with inflection
		Says "mama"
12–15 mo	Directly localizes to sounds at or below ear level	Responds to his or her name and "no"
	Should localize to sounds above ear level by 13 mo	Follows simple requests
		Expressive vocabulary of three to five words
18–24 mo	Responds to tonal stimuli (warble tones to narrowband noise) at or below 25 dB HL in sound field	Knows body parts
	Responds to speech at or below 10 dB HL in sound field	Expressive vocabulary of 20 to 50 words (uses two-word phrases)
		50 percent of speech intelligible to strangers
By 36 mo	Capable of conditioned play audiometry	Expressive vocabulary of 500 words (uses four- to five-word sentences)
		80% of speech intelligible to strangers
		Understands some verbs

Adapted from Northern, J., & Downs, M. (1991). *Hearing in children* (4th ed). Baltimore: Williams & Wilkins; and Bachmann, K. R., & Arvedson, J. C. (1998). Early identification and intervention for children who are hearing impaired. *Pediatrics in Review, 19*(5).

● **Clinical Pearl:** Central auditory processing evaluation is performed using a test battery approach. Recent results suggest that an abbreviated test battery may be the most efficacious means of screening (Singer et al., 1998).

DIAGNOSTIC CRITERIA AND STUDIES

The degree or magnitude (normal, borderline, mild, moderate, moderate to severe, severe, and profound) and type (conductive, sensorineural, or mixed types) of hearing loss can be accurately established by an audiologist through a

Table 53–3.   PRIMARY CARE PROVIDER HEARING/OTOLOGIC SCREENING PROCEDURES

Age	Recommended Procedures
Neonate to 5 mo	Otoscopic inspection
6 mo to 3 y	Otoscopic inspection
	Tympanometry including an ipsilateral acoustic reflex at 1000 Hz*
	Observation of speech-language development
3 y and up	Same as above plus air-conduction screening with hand-held pure-tone screener or screening audiometer if available. Screening should be performed at 1000 Hz, 2000 Hz and 4000 Hz at 20 dB.

*These tests combined with otoscopy provide an objective means to evaluate middle ear status (ASHA, 1990). Recent studies suggest that including an ipsilateral acoustic reflex at 1000 Hz using an absolute acoustic-immittance device has high sensitivity and specificity for detection of middle ear effusion (Sells et al., 1997).

variety of testing techniques selected to be appropriate for the child's developmental level. Testing should be performed in a sound-treated room meeting American National Standards Institute (ANSI) requirements (ANSI, 1991). The audiologist will provide the primary care provider with a graphical representation of the test findings, the audiogram. An audiogram and symbol key are presented in Figure 53-2.

In conventional puretone audiometry, hearing is tested across the speech frequency range of 250 to 8000 Hz. An air-conducted puretone signal is delivered through earphones. Figure 53-2 also shows the different magnitudes of hearing loss. The magnitude of hearing loss will be determined by the air conduction results. An "O" indicates the hearing for the right ear at each frequency and an "X" indicates the hearing for the left ear. Different symbols may be used if modifications in standard testing techniques are required. The sensorineural reserve is measured by a bone-conducted signal presented by a bone oscillator placed on the mastoid. A variety of different symbols could be used by the audiologist, depending on the means by which results were obtained ($<$, $>$, [,]). A difference of more than 10 dB at a particular frequency is called an air-bone gap. An air-bone gap may represent impairment in the conductive system of the ear.

The audiologist will also provide a written interpretation of the findings with specific recommendations and referrals. Many audiologists will include additional information about the associated communication handicap. Table 53-4 provides a useful guide for understanding the audiometric results as they would be described in a report, including the possible test outcomes and the associated findings.

In the event that a child has not achieved the level of development needed for conventional puretone audiometry (usually age 3.5 years), the audiologist will use specialized behavioral or physiologic tests, as provided in Table 53-5. The audiologist's report will state the alternative procedure used and any limitations of the findings.

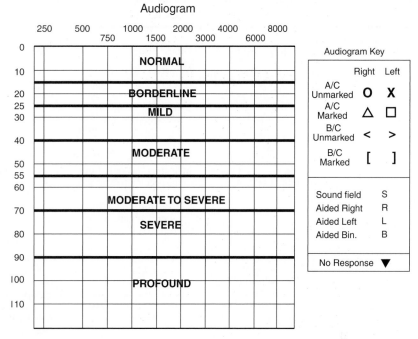

Figure 53–2 ■ Standard audiogram form showing degrees of hearing loss.

▲ **Clinical Warning:** To obtain accurate interpretation of a child's auditory status and communication impairment, testing must be performed by a licensed audiologist.

The audiologist selects the most appropriate diagnostic audiologic evaluation according to the child's developmental age. The primary care provider can expedite this process by referring children as indicated in Table 53-5. According to the guidelines issued by the Agency for Healthcare Policy and Research (Stool et al., 1994), children with persistent or recurrent middle ear effusion for 4 months require the following:

• Ongoing audiologic monitoring
• Speech and language evaluation

• Referral to otolaryngology for possible placement of tympanostomy tubes

The low rate of adherence to these guidelines continues to result in delayed referrals, hearing loss, and complications, including speech delays (Hsu, Levine, & Giebink, 1998).

▲ **Clinical Warning:** Given the detrimental impact of fluctuating hearing losses during the sensitive period for language learning, this 4-month waiting period should be considered as an upper limit. In infants and children younger than 3 years, referral for audiologic monitoring should begin after 6 to 8 weeks of persistent or recurrent otitis media with effusion. The primary care provider and the

Table 53–4. INTERPRETATION GUIDE FOR RESULTS OF CONVENTIONAL (PURETONE, AIR-CONDUCTION) AUDIOMETRIC TESTING

Outcomes of Testing	Associated Findings*	Comments
Hearing within normal limits with no air-bone gaps	Normal auditory function	
Hearing within normal limits, but with air-bone gaps	Conductive component in the presence of normal hearing	Can occur in cases of otitis media in a child with bone conduction thresholds close to 0 dB HL; can also occur after head trauma
Hearing loss with no air-bone gaps	Sensorineural hearing loss	Evaluate for genetic etiology
Hearing loss with air-bone gaps but normal bone conduction thresholds	Conductive hearing loss	Typical of middle ear disorders/effusion, especially if hearing loss is in low frequencies
Hearing loss with air-bone gaps and elevated bone conduction thresholds	Mixed, conductive, and sensorineural hearing loss	Combination of pathologies, common in children with Down syndrome
Inconsistent or conflicting results on conventional audiometric testing	Pseudohypacusis, retrocochlear disorder, or central auditory processing disorder	Tests to rule out pseudohypacusis may be indicated, along with ABR or OAE to estimate peripheral hearing. Acoustic reflex decay testing, neurodiagnostic ABR, or CAP evaluation may be required.

ABR = auditory brainstem response; CAP = central auditory processing; OAE = otoacoustic emissions.
*When reviewed in conjunction with case history and results of immitance testing.
Adapted from Bachmann, K. R., & Arvedson, J. C. (1998). Early identification and intervention for children who are hearing impaired. *Pediatrics in Review,* 19(5).

Table 53–5   REFERRAL GUIDE FOR AUDIOLOGIC TESTS

Developmental Age of Child	Preferred Audiologic Tests	Description	Advantages	Disadvantages
Birth to 4 mo	Auditory brainstem response test (ABR)	Measures electrical activity within neural pathways from cochlea through brainstem in response to sounds; can perform brief screening or complete threshold search	Cooperation not required, yields ear-specific information.	Infant must be inactive/asleep during test. Not a true test of hearing; only assesses auditory system through level of brainstem.
	Evoked otoacoustic emissions (EOAE)	Measures "echoes" from the cochlea in response to sound, thought to arise from activity of outer hair cells within cochlea	Short test time, yields ear-specific results. Presence of EOAE consistent with normal auditory function through the level of the cochlea.	If absent, thresholds cannot be estimated. Not a true test of hearing; only assesses auditory system through level of cochlear outer hair cells.
4 mo to 3.5 y	Modified behavioral audiometry (Visual reinforcement, conditioned orientation response, or play audiometry)	Child conditioned to respond in various ways to speech and noise/tonal stimuli presented through loudspeaker or headphones	Depending on age of child and on procedure, may get ear-specific results or frequency-specific results. True test of hearing.	Results sometimes limited in scope and reliability. ABR or EOAE may be needed to cross-check results. (In this age group, ABR may require sedation.)
3.5 years to adulthood	Conventional puretone audiometry	Behavioral responses to speech and puretone stimuli presented through headphones and/or bone-conduction oscillator.	Ear-specific and frequency-specific results; can determine type of hearing loss (conductive vs sensorineural); true test of hearing	None

Adapted from Bachmann, K. R., & Arvedson, J. C. (1998). Early identification and intervention for children who are hearing impaired. *Pediatrics in Review, 19*(5).

family will be able to make informed decisions regarding referral to otolaryngology for the possible placement of tympanotomy tubes if effusion with hearing loss persists for more than 12 weeks.

If sensorineural hearing loss is diagnosed, parents and siblings should also have audiologic evaluations. Genetic counseling is indicated. Second-stage genetic evaluations include vestibular and ophthalmologic evaluations, urinalysis and serum creatinine measurement, viral and serologic studies, temporal bone imaging, electrocardiogram, and thyroid function tests (Smith, Kimberling, Bradley Shaefer, Horton, & Tinley, 1998).

In older children, educational/academic problems warrant audiologic evaluation to rule out a peripheral hearing loss. Unilateral or minimal losses may go undetected until the school years but may cause significant academic delays (Bess et al., 1998). If peripheral hearing is within normal limits and the case history suggests difficulty in processing auditory stimuli, screening for CAPD is indicated.

● **Clinical Pearl:** Pseudohypacusis (functional, or nonorganic, hearing loss) can occur in school-age children and may be associated with a preceding trauma (Radkowski, Cleveland, Friedman, 1998). Primary care providers and audiologists must be vigilant in ruling out pseudohypacusis prior to planning intervention.

MANAGEMENT

Studies have demonstrated that all degrees of hearing loss, including borderline (minimal) and unilateral, require some

consideration for intervention (Bess et al., 1998; Gravel & Wallace, 1998). Table 53-6 indicates the impact of untreated hearing loss of varying degrees on communication and the educational and amplification needs of the hearing-impaired child.

The audiologist is the professional who is most acutely aware of the child's auditory communication needs. With the aid of the speech-language pathologist, a child's complete communicative function can be evaluated, and a treatment plan can be determined. Audiologists can also evaluate and design treatment programs for CAPD, which may involve a combination of approaches ranging from phonologic awareness training to the use of low-level amplification systems.

● **Clinical Pearl:** The primary care provider should take a lead role in advocating for the child with health insurance and school systems. Recommendations made by the audiologist, such as the need for personal amplification, assistive technology, and placement in appropriate educational settings, often can be expedited when the clinician actively participates in the process.

Comprehensive, multidisciplinary early intervention services are mandated by the U.S. federal government through PL 99-457. Primary care providers have the responsibility to inform parents of their rights, advocating for them when needed. The local health department is an excellent source for helping families receive appropriate diagnostic and therapeutic services. A multidisciplinary approach is the best means to evaluate a child suspected of having a hearing loss. As illustrated in Figure 53-3, the primary care provider should act as the case coordinator.

This complete model is most appropriate for the infant and young child. The primary care provider should refer to

TABLE 53–6. IMPACT OF HEARING LOSS AND EDUCATIONAL AND AMPLIFICATION NEEDS

Degree of Hearing Loss*	Associated Auditory Capabilities Without Amplification	Educational Needs	Audiologic/ Amplification Needs
0–15 dB HL (normal hearing)	None	No special needs	None
16–25 dB HL (borderline/minimal)	Up to 10% of speech information lost in noisy situations (eg, classroom)	Preferential seating Inform teachers of potential impact of loss	Audiologic/medical management Trial of low-gain personal FM system in classroom
16–40 dB HL (mild)	Up to 50% of speech information lost May exhibit attention/behavior problems	Preferential seating May require speech/language therapy	
41–55 dB HL (moderate)	50%–100% of speech information lost Language delay/disorder or phonologic disorder	Preferential seating Speech/language therapy or special education	Audiologic/medical management Use of FM system in classroom essential • Personal FM system *or* • Connection to FM system using "boot" on hearing aid Hearing aids: • *Infants and young children:* postauricular (behind-the-ear) • *Teens:* Custom (in-the-ear) unless loss is severe • *If conductive loss and unable to wear conventional aids:* Bone conduction hearing aid
56–70 dB HL (moderate-severe)	100% of speech information lost at normal speaking levels Delayed speech/language development, limited speech intelligibility	Preferential seating Speech/language therapy Special education	
71–90 dB HL (severe)	*If prelingual onset:* Delayed speech/language development, limited speech intelligibility *If postlingual onset:* Deteriorating speech quality/intelligibility	Special classroom setting for the hearing-impaired with caregivers' choice of emphasis (auditory-verbal, total communication, or sign language), *or* educational interpreter	
90+ dB HL (profound)	Sound vibrations felt but not heard Visual communication	Special program for the deaf *or* educational interpreter required in all settings	Hearing aids for speechreading or environmental awareness Alerting and signal devices Possible tactile aid Possible candidacy for cochlear implant

*Average thresholds at 500 Hz through 2000 Hz.

Adapted from Bachmann, K. R., & Arvedson, J. C. (1998). Early identification and intervention for children who are hearing impaired. *Pediatrics in Review, 19*(5).

an audiologist, otolaryngologist, and early intervention center. Each referral should generate recommendations for the child. The primary care provider acts as a case coordinator for the child, ensuring that recommendations are met and acting as liaison to and for the parent. For the older child or adolescent, an initial referral to the audiologist to rule out a communication disorder prior to making any other referrals is often most appropriate.

What to Tell Parents

The primary care provider can strengthen the care and support of the child with a hearing loss and his or her family by following these guidelines:

- Avoid responding to parental concerns with a "wait and see" attitude instead of a referral for audiologic evaluation.
- The suspicion of a hearing loss on the part of the parents or provider is grounds for audiologic referral.
- After ruling out hearing loss or developmental disabilities, consider CAPD when a child is having academic difficulties.
- If CAPD is part of the differential, referral to both a speech-language pathologist and an audiologist is indicated.
- Refer any child with recurrent otitis media for an audiologic evaluation. A clear picture of the degree of communication handicap is extremely helpful in docu-

menting the need for additional referrals, such as otolaryngology, speech-language pathology, and educational evaluation.
- Referral to an audiologist should be made if any of the following are noted:
  - The parent or primary care provider suspects hearing loss.
  - There are significant risk factors for hearing loss (see Table 53-1).
  - The child demonstrates delays in speech-language development (see Table 53-2).
  - The child fails the air-conduction hearing screening at any test frequency (1000 Hz, 2000 Hz, 4000 Hz at 20 dB HL) in either ear.
  - The child fails tympanometry screening (see manufacturer's pass/refer criteria) on three sequential office screenings.
  - The child suffers from repeated episodes of otitis media.

Finally, the primary care provider must keep in mind that children with persistent or recurrent middle ear effusion for 4 months require the following:

- Ongoing audiologic monitoring
- Speech and language evaluation
- Referral to otolaryngology for possible placement of tympanostomy tubes, especially if effusion with hearing loss persists for more than 12 weeks

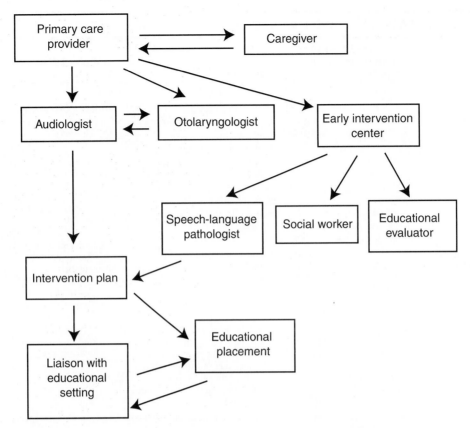

Figure 53–3 ■ Evaluation and management process for the child suspected of having hearing impairment.

These children also require referral for audiologic monitoring. This service should begin after 6 to 8 weeks of persistent or recurrent otitis media with effusion.

COMMUNITY RESOURCES

The following is a list of various resources relating to hearing and hearing impairment.

Boys Town National Research Hospital
555 North 30th Street
Omaha, NE 68131
Internet address: *http://www.boystown.org/Btnrh/Index.htm*

Home of the Center for Hearing Loss in Children, sponsored by the National Institute on Deafness and Other Communication Disorders.
Gallaudet Research Institute
Gallaudet University
800 Florida Avenue, NE-HMB 4th Floor
Washington, DC 20002
Telephone: (202) 651-5575
Internet address: *http://gri.gallaudet.edu*
    This site contains links to information from the demographics and assessment research at Gallaudet University's Research Institute.

National Institute on Deafness and Other Communication Disorders
National Institutes of Health
31 Center Drive, MSC 2320

Bethesda, MD USA 20892-2320
Voice (301) 496-7243
TTY (301) 402-0252
Fax (301) 402-0018
Internet address: *http://www.nih.gov/nidcd*

Early Hearing Detection Intervention Program
Developmental Disabilities Branch
Division of Birth Defects, Child Development, and
    Disability and Health
National Center for Environmental Health
Centers for Disease Control and Prevention
4770 Buford Highway NE, Mailstop F-15
Atlanta, Georgia 30341-3724
Telephone: (770) 488-7360
Fax: (770) 488-7361
Internet address:
http://www.cdc.gov/nceh/programs/cddh/ehdi/ddscreen.htm

    This site gives links to provider information and guidelines for early screening and early intervention for hearing loss.

    Other organizations and websites that may prove helpful to the provider and that give family-focused information include the following:
Audiology Online
Internet address: *http://www.audiologyonline.com*

American Speech-Language Hearing Association
10801 Rockville Pike
Rockville, MD 20852
ASHA Line: (888) 321-ASHA (24 hours a day 7 days a week automated information)

ASHA Action Center: (800) 498-2071
TTY (301) 571-0457
Fax on Demand: (877) 541-5035
Internet address: *http://www.asha.org*

American Academy of Audiology
8300 Greensboro Dr., Suite 750
McLean, VA 22102
Telephone: (703) 790-8466
FAX: (703) 790-8631
Internet address: *http://www.audiology.org*

**Alexander Graham Bell Association for the Deaf and
    Hard of Hearing**
3417 Volta Place, N.W.
Washington, DC 20007-2778
Voice: (202) 337-5220
TTY: (202) 337-5221
Fax: (202) 337-8314
Internet address: *http://www.agbell.org*

REFERENCES

American Academy of Pediatrics Joint Committee on Infant Hearing. (1995). Joint Committee on Infant Hearing 1994 Position Statement. *Pediatrics, 95,* 152–156.

American National Standards Institute (ANSI). (1991). *Maximum permissible ambient noise levels for audiometric test rooms. ANSI S3.1-1991.* New York: Author.

American Speech-Language Hearing Association. (1990). Guidelines for screening for hearing impairment and middle ear disorders. *ASHA, 32*(Suppl. 2).

American Speech-Language Hearing Association Task Force on Central Auditory Processing Disorders Consensus Development. (1996). Central Auditory Processing: Current status of research and implications for clinical practice. *American Journal of Audiology 5*(2), 41–54.

Bachmann, K. R., & Arvedson, J. C. (1998). Early identification and intervention for children who are hearing impaired. *Pediatrics in Review, 19*(5), 155–165.

Bess, F. H., Dodd-Murphy, J., & Parker, R. A. (1998). Children with minimal sensorineural hearing loss: Prevalence, educational performance and functional status. *Ear and Hearing, 19,* 339–354.

Bluestone, C. D. (1998). Epidemiology and pathogensis of chronic suppurative otitis media: Implications for prevention and treatment. *International Journal of Pediatric Otorhionolaryngology, 42,* 207–223.

Borgstein, B. M., & Raglan, E. (1998). Parental awareness and the detection of hearing loss. *Pediatr Rehabil, 2,* 165–172.

Diefendorf, A. O., Bull, M. J., Casey-Harvey, D., Miyamoto, R., Pope, M., Renshaw, J. J., Schreiner, R., & Wagner-Escobar, M. (1995). Down syndrome; A multidisciplinary perspective. *Journal of the American Academy of Audiology, 6,* 39–46.

Erenberg, A., Lemons, J., Sia, C., Trunkel, D., & Ziring, P. (1999). Newborn and infant hearing loss: Detection and intervention. American Academy of Pediatrics. Task Force on Newborn and Infant Hearing, 1998-1999. *Pediatrics, 103,* 527–530.

Fortnum, H., & Davis, A. (1998). Epidemiology of permanent childhood hearing impairment in Trent Region, 1985-1993 [Published erratum appears in Br J Audiol 1998;32:63]. *British Journal of Audiology, 31,* 409–446.

Gravel, J. S., & Wallace, I. F. (1998) Language, speech, and educational outcomes of otitis media. *Journal of Otolaryngology, 27*(Suppl. 2), 17–25.

Hsu, G. S., Levine, S. C., & Giebink, G. S. (1998). Management of otitis media using Agency for Health Care Policy and Research Guidelines. *Otolaryngol Head Neck Surg, 118,* 437–443.

Jacobson, J. T. (1995). Hereditary syndromes. Guest Editorial. *Journal of the American Academy of Audiology, 6.*

Kittrell, A. P., & Arjmand, E. M. (1997). The age of diagnosis of sensorineural hearing impairment in children. *International Journal of Pediatric Otorhinolaryngology, 40*(2–3), 97–106.

Kountakis, S. E., Psifidas, A., Chang, C. J., & Stiernberg, C. M. (1997). Risk factors associated with hearing loss in neonates. *American Journal of Otolaryngology, 18,* 90–93.

Lee, D. J., Gomez-Martin, O., & Lee, H. M. (1996). Prevalence of childhood hearing loss. The Hispanic Health and Nutrition Examination Survey and the National Health and Nutrition Examination Survey II. *American Journal of Epidemiology, 144,* 442–449.

Lee, D. J., Gomez-Martin, O., & Lee, H. M. (1998). Prevalence unilateral hearing loss in children: The National Health and Nutrition Examination Survey II and the Hispanic Health and Nutrition Examination Survey. *Ear Hear, 19,* 329–332.

Maxon, A. B., White, K. R., Behrens, T. B., & Vohr, B. R. (1995). Referral rates and cost efficiency in a universal newborn hearing screening program using transient-evoked otoacoustic emissions. *Journal of the American Academy of Audiology, 6,* 271–277.

Mehl, A. L., & Thomson, V. (1998). Newborn hearing screening: The great omission. *Pediatrics, 101,* 1–6.

Niskar, A. S., Kieszak, S. M., Holmes, A., Esteban, E., Rubin, C., & Brody, D. J. (1998). Prevalence of hearing loss among children 6 to 19 years of age: The Third National Health and Nutrition Examination Survey. *Journal of the American Medical Association, 279,* 1071–1075.

Northern, J., & Downs, M. (1991). *Hearing in children* (4th ed.). Baltimore: Williams & Wilkins.

Radkowski, D., Cleveland, S., & Friedman, E. M. (1998). Childhood pseudohypacusis in patients with high risk for actual hearing loss. *Laryngoscope, 108,* 1534–1538.

Robertson, C. M., Cheung, P. Y., Haluschak, M. M., Elliot, C. A., & Leonard, N. J. (1998). High prevalence of sensorineural hearing loss among survivors of congenital diaphragmatic hernia. Western Canadian ECMO Follow-up Group. *American Journal of Otolaryngology, 19,* 730–736.

Rosenfeld, R. M., Goldsmith, A. J., & Madell, J. R. (1998). How accurate is parent rating of hearing for children with otitis media? *Archives of Otolaryngology-Head and Neck Surgery, 124,* 989–992.

Sells, J. P., Hurley, R. M., Morehouse, C. R., & Douglas, J. E. (1997). Validity of the ipsilateral acoustic reflex as a screening parameter. *Journal of the American Academy of Audiology, 8,* 132–136.

Singer, J., Hurley, R. M., & Preece, J. P. (1998). Effectiveness of central auditory processing tests with children. *American Journal of Audiology 7,* 73–84.

Smith, S. D., Kimberling, W. J., Bradley Shaefer, G., Horton, M. B., & Tinley, S. T. (1998). Medical genetic evaluation for the etiology of hearing loss in children. *Journal of Communication Disorders, 31,* 371–388.

Sorri, M., Maki-Torkko, E., Jarvelin, M. R., & Oja, H. (1997). Prevalence figures for mild hearing impairments can not be based on clinical data. *Acta Otolaryngologica, 117,* 179–181.

Stewart, M. G., Ohlms, L. A., Friedman, E. M., Sulek, M., Duncan 3rd, N. O., Fernandez, A. D., & Bautista, M. H. (1999). Is parental perception an accurate predictor of childhood hearing loss? A prospective study. *Otolaryngol Head and Neck Surgery, 120,* 340–344.

Stool, S., Berg, A., Berman, et. al. (1994). *Otitis media with effusion in young children. Clinical practice guideline.* Number 12. AHCPR Publication N0, 94-0622, Rockville, MD: Agency for Health Care Policy and Research, Public Health Service, U.S. Department of Health and Human Services.

United States Department of Health and Human Services-Public Health Service 1999. Healthy People 2010, Draft for Review and Public Comment. Available at: *http://www.health.gov/healthypeople/Document/default.htm*

Van Naarden, K., Decoufle, P., & Caldwell, K. (1999). Prevalence and characteristics of children with serious hearing impairment in metropolitan Atlanta, 1991-1993. *Pediatrics, 103,* 570–575.

Vatianene, E., & Karjalainen, S. (1998). Prevalence and etiology of unilateral sensorineural hearing impairment in a Finnish childhood population. *International Journal of Pediatric Otolaryngology, 43,* 253–259.

Vohr, B. R., Carty, L. M., Moore, P. E., & Letourneau, K. (1998). The Rhode Island hearing assessment program: Experience with statewide hearing screening (1993-1996). *Journal of Pediatrics, 133,* 353–357.

Yoshinaga-Itano, C. (1998). Early identification and intervention: It does make a difference. *Audiology Today, Special Issue,* 11.

Yoshinaga-Itano, C., & Apuzzo, M.L. (1998). The development of deaf and hard of hearing children identified early through the high-risk registry. *American Annals of the Deaf, 143,* 416–424.

Yoshinaga-Itano, C., Sedey, A. L., Coulter, D. K., & Mehl, A. L., (1998). Language of early and later identified children with hearing loss. *Pediatrics, 102,* 1161–1171.

A P P E N D I X   53–1

Universal Hearing Screening Program: A Collaborative Effort Between Saint Francis Hospital, Department of Communication Disorders, SUNY New Paltz Department Of Communication Disorders, and Vassar Brothers Hospital

Program Goal

To perform hearing screenings at Vassar Brothers Hospital (VBH) to target the well-baby nursery population of approximately 3000 infants.

Program Coordination

Oversight of the program is provided by an audiologist and a speech-language pathologist from SUNY New Paltz Department of Communication Disorders and Saint Francis Hospital, Department of Communication Disorders.

- SUNY New Paltz provides graduate students from the Department of Communication Disorders to be trained to perform screenings Monday through Thursday.
- Volunteer Services at Vassar Brothers Hospital provides individuals to perform screenings for Friday, Saturday, and Sunday.
- SUNY New Paltz and Saint Francis Departments of Communication Disorders will provide NYS licensed, ASHA-certified audiologists to supervise the screening process. The Directors of Speech and Hearing Programs in State Health and Welfare Agencies, Inc. (DSHPSHWA) has developed a position statement for audiologists to supervise, manage, or coordinate infant screening programs (Penn & Abbott, 1997). Per ASHA guidelines, graduate students will be supervised at least 50% of the time.

Equipment and Supplies

An automated ABR screener owned by Vassar Brothers is used to perform the screenings in the well-baby nursery. Additional supplies are purchased by the hospital at a cost of $9.50 per infant for the disposable earphones. An infant formula company subsidizes supply costs.

Implementation

Hearing screenings are performed prior to infant discharge from the hospital. Average daily census of the well-baby nursery is approximately 20 infants. Screening personnel are available each day to perform screenings, specifically in the early evening hours. Supervising audiologists are available for program oversight. Results of the screening, recommendations, and date of rescreening are placed in the patient's medical record, recorded on the patient's immunization record, and forwarded to the primary care provider.

Rescreening

On a twice-monthly basis, any infant missed by the screening process or requiring a repeat screen is encouraged to attend a free walk-in hearing-screening clinic. A certified and licensed audiologist conducts these screenings.

Referral Protocol

Any infant who fails the hearing screening twice is referred for a diagnostic evaluation to Saint Francis Hospital Communication Disorders Department. The evaluation appointment will be made at the time the infant fails the second hearing screening. Supportive counseling and literature will be provided to the parents by an audiologist at this time.

Funding

Potential funding sources are contacted on an ongoing basis by support staff at VBH.

Data Collection

Data collection occurs through the database system within the hearing screener and is reported to the Department of Pediatrics quarterly.

Public and Patient Education

An informational video about hearing screenings is presented on the VBH in-house television station. In addition, an informational brochure is provided to parents in their patient handbook.

Reprinted with permission from:
Stella C. Laufer Turk, MS, CCC-A
SUNY New Paltz

Leslie Talty, MS, CCC-SLP
Saint Francis Hospital

Chronic Allergies

• PRADEEP SHARMA, MD

INTRODUCTION

Allergic diseases, which include allergic rhinitis, bronchial asthma, anaphylaxis, and atopic dermatitis, are among the leading causes of office visits to the primary care provider. This chapter discusses practical aspects in diagnosing and managing chronic allergic diseases. Asthma is covered in Chapter 55. Urticaria, contact dermatitis, and anaphylaxis are covered in Chapter 48.

PATHOLOGY

Allergic diseases can lead to acute reactions, such as anaphylaxis, and chronic diseases, such as allergic rhinitis, atopic dermatitis, and chronic urticaria. This is because immunoglobulin E (IgE)-mediated reactions are biphasic, involving early-phase responses (anaphylaxis) and late-phase responses. The late-phase response is associated with activation of endothelial cells, with migration to and infiltration of eosinophils and basophils, leading to mediator release and inflammation.

EPIDEMIOLOGY

Allergic diseases affect approximately 25% of all children. The economic implications are enormous, with health care costs approaching $1.2 billion per year. Another $1.2 billion can be attributed to indirect health care costs. Inclusion of associated diseases, such as asthma, chronic sinusitis, otitis media with effusion, and nasal polyps (all of which are associated with allergic rhinitis), bring the cost close to a staggering $10 billion per year (Malone, Lawson, Smith, Arrighi, & Battista, 1997). The incidence of allergic diseases, especially asthma, is rising. The exact cause for this phenomenon is not known. Morbidity and associated direct and indirect health costs can be reduced through better primary care provider, patient, and family education.

Allergic Rhinitis

Allergic rhinitis is defined as multiple symptoms affecting the upper airways, primarily the nose, as a result of inflammation. This response is primarily due to the interaction of IgE antibody with mast cells. It is difficult to distinguish allergic rhinitis from other forms of rhinitis in which IgE antibody may not be involved.

PATHOLOGY

The spectrum of rhinitis is characterized by inflammation. In allergic rhinitis, inflammation is due to release of mediators of allergy from mast cells. This is a result of allergen binding two adjacent IgE antibodies on the surface of mast cells. These mediators consist of histamine, prostaglandins, and leukotreines. Another concept to understand is the priming effect of the nasal airway. Priming of the nasal passage is caused by inflammation of the nasal mucous membranes. This results in sequentially lower doses of triggers (allergens, irritants, physical) producing the same degree of nasal symptoms that occurred after the initial exposure.

EPIDEMIOLOGY

A positive family history for allergies is present in about 50% to 75% of patients. Allergic rhinitis affects 52 to 55 million Americans (20%–25% of the population). It is responsible for more than 11 million office visits annually (Malone et al., 1997). Allergic rhinitis is responsible for up to 2 million lost school days. The cost to society is about $2.7 billion per year. Allergic rhinitis is hence not a trivial disease. Its costs are high, not only in dollar amounts, but also in quality of life, as described by Juniper's survey (1997) of patients with chronic rhinitis (a majority of whom have allergic rhinitis). In addition to the perception that their health had changed, patients reported that their chronic rhinitis caused changes in their social functioning, altered their perception of energy level, and affected their emotional and mental well-being.

HISTORY AND PHYSICAL EXAMINATION

The child with allergic rhinitis will typically present with a history of sneezing, runny nose, and itchy eyes. With further questioning, the provider may also uncover indications of lethargy, headache, and loss of productivity in school, hobbies, and sports. The clinician should also inquire about any food sensitivities, because these may complicate the evaluation and treatment of the sensitive patient.

● **Clinical Pearl:** The provider should be aware of the relationship that food sensitivities may have with allergic rhinitis. Often the notion that foods can cause problems with rhinitis is ignored although it is not a common problem (Hadley, 1999).

Typical physical findings in allergic rhinitis include the following:

- Pale boggy edematous nasal mucous membranes with hyperplasia of turbinates
- Constant rubbing of the nose (the allergic salute)
- A faint crease over the bridge of the nose (allergic crease)
- Allergic shiners (dark circles under eyes)
- Associated signs of asthma, allergic rhinitis, sinusitis, or atopic dermatitis

DIAGNOSTIC CRITERIA

The common causes for rhinitis in children are allergies and infections, most of which are viral. Allergic rhinitis is further classified as either seasonal allergic rhinitis (SAR) or perennial allergic rhinitis (PAR). A detailed classification of rhinitis is shown in Display 54-1.

Most patients will have rhinorrhoea, consisting of profuse clear, watery nasal discharge. Itchy nose is frequently present. Multiple fits of sneezing that are explosive in character are typical of allergic rhinitis. Allergic rhinitis seldom occurs alone and is often associated with sinusitis, asthma, and atopic dermatitis. These can present as headaches, sinus congestion, coughing, wheezing, and itchy skin with rashes. Nasal obstruction is frequently seen in allergic rhinitis (especially PAR) and can also result from sinusitis, nasal polyps, nasal septal deviation, tumors, and rarely, granulomatous disorders, such as Wegner's granulomatosis (Nathan, Meltzer, Selner, & Storms, 1997). Foreign bodies may also lead to nasal obstruction. The complications of allergic rhinitis can include the following:

- Sinusitis
- Otitis media
- Nasal polyps
- Asthma
- Malocclusion
- Deviations in facial growth

DIAGNOSTIC STUDIES

In most children and young adults, the clinical presentation as just described along with physical findings is sufficient to establish the diagnosis of allergic rhinitis. Allergic rhinitis is associated with an increased number of eosinophils in the nasal mucosa. A nasal smear will reveal a high number of eosinophils. Serum IgE will also be elevated. Laboratory tests are rarely necessary because the history almost always clinches the diagnosis.

If the suspicion of allergies playing a role is high, then a limited number of skin tests can be performed by the allergist to pin down those precise allergens responsible for inflammation. This information may help the provider make specific recommendations for environmental control. Current recommendations of the American Academy of Allergy, Asthma, and Clinical Immunology state that skin tests are preferred to radioallergosorbent tests for allergy testing because skin testing has higher sensitivity, is lower in cost, and provides almost immediate results. However, the yield from skin tests is low in children younger than 3 years. Testing will often be negative in this age group.

MANAGEMENT

Referral Point

Allergic rhinitis can be associated with considerable morbidity and a decrease in quality of life. Allergic rhinitis is also often associated with asthma. The provider may find that an allergy consultation may be helpful. Such consultation is also warranted in situations in which the diagnosis of allergic rhinitis is in doubt. Environmental control measures will be cost-effective only in patients with rhinitis for which the primary etiology is allergy. The indications for referral to an allergist are summarized in Display 54-2. Information that the provider should receive back from the allergist is also listed.

DISPLAY 54–1 • Classification of Rhinitis

Infectious (acute recurring frequent, chronic mostly viral)
Allergic (seasonal or perennial)
Nonallergic, noninfectious (vasomotor)
  Nonallergic rhinitis with eosinophilia (NARES)
  Iatrogenic (eg, rhinitis medicamentosa caused by over-the-counter nasal decongestants)
  Obstruction due to foreign body
  Atrophic (cocaine abuse)
  Hormonal (pregnancy)

DISPLAY 54–2 • Indications for Referral to an Allergist

The primary care provider should refer the patient to an allergist:

- When the diagnosis of allergic rhinitis is in doubt
- When the condition or its treatment is interfering with the patient's performance or causing significant loss at school or work
- When the patient's quality of life is significantly affected
- When there are complications of rhinitis, such as sinusitis, otitis, hearing loss, asthma, or bronchitis
- When the patient requires systemic corticosteroids to control the disease

The allergist consultant should give to the referring provider:

- Identification of specific allergens or other triggers for the patient's condition and education in ways to avoid these triggers
- Clarification of allergic or other etiologic basis for the patient's condition
- Assistance in developing an effective treatment plan, including allergy avoidance, pharmacotherapy, and, if necessary, immunotherapy
- Provision for specialized services, such as preparation of extracts and provision for immunotherapy

Adapted with permission from Joint Commission on Practice Parameters, Practice Parameter on Cooperative Asthma Management. *Journal of Allergy and Clinical Immunology.* Presented by Michael Kaliner at AAAAI meeting in New Orleans, March 1996.

Environmental Control

Environmental control forms the basis of all allergy management. These measures are effective, relatively inexpensive, and most assuredly free of any side effects. The measures should be adopted in all patients proven to be allergic by history and skin tests and in young children for whom suspicion of allergy is high but skin testing is deferred because of age, such as toddlers and infants.

Pollens

Pollens are important allergens for seasonal allergic rhinitis. Pollen grains can travel long distances on air currents. The provider should advise parents that there are several strategies that they can use to help their child manage their allergies. Clinical instructions should advise parents to do the following:

- Monitor pollen counts.
- Keep their child indoors if pollen counts are high or at least limit outdoor trips to rural areas. Rural residents who have seasonal allergies need to be vigilant about their exposure to pollens from nearby woods and fields. Avoid outdoor activities in the morning, because pollen counts are highest early in the day.
- Keep windows closed and run air conditioners when indoors during the warm weather months.
- Keep windows rolled up in cars.
- Avoid lawn mowing and leaf raking. The patient should use a mask if exposure to these activities is absolutely necessary.
- Have the child wear wraparound sunglasses or goggles, if possible, when outdoors.

Dust Mites

The most important component of house dust to which patients may become allergic is the dust mite. These microscopic arachnids can cause allergic rhinitis and asthma and may contribute to the pathogenesis of atopic dermatitis. Dust mites live primarily in mattresses, pillows, blankets, carpets, curtains, and upholstered furniture. Their primary food is shed human epithelial cells. Fecal pellets passed by these mites are the main source of dust mite allergen. The clinician should instruct parents that the following steps should be taken to reduce dust mite allergen levels:

- Use allergy-proof casings on all mattresses and pillows.
- Note that synthetic pillows may not be the best option for allergies, because recent research indicates that levels of dust mite and pet allergens can be found on synthetic pillow surfaces at an eight-fold higher rate than on feather pillows. This finding suggests that the pillow's surface is more important than what is inside the pillow, in part because the material covering synthetic pillows generally is not as tightly woven as the material covering feather pillows. Feather pillows are covered with tightly woven material to prevent feathers from pushing through to the surface. It is suggested that allergen-proofed or tightly woven pillow encasements be used for patients with dust mite and pet allergies, atopic dermatitis, or asthma (Custovic, Woodock, Craven, et al., 1999; Custovic, Hallan, Woodcock, et. al., 2000).
- Wash sheets and pillow slips every 7 days in laundry soap and hot water (130°F). Every 7 to 14 days, wash everything else on the bed (eg, comforters, blankets, and pillows) in laundry soap and hot water (130°F).
- Comforters that cannot be washed should be covered in an allergy-proof casing and dry-cleaned (a process that kills mites). Because of the trouble and expense of dry cleaning every 7 to 14 days, parents may opt to switch from non–machine-washable to machine-washable bedding. Mason and colleagues report that hot tumble drying also can effectively kill mites (1999).
- Wash the child's security blanket and stuffed toys as frequently as bedding.
- If possible, treat carpets every 4 to 6 months with a product such as Acarosan. This compound works to reduce the number of dust mites, leading to a decrease in dust mite allergen levels.
- Remove all carpeting on concrete floors. Such floors tend to trap moisture and promote mite and mold growth. After carpet removal, the concrete needs to be covered with a vapor barrier and washable floor covering, such as vinyl or linoleum.
- Dust mites thrive in high humidity. The provider should instruct parents to maintain their home's indoor humidity at less than 50%. They need to monitor the humidity, using a dehumidifier if necessary.

▲ **Clinical Warning:** Dampness promotes dust mite and mold growth.

● **Clinical Pearl:** Encourage parents to invest in duplicates—at least for the security blanket and the sleep-time stuffed toy. As any parent who has done so knows, frequent hot water washing of much-loved (and, hence, fabric-challenged) items leads to their rapid demise. A little extra expense up-front can save a lot of heartache later. These items should be stored in plastic bags or in the freezer when not in use.

Animals

If house pets have been or are currently present in the home, house dust will contain large amounts of animal antigens. When pets have been recently removed from the home, patients with allergies should follow these steps:

- Vacuum up any pet hair, and wash all walls and floors.
- Steam-clean all carpets and upholstery, and ensure rapid drying by running heat or air-conditioning system.
- Wash or dry-clean all bedding and draperies, even if the pet was not in direct contact with them.

If pets are still in the home, the following steps should be taken:

- Keep pets out of bedrooms at all times.
- Keep pets outdoors as much as possible (properly protected from the effects of direct sun and the elements).
- When pets are indoors, put them in a separate room from the patient (airborne allergen levels increase 100-fold when pets are in the room).
- Remove carpeting from the entire house, if possible. Start by removing bedroom carpeting because it traps pet allergens.
- Use the same precautions with mattresses and pillows as described for dust mites.
- Use a high-efficiency particulate air (HEPA) cleaner to remove airborne allergens (van der Heide, van Aalderen, Kauffman, Dubois, & de Monchy, 1999). Place one in the child's bedroom. Parents should consider using another one in the room in which their youngster spends the most time.

- Use HEPA central furnace filters to prevent spread of the airborne dander throughout the house.
- Open the windows and ventilate the house, because air exchange can decrease airborne pet allergens.
- Wash pets weekly to remove surface allergens. Any pet bedding should also be washed weekly, using laundry soap and hot water (130°F).

Mold

The provider should instruct parents that molds comprise a significant component of their child's allergy exposure. Parents and child need to be advised to do the following:

- Avoid exposure to damp basements, compost piles and bins, fallen leaves, and cut grass, including lawns and hay, barns, and wooded areas. All of these are areas of high mold growth. The patient should wear a face mask if such exposures are unavoidable.
- Prevent high levels of humidity indoors. Measure the indoor humidity with a gauge, and keep it at 35% or less. This can be accomplished with air conditioners in the summer and by preventing overhumidification in the winter.
- Use an exhaust fan to remove humidity produced by showering or cooking. Mold growth can be prevented indoors by products that kill mildew (eg, diluted bleach).
- If using a humidifier, clean it weekly with a bleach solution. The water needs to be changed completely at least every other day.

Pharmacotherapy

Several medications are available for treating the symptoms of allergic rhinitis without attendant sedation effects.

Antihistamines

Antihistamines block the H_1 receptors, preventing the histamine that is released from mast cells from linking up with these receptors (Meltzer, 1995). Antihistamines thus prevent the development of pruritus and rhinorrhoea. They also decrease the number of eosinophils in the nasal mucosa. Although effective, the first-generation antihistamines have a potentially serious side effect of causing drowsiness. This feature is not present in the second-generation antihistamines.

Second-generation antihistamines bind strongly to the H_1 receptors, do not cause somnolence (with the exception of ceterizine), and have no appreciable anticholinergic effects (Meltzer, 1995). The effect of drowsiness in children attending school would favor the use of second-generation antihistamines, such as loratadine (Claritin), fexofenadine (Allegra), or cetirizine (Zyrtec). However, the latter may cause somnolence in about 13% of children (Meltzer, 1995).

● **Clinical Pearl:** Antihistamines are effective first-line agents in the management of mild to moderate allergy symptoms, including rhinitis, sneezing, or itchy eyes, and are useful because they have few side effects (van Cauwenberge, 1998). They are not as effective when nasal obstruction is the main complaint. Children with seasonal allergic rhinitis should be started on antihistamines just before onset of the allergy season. They need to be maintained on antihistamines until the season is over.

Golden and Craig (1999) describe azelastine nasal spray as being a safe and nonsedating alternative to oral antihistamines in treating SAR allergic rhinitis. Similar to inhaled corticosteroids and unlike oral antihistamines, some authors report that azelastine nasal spray may be helpful in treating nasal congestion. Unfortunately, side effects are noteworthy, including bitter taste, headache, and drowsiness. These may make azelastine nasal spray a choice for only selected patients. Azelastine nasal spray has recently been approved by the Food and Drug Administration (FDA) for use in the treatment of SAR in patients 12 years of age and older at a dosage of 1.1 mg/d (two sprays per nostril, twice daily).

Tables 54-1 and 54-2 provide a synopsis of the dosage and effects of first- and second-generation antihistamines. The reader is referred to a conventional pharmacology text if more in-depth information is desired.

Decongestants

Alpha-adrenergic decongestants, such as phenylephrine (pseudoephederine), can be used either alone or in combination with antihistamines. They are helpful for very short-term use in cases in which allergic rhinitis is associated with nasal obstruction.

▲ **Clinical Warning:** The provider should discourage prolonged topical use of alpha-adrenergic agents, such as phenylephrine, because they can lead to rhinitis medicamentosa (rebound congestion). Overdose can produce medically significant blood pressure increases and can stimulate the central nervous system to dangerous levels.

Intranasal cromolyn sodium is a mast cell stabilizer. It acts by reducing the release of allergy mediators. It is helpful in cases of mild to moderate allergic rhinitis. Intranasal cromolyn sodium has the fewest adverse effects among antiallergic agents (Naclerio, 1998). However, for it to be effective, it has to be sprayed into the nose three to four times daily.

Intranasal steroids are potent anti-inflammatory agents. They decrease the population of inflammatory cells in the nasal mucosa and reduce levels of mediators of allergy and cytokines. They may be used as the primary drug for patients with moderate to severe SAR or PAR (van Cauwen-

Table 54–1. FIRST-GENERATION ANTIHISTAMINES

Antihistamine	H_1 Blockade	Sedation	Anticholinergic Effects
Ethanolamines (diphenhydramine [Benadryl])	+++	++	++
Alkylamines (chlorpheniramine [Chlor-Trimeton])	+++	+	++
Piperazines (hydroxyzine [Atarax])	+++	++	++
Piperadines (azatadine)	+++	++	++
Ethylenediamine (tripelennamine)	+++	++	++

Table 54–2. SECOND-GENERATION ANTIHISTAMINES

Antihistamine	H₁ Blockade	Sedation	Anticholinergic Effects	Dose and Route
Fexofenadine (Allegra)	+++	−	−	12 y and older: 60 mg b.i.d. PO*
Loratadine (Claritin)	+++	−	−	6 y and older: 5–10 mg/d PO
Cetirizine (Zyrtec)	++++	−	−	2 y and older: 5–10 mg/d PO
Azelastine (Astelin)	+++	+	−	Topical nasal spray
				12 y and older: 2 sprays each nostril b.i.d. as needed

b.i.d. = twice daily; PO = by mouth.
*Application for approval for use in children 3 y and older is before the Food and Drug Administration.

berge, 1998). Intranasal steroids are preferred to antihistamines, including topical alpha-adrenergic agents, in any patient with nasal obstruction. Antihistamines may be added or used preferentially in patients whose symptoms are itchy eyes and sneezing fits.

▲ **Clinical Warning:** Children using intranasal steroids should be monitored for growth, and their growth should be charted. Recent evidence suggests that moderate to high doses of topical steroids may result in reduced growth velocity in children. This evidence prompted the FDA to issue an advisory regarding this subject in October of 1998.

● **Clinical Pearls:**

- Proper instruction should be given to the child using intranasal steroids. The spray should not be directed toward the septum but, rather, laterally. The patient should pretend to aim the tip of the nozzle in the nose toward the eye on the same side.
- Because steroids can take 4 to 6 weeks to take effect, the child who has a definite pattern of SAR or PAR should begin using the topical nasal steroid medication 4 weeks before the time when symptoms normally start.

Local irritation of the mucous membranes and mild epistaxis are the most noticed side effects with intranasal steroids. Some patients complain about the strong floral fragrance associated with some preparations, including beclomethasone (Vancenase, Beconase), fluticasone (Flonase), and mometasone (Nasonex). Intranasal steroids come in either an aqueous solution or a dry aerosol powder. The choice of one over the other is based primarily on patient and provider preference. Table 54-3 presents information on

various intranasal steroid preparations. The reader is referred to a conventional pharmacology text if more in-depth information is desired.

▲ **Clinical Warning:** The provider should keep in mind that there is a great deal of reluctance by a significant number of young children toward accepting any intranasal medication. Parents should be made aware of this possibility and told that this reluctance is normal for the child's age and should not be construed as treatment resistance.

Allergy Immunotherapy

If eye and nose symptoms continue despite aggressive environmental control measures and adequate pharmacotherapy, allergy immunotherapy should then be considered in conjunction with an allergy consultation. Allergy immunotherapy is effective for allergens for which standardized extracts are available. These include dust mites, grass and ragweed pollens, cat antigens, and to a lesser degree, tree pollens. Durham and colleagues (1999) report that 3 to 4 years of immunotherapy for grass-pollen allergy leads to an extended clinical remission characterized by a conversion in immunologic response to IgE-mediated SAR.

▲ **Clinical Warnings:**

- The risks versus benefits should be explained to the patient, as well as frequency and duration of allergy injections. It is also advisable to obtain informed consent before initiating immunotherapy.
- If allergy immunotherapy is to be instituted at the primary care provider's office, the office and staff should be equipped and trained for managing anaphylaxis.

Table 54–3. INTRANASAL CORTICOSTEROIDS

Medication	Dosage per Actuation	Formulation Aqueous/MDI	Dosage
Beclomethasone (Vanceril, Beconase)	42 mcg/84 mcg	AQ/MDI	6 y and older: 1–2 sprays each nostril b.i.d.
Budesonide (Rhinocort)	32 mcg	MDI	6 y and older: 2 sprays each nostril per day
			Not for use in nonallergic rhinitis
Flunisolide (Nasarel)	25 mcg	AQ	2 sprays each nostril per day
Fluticasone (Flonase)	50 mcg	AQ	2 sprays each nostril per day
Mometasone (Nasonex)	50 mcg	AQ	2 sprays each nostril per day
Triamcinolone	55 mcg	AQ/MDI	2 sprays each nostril per day

AQ = aqueous; b.i.d. = twice daily; MDI = metered dose inhaler.

Allergy immunotherapy leads to a reduction of allergen-specific IgE antibodies. Outcomes observed with IgE antibody reduction include decreases in the severity and frequency of symptoms and a decrease in the amount of rescue medications needed, such as antihistamines. Allergy immunotherapy can be discontinued after 4 to 5 years. IgE antibodies usually do not rise to preallergy immunotherapy levels, suggesting long-term benefit (Bousque & Demoly, 1996).

Management of Allergic Conjunctivitis

Allergic conjunctivitis is usually associated with allergic rhinitis. Although vision is not normally affected, symptoms can make the patient quite uncomfortable. In addition to avoidance of allergens, symptomatic medications, such as oral antihistamines, can be effective. Saline eye drops have the advantage of being both nontoxic and inexpensive. They are effective in 30% to 35% of patients and when used in conjunction with other eye drop remedies, can decrease the amount of medication required for symptom control. Topical antihistamines and mast cell stabilizers, such as levocabastine (Livostin), olopatadine (Patanol), or cromolyn sodium eye drops, may also be helpful (Joss & Craig, 1999).

▲ **Clinical Warning:** Corticosteroids should be considered an extreme intervention and therefore reserved for only the most severe and refractory instances. Topical corticosteroids should only be used for a limited time. If severity of symptoms suggests that topical corticosteroid medication is needed, the provider should consult first with an ophthalmologist (Joss & Craig, 1999).

Atopic Dermatitis

PATHOLOGY

Atopic dermatitis is a chronic, itchy rash affecting approximately 3% to 5% of all children (Williams, 1999). The exact etiology of atopic dermatitis is as yet not fully understood. It is an immunologic event involving both type 1 (IgE) and type 4 (cellular) immune mechanisms. IgE antibody levels tend to be high in these patients. There is evidence that cell-mediated immunity may be affected, because patients with atopic dermatitis are prone to viral and fungal infections. There may also be some loss of delayed skin reactivity (one of a measure of type 4 immune reactions) to *Candida*, to which most people will show a delayed skin response upon testing with an appropriate antigen. Dust-mite sensitivity may be associated with atopic dermatitis. Histamine is most certainly involved in the genesis of atopic dermatitis. Other mediators involved include prostaglandins, neuropeptides, and kinins. Triggers may include foods; dust mites; seasonal inhalants, such as pollens; and viral and bacterial infections.

EPIDEMIOLOGY

Although it is rare in infancy, about 60% of children who have atopic dermatitis will develop the rash during the first year of life (Kusonoki, Asai, Harazaki, Korematsu, & Hosoi, 1999). In about 33% of all affected children and in about 75% with a positive family history of allergy, atopic dermatitis will be associated with asthma and allergic rhinitis (Williams, 1999; Kusunoki et al., 1999). Many reports in the current literature point toward an increasing incidence of atopic dermatitis in children worldwide. There does not appear to be any ethnic or racial incidence favoring any one particular population of children. Kusunoki and colleagues (1999) report that they have found that an infant's exposure to the drying effects of winter weather very early in infancy (such as with babies born in the fall and winter months) was correlated with atopic dermatitis. This nonallergic etiologic factor could serve as a trigger for the IgE-mediated development of atopic dermatitis.

HISTORY AND PHYSICAL EXAMINATION

Itching is the initial symptom, probably due to histamine release. It is often stated that atopic dermatitis is an itch that rashes rather than a rash that itches. Inflammation of the skin is a key feature. This is why the term eczema was coined. The word eczema means "to boil over." Inflammation causes erythema and scaling with crusts. There is usually underlying chronic inflammation beneath the acute inflammation, leading to lichenification (thickening of skin and accentuated skin markings). Eczematous distribution varies with age. In infants, it may involve the trunk and limbs, sparing the diaper area. In older children, the rash involves the flexural surfaces, including the antecubital and popliteal fossas. However, Tada, Yamasaki, Toi, Akiyama, and Arata (1999) reported a higher incidence of face, neck skin fold, and upper trunk distribution in their sample of 87 Japanese adults. Whether this presentation variant was peculiar to their sample or is an ethnogeographic variation is not yet clear.

More than half of children with atopic dermatitis will show near total resolution at puberty, with the rest showing improvement. A small subset of patients, however, will continue to suffer from atopic dermatitis well into their adult lives. Secondary skin infection of affected areas with *Staphylococcus aureus* may sometimes be seen during phases of acute inflammation.

DIAGNOSTIC CRITERIA AND STUDIES

The major criterion for diagnosis is pruritus along with rash involving the typical locations. Other findings are a personal history of allergy, such as allergic rhinitis, or asthma. A positive family history for allergy is frequently seen.

The differential diagnoses for atopic dermatitis must be considered when diagnosing this disorder. Seborrheic dermatitis has to be distinguished. The rash here involves the inguinal creases, diaper area, and scalp (cradle cap). Irritant or allergic contact dermatitis may masquerade as atopic dermatitis. Location may be a key distinguishing feature. Typical atopic dermatitis spares the diaper area, whereas seborrheic and irritant dermatitis may involve it. Rarely, atopic dermatitis may have to be distinguished from rashes associated with immunodeficiencies, such as Wiskott-Aldrich syndrome and ataxia-telangiectasia.

A laboratory workup or allergy workup including skin tests is generally not necessary.

MANAGEMENT

Infants should be bathed with a mild soap, such as Dove or Caress. Their skin should be lightly patted rather than rubbed dry. This should be immediately followed by application of a rich emollient lubricant, such as Eucerin cream, Keri lotion, Lubriderm lotion, or Lacticare lotion.

● **Clinical Pearl:** In stubborn cases, a greasier preparation, such as Eucerin, should be chosen over less greasy preparations such as Lacticare. The latter may suffice in the patient with mild disease.

Pruritus in atopic dermatitis can be especially frustrating. Common sense measures, such as cutting nails short, avoiding rubbing dry after bathing, and using cotton clothes, may go a long way in reducing itching, thus breaking the itch cycle.

Low- to medium-strength, nonhalogenated corticosteroid creams should work well in all but the most stubborn of cases. The creams should be applied locally over affected areas in a sparing manner, up to twice daily. Hydrocortisone 1% to 2.5% is effective. If the preparation chosen proves noneffective, then the provider can prescribe midpotency preparations, such as mometasone (Elocon) 0.1%.

▲ **Clinical Warning:** Higher potency, halogenated creams, such as betamethasone 0.05% or desoximetasone 0.25%, should be necessary for only the most stubborn cases. These preparations should not be applied to the face or other occluded areas, such as neck or groin, owing to the possibility of causing dermal atrophy. This outcome is particularly distressing if the face is involved.

Even though histamine release occurs in atopic dermatitis, the role of antihistamines is limited to their mild antipruritic effect, which includes sedation, especially if the first-generation antihistamines are used. Hydroxyzine (Atarax) may be helpful, especially if given at bedtime. It has mild antipruritic properties. Mild sedation may also lead to less itching and trauma to the skin at night.

Antibiotics may be necessary if the rash is acute and there is evidence of a secondary infection.

Allergy workup or allergy immunotherapy is not necessary in patients with atopic dermatitis.

● **Clinical Pearl:** Because of the association of atopic dermatitis with dust-mite allergy, in difficult cases, skin tests and patch tests for this allergy may be done, and if positive, dust mite control measures may be helpful. Allergy workup may be considered in cases in which allergic rhinitis and persistent asthma coexist with atopic dermatitis. Allergy immunotherapy may be instituted in cases of allergic rhinitis and asthma that require it, but it should not be used to treat atopic dermatitis alone.

What to Tell Parents

It is important that parents' expectations be realistic. Consistency with basics, such as dry skin care and anti-itch measures, should be emphasized. Parents and children should be told that flare-ups will occur despite consistency. Close follow-through on the guidelines presented here should generally prove helpful to the successful management of their child's atopic dermatitis.

COMMUNITY RESOURCES

The following resources provide information for clinicians, patients, and their families.

Allergy and Asthma Network-Mothers of Asthmatics, Inc.
2751 Prosperity Avenue, Suite 150
Fairfax, VA 22031
Telephone: (800) 878-4403
Fax: (703) 573-7794
Internet address: *http://www.aanma.org/index.html*

Allergy and Asthma Specialists
29 Fox Street
Poughkeepsie, NY 12601
Telephone: (914) 454-1234
Fax: (914) 454-1898
Internet address: *http://www.aaspc.org*

American Academy of Allergy, Asthma and Immunology
611 East Wells Street
Milwaukee, WI 53202
Telephone: (414) 272-6071
Internet address: *http://www.aaaai.org*

American Academy of Dermatology
930 N. Meacham Road
Schaumburg, IL 60173
Telephone: (888) 462-DERM
Internet address: *http://www.aad.org*

American Academy of Pediatrics
141 Northwest Point Boulevard
Elk Grove Village, IL 60007-1098
Telephone: (847) 228-5005
Fax: (847) 228-5097
Internet address: *http://www.aap.org*

American College of Allergy, Asthma and Immunology
85 West Algonquin Road, Suite 550
Arlington Heights, IL 60005
Internet address: *http://www.allergy.mcg.edu/about.html*

Food Allergy Network
10400 Eaton Place, Suite 107
Fairfax, VA 22030-2208
Telephone: (800) 929-4040
Internet address: *http://www.foodallergy.org*

Food and Drug Administration
Telephone: (888) INFO-FDA
Internet address: *http://www.fda.gov*

National Jewish Medical and Research Center
1400 Jackson Street
Denver, CO 80206
Telephone: (303) 388-4461
Internet address: *http://www.njc.org*

Information on Common Skin Diseases
From the web site of the National Skin Centre, Singapore
Internet address: *http://www.nsc.gov.sg/commskin/skin.html*

Information on Food Allergy Versus Food Intolerance
From the web site of the Canadian Lung Association
Internet address: *http://www.lung.ca/asthma/nutrition/intolerance.html*

Information on Sinusitis
A web site by Wellington S. Tichenor, MD
Internet address: *http://www.sinuses.com*

Links of Interest in Immunology and Allergology
From the web site of the Illinois State Academy of Science
Internet address: *http://www.il-st-acad-sci.org/health/immunol.html*

REFERENCES

Bousquet, J., & Demoly, P. (1996). Specific immunotherapy for allergic rhinitis in children. *Journal of Allergy and Clinical Immunology, 8,* 145–150.

Custovic, A., Woodcock, H., Craven, M., et. al. (1999). Dust mite allergens are carried on not only large particles. *Pediatric Allergy and Immunology, 10*(4), 258-260

Custovic, A., Hallam, C., Woodcock, H., et. al. (2000) Synthetic pillows contain higher levels of cat and dog allergen than feather pillows. *Pediatric Allergy and Immunology, 11*(2), 71-73.

Durham, S. R., Walker, S. M., Varga, E. M., Jacobson, M. R., O'Brien, F., Noble, W., et al. (1999). Long-term clinical efficacy of grass-pollen immunotherapy. *New England Journal of Medicine, 341,* 468–475

Golden, S. J., & Craig, T. J. (1999). Efficacy and safety of azelastine nasal spray for the treatment of allergic rhinitis. *Journal of the American Osteopathic Association, 99*(7 suppl), S7–12.

Hadley, J. A. (1999). Evaluation and management of allergic rhinitis. *Medical Clinics of North America, 83,* 13–25.

Joss, J. D., & Craig, T. J. (1999). Seasonal allergic conjunctivitis: Overview and treatment update. *Journal of the American Osteopathic Association, 99*(Suppl. 7), S13–S18.

Juniper et al. (1997). Measuring health-related quality of life in rhinitis. *Journal of Allergy and Clinical Immunology, 99*(2), S742–S749.

Kusunoki, T., Asai, K., Harazaki, M., Korematsu, S., & Hosoi, S. (1999). Month of birth and prevalence of atopic dermatitis in schoolchildren: Dry skin in early infancy as a possible etiologic factor. *Journal of Allergy and Clinical Immunology, 103,* 1148–1152.

Malone, D. C., Lawson, K. A., Smith, D. H., Arrighi, H. M., & Battista, C. (1997). A cost of illness study of allergic rhinitis in the United States. *Journal of Allergy, Asthma and Clinical Immunology, 97,* 22–27.

Mason, K., Riley, G., Siebers, R., Crane, J., & Fitzharris, P. (1999). Hot tumble drying and mite survival in duvets. *Journal of Allergy and Clinical Immunology, 104*(2 Pt 1), 499–500.

Meltzer, E. O. (1995). An overview of current pharmacotherapy in perennial rhinitis. *Journal of Allergy and Clinical Immunology, 95,* 1097–1110.

Naclerio, R. M. (1998). Optimizing treatment options. *Clinical and Experimental Allergy, 28*(Suppl. 6), 54–59.

Nathan, R. A., Meltzer, E. O., Selner, J. C., & Storms, W. (1997). Prevalence of allergic rhinitis in the United States. *Journal of Allergy, Asthma, and Clinical Immunology, 99,* 808–812.

Tada, J., Yamasaki, H., Toi, Y., Akiyama, H., & Arata, J. (1999). Is the face and neck pattern of atopic dermatitis in Japan a special variant? *American Journal of Contact Dermatitis, 10,* 7–11.

van Cauwenberge, P. (1998). Management of rhinitis: The specialist's opinion. *Clinical and Experimental Allergy, 28*(Suppl. 6), 29–33.

van der Heide, S., van Aalderen, W. M., Kauffman, H. F., Dubois, A. E., & de Monchy, J. G. (1999). Clinical effects of air cleaners in homes of asthmatic children sensitized to pet allergens. *Journal of Allergy and Clinical Immunology, 104*(2 Pt 1), 447–451.

Williams, H. C. (1999). Epidemiology of atopic dermatitis: Recent advances and future predictions. *Current Problems in Dermatology, 28,* 9–17.

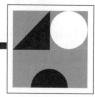

Chronic Pulmonary Diseases

- SUZETTE GJONAJ, MD; CAROL GREEN-HERNANDEZ, PhD, FNP-C;
DANIEL Z. ARONZON, MD, FAAP; JEAN LAVELLE, RN, MSN, FNP;
MARDHIE COLEMAN, RN, PhD(c); HENDRIKA MALTBY, RN, PhD, FRCNA;
LINDA KRISTJANSON, RN, PhD; and SUE ROBINSON, RN, MSC, PhD(c)

P A R T 1

Chronic Lung Diseases: Asthma and Cystic Fibrosis

- SUZETTE GJONAJ, MD; CAROL GREEN-HERNANDEZ
PhD, FNP-C; and DANIEL Z. ARONZON, MD, FAAP

INTRODUCTION

The lung is a remarkable organ that primarily serves as a unit of gas exchange. Asthma and cystic fibrosis (CF) are chronic lung diseases frequently seen in the pediatric population. Either of these lung diseases can impact a child's pulmonary function and, especially in the case of CF, other organ systems. This chapter provides pediatric primary care clinicians with content on the diagnosis and management of asthma and comanagement (with pediatric pulmonologists) of CF. It will examine quality of life issues, because children with these diseases face many challenges.

ASTHMA

Asthma, a chronic disorder of the airways, is characterized by inflammation that leads to hyper-responsiveness of the airways. Airflow limitation results from bronchoconstriction, mucus plugs, and increased inflammation (U.S. Department of Health and Human Services, 1997). Airflow limitation is reversible or partially reversible. Upon receiving a bronchodilator, pulmonary function improves to normal or near normal. Left untreated or undertreated, remodeling of the airways occurs with permanent changes (Laprise, Laviolette, Boutet, & Boutet, 1999).

Pathology

Although asthma exacerbations are episodic, the pathologic feature of the disease is chronic airway inflammation. Attacks often present with symptoms of coughing, wheezing, chest tightness, and difficult breathing. Histologic features of asthma include subepithelial fibrosis, collagen deposition, epithelial shedding, goblet cell metaplasia, smooth muscle hypertrophy, and infiltration of the submucosa by eosinophils (Djukanovic et al., 1990). Mucosal edema often results from microvascular leakage and hypersecretion of mucus from goblet cells, thereby causing mucus plugging of the peripheral airways and focal atelectasis.

Six risk factors exist for the pathogenesis of asthma:

- *Respiratory infections.* Rhinoviruses, respiratory syncytial virus (RSV), and influenza and parainfluenza are the most common responsible viruses. Evidence has shown that respiratory illnesses in childhood may predispose to airway reactivity. Fifty percent of children with RSV bronchiolitis continue to have airway hyper-responsiveness and abnormal pulmonary function tests (Rooney & Williams, 1971; Welliver, 1995; Sigurs et al., 1995). Recent long-term studies have shown that wheezy infants may have narrower peripheral airways, predisposing them to wheeze with viral infections (Martinez et al., 1995). These children, however, may "outgrow" wheezing as they grow older and their airways enlarge.

- **Clinical Pearl:** In children, the most common trigger for an asthmatic episode is a viral illness.

- *Parental smoking and other indoor environmental pollutants.* Maternal smoking during the perinatal period or thereafter (Murray & Morrison, 1986; American Academy of Pediatrics [AAP], 1999) and other indoor pollutants, such as wood stove smoke and dust mite exposure, have been shown to increase the severity of symptoms in children with asthma. Response to parental smoking is worse in males and older children with asthma (Murray & Morrison, 1989). The duration of the fetus's exposure and the number of cigarettes the mother smokes also play a role. Intrauterine exposure to cigarette smoke increases immunoglobulin E levels in the fetus and airway responsiveness at birth. These factors place the infant at risk for developing atopy and asthma in childhood (Young et al., 1991).

- *Atopy.* Most patients with asthma exhibit atopy (Gergen & Turkeltaub, 1992). Exposure to inhaled allergens in early life increases the risk of developing asthma. Studies show a correlation between the level of exposure to dust mites in early infancy and the age at which wheezing subsequently develops (Sporik, Holgate, Platts-Mills, & Cogswell, 1990). The link between food allergy and asthma is controversial. It is rare for a pulmonary reaction to occur secondary to food allergen exposure.

- *Genetics.* Evidence suggests that genetic factors play a role in asthma. One or both parents with asthma have a greater risk of having an asthmatic child than when neither parent is affected (Horwood, Fergusson, Hons, & Shannon, 1985). Seventeen percent of parents and 8% of siblings of asthmatic children have asthma themselves (Sibbald, Horn, Brain, & Gregg, 1980).

▲**Clinical Warning:** Infants of mothers who are heavy smokers have an increased incidence of wheezing and nonwheezing lower respiratory illnesses, even if they do not attend day care. Children with atopic dermatitis are more likely to develop asthma if their mother is a smoker.

- *Air pollution.* Controversy exists as to whether a child's exposure to sulphur dioxide (SO_2) and consequent decreased oxygen (O_2) and increased ozone levels lead to exacerbation of asthma symptoms. Epidemiologic evidence, however, demonstrates increased incidence in regions and countries with decreased air quality (1999) AAP.
- *Socioeconomic factors.* Individuals of African American heritage and lower socioeconomic status have a higher incidence of asthma. It appears that this may be due to the environmental factors associated with poverty and inner-city living (Weitzman, Gortmaker, & Sobol, 1990).

Epidemiology

Asthma is a common pediatric disease. Its incidence and prevalence are increasing throughout the world despite the improved understanding of its pathogenesis. The prevalence of asthma in the United States has increased from 31 per 1000 in 1980 to 54 per 1000 in 1994 (Centers for Disease Control and Prevention [CDC], 1998). Both incidence and prevalence are higher in African Americans compared with Caucasians (CDC, 1998; Lang & Polansky, 1994). Trend in mortality also increased by 6.2% per year during the 1980s (Weiss & Wagnerer, 1990). This trend continued into 1990s, with a higher mortality among individuals of African American heritage (Oliverti, Kercsmar, & Redline, 1996). Unlike other racial and ethnic groups, lifetime incidence of asthma and associated emergency care in African Americans does not change with improved socioeconomic status. Reasons for this epidemiologic fact are not yet clear (Miller, 2000).

Estimated health care costs (inpatient and outpatient) associated with asthma exceed $4 billion per annum (Taylor & Newacheck, 1992). Developed countries have a higher prevalence than third world countries, with less than 1% in some developing countries versus greater than 20% in some developed countries (Valacer, 2000; Newacheck & Halfon, 2000).

History and Physical Examination

When examining the child, the provider should obtain a careful history, paying attention to the following recurrent signs and symptoms:

- Wheezing
- Cough, especially worse at night
- Difficulty breathing
- Chest tightness
- Sinusitis
- Allergic rhinitis or atopic dermatitis
- Symptoms of wheezing, chest tightness, shortness of breath, or cough worsening when exposed to airborne allergens or irritants or during or after exercise (AAP, 1999).

In addition, the provider should document a family history of asthma, allergies (including atopic skin disease), sinusitis, or rhinitis (AAP, 1999).

The clinician should ask whether symptoms tend to worsen when the child is exposed to exercise, viral infections, animals with fur, dust mites, tobacco smoke, pollen, changes in temperature, strong emotional expression (laughing or crying hard), or exposure to aerosolized chemicals. The provider also should ask about self-treatment, including over-the-counter herbal remedies or asthma, cough, or cold medications. Display 55-1 provides a format for taking a comprehensive history for asthma.

▲**Clinical Warning:** Most children older than 3 years with asthma are atopic, so the provider should obtain a comprehensive environmental history. A sample format for an environmental history can be found in Display 55-2.

Physical examination should include observation of the child's pulse rate and rhythm, resting respiratory rate, signs of respiratory distress, evidence of cyanosis in lips and nail beds, signs of nail clubbing, and use of accessory muscles and chest circumference. The provider should auscultate the heart and examine the abdomen. He or she should inspect the skin for signs of atopic skin disease (AAP, 1999).

The provider can perform chest percussion in the older toddler and older children in general. Hyper-resonance indicates air entrapment, while any areas of percussed dullness can be mapped out for discerning mucous plugs versus areas of consolidation. If the provider suspects the latter, he or she should assess for "e" to "a" changes over the areas of dullness. The provider needs to pay special attention to the I:E ratio, normal being 2:1. He or she should auscultate over each lung area for a complete respiratory cycle, being careful to listen for full end-expiratory sounds.

● **Clinical Pearl:** Expiratory phase prolongation is one of the earliest signs of bronchial narrowing.

Diagnostic Criteria

The provider must consider many differential diagnoses before making the final determination that the patient has asthma. Display 55-3 provides the differential diagnosis for the conditions that are most closely associated with recurrent wheezing symptomatology in children. Because many of these problems present with similarities on physical examination, the clinician must carefully weigh these findings in tangent with diagnostic studies and laboratory tests.

Clinicians should note that in children younger than 5 years, wheezing may occur with acute upper respiratory infections. These patients are often diagnosed as having bronchitis, bronchiolitis, or pneumonia, with the result that

---

DISPLAY 55–1 • Format for a Comprehensive History in the Diagnosis of Asthma

Features to Note in an Asthma History

Nature of symptoms (wheeze, cough, chest tightness, dyspnea)

Pattern of symptoms (seasonal, diurnal variation, severity, frequency, triggering factors)

Frequency of hospitalizations, pediatric intensive care unit admissions, emergency room visits

Previous and current drug therapy, including over-the-counter drugs

Atopic history and environmental history

Impact of disease on child (school performance and attendance)

Family history

General medical history

- History of smokers (including family members and patient)
- Heating system (forced air, wood burning stove, kerosene heater)
- Humidity of home (> 50% allow dust mites to thrive)
- Presence of carpets, fabric upholstery, uncovered mattress, and pillow are sites where dust mites live
- Presence of animals (cats, dogs)
- Use of humidifiers (source of mold spores)
- Seasonal worsening of symptoms (trees, grasses, weeds)

they do not receive appropriate therapy for what is in reality asthma. Providers should follow the diagnostic criteria listed in Display 55-3, with the exception that spirometry is not feasible in these young patients (AAP, 1999).

● **Clinical Pearl:** A diagnosis of asthma is not required to begin treatment with asthma therapy. If effective, a trial plan using asthma medications will assist the pediatric provider in making the diagnosis of asthma (AAP, 1999).

In children 5 years old and younger who have wheezing in association with an acute upper respiratory viral infection, two general patterns of asthma occur:

- Symptom remission during the preschool years
- Persistence of asthma, continuing throughout childhood (AAP, 1999)

Diagnostic Studies

Spirometry and peak expiratory flow may show reversible and variable airflow limitation. Pulmonary function tests (eg, body plethysmography) can be done in specialized laboratories in children as young as 3 years (Kanengeiser & Dozor, 1994). Infant pulmonary function tests can be done in specialized laboratories, but in most cases, such testing is expensive and impractical. A more useful approach for the primary care provider is to test the effectiveness of bronchodilators in infants and young children. If a child shows a clinical response to this medication, the provider can presume that the patient has reversibility of bronchoconstriction. In the office, providers may use peak flow meters; however, peak flow has its limitations, as it only evaluates large airway flow. Peak flow is also an extremely effort-dependent test; many children have difficulty performing

DISPLAY 55–3 • Differential Diagnosis of Cough and Wheeze in Infants and Children

Cystic fibrosis and immotile cilia syndrome
Foreign body
Recurrent aspiration
Vascular anomalies
Tracheomalacia
Bronchiolitis obliterans
Immune deficiency states
Bronchopulmonary dysplasia
Left ventricular failure
Mediastinal masses

it. Spirometry can be done in an office setting. If abnormal, the provider can administer a bronchodilator and repeat spirometry to evaluate the patient's response to the bronchodilator.

Chest radiographs also may be useful. Asthmatic lungs may show hyperinflation. Radiographs also may help in narrowing the differential diagnosis by detecting parenchymal disease, congenital anomaly, or foreign bodies.

Management

The goals of asthma management are to minimize or abolish symptoms by selecting appropriate medications and to identify and avoid known triggers. Achieving these goals is important for the child to maximize lung function, minimize exacerbations, prevent limitations on activity, and avoid side effects to medications.

Table 55-1 provides the classification of asthma severity and peak flow and management information. Once asthma has been classified, current therapy follows a "step-wise" approach to asthma treatment. The patient is placed on appropriate medications for that step, and once control is obtained and maintained for about 3 months, there is a step-down in medications to the least required to control symptoms. Table 55-1 also delineates medications and guidelines for their use in asthma therapy.

There are two groups of asthma medications: reliever and controller medications. As Table 55-1 illustrates, patients in step 2 and above will benefit from controller medications.

Controller medications include the following:

- Corticosteroids
- Sodium cromoglycate
- Nedocromil
- Long-acting β2 agonists
- Leukotriene modifiers
- Sustained-release theophylline

The reliever medications include the following:

- Short-acting β2 agonists
- Anticholinergics
- Short-acting theophylline
- Epinephrine injections

Table 55-2 provides a synopsis of controller and reliever medications used in the treatment of asthma. The following discussion provides more in-depth information about these drugs.

Controller Medications

Inhaled Steroids

Since asthma has been recognized as an inflammatory disease, inhaled corticosteroids have played a vital role in its management (Barnes, 1993). Data suggest, however, that inhaled corticosteroids may have significant effects on a child's growth velocity (Witzmann & Fink, 2000).

Inhaled steroids have a broad mechanism of action, which may account for their significant efficacy as a controller medication. Steroids prevent exacerbations of the child's asthma, while decreasing airway hyper-responsiveness, improving pulmonary function tests, reducing asthma severity, and preventing airway remodeling (Vathenen, Knox, Wisniewski, & Tattersfield, 1991).

Table 55–1. CLASSIFICATION, DIAGNOSTIC CRITERIA AND STUDIES, AND MANAGEMENT OF ASTHMA

Classification	Symptoms	Nocturnal Symptoms	Pulmonary Function Tests (PFTs)	Longterm Management	Rescue Management
Step 1: mild intermittent	< one time per week, asymptomatic and normal PEF between episodes	< two times per month	> 80% predicted with < 20% variability	None	As needed: short-acting 2 agonists if symptomatic or before exercise
Step 2: mild persistent	> one time per week, but < one time per day	> two times per month	> 80% predicted with 20%–30% variability	Daily medication of inhaled steroids of 200–500 mcg, cromolyn sodium, nedocromil, leukotriene antagonist, or sustained-release theophylline. If symptoms persist on 500 mcg steroids, then use higher dose steroid, inhaled steroid, or add a long-acting 2 agonist, sustained-release theophylline, or leukotriene modifier	As needed: short-acting 2 agonists
Step 3: moderate persistent	Daily symptoms; daily use of 2 agonist; exacerbations affect activity	> one time per week	> 60%–< 80% predicted, with > 30% variability	Daily medication of inhaled steroids of 800–2000 mcg and a long-acting 2 agonist, sustained-release theophylline preparation, or leukotriene modifier	As needed: short acting 2 agonists
Step 4: severe persistent	Continuous symptoms; limited physical activity	Frequent	< 60% predicted, with > 30% variability	Daily medication of inhaled steroid of 800–2000 mcg or more, and either long-acting 2 agonist or sustained-release theophylline (There may be need for oral corticosteroids long term.)	As needed: short acting 2 agonists

Administration by the inhaled route has aided greatly in the management of asthma. There is high topical anti-inflammatory effect with limited systemic absorption. Long-term use of inhaled steroids reduces airway inflammation and bronchial reactivity (Juniper et al., 1990). Steroids block the late phase of asthma very well. Administration of steroids just prior to exercise does not block exercise-induced symptoms, but regular use does decrease the severity of exercise-induced asthma (Hendricksen & Dahl, 1983).

In Canada and many other countries, as well as in Europe, inhaled steroids are given by metered-dose inhalers (MDI), dry powder delivery systems, or nebulized solutions. This last delivery method is not yet approved for use in the United States, although that is expected to change. The dose of steroids ranges from low dose (200–500 mg/d) to high dose (800–2000 mg/d). One study suggests that doses over 400 mg/m^2 per day may cause

adrenal suppression (Oriftis, Milner, Conway, & Honour, 1990).

▲ **Clinical Warning:** Because of the possible impact inhaled corticosteroids can have on a child's linear growth velocity, the primary care provider should record the patient's height and compare to standard growth charts at each 6-month visit until completion of growth. If there is any question as to the child's growth trajectory, the provider should refer the patient to a pediatric endocrinologist for evaluation (Witzman & Fink, 2000; Littlewood, Johnson, Edwards, & Littlewood, 1988; AAP, 1999).

Some reports indicate that patients may have "catch-up" growth once steroids are discontinued. Other possible side effects of high-dose inhaled steroids include bone resorption and demineralization (Ali, Capewell, & Ward, 1991), cataracts (Karim, Thomson, & Jacob, 1989), and skin atrophy (Capewell, Reynolds, Shuttleworth, Edwards, & Finlay,

Table 55–2. MEDICATIONS USED IN THE TREATMENT OF ASTHMA

Drug	Route	Dosage	Side Effects
Reliever Medications (Short acting β2 agonists)			
albuterol	MDI (90 mcg/puff)	2 puffs 15 minutes prior to exercise or 2 puffs q4h prn	Not recommended for long-term use, can cause tremor, CNS stimulation, headache, insomnia, dizziness, palpitations
albuterol rotahaler	DPI (200 mcg/puff)	1–2 capsules as with MDI	
albuterol	Nebulizer (5 mcg/mL [0.5%] or 0.083% [unit dose vials])	0.05 mg/kg (minimum 1.25 mg and maximum 2.5 mg) mixed with NaCl	May mix with cromolyn or ipratropium; may double during exacerbation
pirbuterol	MDI (200 mcg/puff) Autohaler (200 mcg/puff)	As with albuterol	As with albuterol
terbutaline	MDI (200 mcg/puff)	As with albuterol	As with albuterol
bitolterol	MDI (370 mcg/puff)	As with albuterol	As with albuterol
Systemic Steroids			
prednisolone	Oral (5-mg tabs, 5 mg/5 mL, 15 mg/5 mL)	0.5–2 mg/kg/d, maximum 60 mg/d, for 3–10 d	Short "bursts" are safe, longer courses may cause HPA surpression, growth surpression, cushingnoid state, GI disturbances, muscle weakness
prednisone	Oral (5 mg/5 mL, 1-, 2-, 5-, 10-, 20-, 25-mg tabs)	As for prednisolone	As for prednisolone
methylprednisolone	Oral (2-, 4-, 8-, 16-, 32-mg tabs)	As for prednisolone	As for prednisolone
Long Term Controller Medications			
cromolyn sodium	MDI (1 mg/puff) or nebulizer ampule (20 mg/2 mL)	2–4 puffs t.i.d.-q.i.d. or 1 ampule t.i.d.-q.i.d.	Excellent safety profile; may be given before exposure to allergen or exercise with protection for 1–2 h
nedocromil	MDI (1.75 mg/puff)	2–4 puffs t.i.d.-q.i.d.	As with cromolyn
beclomethasone diproprionate (steroid)	MDI (42 mcg/puff or 84 mcg/puff)	Low dose: 84–336 mcg Medium dose: 336–672 mcg High dose: > 672 mcg	Growth retardation
fluticasone (steroid)	MDI (44, 110, 220 mcg/puff) DPI (50,100 mcg/dose)	Low dose: 88–176 mcg Medium dose: 176–440 mcg High dose: > 440 mcg	As with beclomethasone
triamcinolone (steroid)	MDI (100 mcg/puff)	Low dose: 400–800 mcg Medium dose: 800–1200 mcg High dose: > 1200 mcg	As with beclomethasone
flunisolide (steroid)	MDI (250 mcg/puff)	Low dose: 500–750 mcg Medium dose: 1000–1250 mcg High dose: > 1250 mcg	As with beclomethasone
budesonide (steroid)	DPI (200 mcg/dose)	Low dose: 100–200 mcg Medium dose: 200–400 mcg High dose: 400 mcg	As with beclomethasone
salmeterol (long-acting β2 agonist)	MDI (21 mcg/puff) DPI (50 mcg/dose)	1–2 puffs q12h (MDI) 1 dose q12h (DPI)	May use 1 dose qhs for nocturnal symptoms; not a rescue medication
Sustained-release albuterol	4-mg tablet	0.3–0.6 mg/kg/d, not exceeding 8 mg/d	As with albuterol
theophylline	Liquid, sustained-release tablets, and capsules	Starting dose 10 mg/kg/d to maximum of 16 mg/kg/d	Levels must be monitored may be used qhs for nocturnal symptoms
montelukast (Singulair)	4-, 5- and 10-mg tablets	*2–5 y: 4 mg (chewable tablet) qhs; 6–14 y: 5 mg (chewable tablet) qhs; > 15 y: 10 mg qhs	Headaches
zafirlukast (Accolate)	10- and 20-mg tablets	2–14 y: 10 mg b.i.d. > 14 y: 20 mg b.i.d.	Headaches; take 1 h before or 2 h after meals; warfarin metabolism inhibited
zileuton	300- and 600-mg tablets	> 12 yr: 2400 mg/d daily divided	Monitor hepatic enzymes; inhibits metabolism of warfarin; theophylline, and terfenadine

MDI = metered-dose inhaler; DPI = dry powder inhaler; CNS = central nervous system; HPA = hypothalamic pituitary adrenal; GI = gastrointestinal.
*N.B. Safety and effectiveness in children younger than 2 years have not been established.

1990). *Candida* infection of the oropharynx is rare in children (Shaw & Edmunds, 1986). Risks for *Candida* are decreased further with the use of spacer devices, mouth rinsing after taking the drug, and less frequent dosing schedules (Toogood et al., 1984). Oral steroids are rarely needed in the control of asthma in children. They are extremely useful, however, for short bursts of 4 to 6 days or so, until inhaled steroids can take effect. If a child needs oral steroids, then providers should prescribe the lowest dose possible, preferably on a once daily schedule. There may still be adrenal suppression with alternate-day dosing (Dolan et al., 1987).

Providers should note that not all inhaled steroids are equally potent. Some factors that affect efficacy are topical potency, lipophilicity, receptor binding affinity, and receptor binding half-life. Fluticosone has the greatest topical potency of the corticosteroids, being twice as potent as beclomethasone and about four times more potent than flunisolide and triamcinolone. Fluticasone also has the longest elimination half-life and the greatest adrenal-suppression effect. Because it has the least gastric and pharyngeal absorption, however, its potential for true adrenal suppression may not really be an issue.

Sodium Cromoglycate (Cromolyn)

Sodium cromoglycate (CS) is strictly a preventive drug and has no bronchodilating effects. Because it is an anti-inflammatory agent, it inhibits both early and late phases of asthma. Although CS is expensive, it has few side effects (Murphy, 1988; AAP, 1999). The patient must be an active participant in its use, starting with a four times daily regimen, which then may decrease to three times a day. If used less than three times a day, CS has no effect. CS may be of greater value when it is administered using a nebulizer. It blocks both allergy- and exercise-triggered symptoms well. It also may be used 15 to 20 minutes prior to exposure to allergen or exercise. For seasonal allergy, it is beneficial to start CS several weeks before and continue throughout the expected allergy season. About 66% of patients gain benefit from CS; however, CS is of no value in any child with asthma who is steroid dependent.

Nedocromil

Nedocfomil (NC) has an anti-inflammatory action similar to CS. It inhibits inflammation by blocking the chloride channels, modulating mast cell mediator release, and recruiting eosinophils. NC reduces bronchospasm triggered by cold dry air and exercise. It has been shown to decrease the need for quick-reliever medications, improving peak flow and reducing asthma symptoms. Some adult (Bone et al., 1990) and pediatric (Kemp, 1992) studies show a synergistic effect with inhaled corticosteroids, while other work does not support this effect (Boulet et al., 1990; Goldin & Bateman, 1988). The disadvantage of NC use is that 20% to 30% of users report an unpleasant taste, which may affect a child's willingness to use the medication.

Long Acting b2 Agents

As with the *short-acting* β2 agonists, *long-acting* β2 agents work by relaxing smooth muscles in the airway. They are often used in conjunction with anti-inflammatory medications. Recent studies suggest that this combination is better than doubling the dose of the steroid (AAP, 1999). The combination is used as a controller medication and is often helpful for nocturnal and exercise-induced symptoms. Recent case reports of sudden death while using these long-acting drugs have not been supported in more controlled studies.

Leukotriene Modifiers

This new line of medications blocks the steps that involve cysteinyl leukotrienes in the inflammatory cascade. Montelukast (Singulair) and zafirlukast (Accolate) work by blocking leukotriene D4 receptors, whereas zileuton inhibits the 5-lipoxygenase enzyme, thereby inhibiting the production of various leukotrienes (eg, B4, C4, D4, and E4). A modest increase in forced expiratory volume (FEV_1) by 10% to 15% was seen in clinical trials (Locker, Lavins, & Snader, 1995). In mild to moderate asthmatics, there was a reduction in β2 agonist use. The ease in taking an oral medication once or twice daily is certainly an advantage, as it will enhance compliance. The disadvantages are possible systemic side effects and drug–drug interactions.

Zileuton affects the metabolism of warfarin, theophylline, and terfenadine and can affect liver function. Zafirlukast also affects the metabolism of warfarin and requires liver function monitoring. Zafirlukast and montelukast have both been implicated in unmasking or causing Churg-Strauss syndrome. This syndrome is a vasculitis characterized by peripheral eosinophilia, pulmonary infiltrates, sinus complications, neuropathy, and asthma symptoms (eg, cough).

Theophylline

The use of theophylline is somewhat outdated. Its disadvantages include no sustained decrease in airway hyper-reactivity, high incidence of side effects, and possible behavioral and learning disturbances in some children.

Although theophylline is no longer a first-line medication, it is useful in selected cases. In patients who are inadequately controlled with long-acting β2 agonists and inhaled steroids, the addition of theophylline may be beneficial. For patients who are hospitalized with nocturnal symptoms, a dose at bedtime may help (Barnes, Greening, Neville, Timmers, & Poole, 1982). Patients who are unable to participate in a regimen that includes inhaled medications may tolerate theophylline.

Serum levels of theophylline should be between 12 and 15 mg/L to minimize the risk of side effects. Once therapeutic levels and control of symptoms are achieved, then serum levels should be monitored every 6 to 12 months.

▲ **Clinical Warnings:** If the patient has fever or is on erythromycin, the provider should lower the dose of theophylline by about 50% because the metabolism of theophylline may be affected. Chronic long-term use of theophylline may carry an added risk of mortality.

Reliever Medications
Short Acting β2 Agonists

This class of medications is the most potent of the bronchodilators. Short-acting β2 agonists include albuterol, pirbuterol, bitolterol, fenoterol, metaproterenol, isoetharine, and terbutaline. Their duration of action is between 4 and 8 hours. This class of medications also increases mucociliary clearance and has some anti-inflammatory effects. The typical side effects of these medications include tachycardia, tremor, and hypokalemia. Most children, however, experience few or minimal side effects.

Short-acting β2 agonists should be used as rescue treatment, because studies suggest that there may be down-regulation of receptors with frequent use of these drugs (Lipworth, 1997). Recently, the FDA has approved the use of levalbuterol in patients with asthma. In racemic albuterol, it is the (L)-albuterol that has bronchodilator effects. The (S)-albuterol has no therapeutic benefit and is responsible for the side effects. It appears that levalbuterol has a better therapeutic index than racemic albuterol (Gawchik, Saccar, Noonan, Reasner, & DeGraw, 1999). Whether the increased cost of levalbuterol justifies its decreased rate of side effects, however, remains to be seen. Its niche may be as a short-term reliever in children who have severe side effects with albuterol.

Anticholinergics

Ipratropium bromide has a slower onset of action but a longer duration of action than β2 agonists; however, ipratropium bromide has less bronchodilating properties. In status asthmaticus, the addition of ipratropium bromide provides additional bronchodilation of airways (Rowe, Travers, Holroyd, Kelly, & Bota, 1999). There is no defined role for ipratropium bromide in the maintenance management of asthma. Side effects are not common.

Goals of Asthma Management

The goals of asthma management include the following:

- Minimizing chronic symptoms
- Decreasing exacerbations
- Minimizing use of rescue β2 agonists (see Table 55-2)
- Preventing exercise limitations
- Promoting normal pulmonary function
- Preventing adverse side effects from medications

The child should see the provider every 1 to 6 months, depending on response to therapy (AAP, 1999). During these visits, providers should review therapy goals with the child and parent. They should examine attainment of goals and address concerns. The provider must review the management plan with the patient and family. Children with moderate-to-severe asthma need to monitor their peak flows. The child or parent should perform a return demonstration of peak flow measurement and inhaler use at the time of each office visit. The pediatric provider should then make adjustments in the teaching and treatment plan, based on need (AAP, 1999).

If the patient remains stable for 3 months, then the provider should follow a step down in long-term treatment. If symptoms are not subsequently controlled, the clinician should review content with the parents, teaching them to assess whether the child is using medications as prescribed, while also reviewing proper techniques of medication administration with spacer devices. The provider should review environmental control measures, ensuring that they are in place. If the family indeed understands and is following the management plan, then the provider should consider a step up in preventive medications. The following discussion describes different methods for providing medication to the child with asthma.

Drug Delivery Systems

Inhalation is the preferred route to administer medications in asthma. Inhaled medication can be deposited directly in the airways, where it has a shorter onset of action. The child needs lower doses when inhaling a medication and thus experiences fewer side effects. Three inhalation routes are available:

- Nebulizer
- MDI
- Dry powder

Nebulizer

An advantage of this system is that it does not require patient coordination, so young patients and those who are very ill can easily use it. Its disadvantages are that nebulizers are generally expensive, not very portable (except for the ultrasonic nebulizers), and overall, very inefficient. Up to 60% of the nebulized drug may be lost with this method of administration (Salzman, Steele, Pribble, Elenbaas, & Pyszczynski, 1989). A nebulizer can deliver several short-acting β2 agonists, anticholinergics, cromolyn, and corticosteroids. Of these, corticosteroids are not yet available in the United States for nebulization, although they are available in several other western countries.

Metered-Dose Inhalers

The MDI devices are portable and inexpensive. They require ideal inhalation technique if used without a spacer device. Even with optimum technique, MDIs deposit most of the medication in the oropharynx, with only about 10% reaching the airways. Because of the difficulty in otherwise achieving therapy results, spacer bars are recommended for MDIs.

Spacers and breath-actuated devices increase deposition of drug in the airways. The better spacers have large volumes and the added advantage of reducing oropharyngeal candidiasis. Cromolyn, ipratropium bromide, nedocromil, and a variety of β2 agonists and steroids are available in MDI form.

● **Clinical Pearl:** The provider should review MDI technique with a spacer device at every visit. He or she should encourage its use at every opportunity. The provider should also teach the patient how to use the rolled-up fist as a "built-in" spacer if one is lacking or the child refuses to carry or use it in front of friends.

Dry Powder Inhalers

This line of medications requires less coordination from patients, but an adequate inspiratory flow rate (> 60 L/min) is necessary. This method of delivery may be inadequate in acute exacerbations when the flow rate is reduced. Single- and multiple-dose inhalers are available. A variety of steroids and β2 agonists are available in this form.

What to Tell Parents

Providers should instruct parents and all caregivers that they need to report all asthma episodes to them immediately. Additional office visits may be warranted if instability is noted. In the event that practice coverage is not available, providers should instruct all caregivers to follow up immediately with an emergent provider. In the event that emergency transport to a care center is needed, providers should instruct caregivers to use ambulance rather than private transportation services. Such arrangements are vital should a child's airway be lost while en route for emergent treatment. The goal of therapy must be prevention to minimize the need for emergent intervention, whose positive outcomes cannot always be guaranteed.

Concerns in Infants and Young Children

Infants and young children are prone to have wheezing episodes for a multitude of reasons:

- Increased compliance of their chest wall
- Lower elastic recoil of the lung
- Increased resistance of peripheral airways
- Increased fatigability of the diaphragm muscles

Some infants will be transient wheezers and by ages 3 to 5 years, have no further symptoms (AAP, 1999). This group presents a challenge to providers. The diagnosis of asthma is made on clinical grounds. Viral infections rather than allergen exposure trigger most episodes, the latter of which is seen in the older child. Infant pulmonary function tests can be done; however, they are expensive and difficult to obtain and require specialized laboratories. These problems make infant pulmonary function testing generally impractical.

● **Clinical Pearl:** The diagnosis of asthma is confirmed when the patient responds favorably to a trial of bronchodilators.

An even greater challenge is to administer medications, although these are usually given by nebulizer. If a child needs preventive medications, few data in this population exist about the use of asthma drugs in infants. An effective method of drug delivery can pose another challenge, because parental and caretaker participation in the prescribed regimen typically requires them to give lengthy and multiple nebulized treatments daily. Conversely, they may struggle with giving the child an MDI with a spacer, which may be less effective than in the older child who is often better able to tolerate this method of delivery.

Parents and caretakers need clear teaching about asthma and how to use medications. The provider also should give consistent support and ongoing review about medications and their administration, virus and other episodic illness guidelines, and environmental control measures.

Concerns in Older Children and Adolescents

Older children and adolescents with asthma can present a special challenge for practitioners. These children are developmentally inclined to deny the chronicity of their asthma and to ignore or deny symptoms. They may be angry about their disease, believing that they can ignore symptoms without consequences.

The older child or adolescent may begin smoking, have poor relationships with authority figures, and may abuse their MDIs. With the wide variety of medications and delivery systems available, a mutual decision between provider and patient can assist in developing a partnership that will help the older child or adolescent, while supporting parents in their concerns. In many ways, the older child with asthma behaves as any other adolescent living with chronic disease, whether it be diabetes, cancer, or any other serious health concern. The reader is referred to Chapter 12 for a review of the developmental sequellae of this age category and its meaning in primary care.

Cough

Cough-variant asthma is seen in some patients. These patients may have cough as their only symptom of asthma.

Abnormalities typical of reversible obstructive airway disease include reduced large and small airway flows, increased thoracic gas volumes, and residual volumes that are reversible or partially reversible after a bronchodilator. Although cough is often a challenge to treat, standard asthma management is typically quite successful.

Exercise and Sports Participation

Exercise-induced asthma occurs with most children. A peak in airway obstruction occurs about 15 minutes after exercise begins, but there also may be a delayed phase, occurring a few hours after exercise. Symptoms are more severe when exercising in cold, dry air. The provider should stress the importance of pretreatment with a β2 agonist or cromolyn 15 to 20 minutes before exercise. The clinician needs to emphasize that some children will still need a rescue inhaler with them while exercising. Therefore, the β2 agonist may be a better inhaler choice, especially for youngsters who are unwilling to carry more than one inhaler with them. In any event, pretreatment before exercise may prevent symptoms.

● **Clinical Pearl:** With proper medication, support, and education, most children with asthma can engage in physical activities, including endurance sports. Only patients with the most severe form of asthma need to modify their participation in sports and physical activity (AAP, 1999).

Immunizations

All children and adolescents with asthma should receive influenza prophylaxis. Patients with severe asthma are candidates for the pneumococcal vaccine.

Nocturnal Asthma

Nocturnal asthma is seen in some children. Wheezing and coughing may occur at night or in the early morning. The provider should reassure parents that initial management aims at optimizing overall control of asthma.

▲ **Clinical Warning:** If nocturnal symptoms persist, the clinician should prescribe a nighttime dose of sustained-release theophylline or a leukotriene modifier. Either medication may alleviate the patient's nocturnal symptoms.

Emergencies

Acute exacerbations of asthma are quite common and can be potentially life threatening. Asthma accounts for many emergency room (ER) visits and a large percentage of hospitalizations. Most severe episodes can be prevented if they are recognized early and treated aggressively. The use of β2 agonists and systemic steroids in the early stages of an exacerbation can halt the episode. If the patient is not responding to these medications at home, the provider should refer him or her to an ER for further evaluation and management. Display 55-4 illustrates the pathology of an acute asthma episode.

Patients with an acute asthma episode often present with symptoms of tachycardia, tachypnea, dyspnea, use of accessory muscles, and pulsus paradoxus. Ominous signs include a silent chest on auscultation, cyanosis, respiratory muscle fatigue, and altered level of consciousness and pneumothorax. When treating patients with acute exacerbations, it is necessary to relieve hypoxia and reverse airway obstruction. The approach to this treatment is illustrated in Figure 55-1. Arterial blood gases may be useful in the sick asthmatic in

DISPLAY 55–4 • The Pathology of an Acute Asthmatic Episode

- Triggers: Viral infections, pollutants, allergies, exercise, sinusitis, aspirin
- Airway obstruction: increased airway obstruction, reduced flow rates (FEV1, PEFR), hyperinflation, air trapping, increased resistance, decreased compliance
- V/Q mismatching: some airways overventilated; others underventilated
- Hypoxemia
- Hyperventilation: ABG shows hypoxia (respiratory alkalosis—increased pH and decreased $PaCO_2$). A typical ABG might be 7.48/32/60.
- If the episode progresses: ABG shows respiratory acidosis (increased $PaCO_2$ and decreased pH), demonstrating muscle fatigue and impending respiratory failure (a typical ABG might be 7:36/42/50).

status. Respiratory acidosis can indicate impending respiratory failure.

▲ **Clinical Warning:** A normal pCO_2 with tachypnea is an ominous sign.

The provider does a great service in acknowledging to parents and other caregivers that they recognize that asthma management poses a great challenge. The clinician also should reassure concerned family that the first step in asthma management is to diagnose the disease correctly and then to find the correct line of treatment. The arsenal of medications available helps to individualize the child's treatment so that improved management can lead to tighter control of symptoms.

● **Clinical Pearl:** The pediatric provider should review medications and their delivery at every visit. Patient and family education is an ongoing, never-ending thread that runs through a successful asthma program. The hallmark of every successful asthma regimen is parent, patient, and clinician participation in supporting the child and family living with this disease.

▲ **Clinical Warning:** Parents and caregivers should not forget that asthma mortality still exists.

Teaching and Self-Care

Parents must know that the pediatric provider supports them in dealing with their child's asthma. Parents may be at once fearful and angry. Taking time to sit with them while explaining management information, such as peak flow how-tos or medication use and dosing, is important in helping family members to feel supported, while also enhancing their understanding of what they must do to keep their child healthy. Discussion about potential triggers of asthmatic episodes, including housekeeping practices, wood heat, pets, and smoking materials, must be direct and frank. Providers should encourage parents and caregivers to quit smoking. Because this desired outcome may not occur, the clinician should strongly urge that smoking never take place in the same environment as the child. This includes homes, friends' houses, social settings, and cars. The lingering aftereffects of smoke can trigger an asthmatic episode. Thus, the practitioner also should advise that parents observe for difficult breathing if their child is exposed to a smoker in close quarters. In addition, the practitioner should provide access to community resource information, including local American Lung Association affiliate contacts, because these can help parents to feel less isolated and vulnerable. Examples of such resources are found at the end of this chapter.

CYSTIC FIBROSIS

Cystic fibrosis is an inherited, autosomal recessive disease. It is the most common inherited lethal illness in the Caucasian population. Approximately 1 in 20 African Americans and Caucasians are carriers for CF (CF is rare in Asians). Thirty thousand people have the disease in the United States alone. This life-threatening illness affects multiple organs. Over the past 40 years, median age of survival has increased dramatically from 1 year to presently 31 years in the United States (Morgan et al., 1999). CF affects the sexes approximately equally.

Pathology

The CF gene was discovered in 1989 (Kerem et al., 1989). It is located on the long arm of chromosome 7 and is called the CF transmembrane conductance regulator (CFTR). The discovery of the gene has enabled prenatal testing to be done to detect carriers, which previously was not possible. Since the discovery of CFTR, over 900 known mutations also have

Acute episode unresponsive to treatment at home: ER management
→ Nebulized β_2 agonist with O_2 ± ipratropium bromide.
Steroids: PO or IV
Then:

Responding	Not responding
Discharge home on oral steroids and β_2 agonist	Admit to hospital: Nebulized β_2 agonist may give continuously Nebulized ipratropium bromide; O_2 and IV fluids and corticosteroids.
Re-assess as out-patient.	Re-evaluate; if not responding, add subcutaneous or intravenous (IV) β_2 agonist and IV aminophylline; consider assisted ventilation.

Figure 55–1 ■ Management of an acute exacerbation of asthma.

been discovered (Grody, 1999). Most commercial laboratories test for about 90 of the most common mutations.

The major problem is a defect in exocrine gland function. Abnormal secretions from these glands result in obstruction of and abnormal secretions of apocrine sweat glands. The CFTR gene is extremely large, involving 250,000 base pairs, encoding a protein with 1480 amino acids. The most common mutation is the Δ F508, in which phenylalanine is deleted at position 508 of the CFTR. This mutation occurs in about 70% of patients in the United States (Cystic Fibrosis Genetic Analysis Consortium, 1990), but there are over 900 known mutations. It is thought that CFTR is a cAMP-activated chloride channel. Thus, the defect leads to decreased secretion of chloride into the airway lumen and increased sodium absorption across the airway epithelium. This ultimately causes dehydration of the mucus in the airway, with decreased mucociliary clearance and, hence, obstruction of the organ passages. If needed, the provider should refer to Chapter 5 for more information on counseling and screening for CF (Anderson et al., 1991).

Pulmonary manifestations may not show until weeks, months, or even years after birth. There is inflammation of the airways before colonization by bacteria (Muhlebach, Stewart, Leigh, & Noah, 1999). Abnormally thick, tenacious mucus plugging the small airways initially damages the airways. Changes are usually more bronchial than parenchymal. Bronchiectasis is seen in most patients, even as young as 18 months, and is progressive with age (Thomassen, Demko, & Doershuk, 1987). Bacterial infection then occurs. *Staphylococcus aureus* is frequently seen initially, then *Pseudomonas aeruginosa* (usually the mucoid strain) later (Thomassen et al., 1987). *Burkholderia cepacia* has been isolated in patients with CF, which is associated with a more aggressive decline in pulmonary status (Frangolias et al., 1999). Once *Pseudomonas* is established, it is often difficult if not impossible to eradicate. When there is colonization by bacteria, a vicious cycle of chronic infection, tissue damage, and further obstruction occurs until there is respiratory failure and death.

History and Physical Examination

About half of children diagnosed with CF initially present with respiratory symptoms, predominantly chronic cough and wheezing (Thomassen et al., 1987). Younger patients may present with atelectasis of the right upper lobe. At first the cough may be dry, but with disease progression, it will become more productive. This is especially so with pulmonary exacerbations. The upper airway is also affected, with patients presenting with chronic rhinitis, sinusitis, and nasal polyps. Physical findings include rales, rhonchi, and wheezing.

With disease progression, there will be digital clubbing and a barrel-shaped chest deformity. Radiographic findings initially show hyperinflation and bronchial wall thickening. Subsequently, there will be atelectasis, localized infiltrates, bronchiectasis, pulmonary hypertension, and right ventricular hypertrophy.

Massive hemoptysis due to erosion of the bronchial arteries is serious and life threatening (Coss-Bu, Sachdeva, Bricker, Harrison, & Jefferson, 1997). Recurrence rate is high with significant mortality. In patients with end-stage CF, there is cor pulmonale secondary to chronic hypoxia.

▲ **Clinical Warning:** Providers must refer any child whose history and physical examination are suggestive of CF to an accredited CF center for workup, diagnosis, and management planning. It is imperative for the center's treatment team to

follow the patient and family lifelong to provide the child with consistent treatment, up-to-date technologies, and access to new therapies. In addition, should the child later develop complications of CF, such a center is best equipped to manage them. Consideration for transplantation need is best planned when a patient has continued in a CF practice group.

● **Clinical Pearl:** Providers should refer all parents with a child who is diagnosed with CF for genetics counseling.

The following section outlines the complications of CF by organ system. Management of each of these complications is discussed in the management section itself.

Pulmonary System

Sinopulmonary disease is a serious complication of CF and can include the following problems:

- Colonization by pathogens typical of CF lung disease: *S. aureus* (especially in the younger age group), *P. aeruginosa* (both mucoid and nonmucoid strains), *B. cepacia* (which is quite virulent and can increase mortality), and nontypable *Haemophillus influenzae*
- Endobronchial and parenchymal disease, such as bronchiectasis, bronchitis, bronchiolitis, atelectasis, pneumonias, or cor pulmonale. These may be manifested by wheezing and air-trapping, chronic cough, tenacious mucus production, digital clubbing, radiographic abnormalities (which may objectively be assessed by the Birmingham scoring system at the accredited CF center), and pulmonary function test. Birmingham scoring system indicates abnormalities (progressive loss of lung function).

Other complications of lung involvement in CF can result in the following:

- Pneumothorax and massive hemoptysis
- Chronic sinus disease with or without nasal polyposis
- Allergic bronchopulmonary aspergillosis

Gastrointestinal System

Nutritional and gastrointestinal abnormalities are significant problems that the pediatric provider and family will face in working with the child with CF. These include the following:

- Failure-to-thrive (FTT) due to fat and protein malabsorption (Giglio, Candusso, D'Orazio, Mastella, & Faraguna, 1997)
- Fat-soluble vitamin deficiency (eg, vitamin A and E deficiency, hypoprothrombinemia) for the same reason
- Meconium ileus, meconium ileus equivalent, and meconium plug syndrome
- Exocrine pancreatic insufficiency
- Distal intestinal obstruction syndrome
- Rectal prolapse and intussusception
- Recurrent pancreatitis
- Focal biliary cirrhosis and multilobular cirrhosis, cholecystitis, cholelithiasis, cholestasis, and portal hypertension
- Diabetes mellitus

When pancreatic function is lost, the child with CF will have fat and protein malabsorption. Carbohydrate malabsorption is also a problem to a lesser degree. These problems are manifested by FTT, sometimes despite a voracious appetite. Weight loss; abdominal distention; frequent, pale, oily, foul-smelling stools (steatorrhea); rectal prolapse; edema; and hypoproteinemia are seen as well (Wyllie, 1999). Certain CF mutations are more prone to pancreatitis. It is interesting to note that certain carriers are likely to have pancreatitis as well (Malats & Real, 1999). Up to 40% of all individuals with CF (75% in adults) have endocrine pancreatic abnormalities, exhibiting frank diabetes mellitus (Hardin & Moran, 1999). They usually present with a more insidious, benign clinical course, and rarely develop ketoacidosis. The patients, however, can develop other complications of diabetes, such as retinopathy, nephropathy, and microvascular changes. Refer to Chapter 61 for further discussion of prevention, diagnosis, and management of these problems.

Infants may present with meconium ileus, which is an obstruction of the distal ileum due to inspissated, thick meconium. In abdominal radiographs, the typical finding of distended bowel loops with a characteristic "bubbly" pattern in the distal ileum is diagnostic. There may be associated volvulus, small bowel atresia, microcolon, and perforation with this disorder.

▲ **Clinical Warning:** Providers must rule out CF in any infant with a meconium ileus. In addition, they should be aware that FTT can be an early sign of CF (Giglio et al., 1997).

Older children may develop distal intestinal obstruction syndrome (DIOS) (Freiman & FitzSimmons, 1996), formerly known as meconium ileus equivalent. This recurrent obstruction of the small or large bowel may be partial or complete. It was initially thought to result from use of high-dose enzyme preparations but is more likely to be due to the use of high-dose enzymes or undercontrol of absorption. Decreased fluid intake, changes in diet, discontinuation of pancreatic enzymes, or more recently, high-dose pancreatic enzymes may precipitate DIOS.

Malabsorption of fat-soluble vitamins (A, D, E, K) also occurs. Deficiency of vitamin A can present with xerophthalmia, night blindness, and, in infancy, a bulging fontanelle. Although overt rickets is a rarely seen deficiency of vitamin D, it can present with secondary hyperparathyroidism, decreased bone mineral content, and delayed bone maturation. Prolonged vitamin E deficiency causes spinocerebellar signs and symptoms. Patients may have deficiencies of zinc, iron, and magnesium. Vitamin K deficiency causes deficiency of clotting factors II, VII, IX, and X and hypoprothrombinemia, which may present with severe bleeding.

The liver and gallbladder may be involved in CF as well. The gallbladder is often hypoplastic, and 10% of older patients have gallstones (Shen, Tsen, Hunter, Ghory, & Rappaport, 1995). Multilobular biliary cirrhosis is typical of liver pathology in CF. It often begins focally. Patients who have meconium ileus, severe malnutrition, intrahepatic biliary stasis, and hypoalbuminemia in infancy are at risk of further liver involvement as they get older. Early signs may be thrombocytopenia, but elevation of transaminases may be very mild early in the course of the illness.

Reproductive System

The exocrine implications of long-term CF include endocrine outcomes besides those of the pancreas itself:

- Subfertility in females
- Obstructive azospermia in males, due to absent vas deferens
- Miscellaneous causes

Other Metabolic and Psychological Problems

The complexity of CF can lead to multiple comorbid problems:

- Hypochloremic hypokalemic dehydration
- Chronic metabolic alkalosis
- Arthritis/arthropathy (hypertrophic osteoarthropathy)
- Digital clubbing
- Psychosocial issues

Diagnostic Criteria

Cystic fibrosis can present at any age with a variety of symptoms. Respiratory symptoms include history of repeated pneumonias and sinusitis, respiratory infections, chronic wheezing, and coughing (Thomassen et al., 1987). Gastrointestinal symptoms include FTT, abnormal stool, and recurrent pancreatitis (Wyllie, 1999). Clinical suspicion is extremely important. Presentation with any of the symptoms shown in Table 55-3 requires investigation.

All exocrine glands of the body are affected by CF. Patients exhibit three distinct abnormalities in varying degrees:

1. Abnormal concentrations of inorganic ions are found in secretions from serous glands (eg, elevated chloride and sodium in sweat).

Table 55–3. CLINICAL FEATURES OF PATIENT WITH CYSTIC FIBROSIS

Age (Years)	Clinical Feature (Incidence)
0–2	Steatorrhea (85%)
	Meconium ileus (10%–15%)
	Rectal prolapse (20%)
	Obstructive jaundice
	Hypoproteinemia/anemia
	Bleeding diathesis
	Heat prostration/hyponatremia
	Failure to thrive
	Bronchitis/bronchiolitis
	Staphlococcus pneumonia
2–12	Malabsorption (85%)
	Recurrent pneumonia/ bronchitis (60%)
	Nasal polyps (6%–36%)
	Intussusception (1%–5%)
13+	Aspermia (98%)
	Chronic pulmonary disease (70%)
	Abnormal glucose tolerance (20%–30%)
	Focal biliary cirrhosis (15%–25%)
	Chronic intestinal obstruction (10%–20%)
	Gall stones (4%–14%)
	Diabetes Mellitus (7%)
	Portal hypertension (2%–5%)
	Clubbing
	Recurrent pancreatitis

2. Secretions from mucous glands are extremely viscous, causing obstruction and loss of function of these glands.
3. Endobronchial colonization by specific groups of bacteria occurs.

Diagnostic Studies

The diagnosis of CF is made at an accredited CF treatment center and includes one or more of the clinical features of CF listed on Table 55-1, as well as the following:

- Two positive sweat tests (using the quantitative pilocarpine iontophoresis method with sweat chlorides being > 60), or
- An abnormal nasal transepithelial potential difference, or
- Two CF mutations (although most commercial laboratories test for about 90 of the known mutations)

Newborn screening is also available through the immunoreactive trypsinogen level done on a blood specimen from a heel stick (Harringer et al., 1999). Babies with CF have an increased trypsinogen level.

▲ **Clinical Warning:** Only institutions that are accredited by the Cystic Fibrosis Foundation should do sweat tests, because these centers undergo rigorous evaluation.

The radiologist reading the film at the specialized institution assesses the chest radiograph. Pulmonary function tests show air trapping and airway obstruction, increasing with advancing lung disease (Freiman & FitzSimmons, 1996). During acute exacerbations, vital capacity and flow rates decline markedly, but may improve with inpatient or outpatient therapy. Patients may have a mixed obstructive-restrictive pattern in their pulmonary function tests. Other pulmonary complications include pneumothorax, with an incidence of 2% to 10% and a recurrence rate of 50% on the contralateral side within 6 to 12 months (Shen et al., 1995).

Management

It is essential that parents and child receive treatment at an experienced, accredited CF center with a multidisciplinary team composed of specialist physicians, clinical nurse specialists, nurses, nutritionists, physical therapists, and social workers for initial CF workup and management planning. The team's continued involvement in long-term comanagement with the pediatric primary care provider is essential to achieving the best possible outcomes for the child and family.

Sinopulmonary System

Management of CF should emanate from the team who treats the child at the accredited CF center. The goal of CF pulmonary management is to retard progression of the lung disease. Clearance of the mucus from the tracheobronchial tree is of utmost importance. This is done through airway clearance techniques, such as chest physical therapy, including postural drainage, manual or mechanical percussion (Thairapy vest), vibration (Flutter device) (Homnick, Anderson, & Marks, 1998), and assisted coughing (Malet, Borum, & Fromm, 1991).

Aggressive antibiotic management is also part of the arsenal against lung disease progression. Some centers use antibiotics continuously, while others use antibiotics during acute exacerbations. Antibiotics may be used orally, intravenously, and with a nebulizer (Le Brun et al., 1999). Exacerbations may be treated on an outpatient or inpatient basis at the accredited CF center or, at a minimum, in consultation with the CF treatment team. Antibiotics are usually chosen according to the sensitivities of the bacteria isolated. Combinations of an aminoglycoside and an antipseudomonal penicillin or cephalosporin are often used to decrease the likelihood of bacterial resistance. Nebulized medications also may be useful.

In select patients, the use of bronchodilators may be beneficial. Dornase alfa (Pulmozyme; DNAse) is often used once daily as a mucolytic; it degrades DNA, which is present in large quantities in the sputum of CF patients (Christopher, Chase, Stein, & Milne, 1999). The role of steroids, whether oral or inhaled, is controversial (Oermann, Sockrider, & Konstan, 1999). Because gene therapy is not yet available, the option of lung transplantation (cadaveric or living lung) can be offered to end-stage patients. The 5-year survival rate is 70% in either procedure (Harringer et al., 1999).

In consultation with the CF treatment team, the provider will treat the patient with sinusitis for prolonged courses with antibiotics. If the patient does not respond to this therapy, he or she may need a surgical procedure.

Most patients with pneumothorax require no surgical intervention. If needed, a chest tube can be inserted, with or without a sclerosing agent. Recurrence rate for pneumothorax is high, regardlees of whether surgical intervention was required.

Hemoptysis is often caused by erosion of surface capillaries, and is seen with acute exacerbations. More massive bleeding secondary to erosion of bronchial arteries is life threatening. This latter problem is often recurrent.

Gastrointestinal System

Because 80% to 85% of patients have pancreatic insufficiency, most children are placed on pancreatic enzyme supplements. Once enzymes are started, the pattern of stools becomes more normal in frequency, color, and odor as fat and protein are better absorbed. The dosage of enzymes is adjusted according to the patient's stool and growth pattern.

Patients should have an unrestricted high calorie, fat, and protein diet. The goal should be normal growth (McNaughton, Stormont, Shepherd, Francis, & Dean, 1999). Babies may be breastfed or take elemental formulas, which are easily absorbed. If the child has poor growth and insufficient caloric intake despite good nutritional counseling and attempts at oral supplementation, then enteral feeding should be considered. This may be done by nasogastric tube or gastrostomy tube with high-calorie feeds. Enteral feeding may improve pulmonary status once nutritional status has improved. These patients require supplementation with fat-soluble vitamins. Iron deficiency anemia should be promptly corrected.

▲ **Clinical Warning:** Children with CF require extra fluids with salt supplementation in hot weather.

Patients with diabetes can be treated by modest dietary changes, but many require insulin. With increased life expectancy, these patients should be monitored for vascular complications of diabetes. Hyperosmolar enemas may be successful in treating uncomplicated meconium ileus or DIOS. If this is unsuccessful, then surgical intervention may be needed. In recurrent episodes, increased enzymes, extra fluid intake, high-fiber diet, or a chronic stool softener, such as lactulose, may be helpful.

In patients with abnormal liver function and gallstones, the use of ursodeoxycholic acid (URSO) has resulted in improved liver status and dissolution of gallstones (Malet et al., 1991). Cholecystectomy is done if URSO has failed to dissolve the calculi. If bleeding secondary to varices with portal hypertension occurs, either endoscopic management or surgical intervention is required. Liver transplant can be undertaken with severe liver disease and good pulmonary status (Kelly, 1998). There have been very good survival rates.

Reproductive System

Ninety-eight percent of males are infertile. These patients have absent vas deferens, aspermia, and abnormalities of the seminal vesicle and epididymis (Phillipson, 1998). Females have decreased fertility but can have successful pregnancies without deterioration of pulmonary function (Hilman, Aitken, & Constantinescu, 1996). Favorable outcomes depend on good nutritional status and lung function at the onset of pregnancy. Subfertility is due to thick mucus at the cervix. Patients with CF who wish to avoid pregnancy may use oral contraceptives successfully.

Other Systems

Up to 15% of patients have hypertrophic osteoarthropathy, which presents with long bone pain, arthralgias, joint swelling, effusions, and periostitis (Parasa & Maffulli, 1999). The joints most affected are the knees, wrists, and ankles, with symmetrical involvement. Nonsteroidal anti-inflammatory agents are used quite successfully.

During hot weather (thermal stress) and diarrhea (gastrointestinal losses), patients are prone to dehydration with hyponatremia and hypochloremia. They may also have an associated metabolic alkalosis.

▲ **Clinical Warning:** Because of bleeding tendencies associated with vitamin K deficiency, the pediatric provider should check the prothrombin clotting time regularly if the CF center is not doing so.

What to Tell the Parents

The pediatric provider must remember that CF is a multisystem disease. The course of the illness varies among individuals, even though they may share the identical gene mutation. Frequent complications, psychosocial effects on patient and family, and uncertain prognosis demand the institution of an intensive and aggressive management program.

It is recommended for patients to be followed regularly at the CF treatment center to receive focused, ongoing psychosocial support, education, counseling, maintenance of adequate nutrition and growth, and prevention information, as well as aggressive treatment for pulmonary problems. It is encouraging to note that the survival rate has increased over the past 4 decades and that 33% of patients with CF today are older than 18 years (Dodge et al., 1997).

The pediatric primary care provider must support the child with CF and his or her family throughout childhood for the child to enjoy the best health possible into adulthood. CF is a disease that requires daily medications and, at times, intensive management. The reader is referred to Chapter 49, which will provide information about how to best help the child and family who are dealing with chronic disease. Other chapters, including 25, 26, 28, and 29, may help providers whose patients are having problems growing up with a chronic illness.

The goal is finding a cure for this devastating disease. Human trials testing gene therapy are underway (Chirmule et al., 1999). These studies are using different vectors, such as adenoviruses, adeno-associated viruses, and liposomes, as vehicles for carrying the normal gene into the patient's lungs. Recent work presented at the North American Cystic Fibrosis Conference in 1999 showed the possibility of correcting the fatty acid content of the airway epithelium as a possible cure.

COMMUNITY RESOURCES

Asthma and Cystic Fibrosis

www2.adam.com/dir/Diseases_and_Conditions/Allergies_and_Asthma/Asthma/Asthma.htm

> Ask Adam is a web-based resource that both providers and patients may find helpful for anatomy, pathology, and imaging information.

The American Lung Association (ALA)
1740 Broadway
NY, NY 10019
(212) 315-8700
(800) LUNG-USA or (800) 586-4872.

> The ALA is the oldest voluntary health organization for lung disease in the United States and is a resource for educational materials in English and in Spanish for both provider and families. On the Internet, a site map provides an alphabetical listing of topics available:
> http://www.lungusa.org/site'index/site'map.html

Asthma

American College of Allergy, Asthma, and Immunology
85 West Algonquin Road, Suite 550
Arlington Heights, IL 60005

> The American College of Allergy, Asthma, and Immunology is composed of allergists-immunologists and related health care professionals who do research and provide advocacy and professional and public education.

Allergy and Asthma Network
Mothers of Asthmatics, Inc.
2751 Prosperity Avenue, Suite 150
Fairfax, VA 22031
Phone: (800) 878-4403 or (703) 641-9595

> The Canadian Lung Association is the umbrella group for the 10 provincial Lung Associations in Canada. Information is provided for providers, families, patients, and teachers, with special content for children. Information about children's special summer camps can be found at provincial and national offices. The website is excellent.

The Lung Association's National Office:
The Lung Association
1900 City Park Drive, Suite 508
Blair Business Park
Gloucester, ON K1J 1A3 Canada
Phone: (613) 747-6776
On the internert: *info@lung.ca*

The Journal of the American Medical Association (JAMA) has a special website dedicated to asthma materials for families and providers. The JAMA Asthma Information Center is designed as a professional, produced by JAMA editors and staff and supported by Zeneca Pharmaceuticals. Despite pharmaceutical sponsorship, the site is a good resource for information: *http://www.ama-assn.org/special/asthma/*

Cystic Fibrosis

Cystic Fibrosis Foundation

The CF Foundation is a good resource for provider, family, and patient information about CF. The Foundation can provide information about local support groups, summer camps, and pen pal opportunities:

    6931 Arlington Road
    Bethesda, MD 20814
    Phone (800) 344-4827
    Internet address: *www.cff.org*

Solvay Health Care maintains a web site that provides links to multiple international associations dedicated to CF. This is a resource page that can benefit all associated with CF, from patients and their families to providers: *http://www.cysticfibrosis.co.uk/links.htm*

REFERENCES

Ali, N. J., Capewell, S., & Ward, M. J. (1991). Bone turnover during high dose inhaled corticosteroid therapy. *Thorax, 46*, 160–164.

American Academy of Pediatrics (AAP). (1999). *Practical guide for the diagnosis and management of asthma.*

Anderson, M. P., Rich, D. P., Gregory, R. J., et al. (1991). Generation of cAMP-activated chloride currents by expression of CFTR. *Science, 251*, 679–682.

Barnes, P. J. (1993). Inhaled corticosteroids for asthma. *New England Journal of Medicine, 332*, 868–874.

Barnes, P. J., Greening, A. P., Neville, L., Timmers, J., & Poole, G. W. (1982). Single-dose slow release aminophylline at night prevents nocturnal asthma. *Lancet, 1*, 299–301.

Bone, M. F., Kubik, M. M., Kearny, N. P., et al. (1990). Nedocromil sodium in adults with asthma dependent on inhaled corticosteroids. A double blind, placebo controlled study. *Thorax, 44*, 654–659.

Boulet, L-P., Cartier, A., Cockcroft, D. W., Gruber, J. M., Leberge, F., et al. (1990). Tolerance to reduction of oral steroid dosage in severely asthmatic patients receiving nedocromil sodium. *Respiratory Medicine, 84*, 317–323.

Capewell, S., Reynolds, S., Shuttleworth, D., Edwards, C., & Finlay, A. Y. (1990). Purpura and dermal thinning associated with high dose inhaled corticosteroids. *British Medical Journal, 300*, 1548–1551.

Centers for Disease Control and Prevention. (1998). Surveillance for asthma-United States, 1960–1995. *Morbidity and Mortality Weekly Report, 47*, 1–26.

Chirmule, N., Propert, K., Magosin, S., Qian, Y., Qian, R., & Wilson, J. (1999). Immune responses to adenovirus and adeno-associated virus in humans. *Gene Therapy, 6*(9), 1574–1583.

Christopher, F., Chase, D., Stein, K., & Milne, R. (1999). rhDNase therapy for the treatment of cystic fibrosis patients with mild to moderate lung disease. *Journal of Clinical Pharmacology Therapy, 24*(6), 415–426.

Coss-Bu, J. A., Sachdeva, R. C., Bricker, J. T., Harrison, G. M., & Jefferson, L. S. (1997). Hemoptysis: A 10-year retrospective study. *Pediatrics, 100*(3), E7.

Cystic Fibrosis Genetic Analysis Consortium. (1990). Worldwide survey of the DF508 mutation-Report from the Cystic Fibrosis genetic analysis consortium. *American Journal of Human Genetics, 47*, 354–359.

Djukanovic, R., Roche, W. R., Wilson, J. W., et al. (1990). Mucosal inflammation in asthma. *American Review of Respiratory Disease, 142*, 434–457.

Dodge, J. A., Morison, S., Lewis, P. A., Coles, E. C., Littlewood, J. M., et al. (1997). Incidence, population, and survival of cystic fibrosis in the UK, 1968-95. UK Cystic Fibrosis Survey Management Committee. *Archives of Diseases in Children, 77*(6), 493–496.

Dolan, L. M., Kesarwala, H. H., Holroyde, J. C., et al. (1987). Short-term high-dose systemic steroids in children with asthma: The effect on the hypothalamic-pituitary-adrenal axis. *Journal of Allergy and Clinical Immunology, 80*, 81–86.

Frangolias, D. D., Mahenthiralingam, E., Rae, S., Raboud, J. M., Wilcox, P. G., et al. (1999). Burkholderia cepacia in cystic fibrosis. Variable disease course. *American Journal of Respiratory and Critical Care Medicine, 160*(5 Pt 1), 1572–1577.

Freiman, J. P., & FitzSimmons, S. C. (1996). Colonic strictures in patients with cystic fibrosis: Results of a survey of 114 cystic fibrosis care centers in the United States. *Journal of Pediatric Gastroenterological Nutrition, 22*(2), 153–156.

Gawchik, S. M., Saccar, C. L., Noonan, M., Reasner, D. S., & DeGraw, S. S. (1999). The safety and efficacy of nebulized levalbuterol compared with racemic albuterol and placebo in the treatment of asthma in pediatric patients. *Journal of Allergy and Clinical Immunology, 103*(4), 615–621.

Gergen, P. J., & Turkeltaub, P. C. (1992). The association of individual allergen reactivity with respiratory disease in a national sample: Data from the second National Health and Nutrition Examination Survey, 1976-80 (NHANES II). *Journal of Allergy and Clinical Immunology, 90*, 579–588.

Giglio, L., Candusso, M., D'Orazio, C., Mastella, G., & Faraguna, D. (1997). Failure to thrive: The earliest feature of cystic fibrosis in infants diagnosed by neonatal screening. *Acta Paediatrics, 86*(11), 1162–1165.

Goldin, J. G., & Bateman, E. D. (1988). Does nedocromil sodium have a steroid sparing effect in adult asthmatic patients requiring maintenance oral corticosteroids? *Thorax, 42*, 982–986.

Grody, W. W. (1999). Cystic fibrosis: Molecular diagnosis, population screening, and public policy. *Archives of Pathology and Laboratory Medicine, 123*(11), 1041–1046.

Hardin, D. S., & Moran, A. (1999). Diabetes mellitus in cystic fibrosis. *Endocrinology and Metabolic Clinics of North America, 28*(4), 787–800, ix.

Harringer, W., Wiebe, K., Struber, M., Franke, U., Haverich, A., et al. (1999). Lung transplantation—10-year experience. *European Journal of Cardiothoracic Surgery, 16*(5), 546–554.

Hendricksen, J. M., & Dahl, R. (1983). Effects of inhaled budesonide alone and in combination with low-dose terbutaline in children with exercise induced asthma. *American Review of Respiratory Diseases, 128*, 993–997.

Hilman, B. C., Aitken, M. L., & Constantinescu, M. (1996). Pregnancy in patients with cystic fibrosis. *Clinical Obstetrics and Gynecology, 39*(1), 70–86.

Homnick, D. N., Anderson, K., & Marks, J. H. (1998). Comparison of the flutter device to standard chest physiotherapy in hospitalized patients with cystic fibrosis: A pilot study. *Chest, 114*(4), 993–997.

Horwood, L. J., Fergusson, D. M., Hons, B. A., & Shannon, F. T. (1985). Social and familial factors in the development of early childhood asthma. *Pediatrics, 75*, 859–868.

Juniper, E. F., Kline, P. A., Vanzieleghem, M. A., et al. (1990). Effect of long term treatment with an inhaled corticosteroid (budesonide) on airway hyperrresponsiveness and clinical asthma in non-steroid dependent asthmatics. *American Review of Respiratory Diseases, 142*, 832–836.

Kanengeiser, S., & Dozor, A. (1994). Forced expiratory maneuvers in children aged 3 to 5 years. *Pediatric Pulmonology, 18*, 144–149.

Karim, A. K. A., Thomson, G. M., & Jacob, T. J. L. (1989). Steroid aerosols and cataract formation. *British Medical Journal, 299*, 918.

Kelly, D. A. (1998). Current results and evolving indications for liver transplantation in children. *Journal of Pediatric Gastroenterologic Nutrition, 27*(2), 214–221.

Kemp, J. P. (1992). Nedocromil sodium a new bronchial anti-inflammatory agent. *Today Thor Trends, 10*, 39–42.

Kerem, B., Rommens, J. M., Buchanan, J. A., Markiewicz, D., Tsui, L. C., et al. (1989). Identification of the cystic fibrosis gene: Genetic analysis. *Science, 245*(4922), 1073–1080.

Lang, D. M., & Polansky, M. (1994). Patterns of asthma mortality in Philadelphia from 1969 to 1991. *New England Journal of Medicine, 331*, 1542–1546.

Laprise, C., Laviolette, M., Boutet, M., & Boulet, L. P. (1999). Asymptomatic airway hyperresponsiveness: Relationships with airway inflammation and remodelling. *European Respiratory Journal, 14*(1), 63–73.

Le Brun, P. P., de Boer, A. H., Gjaltema, D., Hagedoorn, P., Heijerman, H. G., & Frijlink, H. W. (1999). Inhalation of tobramycin in cystic fibrosis. Part 1: The choice of a nebulizer. *International Journal of Pharmacology, 189*(2), 205–214.

Lipworth, B. J. (1997). Airway sensitivity with long acting β2 agonists. Is there cause for concern? *Drug Safety, 16*(5), 295–308.

Littlewood, J. M., Johnson, A. W., Edwards, P. A., & Littlewood, A. E. (1988). Growth retardation in asthmatic children treated with inhaled beclomethasone diproprionate. *Lancet, 1*, 115–116.

Locker, R. F., Lavins, B. J., & Snader, L. (1995). Effects of 13 weeks of treatment with ICI204,219 (Accolate) in patients with mild to moderate asthma. *Journal of Allergy and Clinical Immunology, 95*, 839A–845A.

Malats, N., & Real, F. X. (1999). Correction: Mutations of the cystic fibrosis gene in patients with chronic pancreatitis [letter; comment]. *New England Journal of Medicine, 340*(20), 1592–1593.

Malet, P. F., Borum, M., & Fromm, H. (1991). Cystic fibrosis: Another use for urso? *Gastroenterology, 100*(3), 841–842.

Martinez, F. D., Wright, A. L., Taussig, L. M., et al. (1995). Asthma and wheezing in the first six years of life. *New England Journal of Medicine, 332*, 133–140.

McNaughton, S. A., Stormont, D. A., Shepherd, R. W., Francis, P. W., & Dean, B. (1999). Growth failure in cystic fibrosis. *Journal of Paediatric and Child Health, 35*(1), 86–92.

Miller, J. E. (2000). The effects of race/ethnicity and income on early childhood asthma prevalence and health care use. *American Journal of Public Health, 90*(3), 428–430.

Morgan, W. J., Butler, S. M., Johnson, C. A., Colin, A. A., FitzSimmons, S. C., et al. (1999). Epidemiologic study of cystic fibrosis: Design and implementation of a prospective, multicenter, observational study of patients with cystic fibrosis in the U.S. and Canada. *Pediatric Pulmonology, 28*(4), 231–241.

Muhlebach, M. S., Stewart, P. W., Leigh, M. W., & Noah, T. L. (1999). Quantitation of inflammatory responses to bacteria in young cystic fibrosis and control patients. *American Journal of Respiratory and Critical Care Medicine, 160*(1), 186–191.

Murphy, S. (1988). Cromolyn sodium: Basic mechanisms and clinical usage. *Pediatric Allergy Immunology, 2*, 237–254.

Murray, A. B., & Morrison, B. J. (1986). The effect of cigarette smoke from the mother on bronchial responsiveness and severity of symptoms in children with asthma. *Journal of Allergy and Clinical Immunology, 76*, 575–581.

Murray, A. B., & Morrison, B. J. (1989). Passive smoking by asthmatics: Its greater effects on boys than on girls and on older than on younger children. *Pediatrics, 84*, 451–459.

Newacheck, P. W., & Halfon, N. (2000). Prevalence, impact, and trends in childhood disability due to asthma. *Archives of Pediatric and Adolescent Medicine, 154*(3), 287–93.

Oermann, C. M., Sockrider, M. M., & Konstan, M. W. (1999). The use of anti-inflammatory medications in cystic fibrosis: Trends and physician attitudes. *Chest, 115*(4), 1053–1058.

Oliverti, J. O., Kercsmar, C. M., & Redline, S. (1996). Pre- and perinatal risk factors in innercity African-American children. *American Journal of Epidemiology, 143*, 570–573.

Oriftis, K., Milner, A. D., Conway, E., & Honour, J. W. (1990). Adrenal function in asthma. *Archives of Diseases in Children, 65*, 838–840.

Parasa, R. B., & Maffulli, N. (1999). Musculoskeletal involvement in cystic fibrosis. *Bulletin of Hospital Joint Diseases, 58*(1), 37–44.

Phillipson, G. (1998). Cystic fibrosis and reproduction. *Reproduction and Fertility Development, 10*(1), 113–119.

Rooney, J. C., & Williams, H. E. (1971). The relationship between proved viral bronchiolitis and subsequent wheezing. *Journal of Pediatrics, 79*, 744.

Rowe, B. H., Travers, A. H., Holroyd, B. R., Kelly, K. D., & Bota, G. W. (1999). Nebulized ipratropium bromide in acute pediatric asthma: Does it reduce hospital admissions among children presenting to the Emergency Department? *Annals of Emergency Medicine, 34*(1), 75–85.

Salzman, G. A., Steele, M. T., Pribble, J. P., Elenbaas, R. M., & Pyszczynski, D. R. (1989). Aerolsolized metoproternol in the treatment of asthmatics with severe airflow obstruction. Comparison of two delivery methods. *Chest, 95*(5), 1017–1020.

Shaw, N. J., & Edmunds, A. T. (1986). Inhaled beclomethasone and oral condidiasis. *Archives of Diseases in Children, 61*, 788–790.

Shen, G. K., Tsen, A. C., Hunter, G. C., Ghory, M. J., & Rappaport, W. (1995). Surgical treatment of symptomatic biliary stones in patients with cystic fibrosis. *American Surgery, 61*(9), 814–819.

Sibbald, B., Horn, M. E. C., Brain, E. A., & Gregg, I. (1980). Genetic factors in childhood asthma and wheezy bronchitis. *Archives of Diseases in Children, 81*, 63–70.

Sigurs, N., Bjarnason, R., Sigurbergsson, F., et al. (1995). Asthma and immunoglobulin E antibodies after respiratory syncytial virus bronchiolitis: A prospective cohort with matched controls. *Pediatrics, 95*, 500–505.

Sporik, R., Holgate, S. J., Platts-Mills, T. A. E., & Cogswell, J. J. (1990). Exposure to house dust mite allergen (Der p 1) and the development os asthma in children: A prospective study. *New England Journal of Medicine, 323*, 502–507.

Taylor, W. R., & Newacheck, P. W. (1992). Impact of childhood asthma on health. *Pediatrics, 90*, 657–662.

Thomassen, M. J., Demko, C. A., & Doershuk, C. F. (1987). Cystic fibrosis: a review of pulmonary infections and inteventions. *Pediatric Pulmonology, 3*, 334–351.

Toogood, J. H., Baskerville, J., Jennings, B., et al. (1984). Use of spacers to facilitate inhaled corticosteroid treatment of asthma. *American Review of Respiratory Diseases, 129*, 723–729.

U.S. Department of Health and Human Services. (1997). *National Asthma Education and Prevention program, National Heart, Lung, and Blood Institute, National Institutes of Health: Expert Panel Report II: Guidelines for the diagnosis and management of asthma.* Bethesda, MD: Author.

Valacer, D. J. (2000). Childhood asthma: Causes, epidemiological factors and complications. *Drugs, 59*(Suppl 1:1-8), 43–45.

Vathenen, A. S., Knox, A. J., Wisniewski, A., & Tattersfield, A. E. (1991). Time course of change in bronchial reactivity with an inhaled steroid in asthma. *American Review of Respiratory Diseases, 143*, 1317–1321.

Weiss, K. B., & Wagnerer, D. K. (1990). Changing pattern of asthma mortality. Identifying populations at high risk. *Journal of the American Medical Association, 264*, 1683–1687.

Weitzman, M., Gortmaker, S., & Sobol, A. (1990). Racial, social and environmental risks for childhood asthma. *American Journal of Diseases in Children, 144*, 1189–1194.

Welliver, R. C. (1995). RSV and chronic asthma. *Lancet, 346*, 789–790.

Witzmann, K. B. A., & Fink, R. J. (2000). Inhaled corticosteroids in childhood asthma: Growing concerns. *Drugs, 59*(Suppl 1), 9–14; discussion 43–45.

Wyllie, R. (1999). Gastrointestinal manifestations of cystic fibrosis [editorial]. *Clinical Pediatrics (Phila), 38*(12), 735–738.

Young, S., LeSouef, P. N., Geelhoed, G., et al. (1991). The influence of a family history of asthma and parental smoking on airway responsiveness in early infancy. *New England Journal of Medicine, 324*, 1168–1173.

P A R T   2   ▲

A Mother's Perspective of Asthma

- JEAN LAVELLE, RN, MSN, FNP

INTRODUCTION

I have been personally involved in the treatment of pediatric asthma for 20 years. My oldest child, a son, was diagnosed with asthma in the late 1970s, before his first birthday. At that time, the health care community still viewed asthma as a disease of bronchoconstriction. Medical management aimed toward decreasing bronchoconstriction and eliminating environmental triggers. Providers expected parents to master the management of episodic illness in their child when the baseline was wheezing. Now the realistic goal is to have a wheeze-free baseline (National Heart, Lung, and Blood Institute [NHLBI], 1997). Episode prevention is a realistic goal. A shift also has occurred in the last 20 years toward self-management of asthma and its symptoms.

● **Clinical Pearl:** Studies have shown that patient education improves outcomes in asthma (Lieu, Quesenberry, Capra, et al., 1997; Gibson, Shah, & Mammoon, 1998; Stout, White, Rogers, et al., 1998).

Therapeutic goals should focus on changing behavior, not just increasing knowledge (Hanson, 1999). Many of the studies cited make children with asthma participants in the development of a care plan and increase the likelihood that they will respond appropriately when needed. Hopefully, the shift has occurred from a medical management model to one of guided self-management. As a parent of an asthmatic child, I frequently found myself questioning at what point I should call the primary care provider, wondering "Am I overreacting?"

● **Clinical Pearl:** It is difficult to describe the anxiety surrounding knowing when to call. A parent's tendency may be to wait too long, only for clinicians to ask on arrival at the clinic or emergency department, "How long has the child been like this?" or "Why didn't you bring him in sooner?" Frequently, a parent is exhausted from having been up during the night with the sick child. These questions can quickly reduce a parent to tears.

The Guidelines for the Diagnosis and Management of Asthma (NHLBI, 1997) include Asthma Action Plans to assist families in making the decision of when to call the health care provider. Several versions of the form include a delineation of actions to take when peak flow is below the patient's personal best. Green, yellow, and red zones are specified and personalized to the child's own management plan. Written management plans have been shown to reduce the risk of adverse outcomes in asthma (Lieu et al., 1997).

INFANTS

MacDonald (1996) examined mothers of infants with asthma, documenting the feelings of vulnerability of these women. Because the child cannot verbally communicate distress, parents must read the signs the child is giving. Mothers in the study describe eventually overcoming their fears, becoming confident in their ability to read cues. Primary care providers should spend time with parents, suggesting methods of monitoring their child's breathing and when to report change. A useful handout from the NHLBI (1992) is entitled "If Your Infant Has Asthma, You will Have to Take Extra Care." It reviews "dos and don'ts" for parents and caregivers.

Starting in infancy, when an asthma episode occurs, providers should encourage parents to keep a journal of any factors they believe could have precipitated this event. A viral illness is common, but parents should note exposure to any toxins or environmental allergens. Before a child can cooperate with the use of an MDI, nebulizers are recommended for young children with moderate to severe asthma.

The NHLBI (1997) notes that "Tobacco smoke is a major precipitant of asthma symptoms in young children" (p. 4). Families need to eliminate tobacco smoke from the home environment. The Asthma and Allergy Foundation of America notes in its pamphlet entitled "How to Reduce Exposure to Allergens" that other potential allergens to eliminate are dust mites (in bedding and carpets), mold, mildew, animal dander and saliva, and cockroaches. All stuffed toys should be machine washable. In humid climates, the home should have a dehumidifier. Parents should consider a high-efficiency particulate air (HEPA) filter, which has been shown to be effective in removing mold spores, cat dander, and particulate tobacco smoke (NHLBI, 1997). Providers should encourage families when purchasing these filters to be sure they are buying a HEPA filter. These are available in local department stores. In some cases, following these suggested guidelines will not lead to complete relief of symptoms (Gotzsche, Hammarquist, Burr, & Berger, 1998). I remember feeling as though I had somehow done an inadequate job of eliminating these household allergens; after following all the guidelines, my son's asthma still did not improve.

TODDLERS

As children become mobile and verbal, it is possible for them to begin to communicate about their respiratory status. Parents should know the signs that will detect an asthma exacerbation early. For instance, observing that the youngster limits activity may be a clue to a change in status. A dry, persistent clearing of the throat is an early symptom of bronchoconstriction in a toddler too young to use a peak flow meter effectively.

● **Clinical Pearl:** With the toddler's growing independence comes the word "no." Clinicians should caution parents against battling over the use of medication or a nebulizer. Parents may find it useful to associate a pleasurable activity with these interventions. Reading to a child while he or she uses the nebulizer or encouraging another quiet activity, such as coloring, may help to prevent power struggles involving asthma therapy.

PRESCHOOLERS AND SCHOOL-AGE CHILDREN

The Asthma Daily Self-Management Plan proposed by NHLBI (l997) clearly states that asthmatics should be able to participate fully in activities of their choice. The expectation is that children with asthma are not precluded from attending preschool programs because of health concerns.

The American Lung Association has developed a videotape for preschoolers entitled " 'A' is for Asthma." Sesame Street puppets present information about asthma. These programs are made available for school groups.

When a child is to be left regularly at day care or school (including preschool, elementary school, and middle school), the school should have a written management plan for the adults who will care for the child. NHLBI (l997) proposes the use of a student asthma action card or asthma action plan (NHLBI, 1992). Caregivers at school could use such items to remain aware of the triggers that have been identified for this child and what to do if an exacerbation occurs at school.

If parents anticipate that teachers and other caregiving personnel will need to check peak flows while the child is in their care, then they should teach such individuals how to assist the child in obtaining a peak flow reading and recording it. Teachers and other personnel should be aware of changes to make based on the reading (if they need to be made) and who to call in case of an acute exacerbation. If the child needs to restrict an activity, such as a gym class or recess, on the basis of the peak flow readings, the provider should give written instructions. The child may feel more comfortable than caretaking adults in making changes in medications and activity level. Parents may need to insist that the adults in the school or day care learn more about asthma management.

● **Clinical Pearl:** In the absence of a nurse in the building during the school day, Eisenberg, Moe, and Stillger (1993) found that nonmedical personnel who interact with children also can learn the necessary information to help improve asthma care in schools.

The American Lung Association offers a school-based asthma education program called "Open Airways." It is designed over six sessions that include breathing exercises, instruction in how to do a peak flow reading, relaxation techniques, discussion of how to decide when to stay home from school, and when to call the primary care provider. It provides handouts for parents. Two studies have shown that asthma knowledge improves with these programs (Horner, l998; Moe, Eisenberg, Vollmer, et al., 1992). The Asthma and Allergy Foundation of America publishes numerous resources for families and providers to assist children and their families in living with asthma. Their catalogue includes pamphlets, brochures, videos, and CD-ROMs.

As children become cognitively able to understand and socially able to communicate needs, they should become increasingly autonomous in their management plan. In some schools, of course, health care providers will need to sign the necessary forms to allow children to regulate their own participation in gym class, outdoor recess, and other periods of physical exertion. For most schools, primary care providers will need to provide a written prescription to school personnel for medication use. They will need to make decisions as to whether a child can hold these medications in class or must keep them in the nurse's office.

When my son was in school, we found it very difficult to control the triggers in the school environment. Parents must take a proactive role in assisting their child in reducing and eliminating allergens and triggers in school (NHLBI, 1998). Some are obvious, but others are not so clear. For example, most of us would consider chalk dust to be a possible problem. I suggest that every parent walk around a school building during a school day to ascertain their child's exposure to toxins. Are people allowed to smoke tobacco on school grounds? Are animals in classrooms? Does the art teacher use materials with strong odors or fumes? Are there signs of cockroach infestation in the school? What kinds of materials are used to clean and disinfect when children are in the building? Are any plants or fresh flowers in the building (a frequent parent organization fundraiser)? Is the library dusty? Are carpets in the classrooms? Even if none of these are present in the classroom, do children go to other classes for group work where some potential triggers are present?

ADOLESCENTS

The Expert Panel Report (NHLBI, l99l) identified children in the late teen years as a high-risk group for life-threatening asthma episodes. Many factors contribute to this risk. Many teens have been told that someday they will "outgrow" their asthma. If they have not seen improvement or complete relief from symptoms, they may become angry and refuse to participate in their asthma management. Peer pressure and a desire to fit in are other influences. Adolescents may hide asthma from their friends and schoolmates to appear like the rest of their group. Denial and a reluctance to pursue medical attention also play a role (Randolph & Fraser, 1999). The adolescent desire for autonomy also may contribute to skipping peak flow readings and medicine doses. Because many recommended asthma medications are prophylactic drugs, it is difficult to get an adolescent to see the benefit when he or she does not experience immediate gain from taking the medication. As many of their peers begin to experiment with recreational drugs, including tobacco and alcohol, it might prove too difficult for the adolescent not to participate in these activities. One approach would be for the primary care provider to speak frankly with the adolescent (NHLBI, l997), discussing these concerns without the parents present. Doing so will support the teen's need for autonomy and, perhaps, reinforce a sense of responsibility for self-care.

▲ **Clinical Warning:** The dangers of secondhand smoke and the sulfites in beer and alcohol may present real problems for teens.

The American Lung Association and the Asthma and Allergy Association of America have programs specifically designed with teens in mind. On-line chat rooms are available, as are books and videos. Peer-led education groups have been shown to be a good approach to educate teens about asthma (Gibson, Shah, & Mammoon, 1998).

When my son was in grade school, he would go to the nurse's office to take his cromolyn before going outside to recess. A classmate asked him why he frequently left class to go to the nurse's office. "Are you sick?" "No," he replied. "I have asthma." Hopefully, all children will be able to adopt this attitude.

COMMUNITY RESOURCES

Asthma and Allergy Foundation of America
1125 Fifteenth St, NW Suite 502
Washington, DC 20005
(202) 466-7643
(800) 7-ASTHMA
E-mail: info@aafa.org
Internet address: *www.aafa.org*

Free Asthma Action Cards are available; "Resource Guide" lists books, videos, games, and pamphlets written to appeal to separate groups: young children, teens, and adults. The Resource Guide is available in Spanish. Local chapters have support groups. Newsletter is sent to members.

Allergy and Asthma Network/Mothers of Asthmatics
3554 Chain Bridge Rd.
Fairfax, VA 22030-2709
(800) 878-4403

Books, videos, fact sheets, medical supplies (flow meters and holding chambers), and "allergy cookbooks" are available.

National Jewish Center for Immunology and Respiratory Medicine
1400 Jackson St.
Denver, CO 80206
(303) 388-4461
(800) 222-LUNG Can speak with a nurse at this 800 number.
Educational materials: Brochures and pamphlets available.
(800) 552-LUNG: More than 40 recorded messages are
    available.

"Understanding Asthma" is a comprehensive discussion of asthma, allergy, therapy, and monitoring of asthma.

American Lung Association
1740 Broadway
New York, NY 10019-4374
(212) 315-8700
(800) LUNGUSA

"A" is for Asthma" videotape and Sesame Street puppets are available. "Open Airways for Schools" involves trained volunteers who give programs in schools (six sessions) that include breathing exercises, relaxation techniques, medications, peak flow use, and when to call the primary care provider.

Indoor Air Quality Tools for Schools—Done with the EPA

Asthma Information Center
http://www.mdnet.de.asthma

American Academy of Allergy, Asthma and Immunology
611 E Wells St.
Milwaukee, WI 53202
(414) 272-6071
(800) 822-2762
www.aaaai.org

Physician referrals, asthma camps, professional resource center, professional meetings, Journal of the American Medical Association asthma information center are available.
http://www.ama-assn.org/special/asthma
This web site is a resources for patients and professionals; support and information groups are available.

American College of Allergy Asthma and Immunology
85 W Algonquin Rd., Suite 550
Arlington Heights, IL 60005
(847) 427-1200
Fax (847) 427-1200
(800) 842-7777

National Asthma Education and Prevention Program National Heart, Lung, and Blood Institute Information Center
P.O. Box 30105
Bethesda, MD
(301) 592-8573
www.nhlbi.nih.gov/nhlbi.htm
Guidelines for diagnosis and management of asthma are offered.

REFERENCES

Eisenberg, J. D., Moe, E., & Stillger, C. F. (1993). Educating school personnel about asthma. *Journal of Asthma, 30*(5), 351–358.

Gibson, P. G., Shah, S., & Mammoon, H. A. (1998). Peer-led asthma education for adolescents: Impact Evaluation. *Journal of Adolescent Health, 22*, 66–72.

Gotzsche, P. C., Hammarquist, C., Burr, M., & Berger, A. (1998). House dust mite control measures in the management of asthma: Meta-analysis. *British Medical Journal, 317*(7), 1105–1115.

Hanson, J. (1999). Patient education in pediatric asthma. In S. Murphy & H. W. Kelly (Eds.), *Pediatric asthma* (pp. 183–210). New York: Marcel Dekker.

Horner, S. D. (1998). Uncertainty in mothers' care for their ill children. *Journal of School Health, 68*(8), 329–333.

Lieu, T. A., Quesenberry, C. P., Capra, A. M., Sorel, M. E., Martin, K. E., & Mendoza, G. R. (1997). Outpatient management practices associated with reduced risk of pediatric asthma hospitalization and emergency department visits. *Pediatrics, 100*(3), 334–341.

MacDonald, H. (1996). Mastering uncertainty: Mothering the child with asthma. *Pediatric Nursing, 22*(1), 55–59.

Moe, E. L., Eisenberg, J. D., Vollmer, W. M., Wall, M. A., Stevens, V. J., & Hollis, J. F. (1992). Implementation of "Open Airways" as an educational intervention for children with asthma in an HMO. *Journal of Pediatric Health Care, 5*(Part l), 251–255.

National Heart, Lung, and Blood Institute. (1991). *National asthma education Program expert Panel report 1: Guidelines for the diagnosis and management of asthma.* Bethesda, MD: U.S. Dept of Health and Human Services, 1992. DHHSA Publ. No. 91–3042.

National Heart, Lung, and Blood Institute. (1997). *National asthma education program expert panel report 2: Guidelines for the diagnosis and management of asthma.* Bethesda, MD: U.S. Dept of Health and Human Services, NIH Publ. No. 97–4051.

National Heart, Lung, and Blood Institute. (1998). National Asthma Education and Prevention Program. School Asthma Education Subcommittee. *Journal of School Health, 68*(4), 167–168.

National Heart, Lung, and Blood Institute. (1992). *National asthma education Program. Teach your patients about asthma: A clinician's guide.* Bethesda, MD: U.S. Dept of Health and Human Services, Publ. No 92–2737.

Randolph, C., & Fraser, B. (1999). Stressors and concerns in teen asthma. *Current Problems in Pediatrics, 29*, 82–93.

Stout, J. W., White, L. C., Rogers, L., McRorie, T., Morray, B., Miller-Ratcliffe, M., & Redding, G. J. (1998). The Asthma Outreach Project: A promising approach to comprehensive asthma management. *Journal of Asthma, 35*(1), 119–127.

PART 3 ▲

Supporting the Needs of Parents of Children With Asthma

- MARDHIE E. COLEMAN, RN, PhD(c), MRCNA;
  HENDRIKA J. MALTBY, RN, PhD, FRCNA;
  LINDA J. KRISTJANSON, RN, PhD,
  and SUZANNE M. ROBINSON, RN, MSC

INTRODUCTION

The impact of asthma on parents and the extent to which they are able to help their children respond to the demands of this illness are critical components in understanding the social dimension of this disease. This section provides background on the development of an instrument known as the Support Needs Inventory of Parents of Children With Asthma (SNIPAC) tool that providers can use to measure the support needs of parents of children with asthma. It presents directions for gathering and interpreting data collected with this tool. Primary care providers who choose to use this means of collecting information related to family support will find that it enriches any family assessment.

ASTHMA: A COMPLEX DISEASE

Asthma, a complex disease process, involves biochemical, immune, infectious, endocrine, and psychological factors (Anderson, Anderson, & Glanze, 1994). In the United States, asthma affects nearly 15 million people, 1 in 10 children, with 5000 deaths per year (National Institute of Allergy and Infectious Diseases, 1996). In Australia and New Zealand, the incidence has risen from 2:100,000 in 1978, to 1:3 in 1999 for children ages 15 years and younger (Department of Child Welfare, NSW, 1999; International Study of Asthma and Allergies in Childhood, 1992). When one considers that chronic illness, such as asthma, occurs within the family context, the number of individuals that this disease affects is staggering.

Economic, social, and community costs in Australia now total $1.2 billion per year. In the United States, estimates are that children with asthma lose 10 million school days each year, costing approximately $1 billion in lost productivity of their parents. The cost of asthma-related health care in the United States is approximately $6.2 billion (National Institute of Allergy and Infectious Diseases, 1996).

Asthma is more complex than its medical definition suggests. As is true with many other diseases, asthma has a social dimension. Researchers and primary care providers have increasingly recognized that the social and medical dimensions of the illness are linked (Nocon & Booth, 1991). Juniper, Guyatt, Feeny, et al. (1996) reported that children with asthma are troubled not only by symptoms, but by the physical, social, educational, and emotional impairments that they experience in response to their asthma.

Growing evidence has shown that asthma is responsible for a broad range of restrictions, eliciting a variety of emotional and behavioral responses in the child and family. It is known that family responses to illness directly affect the health of family systems (Rolland, 1987; Woods, Yates, & Primomo, 1989). Families represent a significant context for each member's health, responding as an interrelated system to illness in a member. Families living with a chronically ill child must adapt to living in a complex, unpredictable, and changing environment (Donnelly, 1994).

BACKGROUND TO DEVELOPMENT OF THE SNIPAC INSTRUMENT

In examining the needs of English parents of children with asthma, Nocon and Booth interviewed parents of 32 children younger than 10 years (1991). Challenges that families of children with asthma face include frequent hospitalizations, interruptions in education, economic stresses, and restrictions in everyday activities. The researchers also found that the children's asthma required alterations in household arrangements, changes in parents' employment, and limitations on family holidays. Eighteen parents noted that their children's behavior deteriorated, often imposing considerable emotional strain on families. Some reported feeling that they lived their lives in a state of perpetual exhaustion and anxiety related to not knowing when the next acute episode would stop or start. Nocon and Booth concluded that the physical implications of asthma did not totally account for its all-embracing social impact on the lives of families and children with asthma.

Building on this theme, Donnelly (1994) conducted a descriptive study of parents of children with asthma. The children were ages 1 to 5 years and lived on the eastern seaboard of the United States. She reported that families seldom experience one stressor at a time, managing a number of demands from all areas of family life. Some concurrent life stresses reported to reduce a family's ability to adapt are a change of employment status, the birth of another child, and an illness or injury of another family member. Donnelly also concluded that emotional and behavioral responses of parents of asthmatic children require coping strategies for adaptation and adjustment aimed at promoting family health over time.

Little is understood about the families of children who are not in an illness crisis or who are coping well with their disease, as few studies have examined this particular group. Clearly parents must cope with a multitude of social and emotional aspects when their child has asthma, even if that child is not in crisis and is coping well. The following tool was originally developed as a research instrument (Coleman, Maltby, Kristjanson, & Robinson, 1999; Kristjanson, Atwood, & Degner, 1995). Although it continues to be tested, the instrument is provided so that the reader who chooses to may use it in the clinical assessment of parental needs and issues arising when coping with their child who has asthma. The reader is also referred to Part B of this chapter for further validation of parental needs for social support in dealing with a chronically ill child.

THE SNIPAC

The SNIPAC instrument (Appendix 55-1) is structured to elicit two types of information: (1) the extent to which support needs are important and (2) the extent to which support needs have been met (Parents' Fulfillment Scale). The format is straightforward and elicits useful data for the provider at any stage of asthma. The tool is written at a sixth grade reading level and is designed for the child's parents to complete. When combined, the two subscales, Parents' Priority Scale and Parents' Fulfillment Scale, provide information for parents and clinician as to what support(s) the family needs. Items in the first subscale, Parents' Priority Scale, are rated on a scale of one to five, with one being not important and five being extremely important.

Parents answer the second subscale, Parents' Fulfillment Scale, as met, partly met, or unmet. When the provider examines the two scales, he or she should focus on needs that were not met and that parents rated as very to extremely important. The clinician and parents then can collaborate to develop an action plan. In this way, the needs of the parents are met, enabling them to meet the needs of their child. This can result in better management and reduced levels of stress for families dealing with asthma.

Supporting the illness-related needs of parents can be an important component of the provider's treatment of the child with asthma. Supporting the needs of parents may help to control the escalating costs of asthma management, in that it may decrease the economic and social costs to the community associated with provision of care to children with asthma. The provider who uses the SNIPAC as part of the family and cultural assessment can elicit vital information needed for supporting the families of children with asthma. The reader is referred to the Chapter 2 for information on family and cultural assessment.

REFERENCES

Anderson, K. N., Anderson, L. E., & Glanze, W. D. (Ed.). (1994). *Mosby's medical, nursing, and allied health dictionary* (4th ed.). St Louis: Mosby.

Coleman, M.E., Maltby, H.J., Kristjanson, L.J., & Robinson, S.M. (1999). *Development and testing of the support needs inventory tool for parents of children with asthma.* Edith Cowan University: Authors.

Department of Child Welfare, NSW. (1999). *Asthma report.* Sydney: Author.

Donnelly, E. (1994). Parents of children with asthma: An examination of family hardiness, family stressors, and family functioning. *Journal of Paediatric Nursing, 9*(6), 398–408.

International Study of Asthma and Allergies in Childhood (ISSAC) Coordinating Committee. (1992). *Manual for the international study of asthma and allergies in childhood (ISAAC).* Bochum and Auckland: ISAAC Co-ordinating Committee.

Juniper, E., Guyatt, G. H., Feeny, D. H., Ferrie, P. J., Griffith, L. E., & Townsend, M. (1996). Measuring quality of life in children with asthma. *Quality of Life Research, 5*(1), 35–46.

Kristjanson, L. J., Atwood, J., & Degner, L. F. (1995). Validity and reliability of the family inventory needs (FIN): Measuring the care needs of families of advanced cancer patients. *Journal of Nursing Management, 3*(2).

National Institute of Allergy and Infectious Diseases. (1996). *Fact sheet: Asthma: A concern for minority populations.* http://www.niaid.nih.gov/factsheets/minorasthms.htm

Nocon, A., & Booth, T. (1991). The social impact of asthma. *Family Practice, 8*(1), 37–41.

Rolland, J. S. (1987). Chronic illness and the family: An overview. In L. M. Wright & M. Leahy (Eds.) *Families and chronic illness.* Springhouse PA: Springhouse.

Woods, N., Yates, B., & Primomo, J. (1989). State of the science: Supporting families during chronic illness. *Image, 21*, 45–50.

A P P E N D I X   55–1

Support Needs Inventory of Parents of Children With Asthma (SNIPAC)

Please answer both sections of the questionnaire.

SECTION A
Please show how important the following needs are for you as a parent by circling the appropriate number on the questionnaire:

SECTION B
Tick if that need was met, partly met, or not met.

Not important (1), somewhat important (2), Average importance (3), Very important (4), and Extremely important (5).

	Parents' Priority Scale					Parents' Fulfillment Scale		
PERSONAL NEEDS I NEED TO:	RATE FROM 1–5					MET	PARTLY MET	UNMET
1. Have my questions answered honestly	1	2	3	4	5	____	____	____
2. Feel there is help and support	1	2	3	4	5	____	____	____
3. Be assured that the best possible health care is being given to my child	1	2	3	4	5	____	____	____
4. Know that the health care professionals see me as the central person in my child's care	1	2	3	4	5	____	____	____
5. Have trust in the health care team	1	2	3	4	5	____	____	____
6. Meet with other mothers/parents dealing with similar issues	1	2	3	4	5	____	____	____
7. Be involved with a support group	1	2	3	4	5	____	____	____
8. Know that the health care professionals caring for my child are competent	1	2	3	4	5	____	____	____
INFORMATION NEEDS I NEED TO:								
9. Know the long term issues of my child's illness	1	2	3	4	5	____	____	____
10. Know to whom I should direct my questions	1	2	3	4	5	____	____	____
11. Know whom to turn to if conflict situations arise	1	2	3	4	5	____	____	____
12. Know what information to give to extended family about asthma	1	2	3	4	5	____	____	____
13. Know how to handle my child's feelings	1	2	3	4	5	____	____	____
14. Know why things are done to my child	1	2	3	4	5	____	____	____
15. Know what treatment my child is receiving	1	2	3	4	5	____	____	____
16. Know *what* side effects the treatment can cause	1	2	3	4	5	____	____	____
17. Know *when* to expect side effects to occur	1	2	3	4	5	____	____	____
18. Know *what* information to give to my child with asthma (appropriate to his or her age)	1	2	3	4	5	____	____	____
19. Know *how* to give information to my child with asthma (appropriate to his or her age)	1	2	3	4	5	____	____	____
20. Have thorough information about how to care for my child at home	1	2	3	4	5	____	____	____
21. Be told when changes are being made in my child's treatment plans	1	2	3	4	5	____	____	____
22. Be told about people who could help with my concerns	1	2	3	4	5	____	____	____
23. Know where to park when at the hospital/clinic	1	2	3	4	5	____	____	____
24. Know where things are in the hospital	1	2	3	4	5	____	____	____
25. Know where things are in the city	1	2	3	4	5	____	____	____
26. Know *what* information to give to my other children (appropriate to his or her age)	1	2	3	4	5	____	____	____

(Continues)

A P P E N D I X   **55-1**   *(Continued)*

Support Needs Inventory of Parents of Children With Asthma (SNIPAC)

	Parents' Priority Scale					Parents' Fulfillment Scale		

INFORMATION NEEDS
I NEED TO:

27. Know *how* to give information to my other children (appropriate to his or her age)	1	2	3	4	5	____	____	____
28. Know how to handle the feelings of my other children	1	2	3	4	5	____	____	____
29. Know how environmental factors can affect my child	1	2	3	4	5	____	____	____
30. Know exactly what makes my child's asthma worse in the home environment	1	2	3	4	5	____	____	____

COMMUNITY SUPPORT
I NEED TO:

31. Know that the child's teachers have the knowledge to support child at school/day care/after-school care	1	2	3	4	5	____	____	____
32. Know that my child's teachers/day care are able to act appropriately in times of acute episodes	1	2	3	4	5	____	____	____
33. Know that my child's sporting associations are able to act appropriately in times of acute episodes	1	2	3	4	5	____	____	____
34. Know that our friends have the information to support our child when socializing.	1	2	3	4	5	____	____	____

MEDICAL SUPPORT
I NEED TO:

35. Have my child participate in decisions about his or her care (appropriate to his or her age)	1	2	3	4	5	____	____	____
36. Know I can ask questions of the doctors	1	2	3	4	5	____	____	____
37. Have explanations given in terms that are understandable to me	1	2	3	4	5	____	____	____
38. Know what situations I can and cannot control while my child is in the hospital	1	2	3	4	5	____	____	____
39. Know that I am listened to with respect by the health care professionals caring for my child	1	2	3	4	5	____	____	____
40. Feel that health care professionals accept me even if I am angry or upset	1	2	3	4	5	____	____	____

SELF-CARE NEEDS
I NEED TO:

41. Have someone be concerned with my health	1	2	3	4	5	____	____	____
42. Have time to myself	1	2	3	4	5	____	____	____
43. Have time to exercise	1	2	3	4	5	____	____	____
44. Have time to socialize without the child/ren	1	2	3	4	5	____	____	____
45. Have flexible employment opportunities	1	2	3	4	5	____	____	____

LIFESTYLE NEEDS
I NEED TO:

46. Feel encouraged by health care professionals to maintain a normal lifestyle	1	2	3	4	5	____	____	____
47. Have financial assistance to help cope with costs of my child's illness (eg, parking, food, transport, medicine, change to home environment)	1	2	3	4	5	____	____	____
48. Have information to assist with lifestyle planning: a. Seasons b. Holidays c. Air travel d. Social activities	1	2	3	4	5	____	____	____

Are there any other needs in any of the categories that have been missed? _____

CHAPTER 56

Congenital Heart Disease and the Partially Repaired Heart

• CAROLINE TASSEY, MS, CPNP

INTRODUCTION

Care of the child with heart disease can be a challenge for the primary care provider. The variety of structural defects is complex, and the effects of such defects on children range from minimal to life threatening. Specialty management techniques are evolving rapidly. More children with complex heart disease survive longer and have a better quality of life than was true even 15 years ago. While the vast majority of congenital cardiac lesions have few effects on the child's growth and development and require late (if any) intervention, about one third of such lesions have a more significant impact on children and their families. This chapter provides an overview of general clinical problems and management issues that occur in this population, with specific emphasis on the child who requires staged surgical intervention.

ANATOMY, PHYSIOLOGY, AND PATHOLOGY

The most useful way to characterize congenital heart defects is to divide them into defects that increase pulmonary blood flow, decrease pulmonary blood flow, and obstruct systemic blood flow (Display 56-1). Additionally, it helps to know which defects will support a two-ventricle repair and which will require a staged, single-ventricle approach. This classification is far more helpful than classifying defects as cyanotic or acyanotic, because cyanosis is associated with a variety of defects at different physiologic stages. This categorization also is more helpful to the provider in anticipating symptoms and problems.

Blood flow always takes the path of least resistance. When a communicating opening (shunt) exists, blood flows from areas of higher pressure (usually the left side of the heart or aorta) to areas of lower pressure (usually the right side of the heart or the lungs). Pulmonary vascular resistance (PVR) is highest in fetal life and immediately after birth. Maximal shunting occurs once PVR reaches normal, low levels at about 1 to 3 months of age. Occasionally, increased pulmonary blood flow will impair a child's growth or lead to an increased incidence of respiratory infections.

A large ventricular septal defect (VSD) or persistent patent ductus arteriosus may cause congestive heart failure (CHF) once PVR falls. Common atrioventricular canal defects always produce large shunts. This anomaly also is known as an endocardial cushion defect, because it involves the endocardial cushion from which the atrioventricular valves form. Increased pulmonary blood flow causes changes in the endothelial lining and muscle wall of pulmonary vessels, thus increasing resistance to flow. By young adulthood, any large shunt will produce irreversible pulmonary vascular obstructive disease (PVOD). It is uncommon to see irreversible damage before 2 years of age.

▲ **Clinical Warning:** Any shunt that produces symptoms of CHF, is unlikely to close spontaneously, or that causes increased PVR, should be referred for closure of the defect (Garson, Bricker, & McNamara, 1997).

Dilated cardiomyopathy (DCM) is characterized by abnormally depressed contractile function that limits cardiac output. As a result, blood pools in the ventricles, causing progressive dilation. There is minimal compensatory myocardial hypertrophy. This volume load increases ventricular wall stress and oxygen consumption and decreases myocardial efficiency. These changes normally progress gradually.

EPIDEMIOLOGY

Congenital heart disease (CHD) affects about 30,000 infants annually (8 in 1000 live births). It affects more children than childhood cancers or diabetes. The incidence of individual defects varies greatly; VSDs comprise about 23% of all congenital cardiac defects, while more complex lesions constitute only 1% to 2% (Forbess et al., 1995; Allan, Apfel, & Printz, 1998).

With earlier diagnosis, sometimes in fetal life, and the trend toward early, complete repair, chronic hypoxemia and pulmonary vascular disease have become much less common in children with CHD. For example, the infant with Tetralogy of Fallot (TET or TOF), the most common cyanotic cardiac defect, once underwent placement of a palliative shunt in the first months or years of life. Such a child was then at risk for hypercyanotic spells, delayed growth, and neurologic events until definitive surgical correction could be done, usually after age 5 to 6 years. Today, these infants undergo definitive repair in the second half of their first year—sooner if hypercyanotic spells develop. Classic "TET spells" now are seen rarely.

Children whose atrial septal defects must be closed can now have device occlusion during cardiac catheterization, rather than undergoing open-heart surgery. Many complex defects, such as transposition of the great arteries (TGA), which accounts for 5% to 7% of all CHD, and truncus arteriosus, which accounts for 1.4% of all CHD, now are repaired before the newborn leaves the hospital (Spicer, 1994; Garson et al., 1997).

Of most concern to the clinician are patients who require medical management of CHF before surgery, children with DCM, and the growing population with a variety of defects whose surgical options cannot provide two functioning ven-

---

DISPLAY 56–1 • Cardiac Defects

Defects Increasing Pulmonary Blood Flow

Septal defects (VSD, ASD, PDA)
Truncus arteriosus
Endocardial cushion defects (atrioventricular canal defects)
Total anomalous pulmonary venous return

Defects Decreasing Pulmonary Blood Flow

Tetralogy of Fallot
Tricuspid atresia
Pulmonary stenosis
Pulmonary atresia
Ebstein's anomaly

Defects Decreasing Systemic Blood Flow

Aortic stenosis
Coarctation of the aorta
Interrupted aortic arch
Hypoplastic left heart syndrome

Other Defects

TGA (most common cause of cyanosis in the newborn)
Cardiomyopathies

---

tricles. These children require staged surgical palliation to a single-ventricle physiology or cardiac transplant to survive beyond the neonatal period. The best known of these defects is hypoplastic left heart syndrome (HLHS) (Johnston, Chinnock, Zuppan, et al., 1997; Caplan, Cooper, Garcia-Prats, & Brody, 1996; Bove & Lloyd, 1996; Forbess et al., 1995). HLHS is the fourth most common congenital cardiac defect, occurring in 7.4% of all CHD live births; the incidence is much higher if those who die during fetal development are included. HLHS is the most common form of congenital single ventricle (Allan, 1998; Chang, Hanley, Wernovsky, & Wessel, 1998; Garson et al., 1997; Zahka, 1993).

The exact prevalence of DCM in children is unknown. Hypertrophic cardiomyopathy accounts for 20% to 30% of all pediatric cardiomyopathy. DCM may be a result of structural or electrical cardiac abnormalities or may follow acute myocarditis, but 85% to 90% of DCM seen in the pediatric population is idiopathic. Familial DCM accounts for about one third of these cases. Autosomal dominant transmission is most common (Garson et al., 1997). Acquired DCM is the ultimate complication of single ventricle physiology. Heart transplant is the only "curative" treatment.

HISTORY AND PHYSICAL EXAMINATION

Well child visits for the child with a known cardiac disorder should include assessment of common indicators of cardiac compromise. The most strenuous activity for infants is feeding. The infant's daily average number of ounces of formula or episodes of breastfeeding should be noted. Frequent vomiting or diarrhea may represent decreased gut perfusion. Questions for the parents related to feeding include the following:

- Can the infant feed for only short periods before tiring?
- For the experienced parent, is the child's feeding similar to that of siblings when they were babies?

- Is respiratory distress, cyanosis, or diaphoresis ("cold sweats") apparent during feeding or, for the older child, with activity. These symptoms suggest CHF or intermittent systemic desaturation.

● **Clinical Pearl:** An exploration of feeding at visits can provide significant clues to the child's hemodynamic status.

Other issues to explore are as follows:

- What is the infant's respiratory pattern and effort at rest? Resting tachypnea may be the only sign of borderline CHF.
- How many diapers is the infant wetting? Has the parent noted periorbital edema on awakening? Periorbital edema that resolves after awakening (when the child is more active) may be normal.
- Has the child had frequent colds, coughs, or other respiratory illnesses? Does the toddler or older child keep up with playmates? Even children with major hemodynamic defects attempt to participate actively in childhood activities.
- Has fever without other signs and symptoms of illness been a problem? Does the young child complain of frequent stomachaches? Young children often describe chest discomfort or tachycardia as "stomachache."

The provider can question the older child and adolescent directly about chest pain, dizziness, or syncope. While uncommon even in this population, these symptoms can indicate serious decompensation. Older children and adolescents should be asked about palpitations and tachycardia ("heart racing").

The provider should ask about the use of over-the-counter medications and herbal remedies. If the provider is open to alternative therapies, he or she usually can obtain honest information from families. The provider should ask about regular dental visits and the use of subacute bacterial endocarditis (SBE) prophylaxis.

Common physical findings for many defects appear in Table 56-1. Specialized factors in the physical examination of children with large shunts, partially repaired defects, or cardiomyopathy are noted here.

The degree of cyanosis should be observed, as should respiratory rate and work of breathing while the child is undisturbed. Precordial activity is noted; the precordium is palpated for thrill and apical impulse. Heart sounds are auscultated before other physical examination. The characteristics of S_1 and S_2 are noted, as are any murmurs, clicks, or rubs. A gallop rhythm suggests increased failure.

Like all children, those with CHD may have intermittent innocent murmurs. Both physiologic and pathologic murmurs may change in intensity and duration when cardiac output is increased, such as in fever, anxiety, exercise, or agitation.

The lungs should be clear. Rales are rarely heard in infants and young children with pulmonary edema. Tachypnea is a better indicator of increased interstitial lung fluid. Mild to marked intercostal retractions may be seen.

The extremities are examined for clubbing, and peripheral pulses are palpated. Capillary refill and liver size are assessed. A liver that is enlarged because of CHF has a soft edge and cannot be pushed under the rib margin.

Weight and oxygen saturation are obtained. In infants and toddlers, blood pressure is best evaluated after clinical examination. Automated equipment is satisfactory for screening, but accurate pressures require auscultation (Gessner & Victoria, 1993).

Table 56–1. COMMON CARDIAC DISORDERS AND THEIR MANAGEMENT

	Presentation/ Physical Findings	Age at Repair	Primary Care Management	Long-Term Issues
ASD	Almost always asymptomatic in childhood; child may have impaired growth or frequent respiratory infections (less than 10% of children with ASD). PE: Loud S1; second heart sound does not become single on expiration (fixed split S2); murmur, if present, may not be distinguishable from innocent pulmonary flow murmur.	Depending on location within the septum, may close spontaneously. Surgery 2–15 y; device closure in cath lab is possible for some ASD.	Monitor for signs of CHF, FTT. Regular follow-up with pediatric cardiology until closed. Increased risk of paradoxical emboli with OCPs, pregnancy.	*Unrepaired:* Stroke due to paradoxical emboli; arrhythmias most develop symptoms in middle or later decades when CAD develops. *Repaired:* Residual shunts (leaks around the patch) possible but uncommon. SBE: 6 mo post-repair only for secundum ASD; recommendations vary for other types of ASD— consult cardiologist.
VSD	If small, may be asymptomatic; large VSDs may produce CHF, FTT; signs of CHF usually appear between 1 and 3 mo of age. PE: Small VSD—holosystolic murmur at LLSB; loudest murmur tends to be R/T mod VSD; may palpate precordial thrill. ("VSD murmur" in NB is usually a PDA.) Mod/large VSD— holosystolic murmur, S2 may be increased in intensity; if shunt is large, gallop rhythm may be heard and tachypnea seen; liver may be enlarged.	Small VSDs may close spontaneously but are never closed surgically. Mod and large VSDs producing CHF are usually closed 2–6 mo of age. Mod VSDs close if there is any indication of cardiomegaly, pulmonary hypertension, or valve dysfunction. Device occlusion of some VSDs in cath lab may be available in the near future.	Monitor for signs of CHF, FTT. Regular follow-up with pediatric cardiology until closed (spontaneous closure); regular follow-up through adolescence is recommended (mod/ large open or post-repair).	*Unrepaired:* FTT, CHF; OPVD—Eisenmenger's syndrome; endocarditis. *Repaired:* Residual shunts (leaks around the patch) possible but uncommon; RBBB occurs with some VSD closures. SBE: Always, if unrepaired; until 6 mo post repair if no residual leak.
PDA	May be asymptomatic except for continuous murmur that does not disappear when child is supine. If large, prominent left and right ventricular impulses, bounding peripheral pulses; signs of CHF may appear between 1 and 3 mo of age.	Closure indicated at time of detection. May be closed by insertion of coils in the cath lab (after infancy) or by surgical ligation at any age. In NB period indomethacin may be used to initiate closure.	No cardiology follow-up is needed following ligation without residual flow.	*Unrepaired:* FTT, OPVD. *Repaired:* None. SBE: Before repair and for 6 mo post-repair if no residual leak.
CAVC	Most common defect in Down syndrome; presentation and PE similar to infant with large VSD.	Complete repair by 6–8 mo.	Monitor for signs of CHF, FTT. Regular follow-up with pediatric cardiology into adulthood is mandatory. Children with normal chromosomes should be evaluated for heterotaxy syndrome.	*Unrepaired:* Eisenmenger's syndrome. *Repaired:* Mitral regurgitation (may eventually require surgical valvuloplasty or replacement). Postoperative as well as late heart block may occur. SBE: Always.
Truncus arteriosus	Usually presents in NB as respiratory distress with cyanosis unrelieved by O₂, but may not present until several months of age. PE: Tachypnea, resting tachycardia, S1 with single S2; systolic murmur at USB (may be soft); cyanosis minimal except when crying (NB); signs of CHF 2 wk–2 mo.	Complete repair with artificial conduit from RV to pulmonary arteries in neonatal period is common; some centers place interim shunt with or without PA banding at birth and conduit at 6 mo–2 yr.	Regular follow-up with pediatric cardiology. Often associated with DiGeorge syndrome; consider chromsome testing.	*Unrepaired:* CHF, FTT PVOD, death. *Post-shunt:* Cyanosis; FTT; decreased activity tolerance. *Post-conduit:* Conduit stenosis; growing child will require serial conduits. SBE: Always.

(continues)

Table 56–1.   COMMON CARDIAC DISORDERS AND THEIR MANAGEMENT *(Continued)*

	Presentation/ Physical Findings	Age at Repair	Primary Care Management	Long-Term Issues
TAPVR	Presentation depends on site of venous drainage and adequacy of intracardiac mixing; may present at 2 wk–3 mo with CHF. PE: Mild/severe cyanosis, tachypnea, hyperactive precordium; loud S1, widely split S2, murmur, if present, resembles pulmonary flow murmur; liver is usually enlarged.	NO PGE1. Surgical repair at time of detection.	Regular cardiology follow-up is mandatory into adulthood. PVOD, FTT. Frequent respiratory infections, RAD, ↓ exercise tolerance, discuss with cardiology. Monitor growth (LA and LV tend to be small; cardiac output may be restricted).	*Unrepaired:* Death in NB period if pulmonary veins are obstructed; chronic CHF, *Repaired:* Gradual pulmonary vein stenosis, PHTN.
TET	Presentation depends on severity of right ventricular outflow obstruction. PE NB may be cyanotic without murmur; however, most newborns with TET are not cyanotic. No tachypnea, prominent RV impulse, thrill at ULSB, S1 with single S2; loud SEM at LUSB (during hypercyanotic spells, murmur diminishes or disappears).	Complete repair of tetralogy in the middle of the first year of life is now the norm for the majority of children. Corrective surgery can be done in even the youngest infants if hypercyanotic episodes develop earlier. Today, few of these children are cyanotic for any length of time and will not demonstrate clubbing, squatting, or other signs of chronic right-to-left shunting.	The narrower the pulmonary outflow tract, the more easily desaturated blood will shunt across the VSD and out the aorta. This is the physiology of a hypercyanotic or TET spell; anything that lowers systemic vascular resistance, increases shunting. Pulmonary outflow stenosis is dynamic and worsens over time; once hypercyanotic episodes begin, they will continue. Feed on demand; avoid dehydration. Parents should be taught knee–chest prone positioning to terminate a spell. Some cardiologists use oral propranolol to prevent recurrent TET spells prior to surgery. Long-term pediatric cardiology follow-up is mandatory.	*Unrepaired:* Hypercyanotic (TET) spells; progressive PS; progressive hyperviscosity syndrome; endocarditis. *Repaired:* Pulmonary regurgitation (usually well tolerated); RBBB is present after TET repair; late ventricular arrhythmias; endocarditis. SBE: Always.
Pulmonary atresia	Serious defect. Although flow between the right ventricle and the branch pulmonary arteries can be provided by a conduit, the entire pulmonary vascular bed is usually not normal. Both the proximal and distal branch arteries may be stenotic or tortuous. Systemic-venous collateral vessels may already be present at birth; development of these abnormal shunts may continue even after repair; RV usually small. PE Cyanotic NB; S1 with single S2; +/− murmur	May require PGE1 to provide a source of pulmonary blood flow. Placement of conduit RV-PA in neonatal period or first year of life; often requires multiple interventional procedures to occlude collaterals and to dilate pulmonary vessels as they grow. PA may be associated with hypoplastic RV and may require staged single ventricle repair.	Long-term pediatric cardiology follow-up is mandatory.	*Unrepaired:* If survival beyond infancy, Eisenmenger's syndrome due to presence of collateral vessels; cyanosis, FTT. *Repaired:* Cyanosis, FTT, PVOD. SBE: Always.

(continues)

The examination of patients with DCM should focus on indicators of decreased cardiac output (skin temperature, pallor, peripheral pulses) and right heart volume overload (liver size, tachypnea, lung sounds, increased work of breathing). Neck vein distention and peripheral edema may be seen in older children and adolescents. As noted earlier, lung auscultation rarely reveals rales in infants and small children, even in frank pulmonary edema, but rales may be heard in older children.

Palpation of the precordium may reveal a displaced apical impulse. Heart sounds may be muffled, or there may be a third heart sound (gallop rhythm). DCM usually does not produce a murmur until the left ventricle is dilated sufficiently to distort the mitral valve annulus, producing mitral regurgitation.

Table 56–1. COMMON CARDIAC DISORDERS AND THEIR MANAGEMENT *(Continued)*

	Presentation/ Physical Findings	Age at Repair	Primary Care Management	Long-Term Issues
TGA	Presentation depends on presence or absence of VSD; NB with intact ventricular septum is ductal dependent and will quickly become cyanotic and acidotic as ductus closes; NB with TGA/VSD may present more gradually (even weeks after birth). PE: Resting tachypnea (unlabored); gradually progressive cyanosis; hyperactive precordium. Murmur, if present, is usually soft, systolic.	May require PGE1 with or without atrial septostomy to maintain pulmonary blood flow and provide adequate mixing before surgery. Arterial switch in neonatal period. Only a few newborns will not be candidates for this procedure because of abnormal coronary arteries or complicating structural defects. Atrial switch (Mustard, Senning) if not an arterial switch candidate (second half of first year of life). Monitor postatrial switch individuals for development of CHF.	Functionally, these children have a structurally and physiologically normal heart after arterial switch, but procedure is only 15–20 y old. If awaiting atrial switch, monitor O_2 saturation, weight gain. Long-term pediatric cardiology follow-up is mandatory.	*Unrepaired:* Death in days to months. *Postarterial switch:* Few long-term complications anticipated but late risks unknown; stenosis at surgical anastomosis sites above the semilunar valves and at the coronary ostia. *Postatrial switch:* Atrial arrhythmias; right ventricle failure.
Supra-ventricular tachycardia (SVT)	History is the most important factor in diagnosis. Sudden onset, sudden resolution; regular rate >200–210; H/O palpitations, commonly occurs at rest. Baseline PE should be normal, because underlying structural heart disease is rare; infants may present in CHF; syncope at any age is rare.	Vagal maneuvers, ice to face (most effective in infancy). Adenosine 0.1 mg/kg IV, may be repeated once. Avoid verapamil in children under 8 y. Cardiovert if unstable (0.5–1 J/kg).	SVT is generally well tolerated in infancy and childhood; consult a pediatric cardiologist before initiating drug therapy other than adenosine. Teach parents vagal maneuvers and ice-to-face technique. Recurrence in untreated NBs: 33% will never have another episode. 33% will be free of SVT until late childhood or adolescence. 33% will have recurrent episodes throughout childhood and adolescence.	Medical management: NBs are often placed on digoxin for the first year of life. Pharmacologic management may be postponed in older infants and children unless episodes are recurrent or symptomatic. Treatment may be initiated with digoxin or beta-blockers. Radiofrequency ablation to eliminate ectopic foci and accessory pathways is usually offered to children over 1 y who 1) fail medical management; 2) develop cardiac dysfunction; 3) have WPW; or 4) have episodes (or fear of episodes) that limit participation in normal activities, including sports.
PS	Usually asymptomatic; usually nonprogressive. PE click following S1, varies in intensity with respiration; S2 may be widely split; SEM at LUSB radiating to lung fields. Change in intensity, duration, or timing of murmur indicates increasing severity.	Balloon valvotomy at any age if severe or child is symptomatic.	May be associated with Noonan's syndrome. Regular cardiology follow-up through adolescence.	*Unrepaired:* If severe, decreased exercise tolerance ; cyanosis. *Repaired:* Recurrent stenosis is uncommon. Pulmonary regurgitation. SBE: Always.

(continues)

DIAGNOSTIC STUDIES

Echocardiography is valuable in confirming and providing a detailed picture of clinical diagnoses. It has virtually eliminated the need for invasive cardiac catheterization as a diagnostic aid. Studies in children between 6 and 36 months of age usually require sedation for adequate imaging. Some lesions (eg, aortic stenosis) require serial evaluation and more frequent studies than lesions that progress more slowly or not at all.

▲ **Clinical Warning:** Echocardiographic studies performed in adult laboratories that are unskilled in evaluating congenital

Table 56–1.   COMMON CARDIAC DISORDERS AND THEIR MANAGEMENT (Continued)

	Presentation/ Physical Findings	Age at Repair	Primary Care Management	Long-Term Issues
AS	May occur above or below the valve orifice or be limited to the valve itself; valve usually bicuspid. Presentation depends on severity of obstruction. Infants with critically severe valvar stenosis may present with signs of poor cardiac output or in frank cardiogenic shock; murmur is rare. Older children and adolescents are usually asymptomatic until obstruction is severe; left ventricular outflow tract obstruction that has gradually worsened may first (though rarely) present with sudden death. PE: Systolic ejection murmur (harsh, radiating to carotids, with/without apical ejection click) will be present except in neonates. Click does not vary with respiration; thrill at RUSB, suprasternal notch, or carotids. Change in intensity, duration, or timing of murmur indicates increasing severity.	Critically ill newborns may require PGE1. Surgery for critical neonate Balloon valvotomy at any age for severe valvar stenosis; serial cardiac caths may be needed in growing patient. Subaortic stenosis surgically resected, usually after 10 yr of age to prevent recurrence. Supravalvar stenosis surgically resected by age 3 y. Auscultate murmur at each visit; documenting a "picture" of the murmur may help the noncardiologist compare sounds across visits.	All types of AS are usually progressive. Bicuspid valve alone or in combination with mild valvar AS requires follow-up every 1–2 y with pediatric cardiology; recreational activities need not be restricted, Mod/severe followed more closely; no competitive sports. Supravalvar and subvalvar lesions require long-term cardiology follow-up. Supravalvar stenosis is commonly associated with William's syndrome; consider genetic consultation.	*Unrepaired:* Aortic regurgitation; endocarditis; sudden death. *Repaired:* Subaortic and valvar may recur; aortic regurgitation; may require valve replacement in midlife, endocarditis. SBE: Always.
CoA	Usually discrete narrowing; commonly occurs with other CHD. Presentation depends on age and severity of narrowing—typically asymptomatic. Right arm hypertension may be the first sign. In children and adolescents, pulmonary flow murmur may be heard anteriorly or between the scapulae. Rib-notching on CSR in children first diagnosed after 6 y. Neonates with severe coarctation present within the first 3 wk of life in CHF or cardiogenic shock. PE: In both infants and older children, diminished or absent femoral pulses and blood pressure differential between upper and lower extremities can be found on routine well child screening and are diagnostic; good blood pressure measurements are as accurate as ultrasound at establishing the degree of narrowing.	Repair at time of detection; delayed repair is associated with increased incidence of residual hypertension. Critically ill newborns may require PGE1. Native coarctation usually surgically resected; some centers balloon dilate native CoA.	Long-term pediatric cardiology follow-up is mandatory. These children should have routine comparison of right arm and either leg blood pressures at all well child visits. A blood pressure difference greater than 10–15 mmHg (with arm being higher) suggests recoarctation; discuss with cardiologist Frequently require short-term ACE inhibitors post-operatively for rebound hypertension. (See Table 3 for management issues.) May be associated with Turner's syndrome.	*Unrepaired:* Cardiomyopathy; hypertension; endocarditis; aortic dissection; intracranial hemorrhage; accelerated CAD. *Repaired:* Recoarctation is not uncommon; usually managed with balloon angioplasty during cardiac catheterization; may be stented open; risk of essential hypertension with or without recoarctation. SBE: Always.

Yeager, 1990; Driscoll, 1999; Federly, 1999; Grifka, 1999; Spicer, 1994; Waldman, 1999.
Legend: CAD = coronary artery disease; CHF = congestive heart failure; FTT = failure to thrive; LA = left atrium; LSB = left sternal border; LUSB = left upper sternal border; LV = left ventricle; NB = newborn; OCP = oral contraceptive pills; PA = pulmonary artery; PGE = prostaglandins; PHTN = pulmonary hypertension; POVD = pulmonary vascular obstructive disease; RAD = reactive airway disease; RBBB = right bundle branch block; RUSB = right upper sternal border; RV = right ventricle; SEM = systolic ejection murmur; SLE = systemic lupus erythematosis; TAPVR = total anomalous pulmonary venous return.

cardiac anomalies may be technically inadequate and miss significant cardiac problems, especially in infants and young children (Pelech, 1999).

Magnetic resonance imaging (MRI) has become increasingly important in the follow-up of coarctation and other aortic arch problems that are less easily imaged by echocardiography as the child grows. Children with TET, pulmonary atresia, or systemic-pulmonary shunts may need serial lung perfusion scans to assess growth of the branch pulmonary vasculature and to guide interventions.

A 24-hour rhythm recording (Holter monitor) may be done annually or biennially for children whose defects or surgical repairs pose a risk of late arrhythmias. This can be obtained prior to the cardiology visit so that results are available for discussion. The provider should discuss timing with the cardiology team. Someone skilled in pediatric rhythm analysis should provide rhythm interpretation. For children with suspected arrhythmias, a baseline 12-lead electrocardiogram (ECG) and if possible, a 12-lead ECG obtained during any "events" are useful at the cardiology visit. Holter monitoring is less useful as a diagnostic tool for supraventricular tachycardia (SVT) because events usually are infrequent. Event monitors that can be triggered when symptoms appear are more helpful. Holter monitoring is more useful in the evaluation of bradycardia to assess heart rate variability.

Laboratory tests are not required routinely. If anemia is a concern, the clinician should monitor hemoglobin and hematocrit. Children on angiotensin-converting enzyme (ACE) inhibitors should have a complete blood count, electrolytes, blood urea nitrogen, and creatinine done annually to check for evidence of renal failure and electrolyte disturbance. Anemia status also should be assessed. Drug therapy usually is evaluated by clinical response. The clinician should consult with the cardiology team to determine if regular serum drug levels should be obtained.

For children undergoing staged repair, the provider should assess oxygen saturation using pulse oximetry at each well child visit. Determine whether the cardiology team prefers a specific extremity to be used.

Cardiac stress testing has several uses. The cardiologist may clear individuals with minor defects for competitive sports based on their cardiovascular response to exercise. Testing can identify a hypertensive response to exercise or dynamic recoarctation late after coarctation repair. Some defects, such as aortic stenosis, are more hemodynamically significant during exercise. Testing rarely provokes arrhythmias in individuals with SVT and normal hearts and is not useful in the initial diagnostic evaluation of tachycardia. A team familiar with pediatric cardiac stress testing should perform and interpret testing.

MANAGEMENT

Regular follow-up with a pediatric cardiologist is mandatory for virtually all children with heart disease. Of course, children with progressive lesions or who have undergone some type of intervention obviously will require follow-up. More benign lesions, such as small VSDs or pulmonary stenoses, also require specialized follow-up but less frequently. The cardiologist will be most aware of subtle cardiovascular changes, common and uncommon risks of lesions during development, and new management options. The cardiologist is best able to evaluate and manage the child clinically, avoiding extensive and unnecessary testing. A key premise

of pediatric cardiology is that intervention should precede the development of clinical symptoms. An overview of common defects and their management is presented in Table 56-1.

Anticipatory Guidance

Nutrition

Feeding is one of the most stressful areas for families of children with complex CHD. They need a great deal of support in this process. Feedings take longer than those for healthy children and may need to be given more frequently. All the family's efforts may produce little in the way of weight gain. Parents often express frustration with the feeding process. Because feeding is still primarily a maternal responsibility, mothers are most likely to feel they have failed at this primary task. Breast-feeding mothers experience an additional sense of loss when nursing must be interrupted, particularly if it cannot be reestablished. An empathetic and available primary care provider can support the family, maximize caloric intake, and minimize development of long-term feeding issues.

Children with complex lesions may have difficulty gaining weight from birth. They may have difficulty consuming sufficient calories for adequate growth and development. Tachypnea and tachycardia increase both respiratory and cardiac workload, burning calories and decreasing fluid while increasing caloric needs. Infants with moderate to large shunts may gain normally until 2 to 3 months of age when PVR reaches its nadir. Weight gain velocity may then plateau or even decelerate.

In the first year of life, these infants need 120 to 150 cals/kg/d (Queen & Lang, 1993). Unfortunately, standard formulas or breast milk are not enough to meet this goal. Neonates who have had surgery generally are discharged on high-calorie formula. Most primary care providers feel comfortable overseeing formula supplementation and can see the child frequently enough to monitor growth.

● **Clinical Pearl:** Weekly or biweekly weight checks may be necessary. The provider should give written mixing instructions to the family and advise a minimum daily intake of 100 mL/kg or approximately 3 oz/kg daily.

Commercial formulas may be concentrated to provide 24 to 27 cal/oz by changing the proportion of water to concentrate. This is easiest to do with liquid concentrate, but many families prefer powdered concentrate because of cost. Concentrated formulas should be added gradually over 2 to 3 days to reduce gut stress and prevent diarrhea; alternating old and new strengths at feedings is fine (Gaedeke-Norris & Hill, 1994). The provider should consult with the cardiologist if abdominal distention, distress, or diarrhea develops or if weight gain velocity does not improve.

Additional calories can be added to the concentrated formula with supplements (polycose, fats, rice cereal, or corn syrup). The decision to add supplements should be made only in consultation with the cardiology team. Supplemented formula must provide a normal balance of carbohydrates, fats, and proteins without compromising renal function. The primary care provider can assist the nutritionist in choosing supplements that fit into the family's budget or that are available from local health offices. Display 56-2 describes how to modify infant formulas effectively.

▲ **Clinical Warning:** Some families are unable to mix formula in the correct proportions or do not have reliable

---

DISPLAY 56–2 • Modifying Infant Formulas

To make 24-cal formula:
  Mix 13 oz (1 can) liquid concentrate
  8 oz water
To make 27-cal formula
  13 oz (1 can) liquid concentrate
  8 oz water
  2 Tbsp. + 2 tsp. Polycose powder
         OR
  2 tsp. corn syrup
Breast milk may be enhanced with human milk fortifiers or commercial formula to increase calorie provision.

▲ **Clinical Warning:** To ensure that formula preparation is correct, the provider needs to demonstrate the method for preparing formula, and have the family then return the demonstration. This teaching is important to prevent the infant from being fed formula that is either too high or too low in concentration.

---

access to materials necessary for mixing. Because of the danger of hypertonic dehydration should the infant be fed with formula in incorrect proportions, the provider should advise such families that they must use commercially available, 24 cal/oz formula.

Most mothers who have chosen to breast-feed can continue to pump and store milk during perinatal hospitalization. This milk will be used when enteral feedings begin. Unfortunately, exclusive breast-feeding will not provide adequate calories to the infant with complex cardiac problems. The milk can, however, supplement caloric content while providing the infant with the benefits of breast milk. Refer to Chapter 7 for more information.

Fluid restriction rarely is necessary (Garson et al., 1997). Some fluid restriction is an unintentional result of formula concentration and increases renal solute load. Constipation may become a problem, and obstruction can occur. Sodium restriction rarely is attempted, because low-sodium formulas are not well tolerated (Gessner & Victoria, 1993). As parents begin to introduce solids, however, the provider can educate them about high-sodium foods and snacks. The provider should teach the family to avoid snacks high in salt and to practice a no added salt diet. Apart from calories, dietary supplements are rarely necessary. There is no particular advantage to introducing solids before 6 months of age (Gidding & Rosenthal, 1994).

Babies can be switched to whole milk at 12 months. If caloric supplementation is still needed, Pediasure or whole milk plus Carnation Instant Breakfast (a less expensive option for families without public assistance) provides 30 cal/oz (Queen & Lang, 1993). Families may need help in choosing solid foods for toddlers that maximize caloric intake, such as using bananas instead of applesauce or adding butter to cereals or mashed potatoes.

▲ **Clinical Warnings:**

- Adding solid foods may decrease the infant's caloric intake by decreasing the amount of high-calorie formula taken.
- The provider should consult with the cardiologist before routinely switching to skim milk at 2 years.

Sleep

Parents should anticipate sleep disturbances and behavioral regression for up to 3 weeks after hospitalization or procedures (Wong, 1995; Swanson, 1995). No data suggest that sleep disturbances are associated with any cardiac medications except for propranolol, but parents sometimes raise this issue. Medications with short half-lives like captopril and some antiarrhythmics may require waking the child for a dose, but normally dosing can be adjusted to allow a normal sleep pattern.

Elimination

Chronic diuretic therapy may interfere with toilet training. By 2 years, it may be appropriate to give diuretics twice daily (ie, on awakening and in the late afternoon). Toilet readiness may occur later than in well children (Brazelton et al., 1999).

Immunizations

It is not uncommon for the immunization schedule to be interrupted unnecessarily in children with CHD. Delays in immunization most commonly occur after neonatal surgery, because of unnecessary concerns about vaccine administration in the postoperative period during a series of staged surgeries.

● **Clinical Pearl:** Immunizations recommended for well children should be given to all children with complex CHD during the recommended vaccination periods whenever possible. These children actually may be at increased risk for complications of childhood illnesses for many reasons. There is no indication for modifying the dose of any vaccines for children with chronic cardiac problems, including those who are premature or malnourished (American Academy of Pediatrics [AAP], 2000). If fever is a concern (eg, in the infant with CHF or cardiomyopathy), administration of an antipyretic before and at 4 and 8 hours after vaccine administration should be considered.

Because a febrile response to vaccines may mask acute febrile illness, immunizations probably should not be given within 48 hours before a scheduled surgical date. This contraindication is not absolute, however, and it may be necessary to use an available window of opportunity. Live-virus vaccines may have reduced immunogenicity when given shortly before or for a period after administration of immune globulins.

Although the use of transfusion is minimized in current practice, almost all children who go on bypass for open-heart surgery will have some exposure to blood products. Surgical timing must be considered when planning measles, mumps, and rubella (MMR) and varicella administration. Measles vaccine (MMR or monovalent measles vaccine) should not be administered for 5 to 7 months after such surgery (AAP, 2000). Varicella vaccine should not be given for at least 5 months after surgery. Both vaccines may be given a minimum of 14 days before anticipated exposure to blood products. If the provider plans appropriately, children undergoing staged Fontan repairs can receive MMR and varicella vaccines between their second and third operations. Administration of immune globulins/blood products is not a contraindication to giving oral polio vaccine (AAP, 2000).

Finally, children 2 years and older who have CHF, cardiomyopathy, or asplenia should be vaccinated against pneumococcal disease (AAP, 1997). This includes children with single ventricle physiology who are always at risk for pulmonary dysfunction and ventricular dysfunction.

▲ **Clinical Warning:** Influenza can be devastating for children with cyanotic heart disease or cardiomyopathy. These children also may be on long-term aspirin therapy. They should receive an annual flu shot once they are 6 months old (AAP, 2000). Immunization also should be recommended to family members and other caregivers.

Developmental Milestones

The area of developmental outcomes in children with CHD has not been studied extensively. The only population for which there are prospective data on the connections between perioperative techniques and long-term developmental outcomes is the TGA-arterial switch group (Jonas, 1996; Bellinger et al., 1995, 1997; Uzark, 1998). Their findings, however, have already prompted changes in perioperative management for minimizing neurologic sequellae.*

Motor deficits, particularly gross motor deficits and hypotonia, are apparent in about one third of patients at 1 year of age (Jonas, 1995). These may be related in part to lengthy or serial hospitalizations and procedures. At 4 years old, significantly more children were receiving supportive services (eg, speech pathology, physical or occupational therapy, psychology) than their noncardiac peers (Bellinger, 1997; Gutgesell & Massaro, 1995). Neurocognitive deficits, such as in speech and attention span, also were found (Walsh, Morrow, & Jonas, 1995). The most striking deficits may be in the domain of language, with 30% of these children demonstrating abnormal speech or language development (Bellinger, 1997). These findings suggest that the provider should alert parents that their child may have difficulties in an academic setting.

Parents may fear that emotional or physical outbursts will harm the child (Tong et al., 1998; Swanson, 1995). From the standpoint of behavioral development and discipline, parents should be encouraged to treat their child normally.

● **Clinical Pearl:** Except in the child with unrepaired TOF, crying or tantrums cannot "hurt" the heart, although partially repaired children can look quite blue during such behavior. Parental anxiety is a more significant factor in the child's long-term functional outcome than is severity of disease (Garson et al., 1997).

Child Care

Many families are concerned that their child will not be able to be in day care. After surgery, it is advantageous if the child can be out of day care until the postoperative visit; generally, however, day care is not contraindicated for children with complex CHD. Infants with cardiomyopathy and those who have had a Norwood Stage I single ventricle repair are at greater risk than are other infants for bronchiolitis and respiratory infections. Parents should avoid contact with large crowds and sick visitors and should prevent other children from handling their baby.

Common Childhood Illnesses

Management of common childhood illnesses is much the same as for other children. Children with CHD are not at

greater risk for the complications of these illnesses, but they may look sicker.

Children with single ventricle physiology or cardiomyopathy do not tolerate fever or dehydration well. Because their pulmonary blood flow is heavily dependent on volume loading, any situation that decreases time for cardiac filling (eg, tachycardia) or decreases intravascular volume (eg, dehydration) can compromise their systemic perfusion. Fever should be treated; both acetaminophen and ibuprofen can be used. Many of these children, however, will be on some form of anticoagulation. The provider should consult with the cardiologist if the following occur:

- Treatment with antipyretics is necessary for more than 24 hours.
- Fever is prolonged.
- The child is on diuretics.

Simple antihistamines and cough remedies, such as guanefesin, may be used. Parents should be instructed to avoid combination cold and allergy products, which often contain sympathomimetics, such as pseudoephedrine.

▲ **Clinical Warnings:**

- Sympathomimetics are contraindicated in children with single ventricle physiology or cardiomyopathy because of their effect on heart rate.
- Some brands of children's vitamins contain vitamin K; children taking coumadin should avoid these brands. The provider should teach parents to read medication labels carefully before administering any over-the-counter products to their child.
- Medication doses, whether prescribed or over-the-counter, may need to be adjusted during periods of decreased intake or dehydration. The pediatric cardiologist usually should make adjustments.

Dental Hygiene and Endocarditis

Dental health is particularly important for all children with CHD, and it is a topic often left to the primary care provider to address. Healthy teeth and gums reduce the risk of infection both daily and at the time of procedures. Examination of the mouth and teeth should be a regular part of well child visits. In addition to providing anticipatory guidance about good oral hygiene, adequate fluoride intake, and regular dental visits, the provider should address common problems with parents. These children are at increased risk for dental caries (American Academy of Pediatric Dentistry, 1991). Night feedings may continue longer for these children, and given the heavy emphasis on caloric intake by the health care team, parents may be tempted to put older infants and toddlers to bed with a bottle. They should not do so because of the risk for "baby bottle" syndrome.

So that they will not be alarmed, parents need to know that aspirin therapy may cause gingival bleeding during regular hygiene. An athletic mouth guard would be appropriate for children active in organized sports. Whenever possible, necessary dental treatment should be completed before scheduled surgeries. Finding a dental provider for a child with complex needs can be a problem, particularly if the child will need anxiolysis for the visit. Knowledge of community resources and child advocacy are important primary care functions.

Parents need to understand that poor dental hygiene itself increases the risk of bacteremia and endocarditis. Infective endocarditis results from bacterial invasion of cardiac

---

*The TGA-arterial switch study followed a group of children who underwent true surgical correction shortly after birth and who were never chronically cyanotic; few required further intervention. Outcomes for the HLHS group, who underwent three open-heart surgeries and who were cyanotic for 20 to 36 months, should theoretically mirror the TGA experience and may be worse (Forbess et al., 1995). To the author's knowledge, long-term studies of functional outcomes in this population are not currently under investigation.

endothelium damaged by the turbulent, high-velocity flow of some congenital heart defects. Low-velocity flow defects (eg, secundum atrial septal defects) do not predispose an individual to endocarditis. Bacteremia from poor oral hygiene or oral manipulations that cause bleeding is generally thought to be the precipitating cause of bacterial endocarditis. Any child with a known cardiac lesion and unexplained fever may have infective endocarditis. Fever, the most common symptom, is often low grade. About 10% of children will not have fever. Nonspecific symptoms, such as fatigue, malaise, anorexia, nausea, vomiting, abdominal pain, weight loss, or arthralgia, also may occur. Petechiae and other dermatologic signs usually are not seen in early stages of the disease (Gidding & Rosenthal, 1994). Splenomegaly is the most common physical finding. If endocarditis is suspected, the provider should consult with the child's cardiologist. A team that includes the cardiologist and a specialist in pediatric infectious disease should manage infective endocarditis.

Theoretically, endocarditis can be prevented by reducing the likelihood of bacteria in at-risk patients. For this reason, prophylactic antibiotic therapy is recommended for children with CHD who undergo many dental or surgical procedures involving the mucosal surfaces of the oral, respiratory, gastrointestinal, and genitourinary tracts.

● **Clinical Pearl:** Dental cleaning, tooth extraction, tonsillectomy, and adenoidectomy are the most common procedures in childhood and adolescence that require prophylaxis. Prophylaxis is not recommended for placement of tympanostomy tubes but should probably be used for body piercing.

Because beta-hemolytic streptococci are the most common cause of endocarditis following dental, oral, or respiratory procedures, penicillins are the antibiotics of choice (Display 56-3). Complete recommendations appear in the American Heart Association Scientific Statement on the Prevention of Bacterial Endocarditis (1997) and also may be obtained, along with patient wallet cards, from any local American Heart Association affiliate. Children who are receiving penicillin prophylaxis for rheumatic fever or who are currently taking

or have recently completed a course of amoxicillin for any reason may have penicillin-resistant beta-hemolytic streptococci in their oral cavities. These children should receive prophylaxis with clindamycin or a macrolide antibiotic.

▲ **Clinical Warning:** Sometimes community providers are unaware of the need for SBE prophylaxis for oral lacerations. Prophylaxis can be given up to 2 hours after a mouth or gingival injury (American Heart Association, 1997).

Activity

Like all children, those with CHD require opportunities for physical development, socialization, and play. Schools and community organizations may be overly anxious about the child's heart condition and unnecessarily restrict participation. Parents may be nervous when new opportunities for participation present themselves. Activity recommendations should be individualized in consultation with the cardiologist; attempts should be made to minimize activity restrictions as much as possible.

No activity restrictions are placed on infants, toddlers, and preschoolers (Avery & First, 1996). These children generally will restrict themselves. School-age children almost always can participate in physical education and recreational sports. Schools and coaches often ask for a listing of permitted and nonpermitted activities.

● **Clinical Pearl:** The type of activity is usually less important than permitting children to pace themselves and to drop out of any activity if they experience dizziness, shortness of breath, unusual fatigue, or chest discomfort. These symptoms should resolve promptly with rest.

During adolescence, peer pressure and the increased demands of training make it less likely that the individual athlete will self-pace. At the same time, competitive activity places qualitatively greater demands on the heart.

▲ **Clinical Warning:** Families should discuss with the cardiologist a child's participation in competitive sports at the elementary and junior high school levels. Exercise testing may be needed before making recommendations. Most individuals will not be cleared for participation in competitive sports if they have any of the following:

- Some type of intervention for a cardiac defect
- Any type of cardiomyopathy
- A progressive/recurrent lesion, regardles of whether it has required intervention

Children with single ventricle physiology will have lower exercise tolerance than other children their age, because their ability to increase pulmonary blood flow (and cardiac output) in response to exercise is limited. Pulmonary perfusion probably is not normal in these individuals (Colan, 1989). Blood pressure also may drop during exercise. Those with a pressure-relieving shunt (fenestration) will be bluer with exercise. Maintaining an arterial saturation of 80% usually is required for exercise clearance (American College of Cardiology, 1994; Freed, 1994; Graham, Bricker, James, & Strong, 1994). Good hydration during activity is especially important for this population. Individuals with ventricular dysfunction may be at risk for arrhythmias.

▲ **Clinical Warning:** Individuals who are anticoagulated, have extra cardiac shunts or conduits immediately below the

---

DISPLAY 56–3 • SBE Prophylaxis*

Oral recommendations for dental and upper respiratory procedures for individuals who are **not allergic** to penicillin:

Amoxicilllin	50 mg/kg (maximum dose = 2 g) 1 h before procedure

Oral recommendations for dental and upper respiratory procedures for individuals who **are allergic** to penicillin:

Clindamycin	20 mg/kg (maximum dose = 600 mg)
	OR
Azithromycin or clarithromycin	20 mg/kg (maximum dose = 500 mg) 1 h before procedure

No postprocedure dose is needed.

---

*American Heart Association (1997). Scientific statement. Prevention of bacterial endocarditis: A statement for health professionals. Committee on Rheumatic Fever, Endocarditis and Kawasaki disease of the Council on Cardiovascular disease in the Young. *Journal of the American Medical Association, 277*(2), 1764–1801.

sternum, or who are within 6 months of surgery may not participate in contact sports.

Families should be encouraged to help children explore all their talents and avoid focusing solely on sports. The usual concerns of parents and children are risk of exercise-induced catastrophe and sudden death (Uzark, 1992; Freed, 1994). The risk of such events is actually low for most individuals.

● **Clinical Pearl:** Beginning in the early grades, children should be told in a matter-of-fact way that there will be some limitation on their activities in high school.

Transition to Adolescence and Adulthood

Children who grow up with CHD must cope with an uncertain future. Completing the transitional tasks of adolescence, developing a sense of identity, coping with physical and psychological changes, and establishing independence from the family are all more stressful for individuals with CHD (Tong & Sparacino, 1994). Although most available research on psychosocial adjustment of adolescents and young adults is outdated, some data suggest that adolescents with CHD experience more anxiety and have more negative self-images than peers (Uzark, 1992). Further, surgical scars and short stature may have a negative influence on body image.

Certain occupations will be closed to those with complex repairs or single ventricle physiology: military enrollment, trades requiring heavy labor or sustained exercise (eg, standing for an entire shift), sports, and in some circumstances, farming. Unfortunately, these are typical entry fields for young adults with minimal education or for whom higher professional education is not an option due to poverty or other circumstances. Again, encouraging families to explore all their child's interests and proclivities from an early age is important to maximize adult opportunities.

▲ **Clinical Warning:** Life and health insurance are issues for most individuals with CHD. Federal and state programs cease coverage at 18 to 21 years of age. Most young adults with CHD are functionally normal or near normal; they will not be eligible for Medicaid or Social Security insurance. The provider should counsel parents about the importance of retaining insurance coverage for their adolescents and young adults whenever possible.

Pregnancy and its associated hemodynamic challenges present potential risks to the patient with CHD. Because management and long-term outcomes have changed so substantially over the past decade, limited data on the true risk for children and adolescents who become pregnant are available. Both maternal and fetal mortality in women with pulmonary hypertension approach 50%. There is a small but increased risk of heart defects in the offspring of both men and women with CHD.

▲ **Clinical Warnings:** Pregnancy is absolutely contraindicated in only a few conditions:

- Any lesion with pulmonary vascular obstructive disease (Eisenmenger's syndrome)
- Marfan syndrome with aortic root dilation
- DCM

Counseling about birth control options and reproductive risks should begin at menarche, whether or not the adolescent is sexually active. Too often, the first discussion occurs in the cardiologist's office when the adolescent is already pregnant (Cannobio, 1998). Birth control methods should be tailored to the individual's physiology. Barrier methods are always safe.

● **Clinical Pearls:** Genetic counseling should be part of family planning. Some medications, like coumadin or ACE inhibitors, pose a risk to the developing fetus.

Special Clinical Problems

Single Ventricle Repairs

Single ventricle repairs using the Fontan procedure have been done over the past 30 years for a variety of defects that result in right ventricular hypoplasia (eg, tricuspid atresia, pulmonary atresia, double inlet left ventricle). Until the early 1980s, this repair used a single left ventricle as the heart's only pumping chamber and was done at 2 to 5 years of age. Pulmonary blood flow usually was provided by a palliative shunt until definitive correction could be performed.

Left ventricular hypoplsia, which may include aortic and mitral valve atresia, underdeveloped-to-absent left ventricle, and severely hypoplastic ascending aorta and aortic arch, requires immediate surgical intervention if the infant is to survive. The Fontan cannot be done in the neonatal period when PVR is high, however, and palliative shunts alone cannot provide adequate systemic output for the infant (Jonas, 1995).

During the 1980s, surgeons began attempting staged surgical palliation of infants with functionally absent left ventricle. These infants now undergo a three-stage repair. The most complex and extensive surgical staging is performed shortly after birth. The interested reader should refer to Bove (1998) for further information about staged reconstruction. Table 56-2 provides an overview of physical findings, primary care management, disposition, and long-term issues for single ventricle palliation.

Because the child with this cardiac anomaly may be a candidate for transplantation (Morrow et al., 1997), the reader may find Chapter 66 helpful. Specialized centers in North America do staged repairs and pediatric heart transplantation.

Cardiac Medications

Many children with CHD will not need any cardiac medications. Children with complex defects may be on inotropes, diuretics, and ACE inhibitors both preoperatively and postoperatively. Cardiac medications should not be initiated or discontinued without consultation. Many providers are comfortable adjusting doses as the child grows, however, particularly with digoxin and diuretics. Antiarrhythmics should be adjusted in consultation with the cardiologist. A health care provider who frequently monitors these medications in infants, children, and adolescents should monitor anticoagulation. Usually this person is someone on the cardiology team. The provider needs to be aware of community pharmacies that are willing to compound pediatric medications and to advocate for this service within the community. Parents need to understand that children's acceptance of medication has as much to do with presentation as with taste. New options are available for prothrombin time monitoring, such as the whole blood fingerstick monitor. Families may need help in obtaining insurance reimbursement for this service. Table 56-3 discusses common cardiac drugs used in pediatrics and their management.

Table 56–2.   OVERVIEW OF PRESENTATION AND CONCERNS FOR CHILDREN WITH SINGLE VENTRICLE PHYSIOLOGY

Age	Presentation	Surgical Management	Outcomes	Physical Examination	Primary Care Concerns
Newborn	Progressively cyanotic and acidotic as ductus closes. Hypertrophic maxillary frenulum may be a marker for suspicion of HLHS (Lovell & McDaniel, 1995).	PGE1 to keep ductus open until surgery ECHO to delineate anatomy.			Diagnosis and if necessary transport. The emotional and financial toll on family and child is high (Swanson, 1995). Therefore, it is still common to offer parents three options at diagnosis, and all three are reasonable parental choices. 1. Staged surgical palliation at an experienced center; 2. cardiac transplantation[1]; or 3. compassionate (comfort) care only (Zahka, 1993). Pearson, 1997; Caplan, Cooper, Garcia-Prats, & Brody, (1996). The primary care or obstetric provider may be called on to assist the family in making this decision.
1–2 wk of age	Infant transitioned to extra-uterine life and stabilized; fetal diagnosis and delivery at surgical center may improve outcomes (Kumar, R. K., Newburger, J. W., Gauvreau, K., et al., 1999). Infants who leave the nursery undetected may present at this age with cyanosis and acidosis.	Norwood: Stage I palliation Main pulmonary artery is used to construct a new ascending aorta and arch; original aorta is incorporated into new aorta to provide coronary artery perfusion; PDA ligated; synthetic shunt placed between subclavian artery and right branch pulmonary artery (modified Blalock-Taussig shunt/BT shunt); atrial septum is removed to provide unobstructed pulmonary venous return.	All blood flows through a common atrium and (usually) single ventricle. Centers performing the greatest number of neonatal Norwood palliations have the lowest mortality; mortality at centers performing 200–300 complex surgeries annually (including Norwood) is 20%–30% (Chang, Hanley, Wernovsky, & Wessel, 1998; Bove, 1998; Forbesset al., 1995; Gutgesell, & Massaro, 1995). Survival without neurologic sequelae is greater than 50% (Bove & Lloyd, 1996).	Following Stage I repair, the infant may be cyanotic or exhibit pallor. Baseline O$_2$ saturations 75%–80%: Cyanosis will be more marked when the infant is agitated or crying. The cardiology team should have indicated an acceptable range for oxygen saturation. Peripheral pulses and capillary refill should be normal. Clubbing may develop. Decreased peripheral or femoral pulses may indicate renarrowing of the aortic reconstruction or low systemic output. A continuous shunt murmur should be heard. Other murmurs may be present depending on the child's individual anatomy. The infant's work of breathing is often increased at baseline. The liver edge may be palpable below the costal margin. There should be no periorbital or sacral edema.	Length of stay varies greatly—usually 3–4 wk after birth. Discuss saturations above or below expected range with cardiologist. Risk of recoarctation. Monitor growth. Gross motor delay may be seen. Cardiac catheterization needed prior to next surgery.
6–9 mo of age	See physical examination after Stage I palliation. Saturations will drop as the infant grows because BT shunt is "fixed" and cannot provide adequate blood flow indefinitely. PVR should fall to normal or near normal levels.	Stage II palliation (cavopulmonary shunt; Glenn shunt; hemi-Fontan; BDG₂) Ligation of BT shunt; anastamosis of superior vena cava (SVC) directly to the branch pulmonary arteries.	Venous return from the head and upper body no longer returns to the heart but flows directly to the lungs. Venous return from the lower body returns to the common atrium through the inferior vena cava (IVC). Mortality approaches 0% in many centers (Bove, 1998).	Following Stage II repair, the infant will be cyanotic. Oxygensaturations should range from 85%–92%. Clubbing may develop. Peripheral pulses and capillary refill should be normal. Murmur may or may not be present, depending on the child's specific intracardiac anatomy. There should be no periorbital, facial, or chest edema, which would indicate obstruction of pulmonary blood flow through the SVC or increasing PVR. The liver edge may be palpable.	Length of hospital stay usually less than 1 wk. Cardiac catheterization needed prior to next surgery.

| 2–3 y of age | See physical examination after Stage II palliation. | **Fontan**

Venous blood returning to the heart through the IVC is baffled directly to the pulmonary arteries, either through the atrium or through an extracardiac conduit. A fenestration is usually created between the baffle and the atrium to function as a pressure "pop-off," allowing the right-to-left shunting. | All venous return completely bypasses the heart, and pulmonary blood flow is dependent on volume and gravity (ie, blood is not *pumped* to the lungs).

Mortality at this stage is less than 10%–12% with some centers reporting 1%–2%. (Bove, 1998). | Length of stay varies greatly among centers and depends, in part, on the type of anastomosis used. Families should anticipate at least a 10–14 d stay.

Creating a fenestration has decreased short-term morbidity significantly by reducing the incidence of postoperative pleural effusions. Fenestrations can be closed during cardiac catheterization at a later time.

Because pulmonary blood flow is completely dependent on volume and gravity, pulmonary vascular resistance *must* be low and intravascular volume *must* be normal or slightly above normal. Adequate filling pressures vary among children, and a change of 1–2 mm/HG can have significant impact on children with Fontan physiology. Cardiac output (ventricular filling) is completely dependent on pulmonary venous return. Anything that impacts pulmonary venous return (eg, dehydration, tachycardia, loss of atrioventricular synchrony) can significantly impair cardiac output and tissue perfusion. The oldest survivor is less than 20 y old in 1999 (New England Infant Regional Cardiac Program Database). Overall survival to 5 y is currently 70% (Bove, 1998). |
| Post-Fontan | | | | Monitor for signs of CHF, which could indicate AV valve regurgitation or RV cardiomyopathy.

Monitor for arrhythmias.

Provide appropriate birth control information and genetic counseling. | Interventional caths to close fenestrations; balloon dilation for any aortic recoarctation or to manage rhythm problems may be needed. |

[1] 1/3 of all infants listed die waiting for transplant due to the limited availability of infant hearts; another 1/3 eventually undergo staged palliation; (Morrow et al., 1997; Johnston et al., 1997)

Table 56–3.   COMMON CARDIAC MEDICATIONS*

Drug	Dosing	Availability	Common Pediatric Side Effects	Primary Care Issues
Digoxin	10 mcg/kg/d divided b.i.d.	Tablets: commercial pediatric elixir (50 μg/mL)	Anorexia, nausea, vomiting, diarrhea; instruct parent to report GI illness	GI symptoms most common indicator of toxicity, many cardiologists do not follow levels routinely; adjust dose with macrolide antibiotics.
Beta-blockers	*Propranolol:* 0.5–4 mg/kg/d divided q6–8h *Atenolol:* 1 mg/kg/dose divided b.i.d. *Sotalol:* 80–160 mg/m²	Tablets: Commercial propranolol elixir available 4 mg/mL Oral atenolol solution can be compounded (1 mg/mL) Oral sotalol solution can be compounded (5 mg/mL)	Propranolol: Irritability, sleep disturbances, hypoglycemia (Chavez, 1999); wheezing All: decreased exercise tolerance Sotalol: arrhythmias	Instruct parents to report wheezing, behavior changes, dizziness, palpitations, or syncope, wean to discontinue; does not lower BP in normotensive individuals. Sometimes used in chronic fatigue syndrome and Marfan syndrome.
ACE inhibitors	Captopril: 0.5–1 mg/kg/d divided q8h Enalapril: 0.1–0.5 mg/kg/d divided b.i.d.	Tablets: Oral captopril solution can be compounded (1 mg/mL)	Nonproductive cough; facial flushing; rash	K supplements should not be used concomitantly; avoid dehydration; monitor BP when initiating treatment.
Calcium channel blockers	Verapamil 4–8 mg/kg/d divided t.i.d.	Tablets or SR tablets: oral solution can be compounded (50 mg/mL)	Constipation	
Diuretics	Lasix 1 mg/kg/dose b.i.d.	Tablets: commercial solution available (10 mg/mL)	Dry mouth	Dietary K usually adequate to prevent hypokalemia; adjust dose with GI losses; may impede toilet training.
Amiodarone	5 mg/kg/d divided b.i.d.	Tablets: oral solution can be compounded	Anorexia; nausea, vomiting; arrhythmias	LONG half-life; requires annual ophthalmic exam, liver and thyroid function studies, and pulmonary function testing; treatment always initiated in hospital.
Warfarin	Titrate to maintain INR 2.0–3.0 or 2.5–3.5 (cardiologist will identify range); age, weight not predictive of dose needed; infants may require b.i.d. dosing.	Smallest tablet = 1 mg	Petechiae, bruising, bleeding	Report all new meds, including short-term courses of all antibiotics to cardiologist; notify cardiology if antipyretics are needed for more than 24 h.

*Adapted from Chang, op. Cit. & Tassey, 1997.

Hypoxemia

Hypoxemia is defined as an arterial oxygen saturation under 93%. All children undergoing staged surgical repair and some others will be hypoxemic for at least the first 2 to 3 years of life. Hypoxemia contributes to lower IQ and delayed neuromuscular development (Newburger, Tucker, Silbert, & Fyler, 1983; Newburger et al., 1984; Rogers et al., 1995). Chronic hypoxemia results in polycythemia, which can lead to gallstones, bleeding dyscrasias, cerebrovascular accidents, scoliosis, and brain abscess. Fortunately, these are primarily late effects and should only be seen if an individual is hypoxemic into adolescence or adulthood.

Clubbing may be seen in infants and toddlers with right-to-left shunts but usually resolves after surgery. Polycythemia progresses slowly; symptomatic polycythemia is rare in the young child. Any new symptoms suggesting neurologic disorder in the hypoxemic child should be taken seriously (Walsh et al., 1995).

● **Clinical Pearl:** Computed tomography scan or MRI may be needed to rule out brain abscess or stroke. Preventing anemia or relative anemia decreases the risk of stroke. The hematocrit should be maintained above 40%.

Pulmonary Hypertension/PVOD

Chronically increased pulmonary blood flow or chronic hypoxemia produces changes in the endothelial lining of pulmonary vessels. These changes raise PVR, causing pulmonary hypertension, and progressively limit pulmonary blood flow. Over time, these changes become irreversible. Pressures in the right ventricle rise as it is forced to pump against increasing pulmonary pressure. Right heart pressures will eventually exceed systemic blood pressure. If a shunt (eg, a VSD) is available, deoxygenated blood will take the path of least resistance and flow out to the body. End-stage pulmonary vascular obstructive disease is called Eisenmenger's syndrome. Home oxygen therapy and anticoagulation may provide some benefit. However, there is no effective therapy except heart-lung transplant.

Changes in the pulmonary bed usually are reversible before 2 years of age if normal pulmonary blood flow is restored. Children with Down syndrome are particularly susceptible to early, irreversible changes in the pulmonary bed and can develop PVOD at 6 to 8 months of age. The provider may see Eisenmenger's syndrome in adolescents with unrepaired defects or palliative shunts. Fortunately, earlier and more corrective surgeries have made this occurrence rare in children born after the late 1980s.

Congestive Heart Failure

For children with most structural defects, CHF is rarely a problem. In the infant with a large shunt, CHF may require medical management prior to surgery. Some cardiologists consider CHF an indication for surgery. Some children with single ventricle physiology and most children with DCM live in a state of controlled CHF. Management of CHF is discussed earlier in this chapter and is dealt with in greater detail in Chapter 55.

Procedural Pain and Anxiety

Children with complex CHD must undergo numerous procedures and interventions and will have several hospitalizations in the first years of life. Families should have a standing prescription for EMLA anesthetic cream to use before phlebotomy, intravenous infusion starts, and other needle procedures. Minor procedures requiring sedation, including dental procedures, should be done in a setting where a provider is available who is comfortable managing the child's unique hemodynamics.

Long-Term Complications

Conduction aberration and arrhythmias are the most common long-term problem for all types of CHD. Surgical ventricu-lotomy is avoided whenever possible, but any surgical approach involving the intraventricular septum can damage the conduction system. Late complications of Fontan physiology include atrial arrhythmias, ventricular failure, and de-velopment of arteriovenous collateral vessels. Protein-losing enteropathy and chronic pleural effusions are much less common than in the past but still occur. Symptoms include fatigue, decreased exercise tolerance, cough, and later, dyspnea or muscle wasting with increased abdominal girth. There is an increased risk for venous thrombosis. Liver function abnormalities have been reported in this population.

▲ **Clinical Warning:** Many children with single ventricle physiology use a right ventricle as their systemic ventricle. The right ventricle is not designed to pump against systemic pressures for a lifetime and so may fail.

Most children with single ventricle physiology are placed on afterload-reducing agents to retard or prevent ventricular failure, and many centers routinely anticoagulate Fontan patients with warfarin or aspirin. Atrial arrythmias may require medial management, electrophysiology studies, or radio frequency ablation. Pharmacologic management of arrhythmias is less successful in the postoperative patient than in the child with a normal heart (Kanter & Garson, 1997; Balaji, Johnson, & Sade, 1997).

▲ **Clinical Warning:** The provider should consult with the cardiologist if the child reports any symptoms of palpitations, dizziness, chest discomfort, near syncope, or syncope.

The cardiology team may request 24-hour Holter or event monitoring. A 12-lead ECG obtained during a dysrhythmic episode can be very helpful to the electrophysiologist in planning further tests and treatment. Collateral vessels can be closed as often as necessary by coil embolization during cardiac catheterization. The incidence of adverse neurologic sequellae following completion of staged surgical palliation is 2% to 3% but can include seizures (Rosenkrantz, 1998).

When the Outcome Is Terminal

Despite significant advances in medical and surgical management of CHD and the partially repaired congenital heart, some children live only a short time or are terminally ill while living either at home or in the hospital. The provider must work with such families to improve the quality of the time they have with their child. Referral to counseling, mental health, social service, respite, and home nursing services all may prove helpful (Pearson, 1997).

COMMUNITY RESOURCES

There are many important resources for families of children with congenital heart disorders. Many programs and surgical centers have their own booklets, videos, and websites for families. One recommendation is *The Heart of a Child: What Families Need to Know about Heart Disorders in Children* by C. A. Neill, E. B. Clark, and C. Clark (1992), Johns Hopkins University Press, Baltimore. Pamphlets are available in English and Spanish from the American Heart Association include "If your child has a congenital heart defect," and "Feeding infants with congenital heart disease," "Your child in the hospital," and "What about me? When brothers and sisters get sick," are available from:

Association for the Care of Children's Health
7910 Woodmont Avenue, Suite 300
Bethesda MD 20814
(301) 654-6549
Internet address: *acch@clark.net*

Other important organizations:

CHASER (Congenital Heart Anomalies, Support, Education Research)
Internet address: *CHASER@compuserve.com*

Pediheart, a web site for families
Internet address: *www.pediheart.org*

National Down Syndrome Society
666 Broadway, 8th Floor
New York, NY 10012
(800) 221-4602
(212) 460-9330
E-mail: *info@ndss.org*
Internet address: *www.ndss.org*

National Marfan Foundation
382 Main Street
Port Washintton, NY 11050
(518) 883-8712

REFERENCES

Allan, L. D., Apfel, H. D., & Printz, B. F. (1998). Outcome after prenatal diagnosis of the hypoplastic left heart syndrome. *Heart, 79*, 371–373

American College of Cardiology. (1994). 26th Bethesda conference Jan. 6–7 1994: Recommendations for determining eligibility for competition in athletes with cardiovascular abnormalities. *Journal of the American College of Cardiology, 24*(4), 845–899.

American Academy of Pediatric Dentistry. (1991). *Pediatric dental care. An update for the 90s.* Chicago: Author.

American Academy of Pediatrics. Committee on Infectious Disease. (2000). *2000 red book.* Chicago: Author.

American Heart Association. (1997). Scientific statement. Prevention of bacterial endocarditis: A statement for health professionals. Committee on Rheumatic Fever, Endocarditis and Kawasaki disease of the Council on Cardiovascular disease in the Young. *Journal of the American Medical Association, 277*(2), 1794–1801.

Avery, M. E., & First, L. R. (1996). *Pediatric medicine* (2nd ed.). Baltimore: Williams & Wilkins.

Balaji, S., Johnson, T., & Sade, R. (1994). Management of atrial flutter after the Fontan procedure. *Journal of the American College of Cardiology, 23*, 1209–1215.

Bellinger, D., Jonas, R., Rappaport, L., Wypij, D., Wernovsky, G., et al. (1995). Developmental and neurologic status of children after heart surgery with hypothermic circulatory arrest or low-flow cardiopulmonary bypass. *New England Journal of Medicine, 332*, 549–555.

Bellinger, D., Rappaport, L., Wypij, D., Wernovsky, G., et al. (1997). Patterns of developmental dysfunction after surgery to correct transposition of the great arteries. *Journal of Developmental and Behavioral Pediatrics, 18*, 75–83.

Bove, E. (1998). Current status of staged reconstruction for hypoplastic left heart syndrome. *Pediatric Cardiology, 19*(4), 308-15.

Bove, E. L., & Lloyd, T. R. (1996). Staged reconstruction for hypoplastic left heart syndrome: Contemporary results. *Annals of Surgery, 224*(30), 387–394.

Brazelton, T. B., Christopherson, E. R., Frauman, A. C., Gorski, P. A., Poole, J. M., Stadtler, A. C., & Wright, C. L. (1999). Instruction, timeliness and medical influences affecting toilet training. *Pediatrics, 103*(6), 1353–1358.

Cannobio, M. (1994). Pregnancy after Mustard repair of d-transposition of the great arteries. *Circulation, Suppl:I.*

Caplan, W. D., Cooper, T. R., Garcia-Prats, J. A., & Brody, B. A. (1996). Diffusion of innovative approaches to managing hypoplastic left heart syndrome. *Archives of Pediatrics & Adolescent Medicine, 150*(5), 487–490.

Chang, A. C., Hanley, F. L., Wernovsky, G., & Wessel, D. L. (1998). *Pediatric cardiac intensive care.* Baltimore: Williams & Wilkins.

Chavez, H., Ozolins, D., & Loser, J. (1999). Hypoglycemia and propranolol in pediatric behavioral disorders. *Pediatrics, 103*, 1290–1301.

Colan, S. (1989). Long-term results after repair for congenital heart disease [with annotated bibliography]. *Current Opinion in Cardiology, 4*, 111–117.

Driscoll, D. J. (1999). Left-to-right shunt lesions. *Pediatric Clinics of North America, 46*(2), 355–368.

Federly, R. T. (1999). Left ventricular outflow obstruction. *Pediatric Clinics of North America, 46*(2), 369–384.

Forbess, J. M., Cook, N., Roth, S. J., Serraf, A., Mayer, J. E., & Jonas, R. A. (1995). Ten-year institutional experience with palliative surgery for hypoplastic left heart syndrome. *Circulation, 92*(9 Suppl.), ii 262–266.

Freed, M. (1984). Recreational and sports recommendations for the child with heart disease. *Pediatric Clinics of North America, 31*(6), 1307–1320.

Gaedeke-Norris, M., & Hill, C. (1994). Nutritional issues in infants and children with congenital heart disease. *Nursing Clinics of North America, 6*, 153–163.

Garson, A., Bricker, J. T., & McNamara, D. G. (1997). *The science and practice of pediatric cardiology* (2 vols.). Philadelphia: Lea & Febiger.

Gessner, I., & Victoria, B. (1993). *Pediatric cardiology: A problem oriented approach.* Philadelphia: W.B. Saunders.

Gidding, S. S., & Rosenthal, A. (1994). The interface between primary care and pediatric cardiology. *Pediatric Clinics of North America, 31*(6), 1367–1388.

Graham, T., Bricker, J. T., James, F., & Strong, W. (1994). Congenital heart disease. *Medicine and Science in Sports and Exercise,* S246–S253.

Grifka, R. G. (1999). Cyanotic congenital heart disease with increased pulmonary blood flow. *Pediatric Clinics of North America, 46*(2), 405–426.

Gutgesell, H. P., & Massaro, T. A. (1995). Management of hypoplastic left heart syndrome in a consortium of university hospitals. *American Journal of Cardiology, 76*, 809–811.

Johnston, J. K., Chinnock, R. E., Zuppan, C. W., Razzouk, A. J., Gundry, S. R., & Bailey, L. L. (1997). Limitations to survival for infants with hypoplastic left heart syndrome before and after transplant: The Loma Linda experience. *Journal of Transplant Coordination, 7*(4), 180–184.

Jonas, R. A. (1996). Hypothermia, circulatory arrest and the pediatric brain. *Journal of Cardiothoracic and Vascular Anesthesia, 10*(1), 66–74.

Jonas, R. A. (1995). Advances in the surgical care of infants and children with congenital heart disease. *Current Opinion in Pediatrics, 7*, 572–579.

Kanter, R., & Garson, A. (1997). Atrial arrhythmias during chronic follow up of surgery for complex congenital heart disease. *PACE, 20*[part 2], 502–511.

Kumar, R. K., Newburger, J. W., Gauvreau, K., Kamenir, S. A., & Hornberger, L. K. (1999). Comparison of outcome when hypoplastic left heart syndrome and transposition of the great arteries are diagnosed prenatally versus when diagnosis of these two conditions is made only postnatally. *American Journal of Cardiology, 83*, 1649–1653.

Lovell, M. A., & McDaniel, N. L. (1995). Association of hypertrophic maxillary frenulum with hypoplastic left heart syndrome. *Journal of Pediatrics, 137*(5), 749–750.

Morrow, W. R., Naftel, D., Chinnock, R., Canter, C., Boucek, M., Zales, V., McGiffin, D. C., & Kirklin, J. K. (1997). Outcome of listing for heart transplantation in infants younger than six months: Predictors of death and interval to transplantation. The Pediatric Heart Transplantation Study Group. *Journal of Heart and Lung Transplantation, 16*, 1255–1266.

Newburger, J. W., Silbert, A. R., Buckley, L. P., et al. (1984). Cognitive function and age at repair in children with transposition of the great arteries. *New England Journal of Medicine, 310*, 1495–1499.

Newburger, J. W., Tucker, A. D., Silbert, A. R., & Fyler, D. C. (1983). Motor function and timing of surgery in transposition of the great arteries, intact ventricular septum. *Pediatric Cardiology, 4*, 317.

Pearson, L. (1997). Family centered care and the anticipated death of a newborn. *Pediatric Nursing, 23*(2), 162–178.

Pelech, A. N. (1999). Evaluation of the pediatric patient with a cardiac murmur. *Pediatric Clinics of North America, 46*(2), 167–188.

Queen, P. M., & Lang, C. E. (1993). *Handbook of pediatric nutrition.* Gaithersburg, MD: Aspen.

Rogers, B. T., Msail, M. E., Buck, G. M., Lyon, N. R., Norris, M. K., Roland, J. M., & Gingell, R. L. (1995). Neurodevelopmental outcomes of infants with hypoplastic left heart syndrome. *Journal of Pediatrics, 126*(3), 496–498.

Rosenkrantz, E. R. (1998). Caring for the former pediatric cardiac surgery patient. *Pediatric Clinics of North America, 45*, 907–941.

Spicer, R. L. (1994). Cardiovascular disease in Down syndrome. *Pediatric Clinics of North America, 31*(6), 1331–1344.

Swanson, L. T. (1995). Treatment options for HLHS: A mother's perspective. *Critical Care Nurse, 15*(3), 70–79.

Tassey, C. (1997). Patient guides to cardiac medications (ACE inhibitors, beta blockers, calcium channel blockers, digoxin, diuretics, warfarin). [Brochure], Burlington VT: VT/NH Regional Program in Pediatric Cardiology.

Tong, E. M., Sparacino, P. S., Messias, D. K., Foote, D., Chesla, C. A., & Gilliss, C. L. (1998). Growing up with congenital heart disease: The dilemmas of adolescents and young adults. *Cardiology in the Young, 8*(3), 303–309.

Tong, E., & Sparacino, P. (1994). Special management issues for adolescents and young adults with congenital heart disease. *Critical Care Nursing Clinics of North America, 6*(1), 199–214.

Uzark, K., Lincoln, A., Lamberti, J. J., Mainwaring, R. D., Spicer, R. L., & Moore, J. W. (1998). Neurodevelopmental outcomes in children with Fontan repair of functional single ventricle. *Pediatrics, 101*(4), 620–633.

Uzark, K. (1992). Counseling adolescents with congenital heart disease. *Journal of Cardiovascular Nursing, 6*, 65–73.

Waldman, J. D., Wernly, J. A. (1999). Cyanotic congenital heart disease with decreased pulmonary blood flow in children. *Pediatric Clinics of North America, 46*(2), 385–404.

Walsh, A., Morrow, D., & Jonas, R. (1995). Neurologic and developmental outcomes following pediatric cardiac surgery. *Nursing Clinics of North America, 30*(2), 347–364.

Wong, D. L. (1995). *Whaley and Wong's nursing care of infants and children.* St. Louis, MO: Mosby.

Yeager, S. B. (1990). Pediatric cardiology. In Crapo, J. D., Hamilton, M. A., Edgman, S. (eds.). *Medicine and pediatrics.* Philadelphia: Hanley & Belfus, pp. 60–94. In Zahka, K. G., Spector, M., Hanisch, D. (1993) Hypoplastic Left Heart Syndrome: Norwood operation, transplantation or compassionate care? *Clinics in Perinatology, 20*, 145-154.

Chronic Gastrointestinal Disorders

• HARVEY W. AIGES, MD

INTRODUCTION

Chronic gastrointestinal complaints are a significant part of primary care pediatrics. Abdominal pain, diarrhea, constipation, reflux, and emesis are seen frequently. The pediatric primary care provider must determine whether symptoms are functional (nonorganic) or related to disease in the gastrointestinal tract (organic). This chapter provides information about diagnosis and management of common functional and organic gastrointestinal disorders seen in pediatrics, including irritable bowel syndrome (IBS; neonatal through adolescent presentations), constipation and encopresis, chronic and recurrent abdominal pain, gastroesophageal reflux disease (GERD), peptic ulcer disease, chronic diarrhea and malabsorption, and inflammatory bowel disease. The diagnosis and management of abdominal migraine are discussed in Chapter 51. Munchausen syndrome by proxy can also be the underlying cause of a gastrointestinal tract disorder; this problem is discussed in Chapter 23.

Meticulous history, physical examination, and evaluation of the child's growth and development will usually help the pediatric clinician determine the etiology of symptoms, providing the data needed for developing an appropriate therapeutic plan.

Irritable Bowel Syndrome

Irritable bowel syndrome affects a very large number of children and adolescents, resulting in a dramatic amount of school absenteeism and a significant use of health care resources (Camilleri & Choi, 1997). IBS is a psychophysiologic disorder of disturbed bowel habits and abdominal pain in the absence of demonstrable organic disease.

PATHOLOGY

Mast cells are metachromatic cells found widely throughout the body, including the gastrointestinal tract, where they are found in mucosal tissue. Mast cells are, of course, involved in both allergenic and nonallergenic events that are associated with inflammation. In the gastrointestinal tract, mast cell degranulation can occur as an antigen-mediated event, in which an immunoglobulin E (IgE)-dependent hypersensitivity reaction occurs. Mast cell degranulation is in part what underpins some of the symptomatology of such disorders as IBS, gastroenteritis with or without *Helicobacter pylori* infection, Crohn's disease (CD), and ulcerative colitis (UC) (Thomson & Walker-Smith, 1998).

Although the exact mechanisms of IBS have not been clarified, there has been a significant advance in understanding of the factors involved in producing the myriad symptoms of IBS. These factors include dysmotility, visceral hypersensitivity, smooth muscle abnormalities, and psychogenic reasons. Patients with IBS have a different myoelectrical rhythm, meaning that the action potential of the cells of the intestine differs from that of patients without IBS. This different "signature" allows for abnormal contractions of the bowel in response to various stimuli, such as intestinal hormones, foods, and neurotransmitter substances. Therefore, symptoms can be induced by a large number of endogenous and exogenous stimuli, including infections, medications, teething, and emotional stress.

Patients with IBS have visceral hypersensitivity, meaning that they experience the sensation of fullness and pain at smaller volumes of gas or stool than the general population. These children also have systemic smooth muscle abnormalities, with an abnormal response to urodynamic studies. These patients are also more likely to wheeze when stimulated. All of these abnormalities are associated with autonomic nervous system dysfunction with associated blood pressure and pulse changes. These pathologic sequelae help explain many of the clinical findings associated with IBS (Hanauer, 1996; Rasquin-Weber et al., 1999). Adult patients with IBS have a much higher chance of having a definable psychiatric diagnosis, usually chronic anxiety or depression, than the general population (Trikas et al., 1999). There is considerable evidence that adult patients with IBS also have issues with anger management (Trikas et al., 1999; Welgan, Meshkinpour, & Ma, 2000). Ali et al. (2000) reported that emotional abuse, self-blame, and self-silencing were commonly found in women with IBS.

EPIDEMIOLOGY

It has been estimated that between 22 and 30 million Americans have IBS (Hanauer, 1996). Many patients with IBS never come to medical attention; thus, exact figures of prevalence and incidence are not available. Because IBS is not a disease but a function of one's own body makeup, it may affect patients throughout their lives (Rasquin-Weber et al., 1999). No cultural or socioeconomic factors seem to be involved, although upper middle class patients seem to seek medical attention more frequently for IBS than do lower socioeconomic groups (Hanauer, 1996; Everhart & Renault, 1991).

Other disorders are associated with IBS, at least in the older adolescent and adult patient. These include fibromyalgia, chronic fatigue syndrome, and temporomandibular disorder (Aaron, Burke, & Buchwald, 2000; Yunus, Inanici, Aldag, & Mangold, 2000). Locke, Zinsmeister, Talley, Fett, and Melton (2000) also describe analgesics and food sensitivities as risk factors in adulthood.

HISTORY AND PHYSICAL EXAMINATION

A child with IBS may have any or all of the age-related symptoms and signs of the disorder. Other topics related to chronic gastrointestinal problems in children, including constipation and recurrent abdominal pain, probably are part of the clinical spectrum of IBS. The following discussion presents findings associated with IBS by symptom and age range.

- Stool retention (neonatal period): Infants may strain at stool. The physical examination is normal except for tight anal sphincter noted on rectal examination.
- Colic (1–4 months): The definition of colic is prolonged crying without an obvious reason. IBS is the most common etiology of colic. Other causes of colic can include esophagitis secondary to gastroesophageal reflux (GER) and cow's milk protein allergy, or it can be an early sign of increased spasticity, as seen in cerebral palsy.
- Toddler's diarrhea/chronic nonspecific diarrhea of childhood (6 months–3 years): Toddler's diarrhea is frequent loose, pasty bowel movements (ie, 2–12 per day). Food particles are frequently visible in the stool. The first stool of the morning is usually the most formed, because it has remained in the rectal ampulla overnight, allowing for water resorption. Interestingly, this child does not awake during the night to have a bowel movement, as is often seen with organic etiologies. The salient point of toddler's diarrhea is the strikingly normal appearance, physical examination, mood, appetite, and activity level of the child despite runny stools. The child's growth and development are normal unless inappropriate dietary restrictions have been instituted by the provider or the parents. Flare-ups of toddler's diarrhea may occur spontaneously, but they often follow a stress, such as an episode of gastroenteritis, use of antibiotics, or teething (Kneepkens & Hoekstra, 1996).
- Constipation (3–10 years): Although constipation may occur at any age from birth on, the child with IBS most commonly has clinically significant constipation during this time period. The constipation may take the form of infrequent bowel movements, hard and small-volume bowel movements, or incomplete evacuation of stool produced. This latter occurrence is the hardest to diagnose. The constipation of IBS is considered to be secondary to the patient's inherent dysmotility. The patient may have episodes of stress diarrhea coexisting with the constipation.
- Recurrent abdominal pain (11–18 years): Recurrent abdominal pain and vague abdominal pain are well-described clinical entities in adolescents with IBS in whom periumbilical pain of a recurrent or vague nature is present (Hyams et al., 1996). They are far more common in females, usually near the time of menarche. The patient frequently has a history of normal, daily bowel movements but objectively has large amounts of colonic stool by physical examination or abdominal radiographs. This form of IBS often is associated with intermittent episodes of stress diarrhea (eg, loose bowel movements at the times of school examinations, conflicts with friends) (Thomson & Walker-Smith, 1998).
- Adult form of IBS (adolescence to adulthood): The adult form of IBS, which can be seen as early as preadolescence, has all the gastrointestinal features of IBS, including abdominal pain, constipation, and diarrhea, and is associated with autonomic dysfunction. The patient may experience flushing, rapid changes in pulse and blood pressure (especially in response to cold liquid ingestion), headaches, insomnia, lower back pain, and palpitations. Females especially may complain of urinary frequency and urgency. Urodynamic studies are likely to be abnormal. All of these clinical findings are thought to be related to abnormal smooth muscle responsiveness.

DIAGNOSTIC CRITERIA

The diagnosis of IBS cannot be made by any specific test. However, the diagnosis is highly likely if the patient exhibits all of the following:

- Chronic gastrointestinal symptoms with *normal* growth and development
- Symptoms that are not nocturnal
- Normal physical examination, including negative hemoccult test, blood tests (complete blood count [CBC], erythrocyte sedimentation rate [ESR], serum albumin, iron, total iron-binding capacity [TIBC], amylase, *H. pylori*), radiographs, endoscopies, and biopsies (when indicated)
- Positive family history for IBS

DIAGNOSTIC STUDIES

Invasive studies, such as barium radiographs, esophagogastroduodenoscopy, and colonoscopy, may not be necessary if all other evaluations are normal. In cases in which the results are confusing, the history is unclear, or the growth and development are abnormal, a more complete evaluation will be necessary.

MANAGEMENT

The child with IBS should be seen by the provider every 6 months. This frequency will provide a sound framework for following growth and development while addressing any nutritional, psychosocial, or other concerns of the child and parents. This frequency will also allow for surveillance activities and wellness management, while supporting the development of relationship-centered care.

IBS is not an organic disease, and no specific therapies can cure it because it is a function of the patient's own body makeup. The pediatric provider should direct all management and therapeutic plans toward patient and family education about IBS, helping them learn how to cope with the disorder, and giving symptomatic relief when possible. The primary care clinician's role is critical to patient and family acceptance of the diagnosis. The practitioner can support them in their ability to handle the occasional pain and discomfort experienced with IBS.

Treatment for symptomatic relief may include the following:

- For constipation, younger than 1 year: barley malt extract (Maltsupex); older than 1 year: docusate sodium (Colace) for hard stools, senna (Senokot) for difficulty in passing stools
- For chronic diarrhea: Regular diet; avoidance of very cold liquids, excessive sweets, and chewing gum or

candies. The role of aspirin use is also possibly related to IBS symptomatology, but aspirin should be avoided in all children and adolescents in any case because of its relationship to the pathogenesis of Reye's syndrome.

- For alternating constipation and diarrhea: Fiber (Metamucil or Fibercon)
- For abdominal pain: Treatment for underlying cause (eg, constipation)

▲ **Clinical Warning:** The pediatric provider must be careful to avoid using antimotility agents, such as belladonna, loperamide (Imodium), or diphenoxylate (Lomotil), because they may increase constipation and therefore increase the pain.

● **Clinical Pearl:** Lifestyle changes, including avoiding soda and chewing gum or gummy candies, can be helpful in decreasing gassiness. For the older child and adolescent, note that cigarette smoking increases gassiness because of the air swallowing that is a component of smoking.

The vast majority of children with IBS can be managed solely by the pediatric primary care provider. The provider should consult a pediatric gastroenterologist if endoscopy is needed, if the case is atypical, or if the parents need more reassurance. The provider should become concerned that the diagnosis of IBS is incorrect if the following occur:

- Weight, height, and development slow or diminish.
- Symptoms are nocturnal.
- Blood is seen or found in the stool.
- Stool has positive Wright stain or Charcot-Leyden crystals.
- The ESR is elevated, or serum albumin level is low.

What to Tell Parents

Irritable bowel syndrome is not a psychosomatic illness but a true physiologic entity. IBS is not "all in their head." IBS is part of the patient's individual makeup, and symptoms may be intermittent and lifelong. The patient with IBS does not have organic disease; therefore, there are no dietary or activity restrictions.

The school may need to be made aware of special bathroom needs (especially in the child with chronic diarrhea). The provider may need to assist the family in acquiring these bathroom privileges.

Constipation and Encopresis

The pediatric primary care provider may see a large number of children with a complaint of constipation or encopresis. There are not clear definitions of these two entities in children. However, most people accept constipation as meaning infrequent bowel movements, hard stools, or pain or straining with bowel movements. Encopresis is a more confusing term, but it is generally accepted to mean passage of stool into underwear or clothing of children who are 4 years of age or older. In most cases, the term *encopresis* is used synonymously with *fecal soiling* or *fecal incontinence*. Encopresis may also be associated with urinary incontinence disorders. For more information about the diagnosis and management of this latter problem, the reader is referred to Chapter 63.

PATHOLOGY

After the neonatal period, the vast majority of children with constipation have simple constipation as a result of a functional dysmotility (IBS) or from voluntary withholding. The withholding may be a result of problems with toilet training or fear of defecation secondary to passage of a large or painful stool. If stool retention remains untreated for a prolonged period, the rectal wall becomes stretched, and the rectal vault enlarges. Some children with this problem experience significant anorectal pain, so they will repeatedly defecate small amounts of stool to achieve relief. These children are classically dirty while awake and tend to have very little soiling when sleeping.

Other children may have involuntary leakage of semiliquid stool around a hard stool mass. The child usually claims that he or she has not experienced the urge to defecate. This stage is often termed encopresis. Encopresis may also occur in the nonconstipated child who has severe psychogenic problems or in the child with a neuromuscular disorder.

EPIDEMIOLOGY

The normal frequency of bowel movements is age dependent. In the first 3 months of life, 95% of breast-fed infants have 5 to 40 bowel movements per week, while formula-fed infants have 5 to 25 bowel movements per week. In the second half of the first year, most babies will have 5 to 25 bowel movements per week, while toddlers from 1 to 3 years of age usually have 4 to 20 stools each week. The adult pattern of 3 to 14 bowel movements per week is established by about 4 years of age.

Constipation occurs in about 3% to 8% of children, with no ethnic, racial, or gender differences. It is estimated that 3% of children's ambulatory health visits are for constipation. Fecal soiling occurs in 3% of 4-year-olds, 2% of 6-year-olds, and 1.5% of children between 7 and 11 years of age, with a male predominance of 3:1 to 6:1 (Everhart & Renault, 1991; Baker et al., 1999; Hyams, 1999; Nowicki & Bishop, 1999).

HISTORY AND PHYSICAL EXAMINATION

Causes of pediatric constipation are listed in Display 57-1. Historic points that must be obtained include the following:

- Passage of meconium in the first 48 hours of life (if not, consider Hirschsprung's disease)
- Stool history in first year of life
- History of toilet training (eg, trauma)
- History suggestive of IBS
- Average intake of dietary fiber (eating less than the minimum recommendation is a risk factor for chronic constipation in children; Morais, Vitolo, Aguirre, & Fagundes-Neto, 1999)
- Family history

The provider should perform a complete physical examination, looking for evidence of hypothyroidism, neurofibromatosis, neuromuscular disorders, and anorectal abnormalities.

In particular, the abdominal examination should note muscle tone and abdominal contents. A diastasis recti can be noted by having the child do a sit-up. A diastasis recti will

DISPLAY 57–1 • Causes of Pediatric Constipation

Functional

Irritable bowel syndrome
Dietary changes
Toilet training
Febrile illness
Fear
Withholding

Organic

Neuromuscular disorders: spinal defects, intestinal pseudo-obstruction, and so forth
Congenital defects: Hirschsprung's disease, imperforate anus, anal stenosis, and so forth
Endocrine/metabolic: hypothyroid, hypercalcemia, hypokalemia, diabetes mellitus
Perianal: anal fissure, streptococcal cellulitis, atopic dermatitis
Gastrointestinal: gluten-sensitive enteropathy, cystic fibrosis, obstruction

Drugs/Toxins

Pelvic tumors

---

dissipate the intra-abdominal pressure generated by a Valsalva's maneuver, diminishing the ability to have effective bowel movements.

Gold, Levine, Weinstein, Kessler, and Pettei (1999) reported that pediatric providers often neglect to perform a digital rectal examination in the child with chronic constipation. The digital examination is important, because it can help the clinician to determine whether the patient's constipation stems from a functional or an organic process. This differentiation is important because it may affect what therapy is prescribed.

The digital rectal examination should note rectal tone and rectal contents. A large rectal vault suggests chronic constipation or stool withholding. An anteriorly displaced anus with a posterior rectal shelf (noted on rectal examination) may make defecation difficult.

DIAGNOSTIC CRITERIA

Definitive criteria for diagnosis of constipation or encopresis have not been established. Diagnosis is almost always based on history and physical examination.

DIAGNOSTIC STUDIES

Occasionally, an abdominal radiograph may be needed to assess the amount of stool present in the patient who is difficult to examine or in the adolescent with a very muscular abdomen. If growth and development are abnormal in a child with constipation, then the pediatric provider should consider the following in the differential diagnosis:

- Hypothyroidism
- Gluten-sensitive enteropathy (celiac disease)
- Cystic fibrosis

▲ **Clinical Warning:** If Hirschsprung's disease is a possibility, the pediatric provider should refer the patient to a pediatric gastroenterologist for a more complete evaluation. The best way to diagnose Hirschsprung's disease is by rectal biopsy, but if a biopsy cannot be done or cannot be interpreted accurately, a barium enema or anal manometry should be attempted.

● **Clinical Pearl:** The clinician should also consider referring a child to a pediatric gastroenterologist if a case is truly intractable or if the parents demand more reassurance.

MANAGEMENT

The vast majority of children with constipation or encopresis can be managed solely by the primary care provider. Constipation in children often mandates the use of medication. In many adults with constipation, acceptance of dietary measures, including increasing fiber, is all that is necessary. Failure to treat a child's constipation may result in an increase in problems, which in turn may lead to stool-withholding behavior and fecal soiling.

The addition of increased dietary fiber may also help the pediatric patient with functional constipation (Janicke & Finney, 1999). In some instances, the provider also may find that referring the child and family for mental health evaluation and intervention can be efficacious. Janicke and Finney report that cognitive-behavioral treatment may prove useful when added to dietary interventions for functional constipation in children. Unfortunately, dietary manipulation is infrequently successful and may actually lead to caloric deprivation. The pediatric primary care provider is advised to seek nutritional counseling for the infant or younger child especially to ensure proper caloric provision.

Treatments for constipation can include the following:

- Infants
  - Barley malt extract 5 to 10 mL in formula twice daily
- Children older than 1 year
  - Dioctyl sodium sulfosuccinate 5 to 10 mL/kg once daily (softens stool)
  - Senna 5 to 20 mL daily (laxative, effective in withholding)
  - Bisacodyl (Dulcolax) one to two tablets once daily (or one suppository; irritant)

For clean-out or to manage intractable cases, polyethylene glycol lavage may prove efficacious, although the provider may need to use a nasogastric tube.

The provider should be certain of the following:

- The constipated child does not have hypothyroidism or neurofibromatosis.
- Hirschsprung's disease was considered if there was no history of early passage of meconium or if the child passes ribbon- or snake-like stools.
- In difficult to treat cases, physical examination for diastasis recti or an abnormally placed anus has occurred.

What to Tell Parents

Constipation may be a lifelong problem, but it usually becomes easier to treat with increasing age. Dietary manipulation is infrequently successful in children with constipation. Painful, hard stools are to be avoided to prevent withholding and encopresis. The school should make access to a bathroom easy so that children with constipation do not withhold stool.

Chronic and Recurrent Abdominal Pain

Chronic and recurrent abdominal pain are very common health care problems in pediatric practice. More than one third of children complain of abdominal pain that lasts 2 or more weeks (Lake, 1999). The term *chronic abdominal pain* is defined as discomfort that has lasted longer than 1 month. Recurrent abdominal pain requires three episodes of abdominal pain severe enough to limit activity and occurring for more than 3 months, with symptom-free intervals between the episodes of pain.

PATHOLOGY

Abdominal pain may be visceral (from abdominal viscera), somatic (parietal, from underlying peritoneal irritation or inflammation), or referred from a more distal site. In general, visceral pain is produced by a distention of the wall of a hollow organ, stretching of the capsule of a solid organ, inflammation, or ischemia.

EPIDEMIOLOGY

A small but fairly significant number of children have recurrent abdominal pain—as many as 10% to 15% of school-aged youngsters and 15% to 25% of adolescents (Hyams et al., 1996; Hotopf, Carr, Mayou, Wadsworth, & Wessely, 1998). The majority of these children and adolescents have abdominal pain and defecatory symptoms consistent with a diagnosis of IBS (Hyams et al., 1996).

HISTORY AND PHYSICAL EXAMINATION

Visceral pain tends to be poorly localized, but hepatobiliary, pancreatic, and gastroduodenal disease tend to be felt in the epigastrium. Conversely, small and large bowel disease tend to cause periumbilical symptoms. Abnormalities in the rectosigmoid colon, the urinary tract, and the pelvic organs tend to be felt in the suprapubic area. Peritoneal pain is usually more sharp and constant and is localized to the area of the involved viscera. Signs of peritoneal involvement include voluntary guarding or involuntary rigidity of the overlying abdominal musculature, with or without rebound pain. Causes of recurrent or chronic abdominal pain in children are listed in Display 57-2.

● **Clinical Pearl:** The farther away chronic or recurrent abdominal pain is from the umbilicus, the more likely it is to be an organic problem. In addition, when a child complains of pain in different sites on different days without localization, an organic problem is less likely than if the pain is always in the same area.

DIAGNOSTIC CRITERIA

The differential diagnosis of chronic and recurrent abdominal pain is extensive. It is important that the pediatric

---

DISPLAY 57–2 • Causes of Recurrent or Chronic Abdominal Pain in Children

Gastrointestinal

Gastroesophageal reflux disease	Intestinal obstruction (malrotation, intussusception)
Dyspepsia	Meckel's diverticulum (diverticulitis or intussusception)
Carbohydrate intolerance	Intestinal duplication (enteric cyst)
Irritable bowel syndrome	Mesenteric cyst
Constipation	Pancreatitis
Aerophagia	Biliary colic
Inflammatory bowel disease	Parasites (giardia, ascariasis)
Celiac disease	Allergic enteropathy

Genitourinary

Urinary tract infection	Ureteropelvic junction obstruction
Hydronephrosis	Nephrolithiasis

Gynecologic

Endometriosis	Pelvic inflammatory disease
Ovarian cyst or tumor	Dysmenorrhea
Imperforate hymen	Vaginal atresia

Other

Abdominal migraine	Porphyria
Angioneurotic edema	Familial Mediterranean fever
Abdominal muscle tear	Vasculitis (eg, Henoch-Schönlein purpura)

---

provider keep in mind that more than 90% of such patients do not have an organic etiology for their discomfort. The most common cause of the pain is IBS.

It is often difficult to decide how broad a diagnostic evaluation should be done on a child with chronic or recurrent abdominal pain. If no accompanying features suggestive of more serious disease are present, it is reasonable to refrain from an extensive and expensive workup early in the course of the evaluation. A complete history and physical examination often point the primary care provider in the correct diagnostic direction.

● **Clinical Pearls:**

- Nocturnal symptoms are more likely to be organic.
- Pain associated with tenesmus, systemic symptoms, headaches, or vomiting is more likely to be organic.
- Back pain associated with abdominal pain is infrequent and suggests involvement of a retroperitoneal organ or a process abutting the retroperitoneum (eg, pancreatic disease, biliary disease, or penetrating/perforating peptic ulcer disease).
- Acute organomegaly causes pain by stretching the organ's capsule. If an enlarged organ is nontender, it implies adaptation of the capsule, which suggests chronicity.
- Rebound pain is rarely a helpful finding.
- Children with severe abdominal pain causing them to writhe in agony rarely have an organic disease.

DIAGNOSTIC STUDIES

A helpful screening evaluation includes a CBC with platelets, ESR, urinalysis, serum albumin, serum iron/TIBC, and a study to rule out lactose intolerance.

● **Clinical Pearl:** If the history is suggestive of lactose intolerance, a trial of a lactose-free diet with elimination of symptoms may preclude all additional studies.

MANAGEMENT

The majority of children with chronic and recurrent abdominal pain can be managed solely by the primary care provider. However, in view of its chronicity and frequently the frustration of not finding a specific etiology, the clinician may consider a referral to a pediatric gastroenterologist.

Management is dictated by the underlying cause. In many cases in which the cause seems to be functional, education and reassurance may be the best treatment. The use of a pain diary may be helpful in giving the patient insight into personal triggers for abdominal pain. Points to be included in such a diary include the day and time of the symptom(s) and what life events were occurring at that time.

▲ **Clinical Warning:** Antispasmodics and antimotility agents must be used with caution because they may worsen the symptoms in many cases.

What to Tell Parents

Parents must understand that the pain is real, not in the child's head. If no etiology is found, the pain may continue or recur over a long period of time. Parents should encourage their child to follow normal functions of daily living, including school attendance, play activities, camp, and a normal diet.

Gastroesophageal Reflux Disease

Gastroesophageal reflux is the **effortless** regurgitation of gastric contents. This definition is in contrast to vomiting, which is the forceful, effortful ejection of gastric materials. GER may be projectile.

PATHOLOGY

Gastroesphageal reflux is caused primarily by transient lower esophageal sphincter relaxation, unrelated to swallowing. Other factors implicated are diminished lower esophageal tone, large hiatal hernias, and delayed gastric emptying. Virtually all infants have some degree of GER, but only a small percentage have apparent complications. An infant who spits up but has normal weight gain, has no respiratory problems or apnea, and is not irritable during or after feedings, should be considered to have normal spitting up and not a pathologic process (Nelson et al., 1997).

EPIDEMIOLOGY

During the past 2 decades, GER has been diagnosed much more, but that is because of increased awareness and far more sophisticated technology rather than a true increase in occurrence. Physiologic GER occurs in almost all infants. The prevalence of pathologic GER (GERD) is unknown, but it is clearly much higher in children with neurologic impairments and children with repaired tracheoesophageal fistulae, chronic lung disease (asthma, cystic fibrosis, bronchopulmonary dysplasia), preterm status, and orthopedic abnormalities, such as scoliosis. There does not seem to be racial, ethnic, or gender difference in GERD (Fonkalsrud & Arment, 1996).

HISTORY AND PHYSICAL EXAMINATION

It is most critical to differentiate historically between vomiting (effortful) and GER (effortless). The vast majority of infants with GER will do well with time and conservative management. Vomiting, on the other hand, must be evaluated seriously if it is atypical, intractable, or chronic. Vomiting can signify increased intracranial pressure or may be due to metabolic derangements.

The physical examination is usually not informative. The complications from pathologic GERD can include the following:

- Esophagitis, which can cause irritability (colic) and poor eating, blood loss leading to hematemesis or melana, and esophageal stricture
- Failure to thrive
- Sandifer's syndrome: reflux with arching, torticollis, or seizure-like activity
- Respiratory symptoms, including asthma, apnea, pneumonia, or chronic cough
- Ear, nose, and throat (ENT) symptoms: hoarseness, stridor, recurrent sinusitis, or otitis media
- Dysphagia/odynophagia in older children

DIAGNOSTIC CRITERIA

In the absence of gastrointestinal symptoms, GER should be considered when a child has the following:

- Head tilt, arching of the neck, bizarre head tics, or atypical seizures
- Atypical asthma, chronic cough, or unexplained recurrent pneumonia
- Unexplained hoarseness or stridor
- Unexplained anemia

DIAGNOSTIC STUDIES

There is some controversy over using the myriad of studies available to study GER. In the infant with clinically obvious regurgitation, no studies are needed unless complications occur or if surgery is considered. In nonregurgitant cases, such as GER secondary to respiratory or ENT problems, extended pH monitoring may be helpful. In atypical or complicated cases, other tests, such as esophagoscopy with biopsy, barium studies, or scintigraphy, may be necessary.

MANAGEMENT

The vast majority of children with GER can be managed by the primary care provider. In complicated cases, or in cases in which technology is needed, a pediatric gastroenterologist can assist the clinician in evaluating the patient and planning treatment.

Most infants with GER do not require medical intervention. Overfeeding should be avoided. Thickening the infant's feedings with cereal may reduce regurgitation, but care should be taken not to give the child too much protein. Cereal should not be added to bottles because of the risk of choking. Although studies have shown that prone positioning after feedings and at sleep may decrease GER, this position may be a factor in sudden infant death syndrome, so it should be avoided in the first 6 months of life (Vanderplas et al., 1996).

Pharmacotherapy

Pharmacotherapy may be used in more complicated cases. H_2-receptor antagonists are often used in children with GER. Ranitidine (Zantac), available as a syrup of 15 mg/mL, is used at a dose of 5 to 10 mg/kg per day, administered twice daily. In some cases, the use of gastrointestinal prokinetics may be helpful. Cisapride (Propulsid) can be made as a suspension of 1 mg/mL and given as a dose of 0.2 to 0.3 mg/kg per dose, two to three times daily.

When medications are not adequate in controlling symptoms or when complications are very severe (eg, recurrent apneic episodes), the pediatric gastroenterologist may consider referring the patient for surgical intervention. The Nissen fundoplication is the current procedure of choice.

▲ Clinical Warnings:

- At least one recent study that examined the pharmacokinetics of ranitidine in children with cystic fibrosis suggests that toxicity levels may be reached sooner in these patients (James, Stowe, Farrar, Menendez, & Argao, 1999). The provider should be certain of working closely with both the accredited cystic fibrosis treatment center and pediatric gastroenterologist who comanage the child with cystic fibrosis and GER.
- Cisapride has been reported to cause ventricular arrhythmias, especially when used with macrolide antibiotics or antifungal agents (Cuchiara, 1996). This problem is an infrequent but worrisome complication that has led to a decreased use of this agent.

What to Tell Parents

The primary care provider should reassure parents that most cases of GER are normal and will resolve with time. A small number of children will have chronic GER, requiring more active intervention. It is important that the clinician stress that parents and caregivers not overfeed the child. Finally, the practitioner needs to emphasize that parents and caregivers must avoid smoking near the child. Any exposure to passive smoke inhalation will exacerbate GER.

Peptic Ulcer Disease

Peptic disorders, including gastritis, peptic ulcers, and duodenitis, are responsible in fewer than 5% of children presenting with abdominal pain. Peptic disorders are far less common in pediatrics than in adult primary care practice (Jevon, Dimmick, & Hassall, 1997).

PATHOLOGY

H. pylori is by far the most common cause of chronic gastritis, duodenitis, and peptic ulcer disease in children. Ulcers in children are almost always duodenal. The exact nature by which H. pylori causes peptic disease is unclear, but it does not seem to be related to acid hypersecretion.

Tindberg, Blennow, and Granstrom (1999) report that in their cohort study of 305 Swedish children, H. pylori seropositivity was more likely to be found in children whose parents recalled having had a history of unspecified abdominal pain. In the majority of infected patients, H. pylori causes chronic active (type B) gastritis. Whether or not the child will eventually develop peptic ulcer disease or, even later, a gastric cancer or lymphoma depends on how the individual responds to H. pylori infection (Day & Sherman, 1999; Jones, Day, & Sherman, 1999).

EPIDEMIOLOGY

Peptic disease may be caused by aspirin and nonsteroidal anti-inflammatory drug use. Steroids have not been shown to be an independent cause of ulcer disease. Other etiologies of peptic disease in children include CD, stress (significant illness that causes mucosal ischemia), Henoch-Schönlein purpura, and sickle cell disease (George & Glassman, 1994).

H. pylori infects approximately 50% of the world's population. It is the major cause of gastritis and duodenal and gastric ulcers in both children and adults (Gold, 1999). H. pylori infections occur in children worldwide, but because most information comes from western and other developed countries, little is known about the epidemiology of H. pylori in the developing world. Certainly poverty, poor hygiene, and crowded living conditions play a significant role in transmission (Bardhan et al., 1999). Chronic H. pylori infection has been linked with development of gastric carcinomas in later life (Blecker & Gold, 1999). In tropical climates, peptic ulcer disease also has been shown to be related to parasite infestation (Ameh, 1999).

HISTORY AND PHYSICAL EXAMINATION

Symptoms of gastritis, peptic ulcer, and duodenitis may be similar. Epigastric pain that awakens the child from sleep is typical. Younger children may not be able to localize the pain to the epigastrium and may present with anorexia and irritability. Painless bleeding may be the only manifestation of ulcer disease. On physical examination, epigastric tenderness is suggestive but is an inconsistent finding. Perforation and penetration are less common in children than adults.

DIAGNOSTIC STUDIES

The definitive diagnosis of peptic disorders in children generally is made by the pediatric gastroenterologist. This specialist performs an upper endoscopy to visualize mucosa and obtain tissue biopsies.

▲ **Clinical Warnings:**

- Upper gastrointestinal series radiographs are highly unreliable for the diagnosis of peptic disease. Even when an ulcer crater is seen, barium studies cannot tell if the problem is *H. pylori* related.
- Serology for *H. pylori* titers is used as a screening test by many primary care providers, but the titers are not totally reliable.

● **Clinical Pearl:** Urea breath tests for the presence of *H. pylori* are being used more frequently. They are attractive because of their noninvasive nature. Although the breath test yields less information than endoscopy with biopsy, it may play an important follow-up role in assessing whether therapy has eliminated the infection.

MANAGEMENT

If peptic disease is considered, the primary care provider should manage the case with the assistance of a pediatric gastroenterologist, who will be needed for endoscopy, biopsy, and treatment input. Treatment of peptic disease should be directed to the underlying cause (De Giacome et al., 1997).

In *H. pylori*-related peptic disease, eradication of the infection is appropriate, but an ideal regimen for children has not yet been established (Robinson, Abdel-Rahman, & Nahata, 1997). All protocols for treatment of *H. pylori* infection involve long courses of multiple medications. This means that ensuring parent–child participation in the regimen can present a challenge for the primary provider. Currently, a 2-week course of metronidazole, clarithromycin, and omeprazole seems promising (Dohil, Israel, & Hassall, 1997; Gold, 1999). Follow-up studies (biopsy or urea breath test) need to be done to establish bacterial eradication (Robinson et al., 1997; Moshkowitz et al., 1998; Adeyemi, Danial, Helal, Benedict, & Abdulle, 1999).

▲ **Clinical Warning:** Although several international consensus conferences have been held with the goal of developing a framework for duodenal and gastric disease recognition and management, practical guidelines for *H. pylori* eradication in children are still being determined and study results analyzed (Gold, 1999). It is strongly recommended that the primary care provider work in consultation with the pediatric gastroenterologist when developing, prescribing, and following up on a plan of treatment for peptic ulcer disease in children.

Chronic Diarrhea and Malabsorption

Chronic diarrhea is defined as loss of excessive amounts of fluid and electrolyte through liquid stooling, lasting for more than 2 weeks. Chronic diarrhea is relatively common in children and is usually not caused by serious illnesses. Dietary changes or functional motility problems should be considered before an extensive workup is undertaken (Hanauer, 1996).

PATHOLOGY

The most common causes of chronic loose bowel movements include the following:

- Excessive or new intake of formula or other fluids (water, fruit juice, high-carbohydrate beverages)
- Toddler's diarrhea (IBS)
- Encopresis (overflow diarrhea) (Branski, Lerner, & Lebenthal, 1996)

Excessive or new intake of formula or other fluids can cause frequent, green stools with a high mucus content. These stools may mimic chronic diarrhea but are really starvation stools that occur when a child is not fed food or formula, as may occur when the youngster has an acute gastrointestinal illness. Starvation stools occur when well-meaning caretakers feed only clear liquids in the presence of an acute illness.

▲ **Clinical Warning:** In acute diarrhea, clear liquids should only be used for 12 to 24 hours.

Toddler's diarrhea is defined as frequent, loose, pasty bowel movements seen in children 6 months to 3 years of age. Toddler's diarrhea is the most common manifestation of IBS at this age and probably is related to a functional dysmotility. In toddler's diarrhea, the child is happy, active, hungry, and growing normally, despite the increased number of bowel movements. All laboratory studies are normal.

● **Clinical Pearl:** It is important for the primary provider to remember that appropriate treatment for toddler's diarrhea includes no dietary restrictions. The stools tend to normalize with a high-fat diet. This response is related to the slowing of intestinal motility by intestinal hormones that are released in the face of a high-fat load.

In a few cases, chronic diarrhea may be caused by infection (such as giardiasis), a maldigestive/malabsorptive disease (such as gluten-sensitive enteropathy or cystic fibrosis), or as the result of severe intestinal mucosal damage from a variety of insults, especially in infants younger than 6 months (Talusan-Soriano & Lake, 1996; Trancone, Greco, & Auricchio, 1996).

HISTORY AND PHYSICAL EXAMINATION

The differential diagnosis of chronic diarrhea in children is listed in Display 57-3. It is important that the provider determine the number and consistency of stools. It is most critical to evaluate the growth curves. Chronic diarrhea that affects growth must be fully evaluated. The physical examination is unlikely to help the clinician discover a specific organic cause.

A protuberant abdomen that is associated with loss of subcutaneous fat in the buttocks and thighs suggests malabsorption, as do clinical findings associated with various mineral and vitamin deficiencies. However, these markers

- If the diarrhea is nocturnal, an organic cause should be considered.

DISPLAY 57–3 • Differential Diagnosis of Chronic Diarrhea

Children 0 to 6 Months

Carbohydrate malabsorption (acquired or congenital)
Protein allergy
Excess fluid intake (formula, water, fruit juice)
Infections
Postinfectious syndrome and intractable diarrhea
Cystic fibrosis
Immunodeficiency
Lymphangiectasia
Neuroblastoma
Congenital chloridorrhea
Intestinal villus inclusion disease

Children 7 to 23 Months

Toddler's diarrhea (chronic nonspecific diarrhea)
Celiac disease
Immunodeficiency
Munchausen syndrome by proxy
Autoimmune enteropathy
Protein allergy
Carbohydrate malabsorption
Excessive intake of fruit juice
Cystic fibrosis
Infections
Fat malabsorption
Neuroblastoma

Children Older Than 23 Months

Irritable bowel syndrome
Adult-type lactase deficiency
Encopresis
Inflammatory bowel disease
Excessive intake of fruit juices
Excessive intake of laxatives
Infections
Celiac disease
Munchausen syndrome by proxy

---

only tell the provider what the growth curve already has suggested. A workup is indicated.

● **Clinical Pearl:** Chronic diarrhea associated with normal weight and height velocity is unlikely to be from a serious organic etiology.

DIAGNOSTIC CRITERIA

● **Clinical Pearls:**

- If growth is normal, chronic diarrhea is infrequently organic and rarely serious.
- Before undertaking a major workup, the provider should consider encopresis, dietary change or excess, and IBS as part of the differential diagnosis.

▲ **Clinical Warnings:**

- If the stools contain blood, fat, white blood cells, or sugar, an organic workup is indicated.

DIAGNOSTIC STUDIES

Any child with chronic diarrhea and weight loss should have an evaluation. The stools themselves also may be helpful. Diarrhea with blood suggests an infectious or inflammatory etiology, as does a stool Wright stain that shows many white cells. In these cases, stool cultures and parasite investigation are warranted.

A stool Wright stain that shows eosinophils or has Charcot-Leyden crystals may indicate milk protein allergies. Acidic stools (low pH by dipstick), especially in the presence of reducing substances in the stool, suggest carbohydrate intolerance.

Fatty, malodorous stools indicate a possible maldigestive/malabsorptive disease. Such stools suggest that a 72-hour fecal fat study is necessary. If the 72-hour fecal fat study shows an excess amount of fat, cystic fibrosis and gluten-sensitive enteropathy (celiac disease) are the primary entities to be considered. Cystic fibrosis is diagnosed by a sweat test at an accredited cystic fibrosis treatment institution.

Celiac disease is screened for by the celiac panel, which is a group of blood tests looking for circulating antibodies (antigliadin, antireticulin, and endomysial antibodies). Celiac disease must be absolutely confirmed by a small intestinal biopsy, performed by a pediatric gastroenterologist (Rossi & Tjota, 1998). In all cases where the diagnosis is unclear and organic disease is suspected, referral to a pediatric gastroenterologist for a small intestinal biopsy with duodenal fluid assay is probably indicated.

MANAGEMENT

The primary care provider can appropriately manage most, if not all, of the care for children with chronic diarrhea. The child with cystic fibrosis should be comanaged together with an accredited cystic fibrosis treatment center. The patient with celiac disease or inflammatory bowel disease (IBD) should be comanaged along with a gastroenterologist, who may also be needed for technical support, such as endoscopies and biopsies.

Management of the various etiologies of chronic diarrhea and malabsorption is disease specific. Appropriate management and treatment frequently lead to a cessation of the diarrhea and a marked improvement in weight gain and accelerated linear growth. Because of the specificity of the diseases that generally underlie chronic diarrhea and malabsorption, the primary care provider must refer the child to a pediatric gastroenterologist for evaluation and treatment, with comanagement with the primary care practitioner. The reader is referred to Chapter 55 for information about the diagnosis and comanagement of cystic fibrosis.

▲ **Clinical Warning:** The practitioner should never place a child on a restricted diet unless there is a specific, proven indication.

What to Tell Parents

Most children with chronic diarrhea do not have an organic disease. If the cause of the diarrhea is nonorganic, a regular, appropriate diet is indicated, and normal growth and development will ensue.

Inflammatory Bowel Disease

Crohn's disease and UC are the two major chronic inflammatory diseases of the intestines. These are seen with increasing frequency in adolescence and, occasionally, in children younger than 10 years. CD and UC are distinct entities, but they share many signs and symptoms.

PATHOLOGY

Recent evidence indicates that IBD is part of an abnormal immunologic response to undetermined stimuli. Inflammation in the wall of the bowel and the release of inflammatory mediators account for the wide spectrum of symptoms seen in patients with IBD. Specifically, CD is a transmural inflammation, which can involve any part of the bowel from mouth to anus, and UC is a mucosal disease affecting only the large intestines (Hyams et al., 1996).

EPIDEMIOLOGY

The overall incidence of IBD is increasing in children worldwide. Current estimates are that there are four to six cases of IBD per 1000 children and young adults, with a prevalence rate of 40 to 100 per 100,000 and a peak age of onset between 10 and 30 years of age. Of patients in this age range, 20% are younger than 20, some as young as 1 year (Markowitz, 1996a; Hanauer, 1996).

Crohn's disease is increasing in incidence, while UC seems to be relatively stable. The incidence for both entities is highest in Caucasian children in northwestern Europe and North America and among Ashkenazi Jews. A family history of IBD is present in 10% to 39% of affected children (Markowitz, 1996). There have also been several reports of an association of IBD with ankylosing spondylitis and HLA-B27, but specific tissue typings have not yet been determined. It is likely that several genes are involved in the pathogenesis of IBD.

HISTORY AND PHYSICAL EXAMINATION

The primary provider should obtain a thorough history of appetite, abdominal pain, and bowel habits over time since the onset of symptoms. Any associated, unexplained weight loss must also be explored. The following data points are important:

- Abdominal pain and diarrhea (often with blood)
- Tenesmus and urgency (symptoms of proctitis)
- Delayed growth and sexual maturation
- Anorexia
- Fever
- Extraintestinal manifestations, including destructive perianal disease, arthritis or arthralgia, hepatobiliary disease, eye problems (uveitis or episcleritis), and rashes (eg, erythema nodosum) (Markowitz et al., 1993)

DIAGNOSTIC CRITERIA

The provider should consider IBD in any child with the following symptoms:

- Chronic diarrhea
- Perianal lesions
- Unexplained growth failure or sexual delay
- Joint symptoms
- Fever of unknown origin
- Unexplained hepatobiliary disease

Any child with any of these clinical signs who exhibits laboratory abnormalities, such as an elevated ESR, a decreased serum albumin level, and iron studies that show evidence of chronic inflammation (low serum iron with normal to low TIBC), should have an upper gastrointestinal barium series with small bowel follow-through. The child should also be referred to a pediatric gastroenterologist for an upper and lower gastrointestinal endoscopy. Biopsies should be performed.

MANAGEMENT

The primary care provider and a knowledgeable pediatric gastroenterologist should comanage cases of IBD. The need for occasional endoscopy, the explosion of new concepts and therapies, and the urgent need for surveillance for cancer make it necessary for specialist assistance when caring for the child with either UC or CD.

Complications of IBD can include intestinal obstruction, fistula, intestinal perforation, gastrointestinal hemorrhage, and colorectal carcinoma. Thus, referral to a pediatric gastroenterologist is imperative, providing for therapeutic comanagement that will assist the child in preserving bowel function in as normal a range as is possible.

When CD or UC is diagnosed, management is directed toward (1) reducing the inflammation and diminishing symptoms, (2) maintaining normal growth and development, and (3) maintaining normal functions of daily living (normal sleep, school, and play).

▲ **Clinical Warnings:**

- Growth (length or height and weight) must be monitored closely at each scheduled office visit (Markowitz et al., 1993). At the peripubertal period, monitoring for sexual maturation (ie, Tanner staging) must also be done. These monitoring activities need to continue until final growth is achieved. See Chapter 60 for more information about growth delay and its management.
- Episodes of fever, bilious vomiting, or acute onset of severe abdominal pain must be evaluated promptly. If the patient is taking steroids, the abdominal examination may be difficult to trust. Therefore, any change in symptoms must be considered worrisome and evaluated carefully.
- The risk for colonic carcinoma is related to duration of disease, not severity of symptoms. Therefore, asymptomatic patients also must have surveillance and close follow-up (Markowitz, 1996b).

Medications used to reduce inflammation include the following:

- 5-Aminosalicylates (sulfasalazine [Azulfidine], mesalamine [Asacol, Pentasa, Rowasa]) are effective in mild to moderate disease with few serious side effects.
- Corticosteroids are very effective for moderate to severe disease but at the expense of potential adverse effects, including cosmetic and psychological problems, increased appetite (and, consequently, weight gain), and bone demineralization. In addition, steroids interfere with linear growth. New corticosteroids, such as budesonide, may be able to provide anti-inflammatory activity to the gut without systemic toxicity, but pediatric studies are not available.
- Immunomodulators, including 6-mercaptopurine, are very effective in many patients and have replaced steroids as primary therapy. Immunomodulators may also be used in steroid-dependent and steroid-nonresponding patients (Mahdi, Israel, & Hassal, 1996). When used at doses of 1.5 to 2 mg/kg per day, minimal side effects have been apparent. Other immunomodulators, such as cyclosporine and methotrexate, have been used less extensively but show some promise. These drugs have serious side effects that must be weighed against disease outcomes were they not prescribed. Some of these effects include negative affects on the developing kidney and decreased attention span (and hence capacity for classroom learning) in children.
- Currently, new drugs directed at specific cytokines produced by the inflammatory response in IBD are under investigation. These may revolutionize management of the UC and CD.

● **Clinical Pearl:** Surgery may be used when medical therapy is ineffective or too toxic. In UC, surgery is curative. In CD, surgery is usually a temporary aid, with recurrence likely.

What to Tell Parents

A chronic illness, IBD has a relapsing and remitting course. Treatment in IBD must be meticulously comanaged with a pediatric gastroenterologist. Growth and sexual development must be followed closely. Nutrition is an important part of care. Adequate amounts of calories are most important—not dietary restrictions.

There is a real risk of colonic cancer in both UC and CD. Surveillance is mandatory. With proper management, treatment, and surveillance, patients with IBD can have normal, happy lives with success at school, work, and raising a family—in all aspects of life.

COMMUNITY RESOURCES

International Foundation for Functional Gastrointestinal Disorders (IFFGD)
P.O. Box 17864
Milwaukee, WI 53217
Telephone: (888) 964-2001
Internet address: *http://www.iffgd.org*

This organization is a resource for both provider and parents concerned about managing functional gastrointestinal problems.

Gluten Intolerance Group (GIG)
15110 10th Avenue SW, Suite A
Seattle, WA 98166
Telephone: (206) 246-6652

Fax: (206) 246-6531
E-mail: *gig@accessone.com*
Internet address: *http://www.gluten.net/welcome.htm*

This organization can provide a wealth of information to parents and patients about disorders of gluten intolerance, including celiac disease.

Crohn's & Colitis Foundation of America
386 Park Avenue South, 17th Floor
New York, NY 10016
Telephone: (212) 685-3440
Toll-free: (800) 932-2423
Fax: (212) 779-4098
E-mail: *info@ccfa.org*
Internet address: *http://www.ccfa.org*

This organization can provide patients and their families with information and support in dealing with UC and CD. Hyperlinks to associated resources are helpful. Resources for providers are also available.

Reach Out for Youth with Ileitis and Colitis
84 Northgate Circle
Melville, NY 11747
Telephone: (516) 293-3102
Fax: (516) 293-3103
E-mail: *reachoutforyouth@reachoutforyouth.org*
Internet address: *http://www.reachoutforyouth.org*

This resource provides information and support for children and adolescents living with IBD. Family support and information is a feature.

REFERENCES

Aaron, L. A., Burke, M. M., & Buchwald, D. (2000). Overlapping conditions among patients with chronic fatigue syndrome, fibromyalgia, and temporomandibular disorder. *Archives of Internal Medicine, 160,* 221–227.

Adeyemi, E. O., Danial, M. F., Helal, T., Benedict, S., & Abdulle, A. M. (1999). The outcome of a 2-week treatment of Helicobacter pylori-positive duodenal ulcer with omeprazole-based antibiotic regimen in a region with high metronidazole resistance rate. *European Journal of Gastroenterology and Hepatology, 11,* 1259–1263.

Ali, A., Toner, B. B., Stuckless, N., Gallop, R., Diamant, N. E., et al. (2000). Emotional abuse, self-blame, and self-silencing in women with irritable bowel syndrome. *Psychosomatic Medicine, 62,* 76–82.

Ameh, E. A. (1999). Peptic ulcer disease in childhood in Zaria, Nigeria. *Annals of Tropical Paediatrics, 19,* 65–68.

Baker, S. S., Liptak, G. S., Colletti, R. B., Croffie, J. M., Di Lorenzo, C., et al. (1999). Constipation in infants and children: Evaluation and treatment. A medical position statement of the North American Society for Pediatric Gastroenterology and Nutrition. *Journal of Pediatric Gastroenterology and Nutrition, 29,* 612–626. Erratum: *30,* 109.

Bardhan, P. K., Sarker, S. A., Mahalanabis, D., Rahman, M. M., Hildebrand, P., et al. (1999). *Helicobacter pylori* infection in infants and children of Bangladesh. *Schweizerische Rundschau fur Medizin Praxis, 87,* 1814–1816.

Blecker, U., & Gold, B. D. (1999). Gastritis and peptic ulcer disease in childhood. *European Journal of Pediatrics, 158,* 541–546.

Branski, D., Lerner, A., & Lebenthal, E. (1996). Chronic diarrhea and malabsorption. *Pediatric Clinics of North America, 43,* 307–331.

Camilleri, M., & Choi, M. G. (1997). Irritable bowel syndrome. *Aliment Pharmacol Ther 11,* 3–15.

Cuchiara, S. (1996). Cisapride therapy for gastrointestinal disease. *Journal of Pediatric Gastroenterology and Nutrition, 22,* 259–269.

Day, A. S., & Sherman, P. M. (1999). Understanding disease outcome following acquisition of *Helicobacter pylori* infection during childhood. *Canadian Journal of Gastroenterology, 13,* 229–234.

De Giacome, C., Bawa, P., Franceschi, M., et al. (1997). Omeprazole for severe reflux esophagitis in children. *Journal of Pediatric Gastroenterology and Nutrition, 24*, 528–532.

Dohil, R., Israel, D. M., & Hassall, E. (1997). Effective 2-week therapy for *Helicobacter pylori* disease in children. *American Journal of Gastroenterology, 92*, 244–247.

Everhart, J. E., & Renault, P. F. (1991). Irritable bowel syndrome in office-based practice in the United States. *Gastroenterology, 100*, 998–1015.

Fonkalsrud, E., & Ament, M. (1996). Gastroesophageal reflux in children. *Current Problems in Surgery, 1*, 3–70.

George, D. E., & Glassman, M. (1994). Peptic ulcer disease in children. *Gastrointestinal and Endoscopic Clinics of North America, 4*, 23–37.

Gold, B. D. (1999). Current therapy for *Helicobacter pylori* infection in children and adolescents. *Canadian Journal of Gastroenterology, 13*, 571–579.

Gold, D. M., Levine, J., Weinstein, T. A., Kessler, B. H., & Pettei, M. J. (1999). Frequency of digital rectal examination in children with chronic constipation. *Archives in Pediatric and Adolescent Medicine, 153*, 377–379.

Hanauer, S. B. (1996). Inflammatory bowel disease. *New England Journal of Medicine 334*, 841–848. Erratum in 1996: *335*, 143.

Hotopf, M., Carr, S., Mayou, R., Wadsworth, M., & Wessely, S. (1998). Why do children have chronic abdominal pain, and what happens to them when they grow up? Population based cohort study. *British Medical Journal, 316(7139)*, 1196–2000.

Hyams, J. S. (1999). Functional gastrointestinal disorders. *Current Opinions in Pediatrics, 11*, 375–378.

Hyams, J. S., Burke, G., Davis, P. M., et al. (1996). Abdominal pain and irritable bowel syndrome in adolescents: A community based study. *Journal of Pediatrics, 129*, 220–226.

James, L. P., Stowe, C. D., Farrar, H. C., Menendez, A. A., & Argao, E. A. (1999). The pharmacokinetics of oral ranitidine in children and adolescents with cystic fibrosis. *Journal of Clinical Pharmacology, 39*, 1242–1247.

Janicke, D.M., & Finnev, J.W. (1999). Empirically supported treatments in pediatric psychology: Recurrent abdominal pain. *Journal of Pediatric Psychology, 24(2)*: 115-127.

Jevon, G., Dimmick, J. E., & Hassall, E. (1997). Pediatric gastritis. *Perspectives in Pediatric Pathology, 20*, 35–76.

Jones, N. L., Day, A. S., & Sherman, P. M. (1999). Determinants of disease outcome following *Helicobacter pylori* infection in children. *Canadian Journal of Gastroenterology, 13*, 613–617.

Kneepkens, C. M., & Hoekstra, J. H. (1996). Chronic nonspecific diarrhea of childhood: Pathophysiology and management. *Pediatric Clinics of North America, 43*, 375–390.

Lake, A. M. (1999). Chronic abdominal pain in childhood: Diagnosis and management. *American Family Physician, 59*, 1823–1830.

Locke, G. R., Zinsmeister, A. R., Talley, N. J., Fett, S. L., & Melton, L. J. (2000). Risk factors for irritable bowel syndrome: Role of analgesics and food sensitivities. *American Journal of Gastroenterology, 95*, 157–165.

Mahdi, G., Israel, D. M., & Hassal, E. (1996). Cyclosporine and 6-mercaptopurine for active, refractory Crohn's colitis in children. *American Journal of Gastroenterology, 91*, 1355–1359.

Markowitz, J. (1996a). A primer on pediatric inflammatory bowel disease. *Contemporary Pediatrics, 13*, 25–46.

Markowitz, J. (1996b). A primer on pediatric inflammatory disease. *Contemporary Pediatrics, 13*, 25–46.

Markowitz, J., Grancher, K., Rosa, J., et al. (1993). Growth failure in pediatric inflammatory bowel disease. *Journal of Pediatric Gastroenterology and Nutrition, 16*, 373–380.

Morais, M. B., Vitolo, M. R., Aguirre, A. N., & Fagundes-Neto, U. (1999). Measurement of low dietary fiber intake as a risk factor for chronic constipation in children. *Journal of Pediatric Gastroenterology and Nutrition, 29*, 132–135.

Moshkowitz, M., Reif, S., Brill, S., Ringel, Y., Arber, N., et al. (1998). One-week triple therapy with omeprazole, clarithromycin, and nitroimidazole for *Helicobacter pylori* infection in children and adolescents. *Pediatrics, 102(1)*, e14.

Nelson, S. P., Chen, E. H., Syntar, G. M., et al. (1999). Prevalence of symptoms of gastroesophageal reflux during infancy. *Archives of Pediatrics and Adolescent Medicine, 151*, 569–572.

Nowicki, M. J., & Bishop, P. R. (1999). Organic causes of constipation in infants and children. *Pediatric Annals, 28*, 293–300.

Rasquin-Weber, A., Hyman, P. E., Cucchiara, S., Fleisher, D. R., Hyams, J. S., et al. (1999). Childhood functional gastrointestinal disorders. *Gut, 45(Suppl 2)*, II60–II68.

Robinson, D. M., Abdel-Rahman, S. M., & Nahata, M. C. (1997). Guidelines for the treatment of *Helicobacter pylori* in the pediatric population. *Annals of Pharmacotherapy, 31*, 1247–1249.

Rossi, T. M., & Tjota, A. (1998). Serological diagnosis of celiac disease. *J Pediatr Gastroenterol Nutr, 26*, 205–210.

Talusan-Soriano, K., & Lake, A. M. (1996). Malabsorption in childhood. *Pediatric Review, 17*, 135–142.

Thomson, M., & Walker-Smith, J. (1998). Dyspepsia in infants and children. *Baillieres Clinical Gastroenterology, 12*, 601–624.

Tindberg, Y., Blennow, M., & Granstrom, M. (1999). Clinical symptoms and social factors in a cohort of children spontaneously clearing Helicobacter pylori infection. *Acta Pediatrics, 88*, 631–635.

Trancone, R., Greco, L., & Auricchio, S. (1996). Gluten-sensitive enteropathy. *Pediatric Clinics of North America, 43*, 355–373.

Trikas, P., Vlachonikolis, I., Fragkiadakis, N., Vasilakis, S., Manousos, O., & Paritsis, N. (1999). Core mental state in irritable bowel syndrome. *Psychosomatic Medicine, 6*, 781–788.

Vanderplas, Y., Beili, D., Benhamow, P. H., et al. (1996). Current concepts and issues in the management of regurgitation in infants: A reappraisal. *Acta Pediatrics, 85*, 531–534.

Welgan, P., Meshkinpour, H., & Ma, L. (2000). Role of anger in antral motor activity in irritable bowel syndrome. *Digestive Diseases and Sciences, 45*, 248–251.

Yunus, M. B., Inanici, F., Aldag, J. C., & Mangold, R. F. (2000). Fibromyalgia in men: Comparison of clinical features with women. *Journal of Rheumatology 27*, 485–490.

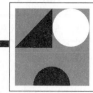

Chronic Dermatology Problems

• GOLDIE GIANOULIS-ALISSANDRATOS, MS, FNP, and ROSE CASSIDY, RN, MS, FNP

INTRODUCTION

The role of the primary care provider in the diagnosis and treatment of dermatologic conditions is increasingly important. This chapter provides a framework for assessing and treating the most common chronic dermatologic disorders seen in the pediatric and adolescent setting, including acne, chronic warts, and molluscum contagiosum. Because it is rarely seen in this setting, psoriasis is not discussed. The interested reader is referred to Common Dermatologic Conditions in *Primary Care* (1999) (the companion volume to this text) or to any standard dermatology reference.

Not every patient with a skin complaint presents in a classic textbook manner. A child may present with skin lesions as the primary complaint, or a lesion may appear as an incidental finding during the physical examination. The prevalence of skin conditions is not easy to estimate. Environmental and social factors influence both the occurrence and detection of the skin condition.

The skin is the largest of all body organs and plays a major role in maintaining the body's homeostasis. The skin serves as a barrier to prevent the loss of important body fluids and the entrance of possible toxic or infectious agents. Skin changes of any variety may be indicative of a primary dermatologic problem, or they may signal the primary care provider to look for an underlying systemic disease. Parents are often only concerned about skin changes themselves and what can be done about them. Unless the issue of the problem underlying the lesion is addressed adequately, parents may not be receptive to the care needed, follow guidelines adequately, or return for follow-up.

● **Clinical Pearl:** Reassurance and a relationship-centered approach between the primary care provider and the patient or family will help improve patient care and reduce patient suffering, disability, and disfigurement from dermatologic problems.

▲ **Clinical Warning:** For any dermatologic complaint, the provider should refer to a dermatology specialist any condition that does not improve within a 2- to 4-month period. If abnormal side effects are reported with any type of treatment, it should be discontinued immediately and the patient referred to a dermatology specialist as deemed necessary.

One of the key aspects in the approach to dermatologic care is the use of standard nomenclature when describing skin lesions. Table 58-1 summarizes the common classification of skin lesions. Standardization of the basic dermatologic terminology allows all practitioners to improve communication and accurate diagnosing of clients. To help prevent confusion in the standard of measurement of lesions, a metric ruler is an essential tool for the provider.

Acne Vulgaris

PATHOLOGY

Acne vulgaris is a condition that affects the pilosebaceous unit that consists of sebaceous glands and hair follicles (Color Plate 1A-E). These units are found on all skin surfaces except for the palms of the hands and the soles of the feet. The development of acne involves four principal factors:

1. Androgen-stimulated sebum production. The main influence of increased sebum production is hormonal. Androgens are essential for the development of acne. No correlation has been found between androgen levels and acne severity (Aizawa, Nakada, & Niimura, 1995).
2. *Propionibacterium acnes*, an anaerobic diphtheroid, colonizes the sebaceous follicles and is transported to the skin surface with the production of sebum. Inflammatory lesions of acne develop when *P. acnes* proliferates and subsequently produces an inflammatory reaction. The severity of the response is variable, and the lesions may present as small superficial papules or pustules with or without cystic nodules.
3. Altered keratinization of the follicular epithelium. Abnormal shedding of the cells that line the sebaceous follicles is a key factor to the pathogenesis of acne. This process is also known as follicular plugging (Arndt, 1995; Fitzpatrick, Johnson, & Wolff, 1997; Schachner, 1998). The result of this process is comedo formation. A whitehead is considered a closed comedo and is formed within a dilated opening. A blackhead is considered an open comedo (Leyden, 1995; Fitzpatrick, Johnson, & Wolf, 1997; Schachner, 1998) and results from the protrusion of the comedonal mass outside of the sebaceous follicle. The black color is due to the oxidation of melanin and sebum in the plugs.
4. Host inflammatory response. Acne breaks sebum into glycerol and free fatty acids; the free fatty acids injure and cause hyperkeratinization and impaired desquamation of the follicular epithelium, leading to plugging and inflammation. *P. acnes* also directly causes inflammation by release of proteolytic enzymes, hyaluronidase, and neutrophil chemotactic factors. If enough inflammation occurs, the contents of the follicle spill out into the dermis, causing an exaggerated host response and an acne cyst (Whitmore, 1995; Fitzpatrick et al., 1997; Schachner, 1998).

EPIDEMIOLOGY

Acne vulgaris is a disorder of the sebaceous gland, sebaceous duct, and hair follicle in areas of high sebaceous den-

Table 58–1.   CLASSIFICATION OF SKIN LESIONS

Type	Appearance	Comments	
Primary Lesions Macule	Flat, well-circumscribed area of any color change within the skin	Measures up to 1 cm in diameter. Area of pigment change is nonpalpable.	 Macule
Patch	Flat, well-circumscribed area of any color change within the skin	Measures greater than 1 cm in diameter. Area of pigment change is nonpalpable.	 Patch
Papule	Solid, raised, circumscribed	Measures less than 1 cm in diameter. Surface may be smooth or rough on palpation.	 Papule
Plaque	Solid, raised, circumscribed	Measures 1 or more cm in diameter. May develop as an individual lesion or a coalescence of papules. Color may range from normal skin color to any color of pigment change.	 Plaque
Nodule	Solid, palpable, possibly freely movable	Measures 1–2 cm in diameter. Extends deeper into the layers of the skin than do papules.	 Nodule
Tumor	Solid, palpable, possibly freely movable	Measures greater than 2 cm in diameter.	 Tumor
Wheals	Elevated, flat-topped, edematous, white or usually pale red	Also known as hives or urticaria. Vary in size. Fluid within the lesion is transitory. Lesions can develop within a few seconds and disappear slowly.	 Wheal

(continues)

Table 58–1. CLASSIFICATION OF SKIN LESIONS *(Continued)*

Type	Appearance	Comments	
Vesicle	Circumscribed, elevated; contain fluid. Color may be clear, turbid, or hemorrhagic.	Also known as a blister. Measures up to 1 cm in diameter. Most often tense.	Vesicle
Bullae	Circumscribed, elevated; contain fluid. Color may be clear, turbid, or hemorrhagic.	Measures greater than 1 cm in diameter. May be flaccid or tense.	Bulla
Secondary Lesions Pustules	Circumscribed elevations of the skin that contain pus	Also known as pimples. Pus is present as a result of the inflammatory nature of the lesion.	Pustule
Scales	Increase in the formation of keratin cells	May vary in size from fine to coarse. Are produced when normal process of keratinization is interrupted. Papulosquamous is used to describe an eruption of scaling papules.	Scales
Crust	Color may vary depending on the exudate; may be yellow, green to greenish-yellow, dark red, or brown.	Develops as a result of the opening and draining of a primary lesion	Crust
Excoriation	Superficial lesions of the epidermis; may be linear or punctate	Commonly known as scratch marks	Excoriation
Fissure	Linear crack that involves the epidermis and sometimes the dermis	Can vary in number and size. Frequently seen in conditions that cause dry skin. Flexural areas are commonly affected.	Fissure

(continues)

Table 58–1.   CLASSIFICATION OF SKIN LESIONS   *(Continued)*

Type	Appearance	Comments	
Erosion	Exudate that may develop into a crust	Results from loss of viable epidermis. Usually heals with no scar.	Erosion
Ulcer	Usually a rounded or irregularly shaped excavation	Results from loss of entire epidermis and some of the dermis. Can vary in diameter and depth. Scar likely to develop when ulcer heals.	Ulcer
Scar	Caused by a deposition of fibrous tissue during the healing process; may become hypertrophic, kelioidal, and even pruritic	Size and shape determined by the preceding damage. Usually tend to become less obvious over time.	Scar
Atrophy	Appears as thin and somewhat transparent epidermis. Dermal atrophy manifests as a depression in the skin.	Loss of epidermis, dermis, or subcutaneous fat	Atrophy

Art from Smeltzer, S., & Bare, B. (1996). *Brunner and Suddarth's textbook of medical-surgical nursing* (8th ed.). Philadelphia: Lippincott-Raven.

sity (the face, back, chest, and upper arms). The face is the site of greatest prevalence. Comedonal, papular, and pustular acne are the most common variants of acne vulgaris. It is an extremely common disorder with a strong genetic predisposition whose peak prevalence occurs during adolescence. Acne affects 90% of males and 80% of females in variable degrees. In males, acne usually starts in early adolescence, is more severe, and resolves in the early to mid 20s. In females, acne usually starts later, is less severe, and lasts longer (late 20s and early 30s). It accounts for the majority of medical visits in this age group to their primary care provider for referrals to the dermatologist (Greydanus, 1997).

Acne has been identified as a contributing factor to psychosocial problems, such as clinical depression, anxiety, and a negative body image (Bergfeld, 1995; Galen, 1997). Successful treatment usually corrects or improves these problems. The treatment plan should be individualized and based on the psychosocial impact the acne poses for the individual.

DIAGNOSTIC CRITERIA

Criteria for diagnosing and treating acne can be guided by staging the acne, as follows:

- Stage 1—comedonal acne: whiteheads and blackheads
- Stage 2—mild to moderate papulopustular acne with comedones
- Stage 3—severe inflammatory acne: large number of papules and pustules. A referral to a dermatologic specialist is recommended when stage 3 acne has not improved within 8 weeks, to minimize scarring.
- Stage 4—severe nodulocystic acne: includes features of all of the previous stages plus nodules and cysts (Galen, 1997; Schachner, 1998). Unless the primary care provider is comfortable and confident with treating stage 4 acne, a referral to a specialist is strongly encouraged.

MANAGEMENT

The diagnosis of acne is fairly straightforward, but treatment involves more than simply writing a prescription. The treatment plan should be a mutual decision made between the primary care provider and the patient or family. Therefore, it is essential that patient motivation be assessed. The management plan should be outlined in detail, with realistic expectations included. An explanation of why acne develops, including a handout on the treatment of acne, should be included with the initial assessment of the patient (Schachner, 1998). Display 58-1 lists suggestions for skin care for patients with acne. Myths about the causes and cures of acne should also be dispelled.

Acne is considered a chronic disease that requires months, if not years, of treatment, with the exception of isotretinoin. Many treatment options are available, and treatment should be tailored to the patient based on the psychosocial impact the acne creates for the individual and treatment costs (Galen, 1997). See Table 58-2 for stage therapy. Scarring, which can be minimized with proper treatment, is the only sequela of acne.

Vehicles of choice for prescribing topical medication should be based on skin type. Gels and solutions are more commonly used on oily skin; creams and lotions are more commonly used on dry skin; and pads or pledgets are more commonly used with combination skin types (oily/dry).

Tretinion (Retin-A) is more effectively used for the treatment of comedonal acne. It is often not covered by insurance plans. However, azaleic acid, which has a mechanism of action similar to tretinoin, is often covered by insurance plans.

Inflammatory acne should be treated with a topical or oral antibiotic in addition to benzoyl peroxide. The advantage of combination topical therapy is that benzoyl peroxide is bacteriocidal, and antibiotics are bacteriostatic. Thus, the chance of developing resistance to the topical therapy is reduced. It is important to inform patients that benzoyl peroxide may cause bleaching of their clothing and of sheets and pillowcases if used at night.

Serious consideration for a referral to a dermatologist is recommended for the treatment of stage 4 acne because of the increased risk of scarring in addition to the difficulty in managing treatment-resistant acne.

■ Acne Keloidalis

Acne keloidalis is a destructive pustulofollicular process that primarily affects the occipital scalp and neck of young African American men (Color Plate 2A-D). Lesions begin as discrete follicular papules or pustules and usually progress to large, nondiscrete keloidal nodules or plaques devoid of hair (Fitzpatrick et al., 1997). The process may be mild or severe enough to cause social isolation during a time in adolescence when socialization is already in turmoil.

PATHOLOGY

The cause of acne keloidalis is unknown. It is thought to be a variant of acne vulgaris (Templeton & Solomon, 1996). Bacteria can be cultured from fluctuant lesions, but it is not clear whether these organisms represent the pathogenesis of acne keloidalis or a superinfection. Close shaving of the occipital scalp and neck hair may cause or even exacerbate acne keloidalis as a result of the hair's growing in curved and breaking through the dermis.

MANAGEMENT

Treatment is paramount in maintaining an individual's self-esteem. Early referral to a dermatologist is key because the treatment can be multifaceted. Display 58-2 summarizes the most common treatments for acne keloidalis. Combination oral and topical antibiotic therapy is the most effective treatment. This dual therapy is also beneficial in preventing the formation of new lesions and is fairly effective in resolving minimally scarred lesions. Oral antibiotics work against the inflammatory pustular lesions. Topical antibiotics (in a drying vehicle of application) are used as adjunctive therapy. Monthly intralesional corticosteroid injections are helpful with the reduction of size and inflammation of the lesions. Large, unresponsive acne keloidalis nodules and plaques usually require surgical excision with close clinical follow-up and prophylactic intralesional corticosteroid injections in the surgical site. The acne skin care information in Display 58-1 should be given to these patients as well.

Chronic Warts

Warts, or verruca, are benign epithelial tumors of the skin and mucosa caused by human papillomaviruses (HPV). The thickening of the epidermis with scaling and an upward extension of the dermal papillae containing prominent capillaries give them their verrucous appearance (Whitmore, 1995).

EPIDEMIOLOGY

Warts occur in healthy children and young adults. Prevalence is estimated at about 5% in adults and 10% in children (Fitzpatrick et al., 1997). Immunosuppressed patients have a significant increase in the development of warts. The highest incidence is estimated in children ages 6 to 12 years.

Although HPV are transmissible viruses, nongenital warts are not considered communicable diseases. In general, person-to-person transmission of warts is possible but not typical.

▲ **Clinical Warning:** Anogenital warts (condyloma acuminata) in children younger than 12 years should raise

---

DISPLAY 58–1 • Patient and Family Education for Acne Skin Care

Advise Patients to Do the Following:

- Wash affected areas daily with a mild, oil-free soap. An antibacterial soap can be used if it does not cause drying or irritation.
- Avoid scrubbing face in an attempt to wash away acne. Avoid picking/popping acne lesions to prevent scarring.
- Avoid excessive sun exposure. Apply an oil-free, noncomedogenic moisturizer with sunscreen (minimum SPF 15) daily.
- Avoid oil-based cosmetics, hair creams, and face creams.
- Any treatment may take up to 2 or 3 months before results are noted. Do not stop treatment without talking to someone first. Preferably, return to site of care where therapy was planned (Galen, 1997).
- Eat a well-balanced diet and maintain adequate hydration. It is a myth that certain foods cause acne.

Table 58–2. STAGE THERAPY FOR TREATMENT OF ACNE VULGARIS

Stage	Initial Therapy	Reevaluate (wk)	Therapy Change if no Response	Therapy Change if Response
I	Retin-A micro 0.1% cream; Retin-A 0.01% gel or 0.05% cream (vehicle of choice based on skin type). Pea-sized drop at bedtime.	8	Increase Retin-A to b.i.d. application or increase the strength of Retin-A. Encourage the use of an oil-free moisturizer *with* sunscreen daily to help decrease any photosensitivity reaction that may occur.	None
II	Retin-A QHS (as in stage I) in addition to benzoyl peroxide 2.5%, erythromycin 2%, or clindamycin 1% every morning (vehicle of choice based on skin type). Azaleic acid is tolerated well by African Americans. Extract comedones PRN using a comedo extractor.	8	Add oral antibiotics, such as tetracycline (500 mg b.i.d.), erythromycin (333 mg t.i.d.), doxycycline (100 mg b.i.d.), trimethoprim/sulfamethoxazole DS (b.i.d.), minocycline (100 mg b.i.d.), or monodox (100 mg b.i.d.).	Taper oral antibiotics by 1 tablet every 4–6 wk for positive results. If a flare occurs, increase oral antibiotic by 1 tablet, reevaluate in 2–4 wk, and if still flaring then restart antibiotic at original dose or change to another antibiotic that was not previously used. Topical therapy should remain unchanged.
III	Start with two different topical medications—one to be applied in the morning and the other to be applied at night. In addition, initiate oral antibiotic therapy as in stage II.	8	May begin isotretinoin (Accutane) (0.5–2 mg/kg per day); however, this is usually reserved for the dermatologist. Note: pregnancy must be excluded prior to starting isotretinoin and at least two contraceptive barriers must be used during the course of therapy. Frequent monitoring of labs and pregnancy testing.	For painful, nodular, cystic lesions, intralesional cortisone injections may be considered. Otherwise, refer to a dermatologist. The recommended dosage is 3–5 mg/cc of triamcinolone for a total of 0.02 cc into each lesion. The same lesion should not be injected more often than every 4 wk. The most common side effect is subcutaneous tissue atrophy and scarring at the site of injection.

b.i.d. = twice daily; PRN = as needed; t.i.d. = three times daily.

suspicion but not indicate child abuse. It is possible that condylomata in children are the result of transmission at birth (Fitzpatrick et al., 1997).

PHYSICAL EXAMINATION AND DIAGNOSTIC CRITERIA

Currently there are more than 60 known types of HPV. Some types are correlated with known clinical manifestations. Common warts, verruca vulgaris, are flesh-colored, hyperkeratotic, or corrugated and dome-shaped. The wart interrupts the normal skin lines, and it can be studded with black puncta. It can sometimes present on a stalk (filiform) or as a cutaneous horn. The cause is usually HPV-2. Common warts can be found on any skin surface, but they are seen most often on the hands (Color Plate 3A). Size varies from 1 mm to clusters of larger than 10 mm.

Plantar warts, verruca plantaris, are hyperkeratotic lesions with a thick surface (Color Plate 3B). They are found on the sole of the foot (especially on the heel), metatarsal head region, and plantar toe. The main differential diagnosis favors corns/calluses. To differentiate a plantar wart, scraping with a scalpel edge will exhibit

---

DISPLAY 58–2 • Treatment of Acne Keloidalis

Topical Antibiotics

Benzamycin gel b.i.d.
Clindamycin solution or pledgets b.i.d.
Erythromycin solution or Erycette pads b.i.d.

Oral Antibiotics

Tetracycline, 500 mg b.i.d.
Doxycycline, 200 mg b.i.d.
Minocycline, 50–200 mg b.i.d.
Cephalexin, 500–1000 mg b.i.d.

---

b.i.d. = twice daily.

punctuate black dots after the keratin is shaved away. These dots represent thrombosed capillaries in elongated dermal papillae. Mosaic verruca results from coalescence of smaller lesions.

Flat warts, verruca plana, are flesh-colored or pale pink lesions 0.5 to 2 mm in size. They have a flat dome, but if examined with a magnifying lens, fine verrucal lines can be seen. They usually occur in clusters, especially on the hands, face, or lower legs.

The venereal wart, condyloma acuminatum, is composed of a soft, moist papule or plaque that may be sessile or pedunculated (Color Plate 3C). It has a verrucous surface with a cauliflower appearance and involves the genitalia, anorectal area, and occasionally the urethra, bladder, and ureter. A commonly used diagnostic test is soaking of the genital area or swabbing the vaginal walls and cervix with 3% to 5% acetic acid (white vinegar). This procedure causes warts to turn white. Although this is not a definitive diagnosis, the procedure helps clarify sites to treat or biopsy. Use of a magnifying lens or colposcopy will enable better visualization. Smaller warts may be hyperpigmented and resemble seborrheic keratosis or melanocytic nevi (moles).

▲ **Clinical Warning:** The high prevalence of HPV types 16, 18, and 31 in cancerous or precancerous lesions of the genitalia suggests a strong association with HPV-induced genital warts and malignancy (Olbricht et al., 1991; Fitzpatrick et al., 1997). Refer to Chapter 41 for more information related to the diagnosis and treatment of venereal warts.

MANAGEMENT

Warts are, in general, benign growths. Overly aggressive treatment can cause increased scarring and permanent pain. Treatment of a few warts may induce a generalized regression of other warts by tripping the body's immune system. It is estimated that up to 65% of all warts will resolve spontaneously within 2 years. The cure rate with treatment is only slightly higher, about 80%.

Verruca vulgaris on the fingers, feet, or limbs can be treated with salicylic acid plasters (keratolytics) at home. The provider needs to instruct the patient to soak the area for 5 minutes in warm water and to dry it thoroughly before applying the plaster. Treatment may continue for up to 12 weeks. If this fails, the clinician can try office cryotherapy, canteridin therapy, trichloroacetic acid, or referral to a dermatology specialist.

▲ **Clinical Warning:** Trichloroacetic acid should not be used on the face.

Verruca plana can be pared periodically or treated with keratolytic agents, such as topical tretinoin, light cryotherapy, or electrodessication. They may be left untreated if not painful. Verruca plantaris can be treated with soaking followed by application of 40% salicylic acid plasters at home, followed by office visits monthly for debulking of lesions. Surgery is very seldom considered because there is a high probability of scar formation.

Condyloma acuminatum are initially treated with a topical application of trichloroacetic acid 60%. They may also be treated with electrosurgery. For recalcitrant lesions, the carbon dioxide laser can be used to melt away the wart and surrounding infected mucosa.

Molluscum Contagiosum

PATHOLOGY

Molluscum contagiosum virus is an unclassified, common pox-virus that infects the skin and mucous membranes. The molluscum contagiosum virus has a propensity to infect follicular epithelium, with the most prominent feature of the lesions being umbilication (Groves, 1996). The disease is generally spread to other people through direct contact. Children with atopic dermatitis tend to be more susceptible to the infection. The incubation period of the virus has been estimated to range from 2 weeks to 2 months.

EPIDEMIOLOGY

Molluscum contagiosum occurs throughout the world and affects people of all ages. Formerly, the majority of the cases were seen in children, but the incidence among sexually active young adults has increased. The severity of the disease is increased in people who are immunocompromised.

▲ **Clinical Warning:** Genital lesions caused by the molluscum contagiosum virus are more than likely to have been sexually transmitted when seen in adults; children with these genital lesions should be carefully evaluated for child abuse.

PHYSICAL EXAMINATION

Lesions caused by the molluscum contagiosum virus can occur anywhere on the body (Color Plate 4A-B). Lesions can range in number from one to hundreds. Lesions have rarely been reported on the palms and soles (Gottlieb & Myskowski, 1994). The eruption begins with flesh-colored or pearly papules; as they progress, they become centrally depressed or umbilicated (Groves, 1996). A white, curdlike core is usually present in the lesion. "Pearly umbilicated papules" is the hallmark description of this disease. Occasionally pruritus or inflammation may be associated with the lesions, but the eruption in general is asymptomatic.

DIAGNOSTIC CRITERIA

The clinical appearance of the eruption is usually characteristic of the disease. However, in cases of doubt, the provider should collect a sample for histologic analysis to confirm clinical suspicion (see directions for pricking of the lesion in the following section). The expressed content is then placed in a jar of formalin and sent to the laboratory for histologic analysis.

● **Clinical Pearl:** Warts are the lesions that are most often confused with molluscum.

MANAGEMENT

The lesions of molluscum usually resolve spontaneously in immunocompetent hosts without any sequelae. If treatment is considered necessary, any of the following methods can be used alone or in combination:

- Cryotherapy with liquid nitrogen can be applied directly to the individual lesions using a cotton wool bud, for a total of 10 to 15 seconds or two 5-second freeze-thaw cycles.
- A vesicant, such as cantharidin (Cantharone), can be applied alone or under occlusion with tape, for 2 to 6 hours. This method may cause a severe inflammatory reaction; therefore, it is important to ensure the medication is dry to the touch before allowing the patient to move around or before occluding it with tape so that it does not spread to normal skin. Instruct the patient or parents to leave the medication on for no longer than 6 hours. If the patient is unable to tolerate the medication because of burning or irritation, then the medication should be washed off immediately. Lesions will usually crust and fall off. Cantharidin should not be used around the eyes.
- The surface of the lesion can be pricked with a #11 blade or a large needle (18 gauge), and then the core can be manually expressed. This will almost guarantee resolution of that lesion. Manual expression can be performed using a comedo extractor or gentle but firm pressure with opposing fingers. A sharp curet may also be used to remove lesions. Anesthesia is generally not warranted.
- Topical applications of tretinoin twice daily can be used in recurrent cases. The strongest dose that does not cause irritation to the patient should be used.

Because one treatment is usually inadequate, the patient should be seen biweekly until no more lesions are present. A final examination may be done 4 to 6 weeks after the last biweekly visit.

● **Clinical Pearl:** The provider should advise the sexually active adolescent patient that lesions are sexually transmissible. It is important for any sexual partner to be examined and treated, if necessary.

COMMUNITY RESOURCES

Provider Resources

American Academy of Dermatology
930 N. Meacham Road
Schaumbury, IL 60173-6016
Telephone: (847) 330-0230
Toll-free: (888) 462-DERM (3376)
Internet address: *http://www.aad.org*

The Academy is also a resource for patient education pamphlets.

American Society for Dermatologic Surgery
930 N. Meacham Rd
Schaumburg, IL 60173-6016
Telephone: (847) 330-9830
Toll-free: (800) 441-2737 (ASDS)
Internet address: *http://www.asds-net.org/index.html*

Patient education on popular treatments and links to other dermatologic sites are also available on the website.

Patient Resources

Acnenet
Internet address: *http://www.derm-infonet.com/acnenet*

General information is provided, including information on treatment and on the social impact of acne, interactive questions and answers, and links to other sites.

Dermnet
Internet address: *http://www.dermnet.org.nz/index.html*

This is a library of information on skin conditions.

REFERENCES

Aizawa, H., Nakada, Y., & Niimura, M. (1995). Androgen status in adolescent women with acne vulgaris. *Journal of Dermatology, 22*, 530–532.

Arndt, K. A. (Ed.). (1995). *Manual of dermatologic therapeutics* (5th ed.). Boston: Little, Brown.

Bergfeld, W. F. (1995). The evaluation and management of acne: Economic considerations. *Journal of the American Academy of Dermatology 32*(Suppl. 3), 52–56.

Fitzpatrick, T., Johnson, R., & Wolff, K. (1997). *Color atlas and synopsis of clinical dermatology* (3rd ed.) (pp. 2–7). New York: McGraw Hill.

Galen, B. A. (1997). Acne vulgaris. *Lippincott's Primary Care Practice, 1*, 88–92.

Gottlieb, S. L., & Myskowski, P. L. (1994). Molluscum contagiosum. *International Journal of Dermatology, 33*, 453–461.

Greydanus, D. (1997). Disorders of the skin. In A. Hoffman & D. Greydanus (Eds.), *Adolescent medicine* (3rd ed.) (pp. 375–380). Stamford, CT: Appleton & Lange.

Groves, R. W. (1996). Poxvirus. In K. A. Arndt, P. E. LeBoit, J. K. Robinson, & B. U. Wintroub (Eds.), *Cutaneous medicine and surgery* (Vol. 2) (pp. 1093–1099). Philadelphia: W.B. Saunders.

Leyden, J. J. (1995). New understandings of the pathogenesis of acne. *Journal of the American Academy of Dermatology, 32*(5 pt 3), S15–25.

Schachner, L. (1998). A fresh look at managing acne. *Contemporary Pediatrics (June Suppl)*, 4–8.

Templeton, S. F., & Solomon, A. R. (1996). Scarring alopecia. In K. A. Arndt, P. E. LeBoit, J. K. Robinson, & B. U. Wintroub (Eds.), *Cutaneous medicine and surgery* (Vol. 2) (pp. 1280–1294). Philadelphia: W.B. Saunders.

Whitmore, E. (1995). Common problems of skin. In L. Barker, J. Burton, & P. Zieve (Eds.), *Principles of ambulatory medicine* (4th ed.) (pp. 1452–1455). Baltimore: Williams & Wilkins.

Chronic Orthopedic Problems

• KEITH P. MANKIN, MD

INTRODUCTION

Orthopedic disorders may be developmental and may lead to longstanding problems involving growth and normal physical activity. As with acute entities, the earlier these problems are recognized, the better they can be treated. Detection may be as early as birth in some cases, but other, more subtle problems may only become clear at major milestones like the onset of ambulation or during periods of rapid growth.

Although many of these entities may require a specialist's evaluation, this chapter describes the role of the primary care provider in diagnosing and helping to instruct and support the family during the long and frustrating clinical course of managing chronic orthopedic problems.

Hip Disorders

Developmental dysplasia of the hip (DDH) is defined as disruption of the normal hip joint alignment and stability. In its most extreme state, the hip or hips may be completely dislocated, with almost no socket formation. Most frequently, there is only mild shallowness of the socket, and the hip may push out of the socket only in a stressed position. Unfortunately, the normal development of the hip depends on normal forces being applied throughout growth. Thus, even a mildly shallow hip may develop into severe hip disease early in adulthood.

EPIDEMIOLOGY

Developmental dysplasia of the hip is more frequent in girls, especially first-born (Weinstein, 1996). It is also associated with conditions that limit the room for the fetus, especially breech position and multiple births. There is a close association between DDH and other molding disorders, such as wryneck and foot deformities. However, there is a clear familial tendency to dysplastic hips, although the exact genetic basis is unknown.

HISTORY AND PHYSICAL EXAMINATION

Early in development, even dysplastic hips tend to be free of symptoms. Because muscle development may be normal, children will not have delayed ambulation except in very extreme cases or in cases associated with neurologic disor-

ders. Later, the child may complain of increased tiredness or stiffness. By the late teens to early adulthood, the hips may be painful, particularly with running and other strenuous activity. This probably indicates the early development of arthritis. Table 59-1 presents data regarding the examination of range of motion, gait, and specific tests for normal hips and early versus late DDH.

At birth, the hips may be innately loose, but the laxity should resolve by 2 to 4 weeks. In the nursery, laxity is felt by pushing the hips outward (Barlow test) or bringing them back to the socket (Ortolani test). Figure 59-1 illustrates these maneuvers. These tests typically elicit an emphatic "clunk." More subtle noises, such as "clicks" or "pops" may represent insignificant ligamentous snapping. Other early signs include leg length discrepancy, as illustrated in Figure 59-2 by the Galleazzi test, asymmetry of thigh folds, as seen in Figure 59-3, or widening of the pelvis. For late physical findings see Table 59-1.

DIAGNOSTIC STUDIES

Because the proximal hip is entirely cartilage for the first 4 to 5 months, early radiographs may not reliably show the condition of the joint. Ultrasound is the most useful imaging modality in younger infants from birth to age 4 or 5 months (Harding et al., 1997). A good ultrasound image demonstrates not only the formation of the ball and socket, but also instability of the joint. To prevent false-positive studies due to the generalized joint laxity that is common in all newborns, ultrasound should be done no earlier than 2 weeks of age, except in extreme cases.

At older ages, the radiographs may show partial or complete migration of the hip from its socket. This is illustrated in Figure 59-4. The socket itself may be very shallow and oversized. Later radiographs may also demonstrate pressure areas, which may represent early arthritis.

MANAGEMENT

If detected early, mild to moderate cases of DDH can be treated in abduction braces, such as the Pavlik harness seen in Figure 59-5. This device directs the hip in a stable position and thus maximizes the child's own developmental potential (Harding et al., 1997). This treatment is most effective under 3 months of age. Multiple diapers (triple or double) may have some benefit early on, particularly while waiting for a consultative appointment, but they do not provide enough stability to maintain a corrective position, so they are not definitive treatment. Beyond 6 months of age, more rigid immobilization, such as casting, and possibly surgical procedures, such as open hip reduction and realignment of

Table 59–1. EXAMINATION OF RANGE OF MOTION, GAIT, AND SPECIFIC TESTS FOR EARLY VERSUS LATE DDH

	Range of Motion	**Gait**	**Tests***
Normal	Symmetric abduction and flexion	Balanced trunk and hip swing	Symmetric thigh folds; femurs equal length
Early DDH < 3 mo	Range of motion symmetric, painless; pelvis may be wide; thigh folds may be symmetric	N/A	Ortolani—reduction with hip flexed abducted Barlow—dislocation with hip flexed, adducted Galleazzi—asymmetry of femur lengths
Late DDH > 18 mo	Decreased range of motion, especially abduction; often painful, thigh fold	Trunk lurch or wide based	Ortolani and Barlow tests negative; Galleazzi more pronounced

DDH = developmental dysplasia of the hip.
  *See Figures 59-1, 59-2, and 59-3.

the bones of the hip and pelvis, more frequently become necessary.

▲ **Clinical Warning:** Because early diagnosis and treatment are essential for a good outcome, the provider should have a low threshold for obtaining ultrasound in any child with an abnormal hip examination or any risk factors (eg, family history, breech presentation, twins). Even without imaging, any child who has a suspicious asymmetry of the hips or demonstrates a gait problem should be referred to an orthopaedist as early as possible.

What to Tell Parents

The most important point to emphasize is the need for long-term observation. Late manifestations of even simple hip dysplasia are unfortunately not common, so children presenting in infancy may need follow-up throughout growth. However, few if any of these children will have special needs beyond yearly or biannual examinations. Children with dysplasia may participate in normal activities without increased risk to their hips. Most treatment is geared toward preventing hip problems (such as arthritis) in adulthood, and childhood functional problems are very unusual.

Knee Disorders

ANATOMY

The knee is not just a simple hinge joint; it is complicated by rotation and translation of the components. The forces across the knee may total up to eight times the body weight in running and on stairs (Simonsen et al., 1995), so even minimal pain or dysfunction can lead to disability. The distribution of force is reliant on muscle balance, bone alignment, and the condition of the soft-tissue stabilizers (ligaments and menisci).

PHYSICAL EXAMINATION

Gait should be assessed, with attention to alignment of the feet, rotation of the legs and thighs, and angulation of the knee itself. The knee should angle slightly inward (7–10 degrees) in stance. The knee is then observed and palpated

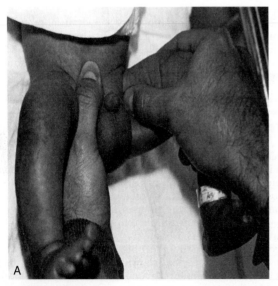
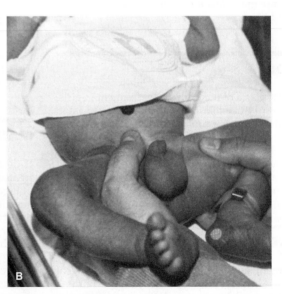

Figure 59–1 ■ Barlow (A) and Ortolani (B) tests for hip instability. The Barlow test pulls the flexed hip towards midline and a posterior force is applied. The Ortolani pushes the flexed hip outward. A palpable "clunk" is felt in a positive test. Adapted with permission from Morrissey, R.T., & Weinstein, S.L. (Eds.). (1996). *Lovell & Winter's pediatric orthopaedics* (4th Ed.). (p. 75). Philadelphia: Lippincott-Raven.

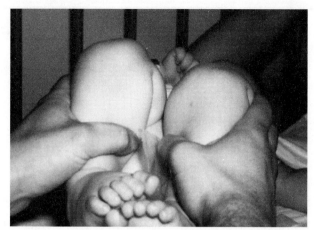

Figure 59–2 ■ The Galleazzi test demonstrates apparent femoral length difference in a child with dislocated hip. The test may be negative if both hips are dislocated. Adapted with permission from Morrissey, R.T., & Weinstein, S.L. (Eds.). (1996). *Lovell & Winter's pediatric orthopaedics* (4th Ed.). (p. 912). Philadelphia: Lippincott-Raven.

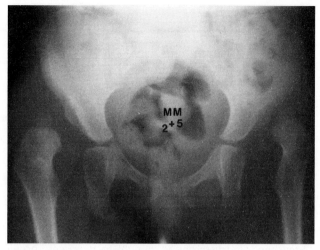

Figure 59–4 ■ Radiograph of a 2-year-old child with bilateral hip dislocation. Note the shallow sockets as well as the abnormal placement of the femoral heads. Adapted with permission from Morrissey, R.T., & Weinstein, S.L. (Eds.). (1996). *Lovell & Winter's pediatric orthopaedics* (4th Ed.). (p. 913). Philadelphia: Lippincott-Raven.

for swelling (or effusion). Normally there is dimpling at the joint lines, so loss of these contours points to fluid in the joint space. The joint lines and bones are palpated for tenderness or bony spurs. The patella is pushed downward to rule out grind pain suggestive of cartilage injury, as described in the following section.

Stability of the knee is tested with simple provocative maneuvers. With the knee at a 30-degree angle, the examiner must first stabilize the femur with one hand while pulling on the tibia with the other hand. The knee is then pushed inward and outward from the side to rule out varus or valgus laxity (collateral ligament injury). With the knee flexed to 90 degrees, the Drawer test is performed by pulling the tibia. The knee is then pushed back to test anterior-posterior laxity. The Lachman test for anterior cruciate instability is performed by pulling forward on the tibia with the knee at 30 degrees flexion. The examiner then needs to push inward and outward on the side of the kneecap in extension and flexion to assess patellar stability.

There are three major causes of nontraumatic knee pain in children (Table 59-2):

- Osgood-Schlatter disease (refer to Chap. 44)
- Osteochondritis dissecans (OCD) of the distal femur
- Patellar disorders

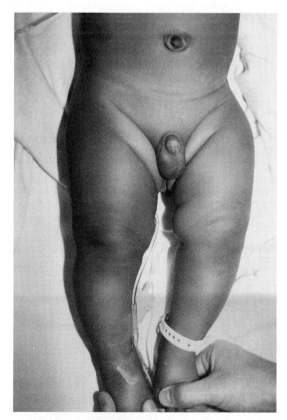

Figure 59–3 ■ Thigh-fold asymmetry in a child with posteriorly dislocated hip. Note also the apparent widening of the pelvis on the left, dislocated side. Adapted with permission from Morrissey, R.T., & Weinstein, S.L. (Eds.). (1996). *Lovell & Winter's pediatric orthopaedics* (4th Ed.). (p. 76). Philadelphia: Lippincott-Raven.

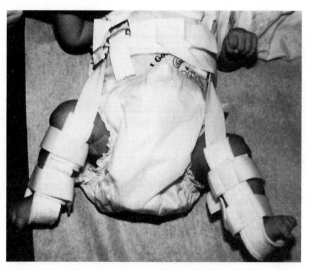

Figure 59–5 ■ The Pavlik harness is a flexible brace used to hold the hips pointing towards the hip socket. This enables the child to develop socket depth. The harness is best used on a child younger than 6 months. Adapted with permission from Morrissey, R.T., & Weinstein, S.L. (Eds.). (1996). *Lovell & Winter's pediatric orthopaedics* (4th Ed.). (p. 922). Philadelphia: Lippincott-Raven.

Table 59–2.   CAUSES OF NONTRAUMATIC KNEE PAIN

Disorder	Ages/Sex	Clinical Findings	Comments
Osgood-Schlatter disease	10–13 y Males predominately	Elevation, tenderness over tibial tubercle	Apophysitis from growth
Osteochodritis dissecans	14–16 y Males predominately	Tenderness over distal femur	Osteonecrosis
Patellofemoral stress syndrome	14–17 y Females predominately	Pain around patella, tilt or subluxation, apprehension	Mechanical mismatch of limb rotation

■ *Osteochondritis Dissecans*

PATHOLOGY

Osteochondritis dissecans is thought to represent chronic fatigue injury or disruption of the blood supply to the bone (Schenck & Goodnight, 1996). The resultant collapse of the bone directly beneath the joint surface can lead to chronic pain or mechanical symptoms, such as snapping or giving way of the knee. Seldom will the pain be severe or acute, although it may crest.

▲ **Clinical Warning:** The risk of chronic cartilage damage without treatment is high, so the provider should have a low threshold for obtaining radiographs of the knee and orthopaedic referral.

EPIDEMIOLOGY

The age range of presentation is from 10 to 16 years, with boys having a higher prevalence for uncertain reasons. As is frequently the case, younger children do best clinically. Older children may have long-term chronic pain and are more likely to need surgery. Young adults may progress to arthrosis or arthritis and may need cartilage transplantation or bony reconstruction. OCD may be bilateral in up to 40% of cases (Schenck & Goodnight, 1996).

PHYSICAL EXAMINATION

The knee may show signs of generalized inflammation, including slight effusion and pain on extremes of motion, especially flexion, but will demonstrate no instability. There is tenderness at the joint line, especially over the distal end of the femur.

● **Clinical Pearl:** The location for findings differentiates OCD from Osgood-Schlatter disease, which is localized on the front of the tibia over the tibia tubercle and represents irritation of the growth center in that location. The provider should refer the patient to a pediatric orthopaedist for diagnosis and management of suspected OCD.

DIAGNOSTIC STUDIES

Radiographs of the knees will show a characteristic defect on the lower end of the femur, usually the lateral side of the medial femoral condyle. A rim of reactive or sclerotic bone, which indicates that the lesion is healing, may surround the area of collapsed bone. There is usually no collapse of the joint itself, except in older teens with large lesions. Figure 59-6 illustrates this finding.

● **Clinical Pearl:** Magnetic resonance imaging (MRI) can be helpful in assessing the extent of the lesion and the degree of cartilage involvement but is not needed for diagnosis. Radiologic studies can help the pediatric orthopaedist in determining prognosis and the need for active therapy in a given case.

MANAGEMENT

Management is normally provided by a pediatric orthopaedist. Bracing or a short period of casting may reduce painful symptoms and help promote healing. Short-term activity modification is also frequently necessary. Surgical intervention, including arthroscopic drilling or bone or cartilage transplants, is seldom required before early adulthood.

What to Tell Parents

Many of these children will present with long-term pain that disrupts their normal activities. Emphasis should be made that a short term of bracing or modification of activity should lead to full recovery.

▲ **Clinical Warning:** A small subset of children may have continuous problems, so the seriousness of this entity must be stressed. After healing of the lesion, continued exercise and fitness are important to prevent recurrence, so the child and parents should understand the level of commitment required. The provider can assist the family by referring the child to a certified athletic trainer, because this health professional specializes in health-maintaining exercise and activities. Alternatively, a physical therapist may be involved, provided he or she specializes in health and fitness.

■ *Patellofemoral Stress Syndrome*

Patellofemoral stress syndrome (PFSS) is sometimes known as chondromalacia patellae (CMP). PFSS is a common disorder of teenagers, occurring late in the adolescent growth spurt and continuing into maturity. Girls are more frequently affected, possibly due to their growth-induced changing distribution of weight and muscle tone.

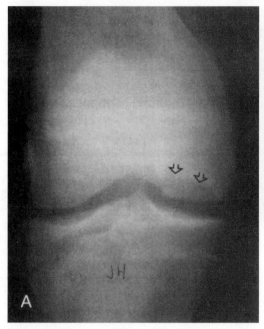

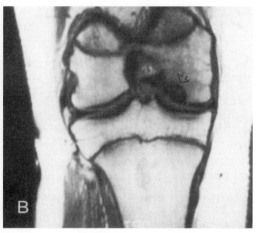

Figure 59–6 ■ Osteochondritis dissecans in the medial femoral condyle (arrows), seen on both radiograph *(A)* and T1-weighted magnetic resonance imaging scan *(B)*. Adapted with permission from Tolo, V.T., & Wood, B. (Eds.). (1993). *Pediatric Orthopaedics in Primary Care.* (p. 180). Baltimore: Williams & Wilkins.

PATHOLOGY

The PFSS appears to arise from an imbalance in the muscles of the front of the thigh, with much stronger pull laterally than medially. This is often accentuated by residual inward rotation of the hip and a relatively externally rotated lower leg. The knee angles more inward (or valgus), leading to increased lateral pull and increased stress on the kneecap itself.

HISTORY AND PHYSICAL EXAMINATION

Although the natural history of PFSS is most often resolution of the symptoms, pain may be extreme enough to significantly limit a young teenager's lifestyle. Fortunately, even minimal intervention may improve the symptoms.

Clinically, PFSS covers a spectrum, ranging from vague discomfort or tiredness in the knees to recurrent dislocation of the kneecap. Children with PFSS are frequently loose-jointed and very flexible.

● **Clinical Pearl:** On walking, the patient with PFSS will have relative external rotation of the lower leg with respect to the thigh, and the kneecap may be observed to swivel or jump at the end of extension (the so-called J-sign).

In flexion, the kneecap will be tilted laterally or even pulled to the outside by muscle forces. There may be tenderness along the borders of the kneecap with apprehension of dislocation on lateral stress. Patellar grind is frequently positive and indicates cartilage injury (or chondromalacia). Feet are generally flat and externally rotated. Hips will most frequently demonstrate increased internal rotation.

DIAGNOSTIC CRITERIA AND STUDIES

The diagnosis of CMP, which is a pathologic diagnosis, is based on clinical, radiologic, or surgical demonstration of cartilage damage.

Radiographs of the knees are not routinely ordered in the initial workup, except to differentiate OCD or Osgood-Schlatter disease. Radiographic studies may show tilt or even lateral subluxation of the kneecap in its groove. Findings can be confirmed on cross-sectional imaging studies, such as computed tomographic (CT) or MRI scans. Radiographic studies are useful for differentiating subluxation from lateral tilt and for ruling out cartilage damage. Study findings govern the treatment approach (Fulkerson, 1994).

MANAGEMENT

Treatment may often be initiated by the primary care provider. Acute-phase management should be aimed initially at reconstituting muscle balance through rest; appropriate applications of moist ice or heat (depending on response to the specific modality) for 20 to 30 minutes at a time, with a full 60 minutes elapsing before reapplying the modality; and exercise of supporting musculature. The kneecap can be centralized with bracing or taping. Referral to an athletic trainer or a physical therapist may assist the youngster in attaining a satisfactory muscle-strengthening response.

Medial shoe supports (arch supports) that will help balance the rotation of the leg segments and decompress the kneecap can be designed by either a podiatrist or an orthopaedist. If all these efforts fail, surgical rebalancing or reconstruction of the kneecap mechanism may be necessary.

● **Clinical Pearl:** Most adolescents will have some level of knee pain from time to time. Those whose pain chronically restricts their activity for greater than 6 months should be evaluated and treated. Referral should be made to an orthopaedist for patients who do not improve rapidly with conservative therapies or for those who have recurrent knee instability.

▲ **Clinical Warning:** Delay in adequate treatment for PFSS may lead to cartilage damage (true CMP), which carries a far worse prognosis.

What to Tell Parents

Although PFSS may be very frustrating at times, it is useful to stress the overall favorable course with growth and therapeutic exercises. Again, emphasis must be placed on the need for continued exercise and fitness throughout adolescence and into adulthood.

Foot and Gait Disorders

The foot reflects muscle balance and nerve function in the infant and growing child; therefore, close attention should be paid to any deformity or perceived malformation. Fortunately, foot abnormalities either are self-limited, remodel with normal growth, or do not lead to any physical disability.

● **Clinical Pearl:** The provider can feel confident in recommending that a child without foot pathology can safely wear garden-variety footwear of any brand. The single most important rule is that the growing child needs to be fitted to a shoe that accommodates normal foot length, with the toes in an "uncurled" position. Generally, the shoe should allow for about one adult thumbnail length's room at the tip of the great toe. This extra room will provide for short-term growth, while also comfortably accommodating the foot. Leather shoes are not preferable to canvas-type shoes, including those that are inexpensive.

PHYSICAL EXAMINATION

The feet should be carefully examined in the newborn nursery and in subsequent well child visits. Note should be made of the position and size of the toes. The presence or absence of a longitudinal arch may be noted, although the arch generally does not form fully until age 6 years.

▲ **Clinical Warning:** The most important examination point is in assessing the flexibility of the foot, particularly rolling inward and outward of the hindfoot. Rigid abnormality of the hindfoot, whether outward into valgus or inward into varus, is most suggestive of a severe foot anomaly, such as vertical talus or clubfoot.

By walking age, the foot position during gait should be assessed. Presence of the arch in both standing and sitting positions should be noted. The alignment of the legs and thighs is very critical to the function of the knee and is best judged in ambulation. Finally, it is essential that the provider assess flexibility of the foot while making careful note of any tender or painful areas.

■ *Flatfoot*

The longitudinal arch of the foot forms around age 6 years, so many children may appear to have flatfoot in early ambulation. In some children, particularly those with generalized ligamentous laxity, the flatness may persist into adulthood. Flatfoot seldom causes severe pain or functional problems, probably owing to improvements in all types of shoes. The days of the "fallen arch" syndrome seem to be past.

PHYSICAL EXAMINATION

Examination of the flatfoot is made to determine if there is a flexible arch that reappears when the foot is unloaded, as seen in Figure 59-7. The provider should note whether there is any bony tenderness suggestive of some other process. The foot should be observed in stance and with the child sitting. In true flexible flatfoot, the arch will be present when the foot is lifted off the ground. These children may show other signs of hyperlaxity, including increased hip rotation, hyperextension of the elbows, and sometimes looseness of the shoulders.

▲ **Clinical Warning:** Although rare, flatfeet may be the first presenting sign of Marfan syndrome or other abnormalities of collagen and soft tissues. Therefore, the spine should be checked for scoliosis, and careful observation of limb lengths must be made. Refer to Chapter 56 for more information on Marfan syndrome.

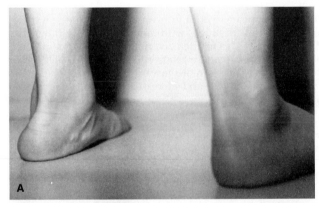
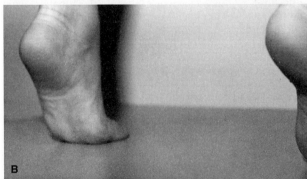

Figure 59–7 ■ Flexible flatfoot. Note how in stance *(A)* the medial arch is flattened to the floor and the foot rolls outward. When the foot lifts off the ground (B), the longitudinal arch reconstitutes. Adapted with permission from Morrissey, R.T., & Weinstein, S.L. (Eds.). (1996). *Lovell & Winter's pediatric orthopaedics* (4th Ed.). (p. 1086). Philadelphia: Lippincott-Raven.

DIAGNOSTIC STUDIES

Radiographs do not add to the diagnostic or treatment plan and are not routinely needed.

▲ **Clinical Warning:** Any flatfoot that has sharp or localizing pain or is rigid may be the cause of bony pathology. In this instance, radiographs should be obtained.

MANAGEMENT

Flexible flatfoot seldom needs treatment, unless the child complains of tiredness or aching in the feet with activity or if there is associated knee pain (see section on knee disorders). At that point, simple arch support with off-the-shelf orthotics may reduce symptoms. No exercise regimens will restore the foot arch. Although there are several surgical procedures described to reconstruct a flatfoot, their indications remain very controversial and probably should be used only in the face of neuromuscular disease, such as cerebral palsy.

■ *Painful Flatfoot*

If the foot has true pain or rigidity, then it is most likely that an acute bony process underlies the loss of the arch (Kumar & Cowell, 1977). The most likely causes of painful flatfoot include the following:

- Accessory navicular, which means that an extra bone is in the midportion of the foot (Fig. 59-8)
- Tarsal coalition, the abnormal connection between two or more foot bones

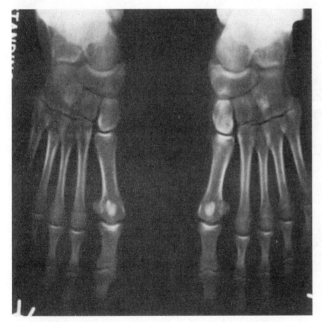

Figure 59–8 ■ Accessory navicular is a cause of painful flatfoot in children. This radiograph shows the accessory bone partially fused with the main body of the navicular on both feet. Adapted with permission from Morrissey, R.T., & Weinstein, S.L. (Eds.). (1996). *Lovell & Winter's pediatric orthopaedics* (4th Ed.). (p. 1100). Philadelphia: Lippincott-Raven.

DIAGNOSTIC STUDIES

Both accessory navicular and tarsal coalition are unusual presentations, with an incidence of approximately 1 in 2500. If untreated, however, either can proceed to disruption of the foot joints and, in severe cases, frank arthritis. Radiographs are diagnostic in almost all cases, although CT or MRI may be needed to see subtle coalitions.

MANAGEMENT

Orthotics can sometimes reduce the symptoms but are never curative. Surgery is often indicated. Under normal circumstances, only painful or rigid flatfoot needs to be evaluated by a pediatric orthopaedist.

Flatfoot can run in families, so the parent's arch alignment may be reflected in the child. It is important that the provider emphasize that pain and foot arthritis are seldom the sequellae of flatfoot in this day and age. To maintain their foot flexibility, children should be urged to wear shoes with some built-in arch support (Theologis, Gordon, & Benson, 1994).

■ *Metatarsus Adductus*

Metatarsus adductus is often erroneously called "one third of a clubfoot." This disorder is almost certainly related solely to in utero molding. The front of the foot may curve inward as much as 30 degrees as it wraps around the shin, and this molding may persist into early childhood (Fig. 59-9). Like other molding abnormalities, the child will outgrow metatarsus adductus, with most of the correction coming by 2 to 3 years after the onset of ambulation (Farsetti, Weinstein, & Ponseti, 1994). Classification of metatarsus adductus is based on the amount of angulation and the rigidity, as shown in Table 59-3.

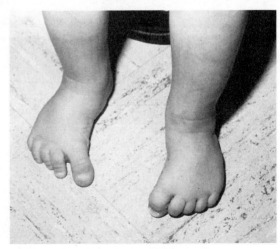

Figure 59–9 ■ Metatarsus adductus is a molding disorder of the forefoot. The back of the foot and the ankle are freely flexible to differentiate from clubfoot deformity. Adapted with permission from Morrissey, R.T., & Weinstein, S.L. (Eds.). (1996). *Lovell & Winter's pediatric orthopaedics* (4th Ed.). (p. 1079). Philadelphia: Lippincott-Raven.

Table 59–3. CLASSIFICATION OF THE AMOUNT OF ANGULATION AND RIGIDITY IN METATARSUS ADDUCTUS

Mild	10- to 15-degree angulation	Correctible past midline
Moderate	15- to 25-degree angulation	Correctible to midline with some difficulty
Severe	>30-degree angulation	Minimally correctible

MANAGEMENT

Most cases of metatarsus adductus are mild to moderate. These respond to stretching by the parents. More severe cases may require corrective shoes or, unusually, casting.

▲ **Clinical Warning:** The provider should refer the patient to a pediatric orthopaedist if the patient's feet do not seem to be responding to stretching regimens.

Metatarsus adductus seldom if ever will result in functional problems, although shoes and the appearance of the foot may be perceived as a difficulty. Maintaining early flexibility is the most important aspect of treatment, so the parents should involve themselves rigorously in stretching of the child's foot. A physical therapist may be assistive in helping parents to set up and follow an effective stretching regimen.

■ *Clubfoot*

It is important that the provider recognize a rigid clubfoot deformity because this foot will require treatment even to approximate normal function. This is one of the orthopaedic entities that require pediatric orthopaedist referral when first diagnosed.

EPIDEMIOLOGY

Clubfoot is reported to have an incidence of 1 in 1000 and to be bilateral in up to 50% of patients (Sullivan, 1996). Boys are affected most commonly. The strong family predisposition points to a possible genetic basis for the disorder (Rebbeck et al., 1993). One-sided disease tends to be more mild and is felt to be a molding disorder like DDH, tibial torsion, and torticollis. Bilateral involvement is generally more rigid and may have a neuromuscular component.

PHYSICAL EXAMINATION

There are three cardinal findings on examination (Fig. 59-10):

- Plantar flexion of the ankle (equinus)
- Rolling inward of heel (varus)
- Toes pointing inward (metatarsus adductus)

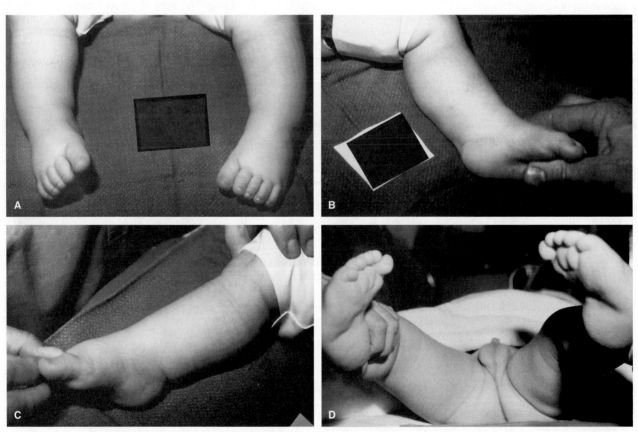

Figure 59–10 ■ Clubfoot or equinovarus deformity in a newborn. Note the cardinal features: *(A)* plantar flexion of the ankle, *(B)* varus of the heel, *(C)* adduction of the forefoot, and *(D)* deep creases in the instep. The deformities are all more or less rigid. Adapted with permission from Morrissey, R.T., & Weinstein, S.L. (Eds.). (1996). *Lovell & Winter's pediatric orthopaedics* (4th Ed.). (p. 1111). Philadelphia: Lippincott-Raven.

All joint components are more or less fixed. Even in a newborn, it may be difficult to correct any or all components. Other findings include marked internal rotation of the shin, small heels, and deep skin folds or clefts in the back of the foot and along the medial border. Presence of these features is felt to worsen the prognosis for correction if aggressive intervention is not made.

DIAGNOSTIC STUDIES

The presence of clubfoot can often be detected in neonatal ultrasound, giving ample opportunity to prepare the parents for the level of care that the child may need. Once the patient is born, clinical findings are more reliable than any imaging. Foot radiographs can be used to assess baseline malalignment and improvement with treatment; however, ossification of the foot bones is very slow, so radiographs may not be interpretable until 2 or 3 months of age. The use of ultrasound or other imaging has not been fully investigated.

▲ **Clinical Warning:** Children with clubfoot have a higher incidence of DDH and neck anomalies, such as those seen in torticollis. Very rigid feet may be associated with other system abnormalities, so the threshold for abdominal ultrasound and other screening techniques should be low.

MANAGEMENT

Even when clubfoot is flexible, the natural history of untreated clubfoot is poor, with severe functional disturbance the norm. For this reason, even relatively mild clubfoot should be assessed early by a pediatric orthopaedist before the infant is 1 month old. Treatment should commence at that point.

All feet except the most rigid (which are associated with other syndromes) are initially treated by stretching and corrective strapping or casting. The casts are changed weekly or biweekly to provide for continuous assessment of the skin and to note progress in correction. A small percentage (< 40%) of patients will respond to casting alone; however, these babies may require long-term bracing or corrective shoes to prevent recurrent deformity (Cooper & Doetz, 1995).

Some patients' feet may require surgical correction through radical soft-tissue releases, typically done at 4 to 6 months of age.

All abnormalities of the feet should be referred as soon as possible to a pediatric orthopaedist. Clubfoot treatment is most effective if instituted at a very early age, and frequently the orthopaedist will assess and begin treatment in the newborn nursery.

The most important point that the provider should stress early on to parents is that clubfeet may never be fully normal in appearance, although the hope is that early treatment will improve function to a significant degree. The affected foot may be a size or more smaller. There may be residual forefoot deformity. Most children with corrected clubfeet can participate in all activities, including high-performance athletics. Residual deformities of the toes and the heel may require late follow-up procedures.

■ *Calcaneovalgus Feet Versus True Congenital Vertical Talus*

Most feet that are seen as out-toeing or everted are flexible feet molded outward in utero. If the back of the foot can be moved fairly easily, the feet do not need specific treatment, although stretching by the parents may help keep them supple. This is illustrated by Figure 59-11.

Rigidly everted feet are significantly more rare than are calcaneovalgus feet. Feet that are rigidly everted may represent a true congenital vertical talus. In this genetic deformity, the foot is rolled outward, and the ankle is fixed in a dorsiflexed or calcaneous position.

MANAGEMENT

Although benign calcaneovalgus deformity of the foot will always resolve, true vertical talus uniformly requires surgical release by 4 to 6 months to enable normal foot positioning and function (Sullivan, 1996).

■ *Torsional and Gait Disturbances*

Although many children will be noted on examination to have intoeing, few will have severe enough disability to require active treatment. In very severe cases, there is frequently an underlying neuromuscular disturbance that accentuates the deformity or limits the normal remodeling processes. The causes of intoeing can be broken down by age at presentation, as follows:

- Metatarsus adductus (refer to section on foot disorders)—newborn
- Internal tibial torsion (ITT)—walking to age 3 years
- Increased femoral anteversion—age 3 to 10 years

■ *Internal Tibial Torsion*

Like metatarsus adductus, ITT is a molding disorder dependent on in utero position and the size of the child. The baby begins to walk with legs positioned as at birth. Ambulation leads to correction. ITT may be more pronounced in early walkers who are younger than 10 months. ITT generally corrects itself by 2 to 3 years of age.

PHYSICAL EXAMINATION

Examination demonstrates a fixed intoeing, usually around 5 to 10 degrees of inward rotation of the foot with respect to the shin. The axis between the malleoli may be pointed inward, whereas in normal legs, it will point out. There may be associated metatarsus adductus. Figure 59-12 illustrates the intoeing position seen in ITT.

MANAGEMENT

Management most frequently involves reassurance and observation. Almost all children will outgrow tibial torsion unless there is a neurologic subtext. For children whose legs

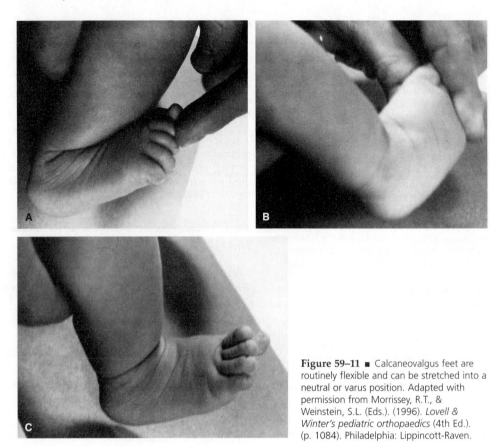

Figure 59–11 ■ Calcaneovalgus feet are routinely flexible and can be stretched into a neutral or varus position. Adapted with permission from Morrissey, R.T., & Weinstein, S.L. (Eds.). (1996). *Lovell & Winter's pediatric orthopaedics* (4th Ed.). (p. 1084). Philadelphia: Lippincott-Raven.

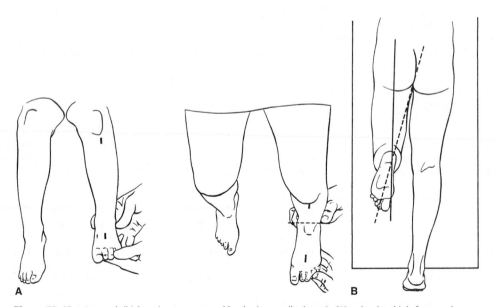

Figure 59–12 ■ Internal tibial torsion as measured by the intramalleolar axis *(A)* or by the thigh-foot angle as seen from above with the child prone *(B)*. Adapted with permission from Morrissey, R.T., & Weinstein, S.L. (Eds.). (1996). *Lovell & Winter's pediatric orthopaedics* (4th Ed.). (p. 1049). Philadelphia: Lippincott-Raven.

roll in more than 40 degrees, night casting or bracing may be necessary.

Most children can be followed to full correction in the primary care setting. Frequently, parents request a specialist's opinion for reassurance of themselves and particularly those around them.

■ *Increased Femoral Anteversion*

ANATOMY AND PATHOLOGY

As part of normal development, the femoral head and neck lie in a plane in front of the femoral shaft. This relationship is termed anteversion. For uncertain reasons, some children have increased anteversion. This phenomenon places the femoral head farther forward than is typical. To seat the hip in the acetabulum, the child must roll the legs inward, leading to classic intoeing.

EPIDEMIOLOGY

Anteversion reaches its peak by age 3 to 4 years. Thus, the intoeing may appear to get worse in early childhood. Girls and boys are involved equally, although girls seem to resolve excess anteversion less quickly. The remodeling process may continue until age 10 or 11 years and is due to improving muscle balance with age.

HISTORY AND PHYSICAL EXAMINATION

When tired, the child will frequently intoe to a greater degree. The provider is advised to ask parents whether they have noticed this phenomenon. It is also important to inquire whether the child finds it most comfortable to sit with their legs rolled behind them, in the so-called w-position. This is not harmful to the hips, and no special effort need be made to prevent this sitting pattern.

Physical examination will show variable intoeing, often changing step-by-step. Range of motion of the hips will demonstrate significantly more internal than external rotation.

▲ **Clinical Warning:** Children who have only minimal external rotation (<10) may be unable to remodel the anteversion and may require treatment.

MANAGEMENT

Treatment rarely is needed for hip anteversion, although parental reassurance is extremely important. The provider should recommend that parents enroll their child in activities that emphasize external rotation of the legs and hips, such as dance, soccer, or ice-skating. These activities maintain flexibility and teach the child the habit of walking with the toes pointing outward. Physical therapy and exercises do not change the course of remodeling but may help maintain flexibility in the hip. Modified shoes do not have any effect on the alignment and function of the hip, so there is no indication for orthotics or "corrective" shoes.

In very rigid anteversion, the child may respond to bracing in light twister cables from the hips to the feet. As with all bracing modalities, cables have not been proven to alter the course of the disorder. In the most extreme cases, surgical correction of the hip alignment through osteotomy may be indicated, although this procedure has a high morbidity and is presented only as a last resort. Almost all children with anteversion can be followed in the primary care setting.

● **Clinical Pearl:** It is important to remind parents that correction will occur very slowly, so improvement must be measured year-to-year rather than day-to-day.

A subset of children may never completely outgrow their anteversion and may show intermittent intoeing into adulthood. However, if they maintain good external rotation of the hips, these individuals should be able to compensate for the minimal residual deformity. They will not have any disability or predisposition to long-term problems, such as hip arthritis.

▲ **Clinical Warning:** The provider should recommend referral to a pediatric orthopaedist if the child cannot compensate because of extreme anteversion or lack of external rotation. Both of these situations may indicate neuromuscular disease and may be indications for more aggressive treatment. Referral to a pediatric orthopaedist may also lead to parental peace of mind.

What to Tell Parents

It is important for the provider to emphasize that the hip is flexible and that the child will be able to compensate for and ultimately outgrow the condition. The clinician may want to point out that many high-performance athletes, particularly in speed sports, have residual anteversion without any disability.

■ *Bowlegs and Knock-knees*

As with so many of the perceived deformities in this chapter, both bowlegs and knock-knees are the result of normal physiologic growth. The key is to identify when a child is beyond normal, both in degree of deformity and in age of presentation, to make sure there is no underlying growth disorder.

PATHOLOGY

Normally, young children begin life with bowlegs (genu varum), a product of their in utero position and molding. Standing and walking remodel and straighten the bones within the first 2 to 3 years, so that by age 3 or 4, the child has grown into a moderate knock-knee or genu valgum alignment (Fig. 59-13). Such alignment in turn slowly corrects to the normal adult alignment of 7 to 10 degrees valgus at the knee (Tolo, 1996).

PHYSICAL EXAMINATION

Examination for bowing or knock-knee deformity consists of observing the child standing upright. If there is genu varum, the ankles should be placed together and the distance

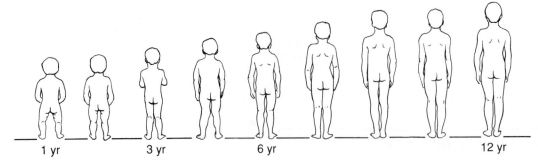

Figure 59–13 ■ The progression of normal knee alignment from moderate varus (bowleg) at age 1 year, through excess knock-knee at 3 years, to normal adult alignment by 6 to 7 years. Adapted with permission from Tolo, V.T., & Wood, B. (Eds.). (1993). *Pediatric Orthopaedics in Primary Care* (p. 254). Baltimore: Williams & Wilkins.

between the knees measured. Conversely, for valgus knees, the knees are placed together and the distance between the ankles measured. A value greater than 5 to 6 in is pathologic and probably needs radiographic evaluation.

● **Clinical Pearl:** As described previously, ITT can cause apparent bowing of the leg, so care should be taken that the foot is pointing forward during these measurements.

▲ **Clinical Warning:** The clinician needs to be sure to note if there is bowing of the shin itself, as seen in Figure 59-14. Particularly with an anterolateral apex, tibial bowing may indicate a more serious disorder, such as neurofibromatosis. Neurofibromatosis is a disease of the nerve sheath, that can

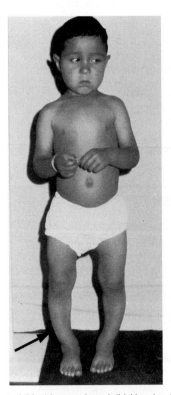

Figure 59–14 ■ A child with anterolateral tibial bowing (arrow), strongly associated with neurofibromatosis. Note that the bow is in the shin itself and not at the knee. Adapted with permission from Morrissey, R.T., & Weinstein, S.L. (Eds.). (1996). *Lovell & Winter's pediatric orthopaedics* (4th Ed.). (p. 84). Philadelphia: Lippincott-Raven.

cause bowing of the shin and fractures that cannot heal (Boero et al., 1997).

DIAGNOSTIC STUDIES

When the deformity is excessive, radiographs should be taken of both legs with the child standing. The radiographs should include the hip joints and the ankles, because assessment of all growth plates may be needed to rule out a systemic developmental disorder.

A child may have excessive bowlegs if ambulation begins before the muscles are developed enough to accept it. This is termed physiologic bowing and is found in heavier children who start walking before age 10 months. Most of these children resolve the bowing within a normal amount of time, but there is a small group of heavier children who take longer. These youngsters must have radiographs to rule out disruption of the growth plate. Otherwise, no specific workup or treatment is needed other than close observation to gauge progress in the remodeling process.

MANAGEMENT

Pathologic processes that can cause persistent or progressive bowing of the knees include the following:

- Rickets, an extremely rare metabolic disorder of vitamin D and calcium function
- Disruption of the tibial growth plate, called infantile Blount disease

A tibial bow, such as is seen in neurofibromatosis, can also be progressive.

Rickets may be the result of dietary restrictions or kidney disease and involves all growth plates (Zaleske, 1996). Further metabolic workup is required to determine the cause. When treated early, the bowing may resolve spontaneously.

Blount disease is defined as growth plate disruption around the knee, most frequently involving the proximal tibia. Children at first appear as physiologic bowers, but with further observation, the bowing increases. Radiographs show beaking of the bone and fragmentation of the medial side of the growth plate (Fig. 59-15). Treatment consists of rigid bracing early and corrective osteotomy in the late stages of the disease. Even after surgery, the process may recur, and many children require further surgical treatment (Doyle, Volk, & Smith, 1996).

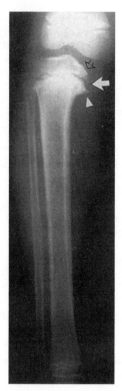

Figure 59–15 ■ Blount disease. Note the fragmentation of the growth plate and the beak of the medial cortex. Adapted with permission from Tolo, V.T., & Wood, B. (Eds.). (1993). *Pediatric Orthopaedics in Primary Care* (p. 257). Baltimore: Williams & Wilkins.

Children who present with knock-knee deformity before the age of 2 years may have bone growth but may also have a developmental disorder, such as metaphyseal dysplasia. These youngsters require radiographs and possibly referral to a pediatric orthopaedist.

▲ **Clinical Warning:** Most children with bowlegs or knock-knees can be followed in the primary care setting, although observation at 3- to 6-month intervals is mandatory. If a child has excessive or progressive deformity, bowlegs after age 3 to 4 years, or bowing earlier than age 2 years, the provider is advised to refer the patient to a pediatric orthopaedist to determine the need for more aggressive interventions.

What to Tell Parents

Almost all of the perceived knee deformities will resolve without any functional problem. It is important to emphasize that the process may move slowly. In the case of bowlegs, this process may even seem to overshoot normal as part of physiologic development.

Spine Disorders

Screening for spinal disorders by the primary provider should start around age 6 to 7 years and should be a regular feature of the well child examination. Care should be made to assess not only the side-to-side alignment, but also the front-to-back shape of the spine. Although most abnormali-

ties will be mild and postural, true spinal deformity can be progressive and disabling, both medically and socially.

■ *Scoliosis*

Scoliosis is the most common spinal deformity. It is defined as a curvature in the side-to-side (or frontal) plane of the spine. The etiology of all deformities of the spine is uncertain. In some rare cases, there are congenital bony deformities that lead to curvature. There is also a close association between scoliosis and connective tissue diseases, such as Marfan syndrome or neurofibromatosis. However, the vast majority of cases are idiopathic, meaning that there is no clear underlying cause. The natural history of scoliosis depends on the rate of the child's growth and the size of the curve.

▲ **Clinical Warning:** A young teenager with a large curve has a much greater chance of progression than an older teen with a small curve. This is the main reason why early detection and close observation of even mild curves are so important.

EPIDEMIOLOGY

The incidence of clinically significant curvature of the spine may be as high as 1 in 200 (Lonstein, 1996). Girls are most frequently involved, although boys may have a more clinically aggressive course. There is a family predisposition. The literature suggests that the disease has some genetic basis.

HISTORY AND PHYSICAL EXAMINATION

Scoliosis does not ordinarily cause pain. Pain or neurologic symptoms, including numbness, weakness, bowel, or bladder dysfunction, are usually indicative of some underlying disorder. The child usually has no presenting complaints, the curve typically being found on routine school or well child screening. There may be a family history of scoliosis. Information about the clinical behavior of scoliosis in other family members may be very important in determining the prognosis.

The spine examination should be done without outer clothing and with the child standing comfortably. The back is assessed for shoulder heights, prominence of the shoulder blade, and any obvious curve of the spine. The child then bends forward to determine if any abnormalities are accentuated. Obvious prominence of the spine can be measured either by angulation of the prominence using a scoliometer, or the height of the prominence in centimeters (Fig. 59-16). A good inspection can yield a clinical impression of scoliosis that is within 5 degrees of that found on radiograph.

● **Clinical Pearl:** It is important to understand that these measurements reflect the rotation and not the curvature of the spine. If the forward bend test is positive, leg lengths should be checked from the anterior superior iliac spine of the pelvis to the medial malleolus, as shown in Figure 59-17. This is necessary because leg-length difference can lead to apparent spinal deformity. Tenderness of the spine or any inflammation of the back should also be noted, because classic spinal anomalies, such as scoliosis, should not be painful.

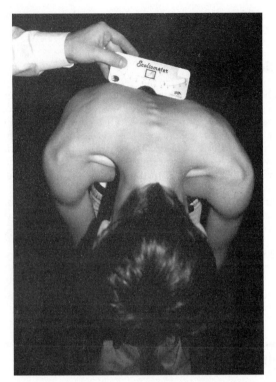

Figure 59–16 ■ Measurement of spinal rotation with the use of a scoliometer on forward bend testing. Adapted with permission from Morrissey, R.T., & Weinstein, S.L. (Eds.). (1996). *Lovell & Winter's pediatric orthopaedics* (4th Ed.). (p. 67). Philadelphia: Lippincott-Raven.

The examiner should evaluate shoulder heights, scapular prominence, and presence of a curve with the patient both upright (Fig. 59-18) and bent forward (Fig. 59-19). Leg lengths are measured because leg-length discrepancy (LLD) may be a nonstructural cause of scoliosis. If there is a rib prominence, the height or angle should be documented with a scoliometer so that a comparison can be made on subsequent examinations.

DIAGNOSTIC CRITERIA AND STUDIES

Radiographs should be restricted to curves that appear significant (greater than 1 cm in scapular height or 5 degrees by scoliometer). Radiographs also should be considered for children with suspected scoliosis if they are about to start a growth spurt. This timing will provide a baseline for later evaluation of the scoliotic condition.

Screening radiographs should be performed with shielding and limited to a single frontal (posteroanterior) view unless there is concern about the front-to-back plane, as described in the section on kyphosis. Figure 59-20 illustrates scoliosis.

MANAGEMENT

Curvatures less than 5 degrees by scoliometer or less than 10 degrees on radiograph are considered to be spinal asymme-

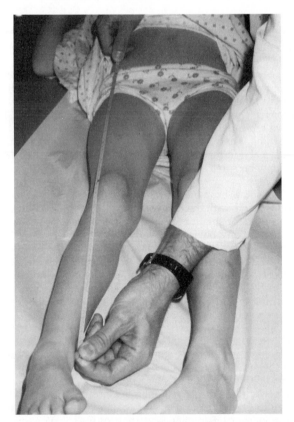

Figure 59–17 ■ Leg length measured from the pelvic crest to the medial side of the ankle. Adapted with permission from Morrissey, R.T., & Weinstein, S.L. (Eds.). (1996). *Lovell & Winter's pediatric orthopaedics* (4th Ed.). (p. 64). Philadelphia: Lippincott-Raven.

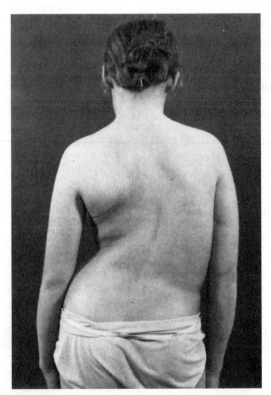

Figure 59–18 ■ Scoliosis in a teenage girl. Note the right thoracic rib prominence. Note also how the body balance shifts towards the apex of the curve. Adapted with permission from Morrissey, R.T., & Weinstein, S.L. (Eds.). (1996). *Lovell & Winter's pediatric orthopaedics* (4th Ed.). (p. 626). Philadelphia: Lippincott-Raven.

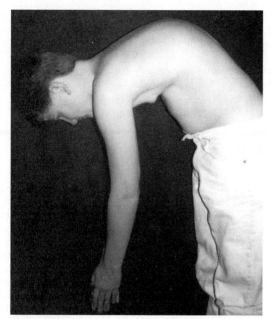

Figure 59–19 ■ Side view of a child with structural kyphosis shows a sharp sagittal curve of the thoracic spine. Adapted with permission from Morrissey, R.T., & Weinstein, S.L. (Eds.). (1996). *Lovell & Winter's pediatric orthopaedics* (4th Ed.). (p. 68). Philadelphia: Lippincott-Raven.

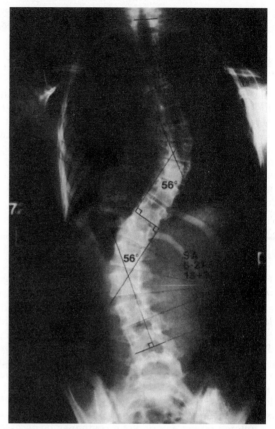

Figure 59–20 ■ Posteroanterior radiograph of a child with scoliosis. Angular measurement by the Cobb technique demonstrates the severity of the curves. Adapted with permission from Morrissey, R.T., & Weinstein, S.L. (Eds.). (1996). *Lovell & Winter's pediatric orthopaedics* (4th Ed.). (p. 630). Philadelphia: Lippincott-Raven.

try, not true scoliosis. Spinal asymmetry can be managed by observation at routine well child visits.

Mild scoliosis (< 20 degrees on radiographic measurement) can be observed closely for signs of progression, but follow-up must be frequent (every 3–4 months) during the adolescent growth spurt.

Progressive curves (a change of more than 6 degrees on repeated radiograph or any change on scoliometer examination) and moderate curves (up to 40 degrees) may require treatment with bracing, either full-time or nighttime (Rowe et al., 1997). Curves greater than 40 degrees frequently require surgical repair.

● **Clinical Pearl:** Exercises, chiropractic manipulation, postural training, electrical stimulation, and admonitions to avoid slouching have not been found to change the course of scoliosis. The clinician can reassure parents and the patient that scoliosis does not typically cause pain. However, physical fitness and weight awareness in the form of a balanced diet and exercise regimen may be helpful in avoiding back pain later in life.

▲ **Clinical Warning:** Referral should be to a pediatric orthopaedist should be based on the age of the patient and the provider's level of comfort with the spinal examination. Any progressive or serious curvature should be referred urgently. A child who presents with pain or neurologic symptoms requires immediate specialist evaluation.

What to Tell Parents

Most scoliosis will be self-limited and will not lead to severe deformity. It is very unusual in a healthy person to have a curve progress to a level that causes health problems, such as pulmonary or cardiac dysfunction. The most likely long-term adverse effect of spinal curvature is back pain, which may be alleviated by good back care, including daily exercises and care with lifting. It is very important that parents and child understand the necessity of these exercises on a lifelong basis.

The psychological issues of scoliosis may be harder to treat than the physical ones. Many children have complex self-esteem and body image problems arising from both the curvature and the treatment. Careful and concerned discussions with parents and child, often done separately, may help alleviate some of the stress. These discussions will help indicate problems that may need to be evaluated by mental health specialists.

■ *Kyphosis*

The front-to-back (or sagittal) plane of the spine may be equally as important as the side-to-side plane in overall appearance. Figure 59-19 demonstrates kyphosis, or round back. Progressive deformity in the upper spine is frequently associated with back pain and bony disruption. This deformity should be distinguished from postural round back, both on the basis of clinical correction and possible radiographic findings. Both the pain and the deformity of progressive kyphosis may respond to bracing and exercises. Surgery is sometimes necessary for severe deformity.

Growth Disorders

■ Leg-Length Discrepancy

Leg-length discrepancy may arise from multiple causes, including traumatic growth disruption, infectious or inflammatory processes, or even tumors. Most cases are limited and are clinically insignificant (Kaufman, Miller, & Sutherland, 1996). LLD may also be a cause of an apparent spinal deformity. If caused by apparent overgrowth of a limb (hemihypertrophy), LLD may be associated with other systemic problems, such as Wilms' tumor, arteriovenous malformation, or neurofibromatosis.

MANAGEMENT

Treatment depends on the clinical setting and the absolute amount of LLD. Children especially will tolerate leg-length differences up to 1.5 to 2 in, even without shoe correction. In older teenagers and early adults, correction by lift inside or outside the shoe may be needed to relieve hip or back pain. A discrepancy of greater than 2 in may require shortening or lengthening of the limb to balance the leg function. In growing children, growth may be selectively arrested to allow the short limb to catch up.

In general, assessment and management need to determine if the LLD is static or progressive. For this reason, long-term follow-up over a period of growth may be necessary.

■ Acute and Chronic Radial Head Subluxation

ANATOMY AND PATHOLOGY

The stability of the proximal radius and ulnar joint is maintained by a ring-shaped restraint called the annular ligament. In rare cases, absence of this ligament from birth may lead to congenital radial head dislocation. In more common situations, the radial head may dislocate fully or partially due to a traction injury. This results in the well-known entity called nursemaid's elbow or pulled elbow syndrome.

The precise pathology of the injury is not completely known, but owing to the marked age predilection of 2 to 4 years, it is probably related to the relative growth of the radius and ulna. By age 2 to 3 years, the radius is relatively shorter at its proximal end than the better developed proximal ulna and olecranon. During a traction event, the radial head in some children can slip under its annular constraint, leading to acute subluxation. It is possible that there is stretching or even microtearing of the ligament as well, which may account for recurrent subluxation.

HISTORY AND PHYSICAL EXAMINATION

Diagnosis of nursemaid's elbow is based on clinical examinations. Most patients have a clear history of a pulling episode and equally clear physical findings. The child will present with pain and unwillingness to use the affected arm. There may be tenderness around the lateral side of the elbow and proximal forearm, and the radial head may be prominent. Elbow flexion and extension may be relatively comfortable, but rotation of the forearm will be extremely painful.

The differential diagnoses for acute elbow dislocation include elbow fracture, infection, congenital radial head dislocation, or, far more rarely, arthritis or neoplasm.

DIAGNOSTIC STUDIES

Diagnostic tests should be reserved for cases that have an unusual or uncertain history, such as fall or other direct blow trauma, or in the child who presents with systemic illness. Furthermore, if the child does not respond to a therapeutic maneuver, a radiograph may document the success or failure of an attempted reduction. Radiographs should include anteroposterior and lateral views of the elbow (as opposed to the distal humerus as in a suspected supracondylar fracture), with imaging of the wrist to rule out complex injury, such as Monteggia fracture dislocation of the radius and ulna. If abnormal, the radiograph will show the radial head pointing away from its articulation with the humerus, as seen in Figure 59-21.

Congenital dislocation is differentiated by abnormal shape of the radial head in addition to the dislocation (Fig 59-22). Congenital dislocation is most often bilateral, so radiographs of the unaffected side may be helpful in suspicious cases.

▲ **Clinical Warning:** All children who present with a history and examination consistent with nursemaid's elbow should have one or two attempts at closed reduction before imaging.

MANAGEMENT

▲ **Clinical Warning:** The provider may want to refer the child with positive radiographs to an orthopedist for reduction.

The reduction technique classically involves rolling the palm up fully (supination), followed by gentle flexion of the elbow. Recent studies suggest that the maneuver can be performed also with the palm facing down (pronation) and may in fact be less painful in this position (McDonald, Whitelaw, & Goldsmith, 1999). Often the professional who is performing the reduction will feel a reduction "clunk," followed by freer and less painful rotation of the forearm. If this successful conclusion occurs, no further evaluation is indicated. The child's arm should be rested in a sling for 2 to 3 days, with return to activities when completely pain free.

If there is no obvious reduction or if the child remains in pain, a second gentle attempt may be undertaken. If there is further concern, radiographs should be performed to rule out persistent dislocation or other occult injury.

● **Clinical Pearl:** Occasionally the elbow remains stiff and sore, despite a documented reduction. This is most likely related to swelling within the elbow joint and should resolve within 3 to 5 days with sling protection.

Referral for radial head subluxation can be reserved for children who have significant pain despite demonstrated reduction, cases that do not reduce within two to three

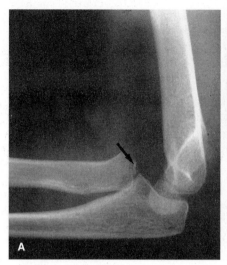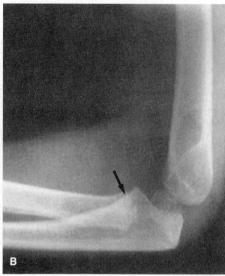

Figure 59–21 ■ Dislocation of the radial head, prereduction *(A)* and postreduction *(B)* lateral radiographs. Note the relation of the radial head with its articulation in the elbow (arrows). Adapted with permission from Morrissey, R.T., & Weinstein, S.L. (Eds.). (1996). *Lovell & Winter's pediatric orthopaedics* (4th Ed.). (p. 1258). Philadelphia: Lippincott-Raven.

attempts, or cases with abnormal physical findings. In addition, recurrent dislocation that recurs more than two or three times should be evaluated by an orthopaedist. Most children will respond to bracing or sometimes a short term of casting. In very extreme laxity or laxity in children older than 3 to 4 years, surgical reconstruction of the ligamentous structure may be indicated.

Summary

Chronic orthopaedic disorders can limit important functions of childhood, but for the most part, they are self-limited and self-improving. Parents and children should be made

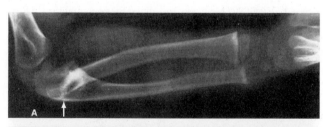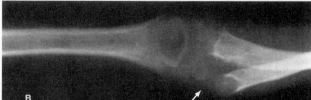

Figure 59–22 ■ Congenital dislocation of the radial head. Note the bony deformity of the chronically dislocated radial head (arrows). Anteroposterior *(A)* and lateral *(B)* views. Adapted with permission from Morrissey, R.T., & Weinstein, S.L., (eds.) (1996). *Lovell & Winter's pediatric orthopaedics, 4th Ed.* Philadelphia: Lippincott-Raven, p. 805.

aware that surgery is rarely needed, regardless of the entity involved. Even if referral is needed, the role of the pediatric orthopaedist is most often to define the condition and the prognosis. The primary care provider needs to function as a partner with the specialist and the family in providing long-term care of these children. This practitioner gives continuity of care in follow-up, offering counseling and education for the child and parents, while providing important feedback and information to the orthopaedic specialist.

COMMUNITY RESOURCES

Resources for Providers

The following sources provide diagnostic and treatment information and valid, relevant links to other sources.

Orthoseek
Internet address: *http://www.orthoseek.com*

Pediatric orthopedics and sports medicine resource authored by orthopaedic surgeons at the following:

Orthogate
Internet address: *http://www.orthogate.org/owl/topics.html*

Web site listing orthopedic web links.

Agency for Healthcare Research and Quality
(formerly the Agency for Healthcare Policy and Research)
Internet address: *http://www.ahrc.gov*

For standards of practice, including practice protocol information.

Orthopedics Today (Medical Matrix)
Internet address: *http://www.slackinc.com/bone/ortoday/othome.asp*

An on-line monthly medical newspaper for orthopedic surgeons.

Resources for Parents

The following sources provide information and support about specific congenital orthopedic problems.

Shriners Hospitals
International Shrine Headquarters
2900 Rocky Point Drive
Tampa, FL 33607-1460
Telephone: (813) 281-0300
Internet address: *http://www.shrinerspfld.org*

> Medical library resource page containing links to orthopedic web sites.

Bearable Times Kids and Teens Club
Internet address: *http://www.bearabletimes.org*

> Resource of the Kids' Hospital Network for hospitalized/homebound children.

MUMS: National Parent to Parent Network
Internet address: *http://www.netnet.net/mums*

> Networking system/support resource for parents.

National Information Center for Children and Youth with Disabilities (NICHCY)
P.O. Box 1492
Washington, DC 20013
Telephone: (800) 695-0285
Internet address: *http://www.nichcy.org*

Southern California Orthopedic Institute
6815 Nobel Avenue
Van Nuys, CA 91405
Telephone: (818) 901-6600
Internet address: *http://www.scoi.com*

Pediatric Internet Directory
Internet address: *http://www.slackinc.com/child/pednet-sn.htm*

REFERENCES

Boero, S., Catagni, M., Donzelli, O., et al. (1997). Congenital pseudoarthrosis of the tibia associated with neurofibromatosis-1. *Journal of Pediatric Orthopedics, 17,* 675–684.

Cooper, D. M., & Doetz, F. R. (1995). Treatment of idiopathic clubfoot: A thirty-year follow-up note. *Journal of Bone and Joint Surgery, 77A,* 1477–1489.

Doyle, B. S., Volk, A. G., & Smith, C. F. (1996). Infantile Blount disease: Long-term follow-up of surgically treated patients at skeletal maturity. *Journal of Pediatric Orthopedics, 16,* 469–476.

Farsetti, P., Weinstein, S. L., & Ponseti, I. V. (1994). The long-term functional and radiographic outcome of untreated and non-operatively treated metatarsus adductus. *Journal of Bone and Joint Surgery, 76A,* 257–265.

Fulkerson, J. P. (1994). Patellofemoral pain disorders: Evaluation and management. *Journal of the American Academy of Orthopedic Surgery, 2,* 124–132.

Harding, M. G., Harcke, H. T., Bowen, J. R., et al. (1997). Management of dislocated hips with Pavlik harness treatment and ultrasound monitoring. *Journal of Pediatric Orthopedics, 17,* 189–198.

Kaufman, K. R., Miller, L. S., & Sutherland, D. H. (1996). Gait asymmetry in patients with limb-length inequality. *Journal of Pediatric Orthopedics, 14,* 339–342.

Kumar, S. J., & Cowell, H. R. (1977). Rigid flatfoot. *Clinical Orthopedics, 122,* 77–84.

Lonstein, J. E. (1996). Scoliosis. In R. T. Morrissey & S. L. Weinstein (Eds.), *Lovell and Winter's pediatric orthopaedics* (4th ed.). Philadelphia: Lippincott-Raven.

McDonald, J., Whitelaw, C., & Goldsmith, L. J. (1999). Radial head subluxations: Comparing two methods of reduction. *Academic Emergency Medicine 6,* 715–718.

Rebbeck, T. R., Dietz, F. R., Murray, J. C., et al. (1993). A single-gene explanation for the probability of having idiopathic talipes equinovarus. *American Journal of Human Genetics, 53,* 1051–1063.

Rowe, D. E., Bernstein, S. M., Riddick, M. F., et al. (1997). A meta-analysis of the efficacy of non-operative treatments for idiopathic scoliosis. *Journal of Bone and Joint Surgery, 79A,* 664–674.

Schenck, R. C. Jr., & Goodnight, J. M. (1996) Osteochondritis dissecans. *Journal of Bone and Joint Surgery, 78A,* 439–456.

Simonsen, E. B., Dyhre-Poulsen, P., Voigt, M., et al. (1995). Bone-on-bone forces during loaded and unloaded walking. *Acta Anatomica (Basel) 152,* 133–142.

Sullivan, J. A. (1996). The child's foot. In R. T. Morrissey & S. L. Weinstein (Eds.), *Lovell and Winter's pediatric orthopaedics* (4th ed.). Philadelphia: Lippincott-Raven.

Theologis, T. N., Gordon, C., & Benson, M. K. (1994). Heel seats and shoe wear. *Journal of Pediatric Orthopedics, 14,* 760–762.

Tolo, V. T. (1996). The lower extremity. In R. T. Morrissey & S. L. Weinstein (Eds.), *Lovell and Winter's pediatric orthopaedics* (4th ed.). Philadelphia: Lippincott-Raven.

Weinstein, S. L. (1996). Developmental hip dysplasia and dislocation. In R. T. Morrissey, & S. L. Weinstein (Eds.), *Lovell and Winter's pediatric orthopaedics* (4th ed.). Philadelphia: Lippincott-Raven.

Zaleske, D. J. (1996). Metabolic and endocrine abnormalities. In R. T. Morrissey & S. L. Weinstein (Eds.). *Lovell and Winter's pediatric orthopaedics* (4th ed.). Philadelphia: Lippincott-Raven.

Chronic Endocrine Disorders

• MARY BETH DAMORE, MD

INTRODUCTION

Chronic endocrine problems run the gamut from mild to severe in the pediatric setting. The long-term implications of an undiagnosed or inadequately managed endocrine disorder can affect a child's quality of life and may even be life threatening. In many instances of endocrine pathology, the primary care provider will need to consult with a pediatric endocrine specialist before embarking on a course of therapy. Often comanagement provides a more optimal management framework for the child with a chronic endocrine problem, whether in pubertal development, growth, or thyroid regulation. This chapter focuses on disorders of pubertal development, growth disorders, and congenital hypothyroidism. Specific indications for specialist consultation and referral and for comanagement are presented.

Disorders of Pubertal Development

ANATOMY, PHYSIOLOGY, AND PATHOLOGY

Normally, the hypothalamic-pituitary-gonadal axis is suppressed in prepubertal children. As a result, the physiology of gonadotropin secretion is one of infrequent, low-amplitude pulses, with a predominance of follicle-stimulating hormone (FSH) relative to luteinizing hormone (LH). Circulating gonadotropins are at a nadir at 6 or 7 years of age but are not completely suppressed. As children approach puberty, there is a change in sensitivity, or disinhibition of the axis, and overriding central nervous system (CNS) control causes episodic pulses of gonadotropin-releasing hormone (GnRH) to be released. As a result, there is an increase in LH and FSH levels, with a relatively greater increase in LH.

The first evidence of the hormonal changes of puberty is episodic LH pulses of high amplitude and short duration. These bursts first occur only during sleep, but with maturity, they also occur regularly throughout the day. The first sign of puberty in girls is generally thelarche, or breast enlargement. Generally gonadarche, or enlargement of the testes, is the first sign in boys.

Variants of Normal Pubertal Development

Three of the most common variants of normal pubertal development are premature thelarche, premature adrenarche, and adolescent gynecomastia.

Premature Thelarche

Premature thelarche is unilateral or bilateral development of breast tissue, which usually occurs during two age periods. The first is 6 months to 2 years. The second is after 6 years. In the earlier type, there is a greater production of ovarian hormones in infancy than later childhood, due to a persistence of infant gonadotropin physiology. Breast development may occur because of hyperresponsiveness or hyperstimulation of breast tissue. In the latter type, the etiology may be breast tissue that is hypersensitive to pubertal estrogen levels or temporarily increased ovarian sex steroid production. Ovarian cysts are identified in some cases, but if present, they do not persist.

▲ **Clinical Warning:** The provider should refer the patient for pediatric endocrine evaluation if there are other signs of rapidly advancing puberty. Clinical concerns that should prompt referral include a rapid tempo of puberty (ie, Tanner III or greater breast development before age 8 years or the appearance of other secondary sexual characteristics), hyperpigmented or enlarged areolae, vaginal discharge or bleeding, an estrogen effect in the perineum (ie, a pale pink vaginal mucosa), or a height acceleration. If it has been obtained, an advanced bone age also warrants referral.

Premature Adrenarche

Premature adrenarche is early development of the androgenic signs of puberty, namely pubic hair, axillary hair, and adult body odor. It most commonly occurs in girls between ages 5 and 8 years.

▲ **Clinical Warning:** Findings that demand immediate endocrine referral include clitoromegaly, phallic enlargement, and growth acceleration.

The development of adrenarche corresponds to levels of dehydroepiandrosterone (DHEA) and dehydroepiandrosterone sulfate (DHEA-S), two of the major androgens produced in the body. Benign premature adrenarche is self-limited and characterized by an elevation of DHEA and DHEA-S only with a normal bone age. The condition may clinically resemble and must be differentiated from congenital adrenal hyperplasia (CAH). CAH is characterized by elevated levels of 17-OH progesterone, 17 pergnenolone, androstenedione, and testosterone along with DHEA, both at baseline and after adrenocorticotropic hormone (ACTH) stimulation, as well as an advanced bone age.

Adolescent Gynecomastia

Adolescent gynecomastia in boys is a benign normal variant. It can be unilateral or bilateral. In general, it begins in stage II or III of puberty and regresses within 2 years. Estimates of the incidence of pubertal gynecomastia range from as low as 4% to as high as 69% (Braunstein, 1993).

▲ **Clinical Warning:** If gynecomastia develops prepubertally, is persistent, exceeds 2 cm, or is of significant concern to the family, an endocrine referral should be made.

Because it is difficult to differentiate benign from pathologic gynecomastia clinically, a complete history, including medication and drug use, and a physical examination, including testicular examination, are critical. Screening blood work includes a serum chemistry profile for assessment of hepatic and renal function and thyroid functions (Braunstein, 1993). If this preliminary workup is negative, referral to a pediatric endocrinologist is indicated, with subsequent measurement of LH, FSH, testosterone, estradiol, prolactin, human chorionic gonadotropin (hCG) (as a screen for tumors), and chromosomes (to rule out Klinefelter's syndrome).

Abnormal Pubertal Development

Abnormal, or precocious, puberty can be divided into three basic classifications: central (or true) isosexual precocity, incomplete isosexual precocity, and contrasexual precocity.

Central Isosexual Precocity

Central means that puberty is driven by a central, hypothalamic source of GnRH. Central precocious puberty occurs when a child develops secondary sexual characteristics that are appropriate for the child's sex in a normal sequence but simply earlier than expected by current standards. Although central precocious puberty is significantly more common in girls than boys, an etiology is found less frequently in girls than boys.

The National Institutes of Health's experience with precocious puberty in 129 children between 1979 and 1983 showed that whereas idiopathic precocious puberty was the most common diagnosis in girls (63%), it was uncommon in boys (6%) (Pescovitz et al., 1986). The majority of boys with central precocious puberty have a history of a CNS disorder, CAH, or chronic exposure to steroids (Neely, 1999). As a general rule, the later the age of onset, the more likely the cause is benign (Lincoln & Zuber, 1998). Display 60-1 presents the differential diagnosis of central isosexual puberty.

Incomplete Isosexual Precocity

Incomplete isosexual precocity, or precocious pseudopuberty, occurs independently of the normal central pathway involving the hypothalamic GnRH pulse generator. It is caused by an abnormal source of gonadotropin or sex steroid, causing premature pubertal development that is appropriate for sex. Display 60-2 presents differential diagnoses for incomplete isosexual precocity.

● **Clinical Pearl:** Exogenous sex steroids can produce the same effects as endogenous sex steroids, and the possibility of ingestion or exposure should be excluded. The list includes oral contraceptives, estrogen creams, phytoestrogens, and supplements, such as DHEA-S and androstenedione (Tham, Gardner, & Haskell, 1998).

Contrasexual Precocity

Contrasexual precocity is the early development of secondary sexual characteristics that are inconsistent with the sex of a child, such as masculinization in girls or feminization in boys. Both masculinization in girls and feminization in boys have three basic causes. Display 60-3 presents differential diagnoses that the provider should consider for either of these presentations.

● **Clinical Pearl:** Consider exogenous androgens as a possibility in children who ingest health food supplements, such as the androgens DHEA-S and androstenedione, and in female athletes who take steroids (Lincoln & Zuber, 1998).

EPIDEMIOLOGY

Data analyzed in a recent cross-sectional study involving 17,077 girls between ages 3 and 12 and followed in various pediatric practices across the United States, suggest that girls are entering puberty at younger ages than previously established norms. Caucasian girls were found to be entering puberty at an average age of 10 years (6 months to 1 year earlier than girls in previous studies), and African American girls were found to be entering puberty at an average age of 8 to 9 years. The African American girls were more physically mature than the Caucasian girls at all ages and for all secondary sexual characteristics (Herman-Giddens et al., 1997).

In response to the data collected by Herman-Giddens et al., (1997), the Lawson Wilkins Pediatric Endocrine Society launched a comprehensive review on this topic (Kaplowitz, Oberfield, & the Drug and Therapeutics and Executive Committees of the Lawson Wilkins Pediatric Endocrine Society, 1999). New guidelines were formulated, proposing criteria deserving pediatric endocrine referral:

- The development of breast tissue or pubic hair before age 7 years in Caucasian girls and before age 6 in African American girls

---

DISPLAY 60–1 ● Differential Diagnoses for Central Isosexual Puberty

Idiopathic (most common)
Acquired causes:
　Inflammation/infection
　Trauma
　Irradiation
Congenital malformations/CNS anomalies
CNS tumors
Chronic sex steroid exposure

CNS = central nervous system.

DISPLAY 60–2 ● Differential Diagnoses for Incomplete Isosexual Precocity (Precocious Pseudopuberty)

Tumors of the ovaries, testes, or adrenal glands
Congenital adrenal hyperplasia
Sex steroid exposure
Hypothyroidism
Hypersecretion of ovarian or testicular sex steroids
　(recently found to be a result of receptor defects)

DISPLAY 60–3 • Differential Diagnoses for Contrasexual Precocity

---

Masculinization in girls can be caused by:

Congenital adrenal hyperplasia, the most common cause of contrasexual precocity
Androgen-producing tumors, which are rare: ovarian arrhenoblastomas, adrenal tumors, and teratomas
Exogenous androgens

Feminization in boys can be caused by:

Estrogen-producing tumors, which are rare: adrenal tumors and teratomas
Exogenous estrogens
Excessive extraglandular aromatase activity

- In Caucasian girls with breast development beginning after age 7 years or African American girls with breast development beginning after age 6, in conjunction with the following conditions:
  - Rapid tempo of puberty with a bone age greater than 2 years ahead of chronologic age and a predicted height (based on bone age) of at least 4 in below their genetic target height or less than 59 in
  - An underlying neurologic problem, such as hydrocephalus, or new CNS findings, such as focal neurologic deficits, headaches, or seizures
  - Behavior-related factors suggesting that the child's or family's emotional state is adversely affected by the progression of puberty and possibility of early menarche

The new Lawson Wilkins guidelines support the currently accepted normal lower limit of 9 years for puberty in boys (Kaplowitz et al., 1999).

Menarche in Caucasian girls in the United States has remained stable over the last 45 years at 12.88 years. In African American girls, on the other hand, the mean age of menarche has apparently decreased from 12.52 years to 12.16 years. This apparent decrease may be related to the move of African Americans toward achievement of optimal health and nutritional status (Kaplowitz et al., 1999).

Why is there a trend toward earlier onset of puberty? The HANES data and the National Growth and Health Study showed similar increases in the heights and weights of Caucasian and African American girls, particularly with increases in age. It is hypothesized that earlier onset of puberty in African American girls may be related in some way to the use of hair products containing estrogen or placenta. A viable etiology for all girls is the more widespread use of certain plastics, insecticides, and pesticides, such as DDT (xenoestrogens), which contain or degrade into substances having estrogen-related physiologic effects (Herman-Giddens et al., 1997; Murkies, Wilcox, & Davis, 1998; Tham et al., 1998).

Recent evidence points to the possible role of serum leptin levels in the initiation of puberty. Leptin, the product of the ob gene, is involved in body composition, specifically fat composition. Studies to date have revealed that a minimum weight for height is necessary for the onset and maintenance of normal menstrual periods. Furthermore, an association has been found between mild obesity and earlier menarche. Palmert, Radovick, and Boepple (1998) found that girls with central precocious puberty had modestly elevated serum leptin levels, compared with the healthy controls, which may be critical in the initiation of puberty in girls.

HISTORY AND PHYSICAL EXAMINATION

The history should begin with noting the age of symptom onset. More importantly, the provider needs to identify the tempo of symptom progression. Review of systems should include questions about the appearance of acne, axillary odor, and axillary and pubic hair. Vaginal discharge in girls should be noted. Headaches and visual disturbances and symptoms of thyroid disease, such as constipation, fatigue, and cold intolerance are also important to note. The possibility of exposure to exogenous hormones, such as oral contraceptives, or androgens, such as DHEA-S or androstenedione, should be raised.

▲ **Clinical Warning:** Earlier onset and faster progression of puberty are more suggestive of a pathologic condition.

Even before examining a child with early development, review of the growth chart is very informative. Evidence of a rapid height acceleration suggests the possibility of true precocious puberty or CAH. The physical examination should include a look at the fundi and visual fields and a neurologic examination, given the possibility of a brain tumor, such as an astrocytoma or craniopharyngioma. The thyroid should be palpated to rule out a goiter. The examination should focus on the presence of acne and axillary hair, with Tanner staging for breasts and pubic hair. Examination of the skin is important, because café au lait spots may be evidence of neurofibromatosis or McCune-Albright syndrome.

● **Clinical Pearls:**

- A family history of early puberty is helpful, because a trend toward earlier development is often simply familial and completely benign.
- Findings that raise the likelihood of true precocious puberty in girls are hyperpigmented areolae and a pale pink vaginal mucosa with a white discharge. A red, glistening mucosa is prepubertal, because it shows no evidence of estrogenization.
- Hirsutism and clitoromegaly point to the possibility of CAH.

DIAGNOSTIC CRITERIA

True precocious puberty is defined as the development of secondary sexual characteristics before 8 years in girls (with a new cut-off of 6 to 7 years proposed by the Lawson Wilkins Pediatric Endocrine Society [Kaplowitz et al., 1999]) or 9 years in boys.

True, or central, precocious puberty can be diagnosed by the demonstration of pubertal levels of gonadotropins and a pubertal response to GnRH stimulation. Both premature thelarche and premature adrenarche are benign, isolated, self-limited conditions that show a prepubertal response to GnRH (Lincoln & Zuber, 1998).

DIAGNOSTIC STUDIES

Laboratory tests for precocious puberty should include the following:

- Gonadotropins (LH and FSH)
- Estradiol or total testosterone
- Thyroxine (T_4) and thyroid-stimulating hormone (TSH)

If CAH is suspected (ie, with evidence of height acceleration, acne, adrenarche, and hirsutism), adrenal hormones studies should be ordered, including the following:

- 17-OH progesterone
- 17 pergnenolone
- DHEA (unsulfonated)
- Androstenedione
- Total testosterone

In all cases of premature thelarche, with or without other signs of puberty, a βHCG should be sent to rule out the possibility of an hCG-producing tumor. If androgen levels are increased and there is a suspicion of CAH, the test of choice is an ACTH-stimulation test. This test shows an elevation of androgens at baseline, with a marked rise in the precursor hormones after stimulation. A pelvic ultrasound can be useful in looking for ovarian tumors, ovarian cysts, and endometrial thickness.

▲ **Clinical Warning:** The provider is advised to consult with a pediatric endocrinologist should any questions arise about ordering or interpreting diagnostic studies. Positive study results warrant an endocrine referral.

MANAGEMENT

The gold standard of treatment for central precocious puberty is GnRH analogues. Not only do these agents decelerate the pace of puberty and even cause regression of secondary sexual characteristics, but they can also improve final height outcome. GnRH analogues offer the advantage of a powerful, sustained suppression of gonadotropins in a convenient monthly depot preparation, without significant side effects (Kauli et al., 1997).

GnRH analogues cause a tonic inhibition of the hypothalamic-pituitary-gonadal axis, causing significant suppression of gonadotropin secretion and consequently a decline in the levels of circulating sex steroids. This slows down growth cartilage activity and ultimately reduces growth velocity and skeletal maturation (Galluzzi, Salti, Bindi, Pasquini, & LaCauza, 1998).

In girls, there is a reduction of breast size and amount of pubic hair within the first 6 months of therapy. If menses were present prior to treatment, they stop. Pelvic ultrasound shows a decreased size of the uterus and ovaries. Potential side effects include recurrent hot flashes and moodiness.

In boys, there is similarly a reduction in testicular size and amount of pubic hair, along with a regression of acne, seborrhea, and frequency of penile erections. With treatment, aggressive behavior gradually diminishes, and self-esteem improves (Styne, 1997).

● **Clinical Pearl:** Target heights may or may not be affected by different treatments (Kaplowitz et al., 1999).

Indications for initiating GnRH analogue therapy include the following:

- Early pubertal development out of proportion to the child's emotional and cognitive development. This takes into consideration embarrassment, distress, or feelings of being different from peers owing to the appearance of secondary sexual characteristics. Perhaps more complicated is the array of physical, emotional, and cognitive issues inherent in the onset of menarche.
- Predicted final height, based on bone age, that is unacceptable to the family. This may involve factors such as self-esteem, socialization, and dating and even the practicality of such activities of daily living as reaching the pedals when driving.

Once therapy is started, children should be evaluated every 3 months, with follow-up visits and LH-releasing hormone stimulation testing to assess the efficacy of gonadotropin suppression. Similarly, the decision to stop treatment depends on the child's psychological ability to cope with and understand the progression of puberty, as well as on the bone age. When an acceptable height is achieved, when the patient and family are satisfied with that height, when the epiphyses are fused, or when a growth velocity of less than 4 cm per year is reached, then therapy is no longer indicated.

Growth Disorders

Normal growth means that the growth velocity is adequate for age. Girls tend to have an earlier, quicker growth spurt than boys. It occurs during Tanner stages II to III and prior to menses. The growth spurt for boys occurs during midpuberty, between Tanner stages III and IV, and usually lasts longer than in girls (Tanner, Whitehouse, & Takaishi, 1966; Tanner & Whitehouse, 1976; Guo et al., 1991). Table 60-1 provides guidelines for normal growth rates categorized by age.

Short stature means height that is below the third percentile for age (Lacey & Parken, 1974). The etiology of short stature can be either normal or pathologic. The most common causes are normal and include constitutional delay of growth and development (CDGD) and familial short stature (FSS) or a combination of the two. Growth hormone (GH) deficiency is an additional cause. These are compared in Table 60-2.

The pathologic causes are more numerous but much less frequent. Pathologic causes of short stature include endocrinologic disorders, gastrointestinal disorders, chromosomal disorders (including Turner syndrome), skeletal dysplasias, intrauterine growth retardation (IUGR) with failure to catch up, various syndromes, chronic disease, and psychosocial dwarfism (Lifshitz, 1996).

● **Clinical Pearl:** Suspicion of an endocrinologic etiology of short stature is strong in the case of suboptimal growth velocity with normal to excess weight gain.

Table 60–1. GUIDELINES FOR NORMAL GROWTH RATES CATEGORIZED BY AGE

Age (y)	Normal Growth Rate (Minimum Number of cm/y)
< 4	7 cm/y
4–6	6 cm/y
6–puberty	4.5 cm/y
Puberty	
Boys (Tanner III–IV)	10.3 cm/y
Girls (Tanner II–III)	9 cm/y

Table 60–2. COMPARISON OF DIAGNOSES FOR SHORT STATURE

	Familial Short Stature (FSS)	Constitutional Growth Delay (CGD)	Growth Hormone Deficiency (GHD)
Growth velocity	Slow during first 6–18 mo, then normal but < 5% after 2–3 y	Slow during first 2–3 y, then normal until a deceleration at 10–14 y, followed by a late pubertal growth spurt	Persistently slow, often apparent at puberty with lack of a growth spurt
Family history	Short stature	Delay in growth and puberty in parents	Variable
Bone age	Equal to chronologic age in simple FSS but is delayed when combined with CGD	2–4 y delayed	Generally delayed, but not as delayed as height age (age for which child's height falls at the 50%)
Final height	Short	Normal	Improved with GH treatment

ANATOMY, PHYSIOLOGY, AND PATHOLOGY

The secretion of GH is controlled mainly by the hypothalamus through the oppositional effects of GH-releasing hormone and somatostatin. At the level of the pituitary somatotropes, GH-releasing peptides function to stimulate GH release. GH is produced by the pituitary in a pulsatile fashion, with the most consistent surges occurring during the slow-wave phases 3 and 4 of sleep. GH produces its biologic effects through the actions of various insulin-like growth factors (IGFs) and insulin-like binding proteins (Rosenfeld et al., 1995).

Deficiencies can occur at various levels, including the production, secretion, and action of GH. Deficiency in GH qualifies as simple GH deficiency. Some children and adolescents are able to produce enough GH hormone after pharmacologic stimulation but have a neurosecretory defect (ie, the average of their own endogenous GH levels, when measured at 20-minute intervals overnight, is subnormal). With bioinactive GH, enough hormone is produced, but it is biologically inactive, unable to produce its desired effect on growth. Finally, defects in the GH receptor, such as in Laron dwarfism, cause GH resistance.

Endocrinologic Causes of Short Stature

Endocrinologic etiologies for short stature include the following:

- GH deficiency
- Hypopituitarism
- Hypothyroidism
- Hypercortisolism

Deficiency in GH is characterized by subnormal growth velocity, often with a drop in 2 percentiles on the curve, due to failure to secrete adequate GH levels in response to provocative stimulation. The incidence of classic GH deficiency is probably about 1 in 10,000. Bone age is generally delayed in GH-deficient children but not as delayed as height (that is, the age for which the child's height would fall at the 50th percentile) (Lifshitz, 1996). Although idiopathic GH deficiency is usually sporadic, it may also be familial (Rimoin, Merimee, & McKusick, 1966).

Hypopituitarism should be suspected in any patient with pathologic short stature who has a history of a disorder affecting the pituitary or any midline defect; medical care warrants involvement of a pediatric endocrinologist. Disorders affecting the pituitary include congenital malformations (particularly agenesis of the corpus callosum), tumors, infection, trauma, surgery, and radiation. All of these raise the possibility of hypopituitarism. GH deficiency may be isolated, but it may occur in conjunction with hypothyroidism, hypocortisolism, and deficiencies of gonadotropins and antidiuretic hormone. Even if hormone screening is initially normal, it is important to follow the pituitary hormone levels regularly, every 3 to 12 months, depending on clinical suspicion of deficiency and CNS defect.

Gastrointestinal Causes of Short Stature

Gastrointestinal etiologies of short stature include the following:

- Nutritional deficiency
- Inflammatory bowel disease
- Celiac disease

Other Causes of Short Stature

Other nonendocrine causes of short stature are related to chronic disease and sometimes occur as an outcome of disease treatment. Such diseases include but are not limited to the following:

- Cancer, with a history of radiation or chemotherapy
- Chronic renal failure
- Significant asthma
- Type 1 diabetes

The provider should consult with the appropriate specialist for clarification of the risk for short stature secondary to chronic disease or treatment effects. Referral to a pediatric endocrinologist for GH therapy is warranted.

EPIDEMIOLOGY

In recent decades, there has been a secular trend toward an increase in the tempo of growth and final adult height. This trend is generally more pronounced in children and adolescents of lower socioeconomic status. Secular trends in growth are important tools in evaluating changes in the status of a population's health, nutritional, and hygienic status. The continued acceleration in growth and maturation seems to indicate an approach toward optimal health (Hauspie, Vercauteren, & Susanne, 1997). This secular trend in the tempo of growth also involves earlier menarche, earlier peak height velocity, and a shortened growth cycle.

HISTORY AND PHYSICAL EXAMINATION

Illustrating previous growth on the growth curve is one of the most important pieces of information in the history. The profoundly low birth weight and length in premature infants may explain their poor growth until about 2 years of age. By that time, catch-up growth should have occurred. A steady tracking at or below but parallel to the fifth percentile with adequate growth velocity could indicate FSS. Growth deceleration during the first 2 to 3 years of life suggests CDGD.

▲ **Clinical Warning:** A height measurement below the third percentile for age, a growth velocity of less than 2 in a year, or a decline across at least 2 growth percentiles suggests the possibility of a pathologic condition and requires referral to a pediatric endocrinologist.

Family history is critical. Often a combination of CDGD and FSS underlies a child's short stature. Parental heights are used to calculate the midparental height. A history of late menarche in the mother or a late growth spurt in the father suggests the possibility of CDGD. Short relatives increase the likelihood of FSS but could also represent adults whose GH deficiency was untreated.

Anthropometric measurements may provide helpful information in the physical examination. Disproportionately short limbs may be seen in achondroplasia, hypochondroplasia, and Turner's syndrome. A disproportionately short spine may be present in spondyloepiphyseal dysplasia or scoliosis. A shortened fourth metacarpal is frequent in Turner's syndrome and pseudopseudohypoparathyroidism. Dentition is usually significantly delayed

in children with untreated hypothyroidism or GH deficiency, whereas mild delays may be present in CDGD. Particular dysmorphic features may diagnose such syndromes as Turner's, Russel-Silver, Williams, and Prader-Willi (Lifshitz, 1996).

Children with CDGD, as well as those with GH deficiency, generally appear younger than their chronologic age. CDGD correlates with delay of puberty. GH-deficient children often retain "cherubic facies" and "baby fat" and therefore appear younger. This is probably related to the lack of GH's effect on increasing lean body mass relative to body fat.

DIAGNOSTIC CRITERIA AND STUDIES

The history, physical examination, growth chart, appropriate laboratory data, and bone age help differentiate among the differential diagnoses. Stimulation testing is the gold standard in diagnosing true GH deficiency. The pharmacologic agents most commonly used are clonidine, L-dopa, arginine, and glucagon. Exercise is a nonpharmacologic stimulus that is used less frequently.

Provocative GH testing has several limitations. It is nonphysiologic and age-dependent. Testing relies on GH assays of variable accuracy and arbitrary definitions of a normal response. Testing effectively diagnoses a child with severe GH deficiency but is not as effective in diagnosing a child with partial GH deficiency. Provocative GH testing is expensive and uncomfortable, and the provocative stimuli may have side effects. Finally, the results are not always reproducible (Rosenfeld et al., 1995).

Comprehensive screening tests include laboratory and radiologic studies. Several laboratory tests need to be obtained, as described in Table 60-3.

A magnetic resonance imaging scan of the brain with contrast, with special attention to the pituitary and hypothalamus, is recommended in patients who fail GH stimulation testing with all GH levels less than 5 ng/mL. It is also warranted if there are any associated midline defects, other pituitary hormone deficiencies, or a particularly abnormal growth curve.

Table 60–3.   DIAGNOSTIC STUDIES FOR SHORT STATURE

Test	Purpose
SMAC	Examines kidney and liver function and looks for acidosis, which could represent renal tubular acidosis or metabolic disease. Calcium, phosphorus, and alkaline phosphatase screen for metabolic bone and kidney disease.
CBC with differential and ESR	Anemia and an elevated ESR can be subtle clues to chronic inflammatory bowel disease, even in the absence of gastrointestinal symptoms.
T_4 and TSH	
IGF-1 and IGF-BP3	Because GH is secreted in periodic surges, random GH levels are not reliable measures of GH secretion. Therefore, markers of GH are used for screening.
In addition, markers of celiac disease: Antigliadan antibodies (IgA and IgG) Endomysial antibodies Antireticulin antibodies	A celiac panel is appropriate if there is poor weight gain, abdominal pain, bloating, or gassiness.
Chromosomes	Any girl with short stature who is prepubertal requires this study to rule out Turner syndrome or Turner mosaicism.
Radiologic test: bone age	A bone age provides critical information for making a diagnosis. In GH deficiency, a bone age will show delay, but not as much delay as a height age will demonstrate.

CBC = complete blood count; ESR = erythrocyte sedimentation rate; GH = growth hormone; IGF = insulin-like growth factor; IGF-BP = insulin-like binding proteins; T_4 = thyroxine; TSH = thyroid stimulating hormone.

MANAGEMENT

● **Clinical Pearl:** FSS requires no treatment. CDGD is characterized by spontaneous catch-up growth later on, and it also requires no treatment. However, if there are psychosocial issues related to physical discrepancies relative to peers, oxandralone provides an option. This nonaromatizable androgen accelerates linear growth and pubertal progression without compromising the final adult height. Because it is not aromatized to estrogen, which is responsible for advancing the bone age, it does not cause the epiphyses to fuse prematurely.

Growth hormone therapy is Food and Drug Administration approved for GH deficiency, Turner syndrome, and chronic renal failure. It has not been definitively proven to be effective in improving the final height of non–GH-deficient children. The general consensus is that GH does improve height velocity during the time it is administered but does not increase final adult height above predicted height (The Drug and Therapeutics Committee of the Lawson Wilkins Pediatric Endocrine Society, 1995).

Rekers-Mombarg et al. (1998) tested three different dosage regimens in children with idiopathic short stature over a 4-year period. They found that although there was an increase in height during the treatment period, there was also an advancement in bone age, suggesting only a modest impact on final height. Similarly, data from Coutant et al. (1997) suggest that GH treatment has a limited effect on final height in short children born with IUGR.

Growth retardation is common in children who are on long-term treatment with high-dose glucocorticoids. Glucocorticoids suppress growth at virtually every level of the hypothalamic-pituitary axis and beyond. Allen et al. (1998) found that GH treatment counterbalanced the growth-suppressing effects of glucocorticoids, with the mean response being a doubling of baseline growth rate. Responsiveness to GH, however, correlated negatively with glucocorticoid dose.

There are few, if any, side effects of GH therapy. Due to the effect of GH on fluid retention, there is a potential risk of pseudotumor cerebri, which resolves after treatment is discontinued. Because GH causes an increase in IGF-I, some authors have expressed concern about an increased risk of malignancy (American Academy of Pediatrics, 1997). However, when such risk factors as previous malignancy and radiation exposure are taken into account, there does not appear to be any increased risk. Although cases of pancreatitis and prepubertal gynecomastia have been described in association with GH, no direct cause-and-effect relation has been documented.

Hypothyroidism has been described as a possible side effect, because GH treatment clearly affects the hypothalamic-pituitary axis. Slipped capital femoral epiphysis may occur as a result of uneven growth rates of the acetabulum and femoral head. Finally, GH therapy may increase the growth of pigmented nevi, but there has been no occurrence of premalignant transformation (The Drug and Therapeutics Committee of the Lawson Wilkins Pediatric Endocrine Society, 1995).

The decision to initiate GH treatment should be made in consultation with the child, the parents, and a pediatric endocrinologist skilled in this area. Medication is administered subcutaneously and should occur with endocrine management. GH therapy generally is administered for 6 to 7 consecutive nights in a dose of 0.3 mg/kg per week for GH deficiency. Dosages for chronic renal failure and Turner syndrome are slightly higher. Dosing three times a week has not proven to be as effective.

▲ **Clinical Warning:** Because of rapid changes in the science and management of growth anomalies, any patient who needs GH therapy should be referred to a pediatric endocrinologist.

Other treatment options have recently become available for treating growth-related conditions. GH-releasing hormone may be beneficial in treating conditions involving hypothalamic dysfunction. Another newly developed pharmaceutical for growth is a GH-releasing peptide called hexarelin. This potent secretagogue was compared with GH-releasing hormone in patients with homozygous α-thalassemia, who often present with abnormalities of endocrine function, such as growth. It evoked a rapid rise in GH in these patients that was significantly higher than that caused by GH-releasing hormone. It may potentially be a beneficial therapeutic agent in treating GH-deficient states (Tolis et al., 1997; Frindik, Kemp, & Sy, 1999).

▲ **Clinical Warning:** The provider should obtain a pediatric endocrinology consultation or referral before making a clinical decision about undertaking treatment with any pharmaceutical agent for GH therapy.

Congenital Hypothyroidism

Over the past 15 to 20 years, routine neonatal screening for congenital hypothyroidism was implemented in industrialized countries. This screening has been remarkably successful in eradicating severe mental deficiency as a result of untreated congenital hypothyroidism.

Screening for congenital hypothyroidism differs from country to country and even from state to state. It involves either a primary TSH screen or a primary T_4 screen with secondary TSH screening on the lowest percentile T_4 values (eg, the lowest 10%).

▲ **Clinical Warnings:**

- Primary TSH screening picks up many newborns who have a normal surge of TSH after delivery but require no treatment. It can miss secondary or tertiary hypothyroidism.
- Primary T_4 screening picks up many premature newborns who have transient hypothyroxinemia of prematurity with a normal TSH. These infants are generally not treated. Primary T_4 screening can miss compensated hypothyroidism.
- Thyroid-binding globulin (TBG) deficiency may present as a false-positive result or as a low total T_4 with a normal TSH. The diagnosis of TBG deficiency is supported by a normal free T_4 and a high T_3 uptake, and it is confirmed by a low TBG level.

● **Clinical Pearl:** A recent Canadian study compared the diagnostic accuracy of the two tests and concluded that in terms of reducing false-positive and false-negative cases, the primary TSH screening is more effective for mass screening than the combined T_4/TSH method (Wang et al., 1998).

ANATOMY, PHYSIOLOGY, AND PATHOLOGY

Normally, the TSH level surges to about 80 mU/L just after delivery. This surge is associated with the clamping of the cord and exposure to a colder environment. During the first 24 hours of life, the TSH declines rapidly and then more gradually to less than 10 mU/L after the first week of life. A genetic basis for congenital hypothyroidism has been demonstrated on the TSH beta gene, the PIT1 gene, and the NIS gene (Tatsumi, Miyai, & Amino, 1998).

● **Clinical Pearl:** Because of the TSH surge in the immediate postpartum period, newborn screening should be performed as close to discharge as possible to avoid false-positive results.

Although gene mutations have been described as causing a few cases of thyroid dysgenesis (Abramowicz et al., 1997; Tatsumi et al., 1998), most cases have no common thread to explain the etiology. The incidence of compensated or transient primary hypothyroidism can be as high as 1 in 10 newborns. The main cause is iodine deficiency (Delange, 1998).

Iodine deficiency has a profound effect on neonatal screening, increasing the rate of false-positives and can cause transient and permanent cases of congenital hypothyroidism. Without iodine deficiency, the frequency of neonatal TSH greater than 10 mU/L is less than 3%. The frequency is 3% to 19.9% in disorders of mild iodine deficiency; 20% to 39.9% in moderate iodine deficiency; and greater than 40% in severe iodine deficiency. Most countries with iodine deficiency implement primary TSH measurement as part of neonatal screening to detect cases of transient and permanent hypothyroidism and to control iodine deficiency (Delange, 1998).

▲ **Clinical Warning:** Neonates seem to be more sensitive to iodine deficiency than adults; they exhibit more frequent elevations in TSH than adults for a similar degree of iodine deficiency.

This may be explained by a low iodine content in the neonatal thyroid, requiring an accelerated iodine turnover rate. This iodine turnover rate is 1% in adults, 17% in iodine-replete neonates, and as high as 62% and 125% in cases of moderate and severe iodine deficiency, respectively. An accelerated iodine turnover rate requires hyperstimulation of TSH (Delange, 1998; Klett, 1998).

Worldwide, iodine deficiency is the most common cause of hypothyroidism. Various organizations, such as the World Health Organization, are sponsoring iodide supplementation programs to help eradicate this most common preventable form of hypothyroidism (Sperling, 1996).

There is increasing evidence that environmental toxins have been implicated in thyroid hormone resistance. The moderate impairment of thyroid function seen in thyroid hormone resistance may cause mild behavioral and intellectual abnormalities, such as attention deficit hyperactivity disorder (Hauser et al., 1998).

EPIDEMIOLOGY

The incidence of congenital hypothyroidism is 1 in 3000 to 1 in 4000 (Klett, 1998). Differences in the incidence of congenital hypothyroidism are more likely due to the type of screening method or to iodine deficiency thyroid disorders than to any ethnic variability. Congenital hypothyroidism results from an absent or defective gland, hypothalamic-pituitary anomalies, or iatrogenic factors. These are presented in Table 60-4.

Congenital hypothyroidism is also seen in conjunction with concomitant anomalies, such as Down syndrome (Chao, Want, & Hwang, 1997). This fact was validated by Roberts et al. (1997), who examined the epidemiology of congenital hypothyroidism and associated birth defects in Atlanta, Georgia, from 1979 to 1992 by linking data from two population-based registries. Ninety-seven infants had been diagnosed with congenital hypothyroidism through newborn screening (1 in 5000 live births); 87 newborns were found to have primary hypothyroidism; and 10 had second-

Table 60-4.   CLASSIFICATION OF CONGENITAL HYPOTHYROIDISM

Thyroid Dysgenesis	Percent of Cases	Prevalence	Subcategory/Pathology
Thyroid dysgenesis	75%	1 in 4000	Agenesis—absent thyroid tissue ($^1/_3$ of cases) Ectopy—thyroid tissue present somewhere between the base of the tongue and the anterior mediastinum Hypoplasia—small gland in the appropriate position
Thyroid dyshormonogenesis	10%	1 in 30,000	Defect in iodide trapping Defect in organification Defect in thyroglobulin Deficiency of iodotyrosine TSH unresponsiveness
Transient hypothyroidism	10%	1 in 40,000	Secondary to iodine deficiency Secondary to drugs (ie, PTU) Secondary to maternal antibodies (ie, Grave's disease) Idiopathic
Hypothalamic-pituitary hypothyroidism	5%	1 in 100,000	Hypothalamic pituitary defect Isolated deficiency of TSH Panhypopituitarism (ie, defects in the PIT1 gene) Thyroid hormone resistance (including abnormalities of hormone binding to the receptor, and abnormalities of the receptor itself)

PTU = propylthiouracil; TSH = thyroid stimulating hormone.
Adapted with permission from Sperling, M. A. (1996). *Pediatric endocrinology.* Philadelphia: W.B. Saunders.

ary hypothyroidism. The inference was made that babies with Down syndrome have a 35-fold increased risk for primary congenital hypothyroidism compared with the general population. Babies with primary congenital hypothyroidism in this study had a 2.2-fold increased risk for major structural abnormalities.

Oakley et al. (1998) reported similar findings in their investigation conducted in Scotland between August 1979 and December 1993. Of 344 babies with elevated TSH levels, 31 (9%) had at least one malformation; 16 had dysmorphic syndromes (including five with Down syndrome); 12 had cardiac anomalies; and 15 had noncardiac malformations.

HISTORY AND PHYSICAL EXAMINATION

Because congenital hypothyroidism is detected on newborn screening by 2 weeks of age, there is usually not enough time for signs or symptoms of the disease to develop. The examiner should ask questions about excessive sleepiness, poor feeding, and constipation. Physical examination should look for an enlarged anterior fontanelle, widely open posterior fontanelle, jaundice, and an umbilical hernia.

DIAGNOSTIC CRITERIA

An initial TSH level greater than 200 mU/L is unequivocally diagnostic and generally represents thyroid agenesis or ectopia. A TSH level that is increased even to 30 to 50 mU/L on the first day of life should be retested, because it could simply represent the normal postnatal surge. The diagnosis of congenital hypothyroidism can be made of a repeated level showing that it is not declining and approaching normal range. There is a subset of infants whose TSH levels decline gradually, taking up to 4 to 6 weeks to reach the normal range; they require no treatment.

DIAGNOSTIC STUDIES

Diagnostic studies include laboratory and radiologic assessments. Laboratory studies include T_4 and TSH levels, which are the minimal diagnostic tests required. A free T_4 level is more accurate, because it eliminates the effect of TBG. Maternal estrogen causes a rise in TBG and thus raises the total T_4 level. It does not affect the free T_4.

Radiographic studies include an I-123 thyroid scan with 4- and 24-hour uptake. This scan is diagnostically helpful, especially in severe cases in which the initial TSH is greater than 200 mU/L, thus proving thyroid agenesis or ectopy (such as a lingual thyroid).

MANAGEMENT

Untreated congenital hypothyroidism can result in severe, irreversible mental retardation. In the first generation of children identified by newborn screening, there was evidence that congenital hypothyroidism had significant intellectual sequelae. Children with severe congenital hypothyroidism (ie, those with a low T_4 level or a marked delay in bone age) showed a loss of 6 to 19 IQ points. Recent studies suggest that this can be ameliorated by earlier diagnosis and treat-

ment (2 weeks instead of 4 to 5 weeks as in the early years of screening) and by using a higher starting dose of levothyroxine (10–15 mcg/kg/d instead of 5–8 mcg/kg/d) (Leger et al., 1997; Van Vliet, 1999).

It has been shown that an initial daily levothyoxine dose of 37.5 mcg/d requires fewer dose changes than a dose of 25 mcg/d. The dose is adjusted based on thyroid function tests in conjunction with the clinical picture. The American Academy of Pediatrics recommends frequent testing of thyroid function, particularly during the first 2 years of life when the brain is developing. Rapid growth may necessitate multiple dosage changes (Vogiatzi & Kirkland, 1997).

Guidelines for endocrine follow-up are monthly for the first year of life, every 2 months for the second year, every 3 months for the second to fifth years, and every 4 months thereafter. Every 6 months is adequate with increasing age as the levothyroxine dose stabilizes. It is important that the provider remain informed of endocrine management results. Conversely, any change in the child's normal level of functioning noted by the clinician, either in the course of well child visits or in treating episodic illness, should be reported to the pediatric endocrine specialist.

What to Tell Parents

Early detection and treatment of congenital hypothyroidism allow for normal prepubertal and pubertal growth, with achievement of normal adult height (Dickerman & De Vries, 1997). The provider can be very reassuring to worried parents that their child with thyroid dysfunction will be able to grow and develop normally. The parents' role in treatment participation includes working with the practitioner and the pediatric endocrinologist in managing the patient's therapy.

COMMUNITY RESOURCES

The Endocrine Society is an excellent resource for print and Web materials, including patient materials, for all endocrine disorders.

The Endocrine Society
4350 East West Highway, Suite 500
Bethesda, MD 20814-4410
Telephone: (301) 941-0200
Toll-free: (800) ENDO-SOC
Fax: (301) 941-0259
http://www.endo-society.org

The American Thyroid Association, Inc.
Townhouse Office Park
55 Old Nyack Turnpike, Suite 611
Nanuet, New York 10954
Fax: (914) 623-3736
Internet address: *http://www.thyroid.org*

The American Thyroid Association is a good resource for print and web materials, including Guidelines for Physicians, which provide up-to-date, approved management criteria for thyroid disorders. Patient materials are also available. The web site also provides links to other approved web sites.

European Thyroid Association
Internet address: *http://www.uwcm.ac.uk/uwcm/md/ETA.html*

Latin American Thyroid Society
Internet address: *http://www.lats.org*

National Institutes of Health
Warren Grant Magnuson Clinical Center
Internet address: *http://www.cc.nih.gov*

Provides up-to-date clinical resources.

Gland Central: Your Hub of Thyroid Health
Internet address: *http://www.glandcentral.com*

This site is approved by the American Thyroid Association and provides valid and reliable patient information.

REFERENCES

Abramowicz, M. J., Duprez, L., Parma, J., et al. (1997). Familial congenital hypothyroidism due to inactivating mutation of the thyrotropin receptor causing profound hypoplasia of the thyroid gland. *Journal of Clinical Investigation, 99,* 3018–3024.

Allen, D. B., Julius, J. R., Breen, T. J., et al. (1998). Treatment of glucocorticoid-induced growth suppression with growth hormone. *Journal of Clinical Endocrinology and Metabolism, 83,* 2824–2829.

American Academy of Pediatrics Committee on Drugs and Committee on Bioethics. (1997). Considerations related to the use of recombinant human growth hormone in children. *Pediatrics, 99,* 122–128.

Braunstein, G. D. (1993). Gynecomastia. *New England Journal of Medicine, 328,* 490–495.

Chao, T., Want, J. R., & Hwang, B. (1997). Congenital hypothyroidism and concomitant anomalies. *Journal of Pediatric Endocrinology and Metabolism, 10,* 217–221.

Coutant, R., Carel, J. C., Letrait, M., et al. (1998). Short stature associated with intrauterine growth retardation: Final height of untreated and growth hormone-treated children. *Journal of Clinical Endocrinology and Metabolism, 83,* 1070–1074.

Delange, F. (1998). Screening for congenital hypothyroidism used as an indicator of the degree of iodine deficiency and of its control. *Thyroid, 8,* 1185–1192.

Dickerman, Z., & DeVries, L. (1997). Prepubertal and pubertal growth, timing and duration of puberty and attained adult height in patients with congenital hypothyroidism detected by the neonatal screening programme for congenital hypothyroidism? a longitudinal study. *Clinical Endocrinology, 47,* 649–654.

Frindik, J. P., Kemp, S. F., & Sy, J. P. (1999). Effects of recombinant human growth hormone on height and skeletal maturation in growth hormone-deficient children with and without severe pretreatment bone age delay. *Hormone Research, 51,* 15–19.

Galluzzi, F., Salti, R., Bindi, G., Pasquini, E., & LaCauza, C. (1998). Adult height comparison between boys and girls with precocious puberty after long-term gonadotrophin-releasing hormone analogue therapy. *Acta Paediatrica, 87,* 521–527.

The Drug and Therapeutics Committee of the Lawson Wilkins Pediatric Endocrine Society. (1995). Guidelines for the use of growth hormone in children with short stature. *Journal of Pediatrics, 27,* 857–867.

Guo, S., Roche, A. F., Foman, S. J., et al. (1991). Reference data on gains in weight, and length during the first two years of life. *Journal of Pediatrics, 119,* 355–362.

Hauser, P., McMillin, J. M., & Bhatara, V. S. (1998). Resistance to thyroid hormone: Implications for neurodevelopmental research on the effects of thyroid hormone disruptors. *Toxicology and Industrial Health, 14,* 85–101.

Hauspie, R. C., Vercauteren, M., & Susanne, C. (1997). Secular changes in growth and maturation: An update. *Acta Paediatr, Suppl 423,* 20–27.

Herman-Giddens, M. E., Slore, E. J., Wasserman, R. C., Bourdony, C. J., Bhapkar, M. V., Koch, G. G., & Hasemeier, C. M. (1997). Secondary sexual characteristics and menses in young girls seen in office practice: A study from the Pediatric Research in Office Settings Network. *Pediatrics, 99,* 505–512.

Kaplowitz, P. H., Oberfield, S. E., & the Drug and Therapeutics and Executive Committees of the Lawson Wilkins Pediatric

Endocrine Society. (1999). Reexamination of the age limit for defining when puberty is precocious in girls in the United States: Implications for evaluation and treatment. *Pediatrics, 104*(4), Part 1 of 2, 936–941.

Kauli, R., Galatzer, A., Kornreich, L., Lazar, L., Pertzelan, A., & Laron, Z. (1997). Final height of girls with central precocious puberty, untreated versus treated with cyproterone acetate or GnRH analogue. *Hormone Research, 47,* 54–61.

Klett, M. (1998). Epidemiology of congenital hypothyroidism. *Journal of Pediatric Endocrinology and Metabolism, 11,* 173–176.

Lacey, K. A., & Parken, J. M. (1974). Causes of short stature. A community study of children in Newcastle-upon-Tyne. *Lancet, 1,* 42–45.

Leger, J., Ruiz, J. C., Guibourdence, J., et al. (1997). Bone mineral density and metabolism in children with congenital hypothyroidism after prolonged L-thyroxine therapy. *Acta Paediatr, 86,* 704–710.

Lifshitz, F. (1996). *Pediatric endocrinology* (pp. 186–187). (3rd ed.). New York: Marcel Dekker.

Lincoln, E. A., & Zuber, T. J. (1998). Management of precocious puberty. *Hospital Practice (Office Edition), 33,* 173–176.

Murkies, A. L., Wilcox, G., & Davis, S. R. (1998). Phytoestrogens. *Journal of Clinical Endocrinology and Metabolism, 83,* 297–303.

Neely, E. K. (1999). Precocious puberty. *International Symposium on A Current Review of Pediatric Endocrinology, April,* 15–25.

Oakley, G. A., Muir, T., Ray, M. et al. (1998). Increased incidence of congenital malformations in children with transient thyroid-stimulating hormone elevation on neonatal screening. *Journal of Pediatrics, 132,* 726–730.

Palmert, M. R., Radovick, S., & Boepple, P. A. (1998). Leptin levels in children with central precocious puberty. *Journal of Clinical Endocrinology and Metabolism, 83,* 2260–2265.

Pescovitz, O. H., Comite, F., Hench, K., et al. (1986). The NIH experience with precocious puberty: Diagnostic subgroups and response to short-term luteinizing hormone releasing hormone analogue therapy. *Journal of Pediatrics, 108,* 47–54.

Rekers-Mombarg, L. T. M., Massa, G. G., Wit, J. M., et al. (1998). Growth hormone therapy with three dosage regimens in children with idiopathic short stature. *Journal of Pediatrics, 132,* 455–460.

Rimoin, D. L., Merimee, T. J., & McKusick, V. A. (1966). Growth hormone deficiency in man: An isolated, recessively inherited defect. *Science, 152,* 1635.

Roberts, H. E., Moore, C. A., Fernhoff, P. M., et al. (1997). Population study of congenital hypothyroidism and associated birth defects, Atlanta, 1979-1992. *American Journal of Medical Genetics, 71,* 29–32.

Rosenfeld, R. G., Albertsson-Wikland, K., Cassorla, F., et al. (1995). Diagnostic controversy: The diagnosis of childhood growth hormone deficiency revisited. *Journal of Clinical Endocrinology and Metabolism, 80,* 1532–1540.

Sperling, M. A. (1996). *Pediatric endocrinology* (pp. 157–161). Philadelphia: W.B. Saunders.

Styne, D. M. (1997). New aspects in the diagnosis and treatment of pubertal disorders. *Pediatric Clinics of North America, 44,* 505–529.

Tanner, J. M., & Whitehouse, R. H. (1976). Clinical longitudinal standard for height, weight, height velocity, weight velocity, and stages of puberty. *Archives of Disease in Childhood, 51,* 170–171.

Tanner, J. M., Whitehouse, R. H., & Takaishi, M. (1966). Standards from birth to maturity for height, weight, height velocity, and weight velocity in British children. *Archives of Disease in Childhood, 41,* 613–616.

Tatsumi, K., Miyai, K., & Amino, N. (1998). Genetic basis of congenital hypothyroidism: Abnormalities in the TSHbeta gene, the PIT1 gene, and the NIS gene. *Clinical Chemistry and Laboratory Medicine, 36,* 652–659.

Tham, D. M., Gardner, C. K., & Haskell, W. L. (1998). Potential health benefits of dietary phytoestrogens: A review of the clinical, epidemiological, and mechanistic evidence. *Journal of Clinical Endocrinology and Metabolism, 83,* 2223–2235.

Tolis, F., Karydis, I., Markousis, V., Karagiorga, M., et al. (1997). Growth hormone release by the novel GH releasing peptide hexarelin in patients with homozygous B-thalassemia. *Journal of Pediatric Endocrinology and Metabolism, 10,* 35–40.

Van Vliet, G. (1999). Neonatal hypothyroidism: Treatment and outcome. *Thyroid, 9,* 79–84.

Vogiatzi, M. G., & Kirkland, J. L. (1997). Frequency and necessity of thyroid function tests in neonates and infants with congenital hypothyroidism. *Pediatrics, 100,* E6.

Wang, S. T., Pizzolato, S., & Demshar, H. P. (1998). Diagnostic effectiveness of TSH screening and of T4 with secondary TSH screening for newborn congenital hypothyroidism. *Clinica Chimica Acta, 274,* 151–158.

Diabetes Mellitus

• CAROL GREEN-HERNANDEZ, PhD, FNP-C, and PAVEL FORT, MD

INTRODUCTION

Diabetes in childhood is a devastating diagnosis for the patient and family, and carries the potential for an altered quality of life and a decreased life span. However, such outcomes need not always occur. This chapter provides information about the diagnosis and management of several variants of diabetes, including type 1 and nonautoimmune variants, type 2 of adolescence, and maturity-onset diabetes of the young (MODY, or type 3). Strategies are emphasized for developing and maintaining a successful partnership with the patient and family in all aspects of primary care. The essentials for successful comanagement of the patient with a pediatric endocrinology team specializing in diabetes are highlighted.

ANATOMY, PHYSIOLOGY, AND PATHOLOGY

Type 1 diabetes mellitus has several variants, including autoimmune type 1 diabetes, nonautoimmune diabetes of infancy, and idiopathic forms of the disease. These each are physiologically different from type 2 diabetes of adolescence, and each of these in turn differs from the autosomal dominant MODY (type 3).

Type 1 Diabetes Mellitus

Autoimmune Type 1 Diabetes Mellitus

Type 1 diabetes is highly correlated with absence of insulin secretory reserve, secondary to beta cell destruction. Type 1 disease is an autoimmune process that is associated with genetic polymorphism in the HLA class II region and also involves component regions of classes I and III (Chervonsky et al., 1997; Ma et al., 1997; Dorman, 1997; Lan et al., 1998; Juneja, 1999). Type 1 diabetes is characterized by destruction of beta cells by glutamic acid decarboxylase antibodies and is therefore classified as immune-mediated diabetes. Autoimmune type 1 diabetes eventually leads to significant infiltration of islet cells by T cells, leading to their scarring and, ultimately, destruction of functioning beta cells for months to years.

Other factors are interwoven with the autoimmune component of type 1 pathogenesis. These factors include the child's genetic background, the perinatal experience, birth weight (both high and low) (Minior et al., 1998), and early exposure to environmental triggers for disease (Klemetti et al., 1998). In addition, the genes and alleles for type 1 appear to differ from population to population (Akerblom, 1998; Dorman, 1997).

The thymus appears to play a dual role: Insulin-like growth factor II (IGF-II) is involved in T-cell development and T-cell negative selection. It is conceivable that defective thymic censorship of the antigen-antibody to insulin may be an important factor in the pathogenesis of type 1 diabetes (Geenen et al., 1998; Like et al., 1982).

The role of environmental triggers in type 1 development is similarly confusing. It is not yet clear whether only one significant exposure to a trigger is enough for ensuing pathogenesis or whether several exposures to a variety of triggers are required (Greenbaum et al., 1999). The question begs to be asked: Do different populations require different triggers, depending on genetic predeterminants? What is clear is that type 1 diabetes is multigenic, its pathogenesis being an outcome of environmental triggers interfacing with a genetically susceptible host.

Clearly, environmental chemical toxins can play an important role in beta cell destruction. Nitrosourea compounds, rodenticides, and streptozocin have all been demonstrated to cause immune-mediated type 1 diabetes (Kaufman, 1997). Fetal exposure to nitrites and nitrates in food and water also have been hypothesized as causative agents of beta-cell destruction (Dorman, 1997).

In recent years, one oft-debated environmental trigger is nutrition. Both cow's milk and meat proteins have been implicated. Several studies have examined the role of cow's milk exposure and type 1 pathogenesis in young children (Dorman, 1997; Saukkonen et al., 1998; Dahlquist, 1998). Saukkonen and colleagues found that Finnish children who express type 1 disease have higher levels of cow's milk antibodies and decreased IgM antibodies to cow's milk formula than sibling controls matched for HLA-DQB1 genotype. The researchers' findings suggest that genetically susceptible children who are exposed to cow's milk itself in their first year of life are at greater risk for later type 1 diabetes.

Population-based studies in diverse cultures and ethnic groups suggest that an environmental trigger may be operant in the growing worldwide incidence of type 1 diabetes (Diabetes Epidemiology Research International Group, 1988, 1990; Green et al., 1992; Karvonen et al., 1993; Dahlquist & Mustonen, 1994; Dorman et al. 1996; Perez-Bravo et al., 1996; Dahlquist, 1998). For example, there is growing speculation that the increasing incidence of type 1 disease among Japanese children may involve an increased propensity for including meat products in the diet. This dietary change is a marked one, compared with the traditional eating habits of previous generations (Dahlquist, 1998). Nevertheless, more work needs to be done in different population groups before a more definitive statement regarding type 1 triggers and disease incidence can be made.

Nonautoimmune Diabetes of Infancy

Because nonautoimmune diabetes of infancy does not differ from type 1 in clinical presentation, the infant presenting in a ketoacidotic state may be misdiagnosed as having type 1 disease. In fact, they are two different and distinct entities. Nonautoimmune diabetes of infancy does not include destruction of beta cells among its sequelae.

Several forms of nonautoimmune diabetes of infancy have been described, including diabetes secondary to congenital agenesis of the pancreas and diabetes occurring as part of the autosomal recessive syndrome of polycystic kidney disease (Zerres et al., 1994). The most frequently seen variant is transient neonatal diabetes mellitus (TNDM). TNDM is still a rare occurrence. The pathogenesis of TNDM is not known, although it may be a logical result of immature beta cell function. This is the reason it is termed *transient*. In transient disease, the infant will mature out of the temporarily diabetic state (Attia et al., 1998).

Transient neonatal diabetes mellitus has been described as developing spontaneously in normal and in low birth weight infants. TNDM has also been observed to occur in infants from the same nuclear family (Attia et al., 1998; Karl & Heiner, 1995). Common features in TNDM presentation include very young age (typically between 1 and 2 months) and diabetic ketoacidosis. Obviously, the latter occurrence may lead the provider to assign a preliminary diagnosis of type 1 diabetes to the child. Unlike in true type 1 disease, insulin therapy usually can be discontinued after a couple of months, although Karl and Heiner reported a case that required insulin therapy for 18 months. Insulin treatment is no longer necessary when the infant's innate beta cell function has matured enough to take on the task of endogenous insulin production. TNDM generally has no further consequences once endogenous beta cell function ensues. However, diabetes recurrence in previously stabilized children has been reported (Attia et al., 1998; Karl & Heiner, 1995).

▲ **Clinical Warning:** On the off-chance that the diabetes recurs later in childhood, infants treated for TNDM should continue to be monitored for diabetes.

● **Clinical Pearl:** Adequate diabetes prevention strategies should be taught to these children and their families for lifelong prevention and delay of later diabetes (Hahl et al., 1998; Knip, 1998).

Idiopathic Type 1 Diabetes Mellitus

Like immune-mediated type 1 disease, idiopathic diabetes is characterized by absence of insulin secretory reserve. As in TNDM and autoimmune type 1 diabetes, patients with idiopathic type 1 diabetes are subject to ketoacidosis (American Diabetes Association [ADA], 1997b). Permanent insulinopenia that is not associated with an autoimmune disease process is rare (Kaufman, 1997).

Diabetes that results from cystic fibrosis (CF) exemplifies nonimmune-mediated type 1 disease, yet it also shares features with type 2 diabetes. Ketoacidosis is a rare event in diabetes of CF, although it may be present at the time of diagnosis in cases in which prolonged hyperglycemia was unrecognized (Moran et al., 1998).

Type 2 Diabetes Mellitus

Traditional models of diabetes classification place type 2 disease firmly in adulthood. This is no longer true; diagnosis of adolescents and occasionally younger children with type 2 disease is becoming increasingly commonplace. Type 2 diabetes is a polygenic disease that occurs as an outcome of long-term insulin excess and concomitant insulin resistance. Sometimes this scenario ends with insulin deficiency, because compensatory hyperinsulinemia cannot override insulin resistance. At levels of 140 mg/dL or more, glucose is toxic to beta cells and to target tissues where insulin works.

Unlike type 1 disease, the insulin deficiency of type 2 disease is not absolute. Exogenous insulin administration cannot override the body's resistance to endogenous insulin at this point in type 2 pathogenesis.

Type 2 disease of adolescence is more common in obese children of color than in their Caucasian peers who are overweight. It is also seen in children of mothers who had gestational diabetes, regardless of race or ethnicity (ADA, 2000a). Obesity plays a central role in the pathogenesis of type 2 diabetes in part because of the metabolic derangements, including excessive insulin secretion, that can accompany obesity (Kaufman, 1997; Scott et al., 1997; Glaser & Jones, 1998; Hanson et al., 1998; Slyper, 1998). The extent of hyperinsulinism and insulin resistance that occur secondary to obesity seems to vary from one ethnic group to another.

Otherwise healthy adolescents with no first-degree family history of diabetes were studied by Arslanian and Suprasongsin (1996). They found that African American adolescents exhibited increased insulin production and decreased insulin sensitivity compared with young Caucasian subjects. Their findings correspond with similar population-based studies of North American adolescents of African, Pima, Ojibwa-Cree, Hispanic, and Japanese heritage (Pettitt et al., 1993; Islam et al., 1995; Haffner et al., 1996; Glaser & Jones, 1998; Dean et al., 1998; Libman et al., 1998; Boyle et al., 1999), as well as Central American youth in Veracruz, Mexico (Aude Rueda et al., 1998).

● **Clinical Pearl:** The outcome of delayed glycolysis and glycogenolysis in infants of very low birth weight (ie, lacking in subcutaneous tissue) means that they face increased risk of insulin resistance and hence type 2 disease in adulthood. The provider needs to be aware of this risk in the patient whose birth weight was very low so as to apprise parents of health-promoting activities that may help their child to delay or avoid type 2 diabetes.

Maturity-Onset Diabetes of the Young

Sometimes referred to as type 3 diabetes, MODY is an autosomal dominant inherited disorder often mistakenly diagnosed as either type 1 or 2 disease. MODY is actually neither, although it is more correctly type 2 than type 1. MODY is a heterogenic disorder of impaired insulin secretion without its absolute absence, characterized by some degree of the insulin resistance syndrome seen in type 2 disease. Mutations of four different genes have been identified in the pathogenesis of MODY (Hattersley, 1998). Further, patients are not predictably from those ethnic groups with a high incidence of type 2 diabetes. Rather, patients with MODY typically are Caucasian, although the subtype for MODY 5 has been well demonstrated in Japan. Hattersley states that there may be a sixth subtype as well (MODY 6).

● **Clinical Pearl:** More subphenotypic variants for MODY will certainly be discovered in coming years. This means that treatment methods will need to be individualized in keeping with each patient's genetic permutation.

Regardless of phenotype, patients with MODY have strong family histories for type 2 disease and sometimes for type 1 disease or even for MODY. They do not demonstrate morphologic evidence of the glutamic decarboxylase antibody of type 1 diabetes. Other characteristics, at least of MODY 1, 2, and 3, include onset before age 25 years and absence of ketosis (Cameron & Batch, 1997). Cortisol, glucagon, and growth hormone levels tend to be normal, as are serum lipids.

There are currently four well-described subphenotypic classifications of MODY (MODY 1, 2, 3, and 4) (Stoffers et al., 1997; Green-Hernandez, 1999a). At this point, MODY 1 and 3 appear to have a central deficiency in insulin secretion. Insulin levels may range from normal or slightly decreased to altogether absent after glucose challenge. Conversely, when faced with a glucose load, the patient with MODY 2 demonstrates a diminished response to signaling for beta cell secretion of insulin, resulting in normal to mild decreases in insulin levels, although hyperglycemia becomes more severe in later life. Microvascular complications are rare in MODY 2. It more typically occurs in early childhood, perhaps even from birth. MODY 2 can thus be confused with early type 1 disease (Cameron & Batch, 1997; Hattersley, 1998).

MODY 3 is more likely to occur in adolescence or early adulthood. Disease presentation is one of mild to moderate hyperglycemia, with the potential to become progressively more severe as the young person grows older. Microvascular complications are an expected outcome if normoglycemia is not achieved in disease management.

MODY 4 appears to occur later than 1, 2, or 3. Stoffers and colleagues (1997) state that in their experience, the average age of onset of MODY 4 is 35 years. Hyperglycemia is variable, depending on patient participation in the diabetic regimen. Thus, microvascular complications are also variable, depending on degree and consistency of patient normoglycemia. Like the other variants, MODY 4 is nonketotic and occurs in families with high diabetes prevalence rates.

Children and adolescents who develop MODY (whether 1, 2, or 3) are generally asymptomatic until after several weeks to months of glucose elevation. Serum glucose can range from impaired glucose tolerance (IGT) to frank fasting hyperglycemia. These youngsters are generally not obese. Just as the incidence of obesity is increasing in the general pediatric population (Slyper, 1998), however, so too is it in the MODY group (Cameron & Batch, 1997; Tattersal, 1982). Unlike in type 1 and type 2 diabetes, environmental factors such as obesity appear to play little role in the pathogenesis of MODY (Hattersley, 1998).

▲ **Clinical Warning:** Consider MODY when a nonobese adolescent presents with elevated blood glucose but without ketosis and has a family history of type 2 diabetes.

Gestational Diabetes Mellitus

Gestational diabetes mellitus (GDM) can occur in the young pregnant adolescent with or without a prior history of obesity. GDM is expressed in response to carbohydrate intolerance in 1% to 5% of pregnant women (Spong et al., 1998). Infants of these pregnancies tend to have higher birth weights and higher incidences of macrosomia, thus placing them at greater risk for subsequent diabetes development. Hispanic women are at increased risk for GDM. The earlier its occurrence in a pregnancy, the greater the risk for GDM in subsequent pregnancies. This is especially true for women who need insulin and who have elevated third trimester glucose values.

Gestational diabetes is not a focus for this text. The reader whose young patient is pregnant and is diagnosed with GDM is directed to examine other resources for the diagnosis and management of GDM, including the works of Coustan & Carpenter (1998) and Langer (1998). The ADA position statement on gestational diabetes outlines current management guidelines for preconception and prenatal care (2000a).

Pathology of Complications of Diabetes

Ketoacidosis

Many children first present with diabetes as a diagnostic outcome of emergency treatment for ketoacidosis. This holds true for both type 1 and type 2 disease. Ketoacidosis is rare in MODY, though it can occur in MODY 2. Insulin deficit underscores ketoacidosis, whether this deficit is relative (as in type 2 and insulin resistance syndrome) or absolute (type 1). Insulin inhibits gluconeogenesis and glycogenolysis. It is needed for ATP synthesis and protein synthesis. Lipogenesis requires insulin bioavailability; its absence leads inexorably to lipolysis. In short, without insulin, glucose could not be taken up by peripheral tissues. Insulin deficiency leads to hyperglycemia. The final outcomes of insulin absence include depletion of hepatic stores of glycogen, muscle breakdown, and release of free fatty acids.

Ketoacidosis results when continued glycogenolysis produces ketone bodies. Dysregulation of the endocrine system's regulatory hormones ensues, including increased cortisol, catecholamine, and growth hormone production. These hormones exacerbate the hyperglycemia. Persistent, profound hyperglycemia leads to osmotic diuresis. Nausea and vomiting may accompany this hormonal dysregulation. As the hyperglycemia deepens, consciousness shifts toward increasing confusion. In a worst-case scenario, profound dehydration and coma occur and, if left untreated or treated too late, lead to brain damage or death (Silink, 1998). Refer to Chapter 47 for an in-depth discussion of the diagnosis and management of ketoacidosis.

Chronic Complications of Diabetes Mellitus

All complications, including nephropathy, neuropathy, and retinopathy, can be prevented or significantly delayed for decades if diabetes is well controlled (Diabetes Control and Complications Trial [DCCT] Research Group, 1993; 1995; Lekakis et al., 1997; Author, 1998; Cooper, 1998; Lovestam-Adrian et al., 1998; Shaw et al., 1998; Aielo, Gardner, King, et al., 1998). Total costs associated with treating the complications of diabetes are astronomical. Direct medical costs in the United States in 1992 alone totaled $44.1 billion. Indirect costs, including work loss, disability, and premature death, totaled $54.1 billion (ADA, 1997a). Because these complications typically occur years and even decades after the diagnosis of diabetes, it may be difficult to explain why the patient should want to participate in a prescribed regimen that is not noted for being much fun.

Vascular changes, including renal and large vessel disease, occur only after many years of poorly controlled diabetes. The average child with diabetes will not demonstrate such changes during early or middle childhood. However, by adolescence, signs of renal complications especially may become apparent in the patient with poorly controlled diabetes. Similarly, retinopathy may begin to be seen in adolescence if chronic hyperglycemia has been a part of the child's management pattern.

Histopathologic changes lead to thickening of glomerular basement membrane. This change is seen in all patients with diabetes mellitus and can lead to persistent microalbuminuria. Left unchecked, microalbuminuria will eventually evolve into albuminuria and nephropathy. In keeping with this phenomenon, nearly all individuals with type 1 diabetes eventually develop nonproliferative retinopathy. Of these, approximately 30% of patients go on to develop vision-threatening retinal diseases (VTRDs), including neovascularization and maculopathies, as outcomes of their disease (Gilbert et al., 1998). These findings are increasingly being seen in members of the adolescent diabetic population who, in an effort to be model-slim, are not as active in coparticipating in their insulin regimen.

The recent work of Gilbert et al. (1998) points toward a connection between evolving nephropathy and increased risk for VTRDs in patients with type 1 disease. The actual timing of stages at which nephropathy and proliferative retinopathy coexist is not yet clear (Lovestam-Adrian et al., 1998). It is reasonable to believe that patients with persistent hyperglycemia who go on to develop nephropathy and VTRDs have a genetic predisposition to do so. Further, the fact that some patients in poor glycemic control will present with VTRDs but not nephropathic findings points to the multifactorial influences of differing genetic and environmental influences in the pathologic consequences of poorly controlled, long-term disease.

EPIDEMIOLOGY

Type 1 diabetes is found in every country and among most ethnic groups. In the United States alone, 123,000 children have type 1 disease (National Diabetes Data Group, 1995). Of these, about 75% are younger than 18 years at the time of diagnosis (ADA, 2000c). Among adolescents, type 1 prevalence is approximately 1 in 500 (Sperling, 1994; Draznin & Patel, 1998). Whether type 1 or 2, diabetes is on the increase in children worldwide. A change in genetics is not operant, because risk genes are not increasing in children born today, compared with previous generations.

Clearly, lifestyle variables have changed in the past generation and, coupled with other environmental factors, seem to be at the core of the diabetes epidemic. The rushed lifestyle of the adult world is no less obvious than that of children. Hurried lives mean more fast food consumption, with increased simple sugar and fat calories. Many empty calories are consumed in soda and other sugared drinks, including juices, sports drinks, and bottled tea and coffee beverages. Adolescents consume these and other covert sugar in their coffee bar beverages, including lattes and other espresso drinks. Children today are also less active than those of earlier generations, with television and computer games replacing bike-riding and pick-up sports activities for many. Snack food consumption and passive activities are well linked in the literature (Strong et al., 1999). Whether or not the child is at genetic risk, these factors are the antecedents to obesity and, ultimately, type 2 diabetes. The youngest recorded child diagnosed with type 2 diabetes was an obese 5 year-old Pima Indian (Hanson et al., 1998).

For children at risk for type 1 disease, the foregoing factors act as triggers to its genetics, at earlier ages and in a wider population and ethnic base than in earlier generations. First-degree relatives of Caucasian patients share a genetic risk for diabetes development that exceeds that of the general population (6% versus 1%), although more than 20% of children with type 1 diabetes exhibit a positive family history (Dorman, 1997; Altobelli et al., 1998).

As population-based epidemiologic studies increase, more will be learned about variations in the epidemiology of type 1 diabetes in different ethnic groups. It is reasonable to say that type 1 diabetes occurs in different genetically determined individuals as an outcome of different combinations of both genetic and nongenetic risk factors. These combine differently from one child to the next in producing type 1 disease. Beta cell destruction is accelerated by insulin

demand as an outcome of different environmental triggers in a genetically susceptible individual. These triggers include the perinatal environment, living in a cold region, infections experienced, nutritional influences (perinatal and in infancy), and a rapid growth rate during pubescence.

Perinatal triggers may include maternal ingestion of nitrites during pregnancy, such as those found in preserved meats and in some drinking water sources. Maternal smoking can be considered a significant environmental trigger in genetically susceptible fetuses (Dahlquist, 1998). Antepartal stress, as well as later psychological stress, has been implicated in triggering of disease (Thernlund et al., 1995). Neonatal birth weight has also been linked to disease onset, with large-for-gestational age babies being at greater risk for type 1 diabetes, and premature and very low birth weight infants facing a risk for type 2 in adulthood (Dahlquist, 1998; Thompson et al., 1997).

Incidence of type 1 disease is greatest in children of northern European heritage, with Finnish people having the world's highest incidence and Japanese the lowest. Seasonal variations have been identified, with more cases presenting in winter than in warm-weather months (Dahlquist, 1998). Infectious exposure antenatum as well as during the clinical year preceding diabetes onset is also a feasible trigger of disease. Rubella was at one time a significant antecedent to type 1 onset, but it is now rare in westernized countries. Coxsackie B virus and other enteroviral exposures have been found to be associated with triggering of type 1 diabetes (Dahlquist, 1998).

Pubescence is a time of significant growth, including increased growth hormone release with concomitant impact on serum cortisol levels and insulin secretion and tissue uptake. Several epidemiologic studies conducted in different regions of the world all demonstrate a peak in the incidence of type 1 diabetes during this period. Rapid growth, with sudden and significant growth rate, including being taller than their peers, has been identified in the later pathogenesis of type 1 in genetically susceptible youth (Blom et al., 1992; Dahlquist, 1998; Tolis et al., 1997).

HISTORY AND PHYSICAL EXAMINATION

Questions specific to screening for diabetes can be found in Display 61-1. Information related to the physical examination is presented in Display 61-2.

DIAGNOSTIC CRITERIA

A suspected diagnosis of diabetes mandates further investigation by the primary care provider. The clinician should consider a diagnosis of diabetes when a patient presents with any of the findings outlined in Display 61-3.

DIAGNOSTIC STUDIES

The following discussion relates to diagnostic testing for type 1 disease and for type 2 diabetes in adolescents. The reader is referred to current endocrine resources or current ADA guidelines for testing in suspected GDM.

The means for diagnosing diabetes have been modified from previous recommendations (ADA, 1997b, 2000c). These include preferential diagnosis through fasting plasma glu-

---

DISPLAY 61–1 • History Questions in Screening for Diabetes

- Do you have a family history of diabetes?
- If yes, then is it type 1 or type 2, and in whom?
- Do you have classic symptoms (ie, polydipsia, polyphagia, unexplained weight loss)?
- Are you a member of an ethnic group having a high incidence of diabetes (Native North American, African American, Asian, Hispanic)?
- What was your birth weight and, if known, approximate gestational age?
- In female of childbearing age: do you have a history of gestational diabetes; delivering an infant over 9 lb; or toxemia, stillbirth, polyhydramnios, or other complications associated with a pregnancy?
- Do you have lifestyle stress?
- Have you had a recent stressful event (positive or negative)?
- What is your weight history (loss or gain)?
- Do you have a history of diabetes treatment? If yes, diet prescription, medications, self-management training, glucose self-monitoring?
- Do you have a history of complications, including ketoacidosis and hypoglycemia?
- List your diet (including fluids) history for food types, amounts, and how prepared in a typical day. Include condiments and all snacks consumed.
- List aerobic and anaerobic exercise, noting type, amount of time, and frequency.
- What is your sleep–rest history (insomnia, nightmares)?
- Do you have visual changes (blurring, diplopia, floaters)?

- Do you have numbness, tingling, or burning in the hands or feet? This is a bilateral rather than unilateral neuropathy in diabetes and, although primarily sensory, motor nerve fibers may be involved. In more extreme cases polyneuropathy may progress from severe pain to anaesthesia, and:
- Are motor manifestations, including muscle weakness progressing to atrophy, with poor hand grasp or footdrop evident?
- Do you have unexplained indigestion or abdominal pain?
- Do you have unexplained diarrhea?
- Have you had infections, including urinary tract infections and candidiasis?
- Have you had intertriginous infections/irritations (in skinfold areas of the obese; under the female breasts, crural areas in men)?
- Have you had vaginitis?
- Do you have a history of chronic disease, including hypertension, endocrine, or autoimmune disease?
- Do you have atherosclerosis risks, including diet, obesity, smoking, dyslipidemia, family history?
- What medications do you take, prescribed and over the counter?
- List your recreational drug use, including tobacco and alcohol (amounts and frequency).
- Do you have any other ethnic, psychosocial, socioeconomic, educational, or lifestyle considerations that could affect the provider and patient in their management of diabetes?

---

cose (FPG), although other blood test analyses can also be used.

- Testing is not recommended for type 1 disease in patients who are healthy and who do not carry autoimmune risk.

- Testing should be considered more frequently in all patients, including those who are younger than 45 years and who:
  - Are obese (at or greater than 120% of desirable weight or with a body mass index at or greater than 27 kg/m^2)

DISPLAY 61–2 • Physical Examination for the Patient With Diabetes

- Length/height and weight, with comparison to norms
- Sexual maturation staging (during prepubertal stage of development)
- Blood pressure (may need to obtain orthostatic measurements as well) and comparison to age-related norms
- Eyeground examination (preferably dilated, done by an ophthalmologist or licensed optometrist skilled in diabetes assessment) for signs of maculopathies and retinopathies:
  - Retinal hemorrhages
  - Scattered hard exudates
  - Cotton-wool exudates (generally in concert with severe hypertension)
- Oral examination (eg, *Candida*)
- Thyroid auscultatin and palpation
- Cardiac examination (eg, S$_4$)
- Abdominal examination (eg, hepatomegaly)
- Examination of pulses by palpation and auscultation
- Hand and finger examination
- Thorough skin examination (including insulin injection sites if applicable)

- Neurologic examination, including assessing for a positive Romberg sign (sometimes presents as swaying, destabilized pattern; type 2, adolescent and older)
- Sensory stimulation changes (peripheral neuropathy and, if indicated by history, abdominal; type 2, adolescent and older)
- Vibratory sense changes (peripheral neuropathy and, if indicated by history, abdominal; type 2, adolescent and older)
- Foot examination, looking for evidence of foot ulcers or infection not otherwise explained (type 2, adolescent and older)
- Deep tendon reflex measurement (may be decreased, especially in presence of PN); absence of ankle reflexes early sign
- Gait analysis (may be unstable, especially in presence of peripheral neuropathy)
- If primary or differential diagnosis includes another endocrine disorder, such as pheochromocytoma, Cushing syndrome, acromegaly, or hemochromatosis or pancreatic disease, secondary diabetes possible in these patients (ADA, 2000b)

PN = peripheral neuropathy.

DISPLAY 61–3 • Diagnostic Criteria for Diabetes Mellitus

- Fasting plasma glucose (FPG) should be measured after > 8 hours of caloric fasting; elevation ≥126 mg/dL (7 mmol/L).
- Patients in the higher FPG ranges usually present with the classic symptoms of polydipsia, polyuria, and unexplained weight loss.
- Casual plasma glucose (ie, taken at any time of day, regardless of meal timing) is ≥ 200 mg/dL (11.1 mmol/L) plus symptoms.
- Oral glucose tolerance test (OGTT) is **not** recommended for routine use. If these data are obtained, then a level ≥200 mg/dL at 2 hours should be investigated using an equivalent 75-g anhydrous glucose/water load.
- Weight loss is common in type 1 but less so in type 2 disease, especially in people with preexisting obesity.
- A patient who presents with FPG between 110 and 126 mg/dL can be classified as having impaired glucose tolerance (IGT). The OGTT should not be routinely used in the average clinical setting. If this value is obtained, its level at 2 hours continues to be classified as IGT if it is between 140 and 200 mg/dL.
- FPG values:
  - *FPG < 110 mg/dL = normal
  - *FPG ≥ 110 and 126 mg/dL = IGT
  - *FPG ≥ 126 = conditional diagnosis of diabetes

The above should be reconfirmed on a different day through repeat testing in any patient presenting without symptoms of hyperglycemia accompanied by acute metabolic decompensation.

Sources: Expert Committee, 1997; ADA, 2000.

- Report a first-degree relative who had diabetes
- Are members of an ethnic group with high risk for diabetes (Native North American, or African, Asian, or Hispanic North American)
- And in adolescents who:
  - Were diagnosed with GDM or delivered a baby over 9 lb
  - Have high blood pressure (at or greater than 140/90 mmHg) (Young et al., 1998; ADA, 2000c)
  - Have low-density lipoprotein cholesterol at or under 135 mg/dL or triglyceride at or exceeding 250 mg/dL
  - Were found previously to have either IGT or impaired fasting glucose (ADA, 1997b; 2000c)
- The clinician should consider for testing any child with a history of:
  - FTT, especially in the absence of abuse or neglect
  - Delayed psychomotor development in which no other cause is operant

If information is needed about FTT or delayed psychomotor development, the reader should refer to Chapters 18 and 23.

MANAGEMENT

Whether type 1 or type 2, diabetes is characterized by consistent elevation of blood glucose; type 2 disease also involves insulin resistance. Clinical diagnosis, appropriate treatment options, and primary care management ideally lead to normalization of blood glucose and, if possible, improved glucose response to endogenous insulin in type 2 diabetes. The goal of treatment is not so much to control the disease but rather to prevent or decrease complications arising from the damaging effects of chronic hyperglycemia. The DCCT Research Group (1993) provided firm evidence that optimal control of blood glucose, defined as HbA$_{1c}$ of 7.4% or less, can delay or prevent long-term complications of diabetes. The ADA 1997 Report from the Expert Committee on the Diagnosis and Classification of Diabetes Mellitus goes a step further, setting an adult target fasting goal of 80 to 120 mg/dL, bedtime glucose level of 100 to 140 mg/dL, and glycosylated hemoglobin (HbA$_{1c}$) of < 7.0%. Any level of improved control will decrease complication rates. Sound management plans arise from appropriate treatment options; more individualized plans of care can maximize positive outcomes for a patient. Various treatment options are appropriate in different clinical circumstances.

When symptoms of polydipsia, polyuria, and polyphagia occur, often accompanied by weight loss and, acutely, dehydration, the diagnosis of type 1 diabetes must be considered. Because the patient with this symptom array typically presents in ketoacidosis, management is emergent initially. Refer to Chapter 47 for information on the diagnosis and management of ketoacidosis. Once the ketoacidosis is reversed, then workup and management should follow ADA guidelines (2000c), with pediatric endocrinology consultation.

When symptoms of polydipsia, polyuria, and polyphagia present, current diagnostic guidelines support making a clinical diagnosis of type 2 based on a single blood glucose measurement. This is true even in the absence of weight loss, which is more typical in type 1 than in most variants of type 2 disease. The glucose test need not be fasting. Specifics for each kind of glucose measurement should correspond with the values presented in Display 61-4 (ADA, 1997b, 2000c;

DISPLAY 61–4 • Laboratory Evaluation and Criteria for Diagnosing Diabetes

---

- Fasting lipids (total cholesterol, high-density lipoprotein cholesterol, triglycerides, and low-density lipoprotein cholesterol)
- Serum creatinine, if proteinuria is present
- Urinalysis for glucose, ketones, protein, and sediment
- Microalbuminuria (timed specimen, or the albumin to creatinine ratio) in pubertal and postpubertal patients with type 1 diabetes after 5 years of disease and in all patients with type 2 diabetes
- Thyroid function tests in all patients with type 1 disease
- Fasting plasma glucose (FPG) at 8 or more hours of ≥ 126 mg/dL, or
- 2-hour plasma glucose ≥ 200 mg/dL during a 75-g oral glucose tolerance test (OGTT), following World Health Organization guidelines; OGTT not recommended for routine clinical analysis
- Random plasma glucose in an undiagnosed symptomatic child for diagnostic purposes
- Unless patient is in metabolic decompensation, repeat the glycemic measure used on a different day to confirm the diagnosis.
- Glycohemoglobin (GHB; HbA$_{1c}$)

Sources: Report of the Expert Committee, 1997; ADA, 2000.

Limbach, 1998). If diabetes is not confirmed but is still suspected, then the provider can obtain an oral glucose tolerance test (ADA, 2000c).

Whether type 1 or type 2 disease is present, the primary care provider must recognize the importance of ethnic and cultural influences when discussing treatment options. This recognition begins before planning interventions. Food customs and eating rituals differ from family to family. Specific ethnic or lifestyle habits greatly influence diet and meal planning. Similarly, cultural beliefs and values surrounding the body and perceived self-harm will influence the child's and family's levels of participation in self-monitoring and medical therapies. Presenting realistic diabetes treatment options mandates that the primary care provider inquire about and respect cultural influences, customs, beliefs, and values. This perspective is especially important when a family's cultural, religious, or ethnic background, or even lifestyle, differs from that of the provider. Chapters 1 and 2 provides a framework for the clinician to examine personal values and for collecting patient data related to cultural and family assessments.

Goals of therapy and management of young children, especially those of preschool age, differ from goals in older children and adolescents. With their unpredictable physical activity, dietary intake, and increased sensitivity to insulin, young children often steer a course between high and low blood glucose. Overzealous treatment may result in frequent hypoglycemic reactions, even convulsions. Studies have demonstrated the detrimental effects of severe hypoglycemia on cognitive function in children with diabetes, specifically deficits on perceptual, motor, memory, and attention tasks (Rovet & Ehrlich, 1999). Hypoglycemic episodes can go undetected during the night, so-called nocturnal hypoglycemia (Beregszaszi et al., 1997). Therefore, most pediatric endocrinologists aim at preprandial glycemic values between 100 and 200 mg/dL in preschool children and between 90 and 140 mg/dL in older patients (Kiess et al., 1998).

▲ **Clinical Warning:** It is important that the parents of a young child with diabetes understand the dangers of hypoglycemia. The provider must ascertain that they are able to monitor their child's blood glucose at least four times a day or more and at an additional time of once a week at 2:00 AM. Glycosylated Hgb values in young patients may be maintained at higher levels than those recommended for older, school-age children. An HbA_{1c} between 7% and 8.5% is quite acceptable for young children with diabetes.

Newer pharmacologic interventions and insulin delivery systems can be combined to achieve these therapeutic goals. Certified Diabetes Educators (CDEs) have curricula and teaching tools for empowering each person to control their diabetes effectively. As their knowledge base expands, both patient and provider must overcome reluctance to inject insulin and self-test glucose several times per day, while continuing to update their understanding of this disease.

Goals of Diabetes Management for All Treatment Options

The following current standards of practice can frame a plan of care that supports the patient with diabetes in obtaining optimal metabolic control. After young childhood, hyperglycemia must be eliminated to control the progression of diabetes and to delay or prevent complications, including microvascular and macrovascular problems. These two problems are discussed later in this chapter.

The *immediate* treatment goals of diabetes management include the following:

- Achievement of optimal glycemic control based on HbA_{1c} up to 8.5%, with preprandial glycemic values between 100 and 200 mg/dL in preschool-age children (Kiess et al., 1998)
- HbA_{1c} of 7.4% or less, with preprandial glycemic values between 90 and 140 mg/dL in older children and adolescents
- Absence of hypoglycemic episodes requiring assistance to treat, including nocturnal hypoglycemia

The *overall* goals of diabetic management for all children and adolescents include the following:

- Providing for normal growth and development to the greatest extent possible
- Normalizing the activities of childhood, such as sports, camping, and peer group functions
- Correction of metabolic irregularities
- Achieving the glycemic range for age, as just discussed, to prevent consequent end organ damage due to microvascular and macrovascular complications

Achievement of these goals depends on maintaining the target blood glucose level. If frequent high and low blood sugar levels are encountered in the face of desirable HbA_{1c}, efforts must be made to smooth out glycemic control within the age-related parameters just discussed. Patient self-monitoring of blood glucose (SMBG) is critical to the success of this effort, whether by the parent or caregiver of the young child or by self-monitoring in the older child and adolescent. Lifestyle assessment is an important first step in creating effective interventions for managing blood glucose.

Lifestyle Assessment and Intervention

The importance of understanding the child's activities of daily life cannot be overstated. Included in this assessment are family meal planning; the child's hours of sleep, school, and activity; and variations in activities on a day-to-day, weekly, and seasonal basis. The provider also needs to assess the parents' educational level and employment, composition and involvement of the rest of the household, and potential for community support. Cultural and ethnic practices and religious beliefs may play an important role in health decisions, food choices, times of ritual fasting, and celebrations. Family habits and customs also may affect the child's eventual self-management of diabetes. Ascertaining insurance status is important, because this often determines patient access to both primary care and specialty providers, support services, medication, and supplies (Songer et al., 1997). Chapter 1 provides a guideline for obtaining cultural and family assessment data.

A certified diabetes educator (CDE) can assist the primary care provider in developing successful intervention strategies for parent and patient teaching. The CDE is a nationally accredited role for professionals who have completed an extensive course of study through the ADA. Most commonly, the CDE is a professional nurse (either BSN or MSN), a physician (MD or DO), a nutritionist (RD), or a social worker (MSW). The CDE has emerged as the recognized consultant for and provider of diabetes education. As a source of knowledge to the patient and the provider, CDEs are increasingly drawn into the patient–provider relationship. CDE services now are more often treated as reimbursable by third-party payers. Further information about the CDE as a resource is provided in the Community Resources section of this chapter.

Whether the sources of information and teaching are the provider, a CDE, or both, it is important that information be given that will support the parents in managing their child's care in a systematic manner. This information includes but is not limited to the following:

- Understanding the rationale for glycohemoglobin (GHB) testing
- The relationship of meal planning, food, and exercise control to glycemic control
- Parental or caregiver SMBG; goal is for the older child to self-manage
- Mode of action and side affects of medications
- Sick-day management; signs and symptoms of hypoglycemia and hyperglycemia and their management
- Possible acute and chronic complications

Taken as a whole, this information constitutes "survival skills" for the person with diabetes.

Glycohemoglobin Testing

Glycohemoglobin testing helps the provider to determine a patient's blood glucose for the 90- to 120-day span prior to testing. A minor hemoglobin, GHB constitutes only 4% to 8% of the total hemoglobin. Three components of GHB are said to be glycosylated: A_{1a}, A_{1b}, and A_{1c}. A_{1c} is the most commonly measured GHB. If A_{1a} is measured, its value is computed at 2.4% higher than A_{1c}.

Analysis of GHB is useful because this component of the red blood cell's hemoglobin combines with some of the bloodstream's glucose load. This process is called *glycosylation* and is irreversible. A patient's GHB level depends on how much glucose was available in the bloodstream over the 100- to 120-day lifespan of the red blood cell. This determination is only an average of that glucose level, because red blood cells undergo a constant cycle of old cell destruction and new cell generation (Pagana & Pagana, 1998).

Certain conditions can interfere with GHB determination, including sickle cell anemia, chronic renal failure, and pregnancy. False elevations of the GHB can occur whenever the lifespan of the red cell is lengthened, as in thalassemia (Pagana & Pagana, 1998). Hemolytic anemia will decrease the GHB, possibly due to increased red cell turnover. Conditions that will increase the GHB include the following:

- New diabetes
- Poor diabetic control
- Chronic renal failure
- Hemodialysis
- Iron-deficiency anemia
- Splenectomy
- Pregnancy (Pagana & Pagana, 1998)

Several assays exist for determination of GHB. Different assays may have different normal ranges. Providers must be aware of assays available at a given practice site.

● **Clinical Pearl:** The GHB should be assayed every 3 months (ADA, 1998, 2000c).

Home Glucose Monitoring

The ADA (1996) recommends that all patients who take insulin also self-monitor their blood glucose levels. This activity is especially important in all pregnant adolescents who have diabetes, regardless of type. The provider should teach SMBG to parents and any caregivers responsible for monitoring the child's glycemic status. As patients get older, they should be encouraged to take on this responsibility. SMBG is especially important in any child whose disease is unstable or who has a tendency toward hypoglycemia that occurs without forewarning, as is not uncommon in type 1 in childhood. SMBG should also be taught to children with type 2 and their parents, to those who are taking antidiabetic medication, to those whose glycemic control is "tight," and in cases of ketoacidosis history. All patients who manage their disease through intensive insulin regimens must use SMBG as part of their therapy. This latter group includes individuals who are on an insulin pump or who self-inject their insulin multiple times daily.

Many glucometers are available for home monitoring of blood glucose. Inserts packaged with these machines provide excellent directions on how to obtain a specimen and how to use the meter for its analysis and interpretation. Parents should be encouraged to bring their child's meter to the provider for one-on-one support and teaching about specimen collection and meter use. CDEs also are a good resource for up-to-date information related to meter choice and use. The parent should be encouraged to purchase a glucose meter that requires only a short wait for results (less than 45 seconds) and that has a memory. The availability of a computer program for memory entry is helpful. Memory stores readings, which, providing the equipment is available at the provider's office, can then be used to off-load blood glucose data.

The provider should teach the child's family to intervene for high or low readings, based on a prescribed sliding scale for those values. The parents and, if old enough, the child should also be taught to record in a time log all blood glucose values, activities, foods and amounts eaten, and type and dosage of insulin given. Ask the parent and child to bring both the log and the glucometer to the provider's office at each visit.

Instruct the family to check their child's urine for ketones if the SMBG reading is 300 or greater or if the child is ill. This is especially important if the child is vomiting or has diarrhea or both.

▲ **Clinical Warning:** Vomiting and diarrhea and a blood sugar level of 300 or greater place a child at risk for ketoacidosis.

Treating Type 1 Diabetes

The treatment of a child with type 1 diabetes is a major challenge for the primary care provider. The mainstays of therapy are insulin administration, proper food intake, and exercise. It is imperative that the clinician develop the management plan in collaboration with the comanaging pediatric endocrine group.

Insulin is given to correct the metabolism of carbohydrates, protein, and fat. However, treatment with insulin must be individualized (Becker, 1998). In concert with the comanaging endocrine group, the provider must decide what type and dosage of insulin are best for a particular patient. The clinician must also consider mode of treatment (ie, conventional versus intensive insulin therapy). Intensive insulin therapy means that the patient injects multiple daily doses of short-acting insulin or uses a pump for continuous insulin infusion. This therapy is generally reserved for older children or adolescents who are mature and self-directed, who do not have a history of repeated hypoglycemia, and who have hypoglycemic self-awareness. These traits are necessary because intensive diabetes therapy in children with type 1 disease carries an increased risk of hypoglycemia (Hershey, Bhargava, Sadler, White, & Craft, 1999).

The introduction of human insulin produced by DNA recombinant technique has expanded the availability of insulin preparations. More recently, a rapid-acting lys-pro insulin (lispro) under the brand name Humalog has been successfully used in patients with diabetes mellitus. Because of its very rapid onset, this insulin has proven to be more beneficial in preventing the transient diurnal hyperglycemia that is often seen in patients taking Humulin (NPH) and regular insulins (Crowne et al., 1998; ADA, 2000c). Lalli et al. (1999) found that combining lispro and NPH at mealtime proved more beneficial than NPH plus regular insulin, with improved blood glucose over a 24-hour period and concomitant improvement in the HbA_{1c}. The improvement can be maintained long term. Intensive therapy with lispro and NPH results in less frequent hypoglycemia and better awareness and counter-regulation of hypoglycemia.

The future of insulin therapy may include some combination of a single daily injection of a long-acting insulin analog, such as glargine. Glargine is now in phase III clinical trial. Because once-daily injection of this proposed insulin analog will still not provide for 24-hour basal insulinemia in most patients, it is anticipated that aerosolized insulin will need to be added to the glargine at up to three points in the day. This therapy is not yet available, but when it is, it undoubtedly will prove more salient as an improved method for medication administration (Rosskamp & Park, 1999).

It is reasonable to expect that the endocrinologist will routinely start children and adolescents on a combination of intermediate human insulin (Humulin NPH or Lente) and short-acting Humalog insulin before breakfast, and again before supper. If morning blood glucose levels run high, the accepted practice is to split the evening dose of insulin by moving intermediate insulin to the bedtime hours. This plan is discussed in greater detail in the next section.

Humalog insulin has proven to be especially helpful in young children with diabetes. Young children's appetites normally may vary, and they typically cannot be forced to eat. In such cases, dosage of Humalog can be adjusted retrospectively to accommodate the amount of food ingested. Humalog may by given immediately after the meal because of its rapid onset of action. At the other end of the treatment spectrum, the duration of Humalog insulin is less than that of classic regular insulin. This is of benefit to clinical management because there is consequently less chance for hypoglycemia. Only rarely will children with diabetes need to be switched to other insulins, such as ultralente.

▲ **Clinical Warnings:**

- Long-acting insulins may have an unpredictable effect on blood glucose levels in young children.
- Because of the risks associated with unrecognized hypoglycemia (and of hyperglycemia), every patient taking insulin should be advised to wear a diabetes identification bracelet. Applications for this tag are readily available in pharmacy settings.

Initiating Insulin Therapy

The purpose of all diabetes therapies is achievement of as close to normal glycemia as possible without hypoglycemia. Insulin is required for a patient's life maintenance and should be prescribed in a proactive manner that directly involves the parents and, if old enough, the child in decision making and management.

The primary care provider must assess each child and family on an individual, case-by-case basis. It is essential that the primary provider remember that the patient with type 1 diabetes requires insulin at all times and will have additional insulin requirements at times of illness and fasting. Withholding insulin in the child with type 1 disease who is vomiting can be a fatal mistake. Lack of insulin in type 1 allows the liver to produce ketones, precipitating illness and nausea and risking diabetic ketoacidosis, as outlined in Display 61-5.

The provider must be in daily contact (until therapy seems stabilized) with the parent(s) responsible for glucose monitoring and insulin administration, both at the time of initiation of therapy and thereafter whenever the dosage is changed. In the patient with newly diagnosed type 1 diabetes, the provider should calculate the dose of insulin in conjunction with the comanaging pediatric endocrinologist. One approach has been to start all newly diagnosed patients on a combination of NPH and lispro insulins, given before breakfast and before dinner.

By anticipating peaks and troughs of blood glucose based on home glucose monitoring results, the provider can work

---

DISPLAY 61–5 • Diagnosis and Deposition of Diabetic Ketoacidosis (DKA) and Nonketotic Hyperosmolar Syndrome (NKHS)

DKA

- DKA is a medical emergency usually associated with type 1 but can (rarely) occur in type 2.
- Suspect DKA in adolescents and in any patient with type 1 who withholds insulin.

▲ **Clinical Warning:** Assess for underlying infection in all cases of DKA.

- Symptoms (most common) include polyuria, polydipsia, vomiting (with or without abdominal pain and weakness).
- Laboratory tests may reveal hyperglycemia, though not always profoundly so; leukocytosis; hypertriglyceridemia, and anion gap acidosis. A serum pH of 7.25 or less and the presence of serum ketones are typical criteria for diagnosis of DKA.

NKHS

- NKHS occurs predominantly in patients with type 2 diabetes.
- NKHS is characterized by hyperglycemia (serum glucose levels often exceed 600 mg/dL), absence of serum ketones, and dehydration as evidenced by weight loss and often azotemia.
- Coma can occur in both DKA and NKHS.
- Mentation changes are common to both DKA and NKHS.
- Like DKA, underlying infection is common in NKHS.
- Intravenous insulin is usually required for treatment of profoundly dehydrated patients, as absorption from muscle and subcutaneous tissue is unpredictable.
- Lactic acidosis can compound either condition and increases the risk of death.
- Very mild DKA or early NKHS can sometimes be managed on an outpatient basis by an experienced primary care provider who is knowledgeable about diabetes.

with the parents and, if possible, the child to achieve smoother glycemic control. Insulin adjustments should be made after a pattern of insulin response is clear. Adjustments are made over a period of 3 or more days, within the context of a patient's diet, SMBG levels, and exercise management. Once a dose is established, teaching, guidance, and support must be provided to parents and caregivers responsible for glucose monitoring and insulin administration. These activities can be done by a member of the health care team who is skilled in teaching this content. The child can begin a self-management program when mature enough for this important learning. Self-administration teaching should not generally be delayed beyond adolescence (ADA, 2000c).

When beginning insulin therapy, the provider should bear in mind that human insulin brings about a lesser antibody response than nonhuman insulin. Because of modern production methods, however, this response is considered slight and therefore of little true clinical significance. In any event, human insulin is less expensive than pork insulin.

Young children and those who have been diagnosed with type 1 early in its onset typically require 0.5 U of insulin/kg of body weight per 24 hours. The older child or adolescent who has a past history of ketoacidosis may need 1 to 1.3 or even 1.5 U/kg per 24 hours. It is not uncommon that these older patients are somewhat insulin resistant and thus require this larger dosage of insulin. Growth spurts and endocrine-driven sexual maturation underlie much of the insulin resistance seen in these two older age groups.

A typical regimen might include two thirds of the day's total insulin in the morning, before breakfast, and one third before the evening meal. Half of this last dose can be given as rapid or, alternatively, short-acting insulin before supper (or after, as for the very young child with unpredictable appetite), with the remaining half of the evening dose given as an intermediate-acting insulin at bedtime. This latter schedule is especially effective for the patient who has problems controlling high prebreakfast glucose levels, because the bedtime NPH works to modulate blood sugars through the night without the concomitant risk of hypoglycemia during sleep, as would almost certainly occur if either rapid- or short-acting insulin were given at bedtime.

Both the morning and the evening doses of insulin are further broken down into NPH and lispro, in a 3:1 ratio. The dose of lispro insulin can be adjusted up or down, according to blood glucose levels, following a sliding scale format that may be prescribed by the comanaging endocrine practice. Because appetite cannot always be predicted in younger children, especially toddlers and preschoolers, lispro administration can be calibrated according to a sliding scale (according to amount of food consumed) and given immediately *after* rather than before the morning and evening meals. This convenience associated with lispro derives from its very rapid onset and is helpful because young children cannot be forced to eat to accommodate an insulin dosage.

▲ Clinical Warnings:

- The goal is to maintain preprandial blood glucose levels in the 90 to 120 mg/dL range in older children (and 100–140 mg/dL before bedtime) and in the 100 to 200 mg/dL range in preschool children (Kiess et al., 1998).
- Unless the injection is given *immediately* after a meal, the patient should eat immediately after the injection of lispro insulin.

In cases in which a child's prebreakfast SMBG is very high (exceeding the recommended preprandial range), the comanaging endocrine practice may recommend that the dose of before-dinner NPH be moved to bedtime. Again, the provider should be in daily contact with the family whenever insulin is adjusted, until satisfied that the patient's glycemic control is stabilized. Because of the vagaries of individual metabolism and ever-changing growth patterns, compounded by varying daily and school activities, many children experience glycemic variations at midday. A sliding scale can offset glycemic peaks and troughs, providing for some additional short-acting insulin coverage at lunchtime on either a regular or as-needed basis. This dosage component is a typical part of the management plan for some patients. Again, SMBG can provide the clinician with the data needed to make this adjustment. The provider will need to work directly with the school nurse to provide for this management component. Consultation with the comanaging endocrine group will prove helpful as well.

▲ **Clinical Warning:** It is important that the provider individualize the insulin regimen to accommodate the child's physiologic needs, recognizing the metabolic influences of family lifestyle, eating habits, activity patterns, cultural variables, and growth and development.

The target ranges for control are as follows:

- 100 to 200 mg/dL before meals and up to 200 mg/dL after eating in preschool children (Kiess et al., 1998)
- 90 to 140 mg/dL before meals and 80 to 150 mg/dL after eating for older children and adolescents

These targets should be adjusted *upward* if there is a history of recurrent severe or unrecognized hypoglycemia (ADA, 2000c).

Maintaining this therapeutic range can be very difficult. If the child has frequent or severe episodes of symptomatic hypoglycemia, the provider needs to reassess nutritional and activity patterns and the insulin therapy plan. This assessment should be undertaken in tandem with a thorough examination of the child's SMBG, food, and activities log and, if available, the readout of the glucometer's stored SMBG data. Uncovering a pattern for the problem may emerge from this work. The clinician may need to consult with a pediatric endocrine specialty practice to ascertain which part or timing of the child's regimen is responsible for the problem. A pattern of 200 mg/dL or higher requires a similar response from the provider. Patterns of nighttime hypoglycemia require consultation with an endocrinology practice for assistance in evaluating the problem and creating a plan for intervention.

▲ **Clinical Warning:** Untreated nighttime hypoglycemia can have a potentially fatal outcome.

Table 61-1 lists prescribing information for the insulins that are most widely available. Display 61-6 pertains to insulin lispro specifically. Display 61-7 outlines methods for teaching insulin self-administration and injection site rotation. Display 61-8 explains how to draw up insulin.

After initial diagnosis and beginning management of diabetes, many children on insulin therapy experience a so-called honeymoon period in which exogenous insulin requirements become more labile. This outcome of apparent endogenous insulin capacity is short-lived. Parents should be warned of and supported through this period; their child has not been miraculously "cured" of his or her disease. To best support the child and family through this emotionally and metabolically stressful time, the provider should continue multiple-dose insulin therapy. Small doses of diluted

Table 61–1. TYPES OF INSULIN

Insulin Type	Source	Manufacturer/ Brand Name	Onset and Peak Effectiveness	Usual Duration of Action	Notes
Short Acting					
Lispro	Insulin analogue	(Lilly) Humalog	2–15 min/30–90 min	2–4 h	Inject into abdomen to enhance rapid uptake. Consider individual response to site of injection. Dose time based on preprandial SMBG. If > 200, then 20 min before meal. If 150–200, then 10 min before. If < 150, then 5 min before meal. Because of hypoglycemia risk, advise SMBG 2–3 h postmeal. See Display 61-6.
Standard	Beef/pork	(Lilly) Regular Iletin I	0.5–1.0 h/2–4 h	4–6+ h	
Purified pork	Pork	(Lilly) Regular Iletin II; also (Novo Nordisk)			
Human	Recombinant DNA	(Lilly) Humulin R; (Novo Nordisk) Novolin Rb,c			
Intermediate Acting					
Standard	Beef/pork	(Lilly) NPH or Lente Iletin I	1–2 h/6–14 h	16–24+ h	
Purified	Pork	(Lilly) Pork NPH or Lente Iletin II; (Novo Nordisk) NPH Purified (N) or Lente (L)			
Human	Recombinant DNA	(Lilly) Humulin N or Humulin L; (Novo Nordisk) Humulin Nb or Humulin Lb			When given before meals, regular insulins should be injected depending on SMBG before injection, and, as for all insulins, site to be used for injection and individual patient responsiveness to regular insulin. Dose time based on preprandial SMBG: If > 200, then approximately 1 h before. If 150–200, then 45 min before. If < 150, then 30 min before meal.
Long Acting					
Ultralente	Recombinant DNA	(Lilly) Humulin U; Ultralente	4–6 h/10–20 h	24–28+ h	
Mixtures					
NPH/Regular (70/30%)	Recombinant DNA	(Lilly) Humulin 70/30; (Novo Nordisk) Novolin 70/30b,c	30 min	16–24 h	
NPH/Regular (50/50%)	Recombinant DNA	(Lilly) Humulin 50/50			

SMBG = self-monitoring of blood glucose.

DISPLAY 61–6 • Insulin Analogue (Lispro)

Lispro is an insulin analogue that is structurally nearly identical to human insulin, except for reversal of amino acids lysine and proline in beta chain positions 28 and 29. Because of its very rapid peak onset and concomitant duration compared to regular insulin, dosage of intermediate-acting insulin may need readjustment.

Concentrations with abdominal injection are higher than those for deltoid or femoral area sites. It is recommended that this insulin be injected into the abdomen to enhance absorption and rapid uptake. Studies have shown that its absorption rate is consistently faster compared to regular, thus decreasing hypoglycemic risk between meals; however, when it occurs, hypoglycemia may be more pronounced (Ter Braak et al., 1996; Tuominen et al., 1995). Mixing lispro with another insulin will blunt its rapid onset and may cause variability in that onset. If lispro is to be mixed with another insulin, care should be taken to draw it up first, before the other insulin, according to the following:

- When mixed with NPH, the time for lispro peak is increased, while absorption rate (but not bioavailability) is decreased. Blood glucose stabilization is delayed about 7 hours. Ives and Dunn (1997) report that mixing lispro with Ultralente does not produce this delay in absorption. For multiple combination dosing, Torlone et al. (1996) found that 20% to 40% NPH + 60% to 80% lispro before meals improved blood glucose stabilization to an average of 4 hours postprandial.
- If lispro is mixed with either NPH or Lente (human preparations), give within 5 minutes after mixing insulins and within 15 minutes premeal.
- Do not premix lispro with NPH ahead of time for storage, even if refrigerated, because its stability is not known.

▲ **Clinical Warning:** Consult with a diabetes specialty practice before prescribing lispro. Comanagement of the patient's insulinization may be necessary for patient safety. Hypoglycemia is less than for regular insulin. Therefore, advise 15 g rather than the normal 20 g of immediate-acting carbohydrate as treatment for hypoglycemic episode.

DISPLAY 61–7 • Teaching Insulin Self-Administration and Injection Site Rotation

- Use the smallest caliber needle available (currently 29- or 30-gauge), preferably silicon-coated.
- Use a low-dose syringe, with a dose indicator line gauged at 1 unit per line.
- 1-cc, ½-cc, ¼-cc, and ³/₁₀-cc syringes are available for U-100 insulin injection. ¼-cc or ³/₁₀-cc syringes are used for children and for insulin-sensitive adults taking small dosages.
- Needle sizes are ½-in, 28- or 29-gauge and are silicon-coated.
- Assure the patient that the very small-gauged, silicon-coated needle will make insulin administration easier and virtually painless.
- Teach administration using a magnifying device if the patient requires help seeing the lines on the syringe. Encourage magnifier use at home for this patient.
- Select site and pinch tissue to be used.
- Hold the barrel straight up, like a pencil (or at a 45-degree angle if emaciated), and quickly thrust needle bevel side up into site.
- Check for blood by gently withdrawing plunger very slightly and, if none, inject insulin.
- Release the pinch and withdraw needle.
- Teach and encourage self–blood glucose monitoring.
- Teach injection site management to prevent alterations in insulin absorption, as well as lipohypertrophy. Sites should be chosen to ensure uniformity of insulin uptake, including exercise. Site rotation should be done within the same anatomic region. An ideal site is the abdomen, which is also one that is least affected by exercise.

---

insulin may be required, especially in young children. The family's pharmacist can assist in procuring the appropriate dilutant directly from the insulin manufacturer.

Managing Insulin Adjustments

The dosages of insulin required by patients with diabetes are usually fairly constant, despite great variations in many factors that alter insulin action. In both nondiabetic and diabetic children, increased insulin resistance occurs immediately prior to and during puberty. While prepubertal children with diabetes usually require less than 1 unit of insulin per kilogram of body weight per day, requirements are generally increased in adolescents, often up to 1.5 U/kg per day. The duration of diabetes is another factor to be considered in determining the dose of insulin, because newly diagnosed patients with diabetes require less insulin than those whose duration of disease has been longer. This can be explained by a partial remission of endogenous insulin secretion in newly diagnosed children.

Adolescence affects all parts of a child's life, including metabolic control. Rapid growth and developmental stresses can increase the body's demand for insulin. The primary care provider may need to increase insulinization to 1, 1.3, or even 1.5 U/kg per day for the adolescent patient. Close attention needs to be paid to both the SMBG and the GHB, however, because this increased insulin load can precipitate overeating (in the body's attempt to maintain euglycemia), hypoglycemia, or both. This is a very real potentiality in the suddenly inactive teen and the adolescent who has completed pubertal growth.

● **Clinical Pearls:**

- Try to adjust only one insulin component at a time unless all levels are consistently at 200 mg/dL or greater.
- Because it is difficult to control and can affect the rest of the day's glycemic levels, start with the fasting prebreakfast glucose.
- Adjust the basic insulin dose 1 to 2 U at a time.

Higher dosages of insulin may be required during periods of stress, increased food intake, and diminished physical activity. However, true insulin resistance syndrome in a healthy child with diabetes is extremely rare. If a patient's glycemic control is suboptimal despite increasing dosages of insulin, overinsulinization must be considered as a cause of the problem. Alternatively, an adolescent may not be taking insulin injections or the recommended insulin dose as prescribed. Sometimes a patient may require unusually small

DISPLAY 61–8 • How to Draw Up Insulin

- For all new, unused bottles of insulins **except** regular (R), agitate vigorously to loosen storage-induced sedimentation.
- Gently roll the bottle between the hands to avoid foaming.
- Keeping the bottle on a flat surface, wipe off the top of the bottle (unless brand new) with a clean alcohol wipe. Draw up air into the syringe in an amount that equals that of insulin to be withdrawn, put the needle into the bottle's diaphragm, and inject the air into the bottle.
- Keeping the needle in place, invert the bottle while supporting the syringe.
- Keeping the needle below the insulin's surface, pull back on the plunger to fill the syringe with insulin in the amount equal to the previously injected air.
- Carefully observe for air bubbles and, if seen, tap out. Gently pull back and forth on the plunger while moving the needle's bevel out of the insulin to push air out, and then moving it back under when pulling more insulin in. Alternate this with tapping, thus helping to dislodge stubborn bubbles.

dosages of insulin. Although this could be secondary to remaining endogenous secretion of insulin, other conditions, such as hypothyroidism or hypoadrenalism, should be ruled out.

▲ **Clinical Warning:** Thyroid function tests should be part of the routine follow-up of children with diabetes. Patients with autoimmune diabetes are more prone to nontropical sprue and gastric autoimmunity. Appropriate antibody measurements should be obtained as needed (anti-endomyselial and anti-parietal cell antibodies) (Acerini et al., 1998; Vitoria et al., 1998). Refer to Chapter 60 for information about these measurements and their interpretation.

Supplementary Doses

Sometimes supplementary insulin is needed to augment the one- or two-times daily dosages of insulin. Either regular or Humalog can be used to correct high premeal glucose concentrations. Planning how much supplemental insulin to prescribe depends on several factors, including the patient's sensitivity to insulin, meal planning, and exercise patterns.

● **Clinical Pearls:**

- Supplementation is generally made in the range of 1 to 2 U for every 50 mg/dL above the glycemic goal.
- When the FBG is 200 mg/dL or greater, then consider either delaying the meal to occur 60 minutes after regular insulin injection (rather than the more usual 20 to 30 minutes), or use Humalog, whose onset of action is closer to 30 minutes than the approximately 56 minutes of regular insulin.
- If preprandial glucose is less than 60 to 70 mg/dL, decrease the premeal regular insulin by 1 to 2 U, and give immediately before eating. This meal needs to include 10 g of glucose if the patient's SMBG was under 50 mg/dL.
- If supplementation is required for 3 or more days, add 2 U of regular or Humalog to the prebreakfast insulin dose.

Monitor carefully for patient response, especially if Humalog is used.

Remember that hyperglycemia can cause transient or permanent visual blurring. In insulin self-administration, it is crucial that a patient be certain he or she is getting the correct dose. If the provider and patient determine that visual, special learning, or self-management needs exist, then a CDE or a provider from a diabetes specialty practice group should be consulted. Either of these professionals can provide information and teaching about possible alternative insulin delivery systems or assistive devices. These include information about syringe magnifiers for enlarging calibration and spring-loaded devices that can automatically insert an insulin needle with minimal hand pressure.

Anticipatory Insulin Doses

Because diet and exercise are interconnected to insulin need and its metabolic intake, the person(s) responsible for insulin administration should be taught how to adjust the basic insulin dose to accommodate anticipated increased or decreased activity or exercise and meal changes, in conjunction with the advice of the comanaging endocrine practice.

● **Clinical Pearls:**

- Increase regular insulin by 1 to 2 U for every additional 20 g of carbohydrate ingested (eg, birthday or major holiday)
- Decrease regular insulin by 1 to 2 U if meal is smaller than usual.

Exercise information related to glycemic monitoring, diet, and insulin prescription is provided in Display 61-9.

Mixing Insulins

Mixing insulins is an important skill for all parents and caregivers of younger children and all older children who are self-administering their insulin. Mixing insulins provides for a truly individualized treatment plan (Becker, 1998). Should the clinician need to prescribe an insulin plan that requires mixing, the person(s) responsible for its administration needs to be taught how to draw up different insulin preparations safely in a single syringe. Display 61-10 provides information needed by the patient for mixing insulins.

Premixed insulins are available commercially. Providers should familiarize themselves with what is available in their areas. These insulins can be used in some cases because they are based on commonly occurring (but changeable) dose ratios. A frequently used combination ratio of NPH (N) to regular (R) is $2/3$ N to $1/3$ R (ie, a ratio of 70:30). This provides 70 U of N and 30 U of R per 100 U. The patient could take 9 U of a 70/30 preparation, rather than mixing the breakfast dose of 6 U of N and 3 U of R insulins. Other mix ratios are available in many countries.

● **Clinical Pearl:** The use of premixed insulins may not be practical in children whose short-acting insulin (Humalog, regular) is adjusted on a sliding scale but whose intermediate-acting insulin is a constant dose.

Intensive Insulin Therapy

Two methods for improving insulinization can be used in managing diabetes: insulin infusion using a pump and the multiple injection technique. The former is beyond the

---

DISPLAY 61–9 • Managing Metabolic Requirements, Medications, and Exercise

- Self-monitor blood glucose (SMBG) before, during, and after exercise.
- If SMBG > 240 to 300 mg/dL before, the patient should not exercise. Because high glycemic levels indicate severe low insulin bioavailability, the patient is at increased risk for hyperglycemia secondary to exercise.
- Inject R into abdomen 30 minutes before, to avoid increased absorption.
- If planning moderate exercise (eg, 30–45 minutes of bicycling or jogging), decrease the preceding R dose by 30% to 50%. Then if SMBG is normal or low just before activity, add a 10- to 15-g carbohydrate snack.
- Anyone whose glycogen stores may be low is at risk for hypoglycemia during and immediately after exercise. These patients include anyone who takes in 800 or fewer calories/d, those on a low-carbohydrate diet of < 10 g/d, and alcoholics.
- Hypoglycemic risk is greater for patients on insulin than for those taking sulfonylureas. Diet-only therapy is generally not a risk for hypoglycemia from exercise.
- Postexercise hypoglycemia is a special risk after prolonged exercise, such as day-long hiking. Carbohydrate intake needs to be increased for that day. SMBG needs to be done during the night to monitor for postexercise nocturnal hypoglycemia, which can occur 8 to 15 hours later.
- Patients with severe proliferative retinopathy or retinal hemorrhage must avoid activities that will subject them to jarring, such as jogging, strenuous walking, horseback riding, skiing, bicycling, or aerobic dance. Any exercise that requires moving the head below waist level must also be avoided.

DISPLAY 61–10 • How to Mix Insulins

Avoid contaminating a short-acting (regular [R]) insulin with an intermediate-acting insulin (N), which will obviously thus alter the ratio of R:N. The reverse risk of contaminating N with R is not problematic, as N's protamine can bind the R without altering N's efficacy. Mixing insulins mandates the following procedure:

- Gently roll the N bottle between the hands to disperse sediment.
- Cleanse the tops of both bottles, and then draw up and inject air into the N bottle in the amount to be given (eg, 12 U).
- Inject air into the R bottle in the amount that equals that of the insulin to be withdrawn (eg, 6 U).
- Leaving the syringe in place, invert the R bottle, and draw up the desired amount (to the 6 U mark on the syringe).
- Withdraw the needle, and then carefully inject the needle into the N bottle, being careful not to push the plunger in.
- Invert the N and withdraw the desired amount (to the 18 U mark), taking care not to push the plunger into the N.

---

bounds of this text. Providers interested in using this approach with a patient are advised to consult with a diabetes practice experienced in pump therapy.

Intensive insulin therapy using the multiple injection technique is best undertaken when the patient (generally at least the older adolescent), parents, provider, and a consultant diabetes practice are able to work together to manage the patient's glycemic control. This regimen is designed to mimic the nondiabetic balance of meeting glycemic demand with insulinization. A total daily insulin dose is calculated, based on predicted calorie and exercise needs. The complexity of this approach requires careful attention to individual patient variances. The method that this approach entails is beyond the scope of this text. This approach is best achieved with referral to a diabetes practice group familiar with calculating split dose regimens.

Because of the very real risk for hypoglycemia, intensive insulin treatment, despite generating widespread enthusiasm, has not been generally accepted as a mode of therapy in young children with diabetes in this country. It is beyond the scope of this chapter to go into detail about such therapeutic modalities, except to say that such patients should be referred to diabetes centers experienced in such treatments.

Factors Complicating Insulin Therapy

Some patients taking insulin may experience variances in their glycemic control despite a strong management plan.

Both the Somogyi effect and the dawn phenomenon can pose challenges to achieving glycemic control. Somogyi effect is suspected when the patient's glycemic log shows bedtime normoglycemia, 2:00 AM hypoglycemia, and rebound prebreakfast hyperglycemia. Waning of the evening dose of NPH may in part contribute to this event. Thirty-three percent of patients taking evening NPH may experience asymptomatic nocturnal hypoglycemia, which can rebound into morning hyperglycemia in 10% (Green-Hernandez, 1999a). Elevated postbreakfast hyperglycemia that is refractory to treatment can also be a consequence of nocturnal hypoglycemia and may be symptomatic of insulin resistance. Similarly, dawn phenomenon is suspected when the patient's 2:00 AM SMBG is euglycemic but then hyperglycemia is demonstrated between 4:00 and 8:00 AM.

● **Clinical Pearls:**

- Decrease the evening dose of NPH by 2 or 3 U and monitor 2:00 AM SMBG or continue with AM NPH/Humalog (NPH/regular dose), take only Humalog (or regular) for evening (ie, before supper) dose, and move the evening NPH to bedtime. Monitor 2:00 AM SMBG until satisfied that this plan is successful. This realignment may be all that is needed to prevent nocturnal hypoglycemia and the hyperglycemic rebound in the morning, because NPH's peak effects are given full sway to cover the night to early morning period. This latter plan may also mitigate postbreakfast hyperglycemia and the dawn phenomenon.
- Patients whose glycemic management proves challenging may benefit from referral to a diabetes specialty practice for consultation.
- Doses of medications and even the medications themselves are rarely static in diabetes therapy.

▲ **Clinical Warnings:**

- The dawn phenomenon varies from one day to the next. To prevent asymptomatic nocturnal hypoglycemia and its attendant risks, patients who demonstrate nocturnal hypoglycemia should be encouraged to do 2AM SMBG a few or more times per week, depending on individual glycemic responses (Green-Hernandez, 1999a).

- Remember that short-acting insulin generally is not to be used at bedtime. The provider *must* consult with a diabetes practice before using short-acting insulin (regular) at bedtime.

Hypoglycemia

Prevention and timely management of hypoglycemia are important in controlling its dangerous effects and metabolic disruptions after its overcorrection. This is especially true should hypoglycemia become a management pattern. Hypoglycemia is defined as blood glucose at or less than 50 mg/dL, regardless of whether the patient is symptomatic. Symptoms are generally reported when blood glucose levels drop below 40 mg/dL. Seizures and coma can be seen below 20 mg/dL. Frequent treatment to cover high or low blood sugars must be eliminated from diabetes management if the patient is to avoid or delay the complications of this disease. SMBG, meal planning, exercise, and pharmacologic agents are used together to maintain a glucose profile close to normal or at least within optimal ranges at any given point.

The provider must remember that children younger than 6 or 7 years lack the cognitive ability to recognize and respond to symptoms of hypoglycemia. Young children are also at risk for hyperglycemia because of the frequency of episodic illness they experience (eg, viral upper respiratory infections). Knowledge of sick-day management is very important for any diabetic who takes either insulin or oral hypoglycemic or antidiabetic agents. Display 61-11 provides information about symptoms of and clinical considerations for hypoglycemia and its management. Display 61-12 provides information related to sick-day management.

Severe hypoglycemia is generally defined as any hypoglycemic event that requires that the patient receive assistance to reverse the symptoms. Severe hypoglycemia generally occurs at blood glucose levels of 50 mg/dL or less. Severe hypoglycemia is diagnosed when symptoms of hypoglycemia occur, blood sugar is low when symptoms occur, and symptoms resolve with the administration of rapidly absorbed carbohydrate.

Frequent and recurrent hypoglycemia can lead to the development of long-term neurologic sequelae, interfering with cognitive function and decreasing perception of symptoms signaling low blood sugar. Obviously, the outcome of this complication will be an increase in frequency and severity of hypoglycemic events. Many children and adolescents with type 1 diabetes remain asymptomatic until blood glucose is profoundly low. Their first sign of metabolic distress may be changes in mentation or behavior.

▲ Clinical Warnings:

- Children younger than 6 or 7 years lack the cognitive ability to recognize and respond to symptoms of hypoglycemia.
- Hypoglycemia can be protracted in patients taking sulfonylureas or long-acting insulins. If these patients ingest alcohol, hypoglycemia can be both severe and prolonged. Further, these patients may again become hypoglycemic even after normal blood glucose levels are achieved through intravenous dextrose. To provide for patient safety, any individual in this situation should remain hospitalized after dextrose administration so that close professional supervision can be ensured.
- Because severe hypoglycemia is a life-threatening condition, tight control of blood sugars should be attempted with caution in any older child or adolescent who is at risk for severe hypoglycemia.

DISPLAY 61–11 • Signs and Symptoms, Clinical Possibilities, and Management of Hypoglycemia

Signs and Symptoms

- Blurred vision, sweaty palms, slurred speech, hunger, confusion, shakiness, anxiety, combativeness; sometimes tingling and numbness around lips. Symptoms can be misinterpreted as signs of inebriation.
- Nocturnal signs and symptoms can include nightmares, disturbed sleep pattern, sweating, morning hangover. Reportedly up to 80% of patients have no symptoms.

Clinical Possibilities

- Last meal/snack eaten?
- Physical activity?
- Adverse sulfonylurea reaction (too much, or interaction with other medications)
- Other drug effects
- Delayed gastric emptying (gastroparesis)

Management

- 15–20 g simple, rapidly acting carbohydrate, depending on protocol. Symptoms and, if possible to obtain, self-monitoring of blood glucose (SMBG) guide amount to ingest. Repeat carbohydrate within 15 to 20 minutes if blood glucose continues under 60 mg/dL or if symptomatic. Eat a meal of complex carbohydrate and protein afterward.
- The preferred treatment is 3 or 4 B/D glucose tablets. If this is not possible, then some foods that contain 15 g of simple carbohydrate per serving include:
  ½ cup (4 oz) of orange juice
  6 oz of carbonated regular soft drink
  3 sugar cubes or 3 tsp granulated sugar
  7 or 8 Lifesaver candies (quickly crunched—not tooth-friendly)
- The unconscious or seizing patient should be given:
  Glucose gel (comes in a tube; squeeze into the inside of the patient's cheek), or
  Glucagon 1 mg SC, IM, or IV (average response time 6.5 minutes), or
  Glucose 25 g IV (50 cc dextrose 50%) (average response time is 4 minutes)
- Follow-up hospitalization may be warranted.

Source: ADA, 2000; Green-Hernandez, 1999.

DISPLAY 61–12 • Sick-Day Guidelines for Patients Taking Medication for Diabetes

TYPE 1

- Avoid dehydration.
- Continue insulin.
- Check blood glucose every 2 hours.
- Give supplemental doses of regular insulin, using an individualized range developed in concert with diabetes specialist. Supplementation may, for example, be established as 1–2 U of R for every 30 to 50 mg/dL elevation above a prearranged glucose level (140 mg/dL).
- Check urine ketones every 4 hours or sooner if blood sugar > 240 mg/dL
- Use a variety of clear fluids (some with sugar and some without) to maintain blood glucose level, especially if unable to eat. Strive for a caloric intake of 50 g of carbohydrate every 4 hours. Jello and popsicles (regular, not sugar-free), juices, regular soda, crackers, soups, and toast may be tolerated.
- Aim to drink 6 to 8 oz of clear fluids every hour. A sound protocol for vomiting or diarrhea could include replacing fluids and electrolytes with Pedialyte or similar solution.

▲ **Clinical Warning:** Patient should seek medical attention for:
- Continued vomiting or diarrhea, if SMBG exceeds 240 mg/dL, or if urine ketones continue elevated despite 2 or 3 supplemental doses of regular insulin if it is part of the patient's sick-day protocol, or if large amount of ketones or trace to small amounts in urine after 24 hours.

- Vomiting or diarrhea and temperature > 101°F for more than 24 hours.
- Signs of local infection (eg, urinary tract infection; open, purulent draining wound; cellulitis-like symptoms).
- Signs of diabetic ketoacidosis, including extreme fatigue, abdominal cramping, and alterations in normal breathing pattern.

TYPE 2

- Avoid dehydration.
- If taking insulin, take ½ usual insulin dose if unable to eat as usual.
- If on oral agents and unable to eat, withhold agent for 1 hour. If able to eat after that time, take medication and some water. If unable to tolerate, notify provider.
- Monitor SMBG as above for type 1.
- Seek medical attention as above or if illness is profound or protracted.
- Some patients will require insulin. Follow individualized protocol as above.

▲ **Clinical Warning:** If taking an alpha-glucosidase inhibitor or metformin, withhold dose if vomiting or diarrhea occurs. Do frequent SMBGs (every 2 hours or so), following guidelines as directed above. Resume medication when normal gastrointestinal function returns.

All patients with a history of severe hypoglycemia or with established risk factors, all household members, and patient's parents will need instruction in the use of glucagon, which is available by prescription. Glucagon can take up to 30 minutes to reverse the hypoglycemic episode. It is therefore important that the patient and family be able to use other, quicker oral methods for treating severe hypoglycemia. If the patient is conscious, a glass of orange juice with an added tablespoon of sugar can be quickly administered. A roll of hard candies can be kept in the bedside table for rapid access. At least seven or eight of these candies should be quickly crunched and swallowed. If the patient loses consciousness, a family or friend who is trained to do so can administer glucose through glucagon injection or alternatively and if there is no danger of choking, placement of glucose gel into the patient's cheeks.

Parents or caregivers and older children should be instructed in the practice of record-keeping whenever a hypoglycemic event occurs, including time of occurrence, relationship to meals or snacks, exercise, sleep, last medication dosage, and amount taken. Physical state immediately prior to the episode should also be noted. When the patient is next seen by the primary care provider, they can go over the record together. If any kind of pattern is seen to emerge in these episodes, a management plan can be developed that may at least help to mitigate the frequency or severity of these episodes.

● **Clinical Pearl:** Patients should be advised to carry 15 g of carbohydrate with them at all times and to wear an identifying bracelet that alerts others that they are diabetic (ADA, 1998).

Meal Planning

The role of proper nutrition in the management of a child with type 1 diabetes cannot be overemphasized. Food intake can affect the presence or absence of hypoglycemia, the dosage and timing of insulin injections, and, ultimately, the prognosis of the patient. A regular meal pattern is important (Kulkarni et al., 1998). The nutritional requirements of a child with diabetes are similar to those of children without diabetes. In general, the term *diabetes diet* is considered improper because it connotes restriction and denial. Instead, terms such as *meal planning* and *nutritional requirements* are preferable.

The key elements of sound meal planning for a child with diabetes are regular timing and consistency of meals and snacks that synchronize with timing of insulin doses. Nutritional recommendations for patients with type 1 diabetes are periodically issued by the ADA. This resource is described in the Community Resources section of this chapter. There is no one ideal diet, but generally 15% to 20% of calories should be provided as protein, 30% as fat, and the remaining calories as carbohydrate. The intake of carbohydrate can be directed by carbohydrate counting, because the total amount of carbohydrate consumed is more important for glycemic control than is the source of carbohydrate. Fat intake should include 10% as saturated fats, less than 10% as polyunsaturated fats, and the remainder as monosaturated fats. The intake of animal fats should, therefore, be reduced through replacement with vegetable sources (Riley & Dwyer, 1998).

Cholesterol intake should be reduced by limiting the intake of fatty meals and non–fat-free dairy products. The metabolism of both carbohydrates and lipids can be further improved by increased intake of dietary fiber. The protein consumed should be of high biologic quality. Excess protein and fat may have adverse effects on both the renal and cardiovascular systems. Despite the many new developments in the nutritional management of patients with type 1 disease, much remains to be learned about optimal nutrition for diabetes.

● **Clinical Pearl:** Because tastes and food preferences change as part of a child's normal growth and development, the provider should assess nutritional patterns and appetite on an annual basis.

Exercise and Activity

Exercise is an integral part of the management of children with type 1 diabetes. Regular exercise may benefit patients in many ways, such as improving metabolic control of diabetes, raising self-esteem, and ameliorating chronic complications of the disease. If significant weight loss is desired, exercise must be done in conjunction with nutritional modifications to achieve maximal results. Even patients who lose only a small amount of weight on an exercise regimen undergo changes in body composition, such as decreased adipose tissue mass and reduced insulin requirements.

Hypoglycemia is the most frequent and dramatic complication of exercise in an individual with diabetes. This is the result of accelerated glucose use during exercise, without the patient's ability to down-regulate insulin secretion, leading to relative hyperinsulinism. This effect occurs even in patients who are receiving an appropriate amount of insulin and whose diabetes is well controlled. Not only can patients develop hypoglycemia during exercise, but they may become hypoglycemic several hours after exercise is completed. This phenomenon has been named *late onset of postexercise hypoglycemia.*

▲ **Clinical Warning:** The provider must keep in mind the risk for late onset of postexercise hypoglycemia when prescribing an exercise regimen, especially one for the evening hours. Exercise should be avoided if blood glucose is high (usually over 300 mg/dL), especially when accompanied by positive urine ketones. In such cases, exercise may elevate blood glucose further, rather than decrease it.

● **Clinical Pearl:** Patients who have problems with hypoglycemia during exercise should consume an extra 15 to 30 g of carbohydrate before or after every 30 minutes of exercise. If they exercise on a regular basis, the dose of insulin should be modified. For example, a 10% reduction in insulin dosage may be attempted when physical activities are planned.

The provider needs to instruct the patient that exercise can alter the rate of insulin absorption. The patient should take care not to use any anatomic site for insulin injection that is to be used in exercise. For example, a runner or dancer should avoid injecting the thigh prior to exercising. Because everyone responds differently to exercise, some patients may require insulin adjustments, whereas others may not.

Adolescent patients who have retinopathy should be taught to be very selective in their exercise routines and other activities in which they participate. Patients with preproliferative and proliferative retinopathy should avoid all activities that increase intraocular pressure. These include weightlifting and arm wrestling. Activities of daily living, such as lifting or moving objects such as heavy toys or sports equipment, also increase the risk of ophthalmic injury. Isometric exercise should be practiced only if the patient has had proper breath training.

All patients who undertake an exercise program or activities should be advised of the importance of careful foot evaluation before and after the activity. They should also be encouraged to use proper equipment and foot gear and to replace it when needed.

Treating Type 2 Diabetes and MODY

Meal Planning

Because *diet* is an emotionally charged and negative word, the concept of a *meal plan* is easier to accept and discuss. The primary goal of meal planning is control of blood sugar and lipid levels. Meal planning is an important skill for both parent and patient learning, because optimal glycemic control can be accomplished through planning meals. Most adolescents do not plan their meals. Planning includes meal composition, preparation methods, portion size, and condiments added. The provider should ask the parents and child specific questions regarding favorite foods and about any food allergies or sensitivities, such as lactose intolerance, which may appear in adolescence.

● **Clinical Pearl:** Weight loss is a secondary target and is not easily sustained. In teaching meal planning, the provider should first aim at what can be done realistically to aid the patient in self-managing glycemic control. Very modest reductions in weight (3–10 lb) often yield dramatic improvements in glycemic control.

▲ **Clinical Warning:** Juice and crackers are not recommended for bedtime consumption. Snacks containing only carbohydrate will provide only short-term fuel and, in fact, can potentiate higher blood glucose levels. Adding high-fat foods, such as peanut butter, may contribute to fasting hyperglycemia and general lipid excess in adults. Fats are not metabolized rapidly enough to prevent short-term hypoglycemia.

Exercise and Activity

Exercise can have positive effects on glucose control across the lifespan (Eriksson et al., 1997; Erikkson, 1999). Exercise can overcome or reverse many common mistakes in meal planning and eating patterns. Moving from the theoretic recognition of its importance to the daily practice of exercise is one of the most challenging tasks in clinical practice. As discussed in the section dealing with type 1 diabetes, learning healthy lifestyle activities in adolescence can greatly ameliorate the otherwise serious complication of long-term diabetes.

Oral Antidiabetic Medication

Whenever antidiabetic medication is initiated or adjusted, the provider must remain in at least weekly contact with the patient and family until glycemic goals are achieved (ADA, 2000b). The primary care provider must assess each child and family on an individual, case-by-case basis. It is essential that the primary care provider remember that the patient with type 2 diabetes will require insulin when ill or if the blood sugar is very high. It is also important that the provider be familiar with signs and symptoms of nonketotic hyperosmolar syndrome, because the individual whose type 2 disease is in poor control for whatever reason is at risk for this potentially fatal complication (see Display 61-5).

Insulin absence in type 2 diabetes (for whatever reason) will prevent the movement of nutrients to tissues. This occurrence will precipitate metabolic acidosis. Metabolic acidosis results from lack of insulin in the hepatocyte, which alters a metabolic pathway whose outcome is ketone production. Low doses of insulin are required to reverse this pathway. Increases in insulin dosage in patients taking insulin will be required in times of illness or fasting. Guidelines for these adjustments are discussed in the section on treatment of type 1 disease (see Display 61-12).

Oral antidiabetic agents can be very effective in the adolescent with type 2 disease who has endogenous insulin capacity. These agents are prescribed when diet and exercise have not corrected hyperglycemia. Over the past 3 to 5 years, several new agents have become available that can control blood sugar with little or no risk of hypoglycemia. This has made it both reasonable and safe to achieve near-normal HbA_{1c} values in many patients who previously would have required insulin.

The choice of which oral agent to prescribe for a particular individual is based on many factors. Age, adiposity or relative leanness, lipid levels, blood pressure, and degree of hyperglycemia are some of the important considerations to bear in mind.

▲ Clinical Warnings:

- The provider is strongly advised to encourage the adolescent with type 2 disease to adopt a healthy lifestyle, including improved dietary habits and daily exercise. The decision to begin medication should be a last resort in a young person whose disease state may reasonably respond to proactive, nonpharmacologic interventions.
- Because of the risks associated with unrecognized hypoglycemia (and of hyperglycemia), every patient taking an antidiabetic agent should be advised to wear a diabetes identification bracelet. Applications for this tag are readily available in pharmacy settings.

Sulfonylureas increase beta-cell insulin secretion through closure of ATP-sensitive potassium channels. They are usually well tolerated. Major side effects include hypoglycemia and, rarely, allergic reactions. Because they are highly protein bound, sulfonylureas have relatively long durations of action. Sulfonylureas are appropriately used in leaner people (eg, diagnosed with MODY) who have moderate hyperglycemia (FPG < 140 mg/dL; HbA_{1c} < 8). Whether to use a first- or a second-generation agent depends on individual clinical factors. Second-generation sulfonylureas, such as glipizide and glyburide, are generally more potent on a mg/mg basis than first-generation drugs. Hypoglycemia is possible with all sulfonylureas. This problem is less likely with the newer second-generation agents than with the first-generation drugs, such as tolbutamide or chlorpropamide. Fewer side effects are associated with second-generation sulfonylureas.

▲ Clinical Warning: Individuals with a known sulfa allergy should be carefully evaluated before beginning therapy with a sulfonylurea, to avoid allergic response (Clark, 1998).

The primary mode of action of *biguanides* (metformin) is to decrease hepatic glucose production. This class of drugs also acts to increase intracellular glucose metabolism. To a lesser extent, biguanides also inhibit intestinal glucose absorption and may involve insulin sensitivity. Because of their efficacy in controlling glucose overproduction by the liver, biguanides are referred to as antihyperglycemics, as compared with other oral agents that are referred to as hypoglycemics. There is virtually no risk of hypoglycemia when biguanides are used as monotherapy. Metformin monotherapy does not promote weight gain and, in fact, may have favorable effects on lipid levels. This may be a good choice in obese patients with hyperlipidemia. Biguanides have been especially effective in interrupting the uncontrolled response of the liver to increased glucagon production. In rare cases, lactic acidosis has been reported in association with biguanides. These instances include hypotension, hypoxemia, and any other condition that could place a patient at risk for lactic acidosis, although this is very rare with metformin. The risk can be further decreased with careful patient evaluation before its prescription (Clark, 1998).

Alpha-glucosidase inhibitors (eg, acarbose, miglitol) are a reasonable choice in mild hyperglycemia, especially in people with a diet rich in carbohydrates. These drugs are helpful for patients whose fasting blood glucose levels are close to normal but whose postprandial glucose levels are elevated. Their primary mode of action is to decrease carbohydrate absorption from the gastrointestinal (GI) tract. This results in a decrease in the normal postprandial glucose rise because glucose digestion is slowed. Because these agents do not enhance insulin secretion, they do not cause hypoglycemia, even if the patient is fasting. Their ability to enhance glycemic control is additive, making them a reasonable addition to an existing regimen, especially in cases in which postprandial glycemic control is refractory. Acarbose does not inhibit lactose; therefore, lactose intolerance should not be seen due to this agent.

▲ Clinical Warnings:

- When metformin is used as monotherapy, overdosage will not result in hypoglycemia. In this instance, the patient may experience GI symptoms of relatively short duration.
- If metformin is used in combination therapy with other agents, hypoglycemia can occur.
- Treatment of low blood sugars with alpha-glucosidase inhibition requires the use of simple sugar, such as glucose tablets or gel. Table sugar, soda, and fruit juices all contain sucrose and will not be effective in treating this form of hypoglycemia.

When using combination therapy as outlined above, adding acarbose may prove helpful in lowering postprandial glucose levels and overall HbA_{1c}. As a monotherapy, acarbose will not affect lipids, nor will it potentiate hypoglycemia. Hypoglycemia can occur when it is used in combination with other agents secondary to postprandial glucose reduction. As with metformin, significant GI effects can be decreased through slow titration and diet management.

The *thiazolidinedione* agents are the newest class of drugs to be used in treatment of type 2 diabetes. Their primary mode of action is to increase insulin sensitivity of the liver, peripheral and adipose tissues, and skeletal muscle. Two currently available thiazolidinediones are Avandia and Actos. Neither agent has been tested in pediatric populations. Multiple fatalities have been associated with troglitazone (Rezulin), which was the first agent available in this class. Troglitazone was removed from the U.S. market by the FDA in March 2000.

▲ Clinical Warning: Because of general hepatotoxicities associated with the thiazolidinedione class of drugs, it is not recommended that these agents be used in the management of type 2 diabetes in children or adolescents at this time.

Regardless of which oral agent is chosen to be added to a type 2 or MODY regimen, two principles must be kept in mind:

- FPG should be obtained 2 weeks after any dosage change. Continue to adjust the dosage at 2-week increments until the FPG is in the therapeutic range of 80 to 120 mg/dL for older children and adolescents.
- If a single agent does not achieve the desired treatment goals, then a combination of oral agents can be used.

The major classes of oral agents and prescribing information are summarized in Table 61-2. This is not intended to be an exhaustive presentation of each agent. As with any medication, consult the package insert or a recent pharmacotherapeutics text for more detailed prescribing information.

▲ **Clinical Warnings:**

- Any time combination therapy is used, the risk for hypoglycemia is potentiated.
- Sulfonylureas and thiazolidinedione agents can all increase appetite, leading to weight gain and, subsequently, elevated blood glucose levels.

Office Management

Elements of the physical examination for patients with diabetes are shown in Display 61-2. Display 61-13 presents a general office management plan for each scheduled visit. Table 61-3 provides an overview of visit frequency for specific management issues.

The provider's comanagement of diabetes needs to be planned in accordance with the family's ethnic and cultural practices. Both patient and family will be more apt to embrace the healthy planning begun with the help of the

Table 61–2. ORAL AGENTS

Drug/Strength	Dose	Mean Half-Life (Hours)	Duration (Hours)	Notes
Chloropropamide 100 mg, 250 mg	0.1–0.5 g/d	35	24–72	Do not prescribe if risk of hyperglycemia is enhanced, as in renal failure, or in the case of decreased protein or energy stores. It has the highest frequency of side effects of sulfas. Should not be prescribed for elderly. Is associated with alcohol-induced flushing; warn about this side effect.
Acetohexamide 250 mg, 500 mg	0.25–1.5 g/d or in divided doses b.i.d.	6	12–18	Caution in elderly with renal disease.
Tolazamide 100 mg, 250 mg, 500 mg	0.2–1 g/d or in divided doses b.i.d.	7	12–24	Renal failure may cause metabolites to accumulate.
Tolbutamide 250 mg, 500 mg	0.05–3 g in divided doses b.i.d. or t.i.d.	7	6–12	Shortest acting of this class.
Glipizide 5 mg, 10 mg	2.5–40 mg/d or in divided doses b.i.d.	3	12–24	Divide doses > 15 mg. Take 30 min before meals. Adverse reactions range from dizziness to leukopenia, thrombocytopenia, mild anemia, hypoglycemia, dilutional hyponatremia, nausea, vomiting, urticaria, facial flushing, constipation, epigastric fullness, heartburn, weakness, and paresthesia. See package insert. May need to discontinue depending on severity of reaction(s).
Glipizide extended release	5–20 mg/d or in divided doses b.i.d.	4–12	24	Same.
Glyburide 1.25 mg, 2.5 mg, 5 mg	1.25–20 mg/d before breakfast or in divided doses b.i.d. before breakfast and supper	4–13	12–24	Initial dose with breakfast. Monitor closely for first week if substituting for chlorpropamide, due to prolonged retention of chlorpropamide. Refer to package insert for dosing information when changing from insulin to glyburide. Caution in elderly, renal failure, intestinal blockage; use with caution in patients tending to hypoglycemia. Adverse reactions resemble those for other sulfonylureas. Divide doses > 10 mg to maximum 20 mg/d.

(continues)

Table 61–2. ORAL AGENTS *(Continued)*

Drug/Strength	Dose	Mean Half-Life (Hours)	Duration (Hours)	Notes
Micronized/glyburide 1.5 mg, 3 mg	1.0–12 mg/d	4	24	Same as for glyburide. Divide doses > 6 mg.
Glimepiride	Initially 1–2 mg/d with breakfast or first main meal of day. Followed by gradual increases to a maximum of 8 mg/d. Most common maintenance dose ranges from 1–4 mg.	5	24	Dose increase after reaching initial 2-mg dose should be based on serum glucose response at no more than 1–2 mg at 1- to 2-wk intervals. Is thought to cause less insulin secretion than others of this class due to different binding sites on cells, so potential for exacerbating insulin resistance may be less than for other second-generations, though clinical experience has not shown this.
				Adverse reactions resemble those for other sulfonylureas. Effective as monotherapy and, for those with type 2 in secondary beta cell failure (with FBG > 150 mg/dL), has shown efficacy with insulin, decreasing insulin requirement. Encourage daily SMBG. In renal and hepatic insufficiency, start with 1 mg/d. No dosage adjustment needed in elderly, but recommended start with 1 mg and increase carefully.
Repaglinide	t.i.d., taken 15 min before meals	~1	~96	Works by producing insulin when needed (ie, at mealtime).
Metaformin 500 mg, 850 mg	0.5–2.5 g in divided doses b.i.d. or t.i.d.	Unknown, but may be ½–3	6–12	Avoid in anyone lacking normal renal function, in hypotension, hypoxemia, or if predisposed to lactic acidosis (eg, ETOH). Discontinue before dye-cast studies or in dehydration. Expensive.
Acarbose 50 mg, 100 mg	Recommended initial dose is 25 mg (½ tablet) t.i.d., gradually titrate up to 50–100 mg t.i.d. chewed with first bite of meal. Alternatively, can start with 25 mg/d at largest meal (usually supper) for 1 wk, then increase each week by 25 mg to a maximum of 100 mg t.i.d. chewed with first bite of each meal. This seems to decrease gastrointestinal (GI) symptoms.	xx	~3	The major side effect is flatulence secondary to bacterial action in the colon on undigested carbohydrates. Base dosing changes on the postprandial blood sugar. Goal is to decrease this and bring HbA$_{1c}$ into therapeutic range. Benefits include no hypoglycemia or weight change effects, as well as decrease in postprandial insulin secretion and in triglyceride/cholesterol levels in FPGs. Contraindicated in bowel disease, ketoacidosis, any condition that may be worsened by gas formation. See package insert for other, less common adverse effects. Reinforce importance of preprandial SMBG to avoid periprandial hypoglycemia due to too high a dose.
Miglitol 25 mg (50 mg, 100 mg)	Recommended initial dose is 25 mg t.i.d. Alternatively, can start at 25 mg once daily to minimize GI symptoms and gradually increase to t.i.d. Take orally t.i.d. with first bite of each main meal.	About 2		Should not cause hypoglycemia when used as monotherapy. Its effect is additive when used with a sulfonylurea. Contraindications same as for acarbose, as are side effects.

b.i.d. = twice daily; ETOH = ethyl alcohol; FBG = fasting blood glucose; FPG = fasting plasma glucose; SMBG = self-monitoring of blood glucose; t.i.d. = three times daily.

diabetic specialty team if foods normally eaten and ritual events are integrated into the teaching plan (McKenzie et al., 1998; Green-Hernandez, 1999b).

Monitoring for Complications

Information related to monitoring for complications is included with that provided for the physical examination for a patient with diabetes in Display 61-2.

Research efforts are making great progress in helping patients normalize organ damage caused by the disease. For example, Bursell et al. (1999) found that adding 1800 IUs of supplemental vitamin E to the daily diet of people with type 1 diabetes normalized retinal blood flow and creatinine clearance. These and other research findings hold promise for the future of diabetes management.

Until such findings can be replicated and become policy, however, the provider would be wise to remember that poorly controlled diabetes, including persistent hyperglycemia and a history of frequent and profound hypoglycemia, exacts a terrible toll on future organ function. The potential of end organ damage is a very real outcome that the child may face as an older adolescent or adult.

Retinopathy

Proliferative retinopathy can begin as early as after 3 to 5 years of diabetes. Annual eye examinations with pupillary dilation by an ophthalmologist or licensed optometrist skilled in retinopathic assessment, including flicker perimetry, are essential to prevent the complications of diabetic retinopathy (Lobefalo et al., 1997). Clinical funduscopic examination cannot reveal the subtleties of diabetic retinopa-

thy. Children who are 10 years of age or older should be examined by an ophthalmologist or optometrist for an initial dilated, comprehensive eye examination within a 3- to 5-year period following their diabetes onset. As a rule, diabetic eye disease screening is not needed before age 10. All patients with type 2 diabetes must be referred for an initial dilated, comprehensive eye examination shortly following diagnosis. Once initiated, dilated eye examinations for both groups must be done annually and lifelong with increased frequency, should retinopathy be noted (ADA, 2000c; Danne, et al., 1998).

● **Clinical Pearl:** The provider is advised to discuss the importance of ophthalmologic screening with the parents, documenting this advice in the child's chart on an annual basis after that time.

▲ **Clinical Warning:** Any decrease in vision or onset of new floaters should be evaluated immediately by an ophthalmologist or licensed optometrist skilled in assessing diabetic retinae. Panretinal or scatter photocoagulation may be used on patients with high-risk characteristics, including proliferation of new vessels on the disc.

Nephropathy

Diabetes is one of the leading causes of end-stage renal disease (ESRD). Five-year survival for people with diabetes and ESRD approaches only 20% (DCCT Research Group, 1993). In patients with type 1 diabetes, renal disease commonly develops 10 to 20 years after the diagnosis of diabetes. The development of nephropathy is heralded by the onset of microalbuminuria several years before blood pressure or serum creatinine become abnormal. Only Caucasians with

---

DISPLAY 61–13 • **General Management Plan for All at Each Office Visit**

- Length/height and weight; height until maturity, with comparison to norms
- Sexual maturation in the peripubertal period, with comparison to norms
- Parent(s)/caregiver(s) progress in managing the child's diabetes
- Patient's progress in self-management and in goal attainment for diabetes care in the older child/adolescent
- Log of blood glucose levels. Ideally, the patient brings the control device to the office, where the stored glucose determinations can be downloaded. The printout serves two purposes: a valid and reliable record of patient's blood sugars since the last visit; and objective data for the patient's medical record.
- Diet and exercise regimens. These should be examined in tandem with the blood glucose record. Any episodes of hyperglycemia or hypoglycemia should be closely correlated with these, with clarification of whether the patient was ill, had missed a meal, had eaten foods not normally consumed, and so forth.
- Contraception (if indicated)
- Medications, including dosage and frequency

- Lifestyle changes since last visit; biopsychosocial stress in general, and related to diabetes
- Complications of diabetes
- Blood pressure control
- Dyslipidemia (if indicated)
- Were any referrals made at previous appointment? Check whether these were followed up. If not, work with patient to determine whether he or she can follow through on this aspect of the self-care plan.
- Specific knowledge related to diabetes self-care should be reviewed on an as-needed basis. Overall self-management knowledge related to medications, self-administration, diet, exercise, and so forth should be reviewed annually.
- Encourage participation in support groups for diabetes, such as the local affiliate of the American Diabetes Association if available. Also encourage joining this organization's lay group. Patients receive *The Diabetes Forecast* as part of their membership. This excellent publication provides current information related to diabetes and its management. The address appears at the end of this chapter. Encourage patients to avail themselves of any continuing education programs on diabetes offered in their community.

Sources: ADA, 1996b; 2000b.

Table 61–3.   VISIT FREQUENCY

Visit Frequency	Therapy Status	Ask
Every 3 mo	All on insulin	Hypoglycemia or hyperglycemia episodes; cause, frequency, severity; glucose self-monitoring results; insulin and therapeutic regimen adjustments; problems with metabolic emergencies, such as hypoglycemia requiring another's help; self-management of diet; exercise and other goals being met? Also, symptoms of complications, other illnesses; current medications; psychosocial or lifestyle issues.
Every 3–6 mo (depends on treatment goal achievement)	Oral hypoglycemics	As above
More frequent	All categories of diabetes	Self-management or medication problems. Acute complications or exacerbation.
Every 3–6 mo (depends on treatment goal achievement)	Diet and exercise only	Self-management of diet, exercise, and other goals being met? Symptoms of complications; other illnesses, current medications; psychosocial or lifestyle issues. Dental hygiene and prophylaxis.
Annually	All	
Age 9 y and older		

type 2 diabetes seem to be relatively spared excessive rates of nephropathy. Individuals at greatest risk for nephropathy include those of Native North American, Hispanic, Asian, African, and Pacific Island heritage. Kidney disease clusters in families. The incidence of diabetic nephropathy throughout a given practice area will vary considerably with the ethnic composition of the clinic and the family history of the patient.

The DCCT Research Group (1993) showed that optimal control of blood glucose can prevent or delay progression of nephropathy in type 1 diabetes. Alzaid (1996) reported that in type 2 disease, higher glucose/glycosylated hemoglobins are most strongly associated with microalbuminuria.

Microalbuminuria is diagnosed when a urine/creatinine ratio of 30 to 300 mg/g creatinine is seen, or an albumin

excretion range of 30 to 300 mg in a 24-hour urine (Cooper, 1998; Bursell et al., 1999; ADA, 1999). Testing should be done on any patient with type 1 diabetes after 5 years of disease or at puberty (whichever comes first) and annually thereafter. Individuals with type 2 diabetes should be tested at the time of diagnosis and annually thereafter. Control of concomitant hypertension must be a goal in all patients to prevent, mitigate, or delay progression of nephropathy.

▲ **Clinical Warning:** Beta-blockers can mute the adrenergic symptoms of hypoglycemia and decrease the movement of glycogen stores in muscle and liver in response to low blood sugar levels. This is especially true for patients taking insulin and for those with longstanding type I disease. In addition, response to counterregulatory

Examine	Plan	Phone or Office Follow-up
Length/height until maturity and compare with compare with age norms; weight; blood pressure; any part of examination that was abnormal at last visit; fundi (preferably with dilation): refer stat to ophthalmologist or optometrist if new finding; if symptomatic feet, check sensation (using and nails; sexual maturation in the peripubertal period.	Refer to relevant specialist if findings suggest significant ischemia, infection, deformity, ulceration, and so forth. Reinforce diabetic teaching as well as foot care as needed. Refer to pediatric endocrinologist if growth or sexual maturation is delayed.	Daily if new to insulin, and if major change in dose. May need daily visits as well until daily glucose controlled, hypoglycemia risk is low, and patient competent in implementing treatment. Hospitalization may be needed for some.
Any relevant system suggested by history.	As above	May need to be seen or phoned weekly if new to treatment, until blood glucose range is reasonable or is able to manage regimen.
System relating to presented problem.	As above	Phone or office follow-up needed when goals not being met; complications arise or worsen, also following metabolic emergencies, such as hypoglycemia requiring another's help (if on medication); diabetic ketoacidosis; acute illness or appearance/exacerbation of chronic illness, including hypertension.
As above	As above	In-between phone follow-up as needed.
	Obtain laboratory data (see Display 61-4). Comprehensive visual and dilated eye exams by ophthalmologist or optometrist after 3–5 y of diabetes, all over age 10 y. Also, if reports visual/eye changes. Influenza vaccine is recommended for all children with diabetes, age ≥ 6 months, beginning each September (ADA, 2000d). Pneumonoccal vaccine per protocol for children 23 months of age and younger with PCV7, and in all 24-59 months of age if at high risk for invasive infection (AAP, 2000) Annual flu vaccine administered at least 1 month apart (the last before December in the Northern Hemisphere) for children < 9 who have never been vaccinated (ADA, 2000d) Pneumococcal vaccine in the same group, with added emphasis for Native American groups who have a high incidence of DM and invasive pneumococcal disease (ADA, 2000d).	

hormones may be excessive because of the lack of alpha opposition of beta blockade. Patients with endogenous insulin capacity may be at risk for hyperosmolar nonketotic coma (Young & Koda-Kimble, 1995). Extreme caution should be used in persons with longstanding diabetes who may have hypoglycemic unawareness. Beta-blockers will further block normal awareness of and recovery from hypoglycemia because they mask symptoms such as tachycardia. The provider must carefully evaluate the risk for a fatal outcome of masked hypoglycemia when using beta-blockers, whose use in pediatrics is in any event controversial.

There are three methods for microalbuminuria screening, any one of which is acceptable:

1. Measurement of albumin-to-creatinine ratio in a random, spot collection. First-void or morning samples are best.
2. 24-hour collection for albumin and creatinine, allowing for simultaneous measurement of the creatinine clearance
3. Timed specimen (eg, 4 hours, or an overnight collection) for albumin and creatinine

Note that urinary albumin levels can be increased over baseline (thus invalidating the sample results) if the patient has a fever, infection, congestive heart failure (Weston et al., 1997), severe hyperglycemia, or serious hypertension or if the individual has exercised vigorously within 24 hours of specimen collection.

There is a normal variation in day-to-day excretion of albumin. Therefore, a minimum of two or three samples that demonstrate sustained elevation should be collected over a period of 3 to 6 months. Only then can incipient nephropathy be diagnosed (Roy et al., 1998; ADA, 2000b).

Discussion of treatment goals for incipient or overt nephropathy is beyond the scope of this text. It is imperative that the provider consult with the comanaging diabetes specialty practice about any patient exhibiting incipient nephropathy, because intensive diabetic treatment strategies may be able to reverse or at least ameliorate its progression. In addition, referral to a pediatric nephrologist may be needed. Chapter 62 provides management information for nephropathy.

Information about the monitoring of kidney function in diabetes is presented in Display 61-14.

Other Complications

Diabetic neuropathy, including peripheral neuropathy and autonomic neuropathy, atherosclerosis, and orthostatic hypotension, is generally not seen in childhood or adolescence. It typically does not occur until the patient has had poorly controlled diabetes for many years. Diabetic neuropathy is characterized by pain and associated symptoms of numbness and tingling in hands and feet plus deep organ system neuropathy. The goal of pediatric management is the prevention of these complications in the patient's late adolescence or adulthood.

Findings of DCCT data analysis in 1993 indicate that most diabetic complications are the result of prolonged hyperglycemia. High levels of glucose can cause proteins to bind together, creating advanced glycation end-products (AGEs). AGEs have the consistency of overcooked spaghetti. AGEs can interfere with multiple cellular activities, ultimately destroying renal filtration capacitance. They are also implicated in the development of neuropathy and vascularopathy in diabetes (Friedman, 1999; Sugimoto et al., 1999; Osicka et al., 2000). The significance of these problems for the patient's long-term health cannot be underestimated.

● **Clinical Pearl:** Good glycemic control is the most powerful preventive measure for the complications of diabetes. At the very least, such control will delay or inhibit the development of microvascular and macrovascular complications. Macrovascular disease in adolescents with a history of poorly controlled diabetes (whether type 1 or 2) is increasingly common (Strong et al., 1999).

The eventual availability of a pharmacologic intervention holds promise for halting AGEs. Pimagedine, which is currently in clinical trail, may be of help in preventing or slowing AGE development. Previously, the only way to restore normal renal filtration in the face of diabetic nephropathy was through kidney transplantation. Pharmacologic normalization of renal function would mean that the progression of complications, such as renal disease, might be prevented by more than maintaining strict glycemic control only (Smulders, 1998; Bursell et al., 1999; Friedman, 1999; Osicka et al., 2000). In the meantime, the primary care provider must apply a total approach to diabetes management that encompasses all metabolic deficits.

The clinician needs to work intensively with the child and family to help them understand the importance of good clinical control of diabetes. Good control will support healthy growth and development. Perhaps of even greater significance, good glycemic management can help protect the child from the deadly complications of this disease. Microvascular and macrovascular disease, nephropathy, and neuropathies can be delayed or prevented altogether when a sound dia-

---

> **DISPLAY 61–14 • Monitoring Kidney Function in Diabetes**
>
> * Yearly assessment of microalbuminuria, serum creatinine, and 24-hour urinary protein (annually with puberty or after 5 years of disease [type 1]).
> * Creatinine clearance determinations at time of type 2 diagnosis and every year thereafter. The use of albumin/creatinine (A/C) ratio on a spot urine specimen can help screen for early nephropathy. An A/C ratio of < 20 mcg/g does not require confirmation by 24-hour or timed urinary collection. If creatinine clearance < 100 mL/min/1.73 M^2, or if abnormal serum creatinine, then check more frequently.
> * Consider nondiabetic cause of nephropathy if proteinuria occurs soon after diagnosis or if creatinine rises with minimal proteinuria.

---

betic regimen underpins the child's lifestyle. Toward this end, families can model healthy eating and exercise habits, smoking cessation, and avoidance of other substances of abuse, including alcohol and street drugs. Healthy lifelong habits are a powerful means to effective self-management of this serious disease.

The primary care provider should consider adding an angiotensin converting enzyme (ACE) inhibitor to the regimen of an adolescent who has a family history of or demonstrated predilection toward hypertension or early microalbumuria (Chiarelli et al., 1998).

▲ **Clinical Warning:** ACE inhibitors are teratogenic. Adolescent girls should be advised to use a backup form of birth control if they are sexually active. Their parents should simply be advised that ACE inhibitors are teratogenic.

Monitoring for Growth

Height or length and weight measurements should be obtained at the time of diagnosis and at least at every 3-month visit for diabetes office management thereafter. These measurements need to be compared to growth norms for age to determine whether the patient is achieving normal growth (Limbach, 1998; ADA, 2000b). Height measurements must continue at every scheduled visit until final adult height is attained. Persistent hyperglycemia can adversely affect normal growth hormone release. Information related to growth and development stages is described by age group in Chapters 8 to 12 which deal with healthy growth and development, from the newborn through adolescent periods.

Taken in context with the child's HbA_{1c} (which, as earlier discussed, must sometimes be tolerated at a higher level during early childhood), the overall growth velocity informs the clinician that sufficient growth hormone is indeed being released to provide for normal growth. Growth information should be shared with both the primary care provider and the comanaging endocrine team.

Sexual maturation staging must be done at these scheduled quarterly visits during the peripubertal period for the same reason (Limbach, 1998). Tanner staging is presented in Chapter 11. Information related to aberrant growth and puberty can be found in Chapter 60.

Prevention

Bone Mineral Density

Persistent hyperglycemia can lead to bone demineralization in an otherwise healthy, active youngster with diabetes. Because adolescence is a prime time for laying down bone matrix, it is especially imperative that the provider encourage the youth with diabetes to maintain active exercise and healthy eating habits (Pascual et al., 1998).

Oral Hygiene

In addition to tobacco avoidance, at least twice-daily brushing, and daily flossing, the provider should encourage regular dental examinations and prophylaxis. Unless actively engaged in good dental hygiene, individuals with diabetes have a higher incidence of tooth decay and tooth loss than do nondiabetic patients. These problems are magnified if oral hygiene is less than optimal or if the child persists with poor metabolic control (Moore et al., 1998). Further, mandibular bone loss that accompanies persistent hyperglycemia can be a significant factor in the pathogenesis of tooth loss in diabetes (Pascual et al., 1998).

Vaccination for Infectious Disease

All patients should be offered annual influenza vaccination after the age of 6 months. All individuals older than 2 years whose metabolic control has proven difficult or who have other comorbid illness, such as asthma, should be innoculated against pneumonoccal infection at the time of diagnosis.

Age-Specific Prevention and Support Needs: Childhood

Supporting the younger child and his or her family through the diagnostic and management phases of diabetes is developmentally less difficult than with older children and adolescents. Younger children are naturally programmed to be excited by new learning opportunities. The provider should capitalize on this normal developmental phase. Local diabetes association affiliates routinely host family events, often built around fun activities that provide support and lifestyle information. Parents find support from other parents facing the challenges of dealing with diabetes. Children learn that they are not alone. Many youngsters with diabetes find that building a peer group with their fellows can support them as they advance toward and through the difficult teenage years. Their nondiabetic siblings can find support with other such siblings. All participants may find that they are not alone in feeling angry or jealous, while also learning to refocus their feelings in positive ways.

In addition to coordinating family events and learning opportunities, some diabetes association affiliates and endocrine practice groups may coordinate a diabetes summer camp, most typically available as a single 1- or 2-week experience. Camp staff include CDEs and diabetes specialist providers. Camp scholarships are often available. The provider should consider exploring the availability of this service. Camp experience can support the patient in learning lifestyle strategies for enhanced diabetes management in an atmosphere of exceptional peer support. Self-esteem can be enhanced and friendships made. These are both vital to the growing child who is living with diabetes.

Age-Specific Prevention and Support Needs: Older Childhood and Adolescence

The provider must teach the patient and family about comorbid risks of diabetes, from the physical complications discussed in this chapter to the more subtle but no less deadly issues surrounding depression and suicide. Chapter 50 may provide some further guidance to the clinician, as will Chapters 28 and 29.

Older children and adolescents who are especially mature and focused may be good candidates for intensive insulin therapy. Certainly, use of an insulin pump or a regimen of three to four insulin injections per day provides for better metabolic balance. Complications of diabetes can be delayed or avoided outright with blood glucose stabilization, while minimizing or avoiding hypoglycemia.

CONTRACEPTION

Every female patient with diabetes who is of childbearing age should be counseled about contraception, whether or not she is sexually active. The provider is advised to document this advice on at least an annual basis. The adolescent who is contemplating pregnancy or who is already pregnant needs to be advised to strive for optimal blood glucose control. The pregnant adolescent must be referred to the diabetes endocrine group for workup and management criteria.

FITTING IN

Consuming alcohol at parties, smoking cigarettes, and eating junk food are all not uncommon among teenagers and their peers, and are discussed in Chapters 12 and 25. However, these so-called rites of passage can have deadly consequences for the adolescent with diabetes.

Similarly, some adolescents with diabetes are prone to eating disorders, not unlike their nondiabetic peers. The provider would be wise to teach parents to expect at least some degree of rebellion in their adolescent, with tactics ranging from refusal to participate fully in the diabetic regimen to refusal to take some or all of the prescribed medication. For example, adolescent females may cut back on their insulin in an effort to be model-slim. Both boys and girls may play with their insulin dosages to binge drink or to accommodate the same kinds of high-fat and sugary snacks that their nondiabetic friends consume. All of these behaviors place the patient at risk for diabetic ketoacidosis.

▲ **Clinical Warnings:**

- Any patient whose behavior can be likened to "ketosis roulette" or who seems prone to ketotic episodes should be evaluated for nonparticipation in the diabetic regimen. The individual and perhaps the family may benefit from counseling from a qualified mental health professional skilled in working with adolescents who are living with a chronic disease. Any patient who has a chronic problem in dealing with diabetes management issues, including a history of repeated episodes of diabetic ketoacidosis, may require institutionalization for safety.

- Any patient who develops an eating disorder requires immediate mental health intervention. Referral to a child psychiatrist may be warranted, especially if the disorder becomes serious and medication seems to be required. The adolescent may also require emergent institutionalization to provide for stabilization of metabolic dysfunctions while interventions for the eating disorder are begun. The reader is referred to Chapter 22 for more information on this topic.

NOT FITTING IN

Comorbidity with depression and even suicidal ideation are problems facing adolescents, their parents, and providers concerned with diabetes management. Today, most children are at some risk for psychosocial issues as a normal part of growing up. As described in the Chapter 29, children with diabetes face a significantly greater risk for depression and suicide than do most of their nondiabetic peers. The normal stresses and uncertainties of growing up are compounded by being singled out for what they cannot do with their friends, from joining in junk food forays to taking a spur-of-the-moment jog without first testing glucose levels and providing for the proper during-activity snack. These barriers identify the child as being "different"—something most adolescents abhor (Palardy et al., 1998). Unless checked, this labeling can affect the child's self-esteem. In extreme cases, the patient may choose to self-isolate rather than risk participating in social activities that seem to come with strings attached— "No punch at the school dance, remember." "Make sure you eat your snack at the ice rink after a half-hour on the ice." "Just have frozen nonfat yogurt at the hamburger joint after the game." (When everyone else is eating cheeseburgers and milkshakes.)

● **Clinical Pearl:** The provider should spend time at each visit to ascertain how the adolescent is dealing with diabetes in adolescence. The clinician should strive to keep open the lines of communication, especially as adolescents typically close down on communicating with their parents. The practitioner can enhance availability, even if just to listen, using e-mail. Ongoing access to counseling support, including for the short-term, can enhance health and well-being during the difficult adolescent years. Support groups for adolescents living with diabetes can also prove exceptionally valuable to patients who otherwise may feel angry, alone, and vulnerable because of their disease (Olsen & Sutton, 1998; Mortensen, 1998).

What to Tell Parents

Because of the subtleties in management problems that often arise in day-to-day practice, the life-threatening emergencies that can occur with devastating swiftness, and the implications for long-term complications, the primary care provider must work closely with the family, the endocrinologist, and the diabetes team in the shared management of diabetes.

Family input and participation are as essential as those of any other team member. The clinician needs to communicate this clearly to the family, because they are in the best position to articulate what does or does not work in the diabetic regimen (Daneman et al., 1998). The diagnosis of diabetes can be devastating, but close family–provider communication and supportive management can prevent or at least mitigate long-term complications. This is especially important when dealing with the rebellious older child and adolescent who chooses not to participate in the diabetic regimen.

COMMUNITY RESOURCES

Provider Resources

The American Diabetes Association
1701 North Beauregard Street
Alexandria, VA 22311
Telephone: (800) DIABETES [(800) 342-2383]
Internet address: *http://www.diabetes.org*

The leading U.S. organization for diabetes. Primary Care Clinical Practice Guidelines are available from ADA. These provide an introduction for the primary care clinician for using guidelines, with source links, major studies, journal articles, and other resources for treating diabetes. Position Statements are available on a variety of clinical topics, such as "Care of Children with Diabetes in the School and Day Care Setting" and "Preconception Care of Women with Diabetes." These are updated annually. Clinical Practice Recommendations are published annually in the journal *Diabetes Care* and are also available at no charge on the Internet.

American Association of Diabetes Educators
100 West Monroe Street, Fourth Floor
Chicago, IL 6063-1901
Telephone: (312) 424-2426
Internet address: *http://www.aadenet.org*

This organization is a source for up-to-date information about diabetes and how to teach patient and family about its management. It can also supply the clinician with information about how to find a CDE in the local practice area. The website includes a directory of the organizations' 10,000 members, on-line conferences, and legislative updates, including the invaluable "Directory of Legislation and Statutes For Coverage of Diabetes Self-Management Education by Health Insurance." This resource provides information about the status of each U.S. state's mandated insurance coverage for diabetes education, equipment, and supplies.

American Association of Clinical Endocrinologists
1000 Riverside Avenue, Suite 205
Jacksonville, FL 32204
Telephone: (904) 353-7878
Fax: (904) 353-8185
Internet address: *http://www.aace.com*

Juvenile Diabetes Foundation
120 Wall Street
New York, NY 10005
Telephone: (800) JDF-CURE
Fax: (212) 785-9595
Internet address: *http://www.jdfcure.org*

This not-for-profit, voluntary health agency's mission is to support and fund research to find a cure for diabetes and its complications.

Doctor's Guide to Diabetes Information and Resources
Internet address: *http://www.pslgroup.com/DIABETES.htm*

Provider Resources In Canada

Canadian Diabetes Association
15 Toronto Street, Suite 800
Toronto, ON, Canada M5C 2E3
Telephone: (800) BANTING
Internet address: *http://www.diabetes.ca*
The web site provides content in both English and French.

Dietitians of Canada
480 University Avenue, Suite 604
Toronto, ON, Canada M5G 1V2
Telephone: (416) 596-0857
Fax: (416) 596-0603
Internet address: *http://www.dietitians.ca*

This is an association of food and nutrition professionals committed to the health and well-being of Canadians. The web site provides content in both English and French.

Provider Resources in Other Countries

On-Line Diabetes Resources: Organizations and Charities Web Sites
Internet address: *http://www.diabetesmonitor.com/org.htm*

The International Diabetes Federation
1 rue Defacqz
B-1000 Brussels
Belgium
Telephone: 32-2/538 55 11
Fax: 32-2/538 51 14
Internet address: *http://www.idf.org*

This is an umbrella organization of 146 national associations in 121 countries, headquartered in Brussels, Belgium. Every 3 years the federation holds an international gathering of the global diabetes community.

Society for Endocrinology
17/18 The Courtyard, Woodlands, Bradley Stoke
Bristol BS32 4NQ, UK
Telephone: 44 (0)1454 619036
Fax: 44 (0)1454 616071
Internet address: *http://www.endocrinology.org*

This is the major endocrine society outside North America. It publishes the *Journal of Endocrinology, Journal of Molecular Endocrinology, Endocrine-Related Cancer,* and *Clinical Endocrinology.* Full-text versions of the society's review articles and commentaries dating back to January 1996 are freely available on-line. Society membership is not required for procurement.

Patient Resources

ADA patient membership provides a subscription to *Diabetes Forecast.* This leading lay publication is a source of current information, support, and updated medical data for patients and families who are living with diabetes.
Internet address: *http://www.diabetes.org/diabetesforecast*

Kids With Diabetes
PMB 153
9452 Telephone Road
Ventura, CA 93004
Telephone: (805) 671-5059
Internet address: *http://www.kidswithdiabetes.org*

This nonprofit organization provides charitable assistance to families with children who are diabetic. Programs include the Fun for Type 1 Playgroup. This is a monthly support group for kids and families, widely available in or near diabetes treatment centers. There are games, fun activities, and guest speakers at each meeting. The New Kids Program is a resource for parents, offering a helping hand during the critical time immediately following diagnosis. The Teen Mentors Program helps adolescents with diabetes during this difficult developmental period. The Sharps Collection Program helps families to dispose of full sharps safely and easily.

The Charles Ray III Diabetes Foundation
P.O. Box 20862
Raleigh, NC 27619
Telephone: (919) 303-6949
Fax: (919) 303-6949
Internet address: *http://www.charlesray.g12.com*

This foundation encourages people with diabetes to monitor their diabetes carefully by providing glucose meters to those who cannot afford them.

Taking Control of Your Diabetes
1110 Camino Del Mar, Suite C
Del Mar, CA 92014
Telephone: (800) 99-TCOYD
Internet address: *http://www.tcoyd.org*

This is a nonprofit educational and motivational conference and health fair held in various larger U.S. cities. Steven V. Edelman, M.D. (himself a diabetic) leads the organization.

The Joslin Diabetes Center
One Joslin Place
Boston, MA 02215
Telephone: (800) JOSLIN-1
Internet address: *http://www.joslin.org*

The Center is associated with Harvard Medical School, Boston, MA. The Joslin is recognized as a leader in research, treatment, and patient and professional education in diabetes. A useful Internet site search engine is a "Beginners Guide" for individuals new to diabetes. A user-friendly diabetes library is featured, as is information on Joslin programs and their nationwide affiliates. Joslin summer camps for children are a special feature.

International Diabetic Athletes Association
1647 West Bethany Home Road, #B
Phoenix, AZ 85015
Telephone: (800) 898-IDAA
Fax: (602) 433-9331
Internet address: *http://www.diabetes-exercise.org*

This resource provides education about the benefits and risks of exercise.

Diabetes Research and Wellness Foundation
1206 Potomac Street N.W.
Washington, DC 20007
Office Telephone: (202) 298-9211
Helpline Telephone: (800) 941-4635
Subscription Telephone: (888) 321-2219
Fax: (202) 342-2039
Internet address: *http://www.diabeteswellness.net*

This foundation provides free medical alert ID necklaces, diabetes self-management diaries, and educational literature on request. It also publishes the *Diabetes Wellness Letter.*

International Society for Pediatric and Adolescent Diabetes
Internet address: *http://www.ispad.org*

This is a rich resource for children and families living with diabetes. The Society will provide a free copy of a CD-ROM game for children ages 5 to 13. It is meant to educate children with diabetes to manage better their disease. The game features fast-paced exercises, quizzes, and arcade-style games. These are meant to help players learn important information about proper diabetes management. The CD-ROM also includes a glossary of terms, diabetes information sections, and a parent information section. The CD-ROM is narrated in both English and Spanish. A parent or caregiver can obtain it by calling (800) 760-3818.

REFERENCES

Acerini, C. L., Ahmed, M.L., Ross, K.M., et al. (1998). Coeliac disease in children and adolescents with IDDM: Clinical characteristics and response to gluten-free diet. *Diabetic Medicine, 15*, 38–44.

Aielo, L. P., Gardner, T.W., King, G.L., et al. (1998). Diabetic nephropathy (Technical Review). *Diabetes Care, 21*, 143–156.

Akerblom, H. K. (1998). Focusing on childhood diabetes. *Acta Paediatr Supplement, 425*, 1–2.

Altobelli, E., et al. (1998). Family history and risk of insulin-dependent diabetes mellitus: A population-based case-control study. *Acta Diabetologia, 35*, 57–60.

Arslanian, S., & Suprasongsin, C. (1996). Differences in the in vivo insulin secretion and sensitivity of healthy black versus white adolescents. *Journal of Pediatrics, 129*, 440–443.

Attia, N., Zahrani, A., Saif, A., et al. (1998). Different faces of non-immune diabetes of infancy. *Acta Paediatr, 87*, 95–97.

American Academy of Pediatrics (AAP) (2000). Policy statement: recommendations fo the prevention of pneumococcal infections, including the use of pneumococcal conjugate vaccine (Prevnar), Pneumococcol polysaccharide vaccine, and antibiotic prophylaxis (RE 9960). *Pediatrics 106*(2), 362-366.

American Diabetes Association. (1996a). Self-monitoring of blood glucose (Consensus Statement). *Diabetes Care, 19*(Suppl 1), S62–66.

American Diabetes Association. (1996b). Standards of medical care for patients with diabetes mellitus (position statement). *Diabetes Care, 19*(Suppl 1), S8–15.

American Diabetes Association. (1997a). Economic consequences of diabetes mellitus in the U.S. in 1997. *Diabetes Care, 21*, 296–309.

American Diabetes Association. (1997b). Report of the Expert Committee. *Diabetes Care, 20*, 11.

American Diabetes Association (1999). Diabetic nephropathy. *Diabetes Care, 22*(Supplement 1), 66–69.

American Diabetes Association. (2000a). Gestational diabetes mellitus. *Diabetes Care, 23*(Suppl 1).

American Diabetes Association. (2000b). Screening for Type 2 diabetes. *Diabetes Care, 23*(Suppl 1).

American Diabetes Association. (2000c). Standards for medical care for patients with diabetes mellitus. *Diabetes Care, 23*(Suppl 1).

American Diabetes Association. (2000d). Immunization and the prevention of influenza and pneumococcal disease. *Diabetes Care 23*(1), 95-108.

Aude Rueda, O., Libman, I.M., Attimirano, B., et al. (1998). Low incidence of IDDM in children of Veracruz-Boca del Rio, Veracruz: Results of the first validated IDDM registry in Mexico. *Diabetes Care, 21*, 1372–1373.

Author. (1998). Quality control of diabetes care and chronic complications in young people after St. Vincent and Kos: Proceedings of the 4th international workshop on diabetic retinopathy in children. *Hormone Research, 50*(Suppl 1), 1–107.

Becker, D. (1998). Individualized insulin therapy in children and adolescents with type 1 diabetes. *Acta Paediatrica Supplement, 425*, 20–24.

Beregszaszi, M., et al. (1997). Nocturnal hypoglycemia in children and adolescents with insulin-dependent diabetes mellitus: Prevalence and risk factors. *Journal of Pediatrics, 131*(1 Pt 1), 27–33.

Blom, L., et al. (1992). A high linear growth is associated with an increased risk of childhood diabetes mellitus. *Diabetologia, 35*, 528–533.

Boyle, J. P., Engelgau, M.M., Thompson, T.J., et al. (1999). Estimating prevalence of type 1 and type 2 diabetes in a population of African Americans with diabetes mellitus. *American Journal of Epidemiology, 149*, 55–63.

Bursell, S. E., Clermont, A. C., Aiello, L. P., et al. (1999). High-dose vitamin E supplementation normalizes retinal blood flow and creatinine clearance in patients with type 1 diabetes. *Diabetes Care, 22*, 1245–1251.

Cameron, F. J., & Batch, J. A. (1997). Maturity-onset diabetes of the young (MODY): Three case reports and new perspectives. *Journal of Pediatric Endocrinology and Metabolism, 10*, 63–68.

Chervonsky A. V., et al. (1997). The role of Fas in autoimmune diabetes. *Cell, 4*, 17–24.

Chiarelli, F., et al. (1998). Diabetic nephropathy in children and adolescents: A critical review with particular reference to angiotensin-converting enzyme inhibitors. *Acta Paediatrica Supplement, 425*, 42–45.

Clark, C. M. (1998). Oral therapy in type 2 diabetes: Pharmacological properties and clinical use of currently available agents. *Diabetes Spectrum, 11*, 211–221.

Cooper, M. E. (1998). Pathophysiology of diabetic nephropathy. *Metabolism, 47*(12 Suppl 1), 3–6.

Coustan, D. R. & Carpenter, M.W. (1998). The diagnosis of gestational diabetes. *Diabetes Care, 21*(Suppl 2), B5–8.

Crowne, E. C., et al. (1998). Recombinant human insulin-like growth factor-I abolishes changes in insulin requirements consequent upon growth hormone pulsatility in young adults with type 1 diabetes. *Metabolism, 47*, 31–38.

Daneman, D., et al. (1998). Defining quality of care for children and adolescents with type 1 diabetes. *Acta Paediatrica Supplement, 425*, 11–19.

Dahlquist, G., & Mustonen, L. (1994). Analysis of a fifteen year prospective incidence study of childhood onset diabetes: Time trends and climatological factors. *International Journal of Epidemiology, 23*, 1–8.

Dahlquist, G. (1998). The aetiology of type 1 diabetes: an epidemiological perspective. *Acta Paediatrica Supplement, 425*, 5–10.

Danne, T., et al. (1998). Monitoring for retinopathy in children and adolescents with type 1 diabetes. *Acta Paediatrica Supplement, 425*, 5–41.

Dean, H. J., Young, T.K., Flett, B., et al. (1998). Screening for type-2 diabetes in aboriginal children in northern Canada. *Lancet, 352*, 1523–1524.

Diabetes Control and Complications Trial (DCCT) Research Group. (1993). The effect of intensive treatment on the development and progression of long-term complication in insulin-dependent diabetes mellitus. *New England Journal of Medicine, 329*, 977–986.

Diabetes Control and Complications Trial (DCCT) Research Group. (1995). The relationship of glycemic exposure (HbA$_{1c}$) to the risk of development and progression of retinopathy in the Control and Complications Trial. *Diabetes, 44*, 968–983.

Diabetes Epidemiology Research International Group. (1988). Geographic patterns of childhood insulin-dependent diabetes mellitus. *Diabetes, 37*, 1113–1119.

Diabetes Epidemiology Research International Group. (1990). Secular trends in incidence of childhood IDDM in 10 countries. *Diabetes Epidemiology, 39*, 858–864.

Dorman, J. S., McCarthy, B., McCanlies, E., et al. (1996). Molecular IDDM epidemiology: International studies. *Diabetes Research in Clinical Practice, 34*(Suppl), S107–116.

Dorman, J. S. (1997). Molecular epidemiology of insulin-dependent diabetes mellitus. *Epidemiologic Review, 19*, 91–98.

Draznin, M. B., & Patel, D.R. (1998). Diabetes mellitus and sports. *Adolescent Medicine, 9*, 457–465.

Eriksson, J. G., Taimelo, S., & Koipisto, V.A. (1997). Exercise and the metabolic syndrome. *Diabetologia, 40*, 125–135.

Eriksson, J. G. (1999). Exercise and the treatment of type 2 diabetes mellitus. *Sports Medicine, 27*, 381–391.

Friedman, E. A. (1999). Advanced glycosylated end products and hyperglycemia in the pathogenesis of diabetic complications. *Diabetes Care, 22*(Suppl 2), B65–71

Geenen, V., & Lefebvre, P.J. (1998). The intrathymic expression of insulin-related genes: Implications for pathophysiology and prevention of Type 1 diabetes. *Diabetes Metabolism Review, 14*, 95–103.

Gilbert R. E., et al. (1998). Early nephropathy predicts vision-threatening retinal disease in patients with type I diabetes mellitus. *Journal of the American Society of Nephrology, 9*, 85–89.

Glaser, N., & Jones, K. L. (1998). Non-insulin dependent diabetes mellitus in Mexican-American children. *Western Journal of Medicine, 168*, 11–16.

Green, A., Gale, E.A., & Patterson, C.C. (1992). and the EURODIAB ACE Study Group. (1992). Incidence of childhood onset insulin-dependent diabetes mellitus: The EURODIAB ACE Study. *Lancet, 339,* 905–909.

Green-Hernandez, C. (1999a). Diabetes mellitus. In J. Singleton, S. Sandowski, C. Green-Hernandez, et al. (Eds.), *Primary care.* Philadelphia: Lippincott Williams and Wilkins.

Green-Hernandez, C. (1999b). Family and cultural assessment measures in primary care. In J. Singleton, S. Sandowski, C. Green-Hernandez, et al. (Eds.), *Primary care.* Philadelphia: Lippincott Williams and Wilkins.

Green, S. M., Rothrock, S.G., Ho, J.D., et al. (1998). Failure of adjunctive bicarbonate to improve outcome in severe pediatric diabetic ketoacidosis. *Annals of Emergency Medicine, 31,* 41–48.

Greenbaum, C. J., Sears, K.L., Kahn, S.E., 7 Palmer, J.P. (1999). Relationship of beta-cell function and autoantibodies to progression and nonprogression of subclinical type 1 diabetes: Follow-up of the Seattle Family Study. *Diabetes, 48,* 170–175.

Haffner, S. M., et al. (1996). Insulin secretion and resistance in non-diabetic Mexican Americans and non-Hispanic whites with a parental history of diabetes. *Journal of Clinical Endocrinology and Metabolism, 81,* 1846–1851.

Hahl, J., Simell, T., Iloen, J., et al. (1998). Costs of predicting IDDM. *Diabetologia, 41,* 79–85.

Hanson, R. L., et al. (1998). Analytic strategies to detect linkage to a common disorder with genetically determined age of onset: Diabetes mellitus in Pima Indians. *Genetics and Epidemiology, 15,* 299–315.

Hattersley, A. T. (1998). Maturity-onset diabetes of the young: Clinical heterogeneity explained by genetic heterogeneity. *Diabetes Medicine, 15,* 15–24.

Hershey, T., Bhargava, N., Sadler, M., White, N. H., & Craft, S. (1999). Conventional versus intensive diabetes therapy in children with type 1 diabetes. *Diabetes Care, 22,* 1318–1324.

Islam, A. H., et al. (1995). Fasting plasma insulin level is an important risk factor for the development of complications in Japanese obese children: Results from a cross-sectional and longitudinal study. *Metabolism, 44,* 478–485.

Juneja, R. (1999). Type 1 1/2 diabetes: Myth or reality? *Autoimmunity, 29,* 65–83.

Karl, E. V. M., & Heiner, H. (1995). Long term course of neonatal diabetes. *New England Journal of Medicine, 333,* 704–708.

Karvonen, M., et al. (1993). A review of the recent epidemiological data on the worldwide incidence of type 1 (insulin-dependent) diabetes mellitus. *Diabetologia, 36,* 883–892.

Kaufman, F. R. (1997). Diabetes mellitus. *Pediatrics in Review 18,* 383–392.

Kiess, W., et al. (1998). Practical aspects of managing preschool children with type 1 diabetes. *Acta Paediatrica Supplement, 425,* 67–71.

Klemetti, P., et al. (1998). T-cell reactivity to wheat gluten in patients with insulin-dependent diabetes mellitus. *Scandinavian Journal of Immunology, 47,* 48–53.

Knip, M. (1998). Prediction and prevention of type 1 diabetes. *Acta Paediatrica Supplement, 425,* 54–62.

Kulkarni, K., et al. (1998). Nutrition practice guidelines for type 1 diabetes mellitus positively affect dietitian practices and patient outcomes. *Journal of the American Dietetic Association, 98,* 62–70.

Lalli, C., Ciofetta, M., Del Sindaco, P., et al. (1999). Long-term intensive treatment of type 1 diabetes with the short-acting insulin analog lispro in variable combination with NPH insulin at mealtime. *Diabetes Care, 22,* 468–477.

Lan, M. S., et al. (1998). HERV-K10s and immune-mediated (type 1) diabetes. *Cell, 95,* 14–16.

Langer, O. (1998). Maternal glycemic criteria for insulin therapy in gestational diabetes mellitus. *Diabetes Care, 21*(Suppl 2), B91–98.

Lekakis, J., et al. (1997). Endothelial dysfunction of conduit arteries in insulin-dependent diabetes mellitus without microalbuminuria. *Cardiovascular Research, 34,* 164–168.

Libman, I. M., LaPorte, R.E., Becker, D., et al. (1998). Was there an epidemic of diabetes in nonwhite adolescents in Allegheny County, Pennsylvania? *Diabetes Care, 21,* 1278–1281.

Like, A. A., et al. (1982). Neonatal thymectomy prevents spontaneous diabetes mellitus in the BB:W rat. *Science, 216,* 644–646.

Limbach, T. (1998). Childhood insulin-dependent diabetes mellitus:

Initial presentation and management in the nineties. *Mineral and Electrolyte Metabolism, 24,* 326–329.

Lobefalo L., et al. (1997). Flicker perimetry in diabetic children without retinopathy. *Canadian Journal of Ophthalmology, 32,* 324–328.

Lovestam-Adrian, M., et al. (1998). The incidence of nephropathy in type 1 diabetic patients with proliferative retinopathy: A 10-year follow-up study. *Diabetes Research in Clinical Practice, 39,* 11–17.

Ma, L., et al. (1997). Evaluation of TAP1 polymorphisms with insulin dependent diabetes mellitus in Finnish diabetic patients: The Childhood Diabetes in Finland (DiMe) Study Group. *Human Immunology, 53,* 159–166.

McKenzie, S. B., O'Connell, J., Smith, L.A., Ottinger, W.E. (1998). A primary intervention program (pilot study) for Mexican American children at risk for type 2 diabetes. *Diabetes Educator, 24,* 180–187.

Minior, V. K., et al. (1998). Fetal growth restriction at term: Myth or reality? *Obstetrical Gynecology, 92,* 57–60.

Moore, P. A., et al. (1998). Type 1 diabetes mellitus and oral health: assessment of tooth loss and edentulism. *Journal of Public Health Dentistry, 58*(2), 35–42.

Moran, A., et al. (1998). Abnormal glucose metabolism in cystic fibrosis. *Journal of Pediatrics, 133,* 10–17.

Mortensen, H. B. (1998). Practical aspects of managing diabetes in adolescents. *Acta Paediatrica Supplement, 425,* 72–76.

National Diabetes Data Group (1995). *Diabetes in America.* Bethesda, MD: National Institutes of Health. NIH Publication No. 95-1468.

Olsen, R., & Sutton, J. (1998). More hassle, more alone: Adolescents with diabetes and the role of formal and informal support. *Child Care and Health Development, 24,* 31–39.

Osicka, T. M., Yu, Y., Panagiotopoulis, S., et al. (2000). Prevention of albuminuria by amino-guanidine or ramipril in streptozotocin-induced diabetic rats is associated with the normalization of glomerular protein kinase C. *Diabetes, 49,* 87–93.

Pagana, K. D., & Pagana, T. J. (1998). *Mosby's manual of diagnostic and laboratory test reference.* St. Louis: Mosby.

Palardy, N., Greening, L., Oh, J., et al. (1998). Adolescents' health attitudes and adherence to treatment for insulin-dependen diabetes mellitus. *Developmental and Behavioral Pediatrics, 19,* 31–37.

Pascual, J., Argente, J., Lopez, M.B., et al. (1998). Bone mineral density in children and adolescents with diabetes mellitus type 1 of recent onset. *Calcif Tissue Int, 62,* 31–35.

Perez-Bravo, Carrasco, E., Gutierrez-Lopez, M.D., et al. (1996). Genetic predisposition and environmental factors leading to the development of insulin-dependent diabetes mellitus in Chilean children. *Journal of Molecular Medicine, 74,* 105–109.

Pettitt, D. J., Moll, P.P., Knowler, W.C., et al. (1993). Insulinemia in children at low and high risk of NIDDM. *Diabetes Care, 16,* 608–614.

Riley, M. D., & Dwyer, T. (1998). Microalbuminuria is positively associated with usual dietary saturated fat intake and negatively associated with usual dietary protein intake in people with insulin-dependent diabetes mellitus. *American Journal of Clinical Nutrition, 67,* 50–57.

Rosskamp, R. H., & Park, G. (1999). Long-acting insulin analogs. *Diabetes Care, 22*(Suppl 2) B109–113.

Rovet, J. F., & Ehrlich, R. M. (1999). The effect of hypoglycemic seizures on cognitive function in children with diabetes: A 7-year prospective study. *Journal of Pediatrics, 134,* 503–506.

Roy, M. S., Roy, A., & Brown, S. (1998). Increased urinary-free cortisol outputs in diabetic patients. *Journal of Diabetes Complications, 12,* 24–27.

Saukkonen, T., Virtanen, S.M., Karppinen, M. (1998). Significance of cow's milk protein antibodies as risk factor for childhood IDDM: Interactions with dietary cow's milk intake and HLA-DQB1 genotype. Childhood Diabetes in Finland Study Group. *Diabetologia, 41,* 72–78.

Scott, C. R., Smith, J.M., Craddock, M.M., & Pihoker, C. (1997). Characteristics of youth-onset noninsulin-dependent diabetes mellitus and insulin-dependent diabetes mellitus at diagnosis. *Pediatrics, 100,* 84–91.

Shaw, J. E., Gokal, R., Hollis, S., & Boulton, A.J. (1998). Does peripheral neuropathy invariably accompany nephropathy in type 1 diabetes mellitus? *Diabetes Research and Clinical Practice, 39,* 55–61.

Silink, M. (1998). Practical management of diabetic ketoacidosis in childhood and adolescence. *Acta Paediatrica Supplement, 425,* 63–66.

Slyper, A. H. (1998). Childhood obesity, adipose tissue distribution, and the pediatric practitioner. *Pediatrics, 102,* e4.

Smulders, R. A. (1998). Distinct associations of HbA_{1c} and the urinary excretion of pentosidine, an advanced glycosylation end-product, with markers of endothelial function in insulin-dependent diabetes mellitus. *Thromb Haemost, 80,* 52–57.

Songer, T. J., et al. (1997). Health insurance and the financial impact of IDDM in families with a child with IDDM. *Diabetes Care, 20,* 577–584.

Sperling, M. A. (1994). Diabetes in Adolescence. *Adolescent medicine: State of the Art Review, 5,* 87.

Spong, C. Y., Guillermo, L., Kuboshige, J., et al. (1998). Recurrence of gestational diabetes mellitus: Identification of risk factors. *American Journal of Perinatology, 15,* 29–33.

Stoffers, D. A., Ferrer, I., Clarke, W.L., & Habeber, J.F. (1997). Early-onset type-II diabetes mellitus (MODY 4) linked to IPF1. *Nature Genetics, 17*(10), 138–139.

Strong, J. P., Malcom, G.T., McMahan, C.A., et al. (1999). Prevalence and extent of athersclerosis in adolescents and young adults. *Journal of the American Medical Association, 281,* 727–735.

Sugimoto, H., Shikata, K., Wada, J., et al. (1999). Advanced glycation end products-cytokine-nitric oxide sequence pathway in the development of diabetic nephropathy: Aminoguanidine ameliorates the overexpression of tumour necrosis factor-alpha and inducible nitric oxide synthase in diabetic rat glomeruli. *Diabetologia, 42,* 878–886.

Tattersal, R. (1982). The present status of maturity-onset diabetes of young people (MODY). *The Genetics of Diabetes: Proceedings of the Serono Symposia, 37,* 261–270.

Thernlund, G., Dahlquist, G., Hansson, K., et al. (1995). Psychosocial stress and the onset of insulin-dependent diabetes mellitus (IDDM) in children. A case-control study. *Diabetes Care, 18,* 1323–1329.

Thompson, C. H., Sanderson, A.L., Sandeman, D., et al. (1997). Fetal growth and insulin resistance in adult life: Role of skeletal muscle morphology. *Clinical Science, 92,* 291–296.

Tolis, G., Karydis, I., Markousis, V., et al. (1997). Growth hormone release by the novel GH releasing peptide hexarelin in patients with homozygous beta-thalassemia. *Journal of Pediatric Endocrinology and Metabolism, 10,* 35–40.

Vitoria, J. C., Castano, L., Rica, I., et al. (1998). Association of insulin-dependent diabetes mellitus and celiac disease: A study based on serologic markers. *Journal of Pediatric Gastroenterology and Nutrition, 27,* 47–52.

Weston P. J., Glancy, J.M., McNally, P.G., et al. (1997). Can abnormalities of ventricular repolarisation identify insulin dependent diabetic patients at risk of sudden cardiac death? *Heart, 78,* 56–60.

Young, L. A., Kimball, T.R., Daniels, S.R., et al. (1998). Nocturnal blood pressure in young patients with insulin-dependent diabetes mellitus: Correlation with cardiac function. *Journal of Pediatrics, 133,* 46–50.

Young, L. Y., & Koda-Kimble, M. A. (1995). *Applied therapeutics.* Vancouver, WA: Applied Therapeutics.

Zerres, K., Mucher, G., Bachner, L., et al. (1994). Mapping of the gene for autosomal recessive polycystic kidney disease (ARPKD) to chromosome 6p21-cen. *Nature Genetics, 7*(1), 429–432.

Chronic Urinary Problems

• ANN P. GUILLOT, MD, and IDA J. MCNAMARA, BSN, RN

INTRODUCTION

Problems with the genitourinary tract often present in the course of childhood. These range from the acute to the chronic, from the merely annoying to the life threatening, and from the readily treatable to those for which there is no effective treatment. This chapter discusses normal voiding and then presents the diagnosis and primary care management of several common chronic urinary problems.

Normal Voiding

ANATOMY, PHYSIOLOGY, AND PATHOLOGY

Normal physiologic and developmental progression from infancy to later childhood includes the attainment of urinary continence, with the attendant ability to empty the bladder completely and voluntarily. The age of learning to use the toilet reliably is debatable and may depend a great deal on parenting styles. Self-toileting for urination usually occurs some time before the fourth birthday and may occur by the second birthday for some children.

The tasks involved in bladder control are complex. The normal infant voids reflexively, emptying the bladder completely as soon as it begins to fill. The bladder muscle is called the detrusor. In infancy, the detrusor has not yet developed the ability to relax with filling; thus, small volumes of urine produce a rise in pressure, which then triggers voiding. For the first few months of life, infants void about 20 times a day.

During the second year of life, the detrusor begins to relax as it fills with urine, and the interval between voids lengthens out. Voiding is still involuntary. It is not until the next phase of development that the child develops central recognition of the sensation of bladder fullness. This sensation allows activation of the external sphincter, keeping the sphincter closed until voluntary voiding can take place.

Even after the child has developed the ability to recognize the sensation of fullness and maintain continence, the job of voiding is complex. The youngster must get to the toilet, manage clothing removal, and then allow sphincter relaxation at the same time that the detrusor contracts to empty smoothly and completely. The whole process is not developmentally easy, requiring the cooperation of autonomic, sensory, and motor nervous systems and skeletal and smooth muscles.

Primary Nocturnal Enuresis

Primary nocturnal enuresis (PNE) is defined as nighttime bedwetting after daytime continence has been achieved. There may be a genetic component in PNE.

EPIDEMIOLOGY

Normal progress toward full diurnal and nocturnal continence can go awry in many ways. The most common is PNE. Although the exact causes are unknown, many children are affected. About 20% of 5-year-olds wet consistently during sleep. Every year of life, some 15% of affected children outgrow the disorder. There is a very high incidence of positive family history in children who have PNE. Often, children find it helpful to know that other family members have had to deal with nighttime bedwetting and have been able to stay dry as they have grown older.

● **Clinical Pearl:** When there is no history of urinary tract infections (UTIs), the child has never been dry during sleep, and the child has normal voiding function during the day, including staying dry while awake, there is almost never an indication to do further workup looking for anatomic or physiologic abnormalities.

HISTORY AND PHYSICAL EXAMINATION

Often families will seek help for their child to overcome PNE. The initial history and physical examination can be helpful to the child and family, and it gives the primary care provider important information.

The history should clarify the following issues:

- Is the problem primary (has always been present, with no consistent period of dry nights, lasting more than 6 months) or secondary (has recurred after consistent dryness for more than 6 months)?
- Does wetting occur only during sleep (nocturnal enuresis) or also during waking hours (diurnal enuresis)?
- Is there a family history of voiding problems (other affected family members may never have discussed the problem)?
- Is there any history of UTIs or UTI symptoms?

The provider should also note the following:

- The voiding pattern, especially frequency, urgency, or dribbling urinary stream;
- Any history of constipation, because bowel and bladder emptying problems are often associated;
- Whether the child exhibits excessive drinking, especially the need the drink during the night (enuresis is rarely due to polyuria secondary to diabetes mellitus or to a urinary concentrating defect);
- Other neurodevelopmental problems, whether motor or cognitive (most children with PNE do not differ developmentally from their peer group in this respect);
- The family's thoughts and attitudes about the enuresis, because PNE can be a major stressor that may affect many other areas of childrearing.

The physical examination should evaluate the child for the following:

- Growth, using a growth chart and previous and current growth values;
- Blood pressure, using norms for age and height;
- A palpable bladder, which suggests inefficient or incomplete emptying;
- Abnormalities of the external genitalia;
- Anal tone, which may be decreased if sacral innervation is abnormal;
- Lower extremity strength and reflexes, which may be abnormal if lumbosacral innervation is abnormal;
- Abnormalities of the lower back, including pigmentation, hairy patches, dimples, or sinus tracts over the lumbosacral spine (all clues to spinal cord problems).

If the history confirms PNE without any history of UTIs, abnormalities of daytime voiding pattern, excessive thirst, or developmental abnormalities, and if the physical examination is normal, a urinalysis and urine culture should be done to rule out any evidence of UTI, glycosuria, significant proteinuria, or hematuria. If these tests also are normal, the diagnosis of uncomplicated PNE is made.

MANAGEMENT

There are several approaches to caring for this problem. First, the family should understand that it is a common problem and one that many children outgrow spontaneously. If the family and patient desire a more active approach to hurrying the resolution, the most successful treatment is behavioral. This may consist of a reward system (eg, a sticker chart rewarding dry nights) and counseling the child to assume more responsibility for the problem (eg, taking responsibility for changing sheets when they are wet). In addition, some families have had success with a frequent waking program, in which the parent wakes the child several times during the early night to void, until the child can stay dry without prompting.

Moisture monitors, such as the battery-driven bell and pad, have been useful for some children. These work by awakening the child as he or she starts to void, thus conditioning the youngster to wake at the sensation of bladder fullness.

The success rate of focused behavioral programs (with or without monitors) is about 75%. The relapse rate after treatment is stopped (20%) is the lowest of all the therapies (Schmitt, 1997; Monda & Hussman, 1995; Tietjen & Hussman, 1996). These treatments aim to teach the child to

awaken at the sensation of bladder fullness and to avoid reflex voiding. They are therefore the most physiologically normalizing of the therapies, but they require the most effort and motivation on the part of the child and the family to carry out.

Medications, including tricyclics and DDVAP (desmopressin), can be used, but their effectiveness and side effects make them controversial. Imipramine has been used since the 1960s for this purpose and is fairly effective. However, if an overdose is taken, the side effects are lethal. Even at the prescribed dose, the drug may increase blood pressure. Once the drug is stopped, the relapse rate of nocturnal enuresis is high. DDAVP can be used intranasally and/or orally in a dose of 10 to 40 μg at bedtime and is also quite effective. However, there have been case reports of seizures secondary to hyponatremia during use of this drug, and the relapse rate once it is discontinued is very high. It is perhaps best to use DDAVP in the lowest effective dose and only for short-term, intermittent episodes (eg, to maintain continence while at overnight camp) (Robson, 1998).

● **Clinical Pearl:** The new oral form of DDAVP will obviate issues of inconsistent drug delivery, which were sometimes responsible for drug failure with the intranasal preparation. Concerns about side effects and relapse after discontinuation of treatment are unchanged.

It is important that the provider attend to the family dynamics surrounding the continence issue, because it is often a heavily charged one. The clinician must be willing to spend time with both the child and the family to explore the anxiety and discouragement that accompany PNE, no matter what treatment is chosen. The more the child can feel responsible for making progress and the more encouraging the family can be, the better. Chapter 63 offers an in-depth discussion of primary care management of PNE using behavioral therapies.

Secondary Enuresis and Other Forms of Voiding Dysfunction

When the initial history reveals that the child has had a period of dryness for 6 months or more and then starts to have enuresis, or when the child has daytime wetting, the likelihood is much higher that there will be associated physiologic abnormalities and that treatment will be more complicated. Likewise, further diagnostic evaluation is indicated when there are abnormalities in the physical examination, as previously described. There is a greater than 60% chance that children in this category will have associated UTIs, which are often recurrent. This figure has not altered in intervening decades (Dodge, West, Bridgforth, & Travis, 1970; Jones et al., 1972). Children who meet these criteria should have a urinalysis and urine culture. They should generally also have a renal ultrasound and fluoroscopic voiding cystourethrogram (VCUG). If abnormalities are apparent on the imaging studies, the patient should be referred to a pediatric urologist or nephrologist for consultation. If the child is constipated, efforts at treatment should begin. Antibiotic treatment for UTIs can be initiated, and efforts to empty the bladder regularly and completely can also be started.

Voiding dysfunction may be due to abnormalities in the bladder's ability to relax and fill properly. This will lead to urgency incontinence and frequency, which may be treated with an anticholinergic drug, such as oxybutynin. UTIs will complicate and exacerbate bladder irritability. If UTIs are recurrent, antibiotic prophylaxis may be necessary over a several-month period as well.

Bladder or sphincter dysfunction exists when the bladder fills well, but the sensation of fullness is poor and the sphincter does not relax well enough to allow an uninterrupted urinary stream. The bladder may have a very large capacity, but it will be incompletely emptied with each void. The residual urine in the bladder increases the risk of UTI and may add to the risk of bladder irritability or even to the risk of vesicoureteral reflux. The child with bladder or sphincter dysfunction requires behavior modification. Through practice, the child learns to empty the bladder regularly, every 2 hours while awake, taking care to allow time to empty completely. The child may need to use a timer as a reminder to stay on the toilet for 2 to 5 minutes; distraction techniques may be needed for the younger child. To achieve success with this plan, the child's understanding and intent to participate are essential.

▲ **Clinical Warning:** A very small percentage of these children have sustained renal functional damage due to high bladder pressure. If success is not achieved with behavioral management, there may be a need for more intensive management.

● **Clinical Pearls:**

- The conversation about timed voiding and staying on the toilet long enough to empty must take place between the provider and the child.
- The topic can be tremendously frustrating to both child and parents, requiring consistency in approach over a long period of time. The provider should help the parents in enlisting the understanding and support of the school, including teachers and the school nurse, as well as any day care providers.
- If UTIs are present, prophylactic antibiotic treatment may be required. If urgency is part of the picture, an anticholinergic drug may be useful.

Both UTIs and urgency can be associated with enough increase in bladder pressure to cause actual damage to the renal parenchyma. A small percentage of patients with severe bladder dysfunction will progress to end-stage renal failure. Most, however, will be amenable to bladder management and can attain dryness with consistent efforts to control UTIs or urgency, while promoting good bladder emptying. Chapter 63 may provide the reader with other insights into the diagnosis and management of secondary enuresis.

Children who have reflux must be managed appropriately for that disorder, as described in the following section. Those rare patients whose enuresis is caused by true polyuria will share the characteristic of drinking large volumes of liquids, even waking at night to drink. They need to be assessed more fully and, in fact, require referral to a pediatric endocrinologist or a pediatric nephrologist for evaluation.

▲ **Clinical Warning:** Water deprivation tests should not be undertaken casually for these children. Any water deprivation for a truly polyuric child must be done in a carefully monitored setting.

Vesicoureteral Reflux

ANATOMY, PATHOLOGY, AND PHYSIOLOGY

Ordinarily, the ureters pump urine into the bladder, and the junction of the ureter with the bladder tunnels inside the bladder wall long enough to create extrinsic pressure on the ureter. The result is that urine is trapped in the bladder and not allowed to move back up the ureter, even when the pressure inside the bladder is great. When the peristaltic activity of the ureter is poor or when the ureteric tunnel in the bladder wall is too short, the pressure inside the bladder may cause urine to move back up the ureter toward the kidney. This situation is called vesicoureteral reflux (VUR). VUR exerts pressure on the renal parenchyma while also bringing bacteria from the bladder, which may cause renal scarring even when VUR is asymptomatic, especially in the young child.

Although common, VUR decreases in incidence as children grow. Therefore, if VUR is mild or moderate, scarring of the kidneys can be prevented if the patient can be kept free of infection until spontaneous resolution occurs. Some children with the following conditions will require surgical correction of reflux:

- Very severe reflux
- Breakthrough infections in spite of medical management
- Failure of VUR to resolve and continued UTIs after several years of medical management

DIAGNOSTIC STUDIES

Vesicoureteral reflux can be diagnosed only by VCUG. This requires that a urethral catheter be placed and the bladder filled with fluid that can be imaged either by fluoroscopic or radionuclide technique. Renal ultrasound may suggest the presence of reflux if there is waxing and waning distention of the renal pelvis with voiding. However, neither renal ultrasound nor intravenous pyelogram (IVP) can rule out the presence of VUR.

Occasionally, a diagnosis of UTI may be unclear. There may be fever or flank pain without a clearly positive urine culture. In this situation, a renal scan using dimercaptosuccinic acid (DMSA) is the most sensitive test available to find areas of poor renal function characteristic of pyelonephritis. The DMSA scan is also useful in defining areas of renal scarring and has replaced the IVP in most cases for this purpose.

MANAGEMENT

When a child is managed medically for VUR, a urine culture should be done whenever symptoms suggesting UTI are present, including fever. The patient should also have occasional surveillance cultures when not symptomatic (ie, every 1–2 months). Surveillance cultures are especially important if the child is very young or if there is bladder dysfunction. Surveillance cultures may be collected by clean-catch or bag, and are useful if negative. If results are positive or unclear, the culture will need to be repeated promptly by catheterization or suprapubic aspiration. Follow-up imaging should be done annually to monitor for resolution of the reflux and for normal growth of the kidneys (Elder et al., 1997).

▲ **Clinical Warning:** If breakthrough infections occur, if there is bladder dysfunction in a child with reflux, or if spontaneous resolution does not occur, the patient should be referred to a pediatric urologist or nephrologist for consultation.

Children who have had one UTI but who do not have VUR are still at risk for recurrent UTIs. If UTIs are accompanied by fever, they can still cause scarring of the kidneys even without VUR. Even if there is no fever, a UTI can exacerbate bladder dysfunction. Prompt diagnosis and appropriate antibiotics are necessary in either of these cases. Sometimes long-term prophylactic antibiotic treatment is needed. Chapter 40 provides information on the diagnosis and management of UTIs, as well as material that the provider can use with parents and the schools.

Nephritis

Nephritis means inflammation of the kidneys. Acute nephritis is usually heralded by hematuria, hypertension, and abnormalities of kidney function. The child with classic acute nephritis presents with brown urine (gross hematuria and mild to moderate proteinuria), mild edema, high blood pressure, and generalized malaise. The initial management of nephritis includes evaluation of its acute features to discern whether the patient needs acute intervention. Evaluation of the episode's etiology follows. Any acute problems that may arise, including hypertension, hyperkalemia, and uremia, are caused by decreased renal function. Urgent measurement should be done of the serum creatinine, blood urea nitrogen (BUN), and electrolytes. A complete blood count (CBC) will show whether there are associated hematologic abnormalities.

▲ **Clinical Warning:** Because hemolytic uremic syndrome is common in young children with acute nephritis, a CBC should be done promptly.

PATHOLOGY

The etiologies of acute nephritis in childhood divide neatly into those accompanied by a low complement (C3) level and those with a normal C3 level. Therefore, C3 should be measured early in the course of evaluation. If the C3 level is very low, the nephritis will almost invariably be due to acute postinfectious glomerulonephritis (GN), membranoproliferative GN, systemic lupus nephritis, shunt nephritis, or subacute bacterial endocarditis nephritis. If the C3 is normal, the most common types of nephritis are GN and tubulointerstitial nephritis (TIN). Forms of GN that are accompanied by a normal C3 level include IgA nephritis, Henoch-Schönlein nephritis, hemolytic uremic syndrome, and a variety of other forms of vasculitis with proliferative and crescentic GN.

Interstitial nephritis may also present with this clinical picture, although it is not as frequently accompanied by hypertension. Interstitial nephritis is most often related to a drug reaction. The classic finding is eosinophils and polymorphonuclear cells in the urinalysis. However, the distinction between GN and TIN may be difficult to make on clinical grounds alone.

Some children will present with a less acute picture. Gross or heavy microscopic hematuria, proteinuria, hypertension, and renal dysfunction may be present, but the child may not appear acutely ill. In this case, Alport syndrome (called familial nephritis, although not an inflammatory disease) should be considered. A careful family history will be helpful. IgA nephropathy, membranoproliferative GN, crescentic GN, and various types of proliferative GN may also present this way.

HISTORY AND PHYSICAL EXAMINATION

The patient who presents with acute nephritis (glomerular or tubulointerstitial) must be evaluated promptly for renal dysfunction, and the etiologic workup should begin without delay. Taking a careful history for duration of symptoms is one component of this evaluation. The provider needs to inquire about any rash, abdominal pain or joint pathology, any drug exposure, any recent infection (especially streptococcal), and family history of renal disease or deafness (Alport's syndrome). Physical examination needs to include a careful blood pressure evaluation. Significant elevations require early treatment. The examiner should look for rashes (seen in Henoch-Schönlein purpura, systemic lupus erythematosus, streptococcal infections). It is also important that pulmonary edema (seen in fluid overload secondary to GN) and other signs of edema in general be ruled out. The provider also must look for joint abnormalities, as are seen in lupus and Henoch-Schönlein purpura.

DIAGNOSTIC CRITERIA

Laboratory data are required in the diagnosis of acute nephritis. The provider should order the following tests:

- Electrolytes to rule out hyperkalemia, hypernatremia, hyponatremia, and acidosis
- Creatinine and BUN, to evaluate glomerular filtration rate (GFR)
- CBC, to rule out anemia, thrombocytopenia, and aberrations in the white blood cell
- C3 complement and serologic evidence of recent streptococcal infection (eg, Streptozyme assay or a streptococcal antibody screen)
- Antineutrophil cytoplasmic antibody, which may be positive in various vasculitides
- Antinuclear antibody, if signs suggestive of systemic lupus erythematosus are present

MANAGEMENT

Functional impairment, including loss of GFR, abnormal electrolytes, and hypertension, may develop rapidly in acute nephritis. This is true for both GN and TIN. The patient presenting with acute nephritis should be evaluated carefully and followed closely to avoid morbidity associated with these changes, particularly hyperkalemia, hypertension, and volume overload. Any of these may occasionally become severe enough to require emergent medical management or even dialysis.

Patients with acute GN who have a very low C3 level and serologic or culture confirmation of a recent streptococcal infection may initially be assumed to have acute postinfectious GN. The diagnosis can be confirmed clinically by observing the complete resolution of the nephritic syndrome (beginning within several days of onset), the resolution of the hypocomplementemia (by 6 weeks after onset), the return to normal blood pressure, and the resolution of hematuria and proteinuria over a period of several months. Chapter 40 offers a more in-depth discussion of diagnosis and management of acute streptoccocal GN.

▲ Clinical Warnings:

- Patients who do not clearly follow this clinical pattern should be referred for evaluation by a pediatric nephrologist. A small percentage of patients who have acute postinfectious GN will continue to have significant proteinuria and hypertension or will redevelop proteinuria and hypertension after 1 to 3 years. These patients are at high risk for chronic progression of their nephritis and loss of (or never regaining) their renal function. They, too, should be referred to a pediatric nephrologist.
- The patient should be followed consistently over the several months after a resolved episode of acute nephritis to ensure that proteinuria and hypertension are not developing. A monthly or bimonthly check for a year in the primary care provider's office will provide this assurance. All subsequent health supervision visits should continue to include urinalysis and blood pressure evaluation. For those patients whose urinalysis shows proteinuria or who develop hypertension, re-referral for pediatric nephrology evaluation is indicated. Treatment may be necessary to decrease the risk for or rate of progression and loss of renal function.

IgA Nephropathy

IgA nephropathy is the syndrome of acute nephritis with histologic appearance of IgA in the mesangium of the glomeruli. Clinical manifestations associated with this tissue appearance are quite varied and include acute and chronic presentations. A common acute picture in adolescent and young adult patients is that of brown urine, often accompanied by flank pain, variable amounts of renal dysfunction, and hypertension. This picture can be associated with simultaneous upper respiratory infection or with very vigorous exercise. The symptoms may resolve over several days or may last longer. The discomfort may be disabling and may be accompanied by loss of appetite and weight loss. There is a variable amount of proteinuria. In all forms of acute nephritis, patients who have nephrotic-range proteinuria are at much higher risk for progression of their nephritis to chronic loss of renal function. Individuals who remain hypertensive also carry this risk.

Membranoproliferative Glomerulonephritis

Membranoproliferative GN is rare and can have a clinical presentation that looks very much like acute postinfectious GN, or it can present with a more chronic picture, as in the nephritis section. There will be variable amounts of hema-

turia, proteinuria (which may vary from mild to nephrotic range), and hypertension. The C3 will be depressed in 85% of patients and will not rebound into the normal range in the short term (West, 1992). The long-range prognosis is poor if there is heavy proteinuria. The diagnosis must be made by renal biopsy.

The provider should refer the patient with suspected membranoproliferative GN to a pediatric nephrologist for biopsy, diagnosis, and treatment. Treatment should be considered in the child who has either proteinuria or renal dysfunction, because outcomes appear to be significantly better when immunosuppressive treatment is used.

Referral Points for Nephritis

The following instances are clinical reasons for referral to a pediatric nephrologist:

- Acute nephritis
  - Hypertension that is not easily controlled
  - Hyperkalemia
  - Acute loss of renal function, with serum creatinine rising
- Chronic nephritis
  - Persistent hypertension
  - Continued proteinuria
  - Persistent hypocomplementemia after 6 to 8 weeks
  - Decreased GFR or increased serum creatinine
  - Continued gross hematuria

Nephrotic Syndrome

Nephrotic syndrome is defined as heavy proteinuria (> 2 g/d per 1.73 m^2 or urine protein-creatinine ratio > 2.0), hypoalbuminemia (serum albumin < 3.0 g/dL), edema, and hyperlipidemia. The most common cause of new-onset NS in childhood is minimal change NS (MCNS), also referred to as nil disease or lipoid nephrosis. All the names refer to the biopsy appearance of the tissue of affected patients, which looks relatively normal by light microscopy. Electron microscopy reveals flattening of the foot processes of the visceral epithelial cells on the outside of the capillary loops in the glomerulus. However, biopsy is not done in most patients who present during childhood, because the diagnosis is confirmed by response to steroid treatment (Clark & Barratt, 1999).

▲ **Clinical Warning:** Any child who presents with signs of NS should be referred to a pediatric nephrologist for evaluation and treatment advice. The primary care provider must be aware of the management of the course of NS, so that the patient's growth, immunizations, and general health care can be managed appropriately. It is important that the provider work with the nephrologist in the co-management of the patient. Consistency of medical guidance for the parents is crucial in maintaining the child in remission and minimizing steroid use. Chapter 40 presents a more in-depth discussion of MCNS.

Focal Segmental Glomerulosclerosis

Focal segmental glomerulosclerosis is a histologic diagnosis that is seen predominantly in patients who present with NS. In children, the presentation can be quite acute, with severe NS, but the appearance can vary a great deal, and some patients will have much milder proteinuria. Some patients will lack the other features of NS, such as edema and hyper-lipidemia, having only the proteinuria. Other children will have associated hematuria, although usually that finding is mild and microscopic. The provider should refer these patients to a pediatric nephrologist for evaluation and treatment advice.

What to Tell Parents

More than two thirds of patients with MCNS will relapse. Relapses are frequent in many affected children. Much of the monitoring must be done by well-informed parents, working in close alliance with a health care team that is expert in the management of this disease. Good management can minimize the amount of time the patient is in relapse, thereby decreasing the edema that is experienced. Good management can also minimize the total amount of time and cumulative dose of steroid therapy (Clark & Barratt, 1999; Trompeter et al., 1985; Foote, Brocklebank, & Meadow, 1985).

Parents should learn to weigh their child, check urine albumin by dipstick, and record these data on a calendar kept specifically for home management of NS. The dosage of prednisone and any other medications given should be recorded on the same calendar. In addition, information about clinical status can be recorded, including infections, edema, or any side effects of medications. Parents must learn to recognize signs of infection and to seek appropriate care and treatment promptly whenever they see these signs.

A nurse coordinator or clinical nurse specialist and a specialist physician who are comfortable with this recurring, chronic disease should be in communication with the patient and the primary care provider whenever there is a relapse or need for steroid dosage adjustment. The school nurse may need to participate in some parts of the monitoring and in optimizing school participation.

Preventing Infections During Immunosuppression

During periods when the patient is on steroid therapy, varicella presents a serious risk, both for severe varicella infection and for triggering a relapse. Therefore, it is optimal for these patients to have documented varicella immunity or to receive the varicella vaccine. The vaccine must be given when the patient is not in relapse and is not on immunosuppressing medications. Humoral immunity may be demonstrated by varicella-specific IgG. However, this level must be drawn when the patient is not hypoalbuminemic.

Bacterial infections also present great risk for these children. Prior to the availability of steroids and antibiotics, deaths due to NS were primarily caused by overwhelming infection. Currently, mortality risk is much lower, but death still occurs as a result of MCNS in about 0.5% to 1% of patients, usually because of infection. Gram-positive organisms, especially *Streptococcus pneumoniae*, have been discussed frequently as a risk to children with NS. However, there is an equal risk that a gram-negative organism will cause an infection. These infections may occur as peritonitis, pneumonia, or other forms of sepsis. Occasionally, a child with new-onset nephrosis will present with peritonitis as the first sign of NS. The risk of bacterial infection is highest by far during relapse, when the IgG level is quite low.

Regardless of the number of relapses, most children with steroid-sensitive NS will cease having episodes of NS sometime during late adolescence. A few will continue to have relapses into adulthood. When this happens, the relapses will usually continue to be steroid sensitive.

Because of the low incidence of the disease and the need to coordinate care for these children, a pediatric nephrologist should be involved, along with the primary care provider, in their management. The primary care office should be well informed about medication strategies, informing the nephrologist about any intercurrent bacterial or severe viral infections that occur. The nurse coordinator or clinical nurse specialist and the school nurse should also be in communication with each other and the family.

Chronic Renal Insufficiency

Chronic renal insufficiency (CRI) is defined as a GFR less than 75 mL/min per 1.73 m^2. Chronic renal failure (CRF), or end-stage renal disease (ESRD), is defined as a GFR less than 15 mL/min per 1.73 m^2. The incidence of CRF in childhood is not high. Approximately two to five children reach end-stage renal failure each year for every 1 million total population (USRDS, 1999). These children need good primary care and specialty care, and their primary care must differ from that of well children. This section limits the discussion about CRI and ESRD to aspects that are important to the provision of good primary care.

MANAGEMENT

When CRI or CRF occurs, it is necessary to have a well-coordinated team approach to management. This team must include the parents, pediatric nephrologist, primary care provider, nurse coordinator or clinical nurse specialist, nutritionist, social worker, school nurse, educational consultants, and often psychology or psychiatry personnel. It is also helpful to enlist the support of other parents who have had children with similar problems, because the burdens on the family are so great.

Immunizations in Chronic Renal Insufficiency and Post-transplantation

The primary care provider will be responsible for keeping immunizations up-to-date. When a child has CRI, there is an even more compelling need than usual to give all of the immunizations at the earliest recommended age, because the goal is to achieve full immunization status before CRI decreases immune reactivity and before the child is immunosuppressed for transplantation.

It is of critical importance to achieve full immunization status in children before they reach end-stage renal failure. Once the GFR is very low, immune reactivity may be decreased, and response to immunizations may not be optimal. Even so, if a child is on dialysis but not on immunosuppressive treatment, all immunizations may be administered as usual.

▲ **Clinical Warning:** After transplantation of any solid organ or bone marrow, the child will be very immunosuppressed. Live virus vaccines should no longer be administered, because the risk of vaccine-induced disease may outweigh the benefit of immunization. An attenuated or killed virus vaccine can be substituted, if available (eg, enhanced-potency, or Salk, inactive polio vaccine [IPV] instead of trivalent, or Sabin, oral polio vaccine [OPV]). Studies are in progress to evaluate the safety and efficacy of varicella vaccine in the post-transplant population, but varicella vaccine should not be administered routinely to any child on immunosupressive medications until those studies have shown a clear benefit that outweighs risk (American Academy of Pediatrics, 1997).

Other Management Issues

The following signs may be present with CRI or may develop after the diagnosis is known. They are all concerns for affected children and must be monitored during their care:

- Growth impairment
- Anemia
- Nutrition
- Hypertension
- Electrolyte imbalance
- Neurodevelopmental delays and cognitive abnormalities
- Seizures

Table 62-1 outlines the management of these signs.

▲ **Clinical Warning:** It is imperative that the provider use Table 62-1 only after reading the following section, which provides the necessary detail for managing these serious problems.

Table 62–1. MANAGEMENT OF SPECIFIC PROBLEMS ASSOCIATED WITH CHRONIC RENAL IMPAIRMENT AND CHRONIC RENAL FAILURE

Problem	Causes	Treatment	Other Interventions
Growth delay	Increased IGH1-BP (usually normal growth hormone level) Acidosis Hyperparathyroidism Poor nutrition	Correct: • Acidosis so that serum bicarbonate level > 22 mEq/L • Poor nutrition • Hyperparathyroid through Ca-P-vitD-PTH system (see text) Give growth hormone (consult with pediatric urologist or endocrinologist).	Careful repeated measurements are needed with a reliable measuring device.
Nutrition	Anorexia Altered taste/dysgeusia Poor absorption	Give dietary supplementation for adequate calories without electrolyte overload. Caloric need is often elevated.	Provide nutrition counseling. Feeding team assistance is needed for infants. Parents need support, because frustration is very high.
Anemia	Lack of erythropoietin Iron deficiency Decreased red blood cell lifespan	Administer erythropoietin. Provide iron supplementation.	Minimize blood volumes drawn for testing.
Hypertension	Volume overload High renin state	Control sodium and fluid intake. Give antihypertensive medication.	Some drugs will worsen blood pressure.
Developmental delay/learning disabilities	Poor brain growth early in life "Uremic toxins" (unknown)	Careful early and repeated evaluation is required. Provide early intervention physical/ occupational therapy. Offer special education planning.	Consider instituting dialysis or transplanting early.
Seizures	"Uremic toxins" (unknown) Electrolyte imbalance Hypertension Drug neurotoxicity	Dialysis/transplantation is needed. Correct electrolytes. Give antihypertensive medication. Consider changing drugs.	Family history may also contribute.
Acidosis	Poor tubular function	Bicarbonate replacement is needed.	May be improved by use of $CaCO_3$.
Hyperparathyroidism	Poor phosphate clearance Inadequate 1,25-dihydroxy-cholecalciferol production	Decrease dietary P. Give oral calcitrol.	Use P binder—oral $CaCO_3$. May use dihydrotachysterol instead.
Electrolyte/water imbalance	Poor tubular function Poor GFR	Control diet.	Will need nutritionist support and often behavior management therapy.
Medication interactions	Necessary polypharmacy	In consultation with pediatric neurologist when appropriate, adjust dosages as needed.	Avoid unnecessary interactions, especially for acute prescription needs. Consider the whole drug list every time. Encourage parents to use the same pharmacy for every prescription every time so that a stable drug record can be maintained.

Ca = calcium; $CaCO_3$ = calcium carbonate; GFR = glomerular filtration rate; IGF1-BP = insulin-like growth factor-1 binding protein; P = phosphorus; PTH = parathyroid hormone; vitD = vitamin D.

Growth Impairment

Growth impairment occurs in most children with CRI and in virtually all children with CRF. Growth is impaired by acidosis, hyperparathyroidism, poor nutrition, and unique abnormalities of the growth hormone system.

Acidosis must be corrected so that the serum bicarbonate level is greater than 22 mEq/L to allow optimal growth. The calcium-phosphorus-parathyroid system must be corrected. As GFR declines, phosphorus cannot be excreted well. Therefore, dietary phosphorus load must be reduced, either by limiting phosphorus-rich foods or by binding phosphorus in the gut with calcium carbonate ($CaCO_3$) taken orally. As GFR declines, the kidneys no longer convert vitamin D to its active form (1,25-dihydroxycholecalciferol), so the gut cannot absorb Ca^{++} optimally. The active form of vitamin D can be replaced orally as calcitriol or dihydrotachysterol. Both the excess phosphorus and the calcium depletion stimulate parathyroid hormone (PTH) secretion. If PTH secretion is stimulated for a long time, hyperparathyroid bone disease occurs. This includes dimineralization and cystic change and growth retardation and rickets. PTH secretion must be suppressed by careful control of the dietary phosphorus load and administration of $CaCO_3$ and calcitriol.

Even when all of the above abnormalities are corrected, however, children with CRF do not grow well. They seldom have a deficiency of growth hormone, but they often have an excess of a binding protein of the growth hormone mediator IGF1. Measurement of growth hormone, or growth hormone provocative testing, will not be useful. Growth hormone therapy is now Food and Drug Administration approved for children with CRI. In most cases, this therapy will significantly increase the child's growth and eventual height. Growth hormone therapy should be considered early in the course of management of CRI, along with all the other components of management.

Occasionally, growth retardation will be the presenting feature of CRI. When this occurs, linear growth (height) is slowed in proportion to the weight. If CRI occurs after infancy, normal growth often has been documented previously, followed later by no growth or very slow growth. Use of the growth chart (including past growth points) is therefore very important in any child whose growth is in question.

Anemia

Anemia in CRF is primarily caused by failure of the renal interstitium to make erythropoietin (EPO). EPO is the hormone that stimulates the red blood cell line in the bone marrow. A slightly decreased red blood cell lifespan and nutritional deficiencies of iron are common in CRF anemia. EPO thus needs to be replaced, but unfortunately it must be given in injectable form. The usual route is subcutaneous, unless the patient is on hemodialysis or for some other reason, has an intravenous access route in place. EPO is given once or twice weekly as a subcutaneous injection, usually at home by a parent or helper. Iron stores must be maintained and monitored. Often oral supplementation of iron is adequate, but some patients require intravenous iron as well.

Nutrition

Nutrition presents one of the greatest challenges to parents who care for a child with CRI. The child will probably have some degree of anorexia. Many children have almost no appetite at all. Infants with CRI often require tube feedings to achieve adequate nutrition. There are also many dietary restrictions, including total fluid content of the diet, sodium, potassium, and phosphate. All these restrictions severely limit available food choices. Careful long-term counseling by a renal and pediatric dietician is required. Often, a multidisciplinary feeding team (occupational therapist, physical therapist, nutritionist) is needed to help the child learn feeding skills. School personnel must be involved as well to allow participation in school activities while meeting dietary goals.

Often so much of the parents' energy is focused on feeding the child to promote adequate growth that there is a great deal of frustration when nutritional needs change. This occurs as GFR declines, necessitating new restrictions. Changes occur dramatically when the child begins dialysis, depending on the dialysis modality chosen. The most dramatic change occurs with transplantation, when the appetite returns with good renal function; many children at this point tend to eat too much and gain weight very rapidly, especially if they are taking high doses of daily steroids. Parents may find that changing feeding practices presents a huge challenge at these times and can be expected to need a lot of support.

Hypertension

Hypertension occurs in patients who have diminished ability to excrete salt and water. Occasionally, renovascular impairment will also lead to excess renin production and release. A variety of other mechanisms may contribute to this problem as well. The need to limit salt and water intake can be a huge challenge. Some patients will respond well to the use of diuretics, but many will not. About 35% of children with CRI require antihypertensive drugs to maintain blood pressure at less than the 95th percentile for age and size (Baluarte et al., 1994).

Electrolyte Imbalance

Electrolyte excesses and imbalances occur when dietary intake exceeds the person's ability to excrete that substance. The most common excesses encountered are of potassium, sodium, and phosphorus. Deficiencies occur when the person is unable to ingest or absorb the component adequately. The most common deficiencies are those of calcium and iron. Dietary adjustments are required and often must change as the person's GFR declines. Supplements are required for calcium and iron, as noted.

Neurodevelopmental Delays and Cognitive Abnormalities

Neurodevelopmental delays and cognitive abnormalities are a tremendous challenge for these chronically ill children. When GFR is impaired during infancy, brain growth is impaired, and learning is slowed. For this reason, infants with CRF are treated aggressively with nutritional support and are often considered for transplantation at a much younger age and smaller size than was true just 10 years ago.

Seizures

Seizures occur in 4% to 10% of children with CRF (Trompeter, Polinsky, Andreoli, & Fennell, 1986). The causes are varied, but seizures must be controlled with anticonvulsants in consultation with a pediatric neurologist. The reader is referred to Chapter 46 for a discussion of the diagnosis and management of seizures.

Renal Replacement Therapy

The decision to start renal replacement therapy, whether with dialysis or transplantation, is an important one. This determination will be made by the pediatric nephrologist, based on the severity of the child's condition. There is no single factor responsible for the timing of this decision. Generally, renal replacement therapy is begun when any of the features of CRI becomes disabling. That is likely to occur when the GFR has declined to approximately 10 mL/min per 1.73 m^2 or less.

The decision about which form of renal replacement therapy to choose is individualized. Transplantation is often chosen if the patient can have the procedure safely without a period of dialysis preceding the transplant. However, often dialysis is required at least for a while to prepare the patient. The nephrologist will, along with the parents, choose hemodialysis or peritoneal dialysis depending on the difficulties of vascular versus peritoneal access, how capable the parents are at home procedures, and how long the patient is likely to remain on dialysis. Local dialysis capabilities and preferences also play a role, as does the distance the family lives from the pediatric nephrology center.

What to Tell Parents

During childhood, CRF continues to cause varying degrees of cognitive dysfunction, some of which can be reversed by transplantation. Careful multidisciplinary evaluation of neurodevelopmental and educational status is required to optimize learning and development at every age for these children. Again, the status may change dramatically as the GFR declines and as the child undergoes dialysis and transplantation (Fennell, 2000). Therefore, regular reevaluation and replanning must be done. Health care and educational teams must work together to help each other understand how best to optimize the educational environment. It is helpful to remember that these children may have some relatively good times, while it is also clear that they will progress to a later stage when learning will be much harder. Take advantage of every period of good health so that the child's eventual educational outcome can be optimized.

In addition to a well-informed and supported family, good team care involves primary and specialty care. Other members should include the nurse coordinator or clinical nurse specialist, nutritionist, developmentalist, occupational and physical therapists, psychologist, and educators. Each of these professionals can help children who have CRI to achieve as successful a transplantation as possible. The goal of this effort is to help the child live as full and productive a life as possible. This chronic disease never disappears; it is never cured. The child must take immunosuppressive drugs and cope with the medical aspects of having a transplant throughout life. However, successful transition to well-adjusted adult life is possible. When this occurs, all who have participated in the care of these children are ultimately rewarded.

Refer to Chapter 66 for the specifics of preparing the child and family for transplantation, as well as post-transplantation management.

COMMUNITY RESOURCES

National Kidney Foundation (NKF)
30 East 33rd Street, Suite 1100
New York, NY 10016
Telephone: For PNE: (888) WAKEDRY

For other problems: (800) 622-9010 or (212) 889-2210
Fax: (212) 889-9261
Internet address: *http://www.kidney.org*

> This group rovides information for parents and professionals, with many resources and web links available for kidney diseases and disorders. Also, referral services are provided to pediatric nephrologists who specialize in kidney and bladder dysfunction. For PNE, a brochure is available as well as a referral to providers who have indicated a willingness to treat bedwetting. The NKF web site provides valuable links to other pertinent web sites and resources.

American Urological Association
1120 North Charles Street
Baltimore, MD 21201
Telephone: (410) 727-1100
Fax: (410) 223-4370
Internet address: *http://www.auanet.org*

> This is an important resource for parents and primary care providers in locating a qualified pediatric urologist.

American Psychiatric Association
1400 K Street, N.W.
Washington, DC 20005
Telephone: (202) 682-6000
Fax: (202) 682-6850
Internet address: *http://www.psych.org*

> This is helpful for parents or referring primary care providers in locating qualified child or adolescent psychiatrists if coexisting mental health problems, including attention deficit hyperactivity disorder, post-traumatic stress disorder, child abuse, or neglect, are known or suspected.

REFERENCES

American Academy of Pediatrics. (1997). Varicella zoster infections. In G. Peter (Ed.), *1997 Red Book: Report of the Committee on Infectious Diseases* (24th ed.) (pp. 583–585). Elk Grove Village, IL: Author.

Baluarte, H. J., Gruskin, A. B., Ingelfinger, J. R., et al. (1994). Analysis of hypertension in children post renal transplantation: A report of the North American Pediatric Renal Cooperative Study. *Pediatric Nephrology, 8,* 570–573.

Clark, A. G., & Barratt, T. M. (1999). Steroid responsive nephrotic syndrome. In T. M. Barratt, E. D. Avner, & W. E. Harmon (Eds.), *Pediatric nephrology* (4th ed.). Baltimore: Lippincott Williams & Wilkins.

Dodge, W. F., West, E. F., Bridgforth, E. B., & Travis, L. B. (1970). Nocturnal enuresis in 6 to 10 year old children: Correlation with bacteriuria, proteinuria and dysuria. *American Journal of Diseases of Childhood, 120,* 32.

Elder, J. S., Peters, C. A., Arant, B. S., et al. (1997). Pediatric vesicoureteral reflux guidelines panel summary report on the management of primary VUR in children. *Journal of Urology, 157,* 1846–1851.

Fennell, E. B. (2000). End stage renal disease. In K. O. Yeates, M. D. Ris, & H. G. Taylor (Eds.), *Pediatric neuropsychology.* New York: Guilford Press.

Foote, K. D., Brocklebank, J. T., & Meadow, S. R. (1985). Height attainment in children with steroid responsive nephrotic syndrome. *Lancet, 2,* 917–919.

Jones, B., Gerrard, J. W., Shokeir, M. K., et al. (1972). Recurrent UTIs in girls: Relation to enuresis. *Canadian Medical Association Journal, 106,* 127.

Monda, J. M., & Husmann, D. A. (1995). Primary nocturnal enuresis: A comparison among observation, imipramine, desmopressin acetate and bed-wetting alarm systems. *Journal of Urology, 54,* 745–748.

Robson, W. L. (1998). Hyponatremia in children treated with desmopressin. *Archives Pediatric and Adolescent Medicine, 152,* 930–931.

Schmitt, B. D. (1997). Nocturnal enuresis. *Pediatrics in Review, 18,* 183–190.

Tietjen, D. N., & Husmann, D. A. (1996). Nocturnal enuresis: A guide to evaluation and treatment. *Mayo Clinic Proceedings, 71,* 857–862.

Trompeter, R. S., Lloyd, B. W., Hicks, J., et al. (1985). Long term outcome for children with minimal change nephrotic syndrome. *Lancet, 1,* 368–370.

Trompeter, R. S., Polinsky, M. S., Andreoli, M., & Fennell, R. S. (1986). Neurological complications of renal failure. *American Journal of Kidney Diseases, 7,* 318–328.

USRDS. (1999). Pediatric end stage renal disease (ESRD). *American Journal of Kidney Diseases, 34*(S1), 102–113.

West, C. D. (1992). Idiopathic membranoproliferative glomerulonephritis in childhood. *Pediatric Nephrology, 6,* 96–103.

Enuresis and Encopresis

• WILLIAM J. DISCIPIO, PhD

INTRODUCTION

The current state of scientific knowledge about childhood dysfunctions or delays in bladder and bowel training suggests that good standards of pediatric practice should be proactive. The primary care provider needs to be knowledgeable about advances in early interventions, selecting treatments on an empirical footing. There is no longer a sufficient basis for ignoring the problem, treating with "tincture of time," or waiting for the child to "grow out of" a presenting problem of self-limiting or monosymptomatic urinary or bowel incontinence.

Most children are physiologically and psychologically ready for successful toilet training before age 4 years, some as early as 18 months. Cultural and familial determinants of the initiation of toilet training vary greatly, with few to no effects on later continence. Persistent failures to achieve diurnal and nocturnal urinary control may signal a need for medical or psychological intervention. The primary care provider should actively investigate the problem, especially if it is raised as a problem by the family. Similarly, the provider needs to intervene if the child experiences the negative psychological impact of not keeping up developmentally with siblings or peers. Chronic and persistent voiding dysfunction associated with high intravesicle pressure and postvoid residual urine can also contribute to infection, bladder decompensation (trabeculated interior), ureteral reflux, hydronephrosis, and ultimately renal failure.

Although the statistical prevalence of serious systemic or psychiatric disorders is low, the difficult-to-train child may be presenting important but subtle diagnostic cues implicating the interaction of the central and autonomic nervous systems. To find a treatment strategy for what is either a psychophysiologic or functional disturbance, the provider must rule out many different causes for the training lag. Cross-disciplinary consultation or referral may be appropriate from specialists in either pediatric urology or behavioral psychology.

Problems of storage and elimination of waste in children pose medical and secondary psychological adjustment and coping problems. The etiology is multidetermined. Therefore, wetting and soiling must be seen as symptoms to be investigated before an efficacious choice of treatment can be made. Incontinence symptoms in children are generally referred to as enuresis (poor bladder control) and encopresis (poor fecal control). These symptoms are rarely indicative of complete loss of function. Obvious lesions or limitations of the central nervous system (CNS) may be present, such as cerebral palsy, severe mental retardation, autism, psychosis, attention deficit disorder, or seizure disorder. In cases in which no primary physical or severe psychiatric diagnosis is present, a functional, or more accurately stated, psychophysiologic, diagnosis is reached by careful elimination of other differential causes for the incontinence. This chapter provides a framework for differentiating organic from functional causes of incontinence, while guiding the provider in appropriate treatment and referral.

ANATOMY, PHYSIOLOGY, AND PATHOLOGY

Normal Bladder Function

Storage and elimination of urine in the infant bladder is entirely an autonomic function, without inhibitory or volitional control connections to the CNS. The bladder itself is composed of smooth muscle, while the length of the urethra contains an increasing presence of striated muscle as it projects distally from the bladder. As the bladder wall accommodates expansion in the storage process, a trigger threshold of fluid capacity is reached. An afferent neural message is sent through the pudendal nerve to sites at S2, S3, and S4, where a synapse is activated with nerves that innervate efferent muscles. Additional neural pathways connect this reflex with regions in the pons and detrusor motor nucleus. The bladder normally contracts in synchrony with the relaxation of sphincter muscle, expelling urine in one continuous stream. When bladder control persists in this automatic fashion in the absence of physical causes, such as a primary disease affecting the nervous system, the child is said to have a pediatric unstable bladder or bladder displaying uninhibited contractions. This can result in a chronic day or night wetting problem.

Primary Diurnal Enuresis

A child who does not show complete daytime urinary continence often experiences repeated and unexpected contractions of the bladder (primary diurnal enuresis [PDE]). These contractions result in intermittent wetting episodes, with accidents occurring at small capacities. Such a youngster has never been dry for a continuous 3-month period. In the presence of an intact nervous system, the child does not respond to a sensation of a gradient of bladder filling but rather will perceive a sensation of the bladder muscle in contraction. In the young child, the most readily available compensatory response to an uninhibited bladder reflex is a volitional contraction of the external sphincter muscles. The child eventually learns to apply pressure on the perineal area by crossing the legs and squeezing the thighs together or performing a "squatting" maneuver by sitting on the heel of one foot. At best, the child is able to inhibit some but not all of the urine flow, because the compensatory maneuver is initiated only after the bladder has begun an uninhibited contraction.

▲ **Clinical Warning:** Wet underpants or remaining in diapers for protracted periods may contribute to the risk of bacterial migration through the urethra to the bladder. Recurring urinary tract and bladder infections, especially in girls, will in turn exacerbate dyscontrol of the bladder and sphincter muscles.

Primary Nocturnal Enuresis

Bedwetting is a relatively common problem that frustrates children and parents long after daytime continence has been achieved. Although the condition most often appears as a monosymptomatic, nonorganically based problem, the psychological impact and persistence of the problem over many years must and should be addressed with active treatment interventions.

● **Clinical Pearl:** Genetics is now known to play a major role in the etiology of bedwetting. If the provider identifies family members who were symptomatic as children, a reasonable prediction can be made as to the age at which the patient will achieve spontaneous remission.

Many myths have been constructed about the causes and cures of primary nocturnal enuresis (PNE) that are based on coincidence and faulty logic. These myths have evolved because of the pervasive epidemiology of the problem combined with unpredictable spontaneous remission rates. Speculation has therefore included small functional bladder capacity, dietary influences, allergies, and excessive water intake as examples of mechanisms underlying the incontinence. To date, there is no support that any of these factors is explanatory of a single underlying cause. Although early studies have been confirmatory of small functional bladder capacity, the occurrence of bladder retention in some patients can also occur, especially in the presence of a mild daytime unstable bladder component (Shima et al., 1998; Medel, Ruarte, Castera, & Podesta, 1998). These children may have learned an overcorrective maneuver by chronic tightening of perineal muscles to overcome any symptoms of diurnal urine loss.

● **Clinical Pearl:** A retentive pattern of bladder capacity may also be manifested in bowel retention or "sluggish" and inconsistent bowel habits. Loening-Baucke's (1997) study adds evidence to this retentive pattern. He found that remission of nocturnal enuresis occurred by simply treating the subclinical constipation.

Explanatory mechanisms involving bladder storage have explored the notion of small functional bladder capacity interacting with high urine production at night (Rasmussen, Kirk, Borup, Norgaard, & Djurhuus, 1996; Djurhuus & Rittig, 1998). Conclusive evidence on this point has proven to be equivocal. Exceptions to the small functional capacity model are frequent, especially as children get older and often decrease their frequency of voluntary daytime voids because of previously acquired annoyance associated with trips to the bathroom. Norgaard, Djurhuus, Watanabe, Stenberg, and Lettgen (1997) implicated hormonal influences by studying bladder capacity with attention to rate of urine production and urine osmolality. Their findings built on work of a decade earlier, when they documented the presence of an insufficient nocturnal antidiuretic control in some patients with PNE, who were also usually treatment resistant (Norgaard, Pedersen, & Djurhuus, 1985).

Wide-scale distribution of DDAVP, a synthetic form of vasopressin, has shown the drug's dramatic immediate effects on abating PNE. Recurrence of symptoms after the drug is withdrawn is high, however, suggesting that a pharmacogenic solution is not likely to "jump-start" the youngster who may have a vasopressin deficiency.

▲ **Clinical Warning:** Because DDAVP will lower kidney production of urine in all children, validation of a hormonal imbalance is not conclusively proven by the action of this particular medication.

Depth of sleep is another competing controversy in the pursuit of an etiologic model for PNE. Many parents and primary care providers have assumed that the bedwetter sleeps too deeply and therefore cannot respond to full bladder cues to awaken and toilet at night. A contradictory view is apparent when one considers that very few normal children awaken at night to void, and if they do, such awakening might be considered a pathologic symptom of nocturia. In addition, children sleep more deeply than adults. This fact might result in a false conclusion that the child is an abnormally deep sleeper when a parent tries to awaken the child to void and keep the bed dry. For many years, studies monitoring electroencephalograms (EEG) and enuresis showed no relationship between depth of sleep and enuretic events in the absence of a known paroxysmal or primary seizure disturbance (Wolfish, Pivik, & Busby, 1997).

Conversely, increasing numbers of recent scientific reports suggest that a possible deficit in CNS arousal underlies PNE (Kawauchi et al., 1998a; Watanabe, Imada, Kawauchi, Koyama, & Shirakawa, 1997). Clinical observations confirming that arousal factors may be implicated include the tendency for the child with PNE to sleep dry on occasion when going to bed very late or sleeping in a different bed when away from home (eg, at sleepovers or at relatives' houses). Jenkins et al. (1996) and Neveus, Lackgren, Tuvemo, and Stenberg (1998) found that children with PNE were indeed harder to bring to full awakening than a nonenuretic population. PNE has also been classified along the lines of arousability by sleep researchers who propose three distinct clinical groups (Watanabe, 1998; Imada et al., 1998):

- Type I: Detectable change in EEG activity in response to bladder distension and stable cystometrograms
- Type IIa: No detectable change in EEG; stable cystometrograms
- Type IIb: No detectable change in EEG; unstable cystometrograms only during sleep

Kawauchi et al. (1998b) propose that type I may involve an immaturity in the function of the thalamus, while type IIa may implicate the pons or the lower urinary tract. Type IIb most closely resembles a neurogenic bladder profile. Refer to Chapter 62 for more information about the use of medications in managing PNE.

Functional Encopresis

Chronic encopresis is mostly an outcome of functional or behavioral causes for stool retention or inappropriate bowel elimination habits. Physical causes or syndromes are consequently an unlikely reason for a child's encopresis. An exception is Hirshsprung's disease, which is an anatomic basis of stool incontinence. Hirshsprung's disease is often apparent at birth or is identified long before the child is seen for encopresis. Other problems involving the integrity of the rectal sphincter and spinal cord innervation also must be considered before accepting a functional cause for incontinent stool loss. Children with functional encopresis (FEN) do not have identifiable anatomic malformations or neurogenic lesions. Abnormal pudendal nerve function, which often contributes to fecal incontinence in adults, does not appear to be implicated in FEN (Sentovich et al., 1998).

The most common presentation of encopresis is a minor stool loss or staining of the underpants ("skid marks") accompanied by retentive toileting habits. Stool retention results in the compaction of large amounts of hard feces in the lower bowel. The passage of loose stool from farther up the intestine is then allowed to "leak" between the hardened stool and the wall of the lower bowel. Many parents mistake the cause of soiled underpants as being related to poor hygiene or wiping technique.

● **Clinical Pearl:** Dietary intake of fiber is likely to be very poor in these children, contributing to their fecal impaction.

EPIDEMIOLOGY

Primary Diurnal Enuresis

About 1% to 5% of children are believed to experience daytime wetting in the absence of physical findings, including bacterial infection of the lower urinary tracts (Bower, Moore, Shepherd, & Adams, 1996). However, Swithinbank, Brookes, Shepherd, and Abrams (1998) reported that a recent survey of 1176 healthy English school children revealed prevalence estimates as high as 12% for day wetting in children aged 11 to 12 years. Nevertheless, the prevalence is much greater in girls than boys. This sex difference is probably related to higher incidence of chronic urinary tract infections (UTIs) seen in girls with PDE, secondary to the shorter urethral distance in girls, which may carry bacteria to the bladder.

Primary Nocturnal Enuresis

Primary nocturnal enuresis occurs in about 10% of all 5-year-old children who are otherwise normal in all other developmental functions. This estimate would include from 5 to 10 million children in North America. The National Kidney Foundation estimates that 5 to 7 million children age 6 years or older have PNE (1999). The prevalence rates vary among cultures, although the condition is documented among all cultures and racial groups (Kalo & Bella, 1996; Trombetta, Savoca, Siracusano, & Liguori, 1997; Chiozza et al., 1998; Chao et al., 1997; Yeung, 1997; Serel et al., 1997; Popper & Steingard, 1996; Byrd, Weitzman, Lanphear, & Auinger, 1996).

It is estimated that up to 70% of children with PNE have a primary relative who shares that history. There is also a 67% concordance rate for identical twins. Recent discoveries of genetic markers for PNE have clearly established a genetic basis of PNE (Hublin, Kaprio, Partinen, & Koskenvuo, 1998; von Gontard, Eiberg, Hollmann, Rittig, & Lehmkuhl, 1997; von Gontard et al., 1997; Arnell et al., 1997; Eiberg, 1998; von Gontard, Eiberg, Hollmann, Rittig, & Lehmkuhl, 1998).

The most conventional criterion for diagnosing PNE is wetting the bed on average at least two times per month. The number of children remitting without treatment is about 15% per year, which reduces the prevalence to 1% by puberty (Petrican & Sawan, 1998). When considering whether PNE will persist into adulthood, Hjalmas (1997) asserts that, if not treated, 10% of these youngsters will persist with PNE for life.

Special needs children have higher rates of PNE. This is especially true for youngsters diagnosed with attention deficit disorder with hyperactivity (ADHD). PNE in such children may in part be related to a "hyperactive" bladder or to behavioral problems encountered in toilet training. These problems may have emerged because of attentional impediments to efficient learning. Pervasive and chronic hyperactivity of the parasympathetic nervous system may also pay a role in uninhibited bladder contractions (Yakinci, Mungen, Durmaz, Balbay, & Karabiber, 1997). Refer to Chapter 21 for more information on diagnosing and managing ADHD.

● **Clinical Pearl:** It is a good idea to assess for PNE when ADHD is identified (Robson, Jackson, Blackhurst, & Leung, 1997).

Functional Encopresis

Prevalence rates of FEN are frequently underestimates of actual occurrence. This may be a result of mild forms of stool loss going unnoticed or being tolerated by family members. Reasons for this tolerance may be multidetermined and can involve individual family and culture-bound attitudes toward hygiene or the belief that stool loss is not a treatable, medical symptom.

HISTORY AND PHYSICAL EXAMINATION

A well-informed parent or guardian is invaluable in establishing a confirmatory history of PDE, PNE, or FEN. A family history of wetting problems in parents or any primary relative is very helpful in identifying the genetic basis of many forms of functional bowel and bladder disturbances. A thorough but noninvasive routine evaluation for enuresis and encopresis starts with a structured interview, as demonstrated in Displays 63-1, 63-2, and 63-3.

● **Clinical Pearl:** The provider may find that it is difficult to establish the history of the onset and pattern of wetting/soiling episodes reliably in one interview. Follow-up charting of base rates of daytime and nighttime symptom events is often required for a minimum of a 1-week period.

A thorough physical examination should be performed, with urine obtained for analysis and culture. The provider should also order a bladder ultrasound if poor bladder emptying or an unusual urinary stream (eg, intermittent flow) is known or suspected (Lettgen, 1997; Kawauchi, Kitamori, Imada, Tanaka, & Watanabe, 1996; Pippi Salle et al., 1998).

The clinician may find that child and parents have a limited accuracy for recalling soiling episodes. This is common, underscoring the need for the collection of prospective data (van der Plas, Benninga, Redekop, Taminiau, & Buller, 1997). Parents are often not aware of damp or soiled underwear during school hours and do not take note of their presumably trained youngster's daily bowel movement activities.

DIAGNOSTIC CRITERIA

Primary Diurnal Enuresis

Children with PDE wet themselves during the day, in the absence of anatomic, neurologic, infectious, or pharmacologic iatrogenic causes. The differential diagnosis must also rule out causes secondary to family stressors, child abuse, or psychiatric crises (secondary diurnal enuresis). The problem of daytime wetting is usually characterized by small losses of urine throughout the day, although the cumulative loss may be greatest in the late afternoon and evening when the

---

DISPLAY 63–1 • Intake Questionnaire for Nocturnal Enuresis

1. Has your child had nighttime wetting (bedwetting) or wetting after falling asleep at any time about twice a week or more for at least 3 consecutive months?
2. Has your child never been dry for 3 or more months?
3. Did the bedwetting start after you or your child experienced a major life event, such as a divorce, birth of sibling, hospitalization, or any other stressor?
4. Do you think the bedwetting is caused by a medical condition or the effect of drugs your child is taking?
5. Do you think the bedwetting is caused by your child's always being thirsty, resulting in excessive drinking?
6. Do you think bedwetting is caused by something your child eats or by fussy or selective dietary habits?
7. Do you think the bedwetting is caused by deep sleep?
8. Do you think the bedwetting is caused by nightmares, night fears or terrors?
9. Do you think that your child is just too lazy to get out of bed when he or she has to go at night?
10. Does your child usually wet more than once during the night?
11. Does your child help with changing the wet bed?
12. Does your child ever get up on his or her own to go to the bathroom during the night?
13. Does your child have a regular bedtime?
14. Does your child have trouble falling asleep?

Psychological Symptoms

1. Do you think your child is old enough to start treatment for bedwetting?
2. Does stress or other emotional problems seem to bring about or worsen the bedwetting?

3. Does your child try to hide or deny the bedwetting took place?
4. Is it very difficult to awaken your child?
5. Does your child miss going to overnight visits with friends or sleep-away camp because of the bedwetting?
6. Do you use a diaper, pull-ups, or special panty or pad for your child at night?
7. Does your child have his or her own room?
8. Do you think your child really wants to stop bedwetting?

Family Incidence

1. Did anyone in your family (including yourself) or your spouse and his or her family wet the bed?
2. Do you have other children who are or were bedwetters?
3. If someone in the family wet the bed, did the wetting stop before the age of 12 years?

Treatment History

1. Have you tried rewards for a dry bed?
2. Have you tried punishment for a wet bed?
3. Have you tried restricting fluids before bedtime?
4. Have you tried asking your child to retain or hold in urine after feeling a sensation to urinate during the day?
5. Have you tried awakening your child for toileting?
6. Have you tried medication?
7. Have you tried different foods or diets?
8. Have you tried a bell and pad or any kind of a urine sensor or wetting alarm?
9. Has your child been seen by a mental health therapist or received psychological help for bedwetting?
10. Has your child been evaluated or treated by a medical doctor, such as a pediatrician or pediatric urologist, for bedwetting?

---

bladder may be fatigued or liquid intake is at a maximum. The actual incontinent episode is associated with a reflexive partial bladder contraction and is not a result of incompetent sphincter function. "Squatting" maneuvers or obvious physical signs that the child is trying to inhibit a full bladder contraction are evident in 3- to 5-year-olds. Older children show more skill at unobservable urethral striated muscle contraction, keeping their perineal muscles at a chronically high resting potential.

● **Clinical Pearl:** UTIs are not uncommon in PDE, and they may be accompanied by symptoms of dysuria. These include marked urgency or frequency and burning or painful urination. In some cases, an odor may be noted by the parent and changes in mood, irritability, or unexplained fever. On the other hand, UTIs may also be asymptomatic. It would be wise to require periodic cultures, particularly after one episode of documented UTI.

Primary Nocturnal Enuresis

"My child wets the bed" is usually not reported as early as the daytime wetting of the child with PDE, because the latter con-

dition is more socially distressing and may be accompanied by a symptomatic UTI. Many parents wait until at least school age (5 years) or later, when social demands, such as sleep-overs or sleep-away camp, necessitate attention to curing the bedwetting problem. Additional intrafamilial pressures, such as the competition imposed by dry siblings who may be younger than the bedwetter, also drive the need to seek treatment.

The following inclusive evidence confirms the diagnosis of PNE:

- Positive family history for PNE, and
- Persistent bedwetting at least two times per month for several months or 1 year and never dry for 3 months of consecutive nights

Exclusionary criteria for diagnosis include the following:

- Medical or pharmacologic causes
- Presence of psychological or traumatic causes or onset after a 3-month period of dryness (secondary nocturnal enuresis)
- Diagnosis of mental retardation (Spee-van der Wekke, Hirasing, Meulmeester, & Radder, 1998), autism (Taira,

---

DISPLAY 63-2 • Intake Questionnaire for Diurnal Enuresis

1. Has your child had damp underpants or daytime wetting twice a week or more in the past 3 months?
2. Does your child often seem to go to the bathroom after experiencing a strong urge?
3. Does your child seem to hold back urine and not go to the bathroom unless prompted?
4. Does your child often push and strain when trying to urinate?
5. Does your child show signs that he or she has to urinate, such as squirming, dancing, face turning red, squatting, or any movements or posturing?
6. Would your child rather play with friends than take time out for urinating, even when he or she experiences a strong urge to go?
7. Does your child experience pain, discomfort, or burning when urinating?
8. If you ask your child to urinate just after he or she finishes going, will he or she produce an unexpectedly large amount?
9. Do you have other children who are or were daytime wetters?

Urologic History

1. Has your child ever had a urinary tract or kidney infection?
2. Has your child been diagnosed or treated for any bladder, kidney, or urinary tract problem?

Takase, & Sasaki, 1998), or other arrested condition of mental development that has contributed to difficulty in acquiring learned toileting behavior

Functional Encopresis

Functional encopresis is a disturbance of bowel elimination involving the involuntary loss of formed or liquid stool after the age of culturally acceptable limits of toileting training. A pattern of sluggish bowel movement behavior is almost always associated with FEN. The American Psychiatric Association's *Diagnostic and Statistical Manual of Mental Disorders*, fourth edition (1994), describes this subtype as encopresis with constipation and overflow incontinence. A secondary subtype, described as encopresis without constipation and overflow incontinence, involves more volitional behavior that may accompany an additional psychiatric diagnosis of oppositional defiant disorder in young children and conduct disorder in older children. The possibility of a psychotic disorder may also be implicated, as might anxiety syndromes or symptoms associated with severe sexual abuse or sodomy.

The following inclusive evidence confirms the diagnosis of FEN:

• Stool soiling occurring at least once a month and persisting for several months in the absence of diarrhea secondary to a medical condition or inappropriate use of laxatives, stool softeners, or lubricants, such as mineral oil

Exclusionary criteria in the diagnosis of FEN include the following:

• Encopresis secondary to a medical cause, such as Hirschsprung's disease, anal or rectal malformation or

trauma, spinal cord anomalies (mylomeningocele) or spinal cord injury, cerebral palsy, mental retardation, or physical abuse
• Encopresis secondary to side effects of medication, such as antibiotics (Loening-Baucke, 1996)

Functional encopresis may also be considered as a diagnosis from either a primary or secondary perspective. Foreman and Thambirajah's (1996) examination of boys who failed to establish toilet training (primary FEN) provided evidence that these children had a greater likelihood to have developmental delays and PNE. Conversely, boys who displayed a breakdown in previously established toilet training (secondary FEN) were more likely to present with symptoms consistent with an excess of psychosocial stressors. They were also more likely to have the comorbid diagnosis of conduct disorder. The reader should refer to Chapters 21, 23, 26, 27, and 28 for a more in-depth examination of these issues.

DIAGNOSTIC STUDIES

Bladder instability has long been thought to play a central role in the etiology of chronic diurnal enuresis (Chandra, 1998). A mechanistic approach to understanding diurnal enuresis as bladder instability carries considerable intuitive validity because the child seems to be caught off-guard when unexpected bladder contractions occur. These contractions lead to otherwise unexplained symptoms of urgency, frequency, and compensatory squatting maneuvers.

The first empirical evidence for this hypothesis was documented by McGuire and Savastano (1984) and Firlit, Smey, and King (1977) in urodynamic studies that showed uninhibited contractions when filling the bladder using urethral catheters or suprapubic vesicle tubes. The limitations of these urodynamic studies include iatrogenic effects of the intrusive nature of the tests, which may have produced artifactual pathogenic findings. There is also the likelihood that patients selected for comprehensive urodynamic study are the more serious cases who have not responded to conservative treatment, so they may represent an occult neurogenic group. In addition, bladder suppression by pharmacogenic agents, such as oxybutynin often results in improvement of wetting symptoms. The effect is usually only temporary, affording symptom relief but not a final solution to the problem. Because the diurnally enuretic child displays behaviors similar to children with identifi-

---

DISPLAY 63–3 • Intake Questionnaire for Encopresis

1. Has your child soiled or had a bowel movement in his or her underwear one or more times in the past 3 months?
2. Does your child ever skip 1 or more days between bowel movements?
3. Does your child tend to have constipation or hard stools?
4. Do you give your child laxatives, stool softeners, mineral oil, or enemas to help with bowel movements?
5. Has your child been diagnosed or treated for any bowel or gastrointestinal problem?

able neurogenic lesions, this syndrome has been labeled the non-neurogenic neurogenic bladder and the pseudoneurogenic bladder (Hanna et al., 1981) or is referred to in the urologic literature as the Hinman syndrome (Hinman, 1986).

A contrasting and more recent hypothesis to explain diurnal wetting and comorbid chronic UTIs is the focus on the overtightening of the perineal floor as the primary mechanism. Children demonstrating bladder-sphincter dyssynergia while voiding are using the striated sphincter in an inefficient and maladaptive fashion, preventing the free flow of urine through an obstructed urethra. Collateral afferent pathways connect the external urinary sphincter with the bladder, which may result in further disruption of bladder functioning by inhibiting the full contractile reflex of the bladder. A partial bladder contraction will cause postvoid residual urine, a condition often seen in children with the Hinman syndrome. The sequela of postvoid residual urine often optimizes the conditions for bacterial growth, adding to the risk of bacterial infection introduced in chronically wet underpants. Biofeedback treatment raises cognitive awareness of the bladder-sphincter dyssynergia problem. Biofeedback has provided confirmatory evidence that the pelvic floor is a salient factor in cause and cure of the problem (Herndon, McKenna, Connery, & Ferrer, 1998).

Further helpful, relatively nonintrusive diagnostic measures for studying PDE or bladder-sphincter dyssynergia include measurement of the hydrodynamics of the urinary stream (flow study) and electromyographic recordings of the perennial floor during voiding with external skin electrodes. These measures are relative easy to perform when good rapport is established with the child. The parent may be present during these tests, which require the child to be alert and fully cooperative. The tests should follow any urine analyses or culture but may prove helpful even before deciding to perform an intravenous pyelogram (IVP), voiding cystourogram (VCU), or cystometrogram.

● **Clinical Pearl:** Most chronically wetting or soiling children will not require more intrusive methods for diagnosis, such as radiologic studies (IVP, VCU), magnetic resonance imaging, bladder cystoscopy, or rectal manometry (Kawauchi et al., 1996; Pippi Salle et al., 1998).

▲ **Clinical Warning:** Either bladder cystoscopy or rectal manometry or both should be considered only if there is reason to suspect uropathology, such as urethral stenosis, neurogenic bladder, ectopic ureter, or duplicated urethra (Hoebeke, Van Laecke, Raes, Vande Walle & Oosterlinck, 1997; Robson, 1997; Liu, Yeung, Lee, & Ku, 1996). Children with these conditions should be referred to pediatric specialists in urology, nephrology, neurology, or gastroenterology.

Although a child's developing self-esteem and social functioning may be at risk as the child grows older, PNE usually does not have comorbid primary psychiatric components (Friman & Jones, 1998). Psychiatric concerns most often arise with secondary forms of enuresis. A child who has experienced a period of complete and successful toilet training of at least 3 months and resumes wetting may be exhibiting a psychological sequella of faulty stress-coping mechanisms. These faulty mechanisms may follow post-traumatic stress disorder or sexual or physical abuse (Faust, Kenny, & Runyon, 1997). Referral to a mental health professional is warranted. Such referral is especially important if the urologic symptoms are comorbid with signs of behavioral distress, depressive ideation, or poor parenting conditions (Geroski & Rodgers, 1998).

MANAGEMENT

Efficacious treatment options of incontinence are varied. They may be classified as follows:

- Psychological—any methodology aimed at retraining bladder or bowel functioning, assisting the family with behavioral management, or counseling patient and family regarding prognostic and preventive measures and collaborative treatment with the assistance of a behavioral psychologist or urologic nurse specialist
- Medical—all prescriptive pharmacogenic approaches and special instructions concerning advisability of altering intake of fluids; restricting caffeine and carbonated sodas; use of laxatives, stool softeners, and lubricants, such as mineral oil

Conversely, symptoms or treatment response may point toward the need for referral, enlisting the assistance of a medical specialty when birth defects, neuropathology, or comorbid medical or psychiatric conditions are known or suspected.

● **Clinical Pearl:** Referral is an appropriate treatment option if symptoms do not abate after primary medical and prescriptive behavioral interventions have failed.

The child whose only symptom is nocturnal enuresis should be evaluated by both interview and prospective symptom observation. Parents should be asked to chart signs of diurnal urinary problems. These problems include diurnal frequency, retention, and wetting. Busy families often overlook minor occurrences of these symptoms. Children find ingenious ways of hiding or denying these annoying, socially intrusive manifestations. If any symptoms are present, the seven-void program is recommended. Stabilization of daytime voiding habits can contribute to better treatment response in a nocturnal program. Treatment gains and successful participation can lead to positive rewards, not the least of which is continence.

Corrective behavior modification interventions, such as establishing a controlled voiding program, should be suggested by the primary care provider if the initial clinical interview reveals the presence of minor encopretic events (soiling) or retentive bowel habits (skipping one or more days without a bowel movement). Return clinic visits should be scheduled over the full course of active behavioral contingency management. Visits may be spaced at increasingly longer intervals as progress is achieved in alleviating symptoms.

● **Clinical Pearl:** If the program becomes too time-consuming for the clinician to instruct and monitor, referral to a behavioral psychologist may be wise.

The child with diurnal enuresis is most likely to be seen first by the primary care provider. Referrals are often made because family distress is driven by social embarrassment and stigma, rather than because of presentation of "medical" symptoms or distress. The clinician should remember that many children with diurnal enuresis have UTIs. The clinician must also consider whether to treat for an acute event or, if the UTI is not the first one, whether to continue medication prophylactically. Long-term use of antibiotics must be weighed against the possibility of breakthrough infections. Such infections render one medication ineffective and potentially exhaust options for using other agents. Figure 63-

1 presents a diagnosis-to-treatment algorithm that the primary care provider may find helpful in managing or choosing to refer enuresis and encopresis in children.

● **Clinical Pearl:** If an active UTI is confirmed, the first priority is to treat the infection with antibiotic pharmacotherapy. Refer to Chapters 40 and 62 for other examples of appropriate pharmacotherapy, including age-appropriate choices.

Approaches to Bladder Retraining

Psychological approaches to retraining toileting behavior are not recommended during the course of an active infection. However, some form of training or efforts at normalizing voiding and defecating schedules should begin immediately after bacterial growth is arrested and symptoms have abated. A voiding schedule for children ages 5 to 12 years would require about seven voids per day. This frequency is slightly more than the normal rate of two to five voids per day. The increased programmed voiding program is aimed at optimizing bladder emptying by avoiding overdistention and reaching trigger capacity. This is because excessive urine storage may contribute to uninhibited contractions and wetting.

Biofeedback therapy is an appropriate option if there is clear documentation of either a bladder-sphincter dyssynergia or an inability to empty the bladder to completion. The method requires specialized equipment and trained biofeedback therapists who have experience working with children. Elimination of bladder-sphincter dyssynergia is accomplished, in part, by raising awareness of volitional control of the sphincter muscle while reducing overactivity of abdominal muscles. External electrodes are pasted on the perianal skin and abdominal areas, and the child is taught a computer assisted Kegel exercise. Emptying to completion may also be trained by combining electromyographic feedback with pre-and post-voiding bladder sonography and uroflowmetry (Pfister, et al., 1999; Porena, Costantini, Rociola, & Mearini, 2000).

Controlled (Timed) Voiding Regimen

Before prescribing the controlled voiding regimen, the child and family should be fully educated and counseled regarding its rationale. Parents should prompt, not force or coerce, their child into going to the toilet at the programmed times when there may be no internal sensation of fullness or perception of an uninhibited bladder contraction. It is a good idea to construct the schedule with a parent handout showing daily routine home and school activities to which a toileting reminder can be associated. Figure 63-2 presents a sample weekly chart for a seven void per day program.

Integrating toileting reminders into a child's schedule avoids the problem of "timed voiding." Requiring voids by watching the clock may exceed the young child's ability to

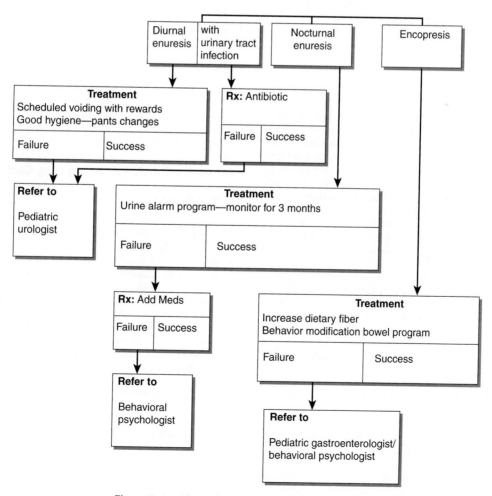

Figure 63–1 ■ Diagnostic, treatment, and referral flow chart.

	M	Tu	W	Th	F	Sat	Sun
Date:							
Getting up							
*Morning break							
*After lunch							
*Afternoon recess							
Getting home							
After supper							
Before bed							

*Usually occurs at school.

Codes:

✔	Void attempts
w	Wets underpants
s	Soils underpants
c	Changes underpants
bm	Has bowel movement

Figure 63–2 ■ Weekly chart for seven-void program.

tell time. Timed voiding is also problematic because it adds time-focused pressure and stress—difficult for anyone, regardless of age. At least three voids are required during school hours. Parents may need to enlist the confidential cooperation of a home-room teacher or school nurse to provide reminders. A system of positive reinforcement for each toileting attempt can be planned with the use of sticker charts for children between 4 and 8 years of age. Older children will require some form of an allowance system (usually monetary). Parents can be told that the rewards are contingent on positive behavior at maintaining the voiding program, not on having dry pants. Dryness itself is only an outcome of successful voiding behavior.

● **Clinical Pearl:** The use of a daily reward system removes the nagging and punitive approaches parents might otherwise use. The contingency reward system gives the child choices in determining the rate and amount of acquiring rewards. Monetary allowances are justified because the child is being asked to perform an additional chore. The parent should not assume that self-care and complex understanding of medical problems will motivate the young child to perform. The child is not to be restricted for going to the toilet at any other time, but extra trips will not earn extra contingent rewards.

▲ **Clinical Warning:** The program should be followed for at least 3 months. Symptoms such as UTIs and wetting need to be monitored daily by the parent's charting. If the family is not able to participate in this self-care regimen or if multiple psychological or medical issues coexist, referral to a pediatric psychologist or psychiatrist may be necessary to help the child

to achieve continence. Conversely, if the family is consistently involved and effective at participating in this regimen but there is no improvement in symptoms after 3 months, further urologic workup may be wise. The provider should refer the child to a pediatric urologist.

Other Methods for Achieving Continence

Urine Alarms

The use of a urine sensor and alarm apparatus for treating PNE has been around for a considerable time (Mowrer & Mowrer, 1938). Use of this method has proven effective in as many as 90% of families who choose to participate in a full course of treatment. The method is labor intensive, disruptive of parent and child sleep patterns, and takes considerable time and patience. Many parents initiate this program on their own but fail because of premature termination of training. The labor- and time-intensive factors may also contribute to the tendency for many providers to delay treatment while awaiting spontaneous remission or to prescribe medication as a primary intervention. The original apparatus (bell and pad) consists of two electrically conductive pads placed between and covered by bed sheets. When the child wets the bed, the auditory alarm connected to the now-completed circuit (urine between the pads) wakes the child and alerts the parent. The youngster is then led from bed to the toilet, where the void is completed.

▲ **Clinical Warnings:**
Although effective, use of the older models of the bell and pad apparatus had serious flaws:

- Too much effort and time to remake the bed at night
- A large urine output required before the system alerts the child and parent
- Of greatest concern, a safety problem related to the strength of the electrical current required to power the alarm. Without expensive optical isolation of the current, the child could receive a shock or develop skin excoriations secondary to low-level electrical leakage.

For these reasons, the provider should screen for and discourage use of older bell-and-pad apparatuses.

State-of-the-art forms of the apparatus now are battery-driven. The alarm unit attaches to the pajama or straps to the wrist. A wire extends from the alarm unit to metal clips which pin to the inside and outside of the underpants. With only a few milliliters of urine in the underpants, the alarm is triggered, sounding like a phone pager. This device poses no electrical danger to the child. The alarm must be unpinned to stop activation of the noise.

Parents must be prepared to use the microalarm system for 2 to 3 months before signs of improvement can be measured or complete dryness attained. Prepubescent children will almost certainly require assistance of one parent during the night; therefore, the parents must be prepared for disturbances in their own sleep patterns. The scientific explanation for the alarm system's effectiveness has not been firmly established. The provider can tell parents only that the alarm provides an arousal cue, which prevents the child from finishing the void in bed. A reasonable but overly simplified explanation is based on an avoidance paradigm of autonomic learning, in which the CNS is provoked into sending inhibitory messages to the bladder to avoid repeated sleep disturbances.

Improvement in self-esteem is often an accompanying outcome when a child and family are successful in achieving continence with the alarm (Schulpen, 1997; Longstaffe, Moffatt, & Whalen, 2000). This active treatment plan involves the child and family in comanagement of PNE. The plan most likely contributes to a good experience and acts as a positive contrast to spontaneous cures or pharmacologic interventions that only require taking a prescribed medication. An enuretic alarm costs the same as a 2-week supply of DDAVP (Schmitt, 1997).

Dry Bed Training

Dry bed training (Azrin, Sneed, & Fox, 1974) combines alarm training, reinforcement techniques, and urine retention control. Unfortunately, the method has proven to be only slightly better than an alarm-alone system (Hirasing, Bolk-Bennink, & Reus, 1996). A precaution is necessary in using a component described as behavioral urine retention training. Because daytime frequency has not been a consistent finding in all children with PNE, the practice of daytime urinary retention ("bladder stretching") may at best add unnecessary stress or at worst may exacerbate an already present problem of high-pressure bladder conditions, bladder trabeculation, or ureteral reflux. Reflux is difficult to diagnosis without imaging techniques. Reflux raises the risk of hydronephrosis or kidney infection if bacterial growth is present in the bladder.

Medication

Medication is used as a first-line treatment by as many as 52% of physicians (Vogel, Young, & Primack, 1996). This practice belies the evidence that sustained outcome after stopping medication is dismal and that side effects are troublesome. Ever since Maclean (1960) found that imipramine, a drug developed to treat depressive illness, had antidiuretic properties in the elderly, its use has been widely applied to treat children with PNE. Imipramine is an anticholinergic agent and a noradrenergic stimulant. It was thought to effect bladder contractility by increasing the threshold capacity. More recently, imipramine has been linked to changing arousal thresholds. Efficacy rates of 60% response while on the drug and 70% recurrence when off the drug are disappointing for a definitive first-line treatment.

▲ **Clinical Warning:** The temporary efficacy of imipramine treatment of PNE must be weighed against the risk of accidental, serious, dose-related cardiac and CNS side effects in children (Rohner, 1975).

Oxybutynin provides an anticholinergic action on the detrusor muscle, which may temporarily result in a reduction of bladder spasms and a secondary gain in bladder capacity in the child with diurnal enuresis with urinary frequency problems. Oxybutynin has not proven efficacious in any form of PNE.

▲ **Clinical Warning:** Therapeutic gains in reducing daytime wetting and frequency are often only temporary. The necessity of increasing dosage levels only adds the risk of side effects, including headache, akathesia, facial flushing, and hypotension. These problems must be weighed against interfering with progress in implementing behavior modification programs for bladder retraining.

More recently, work in Scandinavia has focused on the hormonal pathways controlling the kidney production of urine. Norgaard and colleagues (1985) were among the first researchers to propose that treatment-resistant children showed a hormonal deficiency. Their research focused on a deficiency in the production of plasma arginine vasopressin. This antidiuretic hormone is secreted by normal children and results in reducing urine output to the bladder as the sleep cycle progresses into the night. Introduction of an artificial form of the antidiuretic hormone (DDAVP) showed great promise in abating symptoms during active drug treatment. However, the problem with DDAVP is recurrence of symptoms when the drug is discontinued. Medication can provide an immediate form of relief of bedwetting, but it is not a permanent solution for PNE. Some parents may want to consider medication for temporary solutions like vacations, sleep-overs, or summer camp. As with all medications, the risk of side effects must be considered carefully by parents.

▲ **Clinical Warnings:**

- Although DDAVP is safer than imipramine, there have been increasing numbers of reports of seizure activity, hyponatremia, and cerebral convulsion with DDAVP usage (Schwab, Wenzel, & Ruder, 1996; Robson, Norgaard, & Leung, 1996; Bernstein & Willingford, 1997; Donoghue, Latimer, Pillsbury, & Hertzog, 1998). DDAVP must therefore take its place as a secondary intervention, falling behind the alarm program in outcome and safety. In all likelihood, some children may have faulty antidiuretic hormone production, but they should be assessed for this failure before medication is prescribed. The possibility of using DDAVP in tandem with an alarm training system is also to be considered in

children who are resistant to treatment with alarm training alone.
- Parents are particularly in need of fully informed consent regarding the risk-benefit ratio of medication use. The possible psychological harm resulting from yet another short-term solution or another failure at attaining self-controlled dryness cannot be overestimated.

Incontinence Comorbidity

The problem of FEN may coexist with enuresis (O'Regan, Yzback, Hamberger, & Schick, 1986) or may occur alone. In either case, primary treatment should involve methods of behavior modification. Behavior modification can help in establishing a differential diagnosis of a nonorganic functional disorder if the child responds well to the intervention. Behavior modification can also provide an active, effective treatment for maladaptive bowel habits in the same way that applications to bladder training are efficacious.

When a diagnosis of encopresis with overflow fecal incontinence is established with children approaching school age (chronologic age of at least 4 years), the problem of relieving fecal impaction is the first order of business. Some gastrointestinal specialists advise mild laxatives, such as senna (Senokot), or pediatric enemas, such as children's Fleet, to remove the large collection of fecal material in the lower bowel.

▲ Clinical Warning: A child who has a severe impaction may require an emergency visit or office procedure performed by a gastroenterologist. Whatever method of removal of fecal impaction is chosen, the provider must bear in mind that this is often only a temporary acute care measure. Behavioral treatment plans should be considered for the follow-up need of establishing regular daily bowel movements in the toilet.

A slower but equally effective approach to treating mild impaction may be taken by immediately initiating dietary changes assisted by a behavior modification program of bowel movement attempts. This program requires at least two bowel movement attempts daily, which are monitored and reinforced by parents (Reimeres, 1996). Stark et al. (1997) found that 59 children with retentive encopresis showed soiling decreases of 85% with a combined dietary and behavioral management program. The dietary program aims to increase the quantity of fiber in the child's diet by adding foods including fruits, fresh vegetables, and salads. A small daily quantity (1 teaspoon) of unprocessed wheat or oat bran is also very effective with younger children. It can be made palatable by mixing with applesauce or a favorite cereal. It can also be used as a cooking additive with muffins, breads, and soups.

The provider should reinforce the importance of avoiding repeated use of laxatives. Laxatives pose a risk of dependency and preclude self-controlled learning of normal full bowel sensations and volitional defecating. If lubricants such as mineral oil are used on a routine basis, they are more likely to exacerbate the problem because of increased leakage around entrapped stool formations.

Rectal biofeedback therapy has been reported as unsuccessful in controlled studies in treating anismus as defined by dyssynergic external anal sphincter contraction during attempted defecation (Nolan, Catto-Smith, Coffey, & Wells, 1998; Loening-Baucke, 1996; van der Plas, Benninga, Redekop, Taminiau, & Buller, 1996). Poor results with this method may be attributed to neglect of dietary adjustment and generalization of rectal sphincter training to the home

setting. On the other hand, successful biofeedback interventions have been reported in one case of a postsurgically corrected imperforate anus (Griffiths & Livingstone, 1998).

What to Tell Parents

Setting up a behavioral program is most effective when all adult members who share parenting functions attend at least one meeting, usually the first treatment planning visit. Parents who understand and accept the treatment rationale and who are willing to provide closely monitored toileting prompts, instructions, and rewards for appropriate behavior will have the most efficacious and immediate results. The primary care provider may need to refer inaccessible or discordant families to a mental health or family therapy specialist.

▲ Clinical Warning: A small cottage industry has been active on a national basis, offering behavioral programs for treatment of PNE. These companies are to be viewed critically in relation to using nonprofessionally licensed sales personnel who carry out treatment programs without sufficient medical or psychological consultation. Some companies offer the obsolete bell and pad apparatus at extraordinary rental prices exceeding $1000, in contrast to the number of small battery-operated alarms available for under $100 from mail-order companies.

COMMUNITY RESOURCES

National Kidney Foundation (NKF)
30 East 33rd Street, Suite 1100
New York, NY 10016
Telephone: For PNE: (888) WAKEDRY
For other problems: (800) 622-9010 or (212) 889-2210
Fax: (212) 889-9261
Internet address: *http://www.kidney.org*

A brochure is available, as well as referral to providers who have indicated a willingness to treat bedwetting. This foundation provides information for parents and professionals regarding kidney and urinary tract diseases and referral services to pediatric nephrologists who specialize in kidney and bladder dysfunction.

American Urological Association
1120 North Charles Street
Baltimore, MD 21201
Telephone: (410) 727-1100
Fax: (410) 223-4370
Internet address: *http://www.auanet.org*

This is an important resource for parents and primary care providers in locating a qualified pediatric urologist.

American Psychiatric Association
1400 K Street, N.W.
Washington, DC 20005
Telephone: (202) 682-6000
Fax: (202) 682-6850
Internet address: *http://www.psych.org*

This group is helpful for parents or referring primary care providers in locating qualified child or adolescent psychiatrists if coexisting mental health problems, including ADHD, post-traumatic stress disorder, child abuse, or neglect, are known or suspected. Psychotropic medication prescribed by a child psychiatrist may be very helpful in assisting behavioral enuresis and encopresis treatment programs.

American Psychological Association
750 First Street, N.E.
Washington, DC 20002
Telephone: (202) 336-5500
Internet address: *http://www.apa.org*

This association helps parents and referring primary care providers to locate qualified child or adolescent behavioral or family psychologists to provide behavioral bladder or bowel retraining or to provide treatment of coexisting mental health problems (such as problems with compliance, self-esteem, and intellectual and emotional disturbances), which often accompany secondary enuresis and encopresis.

REFERENCES

American Psychiatric Association. (1994). *Diagnostic and statistical manual of mental disorders* (4th ed.). Washington, DC: Author.

Arnell, H., Hjalmas, K., Jagervall, M., Lackgren, G., Stenberg, A., Bengtsson, B., et al. (1997). The genetics of primary nocturnal enuresis: Inheritance and suggestion of a second major gene on chromosome 12q. *Journal of Medical Genetics, 34,* 360–365.

Azrin, N. H., Sneed, T. J., & Fox, R. M. (1974). Dry-bed training: Rapid elimination of childhood enuresis. *Behavior Research and Therapy, 12,* 147–156.

Bernstein, S. A., & Williford, S. L. (1997). Intranasal desmopressin-associated hyponatremia: A case report and literature review. *Journal of Family Practice, 44,* 203–208.

Bower, W. F., Moore, K. H., Shepherd, R. B., & Adams, R. D. (1996). The epidemiology of childhood enuresis in Australia. *British Journal of Urology, 78,* 602–606.

Byrd, R. S., Weitzman, M., Lanphear, N. E., & Auinger, P. (1996). Bed-wetting in US children: Epidemiology and related behavior problems. *Pediatrics, 98*(3 Pt 1), 414–419.

Chandra, M. (1998) Nocturnal enuresis in children. *Current Opinion in Pediatrics, 10,* 167–173.

Chao, S. M., Yap, H. K. Tan, A., Ong, E. K., Murugasu, B., Low, E. H., et al. (1997). Primary monsymptomatic nocturnal enuresis in Singapore-parental perspectives in an Asian Community. *Annals of the Academy of Medicine, Singapore, 26,* 179–183.

Chiozza, M. L., Bernardinelli, L., Caione, P., Del Gado, R., Ferrara, P., Giorgi, P. L., et al. (1998). An Italian epidemiological multicentre study of nocturnal enuresis. *British Journal of Urology, 81*(Suppl. 3), 86–898.

Djurhuus, J. C., & Rittig, S. (1998). Current trends, diagnosis, and treatment of enuresis. *European Urology, 33*(Suppl. 3), 30–33.

Donoghue, M. B., Latimer, M. E., Pillsbury, H. L., & Hertzog, J. H. (1998). Hyponatremic seizure in a child using desmopressin for nocturnal Enuresis. *Archives of Pediatric and Adolescent Medicine, 152,* 290–292.

Eiberg, H. (1998). Total genome scan analysis in a single extended family for primary nocturnal enuresis: evidence for a new locus (ENUR3) for primary nocturnal enuresis on chromosome 22q11. *European Urology, 33*(Suppl. 3), 34–36.

Faust, J., Kenny, M. C., & Runyon, M. K. (1997) Differences in family functioning of sexually abused vs. nonabused enuretics. *Journal of Family Violence, 12,* 405–416.

Firlit, C. F., Smey, P., & King, L. R. (1977). Micturition urodynamic flow studies in children. *Transactions of the American Association of Genio-Urinary Surgeons, 69,* 8–11.

Foreman, D. M., & Thambirajah, M. S. (1996). Conduct disorder, enuresis and specific developmental delays in two types of encopresis: A case-note study of 63 boys. *European Child and Adolescent Psychiatry, 5,* 33–37.

Friman, P. C., & Jones, K. M. (1998). Elimination disorders in children. In T. S. Watson, F. M. Gresham, et al. (Eds.), *Handbook of child behavior therapy: Issues in clinical child psychology* (pp. 239–260). New York: Plenum Press.

Geroski, A. M., & Rodgers, K. A. (1998). Collaborative assessment and treatment of children with enuresis and encopresis. *Professional School Counseling, 2,* 128–134.

Griffiths, P., & Livingstone, H. (1998). Treatment of encopresis by parent-mediated biofeedback in a child with corrected imperforate anus. *Behavioural and Cognitive Psychotherapy, 26,* 143–152.

Hanna, M. K., Di Scipio, W., Suh, K. K., Kogan, S. J., Levitt, S. B., & Donner, K. (1981). Urodynamics in children. Part II. The pseudoneurogenic bladder. *Journal of Urology, 125,* 534–537.

Herndon, A., McKenna, P. H., Connery, S. C., & Ferrer, F. A. (1998). *Pelvic floor Muscle retraining for pediatric voiding dysfunction using interactive computer games.* Paper presented at the annual meeting of the American Urological Association.

Hinman, F. (1986). Non-neurogenic bladder (the Hinman syndrome) fifteen years later. *Journal of Urology, 136,* 769.

Hirasing, R. A., Bolk-Bennink, L., & Reus, H. (1996). Dry bed training by parents: results of a group instruction program. *Journal of Urology, 156,* 2044–2046.

Hjalmas, K. (1997). Pathophysiology and impact of nocturnal enuresis. *Acta Paediatrica, 86,* 919–922.

Hoebeke, P. B., Van Laecke, E., Raes, A., Vande Walle J., & Oosterlinck, W. (1997). Membrano-bulbo-urethral junction stenosis. Posterior urethra obstruction due to extreme caliber disproportion in the male urethra. *European Urology, 32,* 480–484.

Hublin, C., Kaprio, J., Partinen, M., & Koskenvuo, M. (1998). Nocturnal enuresis in a nationwide twin cohort. *Sleep, 21,* 579–585.

Imada, N., Kawauchi, A., Tanaka, Y., Yamao, Y., Watanabe, H., & Takeuchi, Y. (1998). Classification based on overnight simultaneous monitoring by electroencephalography and cystometry. *European Urology, 33*(Suppl. 3), 45–48.

Jenkins, P. H, Lambert, M. J, Nielsen, S. L., McPherson, D. L., et al. (1996). Nocturnal task responsiveness of primary nocturnal enuretic boys: A behavioral approach to enuresis. *Children's Health Care, 25,* 143–156.

Kalo, B. B., & Bella, H. (1996). Enuresis: Prevalence and associated factors among primary school children in Saudi Arabia. *Acta Paediatrica, 85,* 1217–1222.

Kawauchi, A., Kitamori, T., Imada, N., Tanaka, Y., & Watanabe, H. (1996). Urological abnormalities in 1,328 patients with nocturnal enuresis. *European Urology, 29,* 231–234.

Kawauchi, A., Imada, N., Tanaka, Y., Yamao, Y., & Watanabe, H. (1998a). Effects of systematic treatment based on overnight simultaneous monitoring of electroencephalography and cystometry. *European Urology, 33*(Suppl. 3), 58–61.

Kawauchi, A., Imada, N., Tanaka, Y., Minami M., Watanabe, H., & Shirakawa, S. (1998b). Changes in the structure of sleep spindles and delta waves on electroencephalography in patients with nocturnal enuresis. *British Journal of Urology, 81*(Suppl. 3), 72–75.

Lettgen, B. (1997). Differential diagnoses for nocturnal enuresis. *Scandinavian Journal of Urology and Nephrology, 183*(Suppl.), 48–49.

Liu, K. K., Yeung, C. K., Lee, K. H., & Ku, K. W. (1996). Ectopic ureter as a cause of wetting: The role of laparoscopy in its management. *Australian and New Zealand Journal of Surgery, 66,* 325–326.

Loening-Baucke, V. (1997). Urinary incontinence and urinary tract infection and their resolution with treatment of chronic constipation of childhood. *Pediatrics, 100,* 228–232.

Loening-Baucke, V. (1996). Balloon defecation as a predictor of outcome in children with functional constipation and encopresis. *Journal of Pediatrics, 128,* 336–340.

Longstaffe, S., Moffatt, M.E., & Whalen, J. (2000) Behavioral and self-concept changes after six months of enuresis treatment: A randomized, controlled trial. *Pediatrics, 105,* 935-940.

Maclean, R. E. G. (1960). Imipramine hydrochloride (Tofranil) and enuresis. *American Journal of Psychiatry, 117,* 551.

McGuire, E. J., & Savastano, J. A. (1984). Urodynamic studies in enuresis and the nonneurogenic neurogenic bladder. *Journal of Urology, 132,* 299–302.

Medel, R., Ruarte, A. C., Castera, R., & Podesta, M. L. (1998). Primary enuresis: A urodynamic evaluation. *British Journal of Urology, 81*(Suppl 3), 50–52.

Mowrer, O. H., & Mowrer, W. M. (1938). Enuresis-A method for its study and treatment. *American Journal of Orthopsychiatry, 8,* 436–459.

National Kidney Foundation. (1999). Web site *www.kidney.org*, Patient link "Bedwetting."

Nolan, T., Catto-Smith, T., Coffey, C., & Wells, J. (1998). Randomised controlled trial of biofeedback training in persistent encopresis with anismus. *Archives of Disease in Childhood, 79,* 131–135.

Neveus, T., Lackgren, G., Tuvemo, T., & Stenberg, A. (1998). Osmoregulation and desmopressin pharmacokinetics in enuretic children. *Pediatrics, 103,* 65–70.

Norgaard, J. P., Djurhuus, J. C., Watanabe, H., Stenberg, A., & Lettgen, B. (1997). Experience and current status of research into the pathophysiology of nocturnal enuresis. *British Journal of Urology, 79,* 825–835.

Norgaard, J. P., Hansen, J. H., Nielsen, J. B., Rittig, S., & Djurhuus, J. C. (1989). Nocturnal studies in enuretics. A polygraphic study of sleep EEG and bladder activity. *Scandinavian Journal of Urology and Nephrology, 125*(Suppl.), 73–78.

Norgaard, J. P., Pedersen, E. B., & Djurhuus, J. C. (1985). Diurnal anti-diuretic-hormone levels in enuretics. *Journal of Urology, 134,* 1029–1031.

O'Regan, S., Yazbeck, S., Hamberger, B., & Schick, E. (1986). Constipation a commonly unrecognized cause of enuresis. *American Journal of Diseases of Children, 140,* 260–261.

Petrican, P., & Sawan, M. A. (1998). Design of a miniaturized ultrasonic bladder volume monitor and subsequent preliminary evaluation on 41 enuretic patients. *IEEE Transactions on Rehabilitation Engineering, 6,* 66–74.

Pfister, C., Dacher, J.N., Gaucher, S., Liard-Zmuda, A., Grise, P., & Mitrofanoff, P. (1999) The usefullness of minimal urodynamic evaluation and pelvic floor biofeedback in children with chronic voiding dysfunction. *BJU International, 84,* 1054-1057.

Pippi Salle, J. L., Capolicchio, G., Houle, A. M., Vernet, O., Jednak, R., O'Gorman, et al. (1998). Magnetic resonance imaging in children with voiding dysfunction: Is it indicated? *Journal of Urology, 160*(3 Pt 2), 1080–1083.

Porena, M., Costantini, E., Rociola, W., & Mearini, E. (2000) Biofeedback successfully cures detrustor-sphincter dyssynergia in pediatric patients. *The Journal of Urology, 163,* 1927-1931.

Popper, C. W., & Steingard, R. J. (1996). Disorders usually first diagnosed in infancy, childhood, or adolescence. In R. E. Hales, S. C. Yudofsky, et al. (Eds.), *The American psychiatric press synopsis of psychiatry* (pp. 681–774). Washington, DC: American Psychiatric Press.

Rasmussen, P. V., Kirk, J., Borup, K., Norgaard, J. P., & Djurhuus, J. C. (1996). Enuresis nocturna can be provoked in normal healthy children by increasing the nocturnal urine output. *Scandinavian Journal of Urology and Nephrology, 30,* 57–61.

Reimeres, T. M. (1996). A biobehavioral approach toward managing encopresis. *Behavior Modification, 20,* 469–479.

Robson, W. L. (1997). Diurnal enuresis. *Pediatrics in Review, 18,* 407–412.

Robson, W. L., Jackson, H. P., Blackhurst, D., & Leung, A. K. (1997). Enuresis in children with attention-deficit hyperactivity disorder. *Southern Medical Journal, 90,* 503–505.

Robson, W. L., Norgaard, J. P., & Leung, A. K. (1996). Hyponatremia in patients with nocturnal enuresis treated with DDAVP. *European Journal of Pediatrics, 155,* 959–962.

Rohner, T. J. (1975) Imipramine toxicity. *Journal of Urology, 114,* 402–403.

Schmitt, B. D. (1997). Nocturnal enuresis. *Pediatrics in Review, 18,* 183–190.

Schulpen, T. W. (1997). The burden of nocturnal enuresis. *Acta Paediatrica, 86,* 981–984.

Schwab, M., Wenzel, D., & Ruder, H. (1996). Hyponatraemia and cerebral convulsion due to short-term DDAVP therapy for control of enuresis nocturna. *European Journal of Pediatrics, 155,* 46–48.

Sentovich, S. M., Kaufman, S. S., Cali, R. L., Falk, P. M., Blatchford, G. J., Antonson, D. L., et al. (1998). Pudendal nerve function in normal and encopretic children. *Journal of Pediatric Gastroenterology and Nutrition, 26,* 70–72.

Serel, T. A., Akhan, G., Koyuncuoglu, H. R., Ozturk, A., Dogruer, K., Unal, S., et al. (1997). Epidemiology of enuresis in Turkish children. *Scandinavian Journal of Urology and Nephrology, 31,* 537–539.

Shima, H., Mori, Y., Nojima, M., Miyamoto, I., Chokyu, H., & Ikoma, F. (1998). Lower urinary tract problems in patients with enuresis. *European Urology, 33*(Suppl. 3), 37–40.

Spee-van der Wekke, J., Hirasing, R. A., Meulmeester, J. F., & Radder, J. J. (1998). Childhood nocturnal enuresis in The Netherlands. *Urology, 51,* 1022–1026.

Stark, L. J., Opipari, L. C., Donaldson, D. L., Danovsky, M. B., Rasile, D. A., & DelSanto, A. F. (1997). Evaluation of a standard protocol for retentive encopresis: A replication. *Journal of Pediatric Psychology, 22,* 619–633.

Swithinbank, L. V., Brookes, S. T., Shepherd, A. M., & Abrams, P. (1998). The natural history of urinary symptoms during adolescence. *British Journal of Urology, 81*(Suppl. 3), 90–93.

Taira, M., Takase, M., & Sasaki, H. (1998). Sleep disorder in children with autism. *Psychiatry and Clinical Neurosciences, 52,* 182–183.

Trombetta, C., Savoca, G., Siracusano, S., & Liguori, G. (1997). Prevalence and incidence of enuresis before puberty. *Archivos Espanoles de Urologia, 50,* 1140–1145.

van der Plas, R. N., Benninga, M. A., Redekop, W. K., Taminiau, J. A., & Buller, H. A. (1997). How accurate is the recall of bowel habits in children with defaecation disorders? *European Journal of Pediatrics, 156,* 178–181.

van der Plas, R. N., Benninga, M. A., Redekop, W. K., Taminiau, J. A., & Buller, H. A. (1996). Randomised trial of biofeedback training for encopresis. *Archives of Disease in Childhood, 75,* 367–374.

Vogel, W., Young, M., & Primack, W. (1996). A survey of physician use of treatment methods for functional enuresis. *Journal of Developmental and Behavioral Pediatrics, 17,* 90–93.

von Gontard, A., Eiberg, H., Hollmann, E., Rittig, S. & Lehmkuhl, G. (1997). Genetic heterogeneity in nocturnal enuresis. *American Journal of Psychiatry, 154,* 885.

von Gontard A., Hollmann E., Eiberg, H., Benden B., Rittig, S., & Lehmkuhl, G. (1997). Clinical enuresis phenotypes in familial nocturnal enuresis. *Scandinavian Journal of Urology and Nephrology, 183*(Suppl), 11–16.

von Gontard, A. (1998). Annotation: Day and night wetting in children: A paediatric and child psychiatric perspective. *Journal of Child Psychology and Psychiatry and Allied Disciplines, 39,* 439–451.

von Gontard, A., Eiberg, H., Hollmann, E., Rittig, S., & Lehmkuhl, G. (1998). Molecular genetics of nocturnal enuresis: Clinical and genetic heterogeneity. *Acta Paediatrica, 87,* 487–488.

Watanabe, H. (1998). Nocturnal enuresis. *European Urology, 33*(Suppl. 3), 2–11.

Watanabe, H., Imada, N., Kawauchi, A., Koyama, Y., & Shirakawa, S. (1997). Physiological background of enuresis type I: A preliminary report. *Scandinavian Journal of Urology and Nephrology, 183*(Suppl.), 9–10.

Wolfish, N. M., Pivik, R. T., & Busby, K. A. (1997) Elevated sleep arousal thresholds in enuretic boys: Clinical implications. *Acta Paediatrica, 86,* 381–384.

Yakinci, C., Mungen, B., Durmaz, Y., Balbay, D., & Karabiber, H. (1997). Autonomic nervous system functions in children with nocturnal enuresis. *Brain and Development, 19,* 485–487.

Yeung, C. K. (1997). Nocturnal enuresis in Hong Kong: Different Chienes phenotypes. *Scandinavian Journal of Urology and Nephrology, 183*(Suppl), 17–21.

Neoplasms

• SOMASUNDARAM JAYABOSE, MD

INTRODUCTION

This chapter provides a framework for understanding and interpreting the symptoms and signs in cancer diagnosis. Conditions to be explored include extremity and joint pains, lymphadenopathy, abdominal masses, mediastinal masses, headache and neurologic symptoms, spinal cord compression, and hematologic abnormalities.

Other issues surrounding comanagement of the child with cancer are discussed, including chemotherapy, management of neutropenia, and psychosocial issues surrounding diagnosis and treatment. The remainder of the chapter discusses the most common of the childhood cancers, including the leukemias, brain tumors, neuroblastoma, Wilms' tumor, rhabdomyosarcoma, and the lymphomas.

ANATOMY, PHYSIOLOGY, AND PATHOLOGY

Malignancies in children cause symptoms through various mechanisms. Solid tumors, such as mediastinal tumors and brain tumors, cause symptoms by pressing on adjacent vital structures. Abdominal tumors, such as Wilms' tumor, can remain silent until detected incidentally by a parent or by a care provider. Neuroblastoma frequently manifests with bone pain from disseminated bone metastases. It may also present with ataxia due to paraneoplastic process. Rarely, some cancers, such as rhabdomyosarcoma, may present acutely with metabolic disturbances, such as hypercalcemia.

EPIDEMIOLOGY

Childhood cancer is a rare disease, with only 1% to 2% of all human cancers occurring in children. Its annual incidence is 130 cases per 1 million children (younger than 15 years). In order of frequency, the most common of the childhood cancers include the leukemias, brain tumors, neuroblastoma, Wilms' tumor, rhabdomyosarcoma, and the lymphomas (National Cancer Institute [NCI], 2000). The low incidence and the nonspecific nature of the presenting symptoms make early diagnosis of childhood cancer a challenge to the primary care provider. However, including the neoplastic process in the differential diagnosis of persistent, recurrent, or unexplained symptoms may prevent undue delay in diagnosis.

DIAGNOSTIC CRITERIA AND DIAGNOSTIC STUDIES

Extremity and Joint Pains

Malignant diseases, such as leukemia, lymphoma, neuroblastoma, Ewing's sarcoma, and bone tumors, frequently present as bone or joint pains. Such patients may be mistakenly diagnosed as having rheumatoid arthritis, lupus, Lyme disease, or other rhuematic diseases. Clinical features that are common to both rheumatic and malignant diseases and those that suggest the presence of a malignant disorder are listed in Display 64-1.

▲ **Clinical Warning:** Even in the absence of hematologic abnormalities, children with unexplained (by a previous workup) significant (defined as persistent pain that causes a limp or interrupts normal activity) bone and joint pains or musculoskeletal pains must have a bone marrow aspirate study to rule out leukemia or other malignant disorders.

Lymphadenopathy

Most cases of bacterial lymphadenitis in children respond to oral antibiotics, and viral lymphadenitis usually subsides in 2 to 3 weeks. Thus, an enlarged lymph node measuring greater than 1 cm and persisting and enlarging for more than 2 to 3 weeks requires further evaluation to determine the etiology. A "shotty" lymph node that diminishes in size between intercurrent illnesses probably does not qualify for workup. Initial screening studies should include the following:

- Complete blood count (CBC)
- Erythrocyte sedimentation rate (ESR)
- Titers for Epstein-Barr virus (EBV), cytomegalovirus (CMV), *Bartonella*, and *Toxoplasma*
- Intermediate-strength purified protein derivative
- Plain chest film

Figure 64-1 outlines a plan for investigation of lymphadenopathy. A markedly elevated ESR is usually suggestive of a systemic illness, probably other than a viral infection.

▲ **Clinical Warning:** Presence of neutropenia, thrombocytopenia, mediastinal mass, or hilar lymphadenopathy on plain chest film is very suggestive of malignancy, and such a patient should be further evaluated by a bone marrow aspirate study to rule out leukemia. If the bone marrow aspirate study is negative, a biopsy of the lymph node will be necessary for a definitive diagnosis.

DISPLAY 64–1 • Clinical and Laboratory Features of Rheumatologic and Malignant Conditions

Features Common to Both Rheumatologic and Malignant Diseases
- Musculoskeletal pain
- Fever
- Fatigue
- Weight loss
- Heptomegaly
- Arthritis

Features That Suggest a Malignant Process
- Nonarticular bone pain
- Back pain as a presenting feature
- Bone tenderness
- Night sweats
- Bruising
- Pruritus
- Abnormal neurologic signs
- Anemia, neutropenia, thrombocytopenia
- Elevated serum lactate dehydrogenase
- Abnormal findings on plain skeletal radiograph, bone scan, or abdominal sonogram

Adapted with permission from Cabral, D. A., & Tucker, L. B. (1999). Malignancies in children who initially present with rheumatic complaints. *Journal of Pediatrics*, 134(1), 53–57.

Abdominal and Pelvic Masses

In neonates, more than 85% of abdominal masses are benign. Renal abnormalities, mainly hydronephrosis and cystic dysplasia of kidneys, account for more than 50% of all abdominal masses. In infants and children, fewer than half of all abdominal masses are malignant, and most of the solid renal tumors are Wilms' tumors. Neuroblastomas account for most of the nonrenal solid tumors in the abdomen. Other abdominal tumors include lymphomas and rhabdomyosarcomas. Common pelvic tumors include rhabdomyosarcomas and ovarian tumors. Most of the cystic lesions are benign.

An ultrasound examination is an ideal screening test, because it can differentiate cystic from solid lesions and requires no contrast or sedation. In addition, ultrasound can detect the presence of a tumor thrombus in the renal vein or inferior vena cava in patients with Wilms' tumor. Computed tomography (CT) scan is superior to sonogram in demonstrating retroperitoneal structures, including lymph nodes. Optimal CT imaging requires oral and intravenous contrast, however, and young children need sedation to prevent movement artifacts.

● **Clinical Pearl:** Magnetic resonance imaging (MRI) is superior to CT in visualizing blood vessels, and the additional saggital and coronal views obtained with MRI give better anatomic delineation of the tumor, which may be useful in planning surgery.

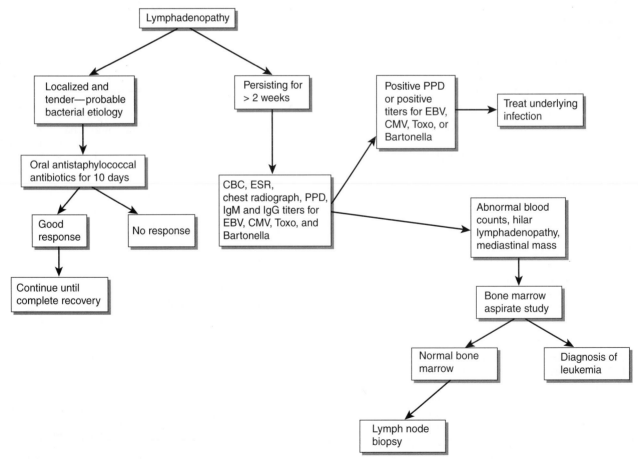

Figure 64–1 ■ Diagnostic approach to lymphadenopathy. CBC = complete blood count; CMV = cytomegalovirus; EBV = Epstein-Barr virus; ESR = erythrocyte sedimentation rate; PPD = intermediate-strength purified protein derivative.

Mediastinal Masses

The differential diagnosis of mediastinal masses is outlined in Display 64-2. Children with anterior mediastinal masses often have tracheal compression and present with wheezing or respiratory distress. These symptoms may be exacerbated in the supine position and mistaken for asthma.

▲ **Clinical Warning:** A child with persistent or recurrent wheezing must be evaluated by a plain chest film before undergoing steroid therapy, because steroids can cause significant shrinkage of a mediastinal lymphoma and improvement in the patient's symptoms, thus falsely reinforcing the diagnosis of asthma.

Anterior mediastinal masses may also compress the superior vena cava, causing some or all manifestations of superior vena cava syndrome. These include orthopnea, headache, dizziness, fainting, plethoric facial swelling, jugular venous distension, papilledema, and pulsus paradoxus.

● **Clinical Pearl:** Plain chest films are adequate to visualize most mediastinal masses. However, in plain chest films, a mass can be easily obscured by an accompanying pleural effusion, giving a false impression of pneumonia with effusion. A CT scan gives better anatomic delineation between the mass, fluid, and the lung parenchyma.

It is sound clinical practice to obtain a CT scan of the chest in cases of large pleural effusion that may be masking a mediastinal mass. Confirmation of diagnosis requires examination of pleural fluid, bone marrow aspirate study, or biopsy of an enlarged cervical lymph node or the mediastinal mass itself.

▲ **Clinical Warning:** Sedation or general anesthesia of a child with anterior mediastinal mass can cause worsening of tracheal compression, resulting in exacerbation of the

respiratory distress and even respiratory arrest. Cases of sudden death in the operating room have been reported because of collapse of the airway and difficulty in intubation. Sedation and general anesthesia should be avoided whenever possible and used only by a team of experienced pediatric anesthesiologists in a tertiary care center.

Headache and Neurologic Symptoms

Brain tumors are the most common solid tumors in children. The possibility of a brain tumor should be considered in any child with unexplained neurologic symptoms or signs. The presenting symptoms and signs of brain tumors may be localizing in nature, such as hemiparesis of hemispheric lesions. Nonlocalizing symptoms are secondary to increased intracranial pressure and include irritability, lethargy, headache, vomiting, and behavioral changes. A more complete list of signs and symptoms of childhood brain tumors is given in Display 64-3.

Spinal Cord Compression

Children who complain of back pain or weakness of lower extremities should be promptly evaluated for spinal cord compression. MRI is the preferred imaging study because it can demonstrate an epidural mass and any intraparenchy-

---

DISPLAY 64–2 • Differential Diagnosis of Mediastinal Masses

Anterior Mediastinum
Leukemia
Non-Hodgkin's lymphoma
Hodgkin's disease
Teratoma
Thymoma
Lipoma
Thyroid tumors

Middle Mediastinum
Lymphoma
Bronchogenic cyst
Pericardial cyst
Esophageal lesions
Metastatic nodes

Posterior Mediastinum
Neuroblastoma
Ganglioneuroblastoma
Ganglioneuroma

Adapted with permission from Steuber, P. & Nesbit, M. E. (1997). Clinical assessment and differential diagnosis of the child with suspected cancer. In P. A. Pizzo & D. G. Poplack (Eds), *Principles and practice of pediatric oncology* (3rd ed.) (p. 129). Philadelphia: Lippincott-Raven.

DISPLAY 64–3 • Signs and Symptoms of Brain Tumors in Children

Increased Intracranial Pressure
- Morning headache
- Vomiting
- Visual disturbances
- Developmental delay
- Regression of intellectual and motor skills
- Lethargy, irritability, anorexia
- Excessive tiredness
- Changes in personality
- Poor school performance

Infratentorial Tumors (Brain Stem, Cerebellum)
- Disturbance of balance or brain stem function
- Ataxia predominantly truncal
- Long tract signs
- Cranial nerve palsy

Supratentorial Tumors
- Subtle loss of consciousness
- Transient focal events
- Grand mal seizures
- Hemiparesis or hemisensory loss

Hypothalamic Tumors
- Loss of growth velocity
- Diabetes insipidus
- Delayed puberty or sexual precocity
- Visual loss

Adapted with permission from Tait, D. M., Bailey, C. C., & Cameron, M. M. (1992). Tumors of the central nervous system. In P. A. Voute, A. Barret, & J. Lemerle (Eds)., *Cancer in children: Clinical management* (3rd ed.). (pp. 184–206). New York: Springer-Verlag.
  Note: None of the more recent pediatric oncology resources have content as comprehensive as that provided in this reference. Symptoms and signs of the disease are not likely to change along with advances in science. The reader should not be concerned about the currency of the reference.

mal spinal cord lesion or compression of the cauda equina. Although rare, neuroblastomas and lymphomas can present with spinal cord compression.

▲ **Clinical Warning:** The provider should treat any suspected spinal cord compression as an emergency, because progression of the lesion can result in irreversible loss of neurologic function. Treatment depends on the underlying diagnosis but usually includes high-dose dexamethasone, laminectomy, radiation therapy, or chemotherapy. Prompt treatment often results in full recovery of neurologic function.

Hematologic Abnormalities

In an otherwise well-looking child, single cytopenia (anemia, thrombocytopenia, or neutropenia) is unlikely to be caused by leukemia.

▲ **Clinical Warning:** If the child is ill with systemic symptoms, leukemia should be considered in the differential diagnosis. Children with neuroblastoma, lymphoma, or Hodgkin's disease may have anemia at presentation. When there is a combination of two or more cytopenias, leukemia must be ruled out by a bone marrow aspirate study. Neutrophilic leukocytosis and microcytic anemia are often seen in Hodgkin's disease.

When bacterial infections cause very high white blood cell (WBC) counts (leukemoid reaction), there is a high percentage of neutrophils and bands. In leukemia, however, a high WBC count is always associated with a very low percentage of neutrophils, because the increase in the WBC count is due to the presence of leukemic cells (blasts) in the peripheral blood.

● **Clinical Pearl:** The higher the WBC count, the more easily one can identify leukemic cells in the peripheral blood.

Referral to the Pediatric Oncologist

A provisional diagnosis of cancer can often be made, or at least strongly suspected, by the primary care provider from the results of the preliminary tests, including certain imaging studies. The definitive diagnosis of cancer, however, frequently requires confirmatory studies, such as bone marrow aspirate study in the case of leukemia or histopathologic examination of the tumor tissue in solid tumors. In addition to routine morphologic examination of the specimen by light microscopy, special studies, such as immunostains, cytogenetics, flow cytometric analysis of tumor-specific antigens, cell ploidy, and molecular biologic studies, are often essential for the definitive diagnosis and assessment of prognosis. These confirmatory tests should be done at the referral center under the direction of a pediatric oncologist.

MANAGEMENT

During the course of their treatment, children with cancer are followed closely by the pediatric oncologist. However, the primary care provider continues to play an important role in the management of the child with cancer. This may include comanaging chemotherapy and other drug administration. The provider will almost certainly manage minor intercurrent illnesses, provide well child care, and offer psychosocial support to the child and the family. In addition, the primary care clinician will follow the patient for several years after the treatment is completed. The provider–patient relationship is important for several reasons, not the least of which is knowing the child and his or her history of illness and response to therapy, which can facilitate an early diagnosis of any late effects of cancer therapy, as described in the following section.

Chemotherapy

The primary care provider can play a significant role in the treatment of the child with cancer. This requires developing a close working relationship with the pediatric oncologist. In some settings, the provider can coparticipate in the patient's cancer therapy, administering selected chemotherapy that has been prescribed by the oncologist. Examples of such agents include vincristine, cytarabine, and dactinomycin. These agents are administered by slow intravenous push through a central venous catheter. In addition, the practitioner may also give intramuscular injections of L-asparaginase and subcutaneous injections of cytosine arabinoside prescribed by the oncologist. These two drugs are commonly used in the treatment of acute lymphoblastic leukemia (ALL). Such participation by the primary provider vastly improves the quality of life for patients and parents by enabling them to receive treatment in a smaller, more familiar setting and by decreasing their visits to an often more distant cancer center.

Side Effects of Chemotherapy

The side effects of chemotherapy can be classified into general and specific. *General* side effects are those that are common to most chemotherapeutic agents. These include nausea, vomiting, mucositis, hair loss, and myelosuppression. These side effects are seen within hours or days from the administration of chemotherapy and are almost always transient. However, the severity of these side effects is variable. For example, vincristine, L-asparaginase, and bleomycin are much less myelosuppressive than most other drugs. Cisplatin, dacarbazine, and mechlorethamine (nitrogen mustard) are among the most emetogenic drugs, while etoposide and bleomycin are only mildly emetogenic. Vincristine seldom causes any nausea or vomiting.

Specific side effects are those that are specific to a particular drug or class of drugs, and they usually involve vital organ systems. Common examples include cardiotoxicity of anthracyclines, nephrotoxicity of platinum compounds, pulmonary toxicity of bleomycin and carmustine (BCNU), and bladder toxicity (hemorrhagic cystitis) of cyclophosphamide and ifosfamide. The reader is referred to Chapters 15, 27, 28, and 49 for more insight into managing care coordination for the child with cancer. Table 64-1 lists the common side effects of the frequently used chemotherapeutic drugs.

Infections

A host of factors, including neutropenia, low immunoglobulin levels, impaired mucosal integrity, and indwelling catheters, compromise the immunity of children with cancer. Lowered immunity makes such children susceptible to serious infections. Gram-negative organisms such as *Pseudomonas aeruginosa, Escherichia coli,* and *Klebsiella pneumoniae* are a particular threat to the neutropenic host. Staphylococcal infections, *Pneumocystis carinii* pneumonia, and cryptococcal meningitis occur in non-neutropenic hosts as well. Coagulase-negative staphylococci are common pathogens in patients with indwelling central lines. Life-

Table 64-1   SIDE EFFECTS OF CHEMOTHERAPY

Drug	Usual Dosage	Special Precautions and Instructions	Adverse Reactions
L-asparaginase (Elspar) IM, IV	$6000/m^2/d$ × three doses per wk for a total of 9 doses in all. High dose: 30,000 U/m^2 or 1000 $U/kg/d$ × 10 d	Do not use solution if it becomes cloudy; IM route is preferred, because IV administration has a higher risk of anaphylaxis.	Anaphylactic shock, hepatotoxicity, pancreatitis, malaise, confusion, lethargy, somnolence
Bleomycin (Blenoxane) especially IV, IM, or SC	$10-20$ U/m^2 once or twice a week	Keep total cumulative dose < 400 U/m^2 to avoid pulmonary toxicity.	Anaphylactoid reaction, in lymphoma patients, pneumonitis → pulmonary toxicity, hyperpigmentation, hyperkeratosis, nail changes, pruritus, phlebitis at injection site
Carboplatin IV (Paraplatin)	360 mg/m^2 q4wk. For renal impairment, adjust total dose using Calvert formula and target AUC.	Avoid aluminum-containing IV infusion sets and needles. Renal effects of nephrotoxic compounds may be potentiated.	Hypersensitivity, nephrotoxicity, peripheral neuropathy
Carmustine (BCNU) IV	$150-200$ mg/m^2 q6wk, given as a single daily dose, or divided into two daily doses, given on consecutive days	Contact with skin may cause brown stain. Pain and burning at injection site, and flushing if infused too quickly. Protect from light.	Pulmonary fibrosis, nephrotoxicity, reversible hepatotoxicity
Cisplatin (Platinol-AQ) IV	100 mg/m^2 q4wk, as a single dose or divided over 5 d. Up to 200 mg/m^2 has been used in investigational protocols.	Ensure adequate hydration to prevent drug from binding to renal tubular proteins. Avoid aluminum-containing IV infusion sets and needles.	Anaphylactoid reaction, nephrotoxicity, various neuropathies, ototoxicity, hypomagnesemia, hypophosphatemia, hypokalemia, hypocalcemia
Cyclophosphamide (Cytoxan) PO, IV	Various regimens	Force fluids. Administer drug early in day as ambulation helps prevent accumulation of drug in bladder.	Hemorrhagic cystitis, interstitial pulmonary fibrosis, amenorrhea, azoospermia, teratogenic, secondary cancer, SIADH
Cytarabine, Ara-C, cytosine arabinoside, IV, SC, or intrathecal	Various regimens. Use preservative-free NS for intrathecal use.		Mucositis, esophagitis, anal ulceration, diarrhea, hepatitic dysfunction, urinary retention
Dactinomycin (Cosmegen) IV	15 mcg/kg/d × 5 d or 45 mcg/kg/d—single dose q3-4wk		Hepatomegaly, mucositis, LFT changes, sensitivity to previously irradiated skin, tissue damage secondary to drug extravasation
Doxorubicin (Adriamycin) IV	Variable	Cumulative dose not to exceed 400 mg/m^2	Cardiotoxicity, mucositis, tissue damage secondary to extravasation, hyperpigmentation of nail beds and skin, skin sensitivity reaction to prior radiation, fever, chills, urticaria
Etoposide (VePesid) IV	100 mg/m^2/d × 3 d q3-4wk	Do not give rapid IV infusion. Solutions should be checked for precipitate before and during administration. Discard if precipitate is seen.	Hypotension, anaphylaxis-like reaction
Fludarabine (Fludara) IV	20 mg/m^2/d × 5 d q4wk	Inadvertent high doses (4 times regular doses) have caused severe neurologic effects, including blindness, coma, and death.	Hypersensitivity, peripheral edema, weakness, agitation, confusion, visual disturbances, peripheral neuropathy, pneumonia
5-fluorouracil (5-FU) IV	Variable	Protect from light.	Hyperpigmentation of skin, nail changes, palmoplantar erythrodysesthesia syndrome, headache, dizziness and blurred vision

(continues)

Table 64–1. SIDE EFFECTS OF CHEMOTHERAPY   *(Continued)*

Drug	Usual Dosage	Special Precautions and Instructions	Adverse Reactions
Idarubicin (Idamycin) IV	8–12 mg/m² daily for 3 d	Precipitation occurs when mixed with heparin.	Cardiotoxicity, tissue damage secondary to extravasation, generalized rash, urticaria
Ifosfamide (Ifex) IV	1.2–2.4 g/m²/d × 5 d	Administer with mesna, and maintain adequate hydration to prevent hemorrhagic cystitis.	Hemorrhagic cystitis, lethargy, somonolence, confusion, disorientation, and hallucination
Mechlorethamine (Mustargen) IV	0.4 mg/kg/course		Vertigo, tinnitus, diminished hearing, metallic taste in the mouth, severe nausea or vomiting
Methotrexate (MTX) PO, IV, IM, intrathecal	20–30 mg/m² PO once or twice a week. High-dose methotrexate 1–12 g/m² IV with leukovorin rescue. Intrathecal maximum dose: 12 mg	Use preservative-free products for intrathecal and high-dose therapy. High-dose MTX should be used only in experienced centers.	Mucosistis, diarrhea, hepatotoxicity, renal failure, cystitis, pulmonary interstitial pneumonitis, urticaria, acne, telangiectasia, photosensitivity, fever, malaise, chills
Mitoxantrone IV	12 mg/m²/d × 2–3 days IV	Incompatible with heparin-containing solutions	Cardiotoxicity, mucositis, urticaria, bluish discoloration of urine
Pegaspargase (PEG-L asparaginase) (Oncaspar) IM	2500 U/m², for children with < 0.6 m², 83 u/kg q2wk	Hypersensitivity reactions; contraindicated in patients with a history of any serious reactions with L-asparaginase	Hypersensitivity reaction, hypotension, hypertension, hepatotoxicity, pancreatitis, malaise, confusion, lethargy, nephrotoxicity, respiratory distress, fever, hyperglycemia
Vinblastine IV (Velban)	6/mg/m²		Constipation, urinary retention, polyurea, peripheral neuropathy, loss of deep tendon reflexes, parasthesias, tissue damage secondary to extravasation
Vincristine IV (Oncovin)	1.5 mg/m² maximum 2 mg	Fatal if given intrathecally	Constipation, ileus, urinary retention, polyuria, numbness, parasthesias, loss of deep tendon, reflexes. SIADH, ophthalmoplegia, extraocular muscle paresis, tissue damage secondary to extravasation

Adapted with permission from McFarland, H. M. et al. (1992). Guide for the administration and use of Cancer chemotherapeutic agents. *Oncology* [special edition] 2, 83–87.

threatening complications include gram-negative sepsis, pneumonias, and disseminated fungal infections.

The Neutropenic Patient With Infection

The risk of serious bacterial and fungal infections is significant when the absolute neutrophil count (ANC) is less than 500/mm³, and it is highest when the ANC drops below 100/mm³. The febrile child with an ANC of less than 500/mm³ should be hospitalized for intravenous broad-spectrum antibiotic coverage and close monitoring for complications, such as septic shock. Display 64-4 presents the clinical features that indicate high risk for life-threatening complications in the neutropenic patient.

▲ **Clinical Warning:** The patient with these risk factors should be managed at a center experienced in the care of immunocompromised patients. Any patient who lacks these high-risk features may be managed by the primary care

provider in consultation with the pediatric oncologist. All patients, however, should be hospitalized and treated with intravenous antibiotics until they are afebrile and the culture results are available to guide further management. Even if the cultures are negative and the patient is afebrile, it is preferable to continue the intravenous antibiotics until the ANC is 500/mm³ or greater.

Ceftazidime is commonly used as the initial empiric therapy (pending culture results), because it provides adequate coverage against most gram-negative organisms. However, it is not very effective in anaerobic and staphylococcal infections, and changes in antibiotic therapy need to be made if there are clinical clues indicating such infections.

▲ **Clinical Warning:** To prevent emergence of vancomycin-resistant *Enterococcus,* the use of vancomycin should be restricted to proven infections with coagulase-negative *Staphylococcus* that are resistant to other antibiotics.

In culture-proven *Pseudomonas* infections, an aminoglycoside, such as gentamycin or tobramycin, should be added to ceftazidime to prevent emergence of resistant organisms. If necessary, imipenem should be substituted for ceftazidime to provide added coverage against anerobic organisms in cases of perirectal abscess, gingivitis, or typhlitis. It may also be preferred in patients who might have resistant organisms because of multiple exposure to previous antibiotic therapy. Refer to the section on fever in the neutropenic child for management information.

The Febrile Non-neutropenic Patient

The non-neutropenic child with a temperature of 102°F or greater warrants careful evaluation, although risk of life-threatening infections is much less than that of the neutropenic child. Physical examination should include a careful search for any evidence of pneumonia or meningitis. Plain chest films and blood cultures from the central line should be done in any patient who does not have a definite focus of infection on physical examination. Indications for hospitalization include ill-looking child, a temperature of 103°F or greater, and radiologic evidence of pneumonia. Outpatient management may be appropriate if the febrile child does not look ill, the temperature is less than 103°F, and there is no evidence of pneumonia. Empiric antibiotic therapy with parenteral ceftriaxone may be used for such a patient pending culture results. Children with implantable subcutaneous catheters (lifeport) are less likely to have central line-related bacteremia compared with those with external catheters.

Respiratory Tract Infections: Otitis Media, Sinusitis, and Pneumonia

In addition to the common bacteria, any gram-positive or gram-negative organism can cause otitis media or sinusitis in immunocompromised children. Oral broad-spectrum antibiotic therapy is sufficient for the non-neutropenic patient. In neutropenic patients, otitis media or sinusitis can be caused by any gram-negative or gram-positive organism.

▲ **Clinical Warning:** Febrile neutropenic patients with otitis media or sinusitis should be treated with intravenous antibiotics until results of blood cultures are available, because clinical evidence of otitis or sinusitis does not rule out the possibility of sepsis.

A CT scan or MRI is more sensitive than plain radiograph in diagnosing sinusitis in immunocompromised children. Sinusitis in patients with severe and prolonged neutropenia is often caused by fungal organisms. If a neutropenic patient with sinusitis does not improve within 72 hours of treatment, aspiration or biopsy of the sinus should be performed to identify the causative organism so that specific therapy can be started.

Pneumonia is one of the common infections in immunocompromised children, and diffuse bilateral pneumonia is one of the main causes of death in children with cancer. The causative organisms may vary depending on the type of pulmonary infiltrate (localized versus diffuse) and the presence or absence of neutropenia.

A localized pulmonary infiltrate in a non-neutropenic patient is usually caused by the same bacteria, virus (respiratory syncytial virus [RSV], adenovirus, influenza), or *Mycoplasma* that cause pneumonia in normal children. Such a patient may be managed by the primary care provider with oral antibiotic therapy if the patient does not look ill and the temperature is less than 103°F. However, less common bacterial agents, such as *Mycobacterium tuberculosis*, atypical mycobacteria, *Legionella,* and fungi (*Cryptococcus, Histoplasma,* and *Coccidioides*) should also be considered in determining the causative organism.

▲ **Clinical Warnings:**

- When the pulmonary infiltrate is diffuse or if the patient is neutropenic, the patient's condition may worsen rapidly, and the risk of mortality is significant. Such a patient should be treated in the intensive care unit at a tertiary care center.
- Whether the infiltrates in the neutropenic patient are localized or diffuse, all organisms should be considered in the etiology:
  - Gram-positive and gram-negative bacteria, including *M. tuberculosis*, atypical mycobacteria, and *Legionella*
  - Viruses, including RSV, CMV, and influenza
  - Fungi, including *Aspergillus* and *Candida*
  - Protozoal (eg, *P. carinii* pneumonia)

● **Clinical Pearl:** Diffuse infiltrates in a non-neutropenic child are more likely to be caused by viruses (RSV, CMV) and *Pneumocystis* than bacterial or fungal organisms.

Infections of the Oral Cavity

Common lesions in the mouth of children receiving chemotherapy include thrush, herpes stomatitis, and gingivitis and periodontitis. Thrush is characterized by whitish plaques with slightly raised and indurated borders caused by unchecked colonization by *Candida albicans.* Mycostatin oral suspension or clotrimazole troches are effective in most patients. Patients who do not respond to these treatments should be treated with oral fluconazole.

Herpes simplex virus (HSV) lesions in the mouth are often multiple and are most commonly seen on the lips and palate. The characteristic finding is a slowly enlarging ulcer (usually measuring greater than 1 cm), with a raised white border and sometimes with small vesicles surrounding the ulcer. The lesions are quite painful, and they affect the patient's oral intake. Empiric treatment with acyclovir should be started as early as possible to prevent more severe stomatitis. Oral acyclovir (20 mg/kg per dose, four times daily) is adequate for mild lesions. Severe herpes stomatitis requires treatment with intravenous acyclovir. HSV lesions are often difficult to differentiate from mucositis induced by chemotherapy or by bacterial or fungal pathogens. Thus, empiric antibiotic therapy in a patient with stomatitis should also cover anerobic organisms.

Esophagitis

Retrosternal pain of a burning nature is indicative of esophagitis. In a non-neutropenic child, this may represent a reflux esophagitis. Children with severe chemotherapy-induced vomiting and those who are ill and bed-ridden for a prolonged period are at high risk for reflux esophagitis.

▲ **Clinical Warnings:**

- Failure to recognize esophagitis promptly may later result in marked esophageal stenosis, requiring treatment with dilatations.
- Esophagoscopy may not be safe in neutropenic patients, because any trauma to the mucosa may aggravate the infection.

Esophagitis in a neutropenic child is commonly caused by *C. albicans* or HSV. Presence of oral thrush suggests *Candida* as the etiology for the esophagitis. Absence of thrush, however, does not rule out *Candida* as the cause of esophagitis. Empiric therapy can be started with oral or intravenous fluconazole and acyclovir. If there is no significant improvement in 2 or 3 days, intravenous amphotericin should be started.

Prevention of Infections in Children With Cancer

Most of the infections in children with cancer are caused by endogenous organisms. Attempts to sterilize the gastrointestinal tract with broad-spectrum antibiotics are not effective in reducing the incidence of infections. In addition, their use may increase the emergence of resistant organisms. Simple hand washing by all hospital personnel and visitors is the most effective prevention against hospital-acquired infections. Strict reverse isolation does not usually add much to hand washing in the prevention of infections. Patients should avoid eating any uncooked food, including fresh vegetables and fresh fruits. High-efficiency particulate air filters may be effective in preventing *Aspergillus* infections (Freifeld, Walsch, & Pizzo, 1997). Chapter 54 provides a discussion about these filters.

Antimicrobials

Trimethoprim-sulfamethoxazole (TMP-SMZ), administered on 3 consecutive days a week, is very effective in preventing *P. carinii* infections and is now routinely prescribed for most children on chemotherapy (El-Sadr, Luskin-Hawk, Yurik, et al., 1999). Children who are allergic to TMP-SMZ may receive biweekly intravenous pentamidine or aerosolized pentamidine.

The prophylactic use of fluconazole has been shown to reduce the incidence of disseminated and mucosal candidiasis (Goodman, 1992). However, it is wise to limit the use of fluconazole to periods of severe and prolonged neutropenia, because its excessive use may encourage the emergence of resistant *Candida* species. Oral acyclovir is effective in preventing reactivation of herpes simplex infections in seropositive bone marrow transplant and in children undergoing intensive chemotherapy for leukemia.

Immunizations: Passive and Active

Irrespective of their history of natural varicella or varicella immunization, children diagnosed with cancer should have their varicella titers tested. Those who do not have adequate titers should receive varicella zoster immune globulin (VZIG) within 96 hours of exposure to chickenpox. Passive immunization with VZIG reduces the incidence of varicella pneumonitis and encephalitis and decreases the mortality rate from between 5% and 7% to 0.5% in patients who are immunocompromised and who have primary varicella infection (Freifeld et al., 1997).

▲ **Clinical Warning:** Live virus vaccines, such as measles, mumps, and rubella vaccine and oral polio vaccine, are contraindicated in children undergoing chemotherapy, although measles vaccine has been safely used in children with human immunodeficiency virus.

Siblings of children on chemotherapy should avoid oral polio vaccine because the vaccine virus is transmissible. Live attenuated varicella virus is still not approved for children who are immunocompromised, although studies have shown that it is safe and 85% protective. However, siblings of children on chemotherapy may receive varicella vaccine.

● **Clinical Pearl:** Patients and siblings of children on chemotherapy may receive inactivated (injectable) polio vaccine.

Although killed vaccines, such as hepatitis B vaccine, and antigens, such as diphtheria-tetanus-pertussis, may be safely administered to immunocompromised children, their immunogenicity may not be optimum. Refer to Chapter 13 for a detailed discussion.

Managing Hematologic Complications of Therapy: Anemia and Thrombocytopenia

Children on cancer chemotherapy are frequently anemic and thrombocytopenic from either chemotherapy or their underlying disease. In most chemotherapy regimens, the nadirs for platelet counts and WBC counts occur 7 to 10 days from the first day of chemotherapy. The counts begin to rise about 10 to 14 days from the completion of therapy. Decrease in the hemoglobin levels is more gradual, because the lifespan of normal red cells is 90 to 120 days.

Red cell transfusions are usually given when the hemoglobin is less than 8 g/dL (hematocrit less than 24%), unless the child is recovering from the chemotherapy and the hemoglobin is expected to rise. When the hemoglobin level falls below 7 g/dL, patients usually have symptoms of anemia, including tiredness, headaches, anorexia, and lack of energy. Transfusion of red cells thus is indicated. One unit of packed red cells (PRBC) is approximately 300 mL. A usual volume used is 15 mL of PRBC per kg of body weight, which will raise the hematocrit by 12% (eg, from 20% to 32%).

● **Clinical Pearl:** One mL of PRBC per kg body weight will raise the hematocrit by 0.8%.

Platelet transfusions are indicated when the platelet count is less than 20,000/mm^3. If there is clinical bleeding (eg, epistaxis or gastrointestinal bleed), any platelet count less than 50,000/mm^3 warrants transfusion. One unit of random platelets (50 mL) per 5 kg of body weight will raise the platelet count by 50,000/mm^3. One unit of single donor platelets (approximately 300 mL) is equal to 6 U of random platelets. Single donor units are preferred for those who receive multiple transfusions.

▲ **Clinical Warning:** Only irradiated blood products should be used in immunocompromised patients. Only CMV-negative blood products should be used for CMV-negative patients undergoing allogeneic stem cell transplantation from a CMV-negative donor.

Use of Growth Factors

Granulocyte-colony stimulating factor (G-CSF, Filgrastim, Neupogen) stimulates the proliferation of the granulocyte precursors, and accelerates their maturation to neutrophils. A course of G-CSF given soon after a cycle of intensive chemotherapy reduces the duration of severe neutropenia, thus reducing the risk of infection and the duration of hospitalization in patients with infection. It is given in doses of 5 mg/kg daily, starting the day after the completion of chemotherapy, and continued until the ANC reaches 5000/mm^3 (which usually takes 10–14 days). It is given as a subcutaneous injection or as an intravenous push through the central line. Blood counts are done twice a week during G-CSF therapy so that treatment can be discontinued once the WBC counts reach high normal values ($> 10,000$).

Continued administration of G-CSF results in extreme leukocytosis ($> 50,000$) and may cause bone pains. G-CSF support is indicated only for patients receiving intensive chemotherapy for solid tumors, acute myeloblastic leukemia, or relapsed ALL. G-CSF is usually not used in newly diagnosed ALL because the chemotherapy is not intensive enough to justify its use. However, most patients with relapsed ALL receive intensive therapy, and G-CSF is used to augment the recovery of neutrophils. There is no risk of G-CSF stimulating the proliferation of leukemia cells.

Erythropoietin is a glycoprotein that stimulates the division and differentiation of erythroid progenitors in the bone marrow. It is given in doses of 150 IU/kg three times per week after myelosuppressive chemotherapy. A modest decrease in the transfusion requirement has been noted in patients receiving erythropoietin (Henry, 1995; Wurnig et al., 1996). However, the cost of erythropoietin exceeds the cost of red cell transfusions (Ortega, Dranitsaris, & Puodziunas, 1998).

Follow-up of the Child Cured of Cancer

Approximately 70% to 80% of all children with cancer are cured by modern therapy. However, a significant percentage of these children have long-term side effects of treatment. Growth and development and reproductive function can be impaired. Cardiac or pulmonary dysfunction and secondary malignancies are also among the common late effects of treatment.

Growth and Development

Prepubertal children receiving 3300 cGy (rads) or more of radiation to the spine for the treatment of brain tumors or Hodgkin's disease have pronounced impairment of linear growth, especially the sitting height. On the other hand, children who get lower doses of radiation (< 3300 cGy), as, for example, for the control of central nervous system (CNS) leukemia, have minimal height loss. Cranial radiation in ALL has minimal risk of growth hormone deficiency (GHD), because the total dose (1800 cGy) and the daily fraction (150

cGy) are low. On the other hand, children receiving radiation for brain tumors (usually < 3000 cGy) have a high risk of GHD. Cranial irradiation for ALL or brain tumors can also cause precocious puberty and decreased adult height. Primary or secondary amenorrhea is seen in one third of patients receiving more than 3000 cGy of radiation for brain tumors (Arlt et al., 1997). Refer to Chapter 60 for information about the management of GHD.

Gonads and Reproductive Function

Alkylating agents (nitrogen mustard, cyclophosphamide, ifosfamide, melphalan, thiotepa, busulfan) cause gonadal damage, particularly in males. Males receiving MOPP regimen (nitrogen mustard, vincristine, procarbazine, prednisone) for Hodgkin's disease have a very high risk of sterility: greater than 90% with six cycles and 50% with three cycles. Overall, the risk of sterility in males treated with alkylating agents for various cancers has varied from 20% to 66% in various studies. On the other hand, the risk of sterility in females from alkylating agents is much lower.

Nervous System

Cranial irradiation and intrathecal chemotherapy can cause a spectrum of neurologic complications ranging from mild learning disabilities to frank leukoencephalopathy. With modern treatment protocols for ALL, most children receive intrathecal methotrexate alone for CNS prophylaxis, and these patients have only a small risk of neurocognitive defects.

▲ **Clinical Warning:** Children who receive cranial irradiation or high doses of systemic methotrexate along with intrathecal methotrexate are at higher risk for neurocognitive sequelae, including learning defects. Infants and young children are more at risk for this complication than older children.

One third of children younger than 5 years receiving cranial irradiation for ALL develop learning difficulties. Children who experience CNS relapse (meningeal leukemia) often receive all three modalities of CNS treatment—systemic methotrexate, intrathecal or intraventricular chemotherapy, and cranial irradiation. Such patients may develop more severe neurologic sequelae, such as leukoencephalopathy, seizures, major motor disabilities, and cranial nerve palsies. Children with malignant brain tumors treated with doses equal to or greater than 54 rads (cGy) of radiation are also at risk for any of these complications.

Cardiac Function

The incidence of clinically evident cardiotoxicity in children has been estimated to be 1.6% from a study of 6493 patients (Krischer et al., 1997). The risk factors for cardiac toxicity include cumulative anthracyclines dose of 550 mg/m^2 or greater, single dose of 50 mg/m^2 or greater, female sex, age younger than 4 years, African American race, length of follow-up, trisomy 21, and exposure to amsacrine (Krischer et al., 1997; Lipshultz et al., 1991).

▲ **Clinical Warning:** Children who have received anthracycline therapy should be screened by echocardiogram every 2 to 3 years until adulthood to identify any late-onset cardiomyopathy. Radiotherapy to the mediastinum or lung fields, as given in Hodgkin's disease or Wilms' tumor, potentiates the cardiotoxicity of anthracyclines. Patients who undergo radiation to the heart are at risk for premature atherosclerosis and coronary heart disease later in life.

Second Malignancies

Children who receive alkylating agents have approximately 1% risk of developing secondary acute nonlymphoblastic leukemia (ANL) within 10 years from diagnosis, although most cases occur within 3 to 5 years. Epipodophyllotoxins (VP-16 and VM-26) have even greater risk of causing secondary ANL, depending on the total dose and schedule of administration (Winick et al., 1993).

Secondary solid tumors have a longer latency period and are almost always caused by radiation therapy. Common secondary solid tumors include bone and soft-tissue sarcomas and non-Hodgkin's lymphoma. The cumulative risk of developing a secondary solid tumor for all children with cancer is 0.9% at 20 years from diagnosis. However, patients with Hodgkin's disease and Ewing's sarcoma have a much higher incidence of second cancers, with actual incidence of 7% at 15 years and 9.2% at 20 years (Marina, 1997).

Pulmonary Toxicity

Both radiation to the lung fields and chemotherapeutic drugs, including bleomycin and BCNU, can cause pulmonary fibrosis with loss of lung volume, compliance, and diffusing capacity. Pneumonia can also result, either alone or in conjunction with pulmonary fibrosis. The incidence and the severity of pulmonary fibrosis depend on several factors: area of the lung irradiated, the cumulative dose of radiation of the offending drug, the age of the patient, and the presence of any preexisting lung conditions, such as asthma. In young children, radiation impairs the growth of the lung parenchyma and chest wall, exacerbating the pulmonary toxicity of radiation or chemotherapy. A radiation dose as low as 1100 to 1400 cGy can cause significant toxicity when given to both lungs. Ten percent of patients who receive bleomycin develop pulmonary fibrosis when the cumulative dose exceeds 400 U/m^2. BCNU in doses greater than 1500 mg/m^2 causes pulmonary toxicity in 50% of patients. Other drugs that can cause pulmonary toxicity include busulfan, cyclphosphamide, and methorexate (Kreisman & Volkov, 1992; Fauroux, Clement, & Tournier, 1996).

Renal Toxicity

Renal toxicity caused by radiation or drugs such as ifosfamide, cisplatin, and carboplatin can be tubular or glomerular and may be transient or irreversible. Tubular dysfunction is characterized by hypokalemia, hypophosphatemia, and hypomagnesemia. Cisplatin and ifosfamide are more nephrotoxic than carboplatin. Renal failure from chemotherapy is usually manifested during or soon after the completion of therapy (Blatt, Copeland, & Bleyer, 1997). Monitoring for chemotherapy-induced renal toxicity should be done during treatment and several months after completion of chemotherapy. This includes questioning for symptoms of chronic renal failure (fatigue, nocturia, edema), measurement of blood pressure, and serum levels of blood urea nitrogen (BUN), creatinine, electrolytes, Ca, PO_4, and Mg. Children who receive radiation to the abdomen and pelvis should be monitored annually until adulthood.

What to Tell Parents

Some of the goals of treatment are to have the child maintain as much normalcy as possible throughout the treatment period and to return to a normal life routine as soon as possible after achieving remission of the cancer. Achievement of these goals depends to a large extent on the nature of the cancer, the intensity and duration of treatment, and the prognosis of cure. School, play activities, and friends comprise a major part of a child's life. The child should return to school as soon after achieving remission as possible. Whether or not the child can participate in physical activities depends on general health, level of nutrition, and hematologic status. Any child who is significantly anemic (hemoglobin < 9 g/dL) should avoid excessive physical activities and competitive sports. Most children are eager to get back to school, even for part of the day. Older children who cannot attend full-time school should receive home-tutoring to make up for lost classes. When the ANC is less than $500/\text{mm}^3$, it may be advisable to keep young children from going to school and any crowded place, such as malls, theaters, and places of worship, and from entertaining friends who have symptoms of any infectious disease.

Any child who has received chemotherapy, radiation treatments, or both is at significant risk for appetite changes. Clearly, nutritional deficits will compromise response to therapy and eventual recovery. The provider is urged to work with the oncology specialty group, including a nutritionist or dietitian who is familiar with cancer in children, to effect a proactive approach to meal and snack planning. If nutritional supplementation is required, the dietary expert can guide planning and provision.

The provider may want to refer the child and family for mental health counseling if further psychosocial support is needed. In addition, the clinician may want to facilitate the child's or family's exposure to cancer support group activities. The Community Resources section at the end of this chapter contains information on national, local, and regional supports.

Discipline

At present, about 70% to 80% of all children with cancer are being cured, and this cure rate is likely to continue to improve. The goal of cancer treatment is not just to cure the child of cancer, but also to have the child return to normal physical and emotional health. It is the responsibility of the provider to help parents and child to achieve this goal. A child who is cured of cancer is likely to be left with severe and incurable emotional and behavior problems, especially if allowed to grow up without any discipline at home during the years of treatment. It is difficult for parents to concentrate on discipline when they are concerned with so many other commitments associated with their child's health care, and because they feel sad and sympathetic toward the child.

Feeling confident about the prospect of cure helps the parents treat the child like a normal child. Despite feelings of shock, sadness, anger, and helplessness in the first weeks after the diagnosis of cancer in their child, it is important for them to become hopeful of cure once remission is achieved. It is also the responsibility of the pediatric provider to emphasize the need to be hopeful of cure, unless dealing with a child who has experienced multiple relapses, who consequently has a very poor prognosis.

Siblings

Well siblings of the child with cancer also have special needs. Normal feelings of envy, jealousy, and rivalry may become exaggerated because of the special attention the ill child receives. They often feel deprived and isolated. Some siblings even feel a sense of guilt for being healthy while the ill child undergoes so much suffering. Overt psychosomatic symptoms seen in siblings can include fearfulness, separation anxieties, poor school performance, preoccupation with their own health, enuresis, depression, withdrawal, sleep disturbances, and antisocial behavior.

The pediatric provider and parents must work together to prevent or minimize the emotional and psychological problems in siblings. From the time of diagnosis, it is important to keep children involved and informed about their sibling's illness, plan of treatment, and prognosis (Perin & Kramer, 1985). Siblings must be encouraged to discuss their feelings openly. They should be told that it is normal to have feelings of jealousy and hostility toward their ill sibling and to feel anger toward their parents.

● **Clinical Pearl:** Parents should try to spend time with their well children at regular intervals. Some youngsters may need professional counseling, especially if there were preexisting psychological or emotional problems.

Common Childhood Cancers

The following section discusses the most common of the childhood cancers. Presented in order of their frequency, these include the leukemias, brain tumors, neuroblastoma, Wilms' tumor, rhabdomyosarcoma, and the lymphomas.

■ Leukemia

Leukemias are the most common form of malignancy in children. ALL accounts for 75% of all cases of childhood leukemias. ANL is less common (20%), and chronic myeloid leukemia is rare (< 5%) (Margolin & Poplack, 1997; Altman, 1997).

■ Acute Lymphoblastic Leukemia

PATHOLOGY

Lymphoid cells express various surface and cytoplasmic markers at different stages of development, and leukemic cells exhibit the markers of the particular stage of lymphocyte development at which the leukemogenesis began. According to the type of markers present on the lymphoblasts, ALL can be classified into various subtypes: B-precursor ALL (pre B-ALL), T-cell ALL, and B-cell ALL. Pre B-ALL is the most common type, accounting for about 83% of all cases of ALL. About 15% are T-cell ALL, and mature B-cell ALL is rare (2%). T-cell and B-cell ALL, once associated with a dire prognosis, now have long-term survival of better than 70% (Pui, 1997).

DIAGNOSTIC CRITERIA

The peak incidence for ALL occurs at approximately 4 years of age, although the disease occurs in all age groups (Margolin & Poplack, 1997; Pui & Evans, 1998). The presenting symptoms and signs of ALL are given in Table 64-2. Most of the symptoms and signs are due to bone marrow failure (neutropenia, anemia, and thrombocytopenia) or to

Table 64–2. CLINICAL AND LABORATORY FEATURES AT DIAGNOSIS IN CHILDREN WITH ACUTE LYMPHOBLASTIC LEUKEMIA

Clinical and Laboratory Features	Percentage of Patients
Fever	61
Bleeding (petechia or purpura)	48
Bone pain	23
Lymphadenopathy	50
Hepatosplenomegaly	68
White blood cell count (/mm^3)	
< 10,000	53
10,000–49,000	30
> 50,000	17
Hemoglobin	
< 7 g/dL	43
7–10 g/dL	45
> 11 g/dL	12
Platelet count (/mm^3)	
< 20,000	28
20,000–99,000	47
> 100,000	25

Adapted with permission from Margolin, J. F. & Poplack, D. G. (1997). Acute lymphoblastic leukemia. In P. A. Pizzo & D. G. Poplack (eds.), *Principles and practice of pediatric oncology* (3rd ed.). (pp. 409–462). Philadelphia: Lippincott-Raven.

leukemic infiltration of the liver, spleen, and lymph nodes. The diagnosis of ALL should be considered in patients who present with generalized bone and joint pains, and a bone marrow aspirate study should be done by a pediatric oncologist to rule out leukemia even when there are no hematologic abnormalities.

DIAGNOSTIC STUDIES

Confirmation of the diagnosis of ALL requires at least 25% blasts on a bone marrow aspirate specimen, although in most patients, the bone marrow shows more than 50% blasts. The lymphoblasts can be differentiated from myeloblasts by morphology, special stains, and immunologic detection of cell surface antigens by flow cytometry.

In addition to CBC, initial evaluation should include a full chemistry profile with electrolytes, BUN, creatinine, uric acid, asparate aminotransferase, alanine aminotransferase, lactate dehydrogenase, Ca, and PO_4. Although tumor lysis syndrome usually does not occur until the treatment is started, patients with a high WBC count may have high hyperuricemia requiring intravenous hydration, alkalinization, and allopurinol.

The two most important prognostic features in ALL are age and WBC count at diagnosis. Patients with T-cell ALL and B-cell ALL also have a greater than 70% chance of long-term survival (Pui, 1997). By means of cytogenetic or molecular genetic methods, chromosomal abnormalities can be detected in the leukemic cells of more than 90% of children with ALL. These genetic markers also have prognostic significance. Infants with t(4;11) and children with t(9;22) have less than a 35% chance of 5-year event-free survival (EFS), whereas children with hyperdiploidy (>50 chromosomes), t(12;21), and t(1;19) have between 70% and 90% 5-year EFS. Patients who remain in continuous remission for more than 5 years are generally considered cured, although there are very rare relapses even after 5 years of remission (Margolin & Poplack, 1997; Pui, 1997).

MANAGEMENT

Chemotherapy for ALL is given in five phases: induction, consolidation, interim maintenance, reintensification, and maintenance, in addition to CNS prophylaxis. With vincristine, prednisone, and asparaginase (and daunorubicin for high-risk patients) and intrathecal methotrexate, 98% to 99% of patients achieve remission within 28 days. The term *remission* indicates absence of clinical or hematologic evidence of disease. The consolidation phase usually consists of cyclophosphamide, cytarabine, 6-mercaptopurine, and intrathecal methotrexate, given over 5 weeks. After a 6-week period of interim maintenance with weekly oral methotrexate and daily oral purinethol, patients receive 6 weeks of reintensification with the same drugs given for induction and consolidation.

Maintenance therapy consists of weekly oral methotrexate and daily oral 6-mercaptopurine, with monthly pulses of intravenous vincristine and oral prednisone. The duration of maintenance therapy is for 2 years for females and 3 years for males. To eradicate any subclinical disease in the CNS, intrathecal methotrexate is given every 2 to 3 months. Selected patients at high risk of CNS relapse and those with CNS disease at diagnosis are usually given cranial irradiation in addition to intrathecal chemotherapy to prevent CNS relapse.

Management of Relapse

Patients with relapse in the bone marrow still have about a 90% chance of achieving complete remission with intensive induction therapy (Pui, 1995). For patients who relapse early (within 18 months from achieving first remission), bone marrow transplantation (BMT) offers a better chance of EFS than chemotherapy alone. For patients who relapse late (>36 months from achieving first remission), BMT is not superior to chemotherapy (Margolin & Poplack, 1997). Allogeneic BMT from an HLA-identical sibling offers better chance of long-term survival than BMT from a matched unrelated donor.

Isolated CNS relapse occurs in fewer than 10% of cases (Margolin & Poplack, 1997). Intensive systemic and intrathecal chemotherapy along with craniospinal irradiation offers long-term survival for two thirds of previously unirradiated children. Testicular relapse is also rare (<5%) (Ritter & Schrappe, 1999). Isolated overt testicular relapse occurring after the completion of chemotherapy has a better prognosis than relapse on therapy (65% versus 50%) (Margolin & Poplack). Testicular relapse is treated with testicular irradiation, followed by more intensive systemic chemotherapy.

■ *Acute Myeloblastic Leukemia/Acute Nonlymphoblastic Leukemia*

PATHOLOGY

The French-American-British (FAB) classification divides acute myeloblastic leukemia (AML), also known as ANL, into seven subtypes:

- M0: Undifferentiated
- M1: Myeloid without maturation
- M2: Myeloid with maturation
- M3: Acute promyelocytic leukemia (APL)
- M4: Myelomonocytic
- M5: Monocytic
- M6: Erythroleukemia
- M7: Megakaryoblastic

M1, M2, M4, and M5 are the most common types, collectively accounting for 80% of all cases of ANL. APL has unique clinical features: characteristic cytogenetic abnormality (t[15;17]), disseminated intravascular coagulation at diagnosis and during induction treatment, and response to retinoic acid therapy. Acute megakaryoblastistic leukemia (M7) usually occurs in children younger than 3 years, especially in those with Down syndrome. About 80% of children younger than 2 years with AML have either M4 or M5 subtypes (Ebb & Weinstein, 1997). Infants and toddlers with M4 and M5 AML are more likely than older children to have high leukocyte counts and a higher incidence of extramedullary leukemia, especially leukemia cutis and CNS (Ebb & Weinstein, 1997).

DIAGNOSTIC CRITERIA

About 15% to 20% all childhood leukemias are AML (ANL). Presenting clinical features are somewhat similar to ALL, except for some uncommon features of ANL: gingival hypertrophy, parotid swelling, and rarely retro-orbital or epidural masses (chloromas). ANL is the predominant type among congenital leukemias (Todd, Weinstein, & Holcombe, 1997).

Secondary ANL, which is ANL that occurs as a late complication of cancer treatment (nitrogen mustard, cyclophosphamide, and etoposide) or after myelodysplastic syndrome, carries a very poor prognosis. Other adverse prognostic factors include age younger than 2 years, WBC count of greater than 100,000/mL, the presence of monosomy 7, M4 and M5 subtypes, and the presence of extramedullary leukemia (other than CNS). Patients whose leukemic cells demonstrate cytogenetic abnormalities of t(8;21) or inv 16 and those with Down syndrome have a very favorable prognosis (Ravindranath et al., 1992; Ravindranath & Taub, 1999).

MANAGEMENT

Approximately 75% to 85% of patients achieve remission with chemotherapy regimens consisting of cytarabine and daunorubicin (Riley, Hann, Wheatley, & Stevens, 1999). Allogeneic BMT from an HLA-identical sibling, done during first remission, offers a 3-year EFS of 52%. Children treated with autologous BMT do not have a significantly better 3-year EFS than those treated with intensive consolidation chemotherapy (38% versus 36%) (Ravindranath et al., 1996).

■ *Central Nervous System Malignancies: Brain Tumors*

Malignancies of the CNS represent 16.6% of all malignancies during childhood, from birth through adolescence. CNS cancer is the second most frequent malignancy seen in pediatrics and the most common of the solid tumors. Approximately 2200 children younger than 20 years are diagnosed with an invasive CNS malignancy in the United States every year (Grovas et al., 1997; NCI, 2000). The following discussion focuses on the most commonly encountered CNS tumors, presented in the order of their frequency.

EPIDEMIOLOGY

Several of the CNS malignancies stand out as more frequently encountered than others. The following list indicates frequency, from greatest to least:

- Astrocytomas, 52%
- Primitive neuroectodermal tumor (PNET) (medullablastoma and pineoblastoma), 21%
- Other gliomas, 15%
- Ependymomas, 9% (Gurney et al., 1999)

Young children have a relatively higher occurrence rate of CNS malignancy in the cerebellum and the brain stem than do older youngsters and adolescents. Brain stem malignancies are almost as frequent as cerebral cancers in patients age 10 years or younger. Cerebellum malignancies are more common than are cerebral malignancies in this age group.

Invasive CNS cancers, especially cerebellar PNET-type tumors (medulloblastoma), brain stem gliomas, and ependymomas, are seen more frequently in boys, in younger children (younger than 10 years), and in Caucasian children. Although tumor type and location are important determinants of survivability, younger children in general tend to experience a more lethal disease course (Grovas et al., 1997; Heideman et al., 1997; NCI, 2000).

The incidence of CNS tumors drops at about age 7 years by 40%, compared with the higher rates seen in infants through 7 years. This drop continues until about age 10. Incidence rates for children ages 11 through 17 years is further decreased. This downward incidence is reported to fall even further by age 18.

Although rates of CNS cancers decrease with increasing age, the overall incidence in the United States continues to increase, with the increase seen over the past generation being a subject of much research. It has been postulated that environmental changes are at least partly responsible, although this reasoning has not been substantiated (Davis, Brownson, Garcia, Bentz, & Turner, 1993; Gurney et al., 1996). It is feasible that the higher incidence is in fact as much an outcome of improved case identification as an outcome of technological advances.

■ *Medulloblastoma*

Medulloblastoma is a primitive, PNET-type, neuroectodermal tumor arising from the cerebellum. Medulloblastoma accounts for 10% to 20% of all primary brain tumors in children (Heidman, Packer & Albright, 1997).

EPIDEMIOLOGY

Most cases of medulloblastoma are seen in the first decade of life, with a peak incidence at 5 years of age (Heideman et al., 1997; Smith et al., 1998; NCI, 2000).

HISTORY AND PHYSICAL EXAMINATION

Presenting symptoms and signs include those of increased intracranial pressure (headache, vomiting, lethargy, and papilledema) and ataxia of the lower extremities. Stiff neck and head tilt may indicate oculomotor paresis or impending herniation.

DIAGNOSTIC STUDIES

A contrast CT or MRI reveals the posterior fossa tumor. Because medulloblastoma has a propensity to spread by subarachnoid seeding, imaging of neuroaxis and cytologic examination of the spinal fluid are essential part of the initial evaluation. Diagnosis is confirmed after surgical removal of the tumor.

MANAGEMENT

Radiation to the craniospinal axis and chemotherapy offer the best chance of survival. Indicators of good prognosis include the following:

- Age older than 3 years
- Total or near-total resection (residual tumor < 1.5 cm^2) of a localized tumor
- No evidence of dissemination

Eighty percent of such patients are free of disease progression at 3 years (Deutsh et al., 1996; Thomas et al., 1995). Children with large residual tumor (>1.5 cm^2) after surgery, neuroaxis dissemination (subarachnoid seeding), or extraneural metastatic disease (bone or bone marrow) are considered to have high-risk medulloblastoma. Such patients have 67% progression-free survival at 5 years (Packer et al., 1994; NCI, 2000).

■ *Ependymoma*

PATHOLOGY, PHYSICAL EXAMINATION, AND MANAGEMENT

Ninety percent of ependymomas arise from the ependymal lining of the ventricular system. The remaining 10% arise from the central canal of the spinal cord. Sixty percent of the intracranial ependymomas occur in the posterior fossa. Similar to the other brain tumors discussed, median age at diagnosis is 5 years (Heideman et al., 1997; Smith et al., 1998). Ependymomas are locally invasive tumors that spread to the adjacent brain. Approximately 10% of patients have spinal subarachnoid dissemination. About 75% of ependymomas are histologically well differentiated, while the remainder are anaplastic in appearance. The histologic grading, however, does not predict outcome (Nazar et al., 1994; Smith et al., 1998).

● **Clinical Pearl:** Presenting signs and symptoms of ependymomas are those of increased intracranial pressure, which are nonspecific and nonlocalizing.

The extent of resection of the tumor markedly influences the prognosis. Patients who have complete resection (gross total resection) have a significantly higher rate of 5-year progression-free survival (82%) than patients who have incomplete resection of the tumor (20%) (Kun et al., 1996). All patients are treated with postoperative radiation therapy. Chemotherapy has not improved the outlook for children whose prognosis is poor.

■ Cerebellar Astrocytoma

PATHOLOGY AND MANAGEMENT

Cerebellar astrocytoma is among the most frequent brain tumors in children and is also one of the most curable. The majority are low grade, slow growing, well circumscribed, and often cystic. Complete excision of the tumor is feasible in about 65% of patients, for whom the expected cure rate is 100% without any additional radiation or chemotherapy. Partial resection, however, gives only a 56% 5-year survival rate (Gurney et al., 1999). It is unclear whether radiation or chemotherapy improves survival rates for patients who have had partial resection of their cerebellar astrocytoma.

■ Low-Grade Supratentorial Astrocytoma

PATHOLOGY, PHYSICAL EXAMINATION, AND MANAGEMENT

Like their cerebellar counterparts, low-grade supratentorial astrocytomas are slow-growing and nonaggressive tumors. They have a benign histologic appearance. Presenting clinical features depend on the location of the tumor and include the following:

- Signs of increased intracranial pressure
- Seizures
- Classic diencephalic syndrome in children younger than 3 years (emesis, emaciation, and euphoria in infants)
- Focal motor deficits
- Monoplegia or hemiplegia
- Chorea
- Dysmetria
- Neuroendocrine abnormalities (growth hormone deficiency, diabetes insipidus, precocious puberty)

As with cerebellar astrocytomas, complete resection of the tumor offers 95% to 100% survival at 5 years and eliminates the need for postoperative radiation therapy (Heideman et al., 1997). The role of radiation and chemotherapy in incompletely resected cases remains uncertain.

■ Optic Glioma

EPIDEMIOLOGY

Gliomas of the visual pathway (optic nerve, chiasm, and optic tract) account for about 5% of all primary CNS tumors in children. Seventy-five percent of all optic gliomas occur in the first decade of life, most of them in the first 5 years of life (Heideman et al., 1997). About 50% of cases are associated with neurofibromatosis (Gurney et al., 1999).

HISTORY AND PHYSICAL EXAMINATION

Slow and progressive visual loss is characteristic of optic gliomas. Young children, however, often present with nonspecific symptoms, such as strabismus, proptosis, nystagmus, and developmental difficulties. Infants with optic glioma may present with spasmus nutans and a clinical triad of head tilt, head bobbing, and nystagmus (either monocular or dissociated asymmetric). Funduscopic examination reveals optic pallor and atrophy in the affected eye. Visual acuity is frequently reduced to less than 20/200. Lesions of the posterior chiasm may involve the hypothalamus, causing hypothalamic dysfunction, including diabetes insipidus and diencephalic syndrome. Figure 64-2 illustrates a case of optic glioma in a 4-year-old boy.

MANAGEMENT

Biopsy has a high risk of worsening the visual loss. Thus, the diagnosis is often made only on the basis of imaging appearance on CT or MRI, especially in children with neurofibromatosis. Excision of the optic nerve tumor is possible in cases in which there is a clear margin between the tumor and the optic chiasm but only at the cost of unilateral blindness. As an alternative, high-dose radiation therapy may be prescribed by the oncologist to reduce the tumor mass, restore vision, and decrease proptosis. However, in young children (younger than 3 years), combination chemotherapy is used to control tumor progression and to delay radiation therapy. Patients with chiasmal tumors have 10-year survival rates of 40% to 85%, compared with 90% to 100% survival for patients with intraorbital tumors (Heideman et al., 1997).

■ Brain Stem Glioma

EPIDEMIOLOGY

Brain stem gliomas constitute 10% to 15% of all primary brain tumors. Two thirds of them are low-grade astrocytomas, and one third are high-grade astrocytomas and

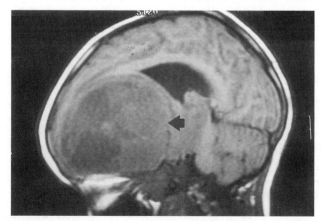

Figure 64–2 ■ Magnetic resonance imaging scan shows a large mass *(arrow)* arising from the optic chiasm. This 4-year-old boy presented with headache, vomiting, and visual disturbances. He underwent a gross total resection. Histologic diagnosis was pilocytic astrocytoma.

glioblastomas. Brain stem gliomas can be divided into five subgroups:

- Diffuse
- Focal
- Cystic
- Dorsal exophytic
- Cervicomedullary

About 85% of all brain stem gliomas are diffuse tumors of the pons and medulla (Heideman et al., 1997).

HISTORY AND PHYSICAL EXAMINATION

Patients with diffuse brain stem glioma of the pons and medulla have rapid progression of symptoms and often present with the clinical triad of long tract signs, multiple cranial nerve palsies, and cerebellar ataxia. Focal tumors have an insidious course and present with isolated cranial nerve deficits and contralateral hemiplegia. Patients with exophytic tumors also have an insidious course with symptoms of increased intracranial pressure. Deficits of cranial nerves VI and VII, long tract signs, and sometimes torticollis are the presenting symptoms of cervicomedullary tumors.

MANAGEMENT

Corticosteroids followed by radiation therapy is the standard therapy for diffuse brain stem glioma. Patients with diffuse brain stem gliomas of the pons and medulla have a very poor prognosis. The 2-year survival rate is 23%, but 3-year survival drops to 11% (Packer et al., 1994; Heideman et al., 1997). However, patients with dorsal exophytic tumors, cervicomedullary tumors, and focal tumors in the midbrain have an excellent chance of survival, because these tumors are amenable to surgery.

■ *Neuroblastoma*

PATHOLOGY

Neuroblastoma is a malignancy involving the cells of neural crest that normally develop into adrenal medulla and sympathetic ganglia. It is the most common extracranial solid tumor in children, occurring predominantly in young children; 36% are younger than 1 year and 79% are younger than 4 years (Brodeur & Castleberry, 1997).

PHYSICAL EXAMINATION AND DIAGNOSTIC CRITERIA

The presenting clinical features of neuroblastoma vary according to the site of primary, regional, or metastatic disease (Table 64-3). The abdomen is the most common site of primary incidence (65%). Children older than 1 year have a higher incidence of adrenal tumors and a lower incidence of thoracic and cervical tumors than do infants younger than 1 (Brodeur & Castleberry, 1997). Figure 64-3A shows a CT scan of the head demonstrating a large cranial mass in a child. Figure 64-3B reproduces abdominal CT findings of a large

Table 64–3. NEUROBLASTOMA: PRESENTING CLINICAL FEATURES

Site of Origin	Presenting Clinical Feature
Primary	
Adrenal gland, abdominal sympathetic chain	Abdominal mass
Posterior mediastinal sympathetic chain	Posterior mediastinal mass detected on routine chest film, spinal cord compression
Pelvic sympathetic chain	Urinary frequency, inability to void
Cervical sympathetic chain	Cervical lymphadenopathy; Horner's syndrome: miosis, narrowing of palpebral fissure, anhidrosis; heterochromia
Olfactory bulb	Esthesioneuroblastoma: unilateral nasal obstruction, epistaxis
Metastatic	
Skin, liver	Subcutaneous nodules, massive hepatomegaly especially in newborn period
Bones	Generalized pain in extremities
Bone marrow	Anemia, thrombocytopenia
Periorbital soft tissue	Proptosis, periorbital ecchymoses—racoon-like appearance
Paraneoplastic	
Vasoactive intestinal peptide	Intractable diarrhea
Autoimmune phenomenon	Opsomyoclonus, ataxia
Prenatal	
	Abdominal or adrenal mass detected on routine prenatal sonogram of the abdomen

abdominal mass in this same patient, which proved to be neuroblastoma.

Stage and Age

The stage of the tumor according to the International Neuroblastoma Staging System and the age at diagnosis are two of the most important prognostic factors. The 3-year EFS rates for various ages and stages are given in Table 64-4.

Genetic Markers

Recently, various genetic markers have been found to have great prognostic significance. Amplification of N-myc (an oncogene), seen in 30% to 40% of advanced stage tumors, is associated with a very poor prognosis. Infants whose tumor cells have a DNA index of greater than 1 (hyperdipoidy) are more likely to have early-stage disease and have a favorable prognosis regardless of stage. Conversely, diploid tumors (DNA index of 1) are associated with less favorable prognosis.

DIAGNOSTIC STUDIES

The primary mass is evaluated by a CT or MRI scan. A biopsy of the tumor tissue is essential for the confirmation of

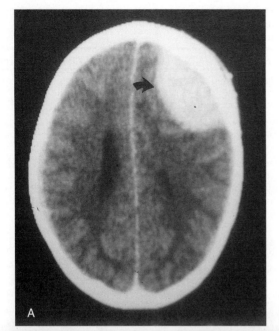

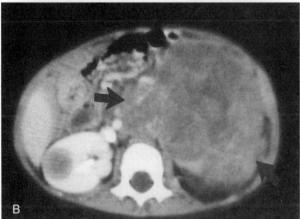

Figure 64–3 ■ This 15-month-old boy presented with a large mass on his frontal bone. On physical examination, a left-sided abdominal mass was palpable. (**A**) Computed tomographic (CT) scan of the head shows a mass *(arrow)* arising from the cranial bone. (**B**) CT scan of the abdomen reveals a large abdominal mass *(arrows)*, which was diagnosed as neuroblastoma by biopsy.

the diagnosis and for obtaining adequate samples for biologic studies, such as N-myc and DNA index. Urinary catecholamines—vanillyl mandelic acid and homovanillic acid—are elevated at the time of diagnosis in more than 90% of patients. The oncologist will follow these levels during and off treatment to monitor the activity of the disease. Investigations aimed at detecting metastases include bilateral bone marrow aspirates and biopsies, bone scans, skeletal surveys, abdominal CTs, plain chest films, and chest CT if the plain films are abnormal (Brodeur et al., 1993).

MANAGEMENT

Current treatment of neuroblastoma is based on the risk of relapse. Patients are assigned to low, intermediate, or high risk using a complex algorithm that takes into account age, stage, N-myc amplification, and DNA index. Low-risk

Table 64–4. PROGNOSIS OF NEUROBLASTOMA ACCORDING TO AGE AND STAGE

International Staging System	3-year Event-Free Survival		
	All Age Groups	Infants (1 yr)	Children 1 yr
Stages 1, 2, and 4S	75%–90%		
Stage 3		80%–90%	50%
Stage 4		60%–75%	15%

Adapted with permission from Castleberry, R. P. (1997). Biology and treatment of neuroblastoma. *Pediatric Clinics of North America, 44,* 919–937.

patients are treated with surgery alone. Intermediate-risk group patients usually undergo chemotherapy and second-look surgery but not irradiation. Patients at high risk of relapse are treated with combination therapy, because it offers a 2-year EFS rate of 50% for these patients at high risk of demise. The oncologist will typically use the following sequence:

- Chemotherapy to achieve remission or a good response
- Second-look surgery to remove any residual tumor
- High-dose (marrow-ablative dose) chemotherapy with autologous stem cell rescue
- Local irradiation to the site of original tumor
- Retinoic acid therapy aimed at differentiation of the tumor cells (Castleberry, 1997)

■ *Nephroblastoma: Wilms' Tumor*

PATHOLOGY

Nephroblastoma, or Wilm' tumor, is a malignant embryonic mixed tumor (International Society of Pediatric Oncology Classification). It is classified into five stages, depending on the extent, infiltration of neighboring organs, metastases, and bilateral involvement. Wilms' tumor has the best prognosis among the malignant tumors seen in childhood. Depending on the histologic grade, the relapse-free survival rate is 80% to 90%.

Classic Wilms' tumor is composed of three histologic elements: persistent blastema, dysplastic tubules, and supporting mesenchyma or stroma. Tumors that show diffuse anaplasia (large nuclei and multipolar mitotic figures) or sarcomatous features, as seen in clear cell sarcoma of the kidney or rhabdoid tumor of the kidney, are considered to have unfavorable histology. However, almost 90% of patients have a tumor with a favorable histology (Green et al., 1994.)

EPIDEMIOLOGY

Wilms' tumor accounts for 6% to 7% of all childhood cancers. It is the most common solid tumor of the kidneys in children, responsible for more than 90% of all malignant renal tumors and is found in all races (Green et al., 1994a; Altman & Quinn, 1998). The annual incidence of Wilms' tumor is eight cases per million Caucasian children in the United States younger than 15 years. Nearly 80% of patients are younger than 5 years. Its incidence in African American children in the United States and Africa is approximately twice that of Caucasian children (Petruzzi & Green, 1997).

HISTORY AND PHYSICAL EXAMINATION

Children with renal tumors usually present with an asymptomatic abdominal mass often detected by the mother or occasionally by the primary care provider. Less common presenting symptoms include gross hematuria (8%–25% of cases), abdominal pain, and fever, which may be associated with hemorrhage into the tumor (8% of cases). Hypertension is present in 25% of patients at diagnosis. About 6% of patients have bilateral Wilms' tumor at presentation (Green et al., 1994a; Grosfeld, 1999). Figure 64-4 reproduces an abdominal CT scan that revealed a left-sided Wilms' tumor.

DIAGNOSTIC STUDIES

Ultrasonography is the initial imaging study of choice. It differentiates solid from cystic masses, and it can detect tumor thrombus in the renal vein and inferior vena cava, a finding of great surgical importance. Plain two-view chest films are adequate to detect pulmonary metastases. A CT or MRI scan of the abdomen provides further anatomic details of surgical importance. Metastatic disease is seen in 10% to 15% of cases at diagnosis; lung is the most common site (85%) followed

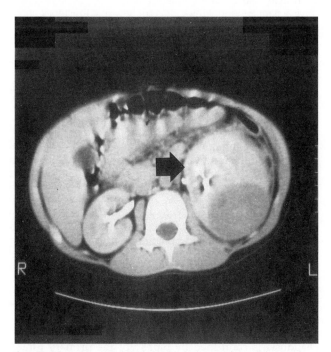

Figure 64–4 ■ Computed tomographic (CT) scan of the abdomen reveals a left-sided intrarenal (Wilms') tumor *(arrow)*. A circumscribed area within the mass represents hemorrhage (demonstrated after surgery). This 5-year-old boy presented with vomiting and abdominal pain. Physical examination did not reveal any abdominal mass. However, the CT scan was done because of microscopic hematuria. Wilms' tumor usually presents as a painless mass. The abdominal pain in this child was probably caused by hemorrhage within the tumor.

by liver (7%) and both liver and lung (8%) (Shochat, 1994; Green et al., 1994a; Grosfeld, 1999).

MANAGEMENT

The approach to management that the pediatric oncologist will take in treating Wilms' tumor depends on the clinicopathologic staging and the histology. Any patient with unilateral Wilms' tumor will undergo nephrectomy of the involved kidney, which allows removal of the entire tumor without spillage in most cases. The tumor may be unresectable if it is large, has infiltrated vital structures, or there is involvement of the inferior vena cava. In these instances, preoperative chemotherapy will be administered by the pediatric oncologist for 4 to 6 weeks to decrease the size of the tumor (Green et al., 1994b; Grosfeld, 1999).

Children who are relapse free at 4 years can be considered cured. Few patients relapse after 2 years from nephrectomy. With current therapy and depending on the tumor's histopathology, upwards of 90% of all children with Wilms' tumor are cured (Grosfield, 1999).

■ *Rhabdomyosarcoma*

Rhabdomyosarcoma is the most common form of soft-tissue sarcoma in children. It occurs at a rate of 4% to 8% of all malignant solid tumors in the pediatric population (Godambe & Rawal, 2000). About half the cases occur before the age of 5 years, and 10% of cases occur before age 1. The site and incidence of primary tumors are as follows:

- Genitourinary tract: 24%
- Extremities: 19%
- Parameningeal: 16%
- Head and neck: 10%
- Orbit: 9%
- Other sites: 22% (Pappo et al., 1995)

Table 64-5 provides information about incidence, site, and presenting symptoms of rhabdomyosarcoma.

PATHOLOGY

Soft-tissue sarcomas in children continue to present a challenge for pathologic classification, which also makes diagnosis and treatment difficult. Embryonal is the most common type of rhabdomyosarcoma, accounting for 60% of cases. Alveolar and undifferentiated histology account for approximately 20% each. Alveolar-type histology is usually associated with a unique chromosomal translocation of the malignant cells, t(2;13). Clinicopathologically, rhabdomyosarcoma can be classified into four groups:

- Group I: Completely resected tumor
- Group II: Grossly resected tumor with the presence of microscopic residue, nodal involvement, or extension into the adjacent organs
- Group III: Incomplete resection or biopsy with gross residual disease
- Group IV: Distant metastases present at diagnosis (Neville et al., 2000)

Table 64–5. SIGNS AND SYMPTOMS OF RHABDOMYOSARCOMA ACCORDING TO THE LOCATION OF TUMOR

Orbit	Exophthalmos, ptosis, swelling of eyelids
Middle ear	Bloody aural discharge, facial nerve palsy, polypoid mass in aural canal
Nasopharynx	Airway obstruction, nasal discharge, polypoid mass in nose, serous otitis media
Oropharynx	Dyspahagia, painful mastication
Neck	Mass, cervical or brachial palsy, pain
Prostate	Urinary obstruction
Bladder	Urinary obstruction, hematuria
Vagina, uterus	Botryoid mass at the vaginal opening
Scrotum, spermatic cord	Mass
Buttocks	Mass
Extremity	Mass lesion, local pain

Adapted with permission from Altman, A. A., & Schwartz, A. D. (1983). The soft tissue sarcomas. In Altman A. A., & Schwartz A. D. (Eds.), *Malignant diseases of infancy, childhood and adolescence* (2nd ed.) (pp. 423–444). Philadelphia: WB Saunders.

Note: None of the more recent pediatric oncology resources have content as comprehensive as that provided in this reference. Symptoms and signs of the disease are not likely to change along with advances in science. The reader should not be concerned about the currency of the reference.

MANAGEMENT

Complete surgical removal of a localized tumor cures 85% of patients. Conversely, metastatic disease at diagnosis is associated with very poor prognosis, with only 20% chance of cure. The site of the primary disease also has prognostic significance. Orbital primary disease has the best prognosis (95% cure), followed by genitourinary, head and neck, extremities, and parameningeal (65%) primary tumors. Chemotherapy is effective against rhabdomyosarcoma, and it is used in all stages. Radiation therapy is indicated for all patients except stage I patients (Cecchetto et al., 2000).

■ *Lymphomas*

■ *Non-Hodgkin's Lymphoma*

PATHOLOGY

A lymphoid cell malignancy, non-Hodgkin's lymphoma (NHL) is divided into three histologic types:

1. Small noncleaved cell
2. Lymphoblastic
3. Large cell lymphomas

An aggressive malignancy of T- or B-lymphocytes, NHL has a varied presentation depending on the site of the origin and the stage of the disease. Lymphomas are the third most common group of malignancies in children, after leukemias and brain tumors. The correlation between histopathology, the cell of origin, the cytogenetic features, and the site of the primary tumor is given in Table 64-6.

EPIDEMIOLOGY

The third leading cause of cancer in children is the lymphomas, at a rate of approximately 15%. Of these, about 60% are NHL, and the remainder are Hodgkin's disease (Grovas et al., 1997; NCI, 2000). NHL has a male predominance, with a 3:1 male-to-female ratio. The incidence of NHL in Caucasian children is twice as much as in African American children (Grovas et al., 1997; NCI, 2000).

HISTORY AND PHYSICAL EXAMINATION

The frequency of the various sites of origin of NHL includes the following:

- Abdomen: 31%
- Mediastinum: 26%
- Head and neck, including the Wadeyer ring and cervical lymph nodes: 29%
- Noncervical nodes: 7%
- Other sites (skin, thyroid, epidural space, and bone): 7% (Sandlund, 1996)

● **Clinical Pearl:** Not infrequently, NHL may first present as cervical lymphadenopathy that is rubbery in consistency and almost always symptomatic.

▲ **Clinical Warning:** Any child with such a presentation should be watched, whether febrile or not. If lymphadenopathy continues for 2 weeks or longer, the provider should refer the patient for evaluation by a pediatric oncologist. It is extremely rare to find lymphadenopathy of lymphoma on routine examination in an asymptomatic child.

Abdominal tumors usually arise at the ileocecal region and may present with pain or abdominal distention. In some cases, the symptoms mimic those of appendicitis or intussusception.

Mediastinal masses present with cough, wheezing, respiratory distress, or as superior vena cava syndrome, symptoms similar to mediastinal Hodgkin's disease. Less common presentations include painless cervical mass, tonsillar mass, and spinal cord compression caused by an epidural mass.

DIAGNOSTIC STUDIES

Diagnosis is confirmed by biopsy of the primary tumor; excisional biopsy may be feasible in some abdominal tumors. Evaluation of the tumor tissue should include flow cytometric analysis of cell-surface (immunologic) markers and cytogenetic studies. CT scans of chest, abdomen, and pelvis help define the extent of the regional disease. A bone scan, gallium scan, and examination of the spinal fluid and bone marrow are necessary to detect metastatic disease.

Table 64–6. HISTOPATHOLOGY OF NON-HODGKIN'S LYMPHOMA: CORRELATION WITH CELL OF ORIGIN AND CLINICAL AND CYTOGENETIC FEATURES

Histologic Type (Frequency)	Cell of Origin	Site of Primary Tumor	Cytogenetic Abnormalities
Small noncleaved cell (50%)	B cell	Abdomen	t(8;14), t(2;8), t(8;22)
Lymphoblastic (33%)	T cell	Mediastinum	
Large cell (17%)	B cell, T cell, or non-B non-T cell	Any site	t(2;5)

DIAGNOSTIC CRITERIA

It is important that the provider refer the patient to a pediatric oncology center for the diagnostic workup.

The staging system for NHL is as follows:

- Stage I: single tumors outside abdomen or mediastinum
- Stage II: single extranodal area with regional lymph node, two or more nodal areas on the same side of the diaphragm, grossly resected intra-abdominal tumor
- Stage III: disease on both sides of the diaphragm, extensive abdominal disease, all mediastinal tumors
- Stage IV: involvement of CNS or bone marrow

MANAGEMENT

Chemotherapy is the mainstay of treatment for NHL. Approximately 80% to 90% of children with early stage disease (stages I and II) and 70% to 80% of children with advanced-stage tumors (stages III and IV) currently can be cured of their disease (Reiter et al., 1995; Magrath et al., 1996; Shad & Mcgrath, 1997; NCI, 2000).

■ Hodgkin's Disease

Hodgkin's disease is a malignancy of lymphoid cells with varied histologic patterns. In children, Hodgkin's disease usually occurs after 12 years of age; it is uncommon in children younger than 10 years.

PATHOLOGY

The finding of EBV genome in the malignant Reed-Sternberg cells suggests a direct role of EBV in Hodgkin's disease. However, there is no risk of transmission of Hodgkin's disease from person to person. The histopathology shows a mixture of various inflammatory cells mixed with the Reed-Sternberg cells and the mononuclear Hodgkin's cells. Four histologic subtypes of Hodgkin's disease have been described. As seen in Table 64-7, these subtypes have different clinical characteristics.

HISTORY AND PHYSICAL EXAMINATION

Children with Hodgkin's disease usually present with a slowly enlarging, painless cervical or supraclavicular lymph node of 3 cm or more in size, which may have a firm, rub-

bery quality. Respiratory symptoms can also be present and include cough, wheezing, and respiratory distress. Respiratory symptoms are caused by an anterior mediastinal mass similar to that seen in Figure 64-5. Systemic symptoms include fever, night sweats, pruritus, and weight loss. Hematologic findings usually show neutrophilic leukocytosis, lymphopenia, anemia, and increased sedimentation rate. Other laboratory features include high serum copper and ferritin levels.

DIAGNOSTIC STUDIES

Definitive diagnosis of Hodgkin's disease is made from the biopsy of the involved lymph node. The extent of the disease is evaluated by CT scans of the neck, chest, abdomen and pelvis, whole body gallium scan, and bone marrow biopsy. Staging laparotomy is rarely done in children, because most children are treated with chemotherapy with or without additional radiation. The extent of the disease is classified

Table 64–7. HODGKIN'S DISEASE: CORRELATION OF HISTOPATHOLOGIC TYPES AND CLINICAL FEATURES

Histopathologic Type (Incidence)	Clinical Features
Nodular sclerosis (50%)	Most common type in adolescents (70%); lower cervical, supraclavicular, and mediastinal nodes commonly involved
Mixed cellularity (25%)	More common in younger patients (< 10 years of age); more likely to present with advanced disease and with extranodal disease
Lymphocyte predominance (20%)	Cervical lymphadenopathy in males; usually localized; most favorable prognosis
Lymphocyte depletion (5%)	Presents as mediastinal mass; > 80% of patients have advanced disease (stage III or IV) at diagnosis

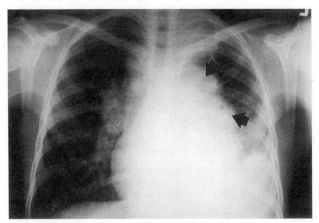

Figure 64–5 ■ Chest radiograph shows an anterior mediastinal mass *(arrow)*, enlarged hilar lymph nodes, and a left-sided pleural effusion. This 12-year-old girl presented with complaints of fatigue, cough, and difficulty in breathing after exercise. Biopsy of an enlarged inguinal lymph node showed Hodgkin's disease—nodular sclerosis type.

into four stages:

- Stage I: disease confined to a single node or extra nodal site
- Stage II: two or more nodes (one organ or site plus one node) on the same side of the diaphragm
- Stage III: disease on both sides of the diaphragm
- Stage IVA: evidence of distant dissemination of disease to one or more organs or tissues (liver, lung, bone, bone marrow, or CNS). B-symptoms may be present at any stage (B systemic symptoms are present [temperature of > 38°C for 3 consecutive days, drenching night sweats, or unexplained loss of about 10% of body weight in the preceding 6 months]) (Hudson & Donaldson, 1997).

MANAGEMENT

Chemotherapy alone remains the mainstay of treatment for early stage disease (stages I and II) in children, with disease-free survival rates of 90% to 100% long-term. A combination of chemotherapy and low-dose radiation therapy offers the best chance of cure for patients with advanced-stage disease (IIB, III, and IV) and for those with large mediastinal masses. The rates for disease-free survival range from 90% to 100% for early stage disease and from 60% to 94% for advanced disease (Hudson & Donaldson, 1997). Treatment-related late effects include sterility, secondary malignancies, cardiac toxicity, and pulmonary toxicity. Radiation therapy can enhance all of the aforementioned chemotherapy-induced toxicities.

COMMUNITY RESOURCES

American Cancer Society
Cancer in Children Resource Center
Telephone: (800) ACS-2345 (24 hours a day)
Internet address: *http://www.cancer.org*

This society provides parents and children with information about cancer causes and risks. Information about prevention, new diagnostic techniques, and current treatment options is provided.

Canadian Cancer Society
Internet address: *http://www.cancer.ca*

Cancer Kids Web Site
Internet address: *http://www.cancerkids.org*

This website for children with cancer is focused on providing a forum for sharing stories. An on-line book store is featured. Prayer is a focus; memorial pictures are posted.

▲ **Clinical Warning:** This site should be prescreened by the provider before recommending to a family, particularly if the family is feeling at all fragile. Although the purpose of the site is to provide on-line support, some families or children may find the emphasis on prayer and memorial items difficult.

CancerNet
Internet address: *http://www.cancernet.nci.nih.gov/index.html*
This on-line resource for providers and families is provided by the National Cancer Institute.

Cancer Information Network
Internet address: *http://www.cancernetwork.com*

The Cancer Network provides educational materials for professionals and for patients and their families. Links to other cancer-related sites are maintained. The mission of this nonprofit organization is improvement of the quality of life of children with cancer. Financial and in-kind assistance, advocacy, support services, education, and prevention activities are available.

Cancer Research Foundation of America
1600 Duke Street
Suite 110
Alexandria, VA 22314
Telephone: (800) 227-CRFA
Internet address: *http://www.preventcancer.org*
The web site provides links to children's health activities.

Eye Cancer Network
Internet address: *http://www.eyecancer.com*

This on-line resource provides information about eye cancers, including visual materials. Links to both professional and patient resources are provided.

Leukemia and Lymphoma Society (formerly the Leukemia Society of America)
Telephone: (800) 955-4572
E-mail: *infocenter@leukemia-lymphoma.org*
Internet address: *http://www.leukemia-lymphoma.org*

The society works through local affiliates. Its purpose is to help in the search for cures for leukemia, lymphoma, Hodgkin's disease, and myeloma. Providers will find educational and support resources appropriate for children and family members, including an innovative "Back to School" program that helps the child to reconnect with peers and school work after the kinds of stressful absences that accompany cancer and its treatment. Links to other cancer sites and resources are provided at this site.

National Brain Tumor Foundation
414 Thirteenth Street, Suite 700
Oakland, CA 94612-2603
Telephone: (510) 839-9777

Toll-free: (800) 934-CURE (2873)
E-mail: *nbtf@braintumor.org*
Internet address: http://*www.braintumor.org*

This organization provides a forum for sharing personal stories. Research activities are highlighted. The web site has a useful feature for parents to contact a foundation nurse for more information.

National Children's Cancer Society
1015 Locust, Suite 600
St. Louis, MO 63101
Telephone: (800) 532-6459
E-mail: pfs@children-cancer.com
Internet address: *http://www.children-cancer.com*

OncoLink
Internet address: *http://www.oncolink.upenn.edu*

The Internet site maintained by the University of Pennsylvania Cancer Center. Like many other sites, it offers an array of provider and patient resources. The site's Children's Art Gallery is particularly poignant, yet full of hope.

Pediatric Cancer Foundation
405 Tarrytown Road, Suite 572
White Plains, NY 10607
Telephone (914) 777-3127
Internet address: *http://www.pcfweb.org*

This organization is a resource for cancer information for both providers and families.

Starbright Foundation
1990 South Bundy Drive, Suite 100
Los Angeles, CA 90025
Telephone: (310) 442-1560
Internet address: *http://www.starbright.org*

This nonprofit organization is a family and child resource for fun educational materials focused on helping children deal with serious illness.

CancerLinks
Internet address: http://*www.cancerlinks.net*

This is a wonderful website because it is specially designed to make searching the World Wide Web for information about cancer faster and easier. Cancer topics are individually linked at the site to sources about disease effects and treatment. The site is regularly updated and contains a tutorial for using links. A Spanish version of the tutorial is also featured.

REFERENCES

Altman, A. (1997). Chronic leukemias of childhood. In P. A. Pizzo & D. G. Poplack (Eds.), *Principles and practice of pediatric oncology* (p. 1319). Philadelphia: Lippincott Raven.

Altman, A. J., & Quinn, J. J. (1998). Management of malignant solid tumors. In D. G. Nathan & S. H. Orkin (Eds.), *Nathan and Oski's hematology of infancy and childhood* (p. 1381). Philadelphia: W.B. Saunders.

Arlt, W., Hove, U., Muller, B., Reincke, M., Berweiler, U., et al. (1997). Frequent and frequently overlooked: Treatment-induced endocrine dysfunction in adult long-term survivors of primary brain tumors. *Neurology, 49,* 498–506.

Blatt, J., Copeland, R., & Bleyer, A. (1997). Late effects of childhood cancer and its treatment. In P. A. Pizzo & D. G. Poplack (Eds.),

Principles and practice of pediatric oncology (3rd ed.) (p. 1303). Philadelphia: Lippincott Raven.

Brodeur, G. M., & Castleberry, R. P. (1997). Neuroblastoma. In P. A. Pizzo & D. G. Poplack (Eds.), *Principles and practice of pediatric oncology* (3rd ed.) (p. 761). Philadelphia: Lippincott Raven.

Brodeur, G. M., Pritchard, J., Berthold, F., et al. (1993). Revision in the interational criteria for diagnosis, staging, and response to treatment. *Journal of Clinical Oncology, 11,* 1466.

Castleberry, R. P. (1997). Biology and treatment of neuroblastoma. *Pediatric Clinics of North America, 44,* 919–937.

Cecchetto, G., Carli, M., Sotti, G., Bisogno, G., Dall'Igna, P., et al. (2000). Importance of local treatment in pediatric soft tissue sarcomas with microscopic residual after primary surgery: Results of the Italian Cooperative Study RMS-88. *Medical Pediatric Oncology, 34,* 97–101.

Davis, J. R., Brownson, R. C., Garcia, R., Bentz, B. J., & Turner, A. (1993). Family pesticide use and childhood brain cancer. *Archives of Environmental Contamination and Toxicology, 24,* 87–92.

Deutsh, M., Thomas, P. R. M., Krischer, et al. (1996). Results of a prospective randomized trial comparing standard dose neuraxis radiation (3600 cGy/20) with reduced neuraxis irradiation (2430 cGy/13) in patients with low-stage medulloblastoma: A combined Children's Cancer Group—Pediatric Oncology group study. *Pediatric Neurosurgery, 24,* 167–177.

Ebb, D. H., & Weinstein, H. J. (1997). Diagnosis and treatment of childhood acute myelogenous leukemia. *Pediatric Clinics of North America, 44,* 847–862.

El-Sadr, W. T., Luskin-Hawk, R., Yurik, T. M., et al. (1999). A randomized trial of daily and thrice-weekly trimethoprim-sulfamethoxazole for the prevention of Pneumocystis carinii pneumonia in human immunodeficiency virus-infected persons. Terry Beirn Community Programs for Clinical Research on AIDS. *Clinical Infectious Diseases, 29,* 775–783.

Fauroux, B., Clement, A., & Tournier, G. (1996). Pulmonary toxicity of drugs and thoracic irradiation in children. *Revue des Maladies Respiratoires, 3,* 235–242.

Freifeld, A. G., Walsch, J. W., & Pizzo, P. A. (1997). Infectious complications in the pediatric cancer patient. In P. A. Pizzo & D. G. Poplack (Eds.), *Principles and practice of pediatric oncology* (3rd ed.) (p. 1102). Philadelphia: Lippincott Raven.

Godambe, S. V., & Rawal, J. (2000). Blueberry muffin rash as a presentation of alveolar cell rhabdomyosarcoma in a neonate. *Acta Paediatrica, 89,* 115–117.

Goodman, J. L., Winston, D. J., Greenfield, R., A., et al. (1992) Controlled trial of fluconazole to prevent fungal infections in patients undergoing bone marrow transplantation. *New England Journal of Medicine, 326,* 845.

Green, D. M., Beckwith, J. B., Weeks, D. A., Moksness, J., Breslow, N. E., & D'Angio, G. J. (1994a). The relationship between microsubstaging variables, age at diagnosis, and tumor weight of children with stage I/favorable histology Wilms' tumor: A report from the National Wilms' Tumor study. *Cancer, 74,* 1817–1820.

Green, D. M., Beckwith, J. B., Breslowm N. E., et al. (1994b). The treatment of children with anaplastic Wilms' tumor. A report from the National Wilms' Tumor Study Group. *Journal of Clinical Oncology, 12,* 2126.

Gurney, J. G., Mueller, B. A., Davis, S., & Schwartz, S. M. (1996). Childhood brain tumor occurrence in relation to residential power line configurations, electric heating sources, and electric appliance use. *American Journal of Epidemiology, 143,* 120–128.

Gurney, J. G., Wall, D. A., Jukich, P. J., & Davis, F. G. (1999). The contribution of nonmalignant tumors to CNS tumor incidence rates among children in the United States. *Cancer Causes and Control, 10,* 101–105.

Heideman, R. L., Packer, R. J., Albright, L. A., et al. (1997). Tumors of the central nervous system. In P. A. Pizzo & D. G. Poplack (Eds.), *Principles and practice of pediatric oncology* (3rd ed.) (p. 633). Philadelphia: Lippincott Raven.

Henry, D. H., & Ables, R I., (1995). Benefits of epoetin alpha therapy in anemic cancer patients receiving chemotherapy. *Journal of Clinical Oncology 13,* 2473.

Hudson, M. M., & Donaldson, S. S. (1997). Hodgkin's disease. *Pediatric Clinics of North America, 44,* 891–906.

Kreisman, H., & Wolkove, N. (1992). Pulmonary toxicity of antineoplastic therapy. *Seminars in Oncology, 19,* 508-520.

Krischer, J. P., Epstein, S., Cuthberston, D. D., et al. (1997). Clinical cardiotoxicity following anthracycline treatment for childhood cancer: The pediatric oncology group experience. *Journal of Clinical Oncology, 15,* 1544–1552.

Kun, L., Burger, P., Kovnar, E., et al. (1996). Childhood intracranial ependymomas: Prospective study of surgery and radiation therapy (RT). *Journal of Neurological Oncology, 28,* 71.

Lipshultz, S. E., Colan, S. D., Gelber, R. D., et al. (1991). Late cardiac effects of doxorubicin therapy for acute lymphoblastic leukemia in childhood. *New England Journal of Medicine, 324,* 808–815.

Magrath, I. T., Adde, M., Shad, A., et al. (1996). Adults and children with small non-cleaved cell lymphoma have similar excellent outcome when treated with the same chemotherapy regimen. *Journal of Clinical Oncology, 14,* 925–934.

Margolin, J., & Poplack, D. (1997). Acute lymphoblastic leukemia. In P. A. Pizzo & D. G. Poplack (Eds.), *Principles and practice of pediatric oncology* (3rd ed.) (p. 409). Philadelphia: Lippincott Raven.

Marina, N. (1997). Long-term survivors of childhood cancer. The medical consequences of cure. *Pediatric Clinics of North America, 44,* 1021–1042.

Nazar, G. B., Hoffman, H. J., Becker, L. E., et al. (1994). Infratentorialependymomas on childhood: Prognostic factors and treatment. *Journal of Neurosurgery, 72,* 408–417.

Neville, H. L., Andrassy, R. J., Lobe, T. E., Bagwell, C. E., Anderson, J. R., et al. (2000). Preoperative staging, prognostic factors, and outcome for extremity rhabdomyosarcoma: A preliminary report from the Intergroup Rhabdomyosarcoma Study IV (1991–1997). *Journal of Pediatric Surgery, 35,* 317–321.

Ortega, A., Dranitsaris, G., & Puodziunas, A. L. (1998). What are cancer patients willing to pay for the prophylactic epoetin alfa? A cost-benefit analysis. *Cancer, 83,* 2588–2596.

Packer, R. J., Sutton, L. N., Elterman, R., et al. (1994). Outcome for children with medulloblastoma treated with radiation and cisplatin, CCNU, and vincristine chemotherapy. Journal of Neurosurgery, 81, 690–698.

Pappo, A. S., Shapiro, D. N., Crist, W. M., et al. (1995). Biology and therapy of rhabdomyosarcoma. *Journal of Clinical Oncology, 13,* 21–23.

Perin, G. M., & Kramer, R. F. (1985). The child and family facing death. In Waechter, E. H., Phillips, J., & Holaday, B. (Eds.). (p. 1333). *Nursing care.* Philaelphia: J. B. Lippincott.

Petruzzi, M. J., & Green, D. M. (1997). Wilms' tumor. *Pediatric Clinics of North America, 44,* 939–952.

Pui, C. (1997). Acute lymphoblastic leukemia. *Pediatric Clinics of North America, 44,* 831–846.

Pui, C., & Evans, W. E. (1998). Acute lymphoblastic leukemia. *New England Journal of Medicine, 339,* 605–615.

Pui, C. (1995). Acute lymphoblastic leukemia. *New England Journal of Medicine, 332,* 1618.

Ravindranath, Y., Abella, E., Krischer, J., et al. (1992). Acute myeloid leukemia (AML) in Down's syndrome is highly responsive to chemotherapy: AML study 8498. *Blood, 80,* 2210.

Ravindranath, Y., & Taub, J. W. (1999). Down syndrome and acute myeloid leukemia: Lessons learned from experience with high-dose Ara-C containing regimens. *Advances in Experimental Medicine and Biology, 457,* 409–414.

Ravindranath, Y., Yeager, A. M., Chang, M. N., Steuber, C. P., Krischer, J., et al. (1996). Autologous bone marrow transplantation versus intensive consolidation chemotherapy for acute myeloid leukemia in childhood. *New England Journal of Medicine, 334,* 1428–1434.

Reiter, A., Schrappe, M., Parwaresch, R., et al. (1995). Non-Hodgkin's lymphoma of childhood and adolescence: Results of treatment stratified for biological subtypes and stage—a report from BFM group. *Journal of Clinical Oncology, 12,* 899.

National Cancer Institute. (2000). *Cancer in children (ages 0-14 and 0-19).* National Cancer Institute SEER Pediatric Monograph cancer statistics review, U.S. Department of Health and Human Services, National Institute of Health, Bethesda, MD.

Grovas, A., Fremgen, A., Rauck, A., Ruymann, F. B., Hutchinson, C. L., et al. (1997). The National Cancer Data Base report on patterns of childhood cancers in the United States. *Cancer, 80,* 2321–2332.

Riley, L. C., Hann, I. M., Wheatley, K., & Stevens, R. F. (1999). Treatment-related deaths during induction and first remission of acute myeloid leukemia in children treated on the Tenth Medical Research Council acute myeloid leukemia trial (MRC AML10). The MCR Childhood Leukemia Working Party. *British Journal of Haematology, 106,* 436–444.

Ritter, J., & Schrappe, M. (1999). Clinical features and therapy of acute lymphoblastic leukemia. In J. Lilleyman, I., Hann, V. Blanchette (Eds.), *Pediatric hematology* (p. 537). London: Churchill Livingstone.

Sandlund, J. T. (1996). Non-Hodgkin's lymphoma. In R. E. Berman, R. M. Kliegman, & A. M. Arvin (Eds.), *Nelson textbook of pediatrics* (15th ed.). Philadelphia: W.B. Saunders.

Shad, A., & Magrath, I. (1997). Non-Hodgkin's lymphoma. *Pediatric Clinics of North America, 44,* 863–890.

Shochat, S. J. (1994). Wilms' tumor: Diagnosis and treatment in the 1990s. *Seminars in Pediatric Surgery, 2,* 59–68.

Smith, M. A., Feidlin, B., Ries, L. A. G., & Simon, R. (1998). Trends in reported incidence of primary malignant brain tumors in children in the United States. *Journal of the National Cancer Institute, 90,* 1269–1277.

Thomas, P. R. M., Deutsch, M., Mulhern, R., et al. (1995). Reduced dose vs standard dose neuraxis irradiation in low stage medulloblastoma: The POG and CCG Study. SIOP XXVII Meeting Abstracts. *Medical and Pediatric Oncology, 25,* 277.

Todd, R., Weinstein, H., & Holcombe, G. (1997). Acute myelogenous leukemia. In P. A. Pizzo & D. G. Poplack (Eds.), *Principles and practice of pediatric oncology* (3rd ed.) (p. 463). Philadelphia: Lippincott Raven.

Winick, N. J., McKenna, R. W., Shuster, J. J., et al. (1993). Secondary acute myeloid leukemia in children with acute lymphoblastic leukemia treated with etoposide. *Journal of Clinical Oncology, 11,* 209.

Wurnig, C., Windhager, R., Schwameis, E., Kotz, R., Zoubek, A., et al. (1996). Prevention of chemotherapy-induced anemia by the use of erythropoietin in patients with primary malignant bone tumors (a double-blind, randomized, phase III study). *Transfusion, 36,* 155–159.

Pediatric Human Immunodeficiency Type 1 Infection

• WILLIAM V. RASZKA, JR., MD, FAAP

INTRODUCTION

Reports of unusual infections, such as *Pneumocystis carinii* pneumonia (PCP) and mucosal candidiasis in previously healthy homosexual men were first published in 1981 (Gottlieb, Schroff, Schanker, et al., 1981). Why patients developed such profound immunodeficiency was not known until 1983 when French and American researchers working independently announced that a retrovirus, now known as the human immunodeficiency virus (HIV), was the etiologic agent that led to the acquired immunodeficiency syndrome (AIDS) (Gallo, Salchuddin, Popovic, et al., 1984; Laurence, Brun-Vezinet, Scuter, et al., 1984). Once primarily a disease of homosexual men, HIV has spread throughout all segments of the human population. In some parts of sub-Saharan Africa, up to 40% of women of childbearing age are HIV infected. The economic and human losses are tremendous. Societies are losing important wage earners, infant mortality rates are rising in the most severely affected areas, and health care systems are strained or overwhelmed. Perhaps HIV will alter human evolution as no disease has since bubonic plague.

Knowledge about and perception of HIV infection have changed dramatically in the past decade. Dismal pessimism, followed by optimism that HIV infection could be "cured," has given way to the notion that with adequate resources, HIV infection can be controlled although not eradicated. New prevention strategies and innovative treatment programs have decreased perinatal transmission rates from 25% to 8% (Connor, Sperling, Gelber, et al., 1994). Powerful combination drug regimens for the treatment of HIV infection have improved AIDS-free survival times in both pediatric and adult patients. Changes in the guidelines for drug development and approval that mandate testing in children have led to expanded access to new and more powerful antiretroviral drug regimens.

Although understanding and management of HIV have improved, enormous challenges remain. Behaviors that lead to an increased risk of HIV infection, such as sexual activity at an early age, multiple sexual partners, and drug use, are notoriously difficult to change. Ensuring that all HIV-infected women of childbearing age are identified and treated appropriately is difficult in the United States and beyond the abilities of most health care infrastructures in developing nations.

PATHOLOGY

HIV, or more appropriately, HIV-1, is a member of the *Lentivirus* genus in the family Retroviridae. Retroviruses contain two copies of single-stranded RNA genome. A unique feature of all retroviruses is their use of reverse transcriptase, an RNA-dependent DNA polymerase, to replicate genetic material. Other primate lentiviruses, such as simian immunodeficiency virus and its subspecies, are similar in structure to HIV but have important genetic and functional differences.

The mature HIV virion consists of three layers: an outer lipid bilayer studded with surface (GP120) and transmembrane (GP41) glycoprotein complexes; a middle layer consisting of matrix, internal capsular, and nuclear capsid proteins; and an internal region, which contains two copies of single-stranded RNA, multiple copies of viral-encoded reverse transcriptase, integrase, and RNAse H. Figure 65-1 illustrates the mature HIV virion.

The HIV-1 genome is organized similarly to that of other retroviruses but is more complex. The 9-kB RNA virus is flanked by long terminal repeat sections, which serve as both promoter and binding sites for host and viral transactivating factors. The genome contains structural (*gag* and *env*) and viral enzyme (*pol*) genes that encode precursor proteins that produce multiple gene products after intracellular processing. The *env* gene encodes surface glycoproteins GP120 and GP41 that are critical for binding to the CD4+ cell receptor. The *gag* region encodes nuclear capsid core and matrix proteins, while the *pol* gene encodes reverse transcriptase, protease, and integrase enzymes. The HIV-1 genome also has at least six other regulatory genes not found in nonprimate retroviruses whose products play critical roles in controlling viral expression, trafficking of viral gene products within the affected cell, and viral infectivity.

The primary binding site for the HIV virion is the CD4+ receptor. Cells that express CD4+ receptors include CD4+ T-cell lymphocytes and cells of the monocyte or macrophage line. While the CD4+ receptor site is a critical binding site, chemokines that function as coreceptors have been identified. All HIV-1 strains use CCR5 or CXCR4, members of the chemokine receptor family, as coreceptors. Lymphocytes from people who do not express CCR5 are relatively resistant to infection, rendering certain population groups inherently more susceptible or resistant to HIV viral infection and replication (Liu et al., 1996; Huang et al., 1996). Globally, the allelelic frequency of CCR5 deletion ranges from 0.5% in African and Asian populations to 20.9% in Ashkanazi Jewish populations (Martinson, 1997).

After binding to the CD4+ receptor complex and other receptors, the HIV virion uncoats and the HIV genome and regulatory enzymes enter the host cell. In the cytoplasm of the host cell, viral-encoded reverse transcriptase transcribes the single-stranded HIV RNA into complementary DNA. Multiple error mechanisms in reverse transcription lead to frequent mutations and significant HIV genomic diversity. In adults with established HIV disease, approximately 10^{10} new CD4+ T-cells are infected each day, making it possible that a mutation will occur at each point along the HIV-1 genome between 10^4 and 10^5 times per day (Perelson, Neumann, Markowitz, Leonard, & Ho, 1996). One consequence

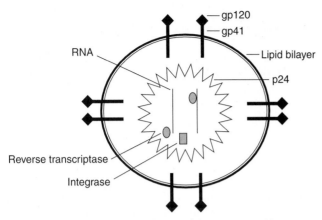

Figure 65–1 ■ Schematic drawing of the mature HIV virion.

of this genomic diversity is the production of antiretroviral-resistant strains.

Once proviral HIV DNA has been synthesized, it is integrated into the host DNA through the actions of viral-encoded integrase. Integrated proviral HIV DNA cannot be eradicated and represents a potential long-lived reservoir for viral persistence. Once integrated, several host transcriptional and viral activation factors stimulate viral replication or transcription. Newly produced proteins and genomic material aggregate near the cytoplasmic side of the cell membrane. One of the last enzymatic steps before budding from the cell membrane involves cleavage of terminal RNA sequences by a viral-encoded protease. Failure to complete this step leads to the production of nonreplicative virions.

Transmission

HIV may be transmitted either as a free virion or as integrated provirus within donated cells. Children become infected with HIV by exposure to infectious human, usually maternal, body fluids. To date in the United States, more than 90% of all pediatric patients with AIDS have acquired their infection perinatally (Centers for Disease Control and Prevention [CDC], 1998b). In 1997, only 9 of 473 pediatric patients diagnosed with AIDS had hemophilia, a coagulation disorder, or had received a blood transfusion, blood component, or tissue. Almost all new cases of HIV infection in children younger than 13 years will be the result of perinatal transmission.

● **Clinical Pearls:**

• HIV transmission associated with casual household contact or closed-mouth kissing is negligible (Courville et al., 1998). Open-mouth ("French") kissing, particularly if the gingiva are inflamed or bloody, very rarely has been associated with transmission.
• Biting very uncommonly results in transmission and only does so after extensive tearing and bleeding.
• Contact with nonbloody saliva, urine, feces, tears, sweat, or biting insects has not resulted in HIV transmission (CDC, 1998d).

Perinatal Transmission

The pathogenesis of perinatally acquired HIV-I infection differs from that of adult infection in several significant ways. The developing immune system of the infant is not as effective at controlling viral replication. After infection, the num-

ber of HIV-1 RNA copies increases dramatically to 10^5 to 10^7 copies/mL (Palumbo et al., 1995; Shearer et al., 1997). Plasma HIV RNA levels decrease very gradually over the first 1 to 2 years of life, but mean plasma HIV RNA levels remain much higher than in adults. The reason for the persistently high viral levels in children is not known. Possible mechanisms include a larger pool of permissive host cells, relatively high thymic mass relative to body size, and an immature host immune response (Wilfert et al., 1994). Similar to adults, in children older than 2 years, plasma viral load at steady state is inversely related to long-term prognosis (Palumbo et al., 1998).

▲ **Clinical Warning:** Perinatal transmission, often called vertical transmission, can occur at any time during pregnancy, at the time of delivery, or after birth.

Failure to detect HIV in infants born to HIV-infected women in the first weeks of life, with subsequent detection of virus in these infants at 1 to 3 months of age, demonstrates that intrapartum transmission occurs (Rogers et al., 1989; Dunn et al., 1995). The overall risk of HIV transmission from an untreated HIV-infected mother to her infant is approximately 25%, with published ranges from 13% to 39% (Connor et al., 1994; European Collaborative Study [ECS], 1992b; Tovo, deMartino, & Gabiano, 1992).

● **Clinical Pearl:** Appropriate antiretroviral therapy in the mother and the infant can decrease the risk of perinatal transmission by approximately two thirds.

Risk factors associated with an increased rate of perinatal transmission include a high maternal plasma copy number of HIV RNA (viral load); low maternal CD4+ lymphocyte cell count or percentage; advanced maternal HIV disease; maternal coinfection, such as chorioamnionitis or syphilis; premature delivery; second born of a twin delivery; prolonged rupture of membranes; and vaginal delivery. Although viral load best correlates with the risk of perinatal transmission, no single factor is predictive of HIV transmission.

Infectious HIV virions have been isolated from breast milk obtained from HIV-infected women. Studies in African populations have demonstrated that up to 30% of perinatal HIV transmission can occur postpartum from breast-feeding (Datta et al., 1994; Leroy et al., 1998). Numerous reports have documented HIV transmission through breast milk to infants born to HIV-negative mothers.

● **Clinical Pearl:** Because of the potential impact of breast-feeding on the overall mother-to-child transmission rate, bottle-feeding is currently recommended for all infants born to HIV-infected mothers in the United States and other industrialized countries (American Academy of Pediatrics [AAP], Committee on Pediatric AIDS, 1998).

In nonindustrialized countries, the issue is more controversial. Currently, the World Health Organization (WHO) recommends that children born to HIV-infected mothers in less developed parts of the world breast-feed, because perinatal morbidity and mortality rates are higher in children who are not breast-fed (HIV and Infant Feeding, 1999).

Sexual Abuse as a Means of Transmission

Sexual abuse is a rare mode of HIV transmission. Of 9136 children reported with HIV or AIDS through December 1996, only 26 had been sexually abused. Of these, 17 had confirmed and 9 suspected exposure to HIV (Lindegren et al., 1998).

Pathogenesis

Variation in the biologic properties of HIV isolates, such as cytotropism, syncytium-inducing capacity, and replication rate, may influence pathogenecity (DeRossi et al., 1993). Cells with integrated HIV DNA may produce huge numbers of HIV virions. The initial viremia leads to seeding of the virus throughout the body. HIV infects lymphoid organs very early in the disease. Follicular dendritic cells trap immune complexes of virus, antibody, and complement in the germinal centers of lymph nodes. This microenvironment is highly conducive to ongoing HIV infection of and replication in CD4+ lymphocytes as they migrate through lymphoid tissue, come into close contact with the follicular dendritic cells, and are activated (Health, 1995). Free virus and latently infected cells may remain sequestered within the lymphoid tissue and serve as a reservoir for persistent viral infection. Host immune responses, particularly the development of HIV-specific cytotoxic T cells, play a critical role in controlling viral replication (Musey et al., 1997). HIV-specific antibodies are detected only after the viremia has declined, suggesting that antibodies are not as critical to controlling viral replication. Why or how high-level viral replication continues despite HIV-specific cytotoxic T-cell lymphocyte production is unclear.

After widespread dissemination and high-grade viremia, the host immune response is effective at reducing the level of viremia. Approximately 6 months after infection in adults, viral load measured by plasma RNA polymerase chain reaction (PCR) reaches a steady state (Pantaleo, Graziosi, Fauci, 1993). This steady state stage may last 10 to 12 years and is often termed the time of *clinical latency*. This concept of immunologic latency is inaccurate. Although the patient experiences few clinical symptoms, rapid CD4+ cell turnover is occurring with high viral replication, and the patient experiences a steady incremental decline in CD4+ lymphocyte cell counts. The half-life of HIV-infected CD4+ cells may only be 2 days, and an estimated 1.8×10^9 cells are destroyed daily (Ho et al., 1995). Maintaining CD4+ lymphocyte cell counts eventually becomes impossible in the face of continued or increased viral replication. The patient's ultimate prognosis depends on how effective the host immune response has been in controlling viral replication. In adults, patients whose host immune response leads to a low level of viral replication and low plasma HIV viral load have a longer life expectancy than those who are unable to control viral replication as well (Mellors et al., 1995). This effect is independent of the CD4+ lymphocyte count.

The exact mechanism by which HIV replication leads to CD4+ lymphocyte cell death is not known. Possible mechanisms include direct lysis; induction of programmed cell death (apoptosis); host-specific immune responses, such as antibody-dependent cellular toxicity mediated by natural killer cells; and disruption of normal immunoregulatory pathways (Ameisen, Estaquier, Idziorek, & De Bels, 1995). Disease progression is associated with degeneration of the germinal center follicle cell network and disruption of lymphoid architecture (Cohen et al., 1995). Destruction of the lymphoid tissue impairs the host's ability to control viral replication effectively, thereby allowing increased viral replication and further destruction of lymphoid tissue. With progressive lymphoid tissue destruction, the host's ability to replace CD4+ lymphocytes is further compromised.

EPIDEMIOLOGY

Understanding the epidemiology of HIV infection is sometimes confusing. Until recently, only AIDS (which is at one end of a continuum of clinical syndromes associated with HIV infection) was a reportable condition. As of December 1997, only 29 states conducted surveillance for HIV infection among children. The CDC has published two separate classification systems for pediatric HIV infection. The 1987 AIDS case definition is used for purposes of surveillance and reporting (CDC, 1987). The CDC has developed a separate classification system to describe the spectrum of HIV disease in pediatric patients (CDC, 1994). Patients are classified into mutually exclusive categories according to three parameters: (1) infection status, (2) clinical status, and (3) immunologic status. CD4+ lymphocyte counts and percentage are used to gauge the degree of immunosuppression. Table 65-1 presents immunologic categories of pediatric HIV infection.

Once classified, an HIV-infected infant or child may not be reclassified in a less severe category even if antiretroviral therapy leads to clinical or immunologic improvement. The expanded definition for AIDS in adolescents and adults, which became effective in 1993, does not apply to individuals younger than 13 years of age (CDC, 1992). AIDS case definitions for children and adults are similar except that lymphoid interstitial pneumonitis and multiple or recurrent serious bacterial infections are AIDS-defining conditions only for children.

The epidemiology of pediatric HIV infection is greatly influenced by the course of the epidemic in childbearing women because the major route of transmission of HIV to children is through perinatal exposure. In most parts of the world, including North America, women of childbearing age (15–44 years) represent one of the fastest growing groups with AIDS. In the United States, women counted for 20% of adult AIDS cases reported in 1996, compared with less than 10% in the 1980s (CDC, 1996). While AIDS case rates have risen in women of all ethnic backgrounds, African American and Hispanic women have higher AIDS case rates than Caucasian women (Whortley & Fleming, 1997). Women with heterosexual contact as the only risk factor for HIV increased

Table 65–1. IMMUNOLOGIC CATEGORIES OF PEDIATRIC HIV INFECTION BASED ON AGE-SPECIFIC CD4+ T-LYMPHOCYTE COUNTS AND PERCENT OF TOTAL LYMPHOCYTES

Immunologic Category	<12 Months		1–5 years		6–12 Years	
	Number/mcL	%	Number/mcL	%	Number/mcL	%
No suppression	≥ 1500	≥ 25	≥ 1000	≥ 25	≥ 500	≥ 25
Moderate suppression	750–1499	15–24	500–999	15–24	200–499	15–24
Severe suppression	< 750	< 15	< 500	< 15	< 200	< 15

Adapted from Centers for Disease Control and Prevention (1994). 1994 revised classification system for human immunodeficiency virus infection in children less than 13 years of age. *Morbidity and Mortality Weekly Report, 43*(RR-12), 1–10.

HIV = human immunodeficiency virus.

from 14% in 1982 to 35% in 1993. Heterosexual contact is now the primary means by which women acquire their infection. Figure 65-2 presents information about perinatally acquired AIDS in the United States between 1980 and 1996.

Pediatric HIV/AIDS has become a leading cause of death in children worldwide. By June 1998, an estimated 2.7 million children worldwide had acquired HIV infection. Of these, more than 1.7 million had progressed to AIDS, and 1.4 million had died (UNAIDS, 1998). Worldwide, more than 1000 children are newly infected with HIV each day. U.S. Bureau of the Census statistics suggest that in many areas, HIV infection has led to increased infant mortality rates and that this effect is expected to increase over the coming decade (Stanecki & Way, 1997). However, significant regional variations exist. Sub-Saharan Africa accounts for the greatest proportion of cases. Although the epidemic began later in Asia and India, the epidemic in this region may overshadow all others because of its large population. HIV infection is well established in Latin America and the Caribbean. Published HIV rates in the Middle East have remained low.

AIDS is the seventh leading cause of childhood mortality in the United States in the age group 1 to 4 years, the fourth leading cause of death among African American children ages 1 to 4 years, and the fifth leading cause of death among Hispanic children. In some areas, such as New York, New Jersey, and Florida, HIV has become one of the top three leading causes of childhood mortality (National Institute of Allergy and Infectious Diseases, 1996). As of September 30, 1997, perinatal transmission of HIV accounted for 7310 (1%) of the 626,334 total AIDS cases in adults and children reported to the CDC by state and territorial health departments (CDC, 1998b). Perinatally acquired pediatric AIDS cases have been reported from 48 states, the District of

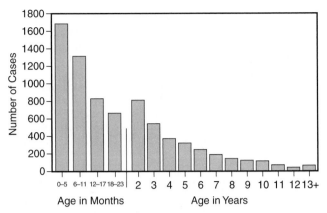

Figure 65–3 ■ Perinatally acquired AIDS Cases by Age at Diagnosis, 1982–1997, in the United States. Adapted from Centers for Disease Control and Prevention. (1997). *HIV/AIDS Surveillance Report 9*, 1–43.

Columbia, Puerto Rico, and the Virgin Islands. Five states or territories account for 64% of all perinatally acquired AIDS cases: New York (27%), Florida (17%), New Jersey (9%), California (6%), and Puerto Rico (5%). The vast majority of cases (85%) were diagnosed in metropolitan areas with populations of more than 500,000 people. Ethnic minorities are overrepresented, because only 14% of cases were in non-Hispanic Caucasian patients (CDC, 1997b). Table 65-2 illustrates these data.

The median age at the time of AIDS diagnosis in children is 17 months. Forty percent of cases are diagnosed in children younger than 1 year, 47% in children ages 1 to 5 years, and 13% in children age 6 years and up. Figure 65-3 demonstrates data for diagnosis of pediatric AIDS by age in the United States between 1982 and 1997.

Contrary to what is happening in many other parts of the world, the number of U.S. children with newly diagnosed AIDS or new perinatally acquired HIV infection is declining. Public health efforts to identify all HIV-infected pregnant women and implementation of zidovudine-based antiretroviral treatment regimens during pregnancy and in the offspring of HIV-infected mothers have led to a substantial decline in the reported incidence of pediatric AIDS cases in the past several years (Simonds et al., 1998). From 1984 through 1992, the estimated number of children with perinatally acquired AIDS diagnosed each year increased, then declined 43% from 1992 to 1996. During this time, declines were similar by race or ethnicity, for different regions of the United States, and in urban and rural areas. The declines were largest among children in whom AIDS was diagnosed at younger ages (CDC, 1998b).

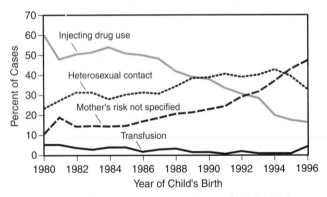

Figure 65–2 ■ Mother's exposure category by year of child's birth for perinatally acquired AIDS, 1980–1996, in the United States. Adapted from Centers for Disease Control and Prevention. (1997). *HIV/AIDS Surveillance Report 9*, 1–39.

Table 65–2.   PEDIATRIC AIDS CASES, PERCENTAGE, AND ANNUAL RATES PER 100,000 POPULATION BY RACE/ETHNICITY REPORTED IN 1997 AND CUMULATIVE TOTALS THROUGH DECEMBER 1997 IN THE UNITED STATES

Race/Ethnicity	Number	%	Rate	Cumulative Total
White, not Hispanic	63	13	0.2	1426
Black, not Hispanic	292	62	4.0	4697
Hispanic	110	23	1.3	1876
Asian/Pacific Islander	3	1	0.1	44
Native American/Alaska Native	2	1	0.4	27

AIDS = acquired immunodeficiency syndrome.
Adapted from Centers for Disease Control and Prevention. (1997). *HIV/AIDS Surveillance Report, 9*, 1–39.

HISTORY AND PHYSICAL EXAMINATION

Infants and children infected with HIV may develop many disparate clinical problems. Some may be directly attributable to HIV infection. Others, such as most infectious disease complications, are the result of HIV-induced immunosuppression. Before widespread maternal HIV testing and antiretroviral use, approximately 50% of children with vertically acquired HIV infection were symptomatic by 8 months and 80% by 2 years of age (Scott et al., 1989). Prospective and retrospective data suggest that two populations of children exist. Approximately 25% of children have rapid progression and death within the first few years, while the remainder survive early childhood and have a clinical course more consistent with adult infection. These children have a mean survival time of more than 9 years (Barnhart et al., 1996).

In adolescents and young adults, the primary viremia associated with HIV infection presents as a mononucleosis-like illness. This illness, called the *acute retroviral syndrome*, is characterized by fever, fatigue, myalgia or arthralgia, adenopathy, pharyngitis, diarrhea, headache, and rash, and it lasts 1 to 2 weeks (Quinn, 1997) Congenital HIV infection is not associated with any distinguishing clinical or morphologic features (Connor et al., 1994). The acute retroviral syndrome is not as well described in infants. Infants may present only with fever or irritability only.

DIAGNOSTIC STUDIES

Lymphoid interstitial pneumonitis/pulmonary lymphoid hyperplasia (LIP/PLH) is a chronic pulmonary disease of unknown etiology characterized by diffuse peribronchiolar lymphoid nodules. LIP/PLH is second only to PCP among pediatric AIDS-defining conditions. Approximately 20% of children present with LIP/PLH as their AIDS indicator disease. Although the incidence has declined slightly, LIP/PLH has remained surprisingly common, even in the era of highly active antiretroviral therapy. The pathogenesis of LIP/PLH is not known. Initially, patients are generally asymptomatic but may have generalized lymphadenopathy. Characteristic clinical features of late disease include tachypnea, cough, wheezing, hypoxemia, and digital clubbing. The most common radiographic findings include a diffuse reticulonodular infiltrate with or without hilar adenopathy. A presumptive diagnosis of LIP can be made based on typical radiographic findings persisting for 2 months that are unresponsive to antimicrobial therapy or, more definitively, by lung biopsy. Although features of LIP/PLH and PCP can be similar, patients with LIP/PLH usually are older, have a more insidious disease onset, and do not have fever or crackles on auscultation.

Diagnosing HIV infection in infants is more complicated than identifying HIV infection in an adult. Immunologic, virologic, and clinical criteria have been published (CDC, 1994). Because maternally derived anti-HIV IgG antibodies may persist for as long as 18 months after delivery, IgG-based serologic assays do not reliably confirm HIV infection in infants less than 18 months old.

● **Clinical Pearl:** Two or more negative anti-HIV IgG antibody test results obtained at greater than 6 months of age, with an interval of at least 1 month between tests, excludes HIV infection in any child of any age without clinical evidence of HIV infection, unless the child is hypogammaglobulinemic or newly infected before the development of an immunologic response.

HIV-specific IgM antibody tests lack sensitivity and specificity and are not available. HIV-specific IgA antibodies have been used to diagnose HIV infection in infants at least 3 months old (Kline et al., 1994). Although used infrequently in the United States, IgA testing is inexpensive and easy to perform, making this a useful tool in many parts of the world. Display 65-1 presents guidelines for making a laboratory diagnosis of HIV in infants and children.

In the United States, nonserologic tests are used for the laboratory diagnosis of HIV infection in infants younger than 18 months. Both HIV culture and PCR are sensitive and specific assays for HIV infection. HIV culture, however, is expensive and time-consuming and is not often used. PCR, which amplifies either HIV RNA from the plasma or proviral DNA from infected mononuclear cells, is currently the diagnostic test of choice. With PCR, HIV infection can be diagnosed definitively in most infants by age 1 month and in virtually all infants by 6 months. A meta-analysis of published data from 271 HIV-infected children showed that 38% had positive HIV DNA PCR test results by 48 hours of age and 93% by the end of the second week (Dunn et al., 1995). In a review of 1209 samples taken at 1 to 36 months of age from 483 HIV-exposed infants, a single PCR assay was 95% sensitive and 97% specific in diagnosing HIV infection (Kline et al., 1994).

DISPLAY 65–1 • Laboratory Diagnosis of HIV Infection in Infants and Children

Laboratory Criteria for Considering a Child HIV Infected

1. Infants younger than 18 months:
   A. Two separate HIV tests by culture, polymerase chain reaction, or p24 antigen* are positive.
   or
   B. The child is HIV antibody-positive and meets criteria for AIDS diagnosis based on the 1987 AIDS surveillance case definitions (CDC, 1987).
2. Children ages 18 months and older:
   A. Repeated HIV-antibody tests by reactive enzyme immunoassay and confirmatory tests (ie, Western blot or immunofluorescence assay) are positive,
   or
   B. The child meets the criteria in 1A.

Laboratory Criteria for Considering a Child HIV Negative

An infant or child is HIV negative (a seroreverter if born to an HIV-infected mother) if the child has the following:

- Two or more HIV antibody tests performed between 6 and 18 months of age or one HIV antibody test after 18 months of age is negative,
  or
- Two separate polymerase chain reaction tests* are negative,
  and
- Child has not had an AIDS-defining condition.

HIV = human immunodeficiency virus; AIDS = acquired immunodeficiency syndrome.

*Both determinations were performed at or beyond 1 month of age and at least one at or beyond 4 months of age.

Adapted from Centers for Disease Control and Prevention. (1994). 1994 Revised Classification System for human immunodeficiency virus infection in children less than 13 years of age. *Morbidity and Mortatlity Weekly Report*, 43(RR-12), 1–10.

● **Clinical Pearl:** To date, maternal or infant zidovudine therapy has not delayed the detection of HIV infection in infants and does not decrease the sensitivity or predictive values of most virologic assays (Conner et al., 1994; Kovacs et al., 1995).

Although the CDC recommends the use of DNA-based PCR tests to diagnose HIV infection, recent data would suggest that RNA-based PCR testing modalities, which are ubiquitous, may be equally sensitive (Steketee et al., 1997). Standard and immune complex dissociated p24 antigen tests are highly specific for HIV infection but are not sensitive compared with other virologic assays and are associated with an unacceptably high false-positive rate in infants younger than 1 month (Nesheim et al., 1997).

Anti-HIV IgG antibody testing reliably predicts HIV infection in children older than 18 months. If anti-HIV IgG antibodies are detected by either enzyme linked immunosorbent assay or enzyme immunoassay, the result should be confirmed using Western blot. This test is a more specific and expensive test that verifies the presence of anti-HIV IgG antibodies to different regions of the HIV virion. The presence of anti-HIV IgG antibodies to different regions of the HIV virion confirms the diagnosis. False-positive Western blots are extremely rare.

▲ **Clinical Warning:** Diagnostic HIV testing should be performed in HIV-exposed infants during the first 48 hours of life, at 1 to 2 months, and at 3 to 6 months (AAP, Committee on Pediatric AIDS, 1998). Umbilical cord blood samples should *not* be used for diagnostic testing owing to unreliable results. Infants with negative virologic test results immediately after birth should be retested at age 1 to 2 months. HIV-exposed children with repeated negative virologic assays at birth and at age 1 to 2 months should be retested again at age 3 to 6 months. No patient should be diagnosed with HIV infection based solely on a single laboratory result. A positive virologic test result indicates probable HIV infection and should be confirmed by a repeated virologic test on a second specimen as quickly as possible.

● **Clinical Pearl:** Any combination of HIV culture, PCR, or p24 antigen testing can be used to confirm infection. HIV infection can be excluded among HIV-exposed children with two or more negative PCR or HIV culture test results if both were performed in infants age 1 month or older and one performed at age 4 months or older (CDC, 1994).

Most public health efforts have focused on the early identification of HIV-infected children born to HIV-infected mothers. However, children who present with recurrent serious bacterial illnesses or even recurrent common childhood diseases (such as otitis media) with other features of immunosuppression, such as at least one invasive bacterial illness or recurrent mucosal candidiasis, should be examined for HIV infection. The provider should not assume that a child is unlikely to be HIV infected because the mother does not have many risk factors. Women who give birth to HIV antibody–positive children often have a history of few sexual contacts.

HIV Encephalopathy

HIV encephalopathy currently accounts for approximately 15% of all pediatric AIDS definition conditions reported to the CDC. The prevalence, severity, and progression remain highly variable and dependent on the age of the child, age at diagnosis, HIV disease stage, and rate of HIV disease progression (ECS, 1990; Englund et al., 1996; Cooper et al., 1998). In patients with HIV encephalopathy, central nervous system (CNS) functions are globally depressed, resulting in defects in cognitive, social, language, and motor skills. Motor and movement disorders but not seizures are common. Children with static encephalopathy continue to gain new skills and abilities but lag behind non–HIV-infected peers. Children with progressive encephalopathy can either fail to gain new milestones or in the worst situation, lose previously acquired skills.

Blood Dyscrasias

Anemia, leukopenia, neutropenia, and thrombocytopenia are common hematologic manifestations of HIV infection in children that are often alleviated by optimal antiretroviral therapy. Normocytic or microcytic anemia may be secondary to chronic disease. Macrocytic anemia is usually a complication of antiretroviral therapy. Leukopenia or neutropenia may be due to the bone marrow toxicity of HIV infection, opportunistic infections, antiretroviral therapy, or other medications, such as trimethoprim-sulfamethoxazole (TMP-SMX). Antiplatelet antibodies, which are detectable in most patients, may lead to thrombocytopenia. Mild thrombocytopenia requires no treatment. More significant thrombocytopenia can be treated with intravenous immunoglobulin (IVIG), steroids, anti-D preparations, or even splenectomy.

Hepatic Changes

Asymptomatic hepatomegaly with or without moderate increases in serum concentrations of hepatic enzymes is a common finding and requires no intervention other than to exclude hepatotrophic viral infection. Persistent proteinuria may be indicative of HIV-induced nephropathy. Malignancies are uncommon among HIV-infected children, accounting for only 2% of AIDS-defining illnesses (CDC, 1997b). The most common cancer is non-Hodgkin's lymphoma. Kaposi's sarcoma is quite rare in children. Comanagement with the HIV specialist should provide the practitioner with the support needed for dealing with hepatic anomalies. Further indications for other specialty referrals should emerge based on the child's findings in concert with comanagement decision making.

Opportunistic and Nonopportunistic Infections

Immunosuppression and the frequent development of opportunistic and nonopportunistic infectious disease complications characterize HIV infection and AIDS. Constitutional symptoms become common as the CD4+ lymphocyte cell count drops beneath approximately 200 cells/mm^3 in adults and children older than 6 years. Opportunistic infections become more prominent as the CD4+ lymphocyte cell count drops beneath 50 cells/mm^3. The precise incidence of many of these infections is poorly defined and influenced by medical care and the prophylactic strategies used. Common infections that occur with increased frequency in HIV-infected children include otitis media, upper respiratory tract infection, and sinusitis.

● **Clinical Pearl:** Aside from a somewhat greater frequency of *Staphylococcus aureus* infections in late-stage HIV disease, the microbiology of upper respiratory tract bacterial illnesses is similar for HIV-infected and non–HIV-infected children.

More serious nonopportunistic bacterial infections also occur more frequently in HIV-infected children. Approximately 20% of patients present with recurrent serious bacterial infections as their AIDS-defining condition (CDC, 1997b).

Pneumococcus is the most common invasive bacterial pathogen in children with HIV infection, accounting for 25% to 50% of episodes (NICHD IVIG Study Group, 1991). Children may develop more severe bacterial illnesses without evidence of severe CD4+ lymphocyte depression (Lichenstein et al., 1998). Potential reasons for the increased risk include neutropenia, hypogammaglobulinemia, and disordered immunoglobulin synthesis. Children with recurrent serious bacterial illness have a worse prognosis than those without recurrent bacterial illness but a better prognosis than those children who present with other AIDS indicator illnesses (Farley et al., 1994).

● **Clinical Pearls:**

• Although TMP-SMX is not used primarily to prevent serious bacterial illnesses, its use does diminish the likelihood of invasive bacterial illness (Spector et al., 1994).

• Monthly infusions of intravenous immunoglobulin are indicated in patients with low serum immunoglobulin levels and recurrent serious bacterial illnesses.

Pneumocystis carinii *Pneumonia*

The most common AIDS indicator disease in pediatric patients, PCP is associated with significant morbidity and mortality. Through June 1997, PCP had been reported in 33% of U.S. children with perinatally acquired HIV infection (CDC, 1997b). Pediatric patients are most often diagnosed at 3 to 6 months of life. Sex, race, and place of residence do not affect PCP incidence rates.

Infants usually present with the sudden onset of fever, cough, tachypnea, and dyspnea. Older children may have a more indolent course. Auscultory findings include decreased breath sounds or crackles. Radiographic features are myriad and most commonly include a diffuse reticulonodular infiltrate. In neonates, the CD4+ lymphocyte count is high compared to adults with PCP but is less than 1500/mL in more than 80% of patients (CDC, 1995). In older children, PCP is rare if CD4+ lymphocyte counts are greater than 200/mL. In patients of all ages, the serum lactate dehydrogenase concentration is often markedly elevated. The diagnosis can be confirmed by demonstration of the organisms in pulmonary fluid specimens.

The treatment of choice is high-dose TMP-SMX with systemic corticosteroids. Patients who cannot tolerate TMP-SMX may be given intravenous pentamidine or if an adolescent with mild disease, oral atovaquone.

All primary care providers should understand the rationale for PCP prophylaxis. Appropriate initiation of PCP prophylaxis is a simple, low-cost intervention that greatly diminishes infant morbidity and mortality. It is one of the most important interventions that a provider can make in the first year of an HIV-exposed child's life (Thea et al., 1996).

▲ **Clinical Warning:** Because of the failure of the guidelines for CD4+ lymphocyte count in reducing the incidence of PCP in pediatric patients, the CDC now recommends that *all* infants born to HIV-infected mothers should be started on PCP prophylaxis at 4 to 6 weeks of age regardless of clinical findings or immunologic testing results (CDC, 1995). PCP prophylaxis is not started until this time because PCP is rare in the first month, and TMP-SMX may displace bilirubin. Table 65-3 gives information for providing initial laboratory testing and management strategies of infants born to HIV-infected mothers.

PCP prophylaxis is continued until HIV infection is excluded or the patient is 12 months old, at which time CD4+ lymphocyte counts and percentage can be used to guide prophylaxis decisions. All children diagnosed with PCP require lifelong prophylaxis. Thrice-weekly SMX is the prophylactic agent of choice. Other agents include dapsone, atovaquone, and nebulized pentamidine. Table 65-4 presents indications for primary PCP prophylaxis. Table 65-5 provides dosing information for this prophylaxis.

Opportunistic Central Nervous System Infections

Opportunistic CNS infections are associated with profound immunosuppression. Patients with *Cryptococcus neoformans* meningitis usually have an indolent course, with complaints of fever, intermittent headache, and vomiting. The diagnosis is confirmed with specialized fungal stains, cryptococcal antigen testing, and culture. Cerebral toxoplasmosis, an uncommon opportunistic infection in children occurring in fewer than 1% of children with AIDS, represents a reactivation of previous infection and presents as fever, headache, seizures, focal neurologic abnormalities, and altered consciousness. Computed tomography or magnetic resonance imaging is usually diagnostic.

Fungal, viral, and parasitic pathogens may cause significant gastrointestinal tract morbidity in HIV-infected patients

---

Table 65–3. INITIAL LABORATORY TESTING AND MEDICAL MANAGEMENT OF INFANTS BORN TO HIV-INFECTED MOTHERS

Category	Medication/Testing	Birth	1 Month	2 Months	4 Months
Antiretrovirals*	Zidovudine	x	x		
HIV testing	Polymerase chain reaction†	x	x		x
	T-cell lymphocytes		x		x
Prophylaxis	TMP-SMX**		x	x	x
Monitoring	Complete blood count	x	x	x	x

TMP-SMX = trimethoprim-sulfamethoxazole; HIV = human immunodeficiency virus.

*Antiretroviral regimens containing zidovudine at a dose of 2 mg/kg per dose every 6 h should be offered to all infants born to HIV-infected mothers, regardless of whether the mother received prophylaxis with zidovudine or not. The prophylaxis is continued until the infant is 6 wk old.

†Any positive polymerase chain reaction test must be confirmed immediately.

**Pneumocystis carinii* pneumonia prophylaxis is initiated at 4–6 wk of life and continued until the patient is proven not to be HIV infected or until at least 12 mo of age (see Table 65-4).

Table 65–4. INDICATIONS FOR PRIMARY PNEUMOCYSTIS CARINII PNEUMONIA (PCP) PROPHYLAXIS BASED ON AGE, HIV STATUS, AND CD4+ LYMPHOCYTE COUNTS

Age	HIV Infection Status	CD4+ Lymphocyte Count (per mL)	CD4+ %	PCP Prophylaxis
Birth to 4–6 wk	Exposed or infected	Not applicable	Not applicable	No
4 wk–12 mo	Exposed or infected	Not applicable	Not applicable	Yes
4–12 mo	Not infected*	Not applicable	Not applicable	No
12–24 mo	Exposed or infected	History of <750 in first 12 mo or <500	<15	Yes
12–24 mo	Not infected	Not applicable	Not applicable	No
2–5 y	Infected	<500	<15	Yes
6–12 y	Infected	<200	<15	Yes

HIV = human immunodeficiency virus.

*HIV infection has been reasonably excluded (ie, with two negative polymerase chain reaction tests in children older than 1 mo with at least one test at 4 mo or older). See Display 65-1.

Adapted from Centers for Disease Control and Prevention (1995). 1995 Revised guidelines for prophylaxis against *Pneumocystis carinii* pneumonia for children affected with or perinatally exposed to human immunodeficiency virus. *Morbidity and Mortality Weekly Report*, 44(RR-4), 1–11.

with advanced disease. Fungal infections of the mouth or esophagus usually respond to topical nystatin, oral amphotericin B, or clotrimazole troches. Cases that are more refractory may require oral fluconazole or itraconazole. Oral or esophageal lesions secondary to viral infections usually respond to specific antiviral therapy. Aphthous ulcers are difficult to treat and may require a short course of topically applied or oral corticosteroids. Both acute and chronic diarrhea may be more common in HIV-infected patients. *Salmonella* and *Giardia lamblia* may be persistent and difficult to eradicate. Cytomegalovirus, *Mycobacterium avium* complex, *Cryptosporidium*, and *Isospora* species may cause chronic diarrhea in patients with low CD4+ lymphocyte counts. Careful microbiologic examination of the stool should be the initial diagnostic step and will guide antimicrobial therapy and management.

Patients with profound immunosuppression may benefit from antimicrobial prophylaxis regimens to prevent either primary or recurrent opportunistic disease. The recommended regimens have been recently reviewed (1998).

MANAGEMENT

Editors' Note: HIV is a very complex disease with a histologic identity that is constantly mutating and changing. Therefore, the reader is advised that specifics of treatment options are evolving and will continue to evolve more frequently than can be predicted by the following information.

▲ **Clinical Warning:** Because of the complexity of HIV management, the provider is advised to refer the patient with HIV to a pediatric HIV specialist for evaluation and comanagement. When adding or changing medications or when in doubt about management specifics, the provider is advised to consult with the comanaging pediatric HIV specialist.

The management of HIV-infected infants, children, and adolescents is complex and evolving rapidly. Patients require careful monitoring to detect clinical and laboratory

Table 65–5 DRUG DOSAGES FOR PNEUMOCYSTIS CARINII PNEUMONIA PROPHYLAXIS IN CHILDREN OLDER THAN 4 WEEKS

Drug	Dose	Route	Dosing
TMP-SMX*	TMP: 150 mg/m² per d SMX: 750 mg/m² per d	Oral	Divided b.i.d. three times/wk on consecutive days
TMP-SMX	TMP: 150 mg/m² per d SMX: 750 mg/m² per d	Oral	Single daily doses three times/wk on consecutive days
TMP-SMX	TMP: 150 mg/m² per d SMX: 750 mg/m² per d	Oral	Divided b.i.d. seven times/wk
TMP-SMX	TMP: 150 mg/m² per d SMX: 750 mg/m² per d	Oral	Divided b.i.d. three times/wk, given on alternate days
Dapsone	2 mg/kg (max 100 mg)	Oral	Once a day
Pentamidine†	300 mg	Nebulized	Every month with Respirgard II inhaler
Atovaquone**	1500 mg	Oral	Once a day

TMP-SMX = trimethoprim-sulfamethoxazole.

†In children older than 5 y.

**In adolescents.

Adapted from Centers for Disease Control and Prevention. (1995). 1995 Revised Guidelines for Prophylaxis against *Pneumocystis carinii* pneumonia for children affected with or perinatally exposed to human immunodeficiency virus. *Morbidity and Mortality Weekly Report,*, 44(RR-4), 1–11.

evidence of HIV disease progression. Social issues are usually complicated and may require enormous amounts of time and public resources. A growing body of evidence suggests that patients cared for by more experienced specialists receive more up-to-date care and have less morbidity (Brosgart et al., 1999; Robbins, 1999). Whenever possible, management of HIV-infected children should be directed by a multidisciplinary team of health care professionals that includes a specialist in the treatment of pediatric and adolescent HIV infection, advanced practice nurses, social workers, psychologists, nutritionists, outreach workers, and pharmacists (AAP, Committee on Pediatric AIDS, 1998). If this is not possible, such a team should be consulted regularly.

Lymphoid Interstitial Pneumonitis/Pulmonary Lymphoid Hyperplasia

Treatment of LIP/PLH is usually chronic and supportive. The mainstays include antiretroviral therapy, antibiotics as needed for superinfections, physical therapy for both continuation of muscle function and pulmonary toilet, and corticosteroids for suppression of inflammation.

For the hospitalized child, the skills of a clinical nurse specialist can be invaluable in providing for coordination of care and for family support and coordination of the entire health care team. This includes postdischarge services, such as visiting nurse and hospice interventions. Similarly, the provider should consider using the skills of the social worker to provide for family support and counseling, including support group activities.

Prevention of Perinatal Transmission

Identification of HIV-infected women before and during pregnancy is critical to providing optimal therapy both for infected women and to prevent perinatal transmission. Prenatal HIV counseling and testing with consent should be the standard of care for all pregnant women in first-world nations (CDC, 1998f; American College of Obstetricians and Gynecologists, 1997).

Cesarean Section

Elective cesarean section decreases perinatal transmission. In a meta-analysis from 15 prospective studies, elective cesarean section reduced transmission by 50% alone and reduced transmission by 87% when used in conjunction with mother–child antiretroviral therapy (International Perinatal HIV Group, 1999). The lessened risk of perinatal transmission, however, must be balanced against the longer hospitalization and increased morbidity associated with cesarean section.

Breast-feeding

Breast-feeding is associated with HIV transmission. In general, HIV-infected women in North America and other first-world regions should refrain from breast-feeding (Morrison, 1999; Latham, 1999). In poverty-stricken areas of the world where safe, nonhuman milk resources are not available for infant feeding, current guidelines indicate that breast-feeding should take place for as short a time as possible (UNAIDS, WHO, and UNICEF, 1997). More than 3 months' duration of breast-feeding is correlated with a significant increase in transmission of HIV DNA (Kuhn & Stein, 1997; Miotti et al., 1999). The importance of early weaning is also suggested by Kreiss' (1997) report that breast-feeding by an HIV-positive

mother for 15 months or longer correlated with CD4 depletion and vitamin A deficiency in her infant. This is especially important if the mother has mastitis, because this condition enhances the transmission of HIV in the nursing infant (Kreiss, 1997; Miotti et al., 1999). Until a safe and effective means is available for pretreating expressed milk from mothers with HIV, it is not universally recommended that mothers with HIV breast-feed their infants (Kreiss, 1997; Morrison, 1999).

In impoverished areas where infant nutrition would otherwise be compromised and because breast-feeding reduces morbidity among these children, the provider must assess for the risk of HIV. This assessment must be balanced with an examination of the availability of safe and affordable formulas and potable water for their reconstitution before formula feeding is recommended (Latham, 1999).

▲ **Clinical Warning:** Because it is also possible that the nursing infant can acquire HIV through vertical transmission should the mother become infected while lactating, the provider should advise all nursing women to avoid high-risk activities during lactation.

Antiretroviral Prophylaxis

No data exist to support the use of zidovudine initiated more than 24 hours after delivery. Single-dose nevirapine therapy in the neonate is currently being explored but is not yet approved for use. If the mother is on a two- or three-drug antiretroviral regimen during pregnancy, some authors advocate continuing those drugs in the infant after delivery as long as at least one of the drugs is zidovudine. However, very little is known about the pharmacokinetics of most other antiretroviral drugs in infants. Only lamivudine and nevirapine have been studied in newborns (Saba, 1999; Luzuriaga et al., 1997). The combination of zidovudine and lamivudine has been well tolerated in HIV-exposed infants.

Based on the results of Pediatric AIDS Clinical Trial Group O76, all pregnant women who are infected with HIV should be offered antiretroviral therapy that includes zidovudine (CDC, 1998e). In healthy women with CD4+ lymphocyte counts greater than 200/mm3, a regimen of oral zidovudine beginning in the second trimester followed by intravenous zidovudine at delivery and oral zidovudine given to the infant after birth reduced the risk of HIV transmission from approximately 25% to 8% (Connor et al., 1994).

Shorter-course, zidovudine-based regimens have also proven effective. Zidovudine started at almost any time during the pregnancy, at delivery, or within the first 24 hours of life in the neonate has been shown to reduce perinatal transmission (Wade et al., 1998).

● **Clinical Pearl:** No special infection control precautions are necessary in the newborn nursery for infants born to HIV-infected mothers. HIV-exposed infants should be given oral zidovudine syrup 2 mg/kg per dose every 6 hours beginning at 8 to 12 hours of life and continuing until 6 weeks of age, regardless of whether the mother received antiretroviral drugs during pregnancy or delivery and regardless of what she is currently taking.

In an African population, in which most children are breast-fed for at least the first 6 weeks of life, the combination of zidovudine and lamivudine started at the onset of labor and continued for 1 week after delivery reduced perinatal transmission by 37% (Saba, 1999). In a Ugandan study recently reported to the press but not yet published, a single dose of nevirapine given to HIV-infected antiretroviral-naive women in labor and to their offspring within 3 days of delivery reduced the perinatal HIV transmission rate to 13% (New York Times, 1999). The implications of this trial may be profound, because the cost of two doses of nevirapine prophylaxis is approximately $4, compared with $268 and $815 for short- and long-term zidovudine prophylaxis regimens. The exact mechanism by which zidovudine or any other antiretroviral reduces perinatal transmission is not known, but in utero exposure to zidovudine has not been associated with any significant toxicity in children followed for up to 4 years following exposure (Culnane et al., 1999; Sperling, 1997).

Less than 5% of HIV-infected pregnant women refuse zidovudine (CDC, 1998g). The strategy of offering antiretroviral therapy to infected childbearing women however, assumes that all HIV-infected pregnant women have been identified. Perinatal transmission could be reduced further if clinicians offered voluntary HIV testing to all women of childbearing age, not just to those thought to be at high risk. Once pregnant HIV-infected women are identified, management is complicated by the conflict between the needs for antiretroviral prophylaxis for the fetus and antiretroviral therapy for the woman (CDC, 1998e). Only zidovudine-based antiretroviral regimens have been shown to decrease perinatal transmission in U.S. trials. However, treatment of HIV-infected adults with zidovudine monotherapy is inappropriate. Hence, many infants will be born to mothers on two- or three-drug regimens.

▲ **Clinical Warning:**

- Because zidovudine use is associated with anemia, a hemoglobin level should be checked at the time zidovudine is initiated and again at 4 to 6 weeks of age.

An approach to the early management of an HIV-exposed infant is outlined in Table 65-3.

▲ **Clinical Warning:**

- PCP prophylaxis should be initiated in all HIV-exposed patients at 4 to 6 weeks of life and continued until HIV infection can be excluded.

Immunizations

Both HIV-exposed and HIV-infected children should be immunized with nonlive vaccines according to the most recent AAP and Advisory Committee on Immunization Practices guidelines. Refer to Chapter 13 for more information.

▲ **Clinical Warning:** Apart from measles, mumps, and rubella (MMR) vaccine, HIV-infected children should *not* be given live-virus vaccines. Infants born to HIV-infected mothers should be immunized with inactivated injectable polio vaccine even if uninfected, because oral polio vaccine may pose a risk to HIV-infected adults in the family. The varicella virus vaccine contains live virus and so is *not* indicated or licensed for use in immunocompromised children. Because measles can cause devastating disease in HIV-infected individuals, patients who are not severely immunosuppressed, as defined in Table 65-1, should be given the MMR vaccine at the recommended times (AAP, Committee on Infectious Diseases and Committee on Pediatric AIDS, 1999). HIV-infected patients, however, still require immunoglobulin prophylaxis after exposure to measles. Because HIV-infected children are at an increased risk of pneumococcal disease, all HIV-infected children should

be immunized with the 23-valent polysaccharide pneumococcal vaccine at 24 months of life (CDC, 1997a).

Revaccination with the pneumococcal vaccine is recommended after 3 to 5 years for children ages 10 years and younger and after 5 years for children older than 10 years. The timing and revaccination strategy will change substantially with the licensure of a conjugated pneumococcal vaccine. HIV-infected children should be given yearly influenza virus vaccinations beginning at 6 months of age.

Growth and Development

Monitoring growth and development is essential for the care of children with HIV infection. Growth failure and neurodevelopmental deterioration may be specific manifestations of HIV infection in children. Parents and children should be educated about the importance of eating a balanced diet. The usefulness of dietary supplements remains unresolved. Most children do not seem to benefit from caloric supplements. Because children lose muscle mass in late-stage disease, stimulants, such as megestrol (Megace) and cyproheptadine (Periactin), may stimulate oral intake; however, they result in an increase in fat rather than lean body mass.

Effective antiretroviral therapy seems the most effective appetite stimulant and the best predictor of adequate growth. A continuing program of regular exercise may increase lean muscle mass and contribute to a sense of well-being. Because HIV-infected children are more prone to a variety of food-borne pathogens, meticulous attention to hygiene is important, particularly late in the disease. HIV-infected children should refrain from eating raw or undercooked animal products.

Other Management Issues

Monitoring the status of lymphoid tissue is an important part of the physical examination. Regression of lymph nodes may suggest either an excellent response to antiretroviral therapy or more advanced disease with loss of functioning lymphoid tissue.

HIV-infected children may acquire and care for pets, but certain precautions should be observed. Gloves should be used for handling any animal waste products. Animals should be examined annually and immunized according to the appropriate schedule. Ill animals should be examined as soon as possible by a veterinarian.

The diagnosis of HIV infection should not be hidden from the child. The American Academy of Pediatrics supports early disclosure and ongoing discussion with the child (AAP, Committee on Pediatric AIDS, 1999). Studies suggest that children who know their HIV status have higher self-esteem than children who are unaware of their status. Parents who have disclosed the HIV status to their children experience less depression than those who do not. The number of HIV-infected children reaching school age will continue to grow. HIV-infected children may attend day care or school and participate in all athletics without any special precautions or notification (Cohen et al., 1997). Health care providers frequently will be asked for guidance by both parents and school officials to ensure confidentiality and optimize educational opportunities.

▲ **Clinical Warning:** HIV-infected adolescents, even those with viral loads below detectable limits, are infectious and should be counseled to avoid unprotected sex and the use of shared needles.

Monitoring Disease Progression

As in adults, HIV RNA PCR assays for HIV and serial CD4+ lymphocyte counts and percentage are used to monitor disease progression, guide antiretroviral therapy, and guide decisions as to when to begin primary PCP prophylaxis in children older than 1 year. Plasma HIV RNA levels indicate the magnitude of HIV replication and its associated rate of CD4+ T-cell destruction, whereas CD4+ T-cell counts indicate the extent of HIV-induced immune damage already suffered. T-cell subsets and HIV RNA viral load should be obtained as soon as possible after a child has a positive virologic test for HIV and every 3 months thereafter. However, providers must keep in mind that the HIV RNA pattern in perinatally infected infants differs from that of infected adults. Infants may maintain high HIV RNA copy numbers for long periods (Palumbo et al., 1995). During the first year of life, the mean HIV RNA level is 185,000 copies/mL (Shearer et al., 1997). Infants may have more than 10 million copies of HIV RNA.

After the first year of life, HIV RNA levels decrease slowly and may not reach adult levels for several years. Although considerable overlap exists in HIV RNA copy number in children younger than 12 months between those who have rapid disease progression and those who do not, generally, a high RNA copy number, particularly in the first week of life, may be associated with more rapid disease progression (Dickover et al., 1998). The data from children ages 30 months and older are similar to data from studies among infected adults, in which the risk for disease progression substantially increases when HIV RNA levels exceed 10,000 to 20,000 copies/mL (CDC, 1998a). Retrospective studies in children that demonstrated that HIV disease progression is directly related to HIV RNA viral load support therapeutic efforts to achieve plasma viral levels as low as possible (Palumbo et al., 1998; Abrams et al., 1998; Valentine et al., 1998).

▲ **Clinical Warning:** Because measurements of HIV RNA levels in even clinically stable individuals can vary significantly over the course of a day or on different days, changes in RNA HIV copy number should be interpreted cautiously and confirmed before being acted on.

Similar to the situation with HIV RNA testing, CD4+ lymphocyte counts in children are age dependent. CD4+ T-lymphocyte count and percentage values in healthy HIV-exposed infants are significantly higher than those observed in unaffected adults and slowly decline to adult values by age 6 years (ECS, 1992a). CD4+ lymphocyte cell counts decline as HIV infection progresses. With continued CD4+ lymphocyte depression, the prognosis worsens (Mofenson et al., 1997). Clinically irrelevant fluctuations in CD4+ lymphocyte count and percentage may occur, particularly with mild intercurrent illness or immunization. Management should not be modified based on a single CD4+ lymphocyte measurement.

● **Clinical Pearl:** In infants and children, a combination of CD4+ lymphocyte cell counts and HIV viral load may be most predictive of disease progression. As expected, children with low CD4+ cell counts and high HIV RNA viral loads have the worst outcome (Mofenson et al., 1997). Changes in these parameters, whether through disease progression or successful initiation of highly active antiretroviral therapy, predict mortality risk (Palumbo et al., 1998).

Antiretroviral Therapy

The use of triple-drug combination therapy now represents state-of-the-art treatment for certain patients with HIV infection. The provider needs to accept the fact that controversies remain over when to start antiretroviral therapy, which initial regimens are likely to be most durable, what constitutes treatment failure, and which salvage regimens are most likely to succeed. Again, close comanagement with the pediatric HIV specialist is warranted.

Several fundamental concepts are key to understanding the principles of antiretroviral therapy. Because ongoing HIV replication leads to immune system damage and progression to AIDS, the goal of therapy is to suppress HIV replication maximally. Combination antimicrobial therapy should be used, because drug resistance emerges rapidly when single-drug regimens are used. Potent combination antiretroviral therapy that suppresses HIV replication to below the levels of detection is important in limiting the potential for selection of HIV variants that are resistant to antiretroviral agents. Resistance is the major factor that limits the ability of antiretroviral drugs to inhibit virus replication and thus delay disease progression. The most effective means to accomplish durable suppression of HIV replication is the simultaneous initiation of combinations of effective anti-HIV drugs with which the patient has not been treated previously and that are not cross-resistant with antiretroviral agents with which the patient has been treated previously (CDC, 1998f).

Most data regarding the clinical efficacy of antiretroviral agents have been from studies of HIV-infected adults.

● **Clinical Pearl:** All antiretroviral drugs approved for treatment of HIV infection may be used in children when indicated—irrespective of labeling notations (AAP, Committee on Pediatric AIDS, 1998).

The agents currently available fall into three major classes:

- Nucleoside reverse transcriptase inhibitors (NRTI), which include zidovudine (AZT or ZDV), didanosine (ddI), stavudine (d4T), lamivudine (3TC), zalcitabine (ddC), and abacavir (ABC)
- Non-nucleoside reverse transcriptase inhibitors (NNRTI), which include nevirapine, efavirenz, and delavirdine
- Protease inhibitors (PI), which include saquinavir, indinavir, retonavir, amprenavir, and nelfinavir

Current preparations in each of these categories, dosing information, and their toxicities are presented in Table 65-6.

Highly active antiretroviral therapy is generally indicated in all HIV-infected children younger than 1 year, in patients with persistently rising HIV RNA levels or falling CD4+ lymphocytes or percentage, in patients with clinical evidence of HIV infection (including the acute retroviral syndrome), and in any child with HIV RNA levels greater than 100,000 copies/mL (CDC, 1998a; Working Group on Antiretroviral Therapy and Medical Management of HIV-Infected Children, 1999). Based on clinical trials in adults, the preferred initial antiretroviral regimen in children includes combination therapy with two NRTI agents and one PI, or two NRTI agents with a single NNRTI agent, such as efavirenz (Working Group on Antiretroviral Therapy and Medical Management of HIV-Infected Children, 1999). Which combination of PI and NRTIs to use is patient specific. Drug combinations depend on whether the child can swallow pills or capsules, what other medications the child may

Table 65–6. PREPARATIONS, DOSES, TOXICITIES, AND SPECIAL INSTRUCTIONS FOR ANTIRETROVIRAL AGENTS APPROVED FOR USE AS OF JULY 1999

Drug	Preparation	Dosing	Toxicities	Notes
Nucleoside Reverse Transcriptase Inhibitors				
Abacavir (ABC)	20 mg/mL solution 300-mg tablets	Children: 8 mg/kg/dose b.i.d. Maximum dose, 300 mg b.i.d.	Common: nausea, vomiting, fever, rash, fatigue Severe: 5% potentially fatal hypersensitivity reaction	Can be given with food Do not restart if hypersensitivity reaction occurs
Didanosine (ddI)	Powder for oral solution, 10 mg/mL 25-, 50-, 100-, 150-mg chewable tablets with buffers	Infants < 90 d: 50 mg/m^2 body surface area q12h Children: 90 mg/m^2 body surface area q12h Adolescents: < 60 kg: 125 mg b.i.d. ≥ 60 kg: 200 mg b.i.d.	Common: diarrhea, nausea, gastrointestinal pain Severe: peripheral neuropathy	Needs to be buffered with antacids Food decreases absorption; give on an empty stomach Multiple interactions
Lamivudine (3TC)	10 mg/mL solution 150-mg tablets	Infants < 30 d: 2 mg/kg/dose b.i.d. Children: 4 mg/kg/dose b.i.d Adolescents: < 50 kg: 2 mg/kg/dose b.i.d. ≥ 50 kg: 150 mg b.i.d.	Common: headache, fatigue, nausea Severe: pancreatitis (rare)	Can be given with food Very well tolerated Prevents emergence of zidovudine (ZDV) resistance
Stavudine (d4T)	1 mg/mL solution 15-, 20-, 30-, 40-mg tablets	Children: 1 mg/kg/dose b.i.d.	Common: headache, gastrointestinal disturbances, rash Severe: peripheral neuropathy and pancreatitis (rare)	Can be given with food Do not give with ZDV (poor effect)
Zalcitabine (ddC)	0.1 mg/mL syrup 0.375-, 0.75-mg tablets	Children: 0.01 mg/kg/dose q8h Adolescents: 0.75 mg t.i.d.	Common: headache, gastrointestinal disturbances, malaise Severe: peripheral neuropathy, pancreatitis, ulcers	Give on an empty stomach Do not give with IV pentamidine or ddC Infrequently used
Zidovudine (ZDV, AZT)	10 mg/mL syrup 100-mg capsules 300-mg tablets	Premature infants: 1.5 mg/kd/dose q12h for 2 wk then 2 mg/kg/dose q8h Neonates: 2 mg/kg/dose q6h Children: 160 mg/m^2/dose q8h Adolescents: 200 mg t.i.d. or 300 mg b.i.d.	Common: hematologic toxicity (granulocytopenia, anemia) Unusual: myopathy, myositis	Can be given with food Should not be given with d4T (poor effect) Substantial bone marrow toxicity may necessitate cessation Many potential drug interactions
Non-nucleoside Reverse Transcriptase Inhibitors				
Delavirdine (DLV)	100-mg tablets	Adolescents: 400 mg t.i.d.	Common: headache, fatigue Severe: rash	Can be given with food Metabolized by hepatic cytochrome p450; multiple drug interactions, including antihistamines, sedative-hypnotics, ergot alkaloid derivatives, rifamycins, azoles, macrolides, and protease inhibitors

(continues)

Table 65–6. PREPARATIONS, DOSES, TOXICITIES, AND SPECIAL INSTRUCTIONS FOR ANTIRETROVIRAL AGENTS APPROVED FOR USE AS OF JULY 1999 *(Continued)*

Drug	Preparation	Dosing	Toxicities	Notes
Efavirenz (DMP-266)	50-, 100-, 200-mg capsules	Children: 10–15 kg: 200/d 15–20 kg: 250 mg/d 20–25 kg: 300 mg/d 25–32.5 kg: 350 mg/d 32.5–40 kg: 400 mg/d >40 kg: 600 mg/d Adolescents: 600 mg/d	Common: skin rash, central nervous system effects: somnolence, confusion, insomnia, abnormal thinking Severe: teratogenic in primates	May be given with food Bedtime dosing recommended Mixed inducer/ inhibitor of cytochrome p450; multiple drug interactions, including antihistamines, sedative-hypnotics, ergot alkaloid derivatives, rifamycins, azoles, macrolides, and protease inhibitors Saquinavir and indinavir dosing may need to be increased
Nevirapine (NVP)	10 mg/mL suspension 200-mg tablets	Infants < 90 d: 5 mg/kg/ dose q.d. for 14 d, then 120 mg/m^2/dose q12h for 14 d, then 200 mg/m^2/dose q12h Children: 120 mg/m^2/d for 14 d, then 120–240 mg/m^2 q12h Adolescents: 100 mg q12h for 14 d, then 200 mg q12h	Common: skin rashes, fatigue, diarrhea, nausea Severe: life-threatening skin rashes (eg, Stevens-Johnson syndrome)	May be given with food Should be discontinued immediately in patients with severe rash or rash with constitutional symptoms Induces hepatic cytochrome p450; potential for multiple drug interactions, including rifamycins, oral contraceptives, digoxin, phenytoin, idinavir, and saquinavir
Protease Inhibitors Amprenavir	15 mg/mL suspension 150-mg gelatin capsules	Children > 4: 22/mg/kg/ dose q12h Adolescents: 1200 mg q12h	Common: nausea, vomiting, diarrhea Severe: severe rashes, Stevens-Johnson syndrome	May be given with or without food but not with a high-fat meal Suspension and capsules are not interchangable for dosing Do not give additional vitamin E supplements Metabolized by cytochrome p450; interactions occur with antihistamines, sedatives, rifampin, antifungals, and others Do not give with efavirenz (decreased effect)

(continues)

Table 65–6. PREPARATIONS, DOSES, TOXICITIES, AND SPECIAL INSTRUCTIONS FOR ANTIRETROVIRAL AGENTS APPROVED FOR USE AS OF JULY 1999 *(Continued)*

Drug	Preparation	Dosing	Toxicities	Notes
Indinavir	200-, 400-mg capsules	Children: 500 mg/m^2/dose q8h Adolescents: 800 mg q8h	Common: nausea, abdominal pain, metallic taste Severe: nephrolithiasis	Give on an empty stomach Maintain excellent hydration Metabolized through cytochrome p450; potential for multiple drug interactions, including antihistamines, cisapride, sedatives, rifampins, macrolides, and protease inhibitors
Nelfinavir	Powder for oral suspension; 50 mg/level gram scoopful 250-mg tablets	Neonates: 10 mg/kg/dose t.i.d. Children: 20–30 mg/kg/dose t.i.d. Adolescents: 750 mg t.i.d.	Common: diarrhea Less common: hyperglycemia, diabetes	May be given with meals or snacks but not acidic food or juice (poor taste) Metabolized in part by cytochrome p450; interactions with antihistamines, sedative-hypnotics, ergot alkaloid derivatives, rifamycins, azoles, macrolides, and protease inhibitors may occur
Ritonavir	80 mg/mL suspension 100-mg capsules	Children: 400 mg/m^2/dose q12h starting at 250 mg/m^2 and increasing over 5 d Adolescents: 600 mg b.i.d. starting at 300 mg b.i.d. and increasing over 5 d	Common: nausea, vomiting, diarrhea, hypertriglyceridemia Severe: pancreatitis, nausea can be severe	Food increases absorption; give with strong-tasting or very cold foods to increase tolerability in children To avoid nausea, slowly increase dose over 5 d Extensively metabolized by cytochrome p450; interactions with antihistamines, sedative-hypnotics, ergot alkaloid derivatives, rifamycins, azoles, macrolides, and protease inhibitors may occur
Saquinavir	200-mg soft gel (Fortovase) and hard gel (Invirase) capsules	Adolescents: hard gel capsules: 600 mg t.i.d. soft gel capsules 1200 mg t.i.d.	Common: diarrhea, abdominal discomfort, headache, skin rash Severe (rare): diabetes	Give within 2 h of a meal to increase absorption Sunscreen is recommended to reduce likelihood of photosensitivity reactions Metabolized by cytochrome p450; interactions with antihistamines, sedative-hypnotics, ergot alkaloid derivatives, rifamycins, azoles, macrolides, anti-convulsants, and protease inhibitors may occur

be taking, and convenience. Display 65-2 presents recommended antiviral regimens for initial therapy in HIV.

▲ **Clinical Warnings:**

- Monotherapy and combinations of NRTI agents that have overlapping toxicities or undesirable viral effects are strongly discouraged.
- Patients on antiretroviral agents need to be monitored closely for evidence of toxicity.
- When referring to and using the information presented in Table 65-6, the provider is advised that pediatric antiretroviral treatment regimens will continue to change and evolve.

The importance of adherence to treatment regimens cannot be overemphasized. Erratic adherence to prescribed regimens with concomitant subtherapeutic levels of antiretroviral medications, particularly PI agents, enhances the development of drug resistance. The primary care provider choosing antiretroviral regimens for children should understand that many factors influence adherence to a therapeutic regimen, including the following:

- Availability and palatability of pediatric formulation
- Complicated and exclusive dosing schedules
- Family understanding and resources
- Potential drug interactions (AAP, Committee on Pediatric AIDS, 1998; CDC, 1998f; Working Group on Antiretroviral Therapy and Medical Management of HIV-Infected Children, 1999)

Each of the antiretroviral drugs used in combination therapy regimens should always be used according to optimal schedules and dosages and with full participation by all caregivers.

DISPLAY 65–2 • Recommended Antiretroviral Regimens for the *Initial* Therapy for HIV-Infected Children

---

Preferred Regimens
- One protease inhibitor plus two nucleoside analogue reverse transcriptase inhibitors
- Efavirenz plus two nucleoside analogue reverse transcriptase inhibitors
- Efevirenz plus nelfinavir and one nucleoside analogue reverse transcriptase inhibitor

Alternative Regimen
- Nevirapine and two nucleoside analogue reverse transcriptase inhibitors

Secondary Alternative Regimen
- Two nucleoside analogue reverse transcriptase inhibitors

Not Recommended
- Any monotherapy
- The following combinations of nucleoside analogue reverse transcriptase inhibitors used alone or in combination with a protease inhibitor
- Stavudine and zidovudine
- Zalcitabine and didanosine
- Zalcitabine and stavudine
- Zalcitabine and lamivudine

Primary indications to change antimicrobial therapy include evidence of virologic, immunologic, or clinical disease progression or intolerable or unmanageable drug toxicities. Failure of the HIV RNA copy number to decrease or drop to undetectable levels after 6 months of therapy should also prompt an antimicrobial treatment regimen change. Treatment failures should prompt an assessment of adherence to the prescribed regimen. The therapy for HIV-infected children who have failed an antiretroviral regimen is difficult. Generally, providers should select at least two new drugs that the patient has not previously used. Refer to Table 65-5 for a review of these agents.

Disease Prevention

Disease prevention has many dimensions. The provider is challenged to educate all patients who are nearing puberty about effective means of preventing sexually transmitted HIV. Obviously, substance abuse should be included in this teaching. Information regarding HIV infection and AIDS, including transmission, implications of infection, and preventive measures, such as abstinence, should be regarded as important components of anticipatory guidance provided by the primary care provider to all adolescent patients. All sexually active adolescents should be counseled about the correct and consistent use of condoms to reduce the risk of infection (AAP, 2000). The reader may refer to Chapters 12, 25, and 41 for more information about these topics.

Although urgently needed, no effective HIV vaccine exists. While the host immune response is not able to eradicate HIV infection, it does reduce replication. Hence, a vaccine that mimics or augments the host immune response might be able to decrease either morbidity or infectiousness. However, the genetic diversity of HIV and the complex biology of HIV–host interaction make vaccine development challenging.

What to Tell Parents

The provider who cares for the child with HIV or AIDS should remember, and remind parents or caregivers, that despite health care needs, the patient is still an infant or a child or an adolescent. All children have needs related to healthy growth and development. The clinician is challenged to help the family meet those needs in the face of significant health concerns. Normal anticipatory guidance, including that related to health maintenance, safety, nutrition, sleep, play and exercise, discipline, and school should be provided at appropriate, age-related intervals as part of well child and adolescent visits. The goal of management is balancing the provider's support of optimum wellness with assisting the child in meeting developmental goals. Concerns related to day-to-day living must be supported within the context of meeting therapeutic goals. Refer to Chapter 49 for other ideas on managing the care of the child with HIV. The chapters that deal with healthy growth and development, as well as Community Resources, may also prove helpful.

School officials, adults associated with activities, and playmates and their families may all need education and support in understanding how to live, play, and learn safely and compassionately with the youngster with HIV. The clinician is referred to the section on Provider Resources at the end of this chapter. These resources can supply answers to often-asked questions and support the practitioner in learning more about management of this chronic condition. Similarly, referring parents, caregivers, and school officials to these community resources may help them in supporting the child's healthy growth and development.

Additional Referral Points and Clinical Warnings

Accidental injuries may result in HIV infection. Prospective studies of health care workers have estimated that the average risk for HIV transmission after a percutaneous exposure to HIV-infected blood is approximately 0.3% and after a mucous membrane exposure, 0.09% (Bell, 1997; Ippolito et al., 1993; Cardo et al., 1997). The risk of HIV infection after percutaneous exposure increases with a larger volume of blood and, possibly, a higher titer of HIV in the source patient's blood. Health care workers who sustain a percutaneous injury with HIV-infected blood should wash the wound with soap and water and consider postexposure prophylaxis. The standard regimen, consisting of 4 weeks of both zidovudine and lamivudine, should be started within the hour if possible (CDC, 1998d). For wounds associated with a greater risk of transmission, indinavir or nelfinavir may be added to the above regimen. The HIV antibody status of the health care worker should be determined at the time of the injury and at 6 weeks, 12 weeks, and 6 months after exposure (CDC, 1998d).

The risk of HIV transmission from a discarded needle in public places appears to be low. Data on the efficacy of postexposure prophylaxis with antiretroviral drugs in children are not available. Some experts recommend that antiretroviral chemoprophylaxis should be considered only in the unusual circumstance in which the syringe is available and is believed to contain fresh blood from an HIV-infected person (AAP, 1997). Testing for the presence of HIV antibody at the time of the injury is similarly controversial, but follow-up testing at 6 to 12 weeks and 6 months after the injury is indicated.

The risks of HIV transmission per episode of receptive penile-anal and receptive vaginal sexual exposures are estimated at 0.1% to 3% and 0.1% to 0.2%, respectively (Mastro & de Vincenzi, 1996). Providers should consider offering postexposure prophylaxis with zidovudine and lamivudine to rape victims who present within 72 hours of the incident (CDC, 1998c).

COMMUNITY RESOURCES

Resources for Patients and Their Families

Community resources are available in formal health care and outside the health care bureaucracy. These resources vary, depending on the region and on numbers of families living with HIV in a particular area. The provider should have a working acquaintance with at least the most common local resources to point parents toward sources of support. Information about what these services can provide and about respite care services is typically balanced by psychosocial support mechanisms. All are needed by these families.

PlanetRx Health Topics: AIDS and HIV
Internet address:
   http://www.planetrx.com/condition/cond_detail/info/
   3_introduction.html

This web site provides a reliable, current starting point for the patient learning about HIV, its management, and strategies for healthy living.

National AIDS Hotline
Telephone: (800) 342-AIDS (2437)

This hotline provides a database of all community-based resources in the United States.

African American AIDS Network
307 South Wabash Avenue
Chicago, IL 60605
Telephone: (312) 786-2226

Educational seminars and technical help are provided.

Minority AIDS Information Network
84 Walton Street NW
Atlanta, GA 30303
Telephone: (404) 651-8187
Fax: (404) 651-8190

Information and technical help for African American youth are provided.

National AIDS Treatment Advocacy Project
580 Broadway, Suite 403
New York, NY 10012
Telephone: (212) 219-0106
Toll-free: (888) 26-NATAP
Fax: (212) 219-8473
Internet address: http://www.natap.org

This project provides patient education about HIV treatments, educational materials.

Resources for Providers

Keeping abreast of the HIV/AIDS literature is a tremendous challenge for all providers, whether generalist or specialist. The following two web sites may be helpful:

HIV/AIDS Treatment Information Service
Internet address: http://www.hivatis.org

This web site includes a library of current and archived treatment guidelines, including Centers for Disease Control and Prevention: Guidelines for the use of antiretroviral agents in pediatric HIV infection. (Internet address: http://www.hivatis.org/guidelines/Pediatric/Text/ped_12.pdf.)

CDC National Center for HIV, STD, and TB Prevention, Divisions of HIV/AIDS Prevention
Fact Sheets
Internet address: http://www.cdc.gov/hiv/pubs/facts.htm

This CDC web page offers information and links to other sites providing current and reliable provider information.

BIBLIOGRAPHY

Abrams, E. J., Weedon, J. C., Steketee, R., et al. (1998). Association of HIV viral load early in life with disease progression among HIV-infected infants. *Journal of Infectious Diseases, 178*, 101–108.

Ameisen, J. C., Estaquier, J., Idziorek, T., & De Bels, F. (1995). Programmed cell death and AIDS pathogenesis: significance and potential mechanisms. *Current Topics in Microbiology and Immunology, 200*, 195–211.

American Academy of Pediatrics. (2000). *2000 Report of the Committee on Infectious Diseases*, p. 344.

American Academy of Pediatrics, Committee on Infectious Diseases and Committee on Pediatric AIDS. (1999). Measles immunization in HIV-infected children. *Pediatrics, 103*, 1057–1060.

American Academy of Pediatrics, Committee on Pediatric AIDS. (1998). Evaluation and medical treatment of the HIV-exposed infant. *Pediatrics, 99*, 909–917.

American Academy of Pediatrics, Committee on Pediatric AIDS. (1999). Disclosure of illness status to children and adolescents with HIV infection. *Pediatrics, 103,* 164–166.

American College of Obstetricians and Gynecologists. (1997). Human immunodeficiency virus infections in pregnancy. *International Journal of Gynaecology and Obstetrics, 57,* 73–80.

Antiretroviral therapy and medical management of pediatric HIV infection and 1997 USPHS/IDSA report on the prevention of opportunistic infections in persons infected with human immunodeficiency virus. (1998). *Pediatrics, 101*(4 Pt 2), 999–1085.

Barnhart, H. X., Caldwell, M. B., Thomas, P., et al. (1996). Natural history of human immunodeficiency virus disease in perinatally infected children: An analysis from the Pediatric Spectrum of Disease Project. *Pediatrics, 97,* 710–716.

Bell, D. M. (1997). Occupational risk of human immunodeficiency virus infection in healthcare workers: an overview. *American Journal of Medicine, 102*(suppl 5B), 9–15.

Brosgart, C. L., Mitchell, T. F., Coleman, R. L., Dyner, T., Stephenson, K. E., & Abrams, D. I. (1999). Clinical experience and choice of drug therapy for human immunodeficiency virus disease. *Clinical Infectious Diseases, 28,* 14–22.

Cardo, D. M., Culver, D. H., Ciesielski, C. A., et al. (1997). A case-control study of HIV seroconversion in health care workers after percutaneous exposure. *New England Journal of Medicine, 337,* 1485–1490.

Centers for Disease Control. (1987). Revision of the CDC surveillance case definition for acquired immunodeficiency syndrome. *Morbidity and Mortality Weekly Report, 36*(supp 11), 1S–15S.

Centers for Disease Control and Prevention. (1992). 1993 revised Classification system for HIV infection and expanded surveillance case definition for AIDS among adolescents and adults. *Morbidity and Mortality Weekly Report, 41*(RR-17), 1.

Centers for Disease Control and Prevention. (1994). 1994 Revised Classification System for human immunodeficiency virus infection in children less than 13 years of age. *Morbidity and Mortality Weekly Report, 43*(RR-12), 1–10.

Centers for Disease Control and Prevention. (1995). 1995 Revised Guidelines for Prophylaxis against *Pneumocystis carinii* pneumonia for children affected with or perinatally exposed to human immunodeficiency virus. *Morbidity and Mortality Weekly Report, 44*(RR-4), 1–11.

Centers for Disease Control and Prevention. (1996). *HIV/AIDS Surveillance Report, 8,* 1–39.

Centers for Disease Control and Prevention. (1997a). 1997 USPHS/IDSA Guidelines for the prevention of opportunistic infections in persons infected with human immunodeficiency virus. *Morbidity and Mortality Weekly Report, 46*(RR-12), 1–46.

Centers for Disease Control and Prevention. (1997b). *HIV/AIDS Surveillance Report 9,* 1–39.

Centers for Disease Control and Prevention. (1998a). Guidelines for the use of antiretroviral agents in HIV-infected adults and adolescents. *Morbidity and Mortality Weekly Report, 47*(RR-5), 39–82.

Centers for Disease Control and Prevention. (1998b). *HIV/AIDS Surveillance Report, 10,* 1–43.

Centers for Disease Control and Prevention. (1998c). Management of possible sexual, injecting-drug-use, or other nonoccupational exposure to HIV, including considerations related to antiretroviral therapy public health service statement. *Morbidity and Mortality Weekly Report, 47*(RR-17), 1–14.

Centers for Disease Control and Prevention. (1998d). Public Health Service guidelines for the management of health-care worker exposures to HIV and recommendations for postexposure prophylaxis. *Morbidity and Mortality Weekly Report, 47*(RR-7), 1–28.

Centers for Disease Control and Prevention. (1998e). Public Health Service task force recommendations for the use of antiretroviral drugs in pregnant women infected with HIV-1 for maternal health and for reducing perinatal HIV-1 transmission in the United States. *Morbidity and Mortality Weekly Report, 47*(RR-2), 1–30.

Centers for Disease Control and Prevention. (1998f). Report of the NIH panel to define principles of therapy for HIV infection. *Morbidity and Mortality Weekly Report, 47*(RR-5), 1–38.

Centers for Disease Control and Prevention. (1998g). Success in implementing public health service guidelines to reduce peri-natal transmission of HIV-Louisiana, Michigan, New Jersey, and South Carolina, 1993, 1995, and 1996. *Morbidity and Mortality Weekly Report, 47,* 688–691.

Cohen, J., Reddington, C., Jacobs, D., et al. (1997). School-related issues among HIV-infected children. *Pediatrics, 100,* 1–5.

Cohen, O. J., Pantaleo, G., Schwartzentruber, D. J., Graziosi, C., Vaccarezza, M., & Fauci, A. S. (1995). Pathogenic insights from studies of lymphoid tissue from HIV-infected individuals [published erratum appears in *Journal of Acquired Immune Deficiency Syndromes Human Retrovirology* 1996 Feb 1;11(2):210]. *Journal of Acquired Immune Deficiency Syndromes Human Retrovirology, 10*(Suppl 1), S6–14.

Connor, E. M., Sperling, R. S., Gelber, R., et al. (1994). Reduction of maternal-infant transmission of human immunodeficiency virus type 1 with zidovudine treatment. *New England Journal of Medicine, 331,* 1173–1180.

Cooper, E. R., Hanson, C., Diaz, C., et al. (1998). Encephalopathy and progression of human immunodeficiency virus disease in a cohort of children with perinatally acquired human immunodeficiency virus infection. Women and Infants Transmission Study Group. *Journal of Pediatrics, 132,* 808–812.

Courville, T. M., Caldwell, B., & Brunell, P. A. (1998). Lack of evidence of transmission of HIV-1 to family contacts of HIV-1 infected children. *Clinical Pediatrics (Phila), 37,* 175–178.

Culnane, M., Fowler, M., Lee, S. S., et al. (1999). Lack of long-term effects of in utero exposure to zidovudine among uninfected children born to HIV-infected women. *Journal of the American Medical Association, 281,* 151–157.

Datta, P., Embree, J. E., Kreiss, J., et al. (1994). Mother to child transmission of human immunodeficiency virus type-1: Report from the Nairobi Study. *Journal of Infectious Diseases, 170,* 1134–1140.

DeRossi, A., Giaquinto, C., Ometto, L., et al. (1993). Replication and tropism of human immunodeficiency virus type 1 as predictors of disease outcome in infants with vertically acquired infection. *Journal of Pediatrics, 123,* 929–936.

Dickover, R. E., Dillon, M., Leung, K. M., et al. (1998). Early prognostic indicators in primary perinatal human immunodeficiency virus type 1 infection: Importance of viral RNA and the timing of transmission on long-term outcome. *Journal of Infectious Diseases, 178,* 375–387.

Dunn, D. T., Brandt, C. D., Kirvine, A., et al. (1995). The sensitivity of HIV-1 DNA polymerase chain reaction in the neonatal period and the relative contributes of intrauterine and intrapartum transition. *AIDS, 9,* F7–F11.

Englund, J. A., Baker, C. J., Raskino, C., et al. (1996). Clinical and laboratory characteristics of a large cohort of symptomatic, human immunodeficiency virus-infected infants and children. *Pediatric Infectious Disease Journal, 15,* 1025–1036.

European Collaborative Study. (1990). Neurologic signs in children with human immunodeficiency virus infection. *Pediatric Infectious Disease Journal, 9,* 402–406.

European Collaborative Study. (1992a). Age-related standards for T-lymphocyte subsets based on uninfected children born to human immunodeficiency virus 1 infected women. *Pediatric Infectious Disease Journal, 11,* 1018–1026.

European Collaborative Study. (1992b). Risk factors for mother to child transmission of HIV-1. *Lancet, 339,* 1007–1012.

Farley, J. J., King, J. G., Nair, P., Hines, S. E., Tressler, R. L., & Vink, P. E. (1994). Invasive pneumococcal disease among infected and uninfected children of mothers with human immunodeficiency virus infection. *Journal of Pediatrics, 124,* 853–858.

Gallo, R. C., Salahuddin, S. Z., Popovic, M., et al. (1984). Frequent detection and isolation of cytopathic retroviruses (HTLV-III) from patients with AIDS and at risk for AIDS. *Science, 224,* 500.

Gottlieb, M. S., Schroff, R., Schanker, H. M. et al. (1981). *Pneumocystis carinii* pneumonia and mucosal candidiasis in previously healthy homosexual men: Evidence for a new severe acquired cellular immunodeficiency syndrome. *New England Journal of Medicine, 305,* 1425–1431.

Heath, S. L., Tew, J. G., Tew, J. G., Szakal, A. K., & Burton, G. F. (1995). Follicular dentritic cells and human immunodeficiency virus infectivity. *Nature, 377,* 740–744.

HIV and infant feeding: A policy statement developed collaboratively by UNAIDS, WHO and UNICEF, 1997. (1999). *Breastfeeding Review, 7,* 14.

Ho, D. D., Neumann, A. U., Perelson, A. S., Chen, W., Leonard, J. M., & Markowitz, M. (1995). Rapid turnover of plasma virions and CD4 lymphocytes in HIV-1 infection. *Nature, 373,* 123–126.

Huang, Y., Paxton, W. A., Wolinsky, S. M., et al. (1996). The role of a mutant CCR5 allele in HIV-1 transmission and disease progression. *Nature Medicine, 2,* 1240–1243.

International Perinatal HIV Group. (1999). The mode of delivery and the risk of vertical transmission of human immunodeficiency virus type 1: A meta-analysis of prospective cohort studies. *New England Journal of Medicine, 340,* 977–987.

Ippolito, G., Puro, V., & De Carli, G. (1993). The risk of occupational human immunodeficiency virus infection in health care workers. Italian Multicenter Study. The Italian Study Group on Occupational Risk of HIV Infection. *Archives of Internal Medicine, 153,* 1451–1458.

Kline, M. W., Lewis, D. E., Hollinger, F. B., et al. (1994). A comparative study of human immunodeficiency virus culture, polymerase chain reaction and anti-human immunodeficiency virus immunoglobulin A antibody detection in the diagnosis during early infancy of vertically acquired human immunodeficiency virus infection. *Pediatric Infectious Disease Journal, 13,* 90–94.

Kovacs, A., Xu, J., Rasheed, S., et al. (1995). Comparison of a rapid non-isotopic polymerase chain reaction assay with four commonly used methods for the early diagnosis of human immunodeficiency virus type 1 infection in neonates and children. *Pediatric Infectjious Disease Journal, 14,* 948–954.

Kreiss, J. (1997). Breastfeeding and vertical transmission of HIV-1. *Acta Paediatrica Supplement, 421,* 113–117.

Kuhn, L., & Stein, Z. (1997). Infant survival, HIV infection, and feeding alternatives in less-developed countries. *American Journal of Public Health, 87,* 926–931.

Latham, M. C. (1999). Breast feeding reduces morbidity. The risk of HIV transmission requires risk assessment—not a shift to formula feeds. *British Medical Journal, 318,* 1303–1304.

Laurence, J., Brun-Vezinet, F., Schutzer, S. E., et al. (1984). Lymphadenopathy-associated viral antibody in AIDS: Immune correlations and definitions of carrier state. *New England Journal of Medicine, 311,* 1269.

Leroy, V., Newell, M. L., Dabis, F., et al. (1998). International multicentre pooled analysis of late postnatal mother-to-child transmission of HIV-1 infection. *Lancet, 352,* 597–600.

Lichenstein, R., King, J. C. Jr, Farley, J. J., et al. (1998). Bacteremia in febrile human immunodeficiency virus-infected children presenting to ambulatory care settings. *Pediatric Infectious Disease Journal, 117,* 381–385.

Lindegren, M. L., Hanson, I. C., Hammett, T. A., et al. (1998). Sexual abuse of children: Intersection with the HIV epidemic. *Pediatrics, 102,* e46.

Liu, R., Paxton, W. A., Choe, S., et al. (1996). Homozygous defect in HIV-1 coreceptor accounts for resistance of some multiply-exposed individuals to HIV-1 infection. *Cell, 86,* 367–377.

Luzuriaga, K., Bryson, Y., Krogstad, P., et al. (1997). Combination treatment with zidovudine, didanosine, and nevirapine in infants with human immunodeficiency virus type 1 infection. *New England Journal of Medicine, 336,* 1343–1349.

Martinson, J. J. (1997). Global distribution of the CCR5 gene 32-base-pair deletion. *Nature Genetics, 16,* 100–103.

Mastro, T. D., & de Vincenzi, I. (1996). Probabilities of sexual HIV-1 transmission. *AIDS, 10*(suppl A), S75–S82.

Mellors, J. W., Kingsley, L. A., Rinaldo, C. R. Jr, et al. (1995). Quantitation of HIV-1 RNA in plasma predicts outcome after seroconversion. *Annals of Internal Medicine, 122,* 573–579.

Miotti, P. G., Taha, T. E., Kumwenda, N. I., Broadhead, R., Mtimavalye, L. A., et al. (1999). HIV transmission through breastfeeding: A study in Malawi. *Journal of the American Medical Association, 282,* 744–749.

Mofenson, L., Korelitz, J., Meyer, W. A., et al. (1997). The relationship between serum human immunodeficiency virus type 1 (HIV-1) RNA level, CD4 lymphocyte percent, and long-term mortality risk in HIV-1-infected children. National Institute of Child Health and Human Development Intravenous Immunoglobulin Clinical Trial Study Group. *Journal of Infectious Diseases, 175,* 1029–1038.

Morrison, P. (1999). HIV and infant feeding: To breastfeed or not to breastfeed: The dilemma of competing risks. Part 1. *Breastfeeding Review, 7,* 5–13.

Musey, L., Hughes, J., Schackter, T., et al. (1997). Cytotoxic-T-cell responses, viral load, and disease progression in early human immunodeficiency virus type 1 infection. *New England Journal of Medicine, 337,* 1267–1274.

National Institute of Allergy and Infectious Diseases (NIAID). *1996 Pediatric AIDS.* NIH NIAID Office of Communications.

Nesheim, S., Lee, F., Kalish, M. L., et al. (1997). Diagnosis of perinatal human immunodeficiency virus infection by polymerase chain reaction and p24 antigen detection after immune complex dissociation in an urban community hospital. *Journal of Infectious Diseases, 175,* 1333–1336.

New York Times. Vol.CXLVIII, no. 51,584. July 15, 1999. Page 1.

NICHD IVIG Study Group. (1991). Intravenous immunoglobulin for the prevention of bacterial infection in children with symptomatic human immunodeficiency virus infection. *New England Journal of Medicine, 325,* 73.

Palumbo, P., Raskino, C., Fiscus, S., et al. (1998). Predictive value of quantitative plasma RNA and CD4+ lymphocyte count in HIV-infected infants and children. *Journal of the American Medical Association, 279,* 756–761.

Palumbo, P. E., Kwok, S., Waters, S., et al. (1995). Viral measurement by polymerase chain reaction-based assays in human immunodeficiency virus-infected infants. *Journal of Pediatrics, 126,* 592–595.

Pantaleo, G., Graziosi, C., & Fauci, A. S. (1993). Immunopathogenesis of human immunodeficiency virus infection. *New England Journal of Medicine, 328,* 327–335.

Perelson, A. S., Neumann, A. U., Markowitz, M., Leonard, J. M., & Ho, D. D. (1996). HIV-1 dynamics in vivo: virion clearance rate, infected cell life-span, and viral generation time. *Science, 271,* 1582–1586.

Quinn, T. C. (1997). Acute primary HIV infection. *Journal of the American Medical Association, 278,* 58–62.

Robbins, G. (1999). Time for a new paradigm: Optimal management of patients with human immunodeficiency virus infection and AIDS. *Clinical Infectious Diseases, 28,* 23–25.

Rogers, M. F., Ou, C. Y., Rayfield, M., et al. (1989). Use of the polymerase chain reaction for early detection of the proviral sequences of human immunodeficiency virus in infants born to seropositive mothers. *New England Journal of Medicine, 320,* 649–654.

Saba, J. (1999). The results of the PETRA intervention trial to prevent perinatal transmission in sub-Saharan Africa. Chicago, IL: 6th Conference on Retroviruses and Opportunistic Infections. Jan 31–Feb 4.

Scott, G. B., Hutto, C., Makuch, R. W., et al. (1989). Survival in children with perinatally acquired human immunodeficiency virus type 1 infection. *New England Journal of Medicine, 321,* 1791.

Shearer, W. T., Quinn, T. C., & LaRussa, P. (1997). Viral load and disease progression in infants infected with human immunodeficiency virus type 1. Women and Infants Transmission Study Group. *New England Journal of Medicine, 336,* 1337–1342.

Simonds, R. J., Steketee, R., Nesheim, S., et al. (1998). Impact of Zidovudine use on risk and risk factors for perinatal transmission of HIV. Perinatal AIDS Collaborative Transmission Studies. *AIDS, 12,* 301–308.

Spector, S. A., Gelber, R. D., McGrath, N., et al. (1994). A controlled trial of intravenous immune globulin for the prevention of serious bacterial infections in children receiving zidovudine for advanced human immunodeficiency virus infection. Pediatric AIDS Clinical Trials Group. *New England Journal of Medicine, 331,* 1181–1187.

Sperling, R. S., Shapiro, D. E., Coombs, R. W., et al. (1997). Maternal viral load, zidovudine treatment and the risk of transmission of human immunodeficiency virus type 1 from mother to infant. Pediatric AIDS Clinical Trials Group Protocol 076 Study Group. *New England Journal of Medicine, 335,* 1621–1629.

Stanecki, K. A., & Way, P. O. (1997). *The demographic impacts of HIV/AIDS-Perspectives from the world population profile: 1996.* U.S. Bureau of the Census, IPC Staff paper No. 86, March 1997.

Steketee, R. W., Abrams, E. J., Thea, D. M., et al. (1997). Early detection of perinatal human immunodeficiency virus (HIV) type 1 infection using HIV RNA amplification and detection. New York City Perinatal HIV Transmission Collaborative Study. *Journal of Infectious Diseases, 175,* 707–711.

Thea, D. M., Lambert, G., Weedon, J., et al. (1996). Benefit of primary prophylaxis before 18 months of age in reducing the incidence of *Pneumocystis carinii* pneumonia and early death in a cohort of 112 human immunodeficiency virus-infected infants. New York City Perinatal HIV Transmission Collaborative Study Group. *Pediatrics, 97,* 59–64.

Tovo, P. A., deMartino, M., & Gabiano, C. (1992). Prognostic factors and survival in children with perinatal HIV-1 infection. *Lancet, 339,* 1249–1253.

UNAIDS. (1998). Report on the global HIV/AIDS epidemic. Available at: *http://www.unaids.org/highband/document/epidemiology/report 97.html.*

Valentine, M. E., Jackson, C. R., Vavro, C., et al. (1998). Evaluation of surrogate markers and clinical outcomes in two-year follow-up of eighty-six human immunodeficiency virus-infected pediatric patients. *Pediatric Infectious Disease Journal, 17,* 18–23.

Wade, N. A., Birkhead, G. S., Warren, B. L., et al. (1998). Abbreviated regimens of zidovudine prophylaxis and perinatal transmission of the human immunodeficiency virus. *New England Journal of Medicine, 339,* 1409–1414.

Whortley, P. M., & Fleming, P. L. (1997). AIDS in women in the United States. *Journal of the American Medical Association, 278,* 911–916.

Wilfert, C. M., Wilson, C., Luzuriaga, K., & Epstein, L. (1994). Pathogenesis of pediatric human immunodeficiency virus type 1 infection. *Journal of Infectious Diseases, 170,* 286–292.

Working Group on Antiretroviral Therapy and Medical Management of HIV-Infected Children. Guidelines for the use of antiretroviral agents in pediatric HIV infection. *www.hivatis.org/guidelines/pedapril415.pdf.* April 15, 1999.

Organ Transplantation

• CAROLINE TASSEY, MS, CPNP

INTRODUCTION

Organ transplant has expanded the treatment options available to children with end-stage disease, structural anomalies incompatible with life, and refractory malignancies. About 2000 infants, children, and adolescents are currently waiting for solid organ transplant (all statistics are from United Network for Organ Sharing [UNOS] and are available on their website at *www.unos.org*). Of these, approximately one third are infants and children younger than 6 years. Bone marrow transplant (BMT) is no longer a treatment of last resource but an increasingly standard treatment for recurrent childhood leukemias. Survival rates for all transplants have increased significantly over the past 10 to 15 years. New techniques, such as partial organ transplant, have expanded recipient options. As a result, the primary care provider can expect to care for one or more children who are awaiting or have undergone transplant. While all these children will be followed by subspecialists and, in varying degrees, by the transplant center, they continue to require good, consistent primary care. This chapter describes the transplant process and transplant-related complications. This information will help the provider in the support and collaborative management of the patient and family.

PATHOLOGY AND EPIDEMIOLOGY

Kidney

End stage renal disease of diverse etiology is the primary indication for renal transplant. Reasons for transplant need include structural anomalies and inborn errors of metabolism. More than 600 pediatric renal transplants were performed in 1997 (Feber et al., 1998; D'Alessandro et al., 1998). Among adolescents on the transplant waiting list, the largest group—43%—are waiting for a kidney (Salvatierra et al., 1997; Feber et al., 1998; Salvatierra et al., 1998). The kidney plays an important role in physical growth. Therefore, kidney transplant in a younger child, before growth has been stunted, improves the chance for attaining normal height (Feber et al., 1998). Refer to Chapter 62 for further detail about the kidneys' role in growth.

Donor kidneys are placed in the abdomen rather than in the retroperitoneal space. Therefore, the size of the graft is not important. Adult kidneys can be used for all but the smallest infants. At 7 to 10 kg, most infants can accept an adult kidney. In fact, survival of infants who receive adult-sized kidneys is higher than those transplanted with size-compatible pediatric kidneys (Salvatierra et al., 1998). Patient survival with an organ from a living related donor (LRD), usually a parent, is 96% at 1 year; 5-year survival is 93%. Graft survival rates are lower (84% and 65%), but graft failure can be managed with dialysis and retransplant.

Cadaver donor transplants are generally less successful. The oldest survivor of a pediatric kidney transplant received an LRD kidney at 14 years of age in 1963. As of 1998, this recipient has had 35 years of continuous graft function. Overall, pediatric renal transplant has been so successful that virtually any child with chronic renal failure should be considered a candidate regardless of age, size, or etiology of renal failure (Salvatierra et al., 1997; UNOS, 1997–1998).

Liver

Indications for liver transplant include congenital malformations, metabolic liver disease, neoplasms without metastases, and liver failure of diverse etiology. Early transplant of the liver-pancreas is also indicated for children with cystic fibrosis whose lung disease is only moderate (Kelly, 1998). About 550 pediatric liver transplants were performed in 1997 (Boucek et al., 1997). The largest number of infants and children up to 10 years of age on the transplant waiting list are waiting for a liver (54% and 45%, respectively) (UNOS, 1999).

The ability to use reduced-size liver transplants by splitting a harvested organ or transplanting only one lobe has reduced waiting time for recipients, improved options for neonates and infants, and allowed the use of LRDs. Neonates under 10 kg can undergo partial liver transplant; the youngest surviving recipient was 12 days old. The current trend is to transplant earlier, before development of significant growth or psychosocial retardation (Zitelli, 1986). Malnutrition is a common complication of chronic liver failure and adversely affects survival after transplant. One-year survival is currently 80%; 5-year survival is 76%. However, longer-term survival should improve with the use of LRD organs (UNOS, 1997–1998).

Heart

Indications for pediatric heart transplant include congenital structural cardiac anomalies and cardiomyopathy, both congenital and acquired. Almost 300 heart transplants were performed in 1997 (Boucek et al., 1997). Infants younger than 1 year account for almost 33% of all heart transplant recipients. Structural congenital heart disease (CHD) is the transplant indication for 75% of these infants. In children up to 10 years of age, CHD and myopathy account for 40% and 60% of transplants, respectively. By adolescence, the most common reason for heart transplant (65%) is cardiomyopathy (Boucek et al., 1997).

Unfortunately, the volume of heart transplants has not changed much since 1990. About one third of listed infants die awaiting a heart (Morrow et al., 1997). The major limiting factor to successful heart transplantation in infants and young children is the limited supply of donors. Further, size concurrence is critical in pediatric heart transplant. The donor heart and great vessels are grafted to the recipient's right atrial appendage and great vessels. If the donor organ is too large, the sternum cannot be closed. The donor heart contains its own functioning sinoatrial node. There is no connection between the recipient's autonomic nervous system and the donor heart.

Early mortality after heart transplant remains high, ranging from 12% to 24%. Survival is best in the adolescent group (80% at 1 year) and worst in the infant group (70% at 1 year), although some centers specializing in infant transplant report better results. The Loma Linda group reports infant survival as 91% at 1 month, 84% at 1 year, 78% at 5 years, and 70% at 7 years (Morrow et al., 1997). By 5 years post-transplant, no age difference is seen in survival rates. Five-year survival is 60% (Boucek et al., 1997; Canter et al., 1997).

Lung

Indications for pediatric lung transplant include congenital pulmonary fibrosis, primary pulmonary hypertension, inborn errors of metabolism, cystic fibrosis, and chronic obstructive pulmonary disease, often secondary to CHD. In the adolescent group, cystic fibrosis is the most common indication for transplant (63%). No single indicator predominates in younger age groups (UNOS, 1997–1998).

Both single-lung and bilateral lung transplants are performed. Size match is not critical. If there is a difference in donor and recipient lung capacity, the transplanted lung will adjust to new surroundings. Sequential single-lung transplant is commonly used for recipients with cystic fibrosis. Children with CHD and pulmonary vascular disease require heart-lung transplantation.

Mortality after lung transplant remains high. One-year survival for all age groups is 70%; 4-year survival is 50% (Boucek et al., 1997). One-year survival for heart-lung recipients is 59%. The longest survival time after pediatric lung transplant is currently 6½ years (UNOS, 1997–1998).

Bone Marrow

Bone marrow transplant is now an accepted therapeutic option for children with a variety of diseases. These include leukemias and other malignancies, as well as several hematologic and immunodeficiency diseases. BMT is the treatment of choice for children who relapse from conventional chemotherapy for mylogenous leukemias in first remission or in chronic phase (Sanders, 1997). Donor marrow is obtained by multiple needle aspirations and infused intravenously into the recipient. The donor's risk is low, although complications from anesthesia and infection have occurred. Donors may be hospitalized overnight. The recipient is pretreated with high-dose chemotherapy and total body irradi-

ation to produce immunosuppression. There are no lower age limits for either recipients or donors, but there are a limited number of pediatric BMT centers.

Mortality remains high. Even in a perfect human leukocyte antigen (HLA)-matched donor-recipient relationship, both acute and chronic graft-versus-host disease (GVHD) can occur. Not all histocompatibility antigens have yet been identified. Five-year event-free survival currently ranges from 38% to 59%, and is dependent on the initial indication for transplant. Children with acute lymphocytic leukemia in second remission who receive allogenic sibling BMT have the lowest mortality (Gordon et al., 1997; Sanders, 1997).

A successful transplant depends on matching the recipient's genetic HLA haplotype with that of a donor. HLA antigens are responsible for the self-specific immune response. HLA antigens vary greatly among individuals. There are three types of BMT. Autologous transplants use marrow previously harvested from the recipient. Syngeneic transplants use marrow harvested from an identical twin. Allogenic transplants are the most common type, using marrow from a donor who has the same histocompatibility antigens as the recipient. Usually, but not always, a sibling, parent, or other relative is the marrow donor.

● **Clinical Pearl:** Donor marrow must be obtained on the day the recipient will acquire it.

Table 66-1 provides a summary of transplant survival rates at 1 year postsurgery.

HELPING THE CHILD AND FAMILY PREPARE FOR TRANSPLANT

Logistical and Practical Issues

Generally, children are considered for transplant when their quality of life begins to deteriorate and their potential lifespan is no more than 1 to 2 years. Most children are already followed by a subspecialist who will make the decision to refer for transplant. Neonates who require heart transplant for complex, single-ventricle defects are listed at birth if the family does not choose or the infant is not a candidate for palliation. Not every child referred for transplant will be listed. Patients and their families undergo extensive medical and psychosocial evaluation by a team consisting of medical specialists, psychologists, clinical nurse specialists, pharmacists, social workers, and others. The family's ability to fol-

Table 66–1. SUMMARY OF CURRENT STATISTICS ON TRANSPLANT SURVIVAL RATES

Type of Transplant	1-Year Survival Rate	1-Year Graft Survival Rate
Heart	82.4%	
Kidney	93.2%	80% (cadaveric graft)
Liver	78.6%	
Lung	68.9%	
Pancreas	89% all recipients	71.9%
Heart-lung	59%	

Data from UNOS Scientific Registry, 1998.

low the post-transplant treatment regimen and to manage the economic and psychosocial impact of the process is an important consideration.

Immunologic testing may suggest that an individual child is unlikely to match with more than 1% to 2% of donors (Stiehm, 1996; Yunis & Dupont, 1993). Children have a poorer chance of being listed if they have active infections, such as human immunodeficiency virus; significant systemic disease, such as diabetes; or chromosomal or genetic abnormalities with poor long-term prognosis.

Once listed, children are designated status I or status II. Status I individuals have priority in the allocation of available organs. To qualify as status I, a child must be hospitalized in the intensive care unit, requiring mechanical ventilation, or intravenous inotropic therapy. Infants younger than 6 months are automatically designated status I. There is no status I for lung (and heart-lung) recipients.

The waiting time for an organ to become available is difficult to predict. Currently, time spent on the list varies significantly from one transplant center to another. For example, patients listed (all organs) at the University of Pittsburgh Medical Center wait 721 days on average, while those listed at the Medical University of South Carolina average a 136-day wait (Langley, 1999). However, new U.S. Department of Health and Human Services regulations may change how donated organs are allocated in the near future. These regulations would establish a national registry and require donated organs to be distributed across the country to the sickest patients. The impact this change will have on pediatric patients waiting for organs remains to be seen.

Transportation time to the transplant center for both the organ and the child can affect waiting time. The window of opportunity between notification that an organ is available and the child's arrival in the operating suite varies by organ. Some families choose or are required to move closer to the transplant center to be ready when an organ becomes available. In reality, this usually means that one parent and the child maintain a residence near the transplant center, while the other parent and any siblings live at home.

Emotional and Ethical Issues

Waiting for an organ is emotionally difficult for families. Parents feel exhilarated when their child is listed, anxious and impatient as they wait, and then depressed while watching their child become sicker and wondering if an organ will become available. They experience relief and excitement when one does, and they also feel guilty, knowing that they are waiting for another parent's child to die. During the long period of waiting for an organ, the primary care provider is a major source of support, counseling, and knowledge of community resources.

The family experiences unique stresses when a family member is considered for donation or becomes the organ donor. Serious complications to the solid (ie, replaced) organ donor are rare, but the risks of surgery, anesthesia, and acute or chronic organ dysfunction do exist. For example, liver function of the partial liver donor is affected in the immediate postoperative period (Tojimbara et al., 1998). The use of minor siblings as organ donors remains an ethical issue, although most primary care providers now accept the parents' right to consent to bone marrow extraction from siblings, including infants older than 6 months, even when the likelihood of successful transplantation is poor (Chan et al., 1996). When a graft is rejected or fails, the sibling or parent donor may experience guilt and distress (Shama, 1998). Sibling donors report higher levels of anxiety and lower levels of self-esteem than nondonor siblings (Packman et al., 1997).

MANAGEMENT

Helping the Child and Family Post-transplantation

Duration of hospitalization after solid organ transplant is 2 to 4 weeks. BMT recipients will be hospitalized for 4 to 6 weeks and will be quite ill during the first 2 to 3 weeks because of the pretransplant conditioning. The transplanted marrow will take 2 to 3 weeks to begin providing effective immunity. Programs have varying requirements for extended stay near the transplant center after discharge. Extended stay is necessary to provide frequent monitoring and close supervision of the immunosuppressant regimen. This period may last for several months. The financial burden for maintaining this second home falls largely on the recipient's family. Family finances and family separation are the biggest parental stressors during the transplant process (Rodrigue et al., 1996). The average cost of pediatric BMT, for example, is $100,000 to $250,000 (Yoder, 1998). Solid organ transplant costs exceed $100,000. Third-party payers will not provide all of the cost of transplant.

It is the primary care provider's responsibility to optimize child and family health during this waiting period. The provider is key in preparing the family for living with an immunosuppressed member. It is very common for families to view transplant as a panacea. They need to understand that transplant is not a cure. For example, although BMT may offer a full return to health, solid organ transplantation trades one chronic illness for another—albeit a more manageable one with a better long-term prognosis.

Vaccinations

Immunosuppression will affect the child's ability to be vaccinated and increase his or her risk when exposed to common contagious diseases. Every effort should be made to complete appropriate vaccination series prior to transplant (vaccination recommendations following the American Academy of Pediatrics 2000 *Red Book: Report of the Committee on Infectious Diseases*; individual transplant centers may have specific recommendations). In particular, hepatitis B vaccination and all live-virus vaccinations (measles-mumps-rubella [MMR], varicella) should be completed if possible. When feasible, immunizations should be given no later than 1 month before transplant to allow an adequate antibody response before immunosuppression. Hepatitis A immunization is not routinely recommended for recipients.

The primary care provider should discuss the immune status of family members and other close contacts. Once the child is immunosuppressed, close contacts may not be immunized with oral polio virus vaccine (Sabin) if the child's polio vaccination series is incomplete. Transmission of the vaccine virus after MMR and varicella immunization has not been documented, so siblings and household contacts can receive these vaccines.

Active disease poses a risk for the immunosuppressed child. Varicella vaccine is recommended for susceptible contacts of immunosuppressed children. If the transplant recipient is at least 2 years old, pneumococcal vaccine should be given at least 2 weeks before transplant. Revaccination after 3 to 5 years is then recommended for children 10 years of age and younger. Yearly influenza immunization should be given to children older than 6 months and their household contacts. All household contacts should be immunized against hepatitis A.

▲ Clinical Warnings:

- Children receiving bone marrow are a special subset of transplant recipients. Their new bone marrow should be functional by 3 months after transplant, although complete recovery of immune function may take up to 1 year. Reimmunization may be necessary, but the effectiveness of immunization varies. Many children acquire the immunity of the donor (American Academy of Pediatrics, 2000). Additional donor immunization with *Haemophilus influenzae* type b, diphtheria toxoid, and pneumococcal vaccine 7 to 10 days prior to harvest and recipient immunization immediately after transplant have been shown to improve recipient antibody response dramatically (Ambrosino, 1998). Donor immunization may be an effective strategy in the future to prevent infections in BMT patients.
- The transplant team should be consulted before proceeding with immunization. Varicella vaccination is currently not recommended for BMT recipients at any time after transplant.

Referral Points and Clinical Warnings

If the child has a tetanus-prone wound in the year after transplant, tetanus immune globulin should be given. Two years after BMT, healthy survivors can receive MMR vaccine, provided they have no evidence of GVHD.

The primary care provider is the child's first line of defense in fighting rejection and infection. Nonspecific symptoms may represent common childhood illnesses or early rejection. Community outbreaks of varicella and other viral syndromes (eg, Epstein-Barr virus [EBV]) pose special risks for the transplant recipient. No immunizations should be administered for the first 3 months after transplantation.

Infants who undergo transplant will not have had an opportunity to complete the recommended immunization series. After 90 days, inactivated vaccines, such as diphtheria and tetanus toxoids and pertussis, hepatitis B, and inactivated polio virus (Salk) may be used as appropriate. However, the child's immune response to these vaccines may be inadequate. If there is any question about the patient's ability to mount a particular immune response, antibody titers should be drawn. Susceptible children who are exposed to measles or varicella should receive passive immunoprophylaxis (immunoglobulin, varicella-zoster immune globulin). Consult with the transplant team if this occurs.

The primary care provider should be aware of the protocol for monitoring immunosuppression and desired drug levels. Management of immunosuppressants is almost always the responsibility of the transplant team. It is important to be aware of common drug interactions that may alter the blood level of immunosuppressants.

▲ Clinical Warnings:

- Erythromycin and other macrolides are commonly used in pediatric practice. All may cause a significant increase in both FK506 and cyclosporine levels. Antiseizure medications, cimetidine, and a variety of other antibiotics can also change the use or excretion of immunosuppressants.
- Echinacea is a common herbal medicine. It can decrease the effectiveness of immunosuppression. Families should be counseled to avoid all prescription and over-the-counter medications unless approved by the transplant team.

Nutrition and growth delay will have been a concern for many of these children prior to transplant. Some will be on low-potassium, low-sodium, or other specific diets for side effects of their immunosuppressant regimen. Parents often need help changing eating behaviors established because of chronic illness, anorexia, or the child's lack of experience with oral feeding. The primary care provider should evaluate the need for calorie supplementation to promote catch-up growth. The provider needs to monitor long-term growth. Growth retardation is common before transplant, but improvements are seen in most transplant recipients, particularly in linear growth (Chinnock & Baum, 1998). Renal transplant recipients and non-Caucasian recipients have the poorest post-transplant improvement in linear growth velocity. These groups may benefit from growth hormone (GH) therapy (Fine, 1997).

Dental hygiene is particularly important for transplant recipients. Examining the mouth and teeth should be a regular part of the well child visit. Oral infections, such as herpes, candidiasis, and mouth ulcers, are complications of immunosuppression. These may occur despite antifungal and antiviral prophylaxis. Gingival hyperplasia is a common side effect of cyclosporine. It is not dose related but occurs because of the individual child's intrinsic susceptibility and the amount of local irritants present. Good oral hygiene reduces plaque and other irritants. Gingivectomy may be necessary, but recurrence is common. Biannual dental examinations are important. Transplant recipients should receive endocarditis prophylaxis for dental care (American Academy of Pediatrics, 1997). Refer to Chapter 56 for guidance in prescribing dental prophylaxis.

Counseling and psychosocial support are essential interventions for both child and family. The primary care provider plays a significant role after transplant in assisting the family to return to a normal lifestyle with an optimal quality of life. Parents are often overprotective after transplant. Most children are ready to return to school and activities within 2 to 3 months. The school nurse may need information and assistance in adapting the child's medication regimen to the school day.

Specific activity limitations vary by organ but are usually short-term. For example, heart transplant recipients may return to normal activities within 6 to 8 weeks of transplant. Children whose physical attributes were affected by their pretransplant condition or treatment often continue to have behavioral difficulties and poorer peer relations after transplant (Vannatta, Zeller, Noll, & Koontz, 1998). Children facing transplant are able to appreciate the life-threatening nature of their illness and its treatment and may demonstrate symptoms of post-traumatic stress disorder after transplant (Stuber, Nader, Houskamp, & Pynoos, 1996). There is a higher incidence of depression and anxiety among pediatric transplant recipients when compared with normal peers (Uzark et al., 1992; Winsorova, Stewart, & Lovitt, 1991). Refer to Chapters 28 and 49 for more information on the topics of depression, anxiety, and living with chronic disease.

The transition to adolescence and adulthood is more difficult for the transplant recipient. Normal adolescent behaviors like experimentation and risk taking may have life-threatening consequences. Failure to engage in their post-transplant regimen is well documented in adolescent recipients and is a major cause of late rejection of heart transplants. There is a 30% mortality rate associated with nonparticipation in the post-transplant regimen (Douglas, Hsu, & Addonizio, 1993). Therefore, family and provider need to monitor shifts in school performance, inconsistent medical follow-up, decreased socialization, and behavioral changes.

The appearance of any of these behaviors should trigger concern about the adolescent's consistency in taking his or her medication.

Managing Post-transplant Complications

The incidence of rejection is greatest in the first 3 months after transplant. Transplant centers maintain close control over the child's care during that period. Once the child has returned to the home community, the team will continue to be involved, but day-to-day management of common childhood problems remains the job of the primary care provider. A transplant coordinator (usually a registered nurse) is available 24 hours a day. A close working relationship with the coordinator facilitates post-transplant care. After the first year, the transplant team's involvement in the patient's care will lessen, but the team will continue to participate in rejection surveillance throughout the child's life.

Rejection and Immunosuppression

Immunosuppressant regimens vary somewhat for individual organs and from one transplant center to another. All immunosuppressants have significant side effects. Short stature or delayed growth, acne, hirsutism, body changes, hypertension, altered fertility, increased pregnancy risks, and insulin-dependent diabetes are all potential consequences of long-term immunosuppression. Display 66-1 presents immunosuppressant agents, side effects, and information about their use, which the provider may find helpful in monitoring this patient.

Rejection, or GVHD, is the primary cause of mortality in the first 3 months post-transplant. GVHD occurs in about 60% of allogenic BMT recipients (Whitington & Balistreri, 1991). It is also seen after liver transplant. Acute disease causes rapidly progressive multisystem organ failure and may reflect transfer of donor-derived EBV RNA. As time passes, the risk of acute rejection and infection decreases, but is never zero (Johnston et al., 1997).

Infection

Ninety percent of overall post-transplant mortality is due to infections. Infection is the leading cause of death between 3 and 12 months after transplant. For example, in the immediate post-BMT period, bacterial and fungal infections are major causes of morbidity and mortality. Because immunosuppressed children are at risk for *Pneumocystis carinii* pneumonia, they will require lifelong prophylaxis, usually with trimethoprim-sulfamethoxazole, once daily, 3 days a week. Immunosuppressed adolescents are at increased risk for sexually transmitted infections.

▲ **Clinical Warning:** Education about safe sex practices and birth control should be an explicit part of well adolescent visits. Pregnancy is not absolutely contraindicated, but it is high risk for both mother and fetus. Annual gynecologic examinations for adolescent women are prudent, whether or not they report being sexually active. The primary provider should have a low threshold for initiating treatment. Chapter 41 can provide the reader with information about how to diagnose and treat these problems.

Post-transplant lymphoproliferative disease (PTLD) is a functional defect in neutrophil function associated with a marked susceptibility to bacterial infection (Avery & First, 1996). PTLD occurs in 10% of all pediatric transplant recipients (American Academy of Pediatrics, 2000). It is caused by EBV; EBV infection produces a loss of natural killer cells (Cao et al., 1998). The highest incidence occurs in recipients of heart transplant.

▲ **Clinical Warning:** Persistent fever, lymphadenopathy, and marked tonsillar or adenoidal hypertrophy should raise suspicion for PTLD and prompt consultation with the transplant team. Gastrointestinal bleeding with EBV infection is strongly correlated with PTLD in liver transplant recipients (Cao et al., 1998). PTLD can be successfully treated with reduction of immunosuppression and administration of antiviral agents. However, there is significant short-term mortality (approximately 20%) and a high risk of developing acute or chronic rejection (Cacciarelli et al., 1998). In pediatric BMT recipients, PTLD is more likely to have a fatal outcome and to be diagnosed postmortem (Lones, Lopez-Terrada, Shintaku, Rosenthal, & Said, 1998).

Kidney

Graft failure immediately post-transplant is most commonly due to acute tubular necrosis or vascular thrombosis. In the first year after transplant, dehydration should be aggressively avoided. This is particularly true for infants who have received adult-sized kidneys (Salvatierra et al., 1998).

Erythrocytosis may develop in some transplant recipients due to anomalies of insulin growth factor secondary to pre-transplant chronic renal failure. Recurrence of the underlying renal disease may occur. Use of recombinant human GH after transplant may help linear growth and improve the ratio of lean-to-fat body mass (Feber et al., 1998; D'Alessandro et al., 1998). However, GH may affect creatinine clearance of the donor kidney. Recipients of GH require monthly renal function testing and annual renal ultrasound. GH therapy does not significantly increase bone mass. Despite routine calcium supplementation, ■ osteopenia and osteoporosis

---

DISPLAY 66–1 • Outpatient Immunosuppressant Agents

Cyclosporine A
- Side effects: nephrotoxicity, hypertension, tremors, paresthesias, seizures, hirsutism, gingival hyperplasia, hepatotoxicity, malignancies
- Erythromycin, fluconazole, diltiazem will increase levels
- Phenytoin, trimethaprim-sulfamethoxazole (TMP-SMX) will decrease levels, metoclopramide phenobarbital

Corticosteroids
- Side effects: hypertension, hyperglycemia, insulin-dependent diabetes mellitus, cushingoid appearance, impaired tissue healing, hypercatabolism
- Some centers discontinue steroid therapy 6 to 12 months after transplant

Azathioprine
- Side effects: hepatotoxicity, glucose intolerance, pancreatitis, stomatitis
- Long-term use increases risk of malignancy

Tacrolimus
- Side effects: nephrotoxicity, neurotoxicity, glucose intolerance, hypertension, gastrointestinal irritability, anemia

are frequent complications after kidney transplantation. Recent research suggests that cyclical treatment with intranasal calcitonin or oral clodronate may increase bone mass density (Grotz et al., 1998).

Liver

Fever, abdominal tenderness, irritability, and fatigue may signal an episode of rejection. Liver function tests will be elevated, but abnormal liver function tests are not specific to rejection. Hepatic vascular thrombosis, atrophy of the biliary tree, and infection may present in a similar fashion (McDiarmid, 1996). The child may develop chronic diarrhea and malabsorption. These symptoms should be discussed with the transplant team. Percutaneous liver biopsy provides a definitive diagnosis.

Heart

Rejection is not usually associated with symptoms until cardiac compromise is severe. The most serious long-term issue after heart transplant is graft coronary artery disease (GCAD). GCAD occurs in 7% to 15% of pediatric heart transplant recipients. The cause is unknown, but development of GCAD appears to be related to the frequency of acute rejection episodes. Hyperlipidemia and viral infection in the postoperative period, particularly cytomegalovirus (CMV) infection, may also be associated with late development of GCAD (Chang, 1998; Canter et al., 1997).

Graft coronary artery disease can be difficult to diagnose. There is diffuse, progressive thickening of the endothelial lining of the coronary arteries; eventually, the lumen is obliterated. Anginal symptoms do not occur, because the transplanted heart is denervated. Noninvasive testing may not reveal signs of impaired myocardial perfusion. Coronary angiography during cardiac catheterization confirms the diagnosis. At minimum, the recipient of a heart transplant undergoes yearly cardiac catheterization and biopsy at the transplant center to assess rejection status and to look for GCAD. There is no effective therapy for GCAD. Retransplantation is the only option.

Lung

Recipients often experience decreased exercise tolerance in the first 6 months after transplant. Pulmonary function testing may show evidence of mild restrictive disease. This generally improves over time (Noyes et al., 1994).

Obliterative bronchiolitis (OB) is the most serious long-term risk after lung transplant, occurring in 20% to 40% of pediatric lung transplant recipients (Spray et al., 1994). There is a positive correlation between frequency of rejection episodes and the development of OB. Postoperative CMV infection, as well as local infections in the transplanted lung, may also play a role. OB involves diffuse, progressive fibrotic changes in the intimal lining that eventually narrow and occlude the bronchioles. Dyspnea and cough are the first clinical signs. Pulmonary function testing will indicate obstruction in the small airways. Chest radiograph may appear normal.

▲ **Clinical Warning:** The provider should discuss with the transplant team any unexplained, persistent cough or symptoms that do not resolve normally after common upper respiratory infections. The team should also be informed promptly of symptoms suggestive of reactive airway disease at any time after transplant. Open lung biopsy is the definitive diagnostic test for OB, but it carries significant risk.

Fortunately, high-resolution computed tomography scan or transbronchial biopsy can often confirm the diagnosis.

The progression of OB may be slowed or arrested with increased immunosuppression. Total lymphoid irradiation has also been used. Unfortunately, retransplantation may be the only effective treatment. Mortality after lung retransplant is high.

Bone Marrow

Growth impairment is commonly seen in children who have undergone total body irradiation in preparation for transplant. Injury to the endocrine glands or the pituitary may result from anticancer chemotherapy, irradiation, and chemotherapy given before transplant. Late effects of treatment include pubertal delay, precocious puberty, and hypothyroidism (Cohen et al., 1998). Refer to Chapter 60 for information on the diagnosis and management of these late effects.

Chronic GVHD is the most common complication after BMT. Histocompatibility differences between the graft (donor) and the host (organ recipient) allow immunocompetent T killer cells from the donor to react against antigens within the host. Chronic GVHD occurs more than 100 days post-transplant and resembles other autoimmune or collagen vascular diseases in its presentation (Avery & First, 1996). Invasive bacterial and fungal infections with common pathogens (*Streptococcus pneumoniae, Candida*) may occur months to years after transplant in these patients. Mortality is 25% to 50%. Maculopapular skin rash is often the first manifestation, followed by fever and diarrhea. Latent viral infections may be reactivated (Engelhard, 1998). The blood count will demonstrate a pancytopenia.

▲ **Clinical Warning:** Contact the transplant team for further evaluation of invasive infections post-BMT. Treatment involves depleting the donor bone marrow of T cells using monoclonal antibodies and complement, then administering thalidomide for 3 to 6 months. Steroids may also be effective (Avery & First, 1996).

Significant late toxicity after BMT treatment also includes avascular necrosis of bone, poor school performance (most often in patients who received cranial irradiation), ocular dysfunction, pulmonary fibrosis, and recurrent malignancy (Gordon et al., 1997; Sanders, 1997).

Teaching and Self-Care

Long-term data on outcomes and quality of life in pediatric transplant recipients are not yet available. Compared with adult transplant recipients, this group is unique from the perspectives of growth, puberty, immune maturation, expectancy for longer life, and infection risk. A good relationship with a consistent primary care provider promotes optimal, family-centered, and age-appropriate participation in self-care. Such a relationship helps in optimizing the long-term quality of life for both child and family.

Post-transplant, the primary provider can continue to provide age-appropriate anticipatory guidance, counseling, and psychosocial support to both the child and family. Priority referral to additional sources for psychological evaluation and counseling may also be necessary. The provider also should be aware of local and national resources that may be helpful to the patient and family.

The primary care provider can be central in preventing problems associated with adolescents' participation in their post-transplant regimen through anticipatory guidance before the transplant. Age-appropriate anticipatory guidance that is tied to a child's drive for independence can help the child and family to prepare for responsible post-transplant management. The provider can also assess the adolescent for capability in taking on some self-care. It is important that parents and clinician work together with adolescents, supporting them as they grow up to meet their normal and acceptable need for regimen control. The ultimate goal is helping both child and family to create a safe plan of care, stressing the teen's responsibility clearly.

COMMUNITY RESOURCES

Most transplant centers have web pages, booklets, and other informational resources for patients and families.

Books and Pamphlets

The Nicholas Effect: A Boy's Gift to the World, by R. Green. O'Reilly and Associates.

Organ Transplants: A Patient's Guide, by H.F. Pizer and the Massachusetts General Hospital Transplant Team. Harvard University Press.

A Will to Live: The Story of a Transplant Kid, by J. Page, J.H. Talbert, and P. Harper. Fawn Grove Press.

Internet Sites

- *http://www.unos.org*
  United Network for Organ Sharing

  Transplant statistics and links to many sites.

- *http://www.stadtlander.com/transplant*

  "An age-appropriate guide to helping your child with a transplant," "What about the siblings?" and "Dealing with your child's medical team," written by pediatric transplant nurses, are available at this site.

- *http://www.ishlt.org*
  International Society for Heart and Lung Transplantation

- *http://www.ktppp.com*
  Kidney Transplant Patient Partnering Program

Organizations

National Transplant Assistance Fund
6 Bryn Mawr Avenue
P.O. Box 258
Bryn Mawr, PA 19010
Telephone: (610) 527-5056
Toll-free: (800) 642-8399
Fax: (610) 527-5210
Internet address: *http://www.transplantfund.org*

This clearing house of information on nonprofit organizations and transplant centers provides fund-raising expertise for families raising money for transplant and offers modest medical assistance grants to families. Web site has links to many patient web sites.

Children's Organ Transplant Association (COTA)
2501 COTA Drive
Bloomington, IN 47403
Telephone: (800) 366-COTA (2682)
Internet address: *http://www.cota.org*

Raises funds for transplant expenses.

National Patient Travel Center
4620 Haygood Road, Suite 1
Virginia Beach, VA 23455
Telephone: (757) 318-9174
Fax: (757) 318-9107
Toll-free Helpline: (800) 296-1217
Internet address: *http://www.PatientTravel.org*

No-cost referral to charitable medical air transport options.

National Association of Hospital Hospitality Houses
P.O. Box 18087
Asheville, NC 28814-0087
Telephone: (828) 253-1188
Toll-free: (800) 542-9730
Fax: (828) 253-8082
Internet address: *http://www.nahhh.org*

Referrals to free or low-cost lodging near medical facilities.

The Transplant Foundation
8002 Discovery Drive, Suite 310
Richmond, VA 23229
Telephone: (804) 285-5115

Financial aid for immunosuppressive drugs.

Many pharmaceutical companies have programs to assist patients who cannot pay for drugs; a comprehensive listing of contacts for these programs can be found at the following Internet address:
http://www.geocities.com/HotSprings/8374/Indigent.html

U.S. Transplant Games
Internet address: *http://www.transplantgames.org*

Presented by the National Kidney Foundation; they take place every 2 years.

REFERENCES

Ambrosino, D. (1998). *Immunizations in stem cell transplantation patients: Evolving issues in pediatric transplantation.* Presented at the 36th annual Infectious Diseases society of America Meeting. November 12–15, 1998. Denver, CO.

American Academy of Pediatrics. (1997). 1997 *Red book: Report of the Committee on Infectious Diseases* (24th ed.). Elk Grove, IL: Author.

Avery, M. L., & First, L. R. (1996). *Pediatric medicine* (2nd ed.). Baltimore: Williams & Wilkins.

Boucek, M. M., Novick, R. J., Bennett, L. E., Fiol, B., Keck, B. M., & Hosenpud, J. D. (1997). The registry of the International Society of Heart and Lung Transplantation: First official pediatric report-1997. *Journal of Heart and Lung Transplantion, 16,* 1189–1206.

Cacciarelli, T. V., Green, M., Jaffe, R., Mazariegos, G. V., Jain, A., et al. (1998). Management of posttransplant lymphoproliferative disease in pediatric liver transplant recipients receiving primary tacrolimus (FK506) therapy. *Transplantation, 66,* 1047–1052.

Canter, C., Nafetel, D., Caldwel,l R., Chinnock, R., Pahl, E., et al. (1997). Survival and risk factors for death after cardiac transplantation in infants. *Circulation, 96,* 227–231.

Cao, S., Cox, K., Esquivel, C. O., Perquist, W., Concepcio, W., et al. (1998). Posttransplant lymphoproliferative disorders and gastrointestinal manifestations of Epstein-Barr virus infection in children following liver transplantation. *Transplantation, 66,* 851–856.

Chan, K. W., Gajewski, J. L., Supkis, D., Pentz, R., Champlin, R., & Bleyer, W. A. (1996). Use of minors as bone marrow donors: Current attitude and management. A survey of 56 pediatric transplantation centers. *Journal of Pediatrics, 128,* 644–648.

Chang, A. C., Hanley, F. L., Wernovsky, G., Wessel, D. L. (1998). *Pediatric cardiac intensive care.* Baltimore: Williams & Wilkins.

Chinnock, R., & Baum, M. (1998). Somatic growth in infant heart transplant recipients. *Pediatric Transplantation, 1,* 55–64.

Cohen, A. R., Zecca, S., Van-Lint, M. T., Parodi, L., Grasso, L., & Uderzo, C. (1998). Endocrine late effects in children who underwent bone marrow transplantation: Review. *Bone Marrow Transplantation, 21*(suppl 2), S64–67.

D'Alessandro, A. M., Pirsch, J. D., Knechtie, S. J., Odorico, J. S., Van der Werf, W. J., et al. (1998). Living unrelated renal donation: The University of Wisconsin experience. *Surgery, 124,* 604–610.

Douglas, J., Hsu, D., & Addonizio, L. (1993). *Late rejection as a major indicator of noncompliance in pediatric heart transplant recipients.* Presented at the 66th Scientific Sessions of the American Heart Association, November 12-15, 1993. Dallas, TX.

Engelhard, D. (1998). Bacterial and fungal infections in children undergoing bone marrow transplantation. *Transplantation, 21*(suppl 2), S78–80.

Feber, J., Cochat, P., Lebl, J., Krasnicanova, H., Stepan, J., et al. (1998). Bone composition in children receiving recombinant human growth hormone after renal transplantation. *Kidney International, 54,* 951–955.

Fine, R. N. (1997). Growth post renal transplantation in children: Lessons from the North American Pediatric Renal Transplant Cooperative Study. *Pediatric Transplantation, 1,* 85–89.

Gordon, B. G., Warkentin, P. I., Standjorn, S. E., Abromowitch, M., Bayerver, E., et al. (1997). Allogeneic bone marrow transplantation for children with acute leukemia: Long term follow up of patients prepared with high-dose cytosine arabinoside and fractionated total body irradiation. *Bone Marrow Transplantation, 20,* 5–10.

Grotz, W. H., Rump, L. C., Niessen, A., Schmidt-Gayk, H., Reichelt, A., & Kirste, G. (1998). Treatment of osteopenia and osteoporosis after kidney transplantation. *Transplantation, 66,* 1004–1008.

Johnston, J. K., Chinnock, R. E., Zuppan, C. W., Razzouk, A. J., Gundry, S. R., & Bailey, L. L. (1997). Limitations to survival for infants with hypoplastic left heart syndrome before and after transplant: The Loma Linda experience. *Journal of Transplant Coordination, 7,* 180–184.

Kelly, D. A. (1998). Current results and evolving indications for liver transplantation in children. *Journal of Pediatric Gastroenterology and Nutrition, 27,* 214–221.

Langley, L. (1999). South Carolina threatens donor organ suit. *Charleston Post & Courier,* March 13, p. 1B.

Lones, M. A., Lopez-Terrada, D., Shintaku, I. P., Rosenthal, J., & Said, J. W. (1998). Posttransplant lymphoproliferative disorder in pediatric bone marrow transplant recipients. *Archives of Pathology and Laboratory Medicine, 122,* 708–714.

McDiarmid, S. V. (1996). Risk factors and outcomes after pediatric liver transplantation. *Liver Transplant, 2,* 5.

Morrow, W. R., Naftel, D., Chinnock, R., Canter, C., Boucek, M., Zales, V., et al. (1997). Outcome of listing for heart transplantation in infants younger than six months: Predictors of death and interval to transplantation. *Journal of Heart and Lung Transplantation, 16,* 1255–1266.

Noyes, B. E., Kurland, G., Orenstein, D. M., et al. (1994). Experience with pediatric lung transplantation. *Journal of Pediatrics, 124,* 261–268.

Packman, W. L., Crittenden, M. R., Schaeffer, E., Bongar, B., Fischer, J. B., & Cowan, M. J. (1997). Psychosocial consequences of bone marrow transplantation in donor and nondonor siblings. *Journal of Developmental and Behavioral Pediatrics, 18,* 244–253.

Razzouk, A.J., Chinnock, R.E., Gundry, S.R., Johnston, J.K., Larsen, R.L., et al. (1996). Transplantation as a primary treatment for hypoplastic left heart syndrome: Intermediate term results. Annals of Thoracic Surgery 62, 1-7.

Rodrigue, J. R., MacNaughton, K., Hoffman, R. G., Graham-Pole, J., Andres, J. M., et al. (1996). Perceptions of parenting stress and family relations by fathers of children evaluated for organ transplantation. *Psychological Reports, 79,* 723–727.

Salvatierra, O., Tanney, D., Mak, R., et al. (1997). Pediatric renal transplantation and its challenges. *Transplantation Reviews, 11,* 51–69.

Salvatierra, O., Singh, T., Shifrin, R., Conley, S., Alexander, S., et al. (1998). Successful transplantation of adult-sized kidneys into infants. *Transplantation, 66,* 819–823.

Sanders, J. E. (1997). Bone marrow transplantation for pediatric malignancies. *Pediatric Clinics of North America, 44,* 1005–1020.

Shama, W. I. (1998). The experience and preparation of pediatric sibling bone marrow donors. *Social Work in Heath Care, 27,* 89–99.

Spray, T. L., Mallory, G. B., Canter, C. B., et al. (1994). Pediatric lung transplantation: Indications, techniques and early results. *Journal of Thoracic and Cardiovascular Surgery, 107,* 990–1000.

Stiehm, E. R. (Ed.). (1996). *Immunologic disorders in infants and children* (4th ed.). Philadelphia: W.B. Saunders.

Stuber, M. L., Nader, K. O., Houskamp, B. M., & Pynoos, R. S. (1996). Appraisal of life threat and acute trauma responses in pediatric bone marrow transplant patients. *Journal of Traumatic Stress, 9,* 673–686.

Tojimbara, T., Fuchinboue, S., Nakajima, I., Koike, T., Abe, M., et al. (1998). Analysis of postoperative liver function of donors in living-related liver transplantation: Comparison of the type of donor hepatectomy. *Transplantation, 66,* 1035–1039.

Uzark, K. C., Sauer, S. N., Lawrence, K. S., et al. (1992). The psychosocial impact of pediatric heart transplantation. *Journal of Heart Lung Transplant, 11,* 1160–1167.

Vannatta, K., Zeller, M., Noll, R. B., & Koontz, K. (1998). Social functioning of children surviving bone marrow transplantation. *Journal of Pediatric Psychology, 23,* 169–178.

Whitington, P. F., & Balistreri, W. F. (1991). Liver transplantation in pediatrics. Indications, contraindications and pretransplant management. *Journal of Pediatrics, 118,* 169.

Winsorova, D., Stewart, S. M., & Lovitt, R. (1991). Emotional adaptation in children after liver transplantation. *Journal of Pediatrics, 119,* 880–887.

Yoder, L. H. (1998). Costs and outcomes of a military bone marrow transplant program. *Military Medicine, 163,* 661–666.

Yunis, E. J., & Dupont, B. (1993). The HLA system. In D. Nathan & F. Oski (Eds.), *Hematology of infancy and childhood* (Vol. 2) (pp. 1692–1728). Philadelphia: W.B. Saunders.

Zitelli, B. J,. Gartner, J. C., Malatack, J. J., et al. (1991). Liver transplantation in children: A pediatrician's perspective. *Pediatric Annals, 20,* 691.

Zitelli, B. J., Malatack, J. J., Gartner, J. C., et al. (1986). Evaluation of the pediatric patient for liver transplantation. *Pediatrics, 78,* 559.

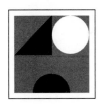

Prenatal Screening/Clinical Warning

In addition to genetic testing, there are some other methods of screening for fetal status during pregnancy. Other most common methods are blood testing, ultrasound imaging, chorionic-villus sampling, and amniocentesis.

Elevations in the maternal serum alpha fetoprotein (MSAFP) have been associated with neural tube defects as far back as the 1970s (Brock & Sutcliffe, 1972). Screening has become routine for this and other indicators (human chorionic gonadatrophin [HCG] and estriol) as the quest for a healthy infant and technology have advanced. According to Alteneder, Kenner, Green, & Pohorecki (1998) there is a high number of false positives which impact the pregnant woman and her partner. For many, the dilemma of making a decision about the outcome of the pregnancy is significant. Also, the anxiety regarding the outcome of the pregnancy and birth is extreme.

Haddow, Polomski, Knight, Williams, Miller, & Johnson (1998) reported that they were able to predict the presence of Down syndrome in the first trimester rather than in the second. However, this has not yet become widespread because of the specialty nature of the testing and the potential risk of pregnancy loss.

Testing for prenatal diagnosis is associated most frequently with maternal age. Testing is usually advised for women over 35 years of age, but only if the outcome would influence the course of the pregnancy. The health care provider plays an important role in supporting the woman and her partner in undergoing testing, and if necessary, in supporting her decision regarding the outcome of the pregnancy.

REFERENCES

Alteneder, R., Kenner, C., Green, D., & Pohorecki, S. (1998). The lived experience of women who undergo prenatal diagnostic testing due to elevated maternal serum alpha-fetoprotein screening. *MCN: The American Journal of Maternal/Child Nursing, 23*(4), 180-186.

Brock, J. & Sutcliffe, R. (1972). Alpha fetoprotein in the antenatal diagnosis of anecephaly and spina bifida. *Lancet 6,* 197-199.

Haddow, J., Palomaki, G., Knight, G., Williams, J., Miller, W., & Johnson, A. (1998). Screening of maternal serum for fetal Down's syndrome in the first trimester. *The New England Journal of Medicine, 338*(14), 955-961.

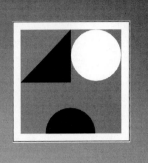

INDEX

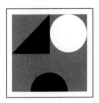

INDEX

Note: Page numbers followed by d, f, and t represent display, figure, and table, respectively.

M

comorbid conditions with, 319
in depression, 313
in diabetes mellitus, 793
diagnosis of, 321
epidemiology of, 320
gender differences in, 319–320
history in, 320–321, 321d
management of, 321–324, 322d
methods for, 320, 321
nonfatal (parasuicidal), 321
of parent, coping with, 308
parent notification of, 323
pathology of, 319–320
physical examination in, 321
physiology of, 319–320
prevention of, 323
repeated, 320, 321, 323
risk factors for, 319–320
school notification of, 323–324
thoughts of, screening for, 154
Sulfasalazine, in inflammatory bowel disease, 730
Sulfisoxazole, in otitis media prevention, 380
Sulfonamides, allergy to, 592
Sulfonylureas, in diabetes mellitus, 786, 787t–788t
Sulfur, in scabies, 604
Sumitriptan, in migraine headache, 639–640, 640t
Sunlight exposure
phytophotodermatitis in, 261
protection against, 605
urticaria due to, 544
Superior vena cava syndrome, in mediastinal masses, 823
Support groups
for adoption, 73
for chronic illness, 625–626
for disability, 213
Support Need Inventory of parents of Children With
Asthma, 699–702
Support services, for chronic illness, 625
Supratentorial tumors, 823d, 834
Supraventricular tachycardia, congenital, 707t
Surfactant therapy, bronchopulmonary dysplasia due to,
201–202
Sutures
skull, of infants, 99–100, 101f
for wound repair
alternatives to, 515
materials for, 514, 514t
removal of, 514
Sweat test, for cystic fibrosis, 409, 692
Swimmer's ear, 380–382, 382t
Swimming
safety in, 111
for toddlers, 124
Sydenham's chorea, 394, 562, 564
in rheumatic fever, 440
Syncope
cardiac, 432–439
in arrhythmias, 435–437, 436f–438f
in cardiac anatomic anomalies, 433
in coronary artery anomalies, 435
diagnosis of, 436–438, 436f–438f
history in, 434–435
in left ventricular outflow obstruction, 435
management of, 438–439
neurocardiogenic, 432–433, 433f
pathology of, 432–434, 433f, 434f

physical examination in, 435
in pulmonary hypertension, 435
spectrum of, 432
in tetralogy of Fallot, 433, 435
exercise-related, 437
Synovial fluid, examination of, in infections, 534
Synovitis, toxic, 533–535, 534f, 534t, 535f, 535t
Syphilis, 159, 487
in pregnancy, 59t
testing for, before adoption placement, 68
Systemic lupus erythematosus, in pregnancy, 60

T

Tachycardia
management of, 439
supraventricular, 707t
Tachypnea
in cardiac disorders, 104
in pneumonia, 415, 416
Tacrolimus, post-transplantation, 867d
Talus, vertical, 747
Tanner stage, of sexual development, 151
Tantrums, 125–126
Tape, skin, for wounds, 515
Tarsal coalition, 745, 745f
Tattoos, 301
Tay-Sachs disease, 48–49
Teaching, patient and family. See Anticipatory guidance
Team approach
to chronic illness, 623–627, 624d
to sexual abuse investigation, 267
Tears
excessive, 656
formation of, 359
in infants, 101
in nasolacrimal obstruction, 363
Tea tree oil, in aromatherapy, 37
Teens. See Adolescents
Teeth
avulsion of, 524
care of
in congenital heart disease, 711–712
in diabetes mellitus, 793
development of, 523t
erosion of, in bulimia nervosa, 252
of infants, 102
injury of, 523–524, 523f
of preschool children, 129
replantation of, 524
of school-age children, 144
of toddlers, 117
Television
drug use promotion in, 289
for preschool children, 139
self-destructive behavior related to, 295–296, 298t
Temperature
bath water, 262
body
high. See Fever
measurement of, in infants, 99
normal, 343
regulation of, 343
Temporomandibular joint disorders, 633–634
Tendon reflexes, in infants, 107

Vagina
candidiasis of, 548, 549
discharge from, 155, 155f
examination of, 484
Vaginitis, 486
streptococcal, 393–394
Validation, in caring relationships, 4
Valproate
in seizures, 554, 555t, 559
in suicidal behavior, 322
Values
clarification of, 9, 15
of families, universal, 13, 13d
Valvular heart disease, in rheumatic fever, 439–441
Vancomycin
in fever, in neutropenia, 351t
in pneumonia, 418, 418t
Vaporizers, in common cold, 330
Varicella, 334–335
immunization for, 156, 163t, 165–166
in cancer chemotherapy, 828
in congenital heart disease, 710
contraindications for, 169t–171t
necrotizing fasciitis in, 546
in pregnancy, 56–57, 59t
Varicocele, 476
Vasculitis
fever in, 344d
in Henoch Schönlein purpura, 448
in Kawasaki disease, 352
urticaria with, 544
Vasoconstrictors, in allergic conjunctivitis, 367, 367t
Vasodilators, in hypertension, 466, 466t
Vaso-occlusive crisis, in sickle cell disease, 500
Vasopressor syncope, 432–433, 433f
Vasovagal (neurocardiogenic) syncope, 432–433, 433f
Vegetarian diet, 138, 147
Venereal Disease Research Laboratory test, for syphilis, 487–488
Venography, magnetic resonance, in headache evaluation, 638
Venom immunotherapy, in insect stings, 590
Venomous bites
centipedes, 608
insects. See Insect bites and stings
spiders, 607–608
Ventricle(s)
left
hypertrophy of, syncope in, 436, 436f
outflow obstruction of, syncope in, 435
right, hypertrophy of, in tetralogy of Fallot, 424
single, 703–704, 713, 714t–715t
Ventricular septal defect, 104, 423–424, 705t
pathology of, 703
in tetralogy of Fallot, 424
Ventriculoperitoneal shunt, failure of, headache in, 633
Verapamil
in congenital heart disease, 716t
in migraine headache, 641, 642t
Vernix, 97
Verrucae. See Warts
Vertebrae. See Spine
Vertigo, benign positional, 631
Vesicants, for molluscum contagiosum, 738

Vesicles
description of, 733t
in enterovirus infections, 338
in herpes simplex virus infections, 338–339, 388–389
in varicella, 334–335
Vesicoureteral reflux, 460–461, 460f, 471–473, 473f, 801–802
Vidarabine, in herpes simplex virus infections, 364–365
Video games, self-destructive behavior related to, 295–296
Vigabatrin, in seizures, 555t
Vinblastine, 826t
Vincristine, 826t
Violence
coping with, 307–308
domestic, 275–281
behavioral indicators of, 275, 276d
child abuse overlap with, 280–281
community resources for, 281
developmental stage and, 275, 275t
diagnosis of, 279–280
dynamics of, 277
epidemiology of, 278
historic perspective of, 276–277
history in, 278–279
against HIV-positive women, 280
management of, 280–281
pathology of, 275–278, 275t, 276d
perpetrators of, 277
in pregnancy, 61
prevention of, 281
psychological abuse in, 277–278
sibling-on-sibling, 281
against undocumented women, 280
in media and entertainment, self-destructive behavior related to, 295–296
Violence Against Women Act, 280
Viral infections. See also specific infections
in adopted children, 71
in athletes, 176
bronchitis, 410
conjunctivitis in, 364–365
oral, pain management in, 194
otitis media, 374
toxic synovitis in, 533–535, 534f, 534t, 535f, 535t
types of, 329
Vision
acuity of, testing of, 360, 653, 654t
of adolescents, 154
assessment of, 360, 653, 654t, 657, 658t
binocular, 368
disorders of
amblyopia, 360, 654
cataract, 369, 371, 657
in cerebral palsy, 224t
community resources for, 658
conjunctival. See Conjunctiva; Conjunctivitis
corneal. See Cornea
in eyelid disorders, 656
glaucoma, 363, 369, 371, 657
in lacrimal system disorders, 656
learning disability in, 655
nystagmus, 101, 654–655
in optic nerve malformations, 658
proptosis, 655
retinal. See Retina; Retinopathy

W

X